FUNDAMENTALS OF HIV MEDICINE 2025 EDITION

FUNDAMENTALS OF HIV MEDICINE 2025 EDITION

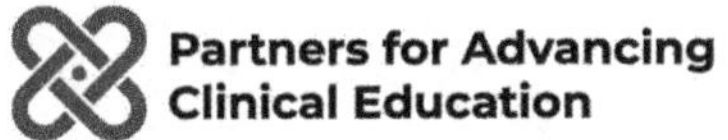

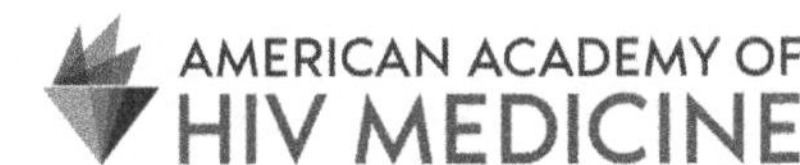

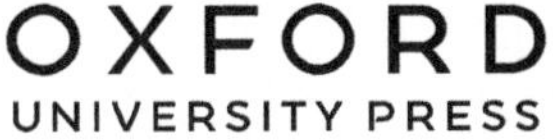

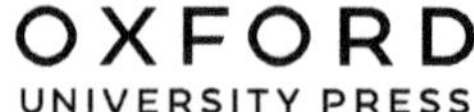

Oxford University Press is a department of the University of Oxford.
It furthers the University's objective of excellence in research, scholarship,
and education by publishing worldwide. Oxford is a registered trade mark of
Oxford University Press in the UK and certain other countries.

Published in the United States of America by Oxford University Press
198 Madison Avenue, New York, NY 10016, United States of America.

CIP data is on file at the Library of Congress

ISBN 978–0–19–781263–1

DOI: 10.1093/med/9780197812631.001.0001

Printed by Marquis Book Printing, Canada

The manufacturer's authorized representative in the EU for product safety is
Oxford University Press España S.A., Parque Empresarial San Fernando de Henares,
Avenida de Castilla, 2 – 28830 Madrid (www.oup.es/en).

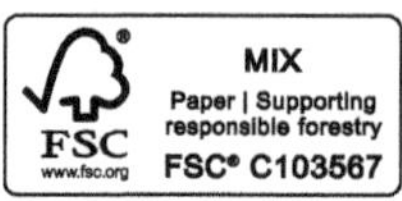

CONTENTS

Overall Learning Objectives vii

Faculty ix

Disclosure of Conflicts of Interest xiii

1. Ending the HIV Epidemic: A Plan for America 1
   Benjamin Sokoloff
2. The Origin, Evolution, and Epidemiology of HIV-1 and HIV-2 5
   Jeffrey T. Kirchner, Emily Min, and Julia Taylor
3. Mechanisms of HIV Transmission 23
   Nancy Aitcheson and Puja H. Nambiar
4. Virology: Life Cycle of HIV 28
   Poonam Mathur and George Lewis
5. Immunology of HIV Infection 36
   Dennis J. Hartigan-O'Connor and Christian Brander
6. HIV Testing and Counseling 48
   M. Elle Saine and Kyle G. Rodino
7. Initial Evaluation of the Patient with HIV: History, Physical Examination, and Laboratory Evaluation 60
   Esteban DelPilar Morales
8. Health Maintenance: Select Topics 71
   Ramiz Kseri
9. Diversity and Health Disparities 79
   Gary F. Spinner
10. HIV Care and Prevention: Special Populations 90
    Catherine Silva, Renata Arrington-Sanders, Zil G. Goldstein, Elizabeth Imbert, Matthew D. Hickey, Olabimpe Asupoto, Alysse G. Wurcel, Abby Davids, Ashley Carvalho, Deliana Garcia, Claire M. Hutkins Seda, and Laszlo Madaras
11. HIV Care Coordination 122
    Margret O. Nelson
12. The Pharmacist's Role in HIV Care 130
    Jennifer Cocohoba
13. Principles and Scientific Basis of HIV Therapy 137
    Neha Sheth Pandit, David E. Koren, and Emily Heil
14. HIV Prevention: Pharmacotherapy and Non-Pharmacotherapy-Based Strategies 153
    Katrina Baumgartner, Christopher M. Bositis, Wyatt Hanft, and Carolyn Chu
15. Antiretroviral Therapy Selection/Decision-Making: Initial and Subsequent Regimens 177
    Saira Ajmal, Zelalem Temesgen, Poonam Mathur, and David E. Koren
16. Antiretroviral Treatment and Stewardship in Hospital Settings 190
    David E. Koren and Yoseph Aldras
17. HIV Drug Resistance: Evaluation and Clinical Management 195
    Carolyn Chu, Avani Dalal, and Robert W. Shafer
18. The HIV Reservoir and Cure and Remission Strategies 218
    Boris Juelg, Rajesh Gandhi, and Nikolaus Jilg
19. Opportunistic Infections 239
    Lisa Y. Armitige, Karen Vigil, and Rita Wilson Dib
20. Immune Reconstitution Inflammatory Syndrome (IRIS) 260
    Dagan Coppock
21. Antiretroviral Therapy for Children and Newborns 266
    Karin Nielsen-Saines
22. Select Topics in the Care of Cisgender Women with HIV 278
    Aasith Villavicencio Paz, Jillian T. Baron, Christina E. Maguire, and William R. Short
23. Aging and HIV 295
    Aroonsiri Howell, John D. Zeuli, and Anchalee Avihingsanon
24. Solid Organ Transplantation in People with HIV 306
    Christine M. Durand
25. Malignancies in HIV 314
    Eva H. Clark and Elizabeth Y. Chiao
26. Understanding and Managing Antineoplastic and Antiretroviral Therapy 359
    Elizabeth M. Sherman and Taylor K. Gill
27. Dermatologic Complications of HIV 363
    Craig Weeks
28. Neurological Complications of HIV Infection 382
    Rodrigo Hasbun and Joseph S. Kass

29. Cardiovascular Disease 404
Jarrett K. Sell and Jonathan J. Nunez

30. Non-Opportunistic Pulmonary Complications 423
Priyanka Chakrabarti

31. Renal Complications 427
Patricia Carr Reese and Umar Farooq

32. Endocrine Disorders and Metabolic Complications in HIV 440
Daniel Lee

33. HIV and Bone Health 451
Roger Bedimo

34. Substance use and HIV 465
Thanh Thuy Truong

35. Psychiatric Disorders and HIV 478
Richa Vijayvargiya and Elizabeth David

36. HIV and Hepatitis Coinfection 489
Karen Vigil

37. Sexually Transmitted Infections 498
Karen Vigil

38. Legal Issues 505
Anna Kastner

39. HIV Healthcare Programs and Insurance Coverage in the U.S. Healthcare System 514
Chauncey McGlathery

Index *521*

OVERALL LEARNING OBJECTIVES

After completing these activities, the participant should be better able to:

- Describe the evolving epidemiology of HIV disease in the United States, with an emphasis on age, gender, sexuality, race/ethnicity, socioeconomic status, emerging subtypes and viral resistance
- Implement appropriate laboratory HIV testing methods for screening and diagnostic HIV
- Adapt pre- and post-testing counseling to best meet individual needs in a variety of situations
- Provide up-to-date HIV care to a broad spectrum of people with HIV, including pediatrics, adolescents, injection-drug users, incarcerated individuals, and an aging population
- Adjust treatment based upon the various comorbidities that are often found in people with HIV, including cardiovascular, renal, and neurologic disease
- Discuss the ethics and legal issues related to caring for people with HIV

FACULTY

LEAD EDITOR

Carolyn Chu, MD, MSc, AAHIVS
Associate Clinical Professor, Department of Family and Community Medicine
Chief Clinical Officer, American Academy of HIV Medicine
Chief Clinical Officer/PI National Clinician Consultation Center
University of California, San Francisco

MANAGING EDITOR

Amy Keller Thyberg, MS
Amy Keller and Associates Consulting, LLC

CO-EDITORS

Roberto C. Arduino, MD
Professor of Medicine
Department of Internal Medicine
Division of Infectious Diseases
McGovern Medical School
The University of Texas Health Science Center at Houston

Philip Bolduc, MD
Associate Professor
Family Medicine and Community Health
University of Massachusetts Chan Medical School
HIV Program and Fellowship Director
Family Health Center of Worcester
Principal Investigator
New England AIDS Education and Training Center

Jarrett K. Sell, MD, FAAFP, AAHIVS
Westside Family Healthcare

William R. Short, MD, MPH, FIDSA, AAHIVS
Associate Professor of Medicine
Associate Professor of Obstetrics and Gynecology
Perelman School of Medicine
University of Pennsylvania

Gary F. Spinner, DMSc, MPH, PA, AAHIVS
Ryan White HIV-AIDS Program
Southwest Community Health Center, Inc.

CONTRIBUTORS

Nancy Aitcheson, MD, MSHP
Clinical Assistant Professor of Medicine
Perelman School of Medicine
University of Pennsylvania

Saira Ajmal, MD
Clinical Assistant Professor
Division of Infectious Diseases
Advocate Christ Medical Center

Yoseph Aldras, MD
Infectious Disease Fellow
Lewis Katz School of Medicine
Temple University

Lisa Y. Armitige, MD, PhD
Co-Medical Director
Heartland National TB Center
Professor of Internal Medicine/Pediatrics/Adult ID
University of Texas Health Center at Tyler

Renata Arrington Sanders, MD, MPH, ScM
Associate Professor
Division of Adolescent and Young Adult Medicine
Department of Pediatrics
Division of Infectious Diseases
Department of Medicine
John Hopkins School of Medicine

Olabimpe Asupoto
Research Assistant I
Division of Geographic Medicine and Infectious Diseases
Department of Medicine
Tulane Medicine

Anchalee Avihingsanon, MD, PhD
Thai Red Cross AIDS Research Centre and Centre of Excellence in Tuberculosis

Jillian T. Barron, MD, MPH
Assistant Professor of Clinical Medicine
Penn Medicine, Division of Infectious Diseases
Medical Director, Penn Community Practice

Katrina Baumgartner, MD, AAHIVS
HIV and Viral Hepatitis Clinical Director
Greater Lawrence Family Health Center

Roger Bedimo, MD
Professor, Department of Internal Medicine
UT Southwestern Medical Center
Division of Infectious Diseases and Clinical Medicine
Infectious Diseases Section Chief, VA
North Texas Health Care System

Christopher M. Bositis, MD, AAHIVS
Associate Clinical Professor
Department of Family and Community Medicine
Clinical Director, National Clinician Consultation Center
University of California, San Francisco

Christian Brander, PhD
ICREA Senior Research Professor
IrsiCaixa AIDS Research Institute
University of Vic, Spain

Patricia Carr Reese, MD, MPH, AAHIVS
Family Physician
Lancaster General Health Physicians – Comprehensive Care
Adjunct Faculty, Family Practice – Obstetrics
Lancaster General Hospital Family Medicine Residency

Ashley Carvalho, MD, MSc
Physician
Full Circle Health

Priyanka Chakrabarti, DO
Staff Physician, Family Medicine
Forward Health

Elizabeth Y. Chiao, MD, MPH
Professor
University of Texas MD Anderson Cancer Center

Eva H. Clark, MD, PhD
Assistant Professor
Department of Medicine
Section of Infectious Diseases
Baylor College of Medicine

Jennifer Cocohoba, PharmD, BCPS, AAHIVP
Professor of Clinical Pharmacy
University of California, San Francisco, School of Pharmacy
University of California, San Francisco, Women's HIV Program

Dagan Coppock, MD, MSCE
Assistant Professor of Medicine
Division of Infectious Diseases
Sidney Kimmel Medical College
Thomas Jefferson University

Avani Dalal, MD
Physician
Albert Einstein Medical Center
Jefferson Health

Elizabeth David, MD
Assistant Professor, Baylor College of Medicine

Abby Davids, MD, MPH, AAHIVS
Physician and Program Director
Full Circle Health

Esteban DelPilar Morales, MD
Physician
Associate Hospital Epidemiologist
Assistant Professor
UMass Chan Medical School
Baystate Health

Christine M. Durand, MD
Associate Professor
Division of Medicine and Oncology
Johns Hopkins University School of Medicine

Umar Farooq, MD, MS, FASN
Associate Professor of Medicine
Division of Nephrology
Penn State University College of Medicine

Rajesh Gandhi, MD
Physician
Director of HIV Services and Clinical Education
Massachusetts General Hospital

Deliana Garcia, MA
Chief Program Officer International and Emerging Issues
Migrant Clinicians Network

Taylor K. Gill, PharmD, BCPS, AAHIVP, FKCHP
Clinical Pharmacist
Ascension Via Christi Hospitals Wichita, Inc.

Zil G. Goldstein, FNP-BC
Associate Medical Director
Callen-Lorde Community Health Center

Wyatt Hanft, MD, MPH
STI Fellow
Department of Family and Community Medicine
University of California, San Francisco

Dennis Joseph Hartigan-O'Connor, MD, PhD
Professor, Department of Medical Microbiology and Immunology
Core Scientist, California National Primate Research Center
University of California, Davis

Rodrigo Hasbun, MD, MPH
Professor of Medicine
The University of Texas McGovern Medical School

Emily Heil, PharmD, MS
Professor
Department of Practice, Sciences, and Health-Outcomes Research
University of Maryland School of Pharmacy

Matthew D. Hickey, MD
Assistant Professor
Division of HIV, Infectious Diseases, and Global Medicine
San Francisco General Hospital
University of California, San Francisco

Aroonsiri Howell, MD
Physician
Department of Geriatric Medicine
Temple University Hospital

Elizabeth Imbert, MD MPH
Associate Professor
Clinical Lead, POP-UP Program, Ward 86
Division of HIV, ID and Global Medicine
San Francisco General Hospital
University of California, San Francisco

Nikolaus Jilg, MD, PhD
Instructor
Division of Infectious Diseases
Massachusetts General Hospital
Harvard Medical School

Boris Juelg, MD, PhD
Associate Professor of Medicine
Harvard Medical School
Division of Infectious Diseases
Massachusetts General Hospital
Ragon Institute of Mass General, MIT and Harvard

Joseph S. Kass, MD, JD, FAAN
Professor of Neurology, Psychiatry and Medical Ethics
Baylor College of Medicine

Anna Kastner, Esq.
Legal Fellow
Sero Project and AIDS Project of Pennsylvania

Jeffrey T. Kirchner, DO, FAAFP, AAHIVS
Medical Director
Caring Communities for HIV
Wilkes-Barre, Hazleton, and Bloomsburg, PA

David E. Koren, PharmD, MPH, BCPS, AAHIVP
Clinical Pharmacist Specialist
Temple University Health System

Ramiz Kseri, MD
Medical Director
Florida Birth-Related Neurological Injury Compensation Association

Daniel Lee, MD
Clinical Professor of Medicine
Owen Health Clinic
University of San Diego Health

George Lewis, PhD
Professor
The Robert C. Gallo, MD Endowed Professor of Translational Medicine
University of Maryland School of Medicine

Laszlo Madaras, MD, MPH, FAAFP, SFHM
Chief Medical Officer
Migrant Clinicians Network
Clinical Assistant Professor of Medicine
Penn State College of Medicine

Christina E. Maguire, PharmD, BCIDP
Infectious Diseases Clinical Pharmacist
Penn Presbyterian Medical Center

Poonam Mathur, DO, MPH
Assistant Professor
Institute of Human Virology
University of Maryland School of Medicine

Chauncey McGlathery
Director of Public Policy
American Academy of HIV Medicine

Emily Min, MD
Staff Physician
Family Health Center of Worcester

Puja H. Nambiar, MD, MPH
Infectious Diseases Specialist
Memorial Sloan Kettering Cancer Center
Assistant Professor of Medicine
Weill Cornell Medical College, New York

Margret O. Nelson
Beth Israel Deaconess Medical Center

Peg O'Byrne Nelson, MSN, RN
Infectious Disease Clinic Nurse
Beth Israel Deaconess Medical Center

Karin Nielsen-Saines, MD, MPH
Professor of Pediatrics
Division of Pediatric Infectious Diseases
David Geffen School of Medicine
University of California, Los Angeles

Jonathan J. Nunez, MD
Associate Professor of Medicine
HIV and Cardiovascular Disease
Penn State Health, Hershey

Neha Sheth Pandit, PharmD, AAHIVP, BCPS
Professor, Infectious Diseases/Pharmacotherapy
Department of Practice, Sciences, and Health Outcomes Research
University of Maryland Baltimore, School of Pharmacy
Clinical Pharmacist, THRIVE Program

Kyle G. Rodino, PharmD
Assistant Professor
University of Maryland
Baltimore School of Pharmacy

M. Elle Saine, MD
Physician Fellow
Hospital of the University of Pennsylvania

Claire M. Hutkins Seda, BA
Director of Communications
Migrant Clinicians Network

Robert W. Shafer, MD
Professor of Medicine
Stanford University

Elizabeth M. Sherman, PharmD
Associate Professor
Barry and Judy Silverman College of Pharmacy
Nova Southeastern University
Clinical Faculty, Division of Infectious Disease
Memorial Healthcare System

Catherine Silva, MD, MHS
Assistant Professor
Department of Pediatrics
Johns Hopkins School of Medicine
Clinical Faculty
Johns Hopkins All Children's Hospital
Adolescent Medicine and Young Adult Specialty Clinic

Benjamin Sokoloff, DO, AAHIVS
Internal Medicine Physician
Cascade AIDS Project | Prism Health

Julia Taylor, MSN FNP
Family Nurse Practitioner
Family Health Center of Worcester

Zelalem Temesgen, MD, FIDSA
Professor of Medicine
Director, Mayo Clinic Center for Tuberculosis
Division of Public Health, Infectious Diseases, and
Occupational Medicine
Mayo Clinic

Thanh Thuy Truong, MD
Addiction Psychiatry
Assistant Professor
Department of Psychiatry and Behavioral Sciences
Baylor College of Medicine

Karen Vigil, MD, FACP, FIDSA
Associate Professor
Department of Internal Medicine
Division of Infectious Diseases
McGovern Medical School
The University of Texas Health Science Center at Houston

Richa Vijayvargiya, MD
Assistant Clinical Professor
Division of Consultation-Liaison Psychiatry
UF Department of Psychiatry

Aasith Villavicencio Paz, MD
Infectious Disease Fellow
Perelman School of Medicine
University of Pennsylvania

Craig S. Weeks, MD
Assistant Clinical Professor of Family Medicine
Central Michigan University
Family Physician
Great Lakes Bay Health Centers

Rita Wilson Dib, MD, MPH
Onco-Infectious Diseases Fellow
Division of Infectious Diseases
McGovern Medical School
The University of Texas Health Science Center at Houston

Alysse G. Wurcel, MD, MS
Associate Professor
Tufts Medical Center
Department of Medicine
Division of Geographic Medicine and Infectious Diseases
Tufts University School of Medicine
Department of Public Health and Community Medicine

John D. Zeuli, PharmD, RPh, BCPS-AQ ID, AAHIVP
Mayo Clinic

DISCLOSURE OF CONFLICTS OF INTEREST

PACE requires every individual in a position to control educational content to disclose all financial relationships with ineligible companies that have occurred within the past 24 months. Ineligible companies are organizations whose primary business is producing, marketing, selling, re-selling, or distributing healthcare products used by or on patients.

All relevant financial relationships for anyone with the ability to control the content of this educational activity are listed below and have been mitigated according to PACE policies. Others involved in the planning of this activity have no relevant financial relationships.

The following faculty for this educational activity have relevant financial relationships to disclose:

Roger Bedimo reports consultant, advisor, or speaker fees from Gilead Sciences, Merck & Co. Janssen Therapeutics, Shionogi, Theratechnologies, and ViiV Healthcare.

Christian Brander reports being a co-founder and stock holder with Aelix Therapeutics.

Joseph Cass reports consultant, advisor, or speaker fees from Cassava Sciences, Inc.

Eva Clark reports royalties or patent beneficiaries from McGraw Hill Publishers.

Jennifer Cocohoba reports being a researcher ViiV Healthcare and a primary investigator for Genetech.

Christine Durand reports being a researcher and paid grant reviewer for Gilead Sciences.

Umar Farooq reports consultant, advisor, or speaker fees from Bayer and being a researcher for Ablative Solutions, Abbot, Remegen, and Roche.

Dennis Hartigan O'Connor reports being an independent contractor and owns stock with Tendel Therapies, Inc.

Rodrigo Hasbun reports research fees for Biomeriaux.

Emily Heil reports being an independent contractor with Wolters Kluwer.

Elizabeth Imbert reports being a researcher for Gilead Sciences.

David Koren reports consultant, advisor, or speaker fees from Gilead Sciences and ViiV Healthcare.

Daniel Lee reports consultant, advisor, or speaker fees from Theratechnologies, being an independent contractor with EMDSerono, and owns stock in Gilead Sciences.

Christina Maguire reports consultant, advisor, or speaker fees from ViiV Healthcare.

Kyle G. Rodino reports being a researcher for DiaSorin and consultant, advisor, or speaker fees from bioMérieux, ClearLabs, and Roche.

Robert W. Shafer reports consultant, advisor, or speaker fees from Gilead Sciences and ViiV Healthcare.

William R. Short reports being a researcher for Gilead Sciences and consultant, speaker, or advisor fees from ViiV Healthcare.

Gary F. Spinner reports consultant, advisor or speaker fees for Gilead Sciences and ViiC Healthcare.

Zelalem Temesgen reports consultant, advisor, or speaker fees and is a researcher from ViiV Healhtcare.

Thanh Thuy Truong reports consultant, advisor, or speaker fees from Takeda Pharmaceuticals.

Karen Vigil reports consultant, advisor, or speaker fees from Gilead Sciences and Viiv Healthcare and research fees from Theratechnologies.

The following faculty for this educational activity have no relevant financial relationships:

Nancy Aitcheson

Saira Ajmal

Yoseph Aldras

Lisa Y. Armitige

Roberto Arduino

Olabimpe Asupoto

Jillian T. Barron

Katrina Baumgartner

Philip Bolduc

Christopher Bositis

Patricia Carr Reese

Ashley Carvalho
Priyanka Chakrabarti
Elizabeth Y. Chiao
Carolyn Chu
Diana Coffa
Dagan Coppock
Avani Dalal
Anny Davids
Esteban DelPilar Morales
Delania Garcia
Rah Ghandi
Taylor Gill
Zil G. Goldstein
Wyatt Hanft
Matt Hickey
Aroonsiri Howell
Claire M. Hutkins Seda
Boris Juelg
Nikolaus Jilg
Anna Kastner
Amy Keller Thyberg
Jeffrey Kirchner
David Koren
Ramiz Kseri
Ann Le
George Lewis
Laszlo Madaras
Chauncey McGathery
Emily Min
Puja Nambiar
Margaret Nelson
Karen Nielsen
Jonathan Nunez
Mathur Poonan
Elle Saine
Jarrett K. Sell
Elizabeth Sherman
Nera Sheth Pandit
Catherine Silva
Benjamin Sokoloff
Julia Taylor
Richa Vijayvargiya
Aasith Villavicencio Paz
Craig Weeks
Rita Wilson Dib
Alysse G. Wurcel

1.

ENDING THE HIV EPIDEMIC

A PLAN FOR AMERICA

Benjamin Sokoloff

LEARNING OBJECTIVES

- Identify the goals of the current nationwide initiative to eliminate new HIV infections in the United States.
- Describe the key strategic pillars upon which this initiative is built to achieve these goals.

KEY POINTS

- Ending the HIV epidemic in the United States is possible; the current goal is to reduce the number of new HIV infections by 75% by 2025 and by 90% by 2030.
- The four key strategies of this initiative are to increase the diagnosis, treatment, and prevention of HIV infection and to respond rapidly to new clusters of HIV transmissions. These strategies are based on robust evidence-based science, medicine, and public health principles.

INTRODUCTION

The management of people with HIV (PWH) has evolved significantly over time, and so has the national response for slowing and eventually ending the HIV epidemic. Throughout its history, the U.S. federal government has responded to emerging epidemics and pandemics with legislative and executive actions with the intent of saving lives and preventing disease. This chapter describes the most recent legislative steps the U.S. government has taken to address the HIV epidemic.

In the first two decades of the 21st century, new HIV infection rates remained stubbornly high and static despite substantial medical advances. With expanding antiretroviral therapy (ART) and pre-exposure prophylaxis (PrEP) options, we now should be able to prevent most new infections. Remaining barriers include limitations of our healthcare systems and implementation challenges. The Ending the HIV Epidemic (EHE) initiative was developed to address these gaps, aspiring to use powerful biomedical and public health tools to end the 40-year epidemic of HIV in the United States. Recent surveillance data give us hopeful signs of early success.

GOALS AND TIMELINE

The EHE initiative is a 10-year plan that aims to reduce the number of new HIV infections in the United States by 75% by 2025, and by 90% by 2030, for a total of 250,000 infections averted over this time period (CDC, 2024a). This translates to a reduction in the incidence of HIV infections to fewer than 3,000 annually. In 2018, the estimated incidence of HIV infections in the United States and dependent areas was 34,800 (CDC, 2021a). EHE goals are in line with the "90-90-90" targets for ending the global HIV/AIDS pandemic as issued by the United Nations Programme on HIV/AIDS (UNAIDS) in 2014. UNAIDS-sponsored modeling predicted that if 90% of PWH were diagnosed, 90% with an established diagnosis were on ART, and 90% of those receiving ART were virally suppressed by 2020, the end of the HIV/AIDS pandemic would be achieved by 2030 (UNAIDS, 2014). Unfortunately, the 90-90-90 goal has been met by only a handful of countries globally. The EHE initiative represents the U.S. government's commitment to these goals and the elimination of HIV/AIDS as a major public health concern.

Over the 10 years of its implementation, the EHE initiative will transition through three phases. The initial phase, which concluded in 2024, focused on cities and regions most heavily affected by HIV based on 2016 and 2017 data. Federal agencies provided supportive funding to various entities in these 40 jurisdictions to implement the four pillars of diagnosis, treatment, prevention, and response (see Figure 1.1). The second phase will seek to expand on the efforts and successes achieved in phase 1 throughout the rest of the country to reach the goal of reducing the infection rate by 90% by 2030. Finally, the third phase of the initiative will focus on improving resources for PWH who are connected to care in order to achieve viral suppression and maintain new infection rates at less than 3,000 per year (Giroir, 2020).

THE FOUR PILLARS (KEY STRATEGIES)

DIAGNOSE

According to Centers for Disease Control and Prevention (CDC) surveillance reports, there were an estimated 1.2 million PWH in the United States at the end of 2019, and 13.3% remained undiagnosed (CDC, 2021b). Undiagnosed individuals account for a disproportionate share of new HIV

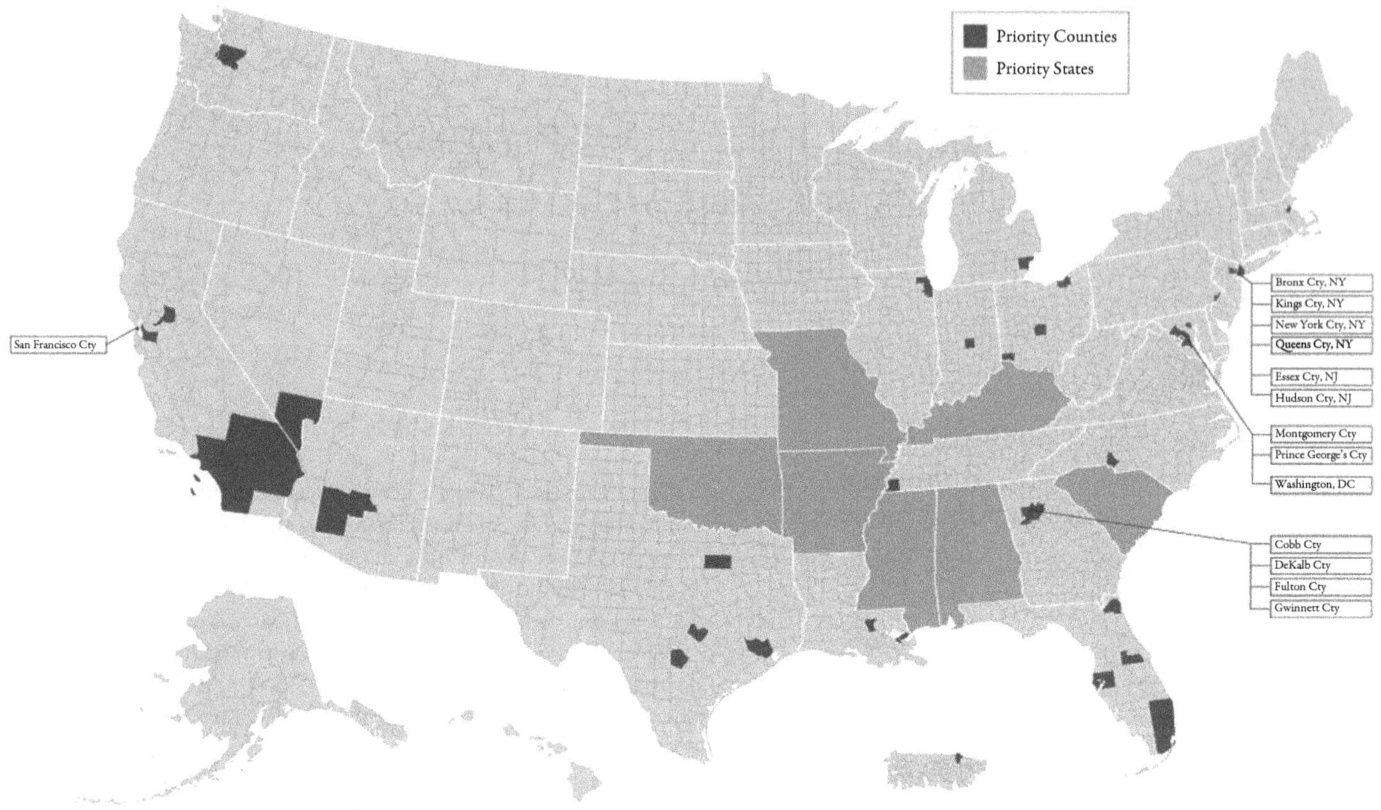

Figure 1.1 Priority jurisdictions for ending the HIV epidemic. SOURCE: https//www.hiv.gov/federal-response/ending-the-hiv-epidemic/jurisdictions/phase-one

transmissions. Therefore, expanding HIV testing efforts to diagnose these individuals is vital not only for their individual benefit but also to halt further HIV transmission. The first pillar of the EHE's key strategies—diagnosis—seeks to address this goal by mobilizing federal and local resources to achieve early diagnosis of all PWH. Several agencies within the Department of Health and Human Services (DHHS), including the CDC, Health Resources and Services Administration (HRSA), National Institutes of Health (NIH), Indian Health Service (HIS), and Substance Abuse and Mental Health Services Administration (SAMHSA), support community structures already in place to increase testing capabilities in both traditional settings (e.g., health facilities providing medical and substance abuse services) as well as nontraditional venues where people congregate (e.g., community festivals, public spaces, and businesses). The overarching goal of this effort is to make HIV testing a noncontroversial, routine event for all adolescents and adults at least once and more often depending on risk factors.

TREAT

Advances in HIV treatment have made it possible for many PWH to live with a well-managed chronic condition rather than a progressive terminal illness. Beyond the profound impact that HIV treatment has on individual health, viral suppression is a powerful intervention that reduces ongoing HIV transmission. Results from the HPTN 052, PARTNER 1, PARTNER 2, and Opposites Attract trials demonstrated that PWH with consistently suppressed viral loads will not transmit HIV to their sex partners by condomless vaginal or anal sex (Bavinton et al., 2019; Cohen et al., 2011; Cohen et al., 2016; Rodger et al., 2019). These studies provide strong support for the role of treatment as prevention (TasP). Yet, as previously reported by the CDC, 6 in 10 HIV transmissions were from PWH who knew about their infection but were either not in care or not virally suppressed despite representing only 37% of PWH (CDC, 2019). This represents a failure of the healthcare system and a key area for significant improvement. The goal of this pillar of the EHE initiative is to increase the proportion of persons with known HIV infection with suppressed viral loads from 69% to 95% by 2030 (CDC, 2024b).

Building on the successes of clinics funded by the Ryan White HIV/AIDS Program, DHHS agencies seek to strengthen and expand local infrastructure and capacity for HIV testing and prevention to complement the traditional role that Ryan White programs play in providing comprehensive HIV care tailored to individual and community needs. In the past few years, the CDC has encouraged a "status neutral" approach to both HIV care and prevention. This means treating the whole person rather than the disease, by offering a full range of healthcare services to encompass HIV treatment, prevention, and general health care. This "one-stop-shop" approach offers a less stigmatizing clinical setting and reduces the risk of missed healthcare opportunities which go beyond only HIV treatment. A status neutral approach introduced in New York City in 2016 led to a 22% decline in new HIV infections by 2019 (CDC, 2024c).

PREVENT

The third pillar of the EHE initiative aims to prevent HIV transmission using PrEP and syringe service programs (SSPs). PrEP in its various forms substantially reduces the risk for HIV acquisition. In 2020 an estimated 1,216,210 people in the United States had an indication for PrEP. However, only 301,033 patients received a prescription for PrEP that same year, representing less than a quarter of eligible candidates. This improved by 2022 to 36% of eligible patients receiving a PrEP prescription (CDC, 2023). A 2024 presentation at the Conference on Retroviruses and Opportunistic Infections (CROI) showed that states in the highest quintile of PrEP coverage for eligible patients had the greatest declines in new HIV infections, even after adjustment for HIV viral suppression among existing PWH, compared to a minor increase in new infections among states in the lowest quintile (Sullivan et al., 2024).

The Ready, Set, PrEP program (readysetprep.hiv.gov) was created by DHHS in 2019 to address one of the barriers contributing to the gap in PrEP prescriptions. With public-private partnerships, the program makes tenofovir/emtricitabine oral tablets available to individuals without prescription drug insurance coverage. To be eligible, an individual: (1) cannot have prescription drug insurance coverage, (2) must have a recent negative HIV test, (3) must have a prescription for oral PrEP, and (4) must live in the United States or its tribal lands or territories. Limitations of this program are that it does not cover costs of medical visits and lab tests, nor does it cover people who are insured, regardless of out-of-pocket cost.

SSPs are community-based prevention programs aimed at providing comprehensive resources to persons who inject drugs (PWID), including access to substance use disorder treatment, needle-exchange services, and infectious diseases screening with linkage-to-care. A meta-analysis of studies conducted in North America and Europe (Aspinal et al., 2014) showed that SSPs contribute to an estimated 58% reduction in incidence of HIV. Because congressional funds cannot be used to purchase needles directly for exchange, the CDC and SAMHSA instead use appropriated funds to support increased access by helping local communities implement SSPs. A recent study demonstrated that PrEP awareness among PWID increased from 25.6% to 35.3% between 2018 and 2022, although PrEP uptake remained flat (Chapin-Bardales et al., 2024). This highlights the importance of integrating co-located PrEP with other medical and social services for PWID.

RESPOND

The final pillar of the EHE initiative aims to strengthen communities' ability to respond quickly to new outbreaks through collaboration between the CDC and local health departments in response to epidemiologic trends and lab surveillance data. These partnerships endeavor to promptly identify clusters of HIV transmission (otherwise known as outbreaks) using real-time molecular techniques with epidemiologic tracing. The end goal is to offer diagnostic, therapeutic, and prophylactic interventions, as appropriate, and to guide the distribution of resources where they are most needed. These partnerships are not limited to health departments and can include local healthcare providers, patients, and advocates.

ASSESSMENT OF INTERVENTION

Federal progress can be visualized at ahead.hiv.gov. Because CDC incidence data lag by 1–2 years, there are few comparative years to assess the effects of EHE thus far. Further, data from early years should be interpreted with careful consideration of the impact from disruptions related to the SARS-CoV-2 pandemic. However, early results may warrant cautious optimism. CDC data show a 12% reduction in HIV incidence among persons aged over 12 years between 2018 and 2022. Among those aged 13–24, new HIV infections declined by 30%, and there were no demographic subsets in which incidence increased. Another notable improvement was a 16% reduction in new infections in the southern United States, which still carries the highest incidence among all geographic regions. In EHE phase I jurisdictions there was a 21% reduction of new infections between 2017 and 2022. However, similar demographic disparities remained (for example, there was no statistically significant decrease in HIV incidence among Hispanic/Latino populations) (CDC, 2024d).

REFERENCES

Aspinal EJ, Nambiar D, Goldberg DJ, et al. Are needle and syringe programmes associated with a reduction in HIV transmission among people who inject drugs: a systematic review and meta-analysis. *Int J Epidemiol.* 2014;43(1):235–248.

Bavinton BR, Prestage GP, Jin F, et al. Strategies used by gay male HIV serodiscordant couples to reduce the risk of HIV transmission from anal intercourse in three countries. *J Int AIDS Soc.* 2019;22(4):e25277.

Centers for Disease Control and Prevention (CDC). Dear colleague: preliminary data on pre-exposure prophylaxis coverage released. HIV. https://www.cdc.gov/hiv/policies/dear-colleague/dcl/20231017.html. Published October 2023. Accessed June 2024.

CDC. Ending HIV transmission. Vital signs. https://www.cdc.gov/vitalsigns/test-treat-prevent/index.html. Published December 2019. Accessed June 2024.

CDC. Estimated HIV incidence and prevalence in the United States, 2015–2019. HIV Surveillance Supplemental Report. 2021;26(1). http://www.cdc.gov/ hiv/library/reports/hiv-surveillance.html. Published May 2021a. Accessed June 2024.

CDC. HIV Surveillance Supplemental Report: estimated HIV incidence and prevalence in the United States, 2018–2022. https://www.cdc.gov/nchhstp/director-letters/cdc-publishes-new-hiv-surveillance-reports.html. Published May 2024d. Accessed June 2024.

CDC. HIV Surveillance Supplemental Report: monitoring selected national HIV prevention and care objectives by using HIV surveillance data United States and 6 territories and freely associated states, 2022. https://stacks.cdc.gov/view/cdc/156511. Published May 2024b. Accessed June 2024.

CDC. Ending the HIV Epidemic in the US (EHE). About Ending the HIV Epidemic in the US. https://www.cdc.gov/nchhstp/director-letters/cdc-publishes-new-hiv-surveillance-reports.html. Published March 2024a. Accessed June 2024.

CDC. Issue brief: status neutral HIV care and service delivery. https://www.cdc.gov/hiv/policies/data/status-neutral-issue-brief.html. Published May 2024c. Accessed June 2024.

CDC. Monitoring selected national HIV prevention and care objectives by using HIV surveillance data—United States and 6 dependent areas, 2021. *HIV Surveillance Supplemental Report*. 2021;26(2). https://stacks.cdc.gov/view/cdc/107935. Published May 2021b. Accessed June 2024.

Chapin-Bardales J, Broz D, Eustaquio P, Feelemyer J, et al. Changes in HIV PrEP awareness and use among PWID in 19 US cities, 2018 and 2022. Conference on Retroviruses and Opportunistic Infections 2024, March 2024: Hazards ahead: the intersection of HIV and substance use. Abstract #1009. https://www.croiconference.org/abstract/changes-in-hiv-prep-awareness-and-use-among-pwid-in-19-us-cities-2018-and-2022

Cohen MS, Chen YQ, McCauley M, et al. Antiretroviral therapy for the prevention of HIV-1 transmission. *N Engl J Med*. 2016;375(9):830–839. https://doi.org/10.1056/NEJMoa1600693

Cohen MS, Chen YQ, McCauley M, et al. Prevention of HIV-1 infection with early antiretroviral therapy. *N Engl J Med* 2011;365(6):493–505. https://doi.org/10.1056/NEJMoa1105243

Giroir BP. The time is now to end the HIV epidemic. *Am J Public Health*. 2020;110(1):22–24.

Rodger AJ, Cambiano V, Bruun T, et al. Risk of HIV transmission through condomless sex in serodifferent gay couples with the HIV-positive partner taking suppressive antiretroviral therapy (PARTNER): final results of a multicentre, prospective, observational study. *Lancet*. 2019;393(10189):2428–2438.

Sullivan PS, Dubose S, Brisco K, Le G, Juhasz M. Association of state-level PrEP coverage and state-level HIV diagnoses, US, 2012–2021. Conference on Retroviruses and Opportunistic Infections 2024, March 2024: Leaning into the success of biomedical HIV prevention #165. https://www.croiconference.org/abstract/association-of-state-level-prep-coverage-and-state-level-hiv-diagnoses-us-2012-2021/

UNAIDS. 90-90-90: an ambitious treatment target to help end the HIV epidemic. https://www.unaids.org/sites/default/files/media_asset/90-90-90_en.pdf. Published October 2014. Accessed June 2024.

2.

THE ORIGIN, EVOLUTION, AND EPIDEMIOLOGY OF HIV-1 AND HIV-2

Jeffrey T. Kirchner, Emily Min, and Julia Taylor

ORIGIN AND EVOLUTION OF HIV-1 AND HIV-2

LEARNING OBJECTIVES

- Discuss the distinct origins of HIV-1 and HIV-2 from simian immunodeficiency viruses (SIVs) and the multiple cross-transmission events from apes to humans.
- Describe the origin of initial HIV infections in South-Central Africa, subsequent viral dissemination to other areas of Africa, and the ultimate global spread of HIV.
- Discuss the diversity of HIV, including viral groups, viral clades, and recombinant forms and their implications for transmission of HIV, as well as treatments and vaccine developments.

WHAT'S NEW?

- Researchers recently identified a new HIV-1 group M subtype called subtype L. This was based on complete genomic sequencing of three non-transmission-linked cases.
- Recombination between different HIV strains continues to drive further diversification of the pandemic. At least 160 distinct circulating forms (CRFs) have now been identified, and this number is increasing.

KEY POINTS

- All strains of HIV-1 and HIV-2 are genetic descendants of SIVs. Initial cross-species transmission of SIVs occurred from consumption of bush meat.
- Phylogenetic studies have determined that HIV-1 emerged from Cameroon into Kinshasa (Democratic Republic of Congo, Africa), and spread westward with urban growth and railway mobility.
- HIV-1 was introduced to Haiti around 1966 before emerging in the United States by 1970. Upon reaching North America, the virus was amplified and established epidemics in Asia, Australia, Europe, and Latin America.
- HIV-1 is divided into four groups based on genetic makeup. These include group M ("Major") and its 12 associated viral subtypes or clades (A–L), which account for approximately 95% of infections globally.
- HIV-2 comprises nine groups (A–I) and is mainly limited to the West. Since its discovery in 1986, cases have been reported in Europe and the United States. Globally, HIV-2 represents approximately 2% of all HIV infections and its prevalence may be declining.
- Genetic diversity of HIV, including recombination between subtypes, may continue to present challenges to the development of a globally effective vaccine.

ORIGIN OF HIV AND ENTRY INTO HUMANS

Human immunodeficiency virus (HIV) is a retrovirus and a member of the lentivirus family. It is characterized by enormous diversity and rapid viral evolution. Simian immunodeficiency virus (SIV) is the zoonotic precursor of HIV. Very strong evidence indicates that the first cross-species transmission of SIV to humans occurred in southeast Cameroon (Sharp and Hahn, 2011). The origin of HIV-1 can be traced to the early 1920s from Cameroon and then to Kinshasa in what is now the Democratic Republic of Congo (DRC). The combination of rapid population growth, migration, changes in sexual behaviors, and the use of unsterilized needles all likely contributed to the rapid spread of HIV-1 in Africa. It is not known specifically how humans acquired SIV. However, based on the recognized biology of these viruses, transmission likely arose from cutaneous or mucous membrane exposure to infected chimpanzee blood or body fluid. Such exposures occur in the context of hunting, butchering, and consuming bush meat (Sharp and Hahn, 2011).

It was first noted in 1999, via genetic sequencing, that the chimpanzee *Pan troglodytes* infected with SIV_{cpz} was likely the primary natural reservoir for HIV-1 (Gao et al., 1999). Later work determined that HIV-1 in humans began with cross-species transmission and recombination of two SIVs (from red-capped mangabeys [*Cercocebus torquatus*] and greater spot-nosed monkeys [*Cercopithecus nictitans*]) to chimpanzees that preyed on these animals (Keele et al., 2006). Keele and colleagues analyzed mitochondrial DNA and viral-specific antibody from 599 fecal samples from chimpanzees. These samples exhibited a strong and broadly cross-reactive western blot profile indistinguishable from that of HIV-1 human controls. To date, serologic evidence for SIV infection has been identified in more than 45 nonhuman primate species (NHPS) (Peeters et al., 2014; Sharp and Hahn, 2011). The genetic diversity of these viral species is complex and includes coevolution of virus–host, cross-species transmission, and viral recombination.

Like HIV, SIV is sexually transmitted in NHPS and can be transmitted perinatally. In contrast to previous thinking, SIV is indeed pathogenic in most NHPS, causing CD4+ T-cell depletion (Keele et al., 2009). Chimpanzees with SIV infection have a 10- to 16-fold increased risk of death compared to those that are uninfected. Fertility and survival of offspring are also decreased in SIV-positive female chimpanzees.

THE DISSEMINATION OF HIV THROUGHOUT AFRICA AND THE WORLD

A study by Faria and colleagues using phylogenetic analysis and "molecular clocks" (that assume that retroviruses mutate over time at a constant rate) confirmed previous work by Hahn and others regarding the initial dissemination routes of HIV-1 in West Africa (Cohen, 2014; Faria et al., 2014; Sharp and Hahn, 2011). It is well established that the first known infections with HIV-1 emerged from Kinshasa (formerly called Leopoldville) in the DRC around 1920. Many refer to Leopoldville/Kinshasa as the "cradle of the AIDS pandemic." From this area, the virus spread somewhat quietly for about 60 years—moving eastward to other communities via migration on railway lines that carried up to 1 million passengers yearly to other areas of Africa. This included the three largest population centers: Brazzaville, Mbuji-Mayi, and Lubumbashi (Cohen, 2014; Faria et al., 2014). Rivers were major travel and commerce routes and are also believed to have facilitated the geographic spread of HIV in these regions (Figure 2.1).

Sexual transmission is the primary mode and driver of new HIV infections and resultant dissemination of the virus. However, unsterilized injections at clinics in Africa also may have greatly contributed to the spread of HIV. According to Jacques Pépin, well-intended public health interventions by authorities in the Belgian Congo from 1921 to 1959 to treat trypanosomiasis, syphilis, yaws, malaria, and leprosy resulted in the administration of millions of injections to residents of these communities. The majority of injections were intravenous and were administered with syringes that clinicians used repeatedly without sterilization of the needles between each

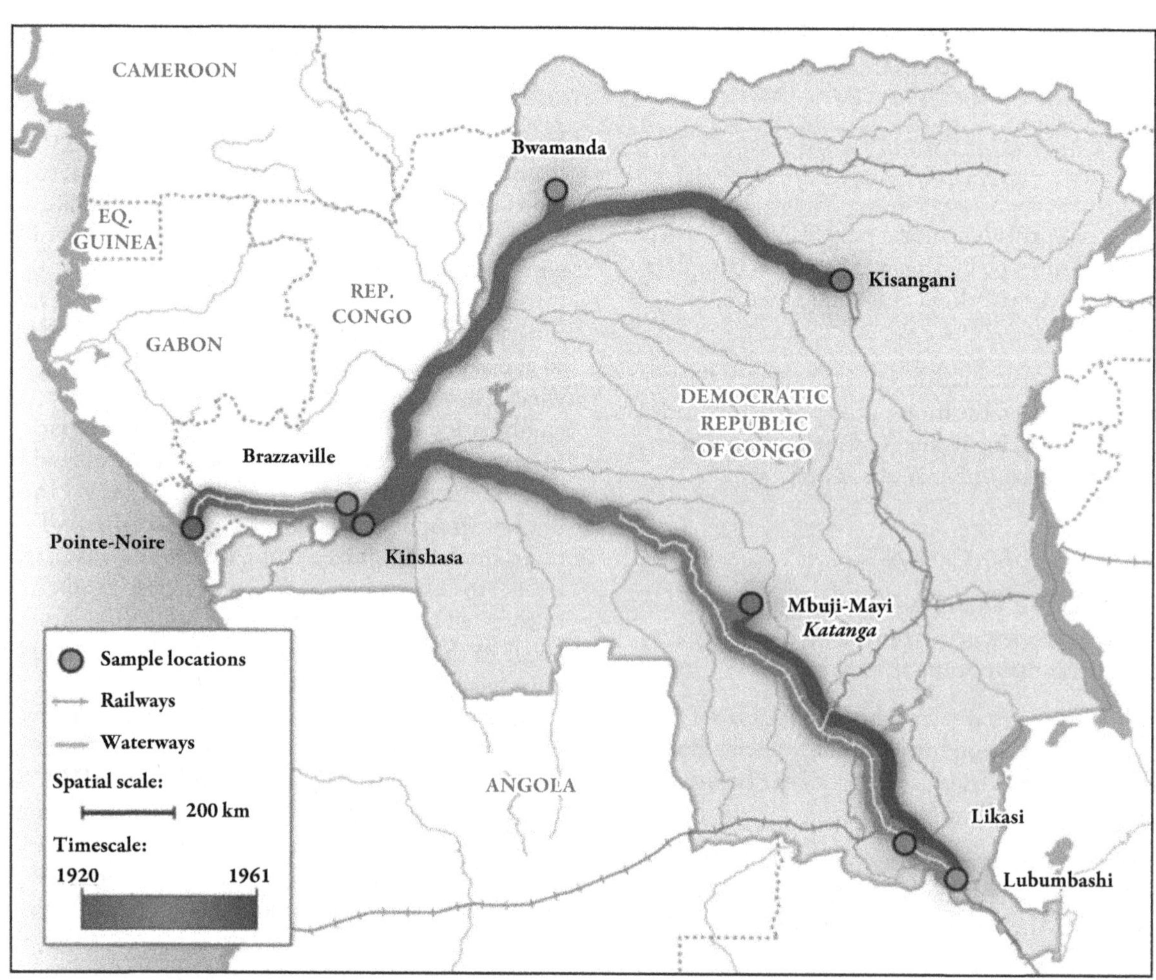

Figure 2.1 Spatial dynamics showing the spread of HIV-1 group 1 from Kinshasa in the Democratic Republic of the Congo via rivers and railways, which were operational until about 1960 SOURCE: Faria NR, et al. *Science*. 2014;346(6205):56–61.

use (Pépin, 2011). Consequently, thousands of individuals may have acquired HIV iatrogenically. Data suggest similar transmission of hepatitis B (HBV) and hepatitis C (HCV) with iatrogenic transmission during public health campaigns (Pépin, 2013).

The epidemic histories of HIV-1 groups M and O were thought to be similar until approximately 1960, when group M infections underwent an epidemiologic transition and exponential increase, outpacing regional population growth (Faria et al., 2014). It is unknown why the growth rate of infections with HIV group M nearly tripled during this time, but likely explanations include virus-specific factors, population growth, and the widespread use of aforementioned public health injection campaigns (Pépin, 2011; Sharp and Hahn, 2011).

Tissues samples collected from two patients in Kinshasa in 1959 and 1960 showed that HIV-1 had diversified into different subtypes much earlier than previously believed. Viral sequencing done on plasma from a sailor who died in 1959 is the oldest case of documented HIV-1 infection (Zhu et al., 1998). Worobey and colleagues subsequently identified HIV-1 from a lymph node specimen obtained in 1960 from a female in Kinshasa (Worobey et al., 2008). The significant genetic difference between these two early HIV specimens demonstrated that diversification of HIV-1 occurred in Kinshasa at least 20 years before the first cases of AIDS were observed in the United States in 1981. As HIV-1 group M spread globally, its dissemination led to population bottlenecks ("founder events") that resulted in different lineages, viral subtypes or clades, and circulating recombinant forms (CRFs) (Peeters et al., 2014).

The initial spread of HIV-1 out of Africa and into the Caribbean region via Haiti occurred sometime between 1960 and 1966. During the early 1960s, approximately 4,500 skilled Haitian workers were employed as teachers or bureaucrats in the newly independent Congo, which had been a colony of Belgium. The presumed source of HIV was these Haitian professionals who returned from working in this part of Africa. Although the first case of AIDS was not reported in Haiti until 1983, there are clinical reports of persons with "AIDS symptoms" going back to 1979 (Junqueira and Almeida, 2016). Work done by investigators using HIV-1 *gag* gene sequences from five Haitian patients with HIV confirmed that HIV-1 subtype B definitely arrived in Haiti by 1966, at least three years before it spread to the United States and then into other countries (see Figure 2.2) (Gilbert et al., 2007). Consequently, these data suggest that HIV-1 was circulating cryptically in the United States for approximately 12 years before the first cases of AIDS were recognized and reported in 1981 (Gottlieb et al., 1981).

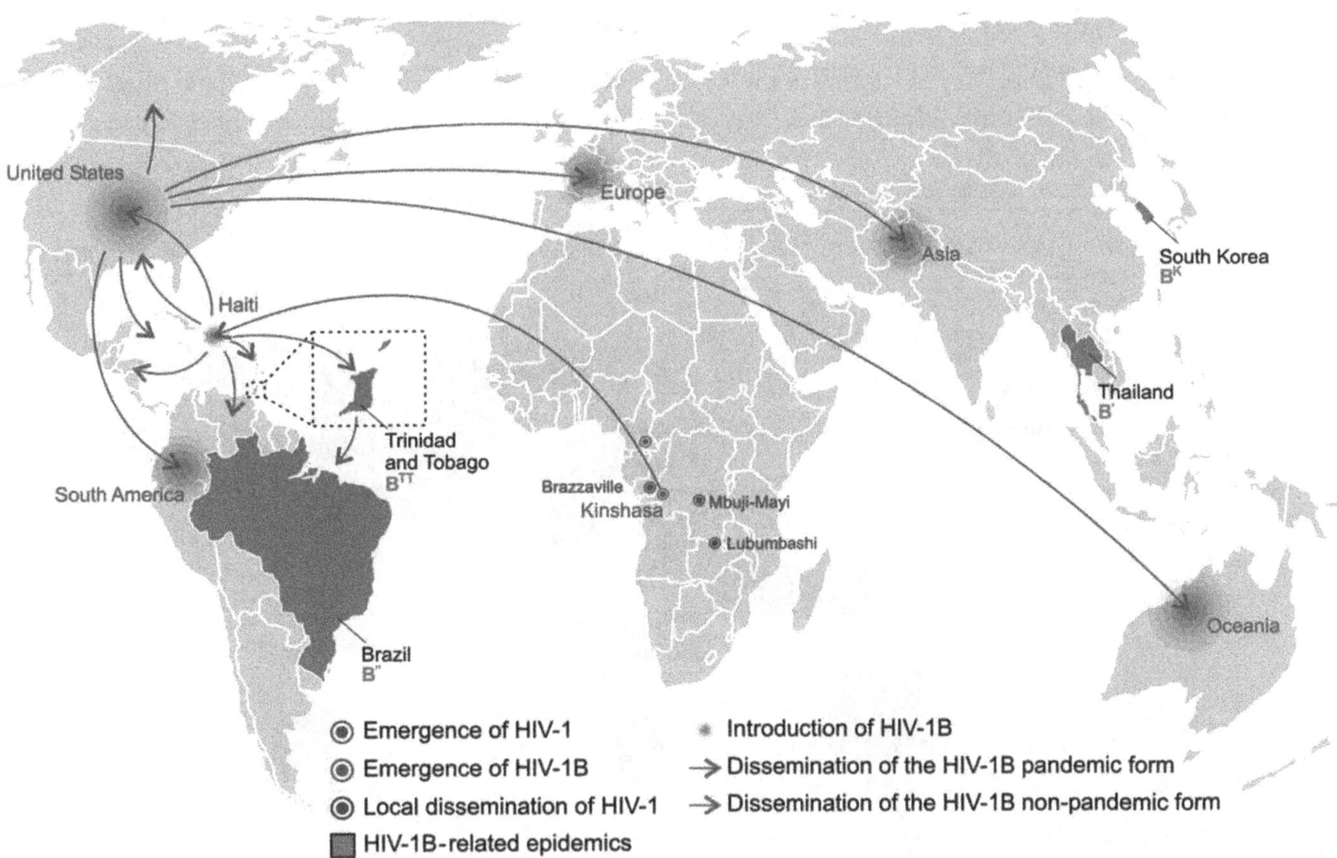

Figure 2.2 Estimated global spatial dynamics of HIV-1 subtype B. Blue lines represent the main dissemination routes of HIV-1 subtype B pandemic form and the main disease epicenters. The epidemic starts in the city of Kinshasa, Democratic Republic of the Congo (Africa). Orange lines represent the direction of the B non-pandemic lineage dissemination. Green regions demarcate the countries where a specific lineage of the HIV-1 subtype B is circulating SOURCE: Junqueira DM, Almeida SE. *Virology*. 2016;495:173–784.

Based on later phylogenetic analyses, it is likely that HIV was in the United States, specifically New York City, "around 1970" (Worobey et al., 2016). The virus was likely spreading slowly among heterosexually active individuals before entering the population of men who have sex with men (MSM), along with people who inject drugs, and then began to be recognized clinically. The actual scientific facts may never be known; however, Pépin believes that the sex trade industry and the blood trade in Port-au-Prince exponentially amplified the number of HIV infections in Haiti and possibly other countries in which blood products were sold, including the United States (Pépin, 2011).

HIV-1 AND HIV-2 GROUPS AND SUBTYPES AND THEIR GEOGRAPHIC DISTRIBUTIONS

HIV-1 is characterized by significant genetic diversification and rapid evolution. The HIV pandemic comprises four distinct lineages that are termed groups M, N, O, and P. Each has resulted from a distinct and independent cross-species transmission event of SIVs infecting African apes. The use of molecular clocks determined that the most recent common ancestor of group M dates to approximately 1920 (Sharp and Hahn, 2011). The four known HIV-1 groups share approximately 50%–60% homology in their nucleotide sequences.

HIV-1 GROUP M

HIV-1 group M (M for "Major" or "Main") was the first lineage discovered and represents the pandemic form of HIV-1. It has a widespread global distribution and accounts for 90%–95% of HIV-1 infections (Sharp and Hahn, 2011). The genetic diversity within HIV-1 group M is the result of subsequent evolution and spread in humans. Based on phylogenic analysis, HIV-1 group M can be further divided into 10 subtypes or clades (A–D, F–H, J, K, and L) and additional sub-subtypes (A1–A4 and F1–F2). The subtypes share 80% homology in their genetic sequences, meaning they differ genetically by approximately 20%. Subtypes and sub-subtypes can form additional mosaic forms through the recombination of different strains inside people with dual or multiple infections. Some CRFs may further achieve epidemic relevance. To date, researchers have now identified about 160 distinct CRFs and unique recombinant strains (Bacque et al., 2021; Elangovan et al., 2021; Mori et al., 2022; www.hiv.lanl.gov/components/sequence/HIV/crfdb/crfs.com). This number has been increasing over time (Switzer et al., 2024).

Globally, subtype C, found mainly in sub-Saharan Africa, represents approximately 50% of HIV-1 infections, although recent data suggest this may be as high as 75% (Faria et al., 2019). This is followed by subtype A (12%), found mainly in central and East Africa and Russia. Subtype B (11%) is the predominant subtype in Europe, the United States, and Oceania and is the most geographically dispersed subtype (Bbosa et al., 2019). The CRFs, most commonly CRF02_AG and CRF01_AE, now account for about 17% of HIV-1 infections worldwide (Elangovan et al., 2021). Subtypes G and D account for 5% and 2% of infections worldwide, respectively (see Figure 2.3 and Box 2.1) (Peeters et al., 2014).

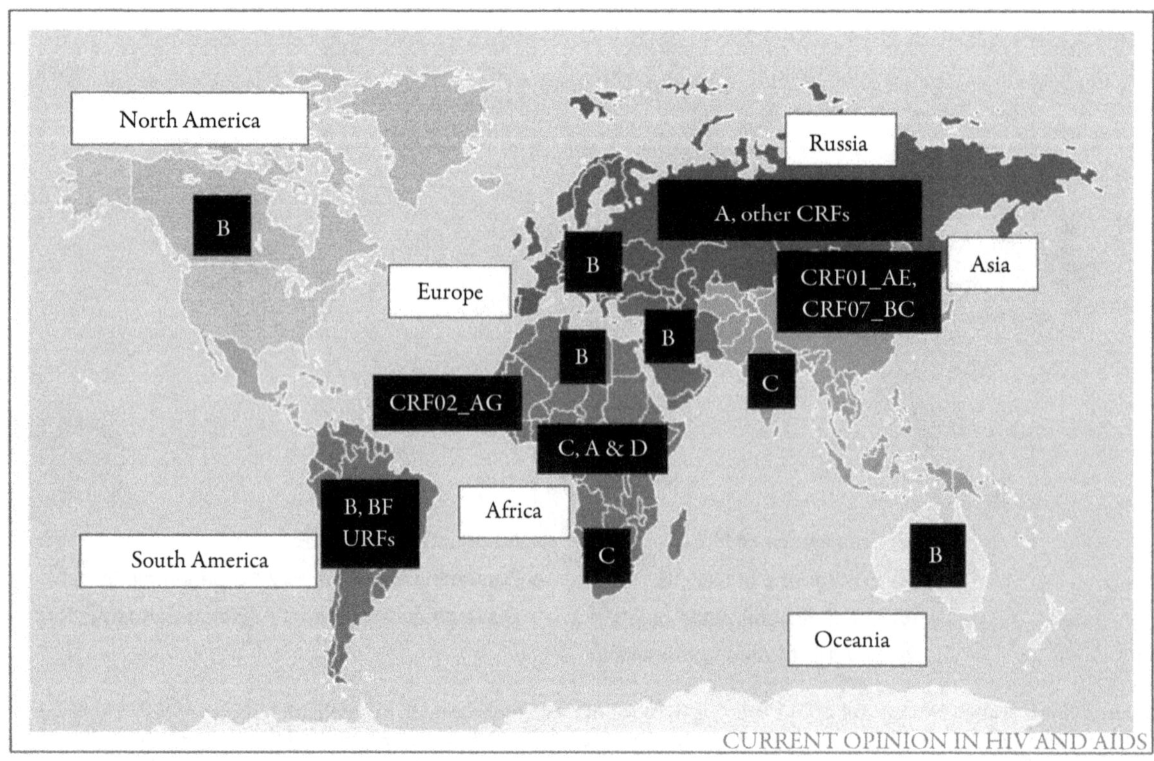

Figure 2.3 Global HIV subtype diversity SOURCE: Bbosa N, et al. *Curr Opin HIV AIDS*. 2019;14:153–560.

Box 2.1 DISTRIBUTION OF HIV-1 SUBTYPES

Historically, the distribution of subtypes followed the geographic patterns listed here:

- *Subtype A*: Central and East Africa as well as Eastern European countries that were formerly part of the Soviet Union
- *Subtype B*: West and Central Europe, the Americas, Australia, South America, and several Southeast Asian countries (Thailand and Japan), as well as northern Africa and the Middle East
- *Subtype C*: Sub-Saharan Africa, India, and Brazil
- *Subtype D*: North Africa and the Middle East
- *Subtype F*: South and Southeast Asia
- *Subtype G*: West and Central Africa
- *Subtypes H, J, and K*: Africa and the Middle East

HIV-1 GROUP N

Group N ("N" for "non-M, non-O," or "new") was isolated in 1995 from a woman in Cameroon who died from AIDS (Pépin, 2011). Fewer than 20 cases of group N infection have been identified, and all except one were from Cameroon. Like group M, it is the result of chimpanzee-to-human transmission. The small number of infections from this group and limited genetic diversity suggest that its introduction into humans did not occur until approximately 1963 (Peeters et al., 2014).

HIV-1 GROUP O

Group O ("O" for "outlier") was first discovered in 1990 in two Cameroonians living in Belgium (De Leys, 1990) and is thought to represent only about 1% of all HIV transmissions. Researchers have determined that group O originated by SIV cross-species transmission from western lowland gorillas and not chimpanzees (D'Arc et al., 2015). Like the other HIV-1 groups, it underwent adaptations to human hosts. Another study found the prevalence of HIV-1 group O in Cameroon to be approximately 0.6%, indicating that the frequency of group O has been stable or perhaps declining during the past few decades. The current distribution of circulating viral strains still does not allow classification as subtypes (Villabona-Arenas et al., 2015). There are also some reports of dual infections with HIV-1 group M and group O but no recombinant forms in patients with coinfection (de Oliveira et al., 2017; Ngoupo et al., 2016). Natural resistance to HIV medications, including integrase inhibitors, has not been identified. This suggests that infection with HIV-1 group O can be effectively treated with antiretroviral therapy in countries in which the virus circulates. Still, group O infections remain challenging with regard to diagnostic and monitoring strategies.

HIV-1 GROUP P

Group P was discovered in 2009, isolated from a Cameroonian woman living in France who had been diagnosed with HIV in 2004 (Plantier et al., 2009). Despite subsequent screening for more infections caused by this group, only two cases have been identified. It is uncertain when group P virus entered the human population; it is estimated to have occurred between 1945 and 1989 (Peeters et al., 2014). In addition, it remains unclear if the source was a chimpanzee or gorilla. The inability to antagonize tetherin protein (human restriction factor) may explain the limited spread of HIV-1 group P in the human population (Sauter et al., 2011). A recent paper suggests that group P is less adaptable and pathogenic than other strains of HIV, leading to what is referred to as a "dead-end infection" (Alessandri-Gradt et al., 2018).

HIV-2

In 1986, a virus that was morphologically similar but antigenically distinct from HIV-1 was found to cause AIDS in persons living in West Africa and was termed HIV-2 (Clavel et al., 1986; Clavel et al., 1987). HIV-2 is approximately 60% identical to HIV-1 at the amino acid level and 48% at the nucleotide level (Meissner et al., 2022). Molecular clock research ascertained that the most common recent ancestor for HIV-2 dates to 1940 and 1945 for the first two groups—A and B, respectively (Pépin, 2011). Since its initial discovery, further phylogenic analysis has identified nine different lineages of HIV-2 (groups A–I) (Fumarola et al., 2022). As with HIV-1, each group represents a different host transfer of SIV from nonprimate species (sooty mangabeys) to humans. However, unlike HIV-1, only groups A and B have spread to humans to any significant degree. The other groups only represent individual human cases. Also, unlike HIV-1, only one recombinant form has been described thus far for HIV-2, known as CRF01_AB (Ceccarelli et al., 2021).

HIV-2 was initially found in parts of West Africa, including Côte d'Ivoire, Guinea-Bissau, Gambia, Mali, Nigeria, Senegal, and Sierra Leone. With widespread immigration, cases were reported throughout other parts of Africa, along with India, Europe (especially Portugal), and the United States (Campbell-Yesufu and Gandi, 2011; Kapoor and Padival, 2022; Peruski et al., 2020). More recent data suggest that HIV-2 prevalence may be declining in West Africa, and a recent paper from Spain also noted a progressive decline in new HIV-2 infections (de Mendoza et al., 2024). This may be due to lower transmission efficacy, decreasing HIV-2 fitness, and competitive exclusion of HIV-1 (Boswell and Roland-Jones, 2019; Ceccarelli et al., 2021).

Of the approximately 38 million people across the globe living with HIV, approximately 2 million are thought to have HIV-2 infection, although this may be an underestimation (Ceccarelli et al., 2021). Moreover, a recent systematic review and meta-analysis of geographic and population distribution of HIV-2 noted a lack of data on new infections and that current surveillance and testing are not adequate to truly assess the total HIV-2 burden or its genetic diversity (Williams et al., 2023). Data from the CDC noted that only about 200 cases of HIV-2 were diagnosed in the United States through 2017 (Peruski et al., 2020)

Clinically, persons with HIV-2 infection traditionally have lower viral loads compared to people with HIV-1 infection (Boswell and Roland-Jones, 2019). There is also less genital shedding in semen and cervical secretions. This likely accounts for decreased infectivity both sexually and perinatally. It has also been observed that persons with HIV-2 infection have a longer asymptomatic phase and a slower decline in CD4+ cells and progression to AIDS than individuals with HIV-1. This is also likely due to lower plasma viral load levels. Treatment of persons with HIV-2 includes some of the same drugs used to treat HIV-1. However, HIV-2 has intrinsic resistance to non-nucleoside reverse transcriptase inhibitors and several protease inhibitors. Based on limited data from clinical trials, ART combinations that include certain integrase inhibitors or protease inhibitors (e.g., raltegravir or lopinavir/ritonavir) paired with a dual nucleoside reverse transcriptase inhibitor backbone appear to be most effective (Rowland-Jones and Gea-Mallorquí, 2024). In the absence of treatment with antiretroviral therapy, a progressive decline in immune function and resultant disease complications, including death, will occur (Boswell and Roland-Jones, 2019; Kapoor and Padvil, 2022; Tzou et al., 2020).

THE FUTURE OF HIV REGIONAL AND GLOBAL GENETIC DIVERSITY

By combining historical, phylogenetic, molecular evolutionary, and epidemiological findings, researchers have been able to reconstruct the history of the AIDS pandemic and many of the unique aspects of HIV-1 and HIV-2. Ongoing research aims to help determine how strains of HIV, including CRFs, continue to spread and colonize new geographic regions and host populations (Switzer et al., 2024; Williams et al., 2023). The progress in understanding the complexity of HIV also raises numerous questions. For example, as there are many other nonhuman primates infected with SIV, should there be concern for future zoonotic lentiviral infections from cross-species transmissions? Will the growing incidence of sexually transmitted infections continue to facilitate the dissemination and adaptation of HIV-1 and HIV-2? Will it be possible to develop a single HIV vaccine that will be effective against all HIV groups and subtypes? For more effective therapies and ideally a vaccine against HIV, it will remain necessary to have up-to-date knowledge of the genetic evolution and diversity of the virus.

RECOMMENDED READING

Pépin J. *The Origins of AIDS*. New York: Cambridge University Press; 2011.

Quammen D. *The Chimp and the River: How AIDS Emerged from an African Forest*. New York: Norton; 2015.

HIV EPIDEMIOLOGY

LEARNING OBJECTIVE

Discuss the global prevalence, and geographic distribution of human immunodeficiency syndrome infections.

WHAT'S NEW

The World Health Organization and Joint United Nations Programme on HIV and AIDS (WHO; UNAIDS) estimate that in 2023, 39.9 million persons worldwide were living with HIV (UNAIDS, 2024). Fewer people acquired HIV in 2022 than in previous decades. An estimated 1.3 million new HIV infections in 2022 marks the lowest number in decades, with significant declines observed particularly in regions with the highest HIV burdens, including Eastern/Southern Africa and Western/Central Africa. The most significant reduction in new HIV infections have been observed among children (aged 0–14 years) and young people (aged 14–24 years), populations which have been the focus of some targeted prevention interventions. In addition, global perinatal HIV programs have prevented 3.4 million new HIV infections in children since 2000.

Despite the significant reduction in HIV incidence, various demographic groups continue to be disproportionately impacted. These include gay men and other men who have sex with men (MSM), people who inject drugs (PWID), transgender persons, and sex workers. In the UNAIDS-identified regions of Eastern/Southern Africa, Western/Central Africa, and Asia and the Pacific, trends of HIV incidence in these demographic groups countered existing progress. In Eastern Europe, the Middle East/North Africa, and Latin America, disproportionate rates of HIV infection contributed to overall regional increases in HIV incidence. Additionally, global conflict and displacement continue to disrupt progress and efforts along the entire HIV care continuum.

KEY POINTS

- UNAIDS identified several demographic subgroups at high risk for HIV infection and in danger of being left behind by the global HIV/AIDS response, including adolescent girls and young women, men who have sex with men (MSM), transgender persons, people who inject drugs, individuals who are incarcerated, and sex workers.
- Criminalization of sex work, same-sex relations, drug use, and HIV transmission, along with humanitarian crises causing mass displacement and healthcare service disruption, contribute to stigma and hamper HIV care and prevention efforts.

OVERVIEW OF THE GLOBAL EPIDEMIC

Since the onset of the global epidemic, the WHO estimates that 85.6 (64.8–113.0) million persons have acquired HIV infection, and 40.4 (32.9–51.3) million have died of AIDS-related illnesses (UNAIDS, 2024). At the end of 2022, an estimated 39 (33.1–45.7) million persons were living with HIV, while 1.3 (1.0–1.7) million persons acquired HIV infection that year, representing a decrease from 1.5 million in 2021. As expected, this has increased from 38.4 million people living with HIV in 2021 and highlights the ever-growing global population of people with HIV needing appropriate healthcare services. An estimated 0.7% of adults aged 15–49 years worldwide are living with HIV, although the burden of the epidemic continues to vary considerably between countries and regions. Eastern and Southern Africa remain the most heavily impacted, representing more than half of all PWH globally (Figure 2.4).

Across all countries, several key demographic subgroups continue to be disproportionately affected by the HIV/AIDS epidemic. UNAIDS has identified six populations at higher risk of acquiring HIV that are in danger of being left behind by the global AIDS response: adolescent girls and young women, MSM, transgender persons, persons who inject drugs (PWID), persons who are incarcerated, and sex workers and their clients. Globally, in 2022, approximately 210,000 adolescent girls and young women acquired HIV, which is half the number recorded in 2010. In the same year, 140,000 adolescent boys and young men acquired HIV, reflecting a 44% decrease since 2010. Fewer new HIV infections in women and increased ART coverage among people with HIV (PWH) collectively led to a 58% decline in the annual number of new infections in children globally between 2010 and 2022, to 130,000. Although this represents notable progress for this key population, other at-risk groups continue to experience significant disparities in HIV infection and related outcomes. In 2022, the risk of acquiring HIV was 14 times higher among persons who inject drugs, 23 times higher among MSM of any age, 9 times higher for sex workers, and 20 times higher for transgender women compared to other adults in the general population (UNAIDS, 2024b).

Unique considerations for each of these populations also vary by region and within countries. For example, in Southern Africa, age-disparate intergenerational sexual relationships and transactional sex place adolescent girls and young women at extremely high risk for HIV; in Eastern Europe and Central Asia, most new HIV infections are associated with PWID; and in Latin America, the Caribbean, Western Europe, and North America, the largest proportion of new HIV diagnoses is among MSM. Notably, the Middle East/North Africa region has experienced the most significant surge of HIV incidence globally during 2010–2022, with a 61% increase driven by infections in MSM, sex workers, and PWID (UNAIDS, 2023a). Varying levels of legislation criminalizing sex work, same-sex relations, drug use/possession, and HIV transmission itself contribute to a culture of stigma that limits engagement in HIV care and prevention efforts, especially in this and other regions experiencing sharp increases in HIV incidence, such as Eastern Europe/Central Asia (49% increase since 2010). Additionally, humanitarian crises contribute to mass displacement and cause disruption in healthcare access and service delivery.

In 2014, the Joint United Nations Programme on HIV/AIDS launched the 90-90-90 initiative. Briefly, it sought to assure that 90% of persons with HIV will be diagnosed, 90% of whom will be started and maintained on antiretroviral

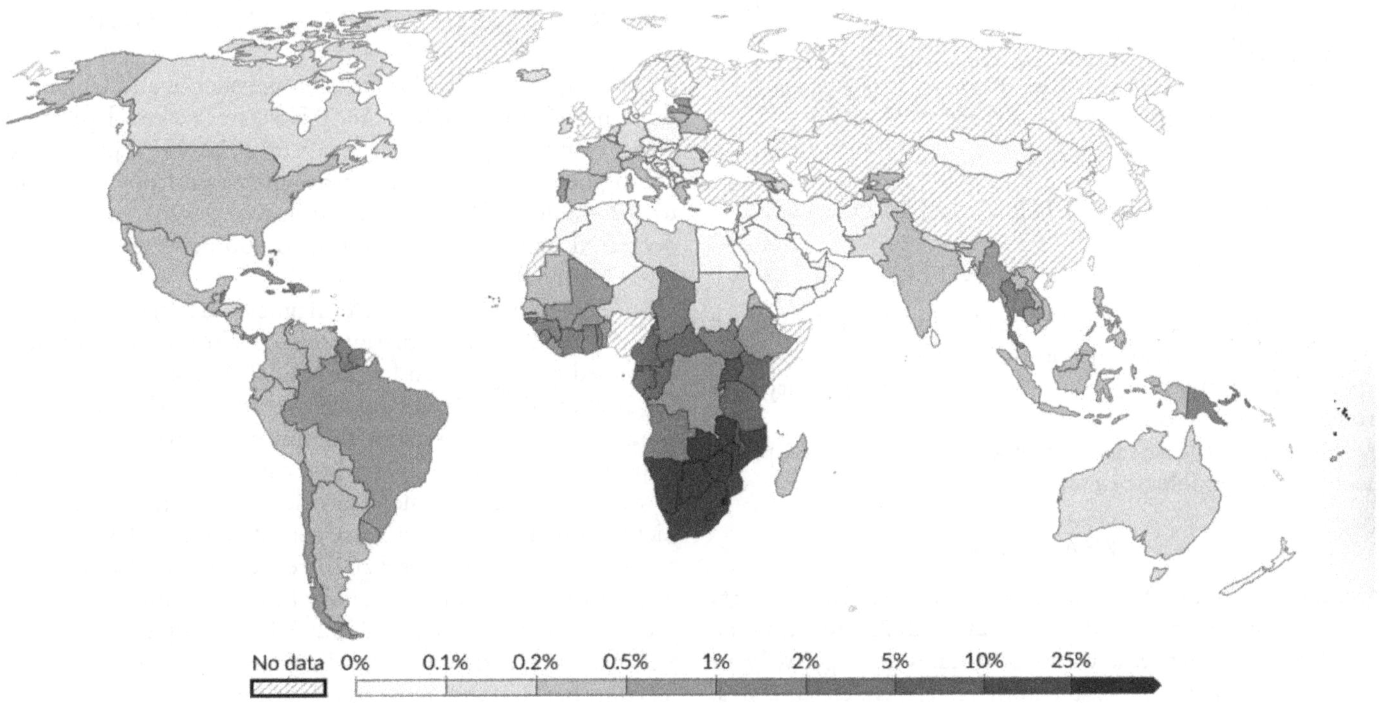

Figure 2.4 Percentage of country populations aged 15–49 years old living with HIV, 2022. SOURCE: Data page: "HIV prevalence," part of the following publication: Max Roserand and Hannah Ritchie, "202/AIDS3 (2023). Data adapted from Joint United Nations Programme on HIV/AIDS. Retrieved from https://ourworldindata.org/grapher/share-of-the-population-infected-with-hiv.

therapy (ART), among whom 90% will be virally suppressed (or an overall viral suppression rate of 73%). The United Nations Member States adopted a more ambitious goal in 2021 of achieving 95-95-95 by 2030, with the goal of ending HIV/AIDS as a global health threat. Currently, Botswana, Eswatini, Rwanda, the United Republic of Tanzania, and Zimbabwe have achieved these targets (UNAIDS, 2023b).

In 2022, considerable progress was seen with these numbers: 86% (73%–98%) of the 29.8 million PWH across the world knew their status. Among them, 89% (75% to 100%) were linked to ART, and of those, 93% (79%–100%) had suppressed viral loads. Looking at it another way, of all PWH, 86% (73%–98%) knew their status; 77% (65%–87%) were accessing treatment; and 71% (61%–81%) were virally suppressed (UNAIDS, 2024a). Data show that programs continue to close global gaps in treatment coverage, with 20.9 million more PWH on treatment in 2021 than in 2020. AIDS-related deaths have decreased by 68% since its peak in 2004, and since 2010, AIDS-related mortality has declined by 57% among women and girls and by 47% among men and boys (UNAIDS, 2024a). However, 9.2 million PWH were not on ART in 2022 and 2.1 million people who were on treatment had not achieved viral suppression in 2022. This was disproportionately represented in Eastern Europe, Central Asia, and the Middle East/North Africa regions. This further highlights the potential effects of anti-HIV discrimination and global conflicts, both natural and manmade, in contributing to disparities in HIV care.

RECOMMENDED READING

UNAIDS. Global HIV & AIDS statistics—2023 fact sheet. unaids.org. https://www.unaids.org/sites/default/files/media_asset/UNAIDS_FactSheet_en.pdf. Published 2024. Accessed September 12, 2024.

UNAIDS. HIV Prevention 2025 road map. Aidsdatahub.org. https://www.aidsdatahub.org/sites/default/files/resource/prevention-2025-roadmap-en.pdf. Published 2022. Accessed June 25, 2024.

OVERVIEW OF THE U.S. EPIDEMIC

LEARNING OBJECTIVE

Describe current demographic trends in HIV in the United States, especially regarding cisgender women, race/ethnicity, specific age groups, region of residence, gender identity, and route of transmission.

Recognize the effects of migration and forced displacement on epidemiologic trends.

WHAT'S NEW

In May 2024, the CDC released new HIV surveillance reports which compiled updated data from 2018–2022 regarding the incidence, prevalence, and mortality rates among PWH in the United States and six territories/freely associated states. Given COVID-19-related disruptions in data collection and reporting, the CDC recommends caution when examining and interpreting information from these surveillance reports.

KEY POINTS

- In 2022, the estimated number of new HIV infections decreased by about 12% compared to 2018, from 36,200 to 31,800. A 30% drop in new HIV infections among young people (13–24 years old) contributed significantly to this decline.
- Significant racial/ethnic disparities continue to exist between racial and ethnic groups with respect to new HIV diagnoses. While there were slight decreases in rates for Black, Asian, and multiracial persons, Black persons are still significantly disproportionately affected. Additionally, rates in Hispanic/Latinx and Native American/Alaska Native persons increased slightly during 2018–2022.
- Between 2010–2014 and 2017–2021, the lifetime risk of HIV diagnosis among Black/African MSM improved from 1 in 2 to 1 in 3.
- The leading mode of HIV transmission continues to be male same-sex sexual contact, although this has decreased by 10% between 2018 and 2022.
- Slowly declining incidence and more rapidly diminishing death rates continue to drive up HIV prevalence and, therefore, demands for a robust HIV provider workforce.
- Recent surveillance data should be viewed with caution, given decreased HIV testing and diagnoses during the height of the COVID-19 pandemic.

OVERALL U.S. HIV PREVALENCE, INCIDENCE, AND DEATHS: EMPHASIS ON KEY POPULATIONS AND PROGRAMS

According to the CDC reports on prevalence and incidence data on HIV and AIDS in the 50 US states and six dependent areas, comparing data from 2019 to 2022, HIV prevalence among persons aged 13 and older increased from 1,189,700 to 1,238,000. HIV incidence within the same time frame decreased by 9% from 35,100 to 31,800 new cases per year (CDC, 2024a).

The decrease in new HIV diagnoses during this period may be attributed to disruptions in clinical services and decreased testing caused by the COVID-19 pandemic. Data for 2020, which coincided with the onset of the pandemic, should thus be interpreted with caution due to the significant impact on access to HIV testing, care, and related services, as well as case surveillance activities in state and local jurisdictions during the surveillance period. Since the COVID-19 pandemic extended beyond 2020, readers should also consider its potential effects on U.S. public health systems when interpreting HIV data for 2021–2022. Additionally, despite CDC and U.S. Preventive Services Task Force recommendations for routine, opt-out, non–risk factor-based HIV screening which have been in place since 2006, AIDS remains relatively common. In 2022, 7,659 persons received an AIDS classification of disease at the time of diagnosis, with the highest rates seen in the Southern United States (52%), followed by the Northeast (13%), West (21%), and Midwest (13%). The high rate of AIDS, despite the widespread availability of effective and well-tolerated ART, highlights the need for improved HIV screening as well as timely linkage to care, ongoing engagement in comprehensive care, and continuous treatment for people with HIV (CDC, 2024b).

Death rates related to HIV have continued to decline slowly following the sharp drop-off with the advent of effective ART in 1996. As expected, with new infections outpacing deaths by approximately 25,000 cases each year, HIV prevalence continues to rise. Two important implications of this are that more clinicians will be needed to care for the growing population of people aging with HIV, and more must be done to prevent HIV transmission by targeting "high-risk" populations with interventions of proven efficacy, such as pre-exposure prophylaxis (PrEP) and treatment as prevention.

THE U.S. HIV CARE CONTINUUM

Since the U.S. Department of Health and Human Services (DHHS) HIV/AIDS Bureau's National HIV/AIDS Strategy (NHAS) release in 2010, many in the HIV treatment community have focused on the HIV care continuum as the leading quality indicator in the U.S. healthcare system's response to HIV (White House Office of National AIDS Policy, 2015). The care continuum highlights new HIV diagnoses among persons estimated to have acquired HIV, effective and timely linkages to care, ongoing engagement and retention in care, and ART-mediated HIV viral suppression (Figure 2.5). Although the NHAS goals (i.e., reducing new HIV diagnoses, increasing access to care, improving health outcomes for persons living with HIV, and reducing HIV-related health disparities) go beyond the care continuum, it nonetheless remains a fundamental indicator of progress not only for the NHAS but also for the newer Ending the HIV Epidemic initiative (see Chapter 1).

As ART has become increasingly potent, less toxic, and easier to take for many people with HIV, the greatest challenges in suppressing what is commonly referred to as "community viral load" (i.e., the collective level of viremia among PWH in a community) now exist primarily in the first three steps of the continuum. By 2022, 87% of PWH were diagnosed; 66% were engaged in some care, and although only 47% were retained in care, 57% were virally suppressed (CDC, 2024c). On the prevention side, the number of adults prescribed PrEP increased significantly from 7,972 in 2014 to an estimated 432,000 in 2022, or 36% of the estimated 1.2 million eligible persons (DHHS, 2023). While these data show progress, significant work remains to fully address the unmet needs of "at-risk" groups and regions. Providing culturally appropriate HIV prevention, testing, and care across a variety of settings, particularly community health centers and other "medical homes" that serve highly affected populations, is critical to further improving outcomes along the care continuum.

EPIDEMIOLOGICAL TRENDS IN CIS WOMEN

Adult cisgender women continue to account for more than half of all people with HIV worldwide and 41.5% of new infections, largely through heterosexual transmission (World Health Organization [WHO], 2023). In sub-Saharan Africa,

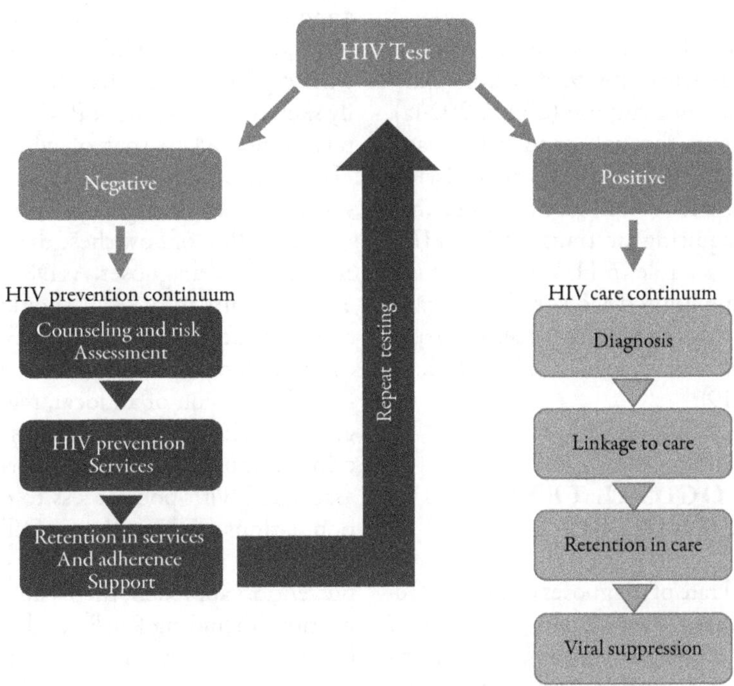

Figure 2.5 HIV testing and care continuum. SOURCE: Adapted from Horn et al. *J Int AIDS Soc.*2016;19(1):21263.

adolescent girls and young women (15–24 years old) comprised more than three-fourths of all new HIV infections in 2022 and were more than three times as likely as their male counterparts to acquire HIV (UNAIDS, 2024c). Conversely, in the United States, women represented only 19% of HIV diagnoses in 2022, or about 6,000 new infections, a disparity likely due to the preponderance of male-to-male HIV transmission in the United States. This was increased from approximately 5,000 new infections among women in 2020, although decreased testing during the COVID-19 pandemic likely influenced these surveillance data.

From 2014 through 2022, compared to other racial/ethnic groups, Black women continued to account for the majority of new HIV diagnoses in the United States: in 2022, they comprised 47% of new HIV infections among ciswomen, despite making up only 14% of the overall female population in the United States (CDC, 2024d). Although this represents an overall decrease from 4,573 to 2,800, the HIV prevalence rate among Black women remains disproportionately high, at 19.2 per 100,000 persons, which is 10 times higher than that of white females (1.9) and 4 times higher than that of Hispanic/Latinx females (4.6).

Factors that increase a woman's risk of acquiring HIV include limited knowledge about HIV, decreased awareness or perception of risk, not knowing partner risk factor(s), and limited awareness or use of HIV PrEP (CDC, 2024c). Ciswomen are under-prescribed PrEP compared to other populations (DHHS, 2023). Women's relationships with their partners play a pivotal role as well: in relationships with intimate partner violence, vulnerability to HIV may be increased due to inconsistent or no condom use (related to fears for personal safety if partners are asked to use condoms). Women with a history of sexual abuse or other traumas may engage in high-risk sexual activity and drug use. This includes exchanging sex for drugs and/or money or encountering challenges when refusing unwanted sex.

The most common mode of transmission for women is high-risk heterosexual contact (64%–92% across various groups), followed by injection drug use (CDC, 2024a). Sexual HIV transmission occurs through condomless vaginal or anal sex. Sexually transmitted infections that disrupt genital mucosa and stimulate a local immune response may increase the likelihood of acquiring or transmitting HIV. Socioeconomic status also plays a role in HIV risk. In states with higher rates of poverty and limited access to health care, women are more likely to use drugs and exchange sex for drugs or money, factors shown to increase the risk of HIV, directly or indirectly (Stoner et al., 2019).

OTHER EPIDEMIOLOGICAL TRENDS BY RACE/ETHNICITY

While the annual number and rate of diagnoses of HIV infection in the United States decreased overall during 2018–2022, this varied widely among different subgroups. Similar to 2014–2018 data, among Native Hawaiians and other Pacific Islanders (NHOPI), new HIV diagnoses increased by 51% during this time frame, with the majority of new cases among NHOPI MSM (although absolute numbers remain relatively low). American Indian/Alaska Native and Hispanic/Latinx diagnoses increased as well. In contrast, rates of new HIV diagnoses among Asians, Blacks, and persons of multiple races decreased slightly, and the rate for white persons remained stable. Although NHOPI makes up <1% of new HIV diagnoses in the United States, HIV may affect this group in ways that are not readily apparent because of their small population size (only 0.09% of the U.S. population in 2022) and a lack of representation in clinical trials or epidemiologic analyses. In addition to societal disadvantages, including poverty and limited access to health care, NHOPI cultural customs, such as not discussing sex across generations, may stigmatize sexuality, especially same-sex relations, and prevent NHOPI from accessing HIV prevention and care services.

The most critical feature to note about current U.S. surveillance data is that Black persons continue to be hardest hit by HIV infections and deaths. Black PWH were vastly overrepresented compared to their percentage of the general population in 2022 (40% vs. 13%). This is also true, but to a lesser extent, for Hispanic/Latinx persons (25% vs. 18%). By comparison, these numbers for white persons are 28% and 60%, respectively. The CDC denotes the rate of difference as an absolute disparity: if Black/African American adults and adolescents had the same rate as white persons of the same age group, then 33 cases of HIV per 100,000 population would have been prevented (Figure 2.6). Additionally, the largest number of new HIV diagnoses exists in Black/African American MSM living in the U.S. South. Figure 2.7 shows how advanced HIV/AIDS has disproportionately affected Black PWH in the United States.

The current highest-risk demographic in the United States is young Black MSM who live in the South; in 2016, the CDC announced that if current demographic trends continue, fully one-half of Black MSM (and one-quarter of Latinx MSM) will acquire HIV in their lifetime. Death rates are also heavily skewed against Black PWH, with a sevenfold higher death rate compared to that of white PWH. Death rates among Hispanic/Latinx persons are almost twice that of white persons, whereas other groups fare the same or better.

Regardless of how these data are examined—whether considering HIV diagnoses, AIDS, or deaths—there is a strikingly excessive burden of HIV shouldered in the United States by communities of color. The 2016 NHAS recognized this in its call to reduce racial disparities, which should be incorporated into the mission of all local, regional, and national HIV programs. Such efforts must address the ongoing stigma, fear, discrimination, homophobia, distrust, and socioeconomic issues associated with poor access to care in these highly impacted populations (White House Office of National AIDS Policy, 2015). The CDC and partners are pursuing a high-impact prevention approach, increasing awareness about testing, prevention (including PrEP), and retention in care among populations disproportionately affected by HIV, particularly gay or bisexual men of color (CDC, 2024d).

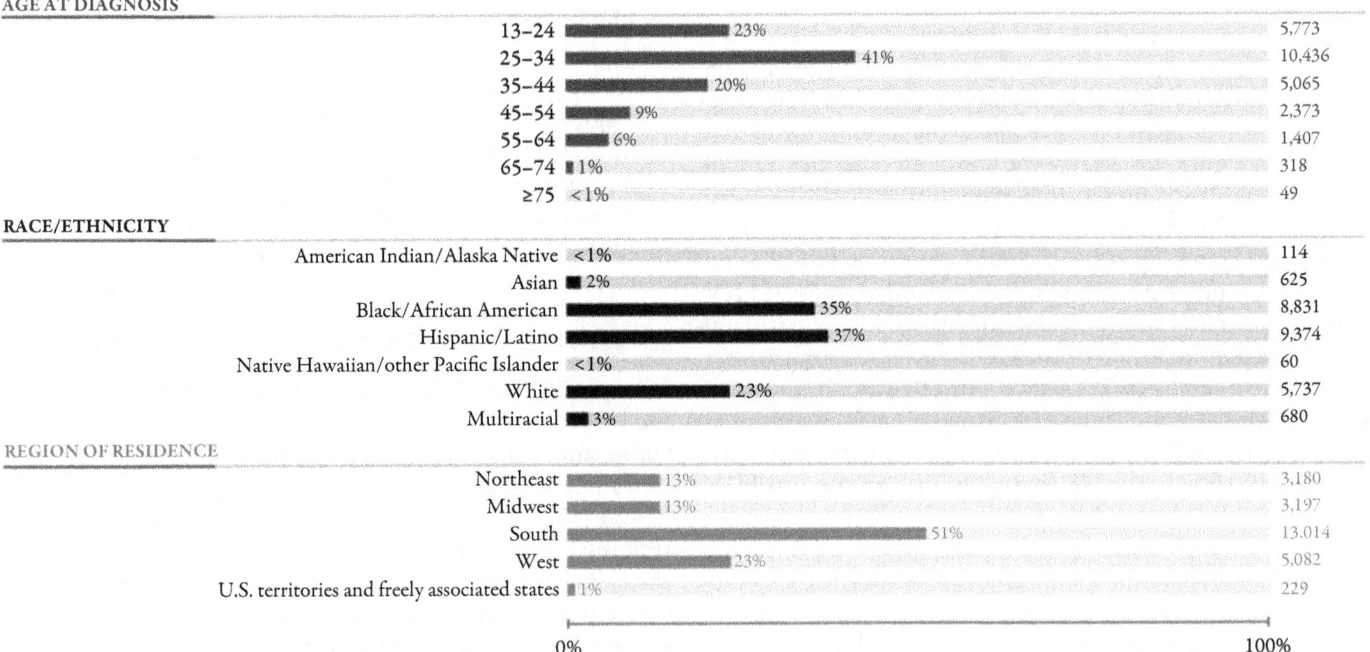

Figure 2.6 Rates and disparities of diagnosis of HIV infection among persons aged ≥13 years, by selected characteristics, 2022—United States. SOURCE: Centers for Disease Control and Prevention. Diagnoses, deaths, and prevalence of HIV in the United States and 6 territories and freely associated states, 2022. May 21, 2024. http://www.cdc.gov/hiv-data/nhss/hiv-diagnoses-deaths-prevalence.html.

EPIDEMIOLOGY IN SPECIFIC AGE GROUPS

In the United States, the epidemiology of HIV varies significantly across different age groups. For instance, new HIV infections have decreased by 12% from 2018 to 2022, with significant reductions among young people. However, racial and ethnic disparities persist, particularly among Black and Hispanic/Latinx communities. Additionally, transgender individuals, especially transgender women, are at high risk for HIV, with significant disparities in testing and access to care due to stigma and social rejection. These variations highlight the need for age-specific strategies in HIV prevention and treatment efforts.

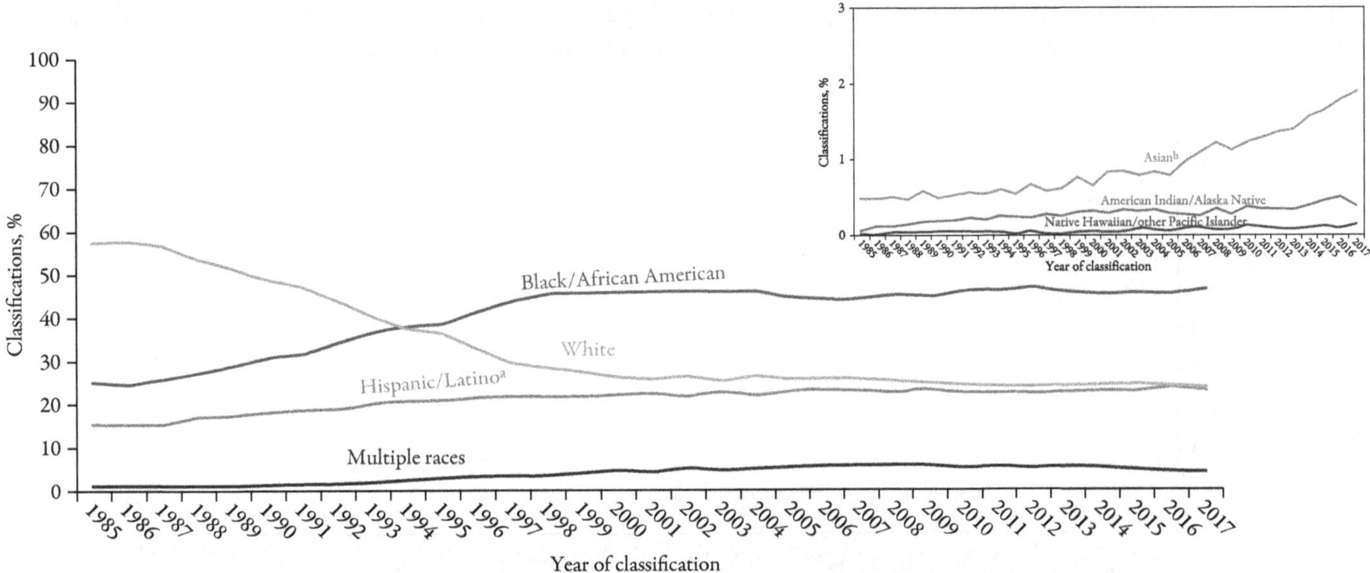

Figure 2.7 Percentages of stage 3 (AIDS) classifications among adults and adolescents with diagnosed HIV infection, by race/ethnicity, 1985–2017, United States and six dependent areas. SOURCE: CDC HIV/AIDS Resource Library Slide Sets. Available at http://www.cdc.gov/hiv/library/slidesets/index.html. Accessed September 22, 2022.

CHILDREN

The reduction of perinatal HIV transmission in the United States is a major success of the current era of ART. Although the CDC has not published a similar graph showing perinatal HIV transmission rates since the beginning of the epidemic, Figure 2.8 shows the dramatic rise and fall in perinatal AIDS diagnoses from 1985 until 2017. In 1992, an estimated 952 pediatric HIV transmissions were reported in the United States. By 2004, the number declined to 177, and in 2019, a total of 32 children received a diagnosis of HIV through perinatal transmission. The overall rate of perinatal HIV infections reported by the CDC decreased from 1.5 per 100,000 live births in 2014 to 1.1 in 2022 (CDC, 2024c). Of note, this is a slight increase from 0.9 in 2018 and does not meet the CDC's goal of <1 new perinatal transmission per 100,000 and <1% among infants exposed to HIV (DHHS, 2024).

Despite the powerful role that ART holds in preventing perinatal HIV transmission, case persistence is tied to factors including uneven prenatal testing coverage related to variable provider perception of patient risk, which may then affect the implementation of third-trimester repeat testing, as recommended for people with higher risk of HIV acquisition. Other factors include an increasing number of pregnancies among people with HIV, with varying amounts of preconception counseling and pre-delivery engagement in care, as well as inadequate viral suppression of persons of childbearing potential known to have HIV. Among all perinatal HIV transmissions during 2016–2019, 58% of birthing parents known to have HIV before or during pregnancy represent gaps in linkage and retention in care and sustained viral suppression. The remainder of individuals who did not test HIV positive until at or after delivery represent missed opportunities to screen and prevent perinatal transmission (Figure 2.9. This highlights the importance of screening all pregnant women for HIV at least once during pregnancy and again in the third trimester, as indicated.

As with adults, HIV disproportionately affects Black children. The rate of perinatal HIV transmission for Black/African-American persons in 2022 was 5.5, which was 5 times the composite rate (CDC, 2024c). While accounting for 58% of diagnoses, they comprised only 14% of the population of U.S. children in 2022, whereas Hispanic/Latinx (16% of HIV diagnoses, 26% of population) and white (13% of HIV diagnoses, 48% of population) children acquire HIV far less often than their population percentages (CDC, 2024b).

ADOLESCENTS AND YOUNG ADULTS

Between 2018 and 2022, persons aged 13–24 years accounted for 18% of newly diagnosed HIV in the United States, while young adults aged 25–34 represented 30% of incident diagnoses (CDC, 2024a), with the highest risk seen in persons 23–24 years old. Young persons with HIV are less likely to seek testing; in 2022, 44% of those with HIV did not know their status, preventing engagement in care and viral suppression and perpetuating increased risk in this age cohort. Encouragingly, the rate of infections in the 13–24-year age group did decrease by 30% between 2018 and 2022, thought to be driven largely by increases in prescriptions of PrEP and HIV testing (CDC, 2024d).

Nevertheless, HIV transmissions remain disproportionately high among Black and Latinx youth. In 2022, of all adolescents and young adults aged 13–24 years diagnosed with HIV infection, the CDC reported that 50% were Black, far outpacing their percentage of the general population. Hispanic/Latinx persons represented an additional 31% of adolescent HIV diagnoses in the same year, a 5% increase from the previous data from 2020, though this may have been impacted by decreased testing during the COVID-19 pandemic (CDC, 2024b). Notably, if Black/African-American persons in the 13–24-year age group had the same rate of HIV diagnoses to their white counterparts, then overall diagnoses would reduce by 45 cases per 100,000.

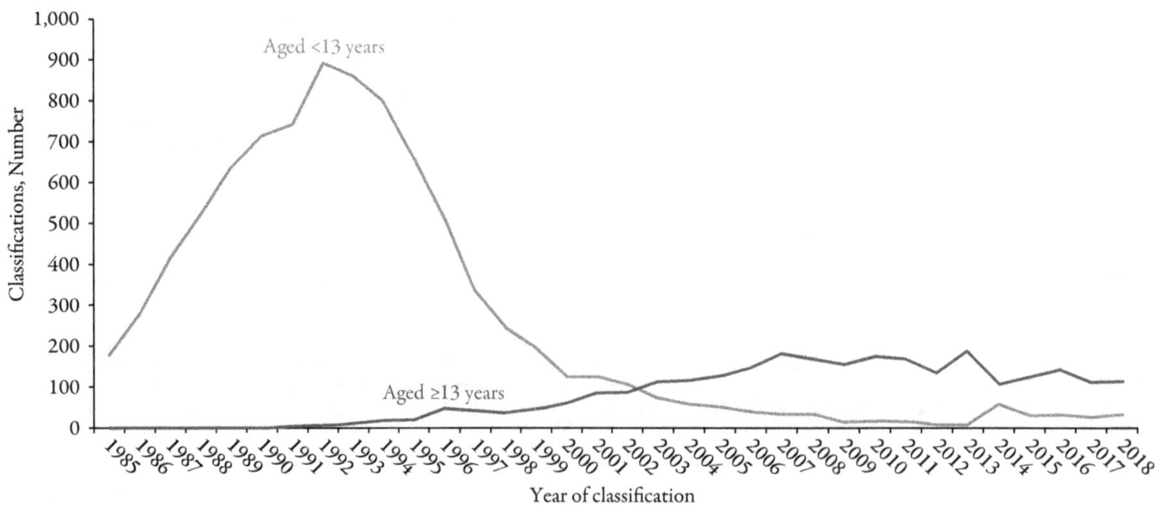

Figure 2.8 Stage 3 (AIDS) classifications among persons with perinatally acquired HIV infection, 1985–2018, United States and six dependent areas. SOURCE: CDC HIV/AIDS Resource Library Slide Sets. Available at http://www.cdc.gov/hiv/library/slidesets/index.html. Accessed September 22, 2022.

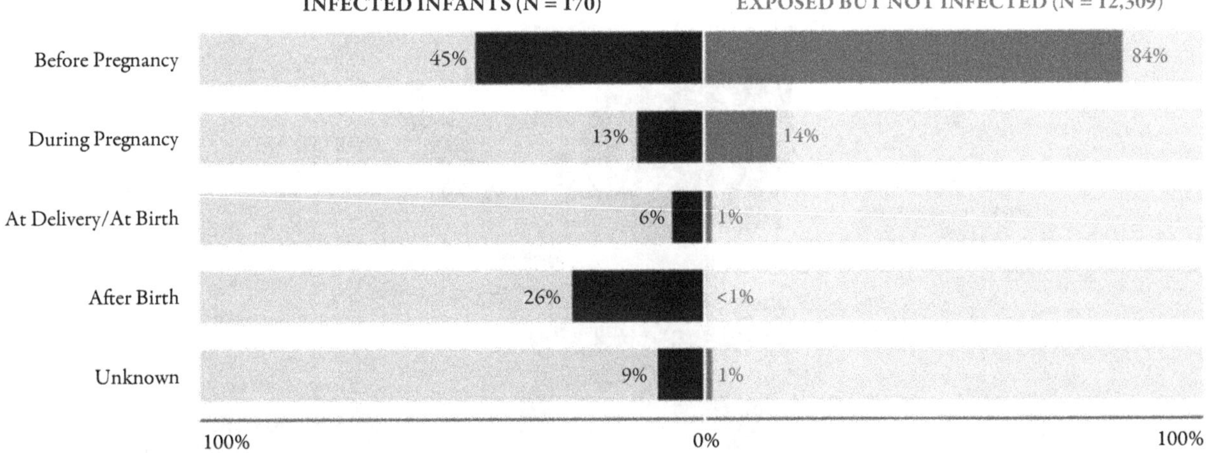

Figure 2.9 Time of maternal HIV testing among children with diagnosed perinatally acquired HIV infection and children exposed to HIV, birth years 2018 to 2021, United States and Puerto Rico SOURCE: Centers for Disease Control and Prevention. Diagnoses, deaths, and prevalence of HIV in the United States and 6 territories and freely associated states, 2022. May 21, 2024. http://www.cdc.gov/hiv-data/nhss/hiv-diagnoses-deaths-prevalence.html.

Male-to-male sexual contact remains the predominant mode of HIV transmission in the adolescent and young adult population, accounting for 81% of new diagnoses. Heterosexual contact is the next most frequent mode of transmission, accounting for approximately 3% among people assigned male at birth and 11% in people assigned female at birth (comprising 85.6% of new infections in this group). Transmissions from injection drug use remain stable at approximately 1% (CDC, 2024b).

As these data suggest, there is a need to address health risk behaviors disproportionately represented in the adolescent/young adult population. This includes providing information and education on condom use, which decreased from 60% in 2011 to 52% in 2021, as well as screening and treatment for substance use disorders, which can contribute to higher-risk sexual encounters. Furthermore, youth who identify as LGBTQ+ are at higher risk for experiencing sexual violence and negative social determinants of health, leading to engagement in survival sex, especially in transgender women. It is crucial for providers to be able to assess for and address these behaviors and risk factors.

HIV AMONG OLDER ADULTS

Many people with HIV enjoy an increased quality of life for longer periods of time as a result of well-tolerated and highly effective ART regimens. As such, there is a steadily increasing prevalence of HIV among all age groups (CDC, 2024a). While incidence rates among adults are generally stable, people aged 55 years and older (the conventional definition of "older adult" with respect to HIV) still accounted for 11.7% of new HIV infections in 2022. Of these 3,722 transmissions in 2022, 2,683 (72%) were in men, mainly through male-to-male sexual contact, and 1,039 (27.9%) were in women, the majority of which were the result of heterosexual contact. This rate decreased compared to 2018, when there were 6,640 new HIV infections (and while increased from 2020, these data were likely incomplete due to COVID-19). It is critical to remember that this older age group remains at significant risk of HIV acquisition and is less likely to receive guideline-based screening (USPSTF, 2019). Additionally, in 2022, when examining persons aged 45 years or older with a new HIV diagnosis, higher percentages (33%) met the criteria for AIDS at the time of initial diagnosis, notably higher than when compared to younger adults with new HIV infection (10.3%–24.5%). In older adults on ART, CD4 cell recovery is generally blunted compared to their younger counterparts; therefore, later HIV diagnoses in more advanced stages of immunosuppression can further contribute to incomplete immune reconstitution. This represents an important opportunity for improved screening, earlier detection, linkage to care, treatment initiation, and decreased transmission.

BY REGION

Regional data on HIV diagnoses is divided between four main regions of the United States: the Northeast, Midwest, South, and West. The rate of diagnoses per 100,000 persons among persons aged ≥13 years by region is shown in Figure 2.10, with the South accounting for 52% of new diagnoses. The South now leads the United States in HIV prevalence as well (533.9 per 100,000 persons), overtaking the Northeast (513.2 per 100,000 persons). Encouragingly, HIV incidence in the South dropped by 16% compared with 2018 data, although other U.S. regions remained the same. Similar regional disparity exists in the estimated percentage of PWH who were diagnosed, with the Midwest (84.7%), West (85.6%), and the South (86.4%) all showing improvements but comparatively lower than in the Northeast (92.3%) (CDC, 2024a). Social determinants of health, such as higher rates of poverty and lower levels of completed education and trust in medical systems, as well as limited public health funding and

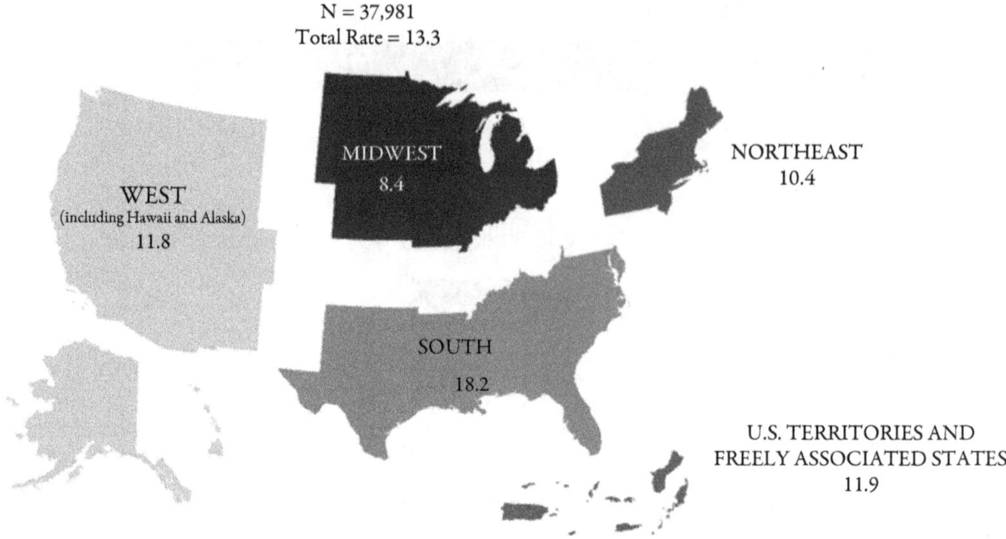

Figure 2.10 Diagnoses of HIV among persons aged ≥13 years, by region, 2022, United States and six territories and freely associated states. SOURCE: Centers for Disease Control and Prevention. Diagnoses, deaths, and prevalence of HIV in the United States and 6 territories and freely associated states, 2022. May 21, 2024. http://www.cdc.gov/hiv-data/nhss/hiv-diagnoses-deaths-prevalence.html.

infrastructure, are all likely factors in the ongoing (though improving) disparity in HIV outcomes in the South.

BY GENDER IDENTITY

Gender identity, or the gender with which a person identifies, is a separate part of identity from sexual orientation. Persons who identify as transgender or additional gender identity (AGI, defined as someone who does not identify as male, female, or transgender) are underrepresented in research studies on HIV treatment interventions and prevention, although representation has recently increased in some larger studies (notably HPTN 091, which seeks to identify strategies incorporating gender-affirming care and HIV-prevention initiatives to improve PrEP acceptance/adherence in transgender women).

Transgender individuals are one of the highest-risk groups in the United States for acquiring HIV. In 2022, the overall prevalence of HIV in transgender women was estimated to be 14.1%, compared to 3.2% in transgender men (Becasen et al., 2019), both significantly higher than the average prevalence rate in U.S. adults (0.3%). In 2022, 41% of new diagnoses in transgender women identified as Black/African American, and 39% identified as Hispanic/Latinx, compared to 13% identifying as white. The majority (44%) resided in the South. One-quarter of transgender women are estimated to have HIV; among Black persons, this figure rises to one-third (previously one-half) (Figure 2.11).

Despite these trends, nearly two-thirds of transgender men and women in the Behavioral Risk Factor Surveillance System from 2014 to 2015 were never tested for HIV. The stigma and social rejection faced by transgender persons lead to significant disparities in housing, education, employment,

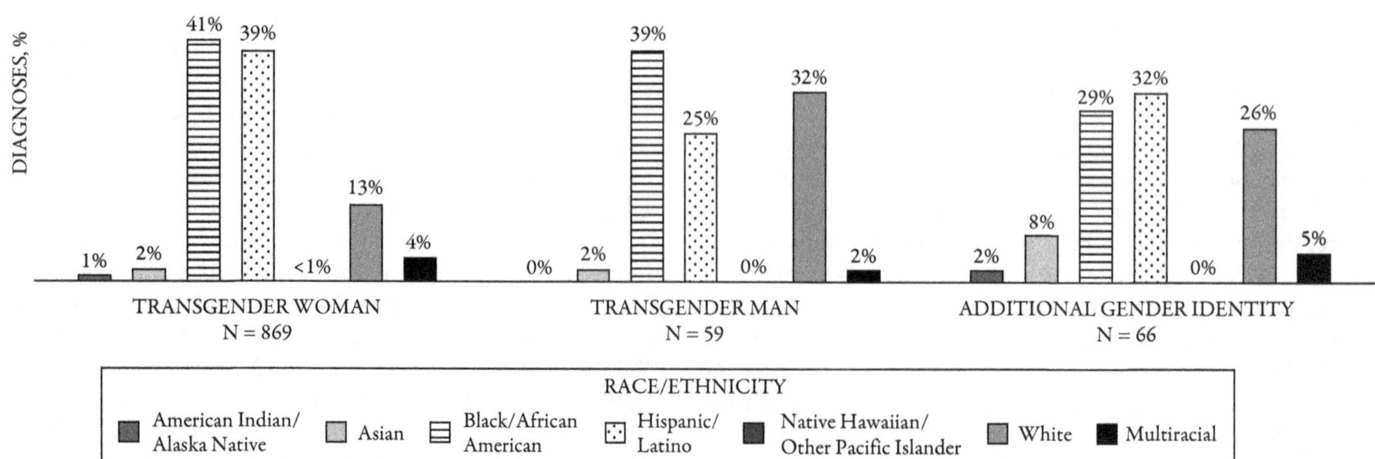

Figure 2.11 Diagnoses of HIV among transgender and additional gender identity persons aged ≥13 years, by gender and race/ethnicity, 2022, United States and six territories and freely associated states. SOURCE: Centers for Disease Control and Prevention. Diagnoses, deaths, and prevalence of HIV in the United States and 6 territories and freely associated states, 2022. May 21, 2024. http://www.cdc.gov/hiv-data/nhss/hiv-diagnoses-deaths-prevalence.html.

and access to health care and preventive services. To obtain further insight, in 2019–2020, the CDC developed the National HIV Behavioral Surveillance Among Transgender Women program, using questionnaires to reach 1,608 trans women (CDC, 2024e). Many respondents described experiencing poverty and housing instability as a result of stigma and social rejection, with economic circumstances forcing them into survival sex and putting them at heightened risk for HIV acquisition. Social interventions such as advocating for safer sexual practices and condom use, advocating for stable housing and employment, increasing PrEP, and addressing the need for gender-affirming and mental health care hold promise in helping to stem the tide of transmissions in this population (CDC, 2024e).

BY ROUTE OF TRANSMISSION

Data from the 2024 Conference for Retrovirus and Opportunistic Infections (CROI) show that male-to-male sexual contact was the leading cause of new infections in the United States during 2010–2021 (Singh et al., 2024). Among persons newly diagnosed with HIV in 2022, an estimated 67% were due to male-to-male sexual contact, 23% to heterosexual contact, 7% to injection drug use, 3% to both male-to-male sexual contact and injection drug use (IDU), and less than 1% to other transmission categories. Encouragingly, there was an overall 10% decrease in HIV incidence from 2018 (23,900 persons) to 2022 (21,400 persons). However, racial disparities in new diagnoses persisted in 2022, as seen in these data: the lifetime risk of HIV diagnosis among Black/African MSM was found to be 1 in 3, improving from the previously reported 1 in 2, compared to that of Hispanic/Latinx MSM (1 in 5, unchanged), Native Hawaiian/other Pacific Islander MSM (1 in 7, increased from 1 in 8), and whites (1 in 15, decreased from 1 in 11) (Singh et al., 2024) (Figure 2.12). Figure 2.13 demonstrates racial, regional, and age disparities among MSM PWH, all following the same trends discussed above. The number of HIV diagnoses among females attributable to IDU and heterosexual contact remained stable (CDC, 2024a).

HIV AMONG IMMIGRANT POPULATIONS

For several years, the CDC has published data on the incidence and prevalence of HIV, AIDS, and HIV-related deaths among Black, Latinx/Hispanic, Asian, Native American, and Pacific Islander persons. These data are summarized in Tables 2.1 and 2.2 (CDC, 2024a), showing the wide range of impact of HIV in these different groups. However, in these data, the CDC does not separate African-born from U.S.-born Black persons, or foreign-born versus U.S.-born Latinx/Hispanic persons, making it difficult to track the HIV epidemic among these different immigrant populations. However, data from the National HIV Surveillance System (NHSS) for Black adults diagnosed between 2008 and 2014 reported that in 2014, African-born Black females had higher rates of HIV infection compared to U.S.-born Black males (1.4 ×), African-born Black males (2 ×), and U.S.-born Black females (5.3 ×) (Demeke et al., 2019). The majority of these cases were attributed to heterosexual contact, and most diagnoses during this time period occurred in the South, where larger proportions of both African- and Caribbean-born Black persons resided. It is worth noting that African-born adults immigrated in large proportions to all four U.S. regions, as opposed to Caribbean-born Black adults who preferentially (95%) immigrated to the South and the Northeast. Finally, in this analysis, more non-U.S.-born Black adults had a late-stage HIV diagnosis compared to U.S.-born Black adults (36.6% vs. 25.8%). These disparities may be attributed to the impact of gender biases, different cultural values between non-U.S.-born and U.S.-born Black adults, delays in accessing health care after migration, stigma associated with

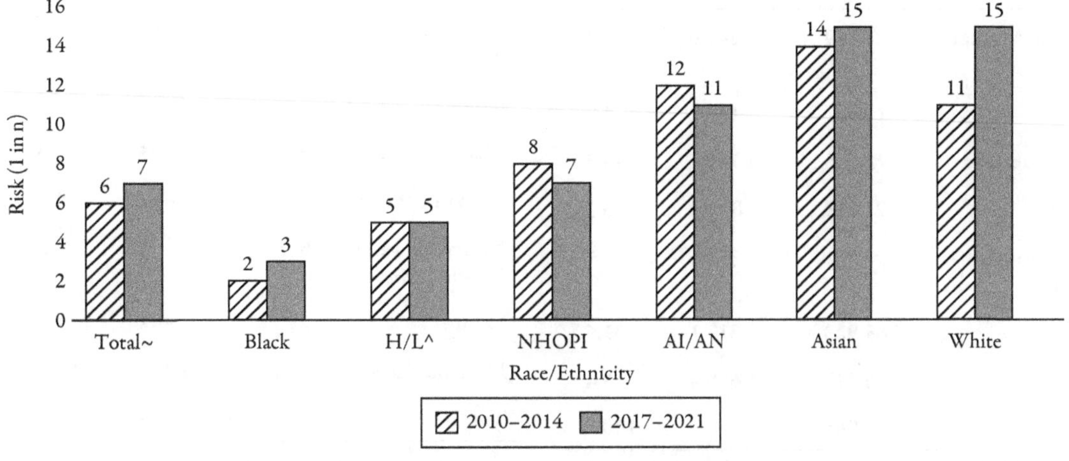

AI/AN = American Indian/Alaskan Native; H/L = Hispanic/Latino; NHOPI = Native Hawaiian/Other Pacific Islander
*Hess, et al. Lifetime risk of a diagnosis of HIV infection in the United States. Ann Epidemiol 2017;27(4):238–243.
“Includes 4,181 multiracial persons for 2017–2021 and 4,572 multiracial persons for 2010–2014

Figure 2.12 Lifetime risk of an HIV diagnosis among MSM by race/ethnicity, 2010–2014 vs. 2017–2021. SOURCE: Singh, Sonia, et al. Estimating lifetime risk of a diagnosis of HIV infection among MSM: United States, 2017–2021. Presented at Conference on Retroviruses and Opportunistic Infections, Denver, CO, March 3–6, 2024.

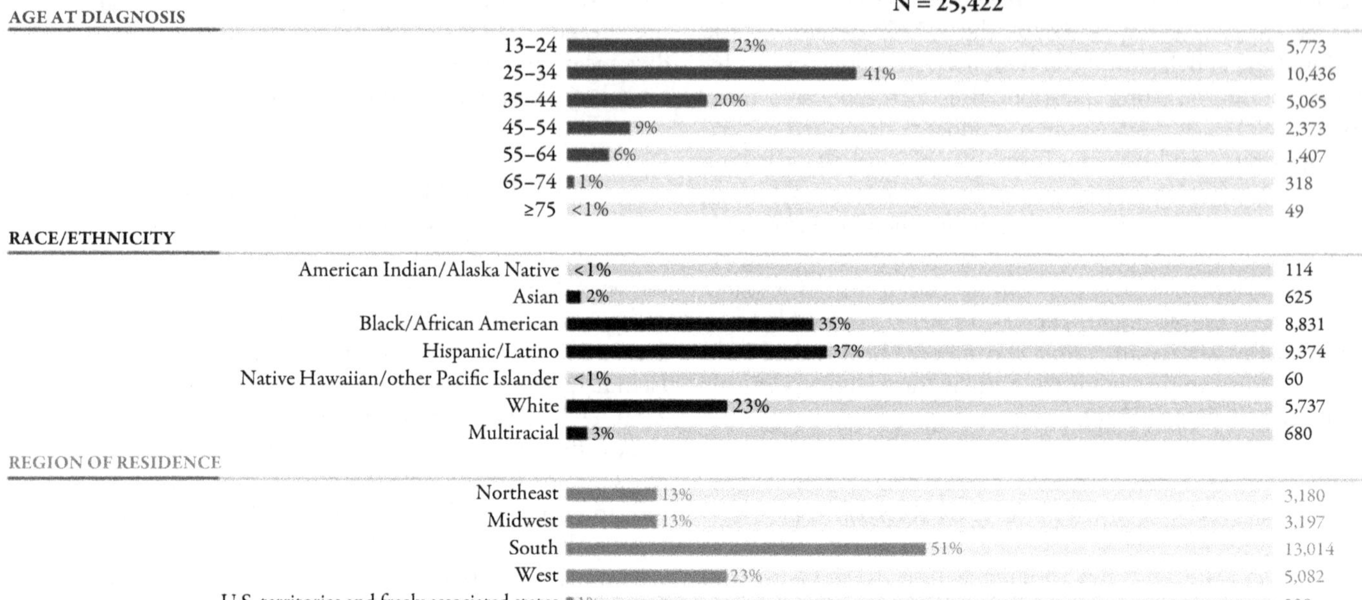

Figure 2.13 Percentages of diagnoses of HIV infection among men who have sex with men, by selected characteristics, 2022, United States and six dependent areas. Note: Data have been statistically adjusted to account for missing transmission category. Male-to-male sexual contact includes persons assigned male sex at birth, regardless of current gender identity, who have had sexual contact with other males, and persons assigned male sex at birth who have had sexual contact with both males and females (i.e., bisexual contact). Hispanic/Latino persons can be of any race. SOURCE: Centers for Disease Control and Prevention. Diagnoses, deaths, and prevalence of HIV in the United States and 6 territories and freely associated states, 2022. May 21, 2024. http://www.cdc.gov/hiv-data/nhss/hiv-diagnoses-deaths-prevalence.html.

HIV, and the possibility of pre-migration HIV acquisition. Nevertheless, non-U.S.-born Black adults were more likely than their U.S.-born counterparts to live for the first three years after a diagnosis of HIV or AIDS, which mirrors findings from prior analyses (Blanas et al., 2013).

Similar findings were elucidated in an NHSS-based analysis during 2010–2017. During this time period, 15.3% of those who received an HIV diagnosis were non-U.S.-born, with a greater proportion found to have AIDS at the time

Table 2.1 ADULTS AND ADOLESCENTS LIVING WITH DIAGNOSED HIV INFECTION BY RACE/ETHNICITY, 2022, UNITED STATES

RACE/ETHNICITY	NUMBER	RATE	%
American Indian/Alaskan Native	2,469	247.0	0.3
Asian	14,337	173.2	1.7
Black/African American	292,655	1,759.7	34.7
Hispanic/Latinx	221,763	868.4	26.3
Native Hawaiian/other Pacific Islander	821	311.6	0.1
White	265,923	313.1	31.5
Multiple races	45,117	1,689.4	5.4
Total	843,085		100

Source: CDC Surveillance Report 2022. Published 2024.

Centers for Disease Control and Prevention. Diagnoses, deaths, and prevalence of HIV in the United States and 6 territories and freely associated states, 2022. HIV Surveillance Report, 2022; vol. 35. http://www.cdc.gov/hiv-data/nhss/hiv-diagnoses-deaths-prevalence.html. Published May 2024. Accessed July 1, 2024.

Table 2.2 DEATHS OF PERSONS WITH DIAGNOSED HIV INFECTION EVER CLASSIFIED AS STAGE 3 (AIDS) BY RACE/ETHNICITY, YEAR-END 2022, UNITED STATES

RACE/ETHNICITY	NUMBER	RATE PER 100,000 POP.	%
American Indian/Alaskan Native	54	2.7	0.4
Asian	86	0.5	0.6
Black/African American	6,035	17.3	42.5
Hispanic/Latinx	2,600	5.2	18.3
Native Hawaiian/other Pacific Islander	5	1.0	<0.1
White	4,303	2.5	30.3
Multiple races	1,125	20.6	7.9
Total	14,208		100

Source: Centers for Disease Control and Prevention. Monitoring selected national HIV prevention and care objectives by using HIV surveillance data—United States and 6 territories and freely associated states, 2022. HIV Surveillance Supplemental Report, 2024; vol. 29 (no. 2). https://www.cdc.gov/hivdata/nhss/national-hiv-prevention-and-care-outcomes.html. Published May 2024. Accessed July 1, 2024.

of diagnosis. When compared to U.S.-born counterparts, more of the non-U.S.-born adults diagnosed with HIV were assigned female at birth and identified as Hispanic/Latinx (Kerani et al., 2020). In those who had known/documented countries of birth, the majority were born in Central America/Mexico, with the greatest percentages of representation from Mexico (22.6%), Haiti (7.5%), and Cuba (5.8%). It should also be noted that in a previous NHSS-based study between 2000 and 2013, a majority of HIV infections in non-U.S.-born persons occurred after immigrating to the United States, as opposed to in their native countries, highlighting the importance of understanding transmission networks (Valverde et al., 2017).

Since January 4, 2010, refugees are no longer tested for HIV infection upon arrival to the United States. However, since 2006, CDC guidelines have recommended universal screening for all persons aged 13–64 years, regardless of risk factors or country of origin (Branson, 2006). Given that the unpredictable and vulnerable conditions of refugee flight and refugee camps create a high risk for HIV transmission, HIV screening of all refugees is encouraged. The CDC-recommended fourth-generation testing algorithm differentiates between HIV-1 and HIV-2, whereas older-generation HIV antibody screening tests generally did not. Therefore, if fourth-generation testing is not available, refugees or immigrants native to or who transited through countries with high HIV-2 prevalence should have specific testing for HIV-2.

Multiple factors contribute to HIV infection among immigrants. Migration within and across national borders in search of work may contribute to increased HIV risk situations. In addition, change in residence can result in loneliness, isolation, and disruption of social, familial, and sexual relationships that can lead to risk-taking behavior (Organista et al., 2004). In 2021, 84 million persons globally were forcibly displaced, 36 million of whom were displaced internationally (WHO, 2022). The risk of HIV increases during conflict in the setting of healthcare system disruptions and gender-based violence. After displacement, it is also important to consider the effects of xenophobia, trauma, and racism and their impacts on the ability and motivation to engage in healthcare.

RECOMMENDED READING

Centers for Disease Control and Prevention. Diagnoses, deaths, and prevalence of HIV in the United States and 6 territories and freely associated states, 2022. May 21, 2024. http://www.cdc.gov/hiv-data/nhss/hiv-diagnoses-deaths-prevalence.html

Centers for Disease Control and Prevention. Estimated HIV incidence and prevalence in the United States, 2018–2022. May 21, 2024. https://www.cdc.gov/hiv-data/nhss/estimated-hiv-incidence-and-prevalence.html

Centers for Disease Control and Prevention. Monitoring selected national HIV prevention and care objectives by using HIV surveillance data United States and 6 territories and freely associated states, 2022. May 21, 2024. https://stacks.cdc.gov/view/cdc/156511

Kerani RP, Satcher JA, Buskin JE, et al., The epidemiology of HIV among people born outside the United States, 2010-2017. *Public Health Rep.* 2020 Sep–Oct;135(5):611–620. doi:10.1177/0033354920942623

World Health Organization. HIV statistics, globally and by WHO region, 2023. July 17, 2023. https://www.who.int/publications/i/item/WHO-UCN-HHS-SIA-2023-01

REFERENCES

Alessandri-Gradt E, De Oliveira F, Leoz M, et al. HIV-1 group P infection: towards a dead-end infection? *AIDS*. 2018;32(10):1317–1322.

Bacque J, Delgado E, Benito S, et al. Identification of CRF66_BF, a new HIV-1 circulating recombinant form of South American origin. *Front Microbiol.* 2021;12:774386.

Bbosa N, Kaleebu P, Ssemwanga D. HIV subtype diversity worldwide. *Curr Opin HIV AIDS.* 2019;14:153–160.

Becasen JS, Denard CL, Mullins MM, et al. Estimating the prevalence of HIV and sexual behaviors among the US transgender population: a systematic review and meta-analysis, 2006–2017. *Am J Public Health.* 2019;109(1):e1–e8.

Blanas DA, Nichols K, Bekele M, et al. HIV/AIDS among African-born residents in the United States. *J Immigr Minor Health.* 2013;15(4):718–724. doi:10.1007/s10903-012-9691-6

Boswell MT, Rowland-Jones SL. Delayed disease progression in HIV-2: the importance of TRIM5a and the retroviral capsid. *Clin Exp Immunol.* 2019 Jun;196(3):305–317. doi:10.1111/cei.13280

Branson BM. To screen or not to screen: is that really the question? *Ann Intern Med.* 2006;145(11):857–859.

Campbell-Yesufu OT, Gandhi RT. Update on human immunodeficiency virus (HIV)-2 infection. *Clin Infect Dis.* 2011;2(6):780–787.

Centers for Disease Control and Prevention (CDC). CDC publishes new HIV surveillance reports. https://www.cdc.gov/nchhstp/director-letters/cdc-publishes-new-hiv-surveillance-reports.html. Published May 21, 2024d. Accessed September 12, 2024.

CDC. Diagnoses, deaths, and prevalence of HIV in the United States and 6 territories and freely associated states, 2022. May 21, 2024b. http://www.cdc.gov/hiv-data/nhss/hiv-diagnoses-deaths-prevalence.html

CDC. Estimated HIV incidence and prevalence in the United States, 2018–2022. May 21, 2024a. https://www.cdc.gov/hiv-data/nhss/estimated-hiv-incidence-and-prevalence.html

CDC. Monitoring selected national HIV prevention and care objectives by using HIV surveillance data United States and 6 territories and freely associated states, 2022. May 21, 2024c. https://stacks.cdc.gov/view/cdc/156511

CDC. Overview and methodology of the national HIV behavioral surveillance among transgender women—seven urban areas, United States, 2019–2020. January 25, 2024e. https://www.cdc.gov/mmwr/volumes/73/su/su7301a1.htm#:~:text=In%202017%2C%20CDC%20established%20the,prevention%20strategies%2C%20and%20HIV%20prevalence

Ceccarelli G, Giovanetti M, Sagnelli C, et al. Human immunodeficiency virus type 2: the neglected threat. *Pathogens.* 2021;10:1377.

Clavel F, Guétard D, Brun-Vézinet F. Isolation of a new human retrovirus from West African patients with AIDS. *Science.* 1986;233(4761):343–346.

Clavel F, Mansinho K, Chamaret S. Human immunodeficiency virus type 2 infection associated with AIDS in West Africa. *N Engl J Med.* 1987;316:1180–1185.

Cohen J. Early AIDS virus may have ridden Africa's rails. *Science.* 2014;346:21–22.

D'Arc M, Ayouba A, Esteban A, et al. Origin of the HIV-1 group O epidemic in western lowland gorillas. *Proc Natl Acad Sci USA.* 2015;112(11): E1343–E1352.

De Leys R. Isolation and partial characterization of an unusual HIV retrovirus from two persons of west-central Africa origin. *J Virol.* 1990;64:1207–1216.

Demeke HB, Johnson AS, Wu B, et al., Differences between US-born and non-US-born Black adults reported with diagnosed HIV infection: United States, 2008–2014. *J Immigr Minor Health.* 2019;21(1):30–38.

De Mendoza C, Lozano AB, Rando A, et al. The incidence of HIV-2 infection is declining: a registry data analysis. *Int J Infect Dis.* 2024;146:107076.

De Oliveira F, Mourez T, Aurélia Vessiere, A et al. Multiple HIV-1/M + HIV-1/O dual infections and new HIV-1/MO inter-group recombinant forms detected in Cameroon. *Retrovirology.* 2017;14(1):1.

Department of Health and Human Services (DHHS). Expanding PrEP coverage in the United States to achieve EHE goals. October 18, 2023. https://www.hiv.gov/blog/expanding-prep-coverage-in-the-united-states-to-achieve-ehe-goals#:~:text=The%202022%20%20preliminary%20data%20%20indicate,compared%20with%2015%25%20of%20females

DHHS. Recommendations for the use of antiretroviral drugs during pregnancy and interventions to reduce perinatal HIV transmission in the United States. January 31, 2024. https://clinicalinfo.hiv.gov/en/guidelines/perinatal/introduction?view=full

Elangovan R, Jenks M, Yun J et al. Global and regional estimates for subtype-specific therapeutic and prophylactic HIV-1 vaccines: a modeling study. *Front Microbiol.* 2021;12:690647.

Faria, NR, Rambaut A, Suchard MA, et al. The early spread and epidemic ignition of HIV-1 in human populations. *Science.* 2014;346(6205):56–61.

Faria, NR, Vidal N, Lourencio J, et al. Distinct rates and patterns of spread of the major HIV-1 subtypes in Central and East Africa. *PLoS Pathog.* 2019;15(12):e1007976.

Fumarola B, Calza S, Renzetti S, et al. Immunological evolution of a cohort of HIV-2 infected patients: peculiarities of an underestimated infection. *Mediterr J Hematol Infect Dis.* 2022; 14(1):e2022016.

Gao F, Bailes E, Robertson DL, et al. Origin of HIV-1 in the chimpanzee *Pan troglodytes troglodytes. Nature.* 1999;397:436–441.

Gilbert MTP, Rambaut A, Wlasiuk G, et al. The emergence of HIV/AIDS in the Americas and beyond. *Proc Natl Assoc Sci USA.* 2007 Nov 20;104(47):18566–18570.

Gottlieb MS, Schanker HM, Fan PT, et al. *Pneumocystis* pneumonia—Los Angeles. *MMWR.* 1981 Jun 5;30(21):1–3.

Junqueira DM, Almeida SE. HIV-1 subtype B: traces of a pandemic. *Virology.* 2016 Aug;495:173–184.

Kapoor AK, Padival S. HIV-2. 2022 Sep 20. In: *StatPearls* [Internet]. Treasure Island (FL): Publishing; 2025 Jan–.

Keele BF, Jones JH, Terio KA, et al. Increased mortality and AIDS-like immunopathology in wild chimpanzees infected with SIV_{cpz}. *Nature.* 2009;460:515–519.

Keele BF, Van Heuverswyn F, Li Y, et al. Chimpanzee reservoirs for pandemic and nonpandemic HIV-1. *Science.* 2006;313(5786):523–526.

Kerani RP, Johnson AS, Buskin SE, et al. The epidemiology of HIV among people born outside the United States, 2010–2017. *Public Health Rep.* 2020;135:611–620.

Meissner ME, Talledge N, Mansky LM. Molecular biology and diversification of human retroviruses. *Front Virol.* 2022;2:872599.

Mori M, Ode H, Kubota M, et al. Nanopore sequencing for characterization of HIV-1 recombinant forms. *Microbiol Spectr.* 2022;10(4):e0150722. doi:10.1128/spectrum.01507-22. Epub 2022 Jul 27. PMID: 35894615; PMCID: PMC9431566.

Ngoupo PA, Sadeu, MB, Alain S, et al. First evidence of transmission of an HIV-1 M/O intergroup recombinant virus. *AIDS.* 2016;30(1):1–8.

Organista K, Hector C, George A. HIV prevention with Mexican migrants: review, critique, and recommendations. *J Acquir Immune Defic Syndr.* 2004;374:S227–S239.

Peeters M, D'Arc M, Delaporta E. The origin and diversity of human retroviruses. *AIDS Rev.* 2014;16(1):23–34.

Pépin J. *The Origins of AIDS.* New York: Cambridge University Press; 2011.

Pe'pin J. The origins of AIDS: from patient zero to ground zero. *J Epidemiol Community Health.* 2013;67(6):473–475.

Peruski AH, Wesolowski LG, Delaney KP, et al. Trends in HIV-2 diagnosis and use of HIV-1/HIV-2 differentiation test—United States, 2010–2017. *MMWR.* 2020;69(3):63–66.

Plantier JC, Leoz, M, Dickerson JE. A new immunodeficiency virus derived from gorillas designated group "P." *Nature Med.* 2009;15:871–872.

Rowland-Jones S, Gea-Mallorquí E. Closing the equity gap in the treatment of HIV-2 infection. *Lancet HIV.* 2024;11(6):e347–e349.

Sauter D, Hué S, Petit S, et al. HIV-1 group P is unable to antagonize human tetherin by Vpu, Env or Nef. *Retrovirology.* 2011;8:103.

Sharp PM, Hahn BH. Origins of HIV and the AIDS pandemic. *Cold Spring Harbor Perspect Med.* 2011;1:1–22.

Singh S, Hu X, Hess K, et al. Estimating lifetime risk of a diagnosis of HIV infection among MSM: United States, 2017–2021. Presented at Conference on Retroviruses and Opportunistic Infections, Denver, CO, March 3–6, 2024.

Stoner MCD, Haley DF, Golin CE, et al. The relationship between economic deprivation, housing instability and transactional sex among women in North Carolina (HPTN 064). *AIDS Behav.* 2019; 23(11):2946–2955.

Switzer WM, Shankar A, Jia H, et al. Kentucky/Ohio response to HIV among PWID workgroup: high HIV diversity, recombination, and superinfection revealed in a large outbreak among persons who inject drugs in Kentucky and Ohio, USA. *Virus Evol.* 2024;10(1):veae015.

Tzou PL, Descamps D, Rhee SY, et al. Expanded spectrum of antiretroviral-selected mutations in human immunodeficiency virus type-2. *J Infect Dis.* 2020;211:1962–1972.

United Nations Programme on HIV/AIDS (UNAIDS). HIV and adolescent girls and young women. https://www.unaids.org/sites/default/files/media_asset/2024-unaids-global-aids-update-adolescent-girls-young-women_en.pdf. Published 2024c. Accessed September 12, 2024.

UNAIDS. New HIV infections data among key populations: proportions in 2010 and 2022. https:// www.unaids.org/sites/default/files/media_asset/new-hiv-infections-data-among-key-populations-proportions_en.pdf. Published 2024b. Accessed September 12, 2024.

UNAIDS. The path that ends AIDS: UNAIDS global AIDS update 2023. https:// thepath.unaids.org/wp-content/themes/unaids2023/assets/files/2023_report.pdf. Published July 13, 2023b. Accessed August 24, 2024.

UNAIDS. UNAIDS data 2023. https://www.unaids.org/en/resources/documents/2023/2023_unaids_data. Published October 31, 2023a. Accessed August 24, 2024.

UNAIDS. UNAIDS World AIDS Day 2024 fact sheet. https://www.unaids.org/sites/default/files/media_asset/UNAIDS_FactSheet_en.pdf. Published July 22, 2024a. Accessed August 24, 2024.

U.S. Preventive Services Task Force (USPSTF). Screening for HIV infection: US Preventive Services Task Force recommendation statement. *JAMA.* 2019;321:2326–2336.

Valverde E, Oster AM, Songli X, et al. HIV transmission dynamics among foreign-born persons in the United States. *J Acquir Immune Defic Syndr.* 2017;76(5):445–452.

Villabona-Arenas CJ, Domyeum J, Mouacha F, et al. HIV-1 group O infection in Cameroon from 2006–2013: prevalence, genetic diversity, evolution, and public health challenges. *Infect Gener Evo.* 2015;36:210–216.

White House Office of National AIDS Policy. National HIV/AIDS strategy for the United States: updated to 2020. https://files.hiv.gov/s3fs-public/nhas-update.pdf. Published online July 2015. Accessed August 24, 2024.

Williams A, Menon S, Crowe M, et al. Geographic and population distribution of human immunodeficiency virus (HIV)-1 and HIV-2 circulation subtypes: a systematic literature review and meta-analysis (2010–2021). *J Infect Dis.* 2023;228:1583–1591.

World Health Organization (WHO). HIV statistics, globally and by WHO region, 2023. July 17, 2023. https://www.who.int/publications/i/item/WHO-UCN-HHS-SIA-2023-01

WHO. Refugee and migrant health. May 2, 2022. https://www.who.int/news-room/fact-sheets/detail/refugee-and-migrant-health#:~:text=Of%20this%20total%2C%20281%20million,into%20refugee%20life%20(2)

Worobey M, Gemmel M, Teuwen DE, et al. Direct evidence of extensive diversity of HIV-1 in Kinshasa by 1960. *Nature.* 2008;455(7213):661–664.

Worobey M, Watts T, McKay R, et al. 1970s and 'patient 0' HIV-1 genomes illuminate early HIV/AIDS history in North America. *Nature.* 2016;539:98–101.

Zhu T, Korber BT, Nahmias AJ, et al. An African HIV-1 sequence from 1959 and implications for the origin of the epidemic. *Nature.* 1998;391(6667):594–597.

3.

MECHANISMS OF HIV TRANSMISSION

Nancy Aitcheson and Puja H. Nambiar

LEARNING OBJECTIVES

Upon completion of this chapter, the reader should be able to:

- Describe the relative risk of HIV transmission based on various types of sexual behaviors/exposures, occupational exposures, drug use–related exposures, and perinatal exposures.
- Discuss the significance of viral load quantity and its relationship to transmission risk.
- Explain the impact of co-occurring sexually transmitted infections on HIV transmission.

INTRODUCTION

With almost 30 years of experience demonstrating that antiretroviral therapy (ART) is highly effective in reducing the transmission of HIV, there is now clear evidence that people with HIV who have an undetectable viral load cannot transmit HIV sexually.

WHAT'S NEW?

- Recent CDC surveillance reports indicate that the estimated number of new HIV infections in 2022 decreased by 12% compared to 2018; increases in pre-exposure prophylaxis use, HIV testing, and viral suppression likely contributed to this trend.
- Breastfeeding guidance for women with HIV has evolved in resource-rich settings; early and sustained maternal ART with virologic suppression, including in the postpartum period, decreases the risk of perinatal transmission.

KEY POINTS

- The risk of HIV transmission to a receptive partner remains higher than that to an insertive one; however, both carry some risk.
- Anything that compromises the integrity of mucous membranes, such as sexually transmitted infections, may increase the risk of HIV transmission.
- For serodifferent couples, keeping the viral load of the person with HIV (PWH) persistently suppressed to an undetectable level eliminates the risk of sexual transmission to the seronegative partner.
- Perinatal transmission is a significant concern in resource-limited countries because of uneven access to early maternal ART.

SEXUAL TRANSMISSION

HIV can be transmitted through infectious body fluids—blood, seminal fluid, vaginal fluid, rectal fluid, and breast milk. Sexual contact is the most common mode of HIV transmission worldwide. In the United States, HIV is mainly transmitted by anal or vaginal sex and less commonly by other modes such as perinatal transmission (during pregnancy, birth, or breastfeeding), needlestick injury, blood transfusion, or organ transplants. In 2022, 67% of all new infections among persons aged 13 years and older were among persons with HIV attributable to male-to-male sexual contact (Centers for Disease Control and Prevention [CDC], 2024a).

Individuals with acute HIV infection with high levels of viremia are at the highest risk of transmitting the virus to others. HIV can be readily found in semen and in vaginal fluid from a person with HIV. There is a strong correlation between high plasma viral load and the amount of virus in genital secretions (Zhang et al., 1998). However, compartmental discordance has been observed (rarely) between levels of HIV in the plasma and genital secretions. Men with HIV on ART with undetectable virus in plasma can infrequently have detectable HIV in their seminal fluid (Zhang et al., 1998).

Condomless anal sex has the highest risk for HIV transmission, with the receptive partner being at higher risk than the insertive partner. The person receiving semen with HIV is believed to be at the highest risk because of the single-cell layer of epithelium lining the rectum, which can be easily disrupted and permit entry of the virus across the rectal mucosa. The insertive partner is also at some risk because HIV can enter the penis through the urethra, the mucosa of nonkeratinized portions of the foreskin, or through cuts, abrasions, or open sores on the penis. Circumcision has been demonstrated to significantly reduce the risk of HIV acquisition but not of transmission (Dosekun and Fox, 2010).

Worldwide, the AIDS epidemic is being driven by new infections occurring in women of childbearing age. During condomless vaginal intercourse, both partners are at risk for HIV, although there is a higher risk of a woman acquiring

HIV from a man with HIV than a man acquiring HIV from a woman with HIV. HIV can enter the body through the vaginal and cervical mucous membrane linings. HIV-1 replicates and persists in the vaginal epithelial dendritic cells (Pena-Cruz et al., 2018), which provides a recognizable mechanism for transmission via the vaginal mucosa. Although the risk of men acquiring HIV through heterosexual vaginal or anal intercourse is lower, HIV is abundantly present in vaginal secretions, and the anatomic sites of potential infection in the penis are the same as those described previously for anal intercourse (Dosekun and Fox, 2010).

Sexually transmitted infections (STIs) have a significant role in HIV transmission. Genital ulcer disease (i.e., syphilis, chancroid, and herpes simplex infections) and infections causing mucosal inflammation (i.e., gonorrhea and chlamydia) have been shown to increase HIV transmission threefold. Trichomonas has been shown to increase the risk of HIV acquisition among women by 50% (McClelland et al., 2007). This increase is most likely due to both heightened infectivity and susceptibility. Open ulcers aid the entry of HIV, and inflammation recruits increased numbers of $CD4^{+}$ cells that serve as targets for HIV. Prevention, early diagnosis, and treatment of STIs thus have the potential to significantly reduce HIV incidence in general, especially for high-risk populations.

Limiting viral replication in genital secretions is a logical approach to preventing HIV acquisition. Data from the pivotal HPTN 052 study showed dramatic reductions in HIV transmission among serodifferent couples in which the seropositive partner was virologically suppressed on ART, along with monthly HIV prevention counseling and regular STI testing and treatment. This unique clinical trial showed that men and women living with HIV had a 96% reduced risk of transmitting the virus to their original linked, HIV-negative sexual partners through early initiation of ART (Cohen et al., 2011). Longer-term follow-up of the study showed a sustained, overall 93% reduction of HIV transmission between linked couples when the seropositive partner was taking ART and had a suppressed viral load (Cohen et al., 2016). The results of this historic study provided irrefutable evidence to support the concept of "treatment as prevention" (TasP).

Taking evaluation of TasP even further, the prospective observational PARTNER-1 (Partners of People on ART: A New Evaluation of the Risks) study, although involving limited follow-up time (median = 1.3 years per couple), showed no linked HIV transmissions with condomless anal and vaginal sex among serodifferent heterosexual and same-sex male couples in which the seropositive partner was virologically suppressed on ART (Rodger et al., 2016). The subsequent PARTNER-2 study reported no phylogenetically linked HIV transmissions over 415 couple-years of follow-up in same-sex male couples reporting condomless anal intercourse, in which the seropositive partners were virologically suppressed and seronegative partners reported no use of pre-exposure prophylaxis (PrEP) (Rodger et al., 2019). An international, prospective observational cohort study (the Opposites Attract study) examining the association between ART and viral load and HIV transmission in serodifferent male couples in Australia, Brazil, and Thailand also reported similar results (Bavinton et al., 2018). Together, the PARTNER and Opposites Attract studies have reported no linked transmissions despite nearly 35,000 acts of condomless anal intercourse between HIV serodifferent male couples not using daily pre-exposure prophylaxis. Transmission risk is likely proportional to viral load even beyond remaining undetectable (<200 copies per mL); a recent systematic review commissioned by the World Health Organization found sexual HIV transmission to be absent in cases involving less than 600 copies per mL and exceedingly rare in cases of less than 1,000 copies per mL (Broyles et al., 2023).

Developing novel approaches for the rapid detection and diagnosis of HIV infection and increasing effective ART coverage are the next important steps in realizing the potential public benefits of these discoveries.

TRANSMISSION IN THE HEALTHCARE SETTING

All persons working in healthcare and other occupational settings with the potential for exposure to infectious blood and body fluids and nonsterile medical equipment or surroundings are at risk for HIV acquisition. The risk of occupational HIV transmission is low and occurs when a healthcare worker has a percutaneous injury or contact with a mucous membrane or nonintact skin with HIV-infected blood, tissue, or other body fluids. The risk of HIV transmission following percutaneous and mucous membrane exposures to HIV-infected blood has been roughly estimated to be 0.2% and 0.09%, respectively. There is no risk of HIV transmission via contact with HIV-infected body fluids with intact skin (CDC, 2024b).

In addition to blood, other bodily fluids, such as cerebrospinal, synovial, amniotic, pleural, peritoneal, and pericardial fluids, are considered potentially infectious. The risk from these fluids remains unknown, owing to the lack of epidemiologic studies in healthcare settings to assess the risk of HIV transmission to healthcare workers from exposure to these specific fluids. Although semen and cervicovaginal secretions have been shown to contain virus-infected cells, they have not been implicated in occupational transmission from patients to healthcare practitioners (HCP). Feces, urine, nasal secretions, sweat, tears, sputum, vomitus, and saliva are not considered potentially infectious unless visibly bloody (Bell, 1997). The major factors influencing the possibility of transmission include type and severity of exposure and magnitude of viremia. A greater risk of transmission was seen with exposures involving a large quantity of blood from source persons living with HIV, deep injuries, and hollow bore needle injuries. Higher titers of HIV in blood (often described as the "inoculum")—as seen in persons with acute HIV infection or uncontrolled HIV—increase transmission risk (CDC, 2024b).

Although uncommon, there have been several documented transmission events from HCP to patients during routine medical or dental care, most likely caused by poor adherence to infection-control procedures. Further, although increasingly less frequent, there have been documented cases of patient-to-patient transmission, most of which involved the use of unsterilized instruments or syringes. The use of universal precautions during all healthcare procedures and encounters cannot be overemphasized. Since 1991, the CDC has investigated all cases of HIV infection reported as acquired occupationally by healthcare workers. Until now, the National HIV Surveillance System recorded 58 confirmed and 150 possible cases of occupationally acquired HIV transmission among healthcare professionals. Among the 58 confirmed cases, the primary route of exposure resulting in infection was percutaneous puncture or cut (49/58 cases), followed by mucocutaneous exposure (5), both percutaneous and mucocutaneous exposure (2), and unknown (2). The majority were nurses (41%), followed by laboratory clinicians (35%), physicians (10%), and other health-related workers (14%). Since 1999, there has been only one case of occupationally acquired HIV (a laboratory technician who sustained a needle puncture while working with high-titer HIV cultures in 2008) (Joyce et al., 2015). In 2024, CDC reported their investigation of 4 new HIV infections among persons with no known HIV risk factors who received platelet-rich plasma with microneedling ("vampire facials") at an unlicensed New Mexico spa, suggesting that HIV transmission was associated with these cosmetic injection services (Stadelman-Behar et al., 2024).

For cases in which risk of HIV transmission can be determined, specific guidelines exist for the use of antivirals for postexposure prophylaxis (PEP). Occupational exposures require urgent medical evaluation and initiation of PEP, ideally within 2–6 hours after exposure. Prospective, well-controlled clinical data supporting PEP do not exist. By extrapolation from well-controlled animal model studies, it has been estimated that PEP reduces the risk of infection by approximately 80%, and that it becomes less effective as time lapses (>72 hours). Currently, the preferred initial occupational PEP regimen involves three or more antiretroviral drugs, namely tenofovir disoproxil fumarate/emtricitabine plus either raltegravir (TDF/FTC + RAL) or dolutegravir (TDF/FTC + DTG). This is due to ease of administration, proven potency when used as treatment among people with established HIV infection, and favorable tolerability. It is recommended to start PEP following exposure to a source person who is known to be living with HIV or for whom there is a reasonably high clinical suspicion of having HIV. If the source person is determined to be HIV-negative, PEP can be discontinued. The recommended duration of PEP is 28 days.

PEP is also recommended for nonoccupational exposures, sometimes referred to as "nPEP." CDC recommendations indicate that nPEP should be used when the source person is known to be living with HIV, and case-by-case determinations should be made for instances when the source person has an unknown HIV status. CDC also recommends evaluating patients requiring nPEP for transition to pre-exposure prophylaxis (PrEP) in the future (CDC, 2021). For both occupational and nonoccupational indications for PEP, administration should not be delayed while awaiting the source person's HIV test results, but rather should be started empirically and discontinued later if the source person's test results are negative (Kuhar et al., 2013).

More detailed information regarding occupational and non-occupational PEP, as well as pre-exposure prophylaxis (PrEP), is provided in Chapter 14, "HIV Prevention: Pharmacotherapy and Non-Pharmacotherapy-Based Strategies."

TRANSMISSION THROUGH THE USE OF INJECTION DRUGS

People who inject drugs (PWID) are at high risk of acquiring HIV if they use and share needles, syringes, or other drug-injection equipment previously used by someone with HIV. Sharing syringes is the second-highest-risk behavior for acquiring HIV. HIV survival in syringes has been associated with volume of blood remaining in the syringe as well as storage temperature. In one study, viable HIV was isolated from 50% of all syringes stored at 4°C for up to 42 days (Abdala et al., 2000).

The high-risk practices of sharing needles and syringes, engaging in risky sexual behavior, drug use, and socioeconomic factors limiting access to HIV prevention and care, as well as to substance use and mental health programs, are some of the ongoing prevention challenges currently identified by the CDC.

The CDC has pursued a systematic prevention approach by distributing funds to health departments for surveillance and by supporting intervention programs such as community PROMISE (Peers Reaching Out and Modeling Intervention Strategies); syringe service programs that provide access to sterile syringes and needles and thereby reduce community transmission of HIV, hepatitis C, hepatitis B virus, and other blood-borne infections; and PrEP and PEP services, among other interventions. Providing comprehensive prevention services and medical and/or substance use disorder treatment referrals for PWID can help increase access to health care and substance use disorder treatment (CDC, 2008).

Individuals who use recreational crystal methamphetamine are at increased risk of acquiring HIV. However, there is no clear evidence that methamphetamine itself increases HIV transmission or acquisition. People who use methamphetamine, in general, report several behaviors associated with HIV transmission, including greater numbers of sex partners, reduced use of condoms, exchange of sex for money or drugs, sex with PWID, and/or a history of STIs. Further, they are more likely to engage in condomless anal or vaginal sex with partners of unknown HIV status. Individuals using other mind/behavior-altering drugs, such as alcohol, can also be at increased risk for HIV infection (CDC, 2021). The risk of HIV transmission involving persons with undetectable viral load who share syringes or other drug-injection equipment is unknown, but likely reduced.

PERINATAL TRANSMISSION

Perinatal transmission of HIV is a unique scenario, as infant exposure to HIV occurs despite the presence of HIV-specific antibodies that are passively transferred from the mother to fetus while in utero. Several factors have been identified that influence the risk of perinatal HIV transmission. High maternal viral load (in blood and the genital tract) at the time of delivery, lower CD4$^+$ T-cell count, and advanced HIV disease have been associated with higher risk of perinatal HIV transmission (Yah and Tambo, 2019).

Universal perinatal HIV counseling and testing, ART for all pregnant women with HIV, scheduled cesarean delivery for women with viremia (HIV RNA >1,000 copies/mL), infant ART (presumptive treatment or ARVs used as prophylaxis), and avoidance of breastfeeding have contributed to the remarkable decline in annual rate of perinatal transmission of HIV to less than 1% in the United States. In the absence of any intervention, transmission rates can vary from 15% to 45%, and despite scaled-up prevention programs, perinatal HIV infection continues in regions of Sub-Saharan Africa (Yah and Tambo, 2019). The most common barriers and challenges described include nondisclosure of HIV status to partners and family, late initiation of ART or medication adherence, limited STI screening, long clinic travel and wait times, and infant-feeding methods.

Pediatric HIV infection is associated with an accelerated course of disease and high mortality. In the absence of ART, only 65% of children with HIV survive until their first birthday, and less than half will reach 2 years of age. In the absence of breastfeeding and with no ART, the risk of perinatal transmission is estimated at 25%. Up to 20% more children can acquire HIV through breastfeeding. Despite the presence of innate factors in human breast milk that display strong HIV inhibitory activity in vitro, up to 44% of HIV infections in children can be attributed to breastfeeding. The risk of acquiring HIV after a single day of breastfeeding is extremely low: 0.00028 per day of breastfeeding (Richardson et al., 2003). However, after ingesting liters of breast milk over a span of several months to years (~250 liters per year), 5%–20% of infants born to women living with HIV will eventually acquire HIV in the absence of any preventive measures (WHO, UNICEF, UNFPA, and UNAIDS, 2008). Elevated levels of HIV particles (cell-free virus) and HIV-infected cells (cell-associated virus) in the breast milk of women living with HIV are associated with an increased risk of HIV transmission during breastfeeding. Although it has been reported that a tenfold increase in cell-free or cell-associated HIV in breast milk is associated with a threefold increase in transmission, it is still unclear whether cell-free virus and/or cell-associated virus are transmitted during breastfeeding. Further, it is not known if the frequency of cell-free and cell-associated HIV transmission varies at different stages of lactation (i.e., colostrum, early breast milk, and mature breast milk).

Recent results from the PROMISE study, a randomized control trial of infant nevirapine prophylaxis versus maternal ART comprising 2,431 mother-child pairs, showed that both strategies were safe and were associated with very low HIV transmission to infants and high rates of infant HIV-free survival (Flynn et al., 2021). Currently, the estimated risk of HIV transmission via breastfeeding from a parent with HIV who is receiving ART and is virally suppressed is estimated to be less than 1%. In early 2023, U.S. perinatal HIV clinical guidelines were updated to support a shift toward shared decision-making regarding infant feeding for mothers who were stably virologically suppressed on ART, due to the well-documented benefits of breastfeeding and increasing advocacy from community members and their providers. A recent clinical report from the American Academy of Pediatrics (AAP) notes that people with HIV may express a desire to breastfeed, and pediatricians should be prepared to offer a family-centered, nonjudgmental, harm-reduction approach to support PWH on ART with sustained viral suppression (<50 copies per mL) who desire to breastfeed (Abuogi et al., 2024). The report also offers specific recommendations regarding duration, exclusivity, frequency of maternal viral load testing, and infant HIV-screening intervals. However, the guidance also continues to state that avoidance of breastfeeding is the only infant feeding option with 0% risk of HIV transmission. Given continued interest on the part of women living with HIV in breastfeeding their infants, further study of HIV transmission through breastfeeding among mothers with viral suppression is warranted, in addition to updated clinical recommendations (especially for infant ARV prophylaxis management) and information-sharing across patient communities and healthcare professionals.

REFERENCES

Abdala N, Reyes R, Carney JM, Heimer R. Survival of HIV-1 in syringes: effects of temperature during storage external icon. *Subst Use Misuse*. 2000;35(10):1369–1383.

Abuogi L, Noble L, Smith C, Committee on Pediatric and Adolescent HIV, Section on Breastfeeding. Infant feeding for persons living with and at risk for HIV in the United States: clinical report. *Pediatrics*. 2024;153(6):e2024066843.

Bavinton BR, Pinto AN, Phanuphak N, et al. Viral suppression and HIV transmission in serodiscordant male couples: an international, prospective, observational, cohort study. *Lancet HIV*. 2018;5(8):e438–e447. https://doi:10.1016/S2352-3018(18)30132-2

Bell DM. Occupational risk of human immunodeficiency virus infection in healthcare workers: an overview. *Am J Med*. 1997;102(5B):9–15.

Broyles LN, Luo R, Boeras D, Vojnov L. The risk of sexual transmission of HIV in individuals with low-level HIV viraemia: a systematic review. *Lancet*. 2023;402(10400):464–471. (published online July 23). https://doi.org/10.1016/S0140-6736(23)00877-2

CDC. HIV transmission. cdc.gov. https:// www.cdc.gov/hiv/causes/index.html. Published January 18, 2024b. Accessed August 2022.

CDC. Recommendations for post-exposure interventions to prevent infection with hepatitis B virus, hepatitis C virus, or human immunodeficiency virus, and tetanus in persons wounded during bombings and other mass-casualty events—United States, 2008. *MMWR*. August 1, 2008;57(RR06):1–19.

CDC. Updated guidelines for antiretroviral postexposure prophylaxis after sexual, injection drug use, or other nonoccupational exposure to HIV—United States, 2016. https:// cdc-hiv-prep-guidelines-2021.pdf. Published 2021. Accessed August 21, 2024.

Centers for Disease Control and Prevention (CDC). HIV surveillance report, 2024. http:// stacks.cdc.gov/view/cdc/156513 l. Published May 21, 2024a. Accessed September 11, 2024.
Cohen MS, Chen YQ, McCauley M, et al. Final results of the HPTN 052 randomized controlled trial: antiretroviral therapy prevents HIV transmission. *N Engl J Med*. 2016;375:830–839.
Cohen MS, Chen YQ, McCauley M, et al. Prevention of HIV-1 infection with early antiretroviral therapy. *N Engl J Med*. 2011;365:493–505.
Dosekun O, Fox J. An overview of the relative risks of different sexual behaviours on HIV transmission. *Curr Opin HIV AIDS*. 2010;5:291–297.
Flynn PM, Taha TE, Cababasay M, et al. Association of maternal viral load and CD4 count with perinatal HIV-1 transmission risk during breastfeeding in the PROMISE postpartum component. *J Acquir Immune Defic Syndr*. 2021;88(2):206–213. https://www.ncbi.nlm.nih.gov/pubmed/34108383
Joyce MP, Kuhar D, Brooks JT. Occupationally acquired HIV infection by healthcare personnel—United States, 1985–2013. *MMWR*. January 9, 2015;63(53):1245–1246.
Kuhar DT, Henderson DK, Struble KA, et al. Updated US Public Health Service guidelines for the management of occupational exposures to human immunodeficiency virus and recommendations for postexposure prophylaxis. *Infect Control Hosp Epidemiol*. November 2013;34(11):1238.
McClelland RS, Sangare L, Hassan WM, et al. Infection with *Trichomonas vaginalis* increases the risk of HIV-1 acquisition. *J Infect Dis*. 2007;195(5):698–702.
Pena-Cruz V, Agosto, Akiyama et al. HIV replicates and persists in vaginal epithelial dendritic cells. *J Clin Invest*. 2018;128(8):3439–3444. https://doi.org/10.1172/JCI98943
Richardson BA, John-Stewart GC, Hughes JP, et al. Breast-milk infectivity in human immunodeficiency virus type 1-infected mothers. *J Infect Dis*. 2003;187:736–740.
Rodger AJ, Cambiano V, Bruun T, et al. Risk of HIV transmission through condomless sex in serodifferent gay couples with the HIV-positive partner taking suppressive antiretroviral therapy (PARTNER): final results of a multicentre, prospective, observational study. *Lancet*. 2019;393(10189):2428–2438.
Rodger AJ, Cambiano V, Bruun T, et al. Sexual activity without condoms and risk of HIV transmission in serodifferent couples when the HIV-positive partner is using suppressive antiretroviral therapy. *JAMA*. 2016;316(2):171–181. http://doi:10.1001/jama.2016.5148
Stadelman-Behar AM, Gehre MN, Atallah L, et al. Investigation of presumptive HIV transmission associated with receipt of platelet-rich plasma microneedling facials at a spa among former spa clients — New Mexico, 2018–2023. *MMWR*. 2024;73:372–376.
WHO, UNICEF, UNFPA, and UNAIDS. *HIV Transmission Through Breastfeeding: A Review of Available Evidence: 2007 Update*. Geneva: World Health Organization; 2008.
Yah CS, Tambo E. Why is mother to child transmission (MTCT) of HIV a continual threat to new-borns in sub-Saharan Africa (SSA). *J Infect Public Health*. 2019;12(2):213–223. http://doi:10.1016/j.jiph.2018.10.008
Zhang H, Dornadula G, Beumont M, et al. Human immunodeficiency virus type 1 in the semen of men receiving highly active antiretroviral therapy. *N Engl J Med*. December 17, 1998;339(25):1803–1809.

4.

VIROLOGY

LIFE CYCLE OF HIV

Poonam Mathur and George Lewis

HIV STRUCTURE AND LIFE CYCLE

LEARNING OBJECTIVE

- Demonstrate and apply knowledge of the established and evolving science of human immunodeficiency virus (HIV) virology, in both the cell and the host.
- Discuss basic HIV virology and its relevance to current and potential drug targets.
- Describe how HIV virology informs therapeutic approaches aimed at various stages of the viral life cycle.

WHAT'S NEW?

Research continues to elucidate details on reverse transcription and integration, which may inform the development of new therapeutic strategies and agents.

KEY POINTS

- HIV is a member of the lentivirus subfamily of retroviruses.
- The HIV life cycle can be divided into two phases: (1) virus entry, reverse transcription, entry into the nucleus, and integration of double-stranded DNA (the provirus); and (2) regulation of production of viral proteins and new infectious virions.
- HIV enters the human cell via the CD4 receptor and chemokine coreceptors, primarily CCR5 and CXCR4.
- The viral genome is transcribed from RNA to DNA by reverse transcriptase and is integrated into the host genome by integrase.
- The HIV genome encodes 15 proteins comprising three categories: structural, regulatory, and accessory.
- After budding from the host cell, the virus matures into its infectious form through cleavage of viral precursor proteins by protease.

VIRAL CLASSIFICATION

HIV is a member of the lentivirus subfamily of retroviruses, differing from HTLV-1 and HTLV-2, which are oncoviruses. Two distinct groups of HIV lentiviruses are pathogenic in humans: HIV-1 and HIV-2, both of which cause immunodeficiency disease. HIV-2 is epidemiologically distinct from HIV-1 and less pathogenic, with a longer asymptomatic phase, slower rate of $CD4^+$ T-cell decline, and lower plasma viral loads. Given these factors, it has historically been associated with lower mortality compared to HIV-1 (Alabi et al., 2003; Berry et al., 1998). Subsequent discussion will focus on HIV-1 infection and pathogenesis.

HIV-1 is subclassified into three groups: M (major), O (outlier), and N (non-M, non-O) (Simon et al., 1998). The vast majority of HIV-1 infections belong to group M, which has at least nine known genetically distinct subtypes (or clades): A, B, C, D, F, G, H, J, and K. Subtype A remains the most prevalent in parts of East Africa, Russia, and the former Soviet Union; subtype B in Europe and the Americas; and subtype C in Southern Africa and India (Bbosa et al., 2019). Occasionally, genetic material from different clades of HIV-1 may recombine within the same host to form hybrid viruses, called *circulating recombinant forms* or *CRFs* (Salminen et al., 1997). Ninety inter-subtype recombinants have been shown to be recurrent among circulating HIV-1, and studies based on nearly full-length genome sequencing have highlighted the growing importance of recombinant variants and subtype C viruses (Bbosa et al., 2019). Subtype C is the most common form of HIV-1 globally, accounting for 46% of infections worldwide (Gartner et al., 2020); it became the most prevalent form by heterosexual transmission that spread from Africa to Europe (Li et al., 2024). It is unclear if subtype C leads to a faster progression to AIDS compared to other subtypes; in addition, the transmission and replication capacity of subtype C in genital and rectal lymphoid cells is under investigation to determine if those characteristics account for its high prevalence worldwide. A list of current CRFs is available at: https://www.hiv.lanl.gov/components/sequence/HIV/crfdb/crfs.comp (Song et al., 2018).

VIRAL STRUCTURE

HIV-1 is an RNA virus, and its basic genomic structure is typical of other retroviruses. The integrated form of HIV is known as the *provirus*, which is flanked at both ends by a repeated sequence known as the *long terminal repeats* (LTRs). The genes of HIV are located in the central region of the

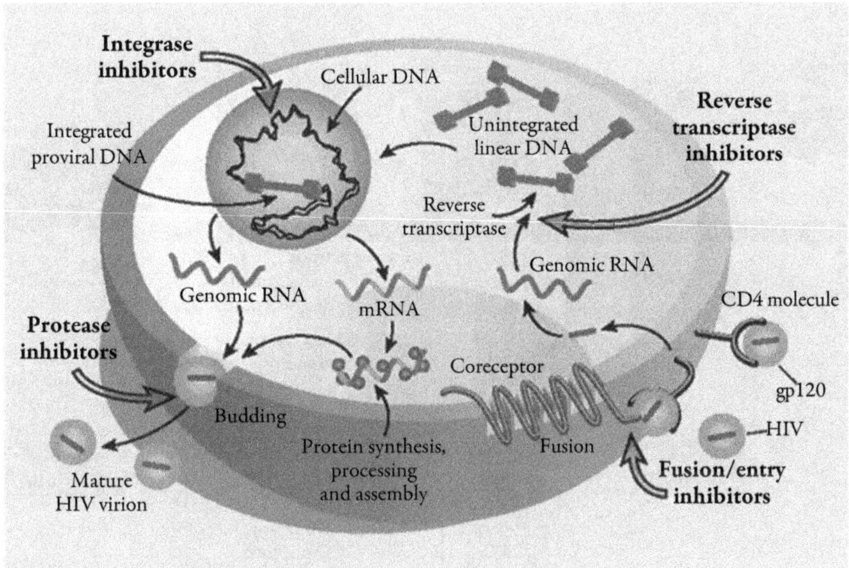

Figure 4.1 HIV life cycle and drug targets. SOURCE: Reproduced from Fauci AS. *Nat Med.* 2003;9(7):834–843, with permission from Macmillan Publishers Ltd.: *Nat Med*, copyright 2003.

proviral DNA and encode 15 distinct proteins divided into three classes: structural proteins (Gag, Pol, and Env), regulatory proteins (Tat and Rev), and accessory proteins (Vpu, Vpr, Vif, and Nef) (Klimkait et al., 1990; Willey et al., 1992). In the mature HIV-1 virion, the inner capsid contains two molecules of single-stranded RNA and key enzymes necessary for infection: reverse transcriptase, integrase, protease, and accessory proteins (Figure 4.1). Recent research has provided insight on the importance of the capsid protein in HIV-1 infection, as the capsid regulates several virus–host interactions in the HIV-1 life cycle (Rossi et al., 2021). The capsid is surrounded by structural matrix protein, itself contained within the viral envelope. Composed of a phospholipid bilayer derived from the host cell, the envelope contains trimers of the viral glycoproteins gp120 and gp41. The exposed surfaces of gp120 exhibit a high level of variability, which enables escape from neutralizing antibodies against circulating virus circulating virus (Tilton and Doms, 2010).

VIRAL ENTRY

The viral envelope contains the necessary proteins for cell fusion and viral entry, initiating infection of the host cell. HIV gains access to its target cells via multiple interactions of viral proteins with receptors on the cell membrane (Figure 4.2). The viral glycoprotein gp120 binds with high affinity to the CD4 receptor, which normally functions as a coreceptor in the activation of helper T cells. CD4 binding induces a conformational change in gp120, exposing its binding sites for coreceptors (either CCR5 or CXCR4) on the host cell surface. Binding of gp120 to the coreceptor exposes the fusion domain of the viral glycoprotein gp41. Then, glycoprotein gp41 inserts its hydrophobic peptide into the target cell membrane, forming a pore through which the viral capsid enters (Tavasolli, 2011). This process is known as *fusion*. Gp41 is a target of drugs that bind to this glycoprotein and prevent formation of the fusion pore. In addition to CD4 T cells, macrophages have become increasingly recognized as a target of HIV-1 infection, playing a role not only in pathogenesis, but also in persistence of infection (Han et al., 2021).

Viral strains vary in their coreceptor usage. Those that bind the chemokine receptors CCR5 or CXCR4 are classified as R5-tropic or X4-tropic, respectively, and some viral strains can use both CCR5 and CXCR4. During HIV transmission and early infection, R5-tropic strains predominate. Individuals who do not express CCR5, by virtue of genetic mutation, are highly resistant to HIV infection by R5-tropic viruses (Reiche et al., 2007). Mutant alleles in the CCR5 gene have also been shown to prevent HIV infection by creating a nonfunctional coreceptor for HIV entry (Liu et al., 1996; Samson et al., 1996).

Drugs that target CCR5 and bind to the coreceptor alter its interaction with gp120. However, these drugs can only be used in persons with HIV (PWH) whose virus has been determined to be R5-tropic. Through evolution within the host, some HIV strains become X4-tropic, rendering them resistant to these agents. There have been a small number of PWH reported to achieve sustained HIV remission (cure) following stem cell transplantation with allogeneic, homozygous CCR5-Δ32 mutated donor cells, and efforts to modify CCR5 receptors to maintain HIV-1 remission in the absence of antiretroviral therapy (ART) are ongoing (Gupta et al., 2019). Downregulation of the CCR5 gene through genetic modification (gene therapy) of $CD4^{+}$ T cells and hematopoietic stem/progenitor cells and autologous transplantation of these cells was proposed over a decade ago as a mechanism for curing HIV without needing to find a donor with the homozygous CCR5-Δ32 mutated donor cells (Deeks et al., 2012, Mitsuyasu et al., 2020).

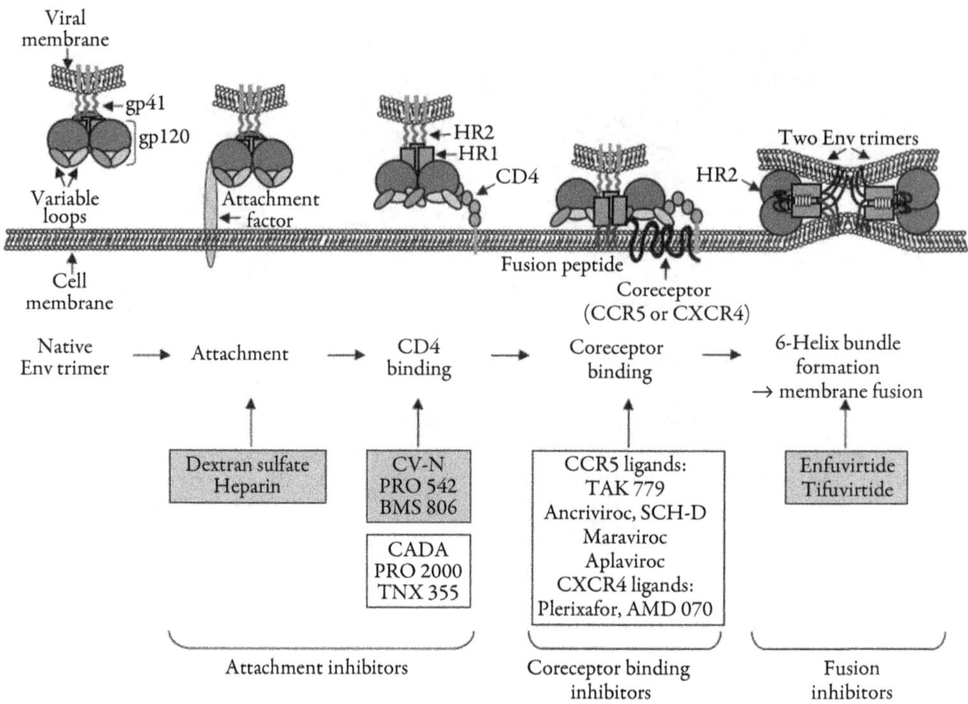

Figure 4.2 HIV entry into cells and drug targets. SOURCE: Reeves J, et al. *Drugs*. 2005;65(13):1747–1766 with permission from Springer Nature.

REVERSE TRANSCRIPTION AND INTEGRATION

After fusion, viral disassembly (which is distinct from and not merely the reverse of viral assembly) occurs before reverse transcription can take place. For HIV-1 to fully establish infection in a susceptible cell, the RNA must undergo reverse transcription into double-stranded DNA and integrate into the host genome (Tekeste et al., 2015). Reverse transcription starts when viral RNA is released into the host cell cytoplasm, shedding associated proteins in a process known as *uncoating*. Recent data show that for the uncoating process to complete and occur efficiently, reverse transcription is required (Burdick et al., 2024). In addition, the long, double-stranded reverse transcription products of the viral enzyme reverse transcriptase (RT) triggers efficient uncoating. RT is a heterodimer composed of a larger, functional subunit (p66) and a smaller, structural subunit (p51). After double-stranded DNA is produced from the viral RNA template (via RT), the host's natural antiviral immunity is activated, and the enzyme APOBEC3G, found in $CD4^+$ T cells and macrophages, terminates the elongating viral DNA by causing hypermutations. However, the HIV protein Vif, which binds APOBEC3G and leads to its degradation, overrides the host's natural immunity, allowing propagation of viral DNA (Table 4.1) (Tavasolli, 2011).

Newly synthesized viral DNA then integrates into the host DNA. Integration is an essential step in sustained propagation of the virus and its progeny; integrase-negative HIV mutants do not integrate and therefore do not produce infectious virions (Wiskerchen and Muesing, 1995). Integration is catalyzed by integrase (IN), in conjunction with the nuclear localization factor Vpr, to form the pre-integration complex. Once in the nucleus, a critical interaction between IN and the host protein LEDGF/p75 directs this complex to the host DNA (Tavasolli, 2011), and IN mediates strand transfer, linking viral and host DNA through covalent bonds. Co-opting host cell proteins, HIV relies on the cell's normal DNA repair mechanism to complete integration.

Integrase strand transfer inhibitors work by blocking the penultimate step of integration by preventing strand transfer to the host DNA. Also, it has been demonstrated in vitro that the RT-IN interaction is biologically significant for reverse transcription (Tekeste et al., 2015), and some IN resistance mutations contribute to loss of viral fitness (Ratouit et al., 2024). Therefore, the interaction between these two enzymes

Table 4.1 **VIRAL ACCESSORY AND REGULATORY PROTEIN FUNCTIONS**

GENE	FUNCTION
Tat	Transcriptional transactivator
Rev	Allows unspliced viral genomes to leave the nucleus
Nef	Downregulates CD4 receptor and major histocompatibility complex class I, alters T-cell activation, aids viral infectivity
Vif	Counters the host restriction factor APOBEC3G
Vpr	Facilitates the nuclear localization of the viral genome
Vpr	Downregulates CD4 receptor, increases viral release

Source: Adapted from Miller et al. *Trends Microbiol.* 1994 Aug;2(8):294–298.

has been a target for development of safe and effective two-drug combination therapies (Llibre et al., 2018).

Reeves JD, Piefer AJ. Emerging drug targets for antiretroviral therapy. *Drugs*. 2005;65(13):1747–1766.

VIRUS PRODUCTION

Once integrated into the host DNA, the viral genome can remain latent or undergo active expression. Active expression is dependent on cellular and viral factors that activate viral promotors, including coinfection with other agents, production of inflammatory cytokines, and cellular activation (Honda et al., 1998). In active infection, viral DNA is first transcribed into mRNA. Some of the early mRNA produced are 2-kb in size and serve as viral regulatory proteins. These mRNAs can be detected by Southern blot analysis (Kim et al., 1989) or polymerase chain reaction within 6 hours of infection (Klotman et al., 1991). Many of the same transcription factors involved in $CD4^+$ T-cell activation also bind to the HIV LTR, promoting expression of the viral genome (Pereira et al., 2000). The resulting mRNA is spliced, processed, and ultimately translated into viral proteins by host cell machinery. In a positive feedback loop, the viral protein Tat (transactivator) promotes further viral transcription by facilitating the elongation of nascent viral transcripts (Kao et al., 1987).

The viral protein gag mediates assembly of progeny virions by packaging genomic RNA within virus particles. Finally, HIV protease catalyzes the cleavage of the gag-pol precursor polyprotein (p55), yielding structural proteins that form the mature virion. HIV protease's activity is modulated by reverse transcriptase, so mutations in reverse transcriptase can affect protease activation (Hsieh et al., 2023). Assembly of mature virus occurs at the cell membrane, and these virus particles exit the cell in a process known as *viral budding*. Budding occurs in areas called *lipid rafts*, located in the cell membrane, composed of high concentrations of cholesterol, sphingolipids, and glycolipids (Liao et al., 2001). HIV-1 generation time in vivo is 2 days, and the half-life of infected $CD4^+$ T cells is 0.7 days (Markowitz et al., 2003). The ubiquitin proteasome system (UPS), which is a major protein degradation mechanism for eukaryotic cellular processes, may also play a critical role in regulation of proteasomal degradation of viral and cellular counterparts during the HIV-1 life cycle, ultimately resulting in a contest for the host or virus survival. However, the coordination and significance of viral protein degradation at different stages of the life cycle remain elusive, warranting further investigation (Rojas and Park, 2019).

RECOMMENDED READING

Fauci AS. HIV and AIDS: 20 years of science. *Nat Med*. 2003;9(7): 834–843.

Moore JP, Kitchen SG, Pugach P, et al. The CCR5 and CXCR4 coreceptors: central to understanding the transmission and pathogenesis of human immunodeficiency virus type 1 infection. *AIDS Res Hum Retroviruses*. 2004;20(1):111–126.

HIV NATURAL HISTORY

LEARNING OBJECTIVE

Discuss the course of HIV infection and its dynamics in the host over time.

WHAT'S NEW?

The natural history of acute infection, viral kinetics and latency, and viral diversity of HIV represent a highly complex and unique interplay of factors and processes; increased understanding of these mechanisms has guided the ongoing development of preventive interventions such as pre- and postexposure prophylaxis, as well as vaccine development.

KEY POINTS

- In mucosal transmission, HIV crosses the epithelial barrier and establishes an expanding infection at the site of entry.
- During acute infection, HIV disseminates to lymphatic tissue throughout the body.
- The rate of fall in plasma viremia with ART reflects the kinetics of different types of infected host cells.
- HIV exhibits remarkable levels of diversity, both globally and within a single host.
- HIV establishes latent infection in a subset of host cells, allowing it to persist despite ART.

ESTABLISHMENT OF INFECTION

In sexual transmission, HIV must first breach the epithelial barrier of the genital or rectal mucosa. This may occur via physical breaks in the epithelium related to trauma or sexually transmitted infections, particularly herpes simplex virus. However, HIV can also cross intact mucosa via specialized dendritic cells in the genital tract or transcytosis in the gastrointestinal (GI) tract (Morrow et al., 2008). Upon crossing the epithelial barrier, the virus encounters multiple potential target cells. The major cellular receptor for fusion and entry of HIV is $CD4^+$ T cells, whose critical role in HIV infection was identified in 1984 (Dalgleish et al., 1984; Klatzmann et al., 1984). Initial infection is propagated by dendritic cells (especially Langerhans cells), components of the innate immune system that deliver HIV to $CD4^+$ T cells; alternatively, the virus may directly infect local $CD4^+$ T cells without the aid of dendritic cells. The initial proliferation of HIV represents a genetic bottleneck in which a large viral inoculum gives rise to a small founder population of infected cells. In heterosexual transmission, infection results from a single viral genotype in 80% of cases, with a preference for the CCR5 coreceptor (Haase, 2010).

The *eclipse phase* refers to the period after mucosal exposure, when the virus remains undetectable in plasma, and lasts approximately 10 days. Once a founder viral population is established at the portal of entry, it must expand locally by rapid migration to regional lymph nodes and dissemination to distant draining lymph nodes via the bloodstream. In a chain reaction of cell-to-cell signaling, termed the *virologic synapse* (Piguet and Steinman, 2007), dendritic and Langerhans cell-type T cells' exposure to HIV induces the recruitment of more plasmacytoid dendritic cells, and ultimately, more $CD4^+$ T cells (Haase, 2010). Therefore, in addition to the role that lymphoid tissue (in particular, dendritic cells) plays in the initial establishment of HIV infection, it is also responsible for the dissemination of HIV infection. These early events may be altered to prevent infection, and they figure prominently in research on microbicides, pre-exposure prophylaxis (PrEP) and postexposure prophylaxis (PEP), and preventive vaccines.

ACUTE INFECTION

Once infection is established in draining lymph nodes, activated $CD4^+$ T lymphocytes become the predominant source of viral replication. Immune activation increases the pool of susceptible activated $CD4^+$ T cells, creating a positive feedback loop. An exponential increase in plasma viremia ensues, and PWH may develop symptoms of acute retroviral syndrome. HIV disseminates and then infects other lymphatic tissues throughout the body. The $CD4^+$ T-cell count in peripheral blood declines markedly, and this is thought to occur through several mechanisms: increased destruction of cells by direct infection by HIV infection, activation of apoptosis, increased lymphocyte turnover, decreased production by reduced thymic output, and redistribution of cells from peripheral blood to lymphoid tissue. A profound depletion of $CD4^+$ T cells also occurs in the gut-associated lymphatic tissue (GALT), causing permanent damage to the gastrointestinal tract. Natural killer (NK) cells also play an important role during acute infection: HIV-1 triggers activation of these cells, which in turn kill infected CD4+ T cells and secrete inflammatory cytokines in an attempt to limit HIV-1 infection (Joshi and Atfield, 2024).

The events in acute infection have long-term consequences for PWH. Activation of $CD4^+$ T cells and HIV RNA replication causes fibrosis to occur in the lymphoid architecture, leading to incomplete immune reconstitution even after initiation of ART (Brenchley et al., 2004). Damage to the GI epithelium and mucosal immune response allows an increase in microbial translocation (Haase, 2010), although changes in the gut microbiome composition differ between men who have sex with men and people who are heterosexual (Noguera-Julain et al., 2016). Over time, microbial translocation also contributes to chronic immune activation and progression to AIDS, which may be mitigated by early initiation of ART (Planchais et al., 2023). Finally, a reservoir of latently infected cells is established which later prevents viral eradication, even with ART use. Important reservoir sites include the GALT, peripheral lymphoid tissues, adipose tissue, and brain microglia. In the rare cases in which HIV is diagnosed during primary (acute) infection, immediate ART may have the potential to attenuate, although not reverse, these changes.

The establishment of the HIV reservoir and viral latency is widely discussed as the barrier to curing HIV (Castro-Gonzalez et al., 2018). Current therapies do not completely eliminate the reservoir after it has been established, since infected cells harbor replication-competent proviruses that are transcriptionally inactive, thus not utilizing the replication enzymes, which are targets for ART. A more detailed discussion of this topic is included in Chapter 18, "The HIV Reservoir and Cure and Remission Strategies."

VIRAL KINETICS AND LATENCY

Plasma HIV RNA levels reflect a dynamic interplay between the infection of susceptible cells and the destruction of infected cells. With the initiation of ART, susceptible host cells are protected from infection. Consequently, the rate of viral load decline following initiation of ART reflects the kinetics of the death of HIV-infected cells (Figure 4.3) (Palmer et al., 2011).

Viral decay occurs in four distinct phases. The viral load declines dramatically in the first phase of 7–10 days, reflecting the clearance of activated $CD4^+$ T cells ($t_{½}$ = 1 or 2 days), with roughly 90% of the decrease in plasma HIV occurring in these first weeks of therapy (Markowitz et al., 2003). The second phase, characterized by a more gradual decline in viral load and an average viral half-life of 14 days (Andrade et al., 2013), correlates with the intermediate half-lives of partially activated $CD4^+$ T cells, macrophages, and possibly dendritic cells. In the third phase, plasma HIV continues to decline, although at levels detectable only by ultrasensitive assays. This phase may represent the decay of latently infected resting $CD4^+$ T cells that are producing HIV, but HIV RNA levels are unobserved since they have fallen below the limit of detection used by most clinical assays (Andrade et al., 2013). It is thought that during this phase, a first reservoir is maintained since there is suboptimal diffusion of ART into lymphoid tissues, allowing the virus to replicate at low levels. However, whether this phenomenon occurs in the majority of individuals on ART is controversial (Dufour et al., 2020). The fourth phase occurs 4–5 years after ART initiation and finally stabilizes at very low levels (<1–5 copies/mL) (Siliciano et al., 2003). Research has focused on the resting memory $CD4^+$ T cell as the source of viral replication during these latter stages. In addition, monocytes, derivative macrophages or dendritic cells, stem cell–like memory T cells, and T follicular helper cells have been shown to play a role in latency establishment (Fukazawa et al., 2015; Garcia et al., 2017; Ta and Anderson, 2022). Despite fully suppressive ART, the proportion of resting $CD4^+$ T cells that are latently infected shows minimal decline over time, yielding an estimated half-life of 44 months (Siliciano et al., 2003). By this estimate, HIV eradication would require more than 70 years of uninterrupted ART.

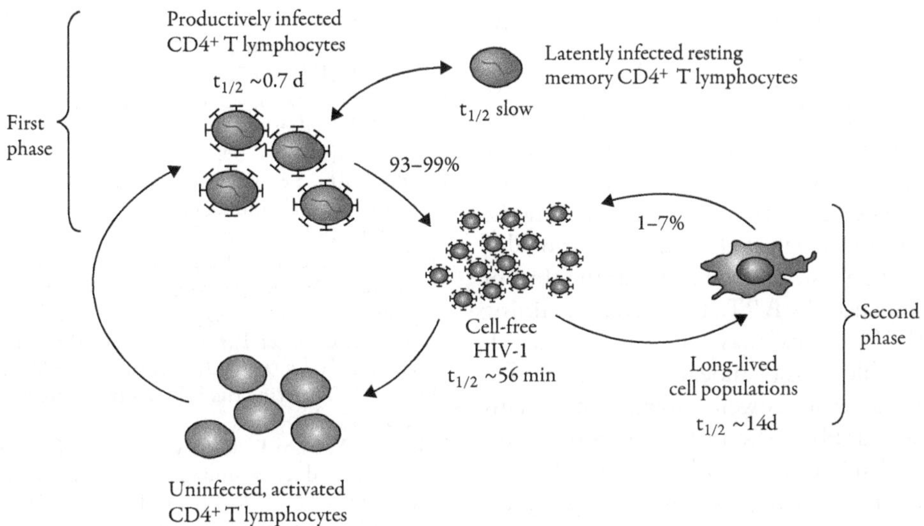

Figure 4.3 Rates of clearance of different cell populations and viral turnover. SOURCE: Simon V, et al. *Nat Rev Microbiol.* 2003;1(3):181–190.

Since HIV latency is the chief obstacle to eradicating HIV, increasing attention has turned to the mechanisms that maintain latent infection. In latent infection, proviral DNA is integrated into the host genome but remains in a transcriptionally silent yet inducible state. Latently infected cells serve as a reservoir for the virus that can reactivate and drive HIV viral loads to pretreatment levels if ART is interrupted (Rouzine et al., 2015). In rhesus macaque models, simian immunodeficiency virus (SIV) established latency in reservoir cells occurs as early as 3 days after infection, before viremia is detected (Whitney et al., 2014). An observational study of two individuals on PrEP who started prophylactic ART an estimated 10 days after infection showed that after ART interruption, HIV viremia recurred despite initiation of ART at one of the earliest stages of acute infection. Therefore, the establishment of the reservoir occurs extremely early after infection (Henrich et al., 2017). Different biological processes, such as host transcription factors, histone deacetylase-mediated epigenetic silencing, and cytokines, have been shown to play a role in HIV latency. The host transcription factors (NF-κB, NFAT, and P-TEFβ) and the viral protein Tat promote the expression of proviral DNA, but they are present at low levels in resting $CD4^+$ T cells, thus maintaining latency. Histone deacetylation and DNA methylation at the HIV LTR alter the local chromatin environment, denying access to the machinery of transcription (Palmer et al., 2011). The establishment of the reservoir is also facilitated by cell-to-cell transmission of HIV rather than cell-free transmission, which is more efficient and does not expose virus particles to the challenges of surviving in the extracellular environment (Pedro et al., 2019).

Unfortunately, initiation of ART early after infection, following the *eclipse phase,* does not preclude the establishment of chronic infection (Henrich et al., 2017). Therapies that promote expression of the proviral genome or activate resting $CD4^+$ T cells have the potential to speed the decay of the latent reservoir. Two animal studies demonstrated robust and persistent latency reversal in mice and SIV models in multiple tissues and peripheral blood by activating the noncanonical NF-κB pathway (Nixon et al., 2020) and by interleukin-15 stimulation combined with $CD8^+$ T-cells depletion (McBrien et al., 2020). NK cells are also being targeted to mitigate the reservoir, given their role in acute infection (Joshi and Atfield, 2024). Further investigations on latency reversal agents are reviewed in more detail in Chapter 18, "The HIV Reservoir and Cure and Remission Strategies."

VIRAL DIVERSITY

During untreated infection, HIV replicates at an extraordinary rate, with roughly 10 billion new virions produced each day. Reverse transcriptase, in contrast to DNA polymerases, lacks proofreading activity (Taylor et al., 2008). As a result, frequent mutations occur in the daughter viral genome, potentially altering the structure and function of viral proteins. HIV recombination is another means of viral diversity and occurs when one person is coinfected with two strains of the virus which replicate within the cell (Taylor et al., 2008). The rapid rate of production, combined with frequent mutations and recombination, leads to the production of diverse quasi-species. Strikingly, the genetic diversity observed in a single individual after six years of HIV infection is roughly equivalent to that observed worldwide in influenza A virus within a given year (Korber et al., 2001). However, the genetic diversity that occurs in acute infection occurs at a much higher rate than in chronic infection. The high number of replication cycles also allows for selection of ARV-resistant variants, with emergence of HIV drug-resistance mutations governed by selection forces and drift (Maldarelli et al., 2013).

Viral diversity presents a unique challenge for producing an HIV vaccine. Historically, vaccines have prevented infection by stimulating antibody or cell-mediated immunity. Both HIV and SIV have been shown to escape from these host immune responses by virtue of their extreme diversity. Broadly neutralizing antibodies (bNAbs) are under investigation for vaccine development. The HIV-1 fusion peptide is a promising vaccine target, but diversity among circulating strains has limited antibodies targeting the peptide to ~60% efficacy (Banach et al., 2023; Du Toit, 2024). An effective HIV vaccine may need to elicit broad immune responses that protect against multiple quasi-species and possibly other HIV subtypes. This could be achieved by developing a vaccine that accommodates fusion peptide diversity while recognizing the HIV-1 envelope backbone (Banach et al., 2023). Additionally, studies suggest that viral diversity is established at the time of infection and is not influenced by ART. Therefore, examining the diversity of the HIV "provirus" may help identify individuals with bNAb-susceptible virus (VanderVeen et al., 2024).

The impact of viral diversity is well known to clinicians engaged in the treatment of HIV. The administration of multiple agents, initially called "drug cocktails," but now known as *combination antiretroviral therapy*, is required to suppress viral replication to levels at which antiretroviral (ARV) drug-resistant strains are unlikely to emerge (i.e., viral diversity underpins the importance of strict adherence to HIV therapy). Similarly, the continuous evolution of HIV has required routine utilization of HIV drug-resistance testing in clinical practice and the continued development of antiretrovirals with novel therapeutic mechanisms.

RECOMMENDED READING

Finzi D, Blankson J, Siliciano JD, et al. Latent infection of CD4+ T cells provides a mechanism for lifelong persistence of HIV-1, even in patients on effective combination therapy. *Nat Med.* 1999;5(5):512–517.

Harris RS, Liddament MT. Retroviral restriction by APOBEC proteins. *Nat Rev Immunol.* 2004;4(11):868–877.

Mehandru S, Tenner-Racz K, Racz P, et al. The gastrointestinal tract is critical to the pathogenesis of acute HIV infection. *J Allergy Clin Immunol.* 2005;116(2):419–422.

Persaud D, Zhou Y, Siliciano JM, et al. Latency in human immunodeficiency virus type 1 infection: no easy answers. *J Virol.* 2003;77(3):1659–1665.

Simon V, Ho DD. HIV-1 dynamics in vivo: implications for therapy. *Nat Rev Microbiol.* 2003;1(3):181–190.

REFERENCES

Alabi AS, Jaffar S, Ariyoshi K, et al. Plasma viral load, CD4 cell percentage, HLA and survival of HIV-1, HIV-2, and dually infected Gambian patients. *AIDS.* 2003;17(10):1513–1520.

Andrade A, Rosenkranz S, Cillo A, et al. Three distinct phases of HIV-1 RNA decay in treatment-naïve patients receiving raltegravir-based antiretroviral therapy: ACTG A5248. *J Inf Dis.* 2013;208(6): 884–891.

Banach B, Pletnev S, Olia A, et al. Antibody-directed evolution reveals a mechanism for enhanced neutralization at the HIV-fusion peptide site. *Nat Commun.* 2023; 14:7593.

Bbosa N, Kaleebu P, Sswemwanga D. HIV subtype diversity worldwide. *HIV and AIDS.* 2019;14(3):153–160.

Berry N, Ariyoshi K, Jaffar S, et al. Low peripheral blood viral HIV-2 RNA in individuals with high CD4 percentage differentiates HIV-2 from HIV-1 infection. *J Hum Virol.* 1998;1(7):457–468.

Brenchley JM, Schacker TW, Ruff LE, et al. CD4+ T cell depletion during all stages of HIV disease occurs predominantly in the gastrointestinal tract. *J Exp Med.* 2004;200(6):749–759.

Burdick R, Morse M, Rouzina I, et al. HIV-1 uncoating requires long double-stranded reverse transcription products. *Sci Adv.* 2024;10(17):eadn7033.

Castro-Gonzalez S, Colomer-Lluch M, Serra-Moreno R. Barriers for HIV cure: the latent reservoir. *AIDS Res Hum Retroviruses.* 2018;34(9):739–759.

Dalgleish AG, Beverly PC, Clapham PR, et al. The CD4(T4) antigen is an essential component of the receptor for the AIDS retrovirus. *Nature.* 1984;312:763–767.

Deeks SG, Autran B, Berkhout B, et al.; International AIDS Society Scientific Working Group on HIV Cure. Towards an HIV cure: a global scientific strategy. *Nat Rev Immunol.* 2012;12:607–614.

Dufour C, Gantner P, Fromentin R. The multifaceted nature of HIV latency. *J Clin Invest.* 2020;130(7): e136227.

DuTroit A. Targeting the HIV-1 Env fusion protein. *Nat Rev Microbiol.* 2024;22:120.

Fukazawa Y, Lum R, Okkoye A. B cell follicle sanctuary permits persistent productive simian immunodeficiency virus infection in elite controllers. *Nat Med.* 2015;21(2):132–139.

Garcia M, Gorgolas M, Cabello A, et al. Peripheral T follicular cells make a difference in HIV reservoir size between elite controllers and patients on successful cART. *Sci Rep.* 2017;7.16799.

Gartner M, Roche M, Churchill M, et al. Understanding the mechanisms driving the spread of subtype C HIV-1. *Lancet.* 2020;53:102682.

Gupta RK, Abdul-Jawad S, McCoy LE, et al. HIV-1 remission following CCR5Δ32/Δ32 haematopoietic stem-cell transplantation. *Nature.* 2019;568(7751):244–248.

Haase A. Targeting early infection to prevent HIV-1 mucosal transmission. *Nature.* 2010;464:217–223.

Han M, Cantaloube-Ferrieu V, Xie M, et al. HIV-1 cell-to-cell spread overcomes the virus entry block of non-macrophage-tropic strains in macrophages. *Lancet HIV.* 2021;8(6):e324–e333.

Henrich T, Hatano H, Bacon O. HIV-1 persistence following extremely early initiation of antiretroviral therapy (ART) during acute HIV-1 infection: an observational study. *PLoS Med.* 2017;14(11):e1002417.

Honda Y, Rogers L, Nakata K, et al. Type I interferon induces inhibitory 16-kD CCAAT/enhancer binding protein (C/EBP) beta, repressing the HIV-1 long terminal repeat in macrophages: pulmonary tuberculosis alters C/EBP expression, enhancing HIV-1 replication. *J Exp Med.* 1998;188:1255–1265.

Hsieh S-H, Yu F-H, Huang K-J. HIV-1 reverse transcriptase stability correlates with Gag cleavage efficiency: reverse transcriptase interaction implications for modulating protease activation. *J Virol.* 2023;97(9): e0094823.

Joshi V, Altfield M. Harnessing natural killer cells to target HIV-1 persistence. *Curr Opin HIV AIDS.* 2024;19(3):141–149.

Kao SY, Calman AF, Luciw PA, et al. Anti-termination of transcription within the long terminal repeat of HIV-1 by tat gene product. *Nature.* 1987;330(6147):489–493.

Kim SY, Byrn R, Groopman J, et al. Temporal aspects of DNA and RNA synthesis during human immunodeficiency virus infection: evidence for differential gene expression. *J Virol.* 1989;63:3708–3713.

Klatzmann D, Champagne E, Chamaret S, et al. T-lymphocyte T4 molecule behaves as receptor for human retrovirus LAV. *Nature.* 1984;312:767–768.

Klimkait T, Strebel K, Hoggan MD, et al. The human immunodeficiency virus type 1-specific protein Vpu is required for efficient virus maturation and release. *J Virol.* 1990;64(2):621–629.

Klotman ME, Kim S, Buchbinder A, et al. Kinetics of expression of multiply spliced RNA in early human immunodeficiency virus type 1 infection of lymphocytes and monocytes. *Proc Natl Acad Sci U S A.* 1991;88:5011–5015.

Korber B, Gaschen B, Yusim K, et al. Evolutionary and immunological implications of contemporary HIV-1 variation. *Br Med Bull.* 2001;58:19–42.

Li X, Tamim S, Trovao N. The emergence and circulation of human immunodeficiency virus (HIV)-1 subtype C. *J Med Microbiol.* 2024;73(5):1–9.

Liao Z, Cimakasky LM, Hampton R, et al. Lipid rafts and HIV pathogenesis: host membrane cholesterol is required for infection by HIV type 1. *AIDS Res Hum Retroviruses*. 2001;17:1009–1019.

Liu R, Paxton W, Choe S, et al. Homozygous defect in HIV-1 coreceptor accounts for resistance of some multiply-exposed individuals to HIV-1 infection. *Cell*. 1996;86:367–377.

Llibre J, Chien-Ching H, Brinson C, et al. Efficacy, safety, and tolerability of dolutegravir-rilpivirine for the maintenance of virological suppression in adults with HIV-1: phase 3, randomised, non-inferiority SWORD-1 and SWORD-2 studies. *Lancet*. 2018;391(10123):839–849.

Maldarelli F, Kearney M, Palmer S, et al. HIV populations are large and accumulate high genetic diversity in a nonlinear fashion. *J Virol*. 2013;87(18):10313–10323.

Markowitz M, Louie M, Hurley A, et al. A novel antiviral intervention results in more accurate assessment of human immunodeficiency virus type 1 replication dynamics and T-cell decay in vivo. *J Virol*. 2003;77:5037–5038.

McBrien JB, Mavigner M, Franchitti L, et al. Robust and persistent reactivation of SIV and HIV by N-803 and depletion of CD8+ cells. *Nature*. 2020;578(7793):154–159.

Mitsuyasu R, Lalezari J, Burke B, et al. Phase I study of gene-modified CD4+ cells and CD34+ cells with or without busulfan in HIV+ adults. [CROI abstract 338]. In: Special issue: abstracts from the 2020 Conference on Retroviruses and Opportunistic Infections. *Top Antivir Med*. 2020;28(1):117.

Morrow G, Vachot L, Vagenas P, et al. Current concepts of HIV transmission. *Curr Infect Dis Rep*. 2008 May;10(2):133–139.

Noguera-Julian M, Rocafort M, Guillen Y, et al. Gut microbiota linked to sexual preference and HIV infection. *EbioMedicine*. 2016;28(5):135–146.

Nixon CC, Mavigner M, Sampey GC, et al. Systemic HIV and SIV latency reversal via non-canonical NF-κB signaling in vivo. *Nature*. 2020;578(7793):160–165.

Palmer S, Josefsson L, Coffin JM. HIV reservoirs and the possibility of a cure for HIV infection. *J Intern Med*. 2011;270(6):550–560. doi:10.1111/j.1365-2796.2011.02457.x

Pedro K, Henderson A, Agosto L. Mechanisms of HIV-1 cell-to-cell transmission and the establishment of the latent reservoir. *Virus Res*. 2019: 265;115–121.

Pereira LA, Bentley K, Peeters A, et al. A compilation of cellular transcription factor interactions with the HIV-1 LTV promoter. *Nucleic Acids Res*. 2000;28(3):663–668.

Piguet V, Steinman RM. The interaction of HIV with dendritic cells: outcomes and pathways. *Trends Immunol*. 2007;28:503–510.

Planchais C, Molinos-Albert L, Rosenbaum P, et al. HIV-1 treatment timing shapes the human intestinal memory B-cell repertoire to commensal bacteria. *Nat Commun*. 2023;14(1):6326.

Ratouit P, Malet I, Soulie C. HIV-1 resistance mutations to integrase inhibitors impair both integration and reverse transcription steps. *Int J Antimicrob Agents*. 2024;63(1):107026.

Reiche EM, Bonametti AM, Voltarelli JC, et al. Genetic polymorphisms in the chemokine and chemokine receptors: impact on clinical course and therapy of the human immunodeficiency virus type 1 infection (HIV-1). *Curr Med Chem*. 2007;14:1325–1334.

Rojas V, Park I-W. Role of the ubiquitin proteasome system (UPS) in the HIV-1 life cycle. *Int J Mol Sci*. 2019;20(12):2984.

Rossi E, Meuser E, Cunan C, et al. Structure, function and interactions of the HIV-1 capsid protein. *Life (Basel)*. 2021;11(2):100.

Rouzine I, Weinberger A, Weinberger L. An evolutionary role for HIV latency in enhancing viral transmission. *Cell*. 2015;160(5):1002–1012.

Salminen MO, Carr JK, Robertson DL, et al. Evolution and probably transmission of intersubtype recombinant human immunodeficiency virus type 1 in a Zambian couple. *J Virol*. 1997;71(4)2647–2655.

Samson M, Libert F, Doranz B, et al. Resistance to HIV-1 infection in Caucasian individuals bearing mutant alleles of the CCR-5 chemokine receptor gene. *Nature*. 1996;382:722–725.

Siliciano JD, Kaidas J, Finzi D, et al. Long-term follow-up studies confirm the stability of the latent reservoir for HIV-1 in resting CD4\+ T cells. *Nat Med*. 2003;9(6):727–728. doi:10.1038/nm880

Simon F, Mauclere P, Roques P, et al. Identification of a new human immunodeficiency virus type 1 distinct from group M and group O. *Nat Med*. 1998;4(9):1032–1037.

Song H, Giorgi E, Ganusov V, et al. Tracking HIV-1 recombination to resolve its contribution to HIV-1 evolution in natural infection. *Nat Commun*. 2018;9:1928.

Ta TM, Malik S, Anderson E, et al. Insights into persistent HIV-1 infection and functional cure: novel capabilities and strategies. *Front Microbiol*. 2022;13:862270. doi:10.3389/fmicb.2022.862270

Tavasolli A. Targeting the protein-protein interactions of the HIV lifecycle. *Chem Soc Rev*. 2011;40(3):1337–1346.

Taylor B, Sobieszczyk M, McCutchan F, et al. The challenge of HIV-1 subtype diversity. *N Engl J Med*. 2008;358(15):1590–1602.

Tekeste SS, Wilkonson TA, Weiner EM, et al. Interaction between reverse transcriptase and integrase is required for reverse transcription during HIV-1 replication. *J Virology*. 2015;89(23):12058–12069.

Tilton JC, Doms RW. Entry inhibitors in the treatment of HIV-1 infection. *Antiviral Res*. 2010;85(1):91–100. doi:10.1016/j.antiviral.2009.07.022

VanderVeen L, Selzer L, Moldt B, et al. HIV-1 envelope diversity and sensitivity to broadly neutralizing antibodies across stages of acute HIV-1 infection. *AIDS*. 2024;38(4):607–610.

Whitney JB, Hill AL, Sanisetty S, et al. Rapid seeding of the viral reservoir prior to SIV viraemia in rhesus monkeys. *Nature*. 2014;512:74–77.

Willey RL, Maldarelli F, Martin MA, et al. Human immunodeficiency virus type 1 Vpu protein regulates the formation of intracellular gp160-CD4 complexes. *J Virol*. 1992 Jan;66(1):226–234.

Wiskerchen M, Muesing MA. Human immunodeficiency virus type 1 integrase: effects of mutations on viral ability to integrate, direct viral gene expression from unintegrated viral DNA templates, and sustain viral propagation in primary cells. *J Virol*. 1995;69:376–386.

5.

IMMUNOLOGY OF HIV INFECTION

Dennis J. Hartigan-O'Connor and Christian Brander

MECHANISMS OF CD4⁺ T-CELL DECLINE

LEARNING OBJECTIVE

Describe the processes contributing to CD4⁺ T-cell decline and immune activation in untreated HIV infection.

WHAT'S NEW

Chronic inflammation in HIV disease contributes to progressive CD4⁺ T-cell loss and may originate in translocation of microbial products across a Th17 cell-deficient mucosal barrier. Sensing of intracellular pathogens, including HIV in abortively infected cells, further contributes to inflammation and CD4⁺ T-cell loss. Collagen deposition in lymph nodes contributes to T-cell loss by interfering with restorative homeostasis.

KEY POINTS

- Cytopathic infection alone is insufficient to explain CD4⁺ T-cell loss in HIV infection.
- Chronic inflammation is strongly associated with CD4⁺ T-cell loss in pathogenic lentiviral infection such as HIV, but is not seen in non-pathogenic infections.
- Abortive infection of T cells leads to their elimination.
- Translocation of microbial constituents and lymph node scarring have been recognized as likely contributors to CD4⁺ T-cell decline.

The prototypic outcomes associated with untreated HIV infection are progressive CD4⁺ T-cell decline, consequent immunodeficiency, and chronic inflammation. In untreated disease, circulating memory CD4⁺ T cells, some of which are virus infected, are both dividing and dying at an accelerated rate (Hellerstein et al., 1999). In addition, CD4⁺ T cells that reside in the gastrointestinal mucosa are important early targets of infection and are decimated early in the disease (Guadalupe et al., 2003; Heise et al., 1994; Veazey et al., 1998). Although direct cytopathic infection contributes to CD4⁺ T-cell loss, many *uninfected* CD4⁺ T cells are also dying in HIV disease; thus, other mechanisms must be invoked to fully explain CD4⁺ T-cell decline. The death of infected cells is likely due to exposure to Tat, gp120, or other toxic proteins (all of which can induce apoptosis) and/or adaptive immune clearance of HIV-infected cells (Lenardo et al., 2002). In addition, abortive infection of T cells (i.e., cells that become infected with the virus but where the virus cannot complete reverse transcription and thus is not productively infected) can lead to massive cell death in tissue. Such abortive infection drives a process known as *pyroptosis*, a form of programmed cell death triggered by danger signals within the abortively infected cell and which is believed to significantly contribute to the loss of CD4⁺ T cells (He et al., 2022; Ke et al., 2017). Pyroptosis is an intensely inflammatory form of cell death due to release of pro-inflammatory cytokines including interleukin-1β (IL-1β)—and so additionally contributes to the inflammatory processes discussed below. HIV can also impair CD4⁺ T-cell regeneration by destroying the immunologic niches required for T-cell homeostasis, by depleting essential hematopoietic progenitor cells and by inhibiting the regenerative process through production of immune mediators (Douek et al., 2003; Grossman et al., 2002).

Chronic inflammation and immune activation have been closely linked to CD4⁺ T-cell decline. For example, pathogenic lentiviral infections, such as HIV infection, and nonpathogenic infections, such as lentiviral infections of many nonhuman primates, are each associated with robust virus replication. Immune activation, however, is observed only in the pathogenic models, suggesting that this mechanism is directly responsible for CD4 decline and disease progression (Silvestri et al., 2003).

In addition, chronic inflammation and CD4+ T-cell decline may be linked in a self-perpetuating cycle involving gut tissue. CD4⁺ Th17 cells are among those cells lost from the gastrointestinal tract in early HIV and simian immunodeficiency virus (SIV) infection (Brenchley et al., 2008; Favre et al., 2009). Th17 cells are important for maintenance of the "mucosal barrier" between gut luminal contents and circulation; when these are depleted, microbial constituents and even whole microbes can migrate from the gut into circulation (a process referred to as *microbial translocation*) (Brenchley et al., 2006; Raffatellu et al., 2008). These proinflammatory microbial products, in particular lipopolysaccharides (LPS) from the outer membrane of Gram-negative bacteria, vigorously activate the immune system, resulting in activation-induced cell death and/or altered homeostasis. This cycle is initiated early in SIV infection (Hirao et al., 2014) and appears to be an important driver of disease progression, as presence of sufficient Th17 cells before infection can limit viral replication (Hartigan-O'Connor et al., 2012;

Ruiz-Riol et al., 2017). Further, the frequency of gut-homing, alpha-4 beta-7 integrin^{hi} CD4$^+$ T cells in blood was correlated with acquisition risk in a cohort of women participating in a CAPRISA-sponsored HIV prevention study in South Africa (Sivro et al., 2018). The pre-infection frequency of alpha-4 beta-7 integrin^{hi} CD4$^+$ T cells was strongly correlated with the rate of CD4$^+$ T-cell decline following HIV infection.

Another increasingly recognized self-perpetuating cycle pertains to the impact of HIV-associated inflammation on lymphoid structures. The inflammatory response generated by HIV results in upregulation of certain countervailing "regulatory" responses, including production of TGF-beta, which stimulates collagen deposition (Estes et al., 2008). Such "scarring" of the lymph nodes, which appears to be irreversible, prevents normal T-cell homeostasis and antigen presentation. The immunodeficiency that results can lead to an excess burden of a variety of microbes, including cytomegalovirus (CMV), gut microbes, and perhaps HIV itself. This microbial burden continues the cycle by causing even more inflammation and scarring (Arthos et al., 2008).

EFFECTS OF HIV ON THE WHOLE IMMUNE SYSTEM

LEARNING OBJECTIVE

Discuss the effects of HIV on immune cells other than CD4$^+$ T cells.

KEY POINTS

- HIV has broad effects on many immune cell types, including many cells that are not infected by the virus.
- HIV disrupts the entire lymphoid system through its effects on secondary lymphoid organs such as lymph nodes and regulatory populations such as T-regs and iNKT cells.

Although HIV is tropic for CD4-expressing cells, many manifestations of HIV infection result from direct or indirect effects on other immune cell types. One example is the high death rate and turnover of CD8$^+$ T cells, as well as numerical depletion of naïve CD8$^+$ T cells, even in the asymptomatic phase of infection (Roederer et al., 1995). HIV also has direct or indirect effects on antigen-presenting cells such as dendritic, B, and NK cells (Ruffin et al., 2017).

One factor that likely mediates some of the effects of HIV on the broader immune system, particularly in late disease, is the destruction of lymphoid tissue architecture. In early disease, as antigen-presenting cells are activated and initiate immune responses within lymph nodes, CD4$^+$ T cells are retained within the nodes while activated CD8$^+$ T cells migrate into circulation, a process that contributes to CD8$^+$ lymphocytosis and inversion of the CD4:CD8 ratio, which can be low in advanced HIV disease (Bishop et al., 1990; Bujdoso et al., 1989). In later disease, there is structural damage to primary and secondary lymphoid organs resulting from fibrotic scarring as well as functional inhibition due to interleukin-10 production (Estes et al., 2008; Harper et al., 2022; Samal et al., 2018). However, naïve T cells, including CD8$^+$ T cells, require access to lymph node paracortical T-cell zones for access to critical homeostatic signals and growth factors, including interleukin-7 (IL-7) (Link et al., 2007). Therefore, lymphoid tissue scarring is presumably one factor that contributes to failure to fully reconstitute CD4$^+$ and CD8$^+$ T cells despite complete virologic suppression.

HIV-1 can also infect myeloid cells including macrophages and dendritic cells, both of which can express CCR5. However, myeloid cells are relatively resistant to *productive* infection (i.e., infection that produces infectious viral progeny) with HIV, as compared to CD4$^+$ T cells (Coleman and Wu, 2009). The relative inability of SIV and HIV-2 to cause productive infection of these cells is mediated by the cellular restriction factor SAMHD1 (Hrecka et al., 2011; Laguette et al., 2011). The viral accessory protein Vpx blocks this cellular response, thus allowing infection. As HIV-1 lacks this accessory protein, it remains unclear as to how this virus might productively infect macrophages (Hrecka et al., 2011; Laguette et al., 2011; Manel et al., 2010).

Surprisingly, it is now appreciated that macrophages and memory CD4$^+$ T cells accumulate in adipose tissue during HIV infection (Damouche et al., 2017; Hsu et al., 2017; Koethe et al., 2018). Replicating virus can be recovered from these adipose tissue-resident cells, indicating that the tissue is a reservoir, though probably a minor one compared to lymphoid tissue. Antiviral effector cells, such as CD8$^+$ T cells and NK cells, are also present in large numbers in adipose tissue (Couturier et al., 2016; Couturier et al., 2015; Damouche et al., 2015; Dupin et al., 2002).

Natural killer T (NKT) cells are also rapidly and selectively depleted in HIV infection (Sandberg et al., 2002; van der Vliet et al., 2002). NKT cells may be broadly divided into those that are CD4$^+$ and those that are CD4$^-$, with the former population secreting both Th1 and Th2 cytokines and likely providing B cell help or carrying out immunoregulatory functions, while the latter produces mainly Th1 cytokines and has stronger cytolytic activity. Interestingly, it was shown that the pre-infection level of CD4$^+$ invariant NKT cells was directly correlated with the peak HIV viral load, suggesting a less effective host response in the presence of more of these immunoregulatory cells (Paquin-Proulx et al., 2021). The CD4$^+$ NKT population is depleted more rapidly in HIV infection than the CD4$^-$ population but is restored more slowly after treatment with antiretroviral therapy (ART) (Li and Xu, 2008). HIV also interferes with the activation of NKT cells by downregulating expression of CD1d (an MHC-related protein that presents glycolipid antigens to NKT cells) on antigen-presenting cells (Hage et al., 2005). This downregulation appears to be mediated mainly by the viral Nef protein (Cho et al., 2005).

There is continued interest in the effect of HIV and other agents of chronic infection on NK cells, particularly subsets with expanded functional capacity, including "memory" NK cells (Hwang et al., 2012; Lee et al., 2015; Lopez-Verges et al., 2011; Sun et al., 2009; Zhang et al.,

2013). Such cells are considered to be innate cells with adaptive features, including more robust and rapid responses to pathogen encounter (Sun et al., 2009). Limited evidence has demonstrated that HIV infection drives expansion of memory NK cells (Zhou et al., 2015). However, NK cells from SIV-infected macaques or those vaccinated with an Ad26-vectored candidate SIV/HIV vaccine can lyse targets pulsed with SIV peptides in an antigen- and NKG2-dependent fashion (Reeves et al., 2015). CMV infection, which is common in people with HIV (PWH), is thought to be the most important driver of memory NK-cell expansion (Brodin et al., 2015; Lopez-Verges et al., 2011; Zhang et al., 2013). People with HIV-CMV coinfection may therefore present unique immunologic features.

MECHANISMS OF CHRONIC INFLAMMATION IN HIV DISEASE

LEARNING OBJECTIVE

Discuss the mechanisms that contribute to chronic inflammation and T-cell activation in HIV disease.

KEY POINTS

- Innate immune responses that result in production of type I interferons are important drivers of inflammation in early infection.
- CMV and other chronic infections are important contributors to T-cell activation in coinfected individuals.
- Early depletion of CD4⁺ T cells from the gastrointestinal mucosa likely contributes to chronic, persistent immune activation.

It was first demonstrated 25 years ago that T-cell activation was associated with shorter survival in advanced HIV disease (Giorgi et al., 1999). One might imagine that chronic T-cell activation is simply the inevitable consequence of ongoing viral replication, and that more T-cell activation is indicative of more active disease. However, it is clear from studies of nonpathogenic lentiviral infections that chronic, high-level virus replication can occur without eliciting massive immune activation (Silvestri et al., 2003). In the natural hosts of SIV, rapid reduction of initial immune activation appears to protect against subsequent CD4⁺ T-cell decline and disease progression. HIV-associated inflammation is associated with a transformation of "immunometabolism" to greater dependence on aerobic glycolysis, which is partly dependent on mTORC1 activation (Sáez-Cirión and Sereti, 2021). This transformation can be imaged using positron emission tomography (PET) scanning to reveal upregulation of the glucose transporter, GLUT1, and resultant accumulation of FDG tracer in PWH ranging from the successfully ART suppressed to late presenters experiencing opportunistic infection (Brust et al., 2006; Hammoud et al., 2019).

The virion itself elicits innate immune responses via activation of toll-like receptors (TLRs) 7, 8, and 9 within antigen-presenting cells. TLR engagement results in production of type I interferons, including IFN-α. A spike of IFN-α production is observed in acute HIV and SIV infection, which doubtless shapes the ensuing adaptive immune responses (Favre et al., 2009; Stacey et al., 2009). Viral proteins such as Tat and Nef have been shown to have pro-inflammatory effects with consequences that can even affect neurogenesis and other brain functions (Decrion et al., 2005; Fan et al., 2016). After the first two weeks of infection, the induction of adaptive immunity contributes to T-cell activation, although many of these activated T cells are specific for CMV and other chronic pathogens, rather than HIV (Doisne et al., 2004; Papagno et al., 2005). Less appreciated is the fact that host genetics, in addition to controlling the adaptive immune response, may modulate the intensity of inflammation induced by these pro-inflammatory influences. Subjects in a Zimbabwean cohort having an interleukin-10 (IL-10) promoter mutation associated with lower inflammation experienced reductions in both mortality and CD4⁺ T-cell loss (Erikstrup et al., 2007). Finally, lymphopenia itself can lead to T-cell activation; for example, resting T cells spontaneously become activated and proliferate when introduced into T-cell-deficient hosts (Srinivasula et al., 2011; Surh and Sprent, 2008). Thus, the progressive loss of CD4⁺ T cells can be both a consequence and cause of immune activation (Jones et al., 2009; King et al., 2004).

In addition to these general effects of lymphocyte depletion, the field has discovered the implications of early and profound lymphocyte depletion from the gastrointestinal mucosa (Heise et al., 1994; Veazey et al., 1998). Among the lymphocytes lost in early infection are CD4⁺ Th17 cells, which have an important structural role in maintenance of the tight junctions between intestinal epithelial cells (Brenchley et al., 2008; Favre et al., 2009; Pandiyan et al., 2016). Loss of these cells contributes to a breakdown in the physical barrier separating the gut lumen from general circulation, which allows bioactive microbial products such as lipopolysaccharides (LPS) into the blood, while maintenance of sufficient Th17 cells is associated with reduced viral replication (Brenchley et al., 2006; Hartigan-O'Connor et al., 2012; Ruiz-Riol et al., 2017). Mucosal barrier breakdown and pro-inflammatory processes such as tryptophan catabolism, in turn, are associated with disturbance ("dysbiosis") of the gut-resident microbial community (Vujkovic-Cvijin et al., 2013; Vujkovic-Cvijin et al., 2020). Persistent microbial dysbiosis drives further immune dysregulation and inflammation in part via loss of peroxisomal proliferator-activated receptor-α (PPARα) signaling (Crakes et al., 2019; Guillén et al., 2019). In animal models, partial reversal of dysbiosis with *Lactobacillus plantarum* leads to recovery of the epithelium due to PPARα activation and restoration of mitochondrial structure and fatty acid β-oxidation (Crakes et al., 2019).

Occult and symptomatic opportunistic infections also contribute to chronic inflammation in HIV disease. In particular, the prevalence of CMV coinfection among PWH is at least 90% (Berry et al., 1988; Lang et al., 1989). Furthermore,

CMV infection has been associated with T-cell activation in HIV-negative people (Lenkei and Andersson, 1995). Indeed, CMV-specific T cells can account for more than 10% of the circulating memory T-cell pool in seropositive individuals, suggesting that CMV replication can have a major influence on the immune system even in healthy individuals who are not immunocompromised, as well as in the growing population of elderly PWH (Margolick et al., 2018; Sylwester et al., 2005). A pilot study tested the possibility that chronic immune activation in HIV disease could be reduced by treatment of CMV infection, randomizing 30 individuals on ART to treatment with valganciclovir or placebo (Hunt et al., 2011). A significant 20% reduction in the percentage of activated $CD8^+$ T cells was demonstrated in the valganciclovir group, suggesting that CMV infection is a significant contributor to T-cell activation in treated HIV- and CMV-coinfected individuals (Maidji et al., 2017).

IMMUNOLOGIC EFFECTS OF ANTIRETROVIRAL THERAPY AND THE ROLE OF PERSISTENT IMMUNE DYSFUNCTION DURING THERAPY ON CLINICAL OUTCOMES

LEARNING OBJECTIVE

Discuss the effect of antiretroviral therapy (ART) on immune function.

KEY POINTS

- A small but clinically important subset of PWH exhibit suboptimal CD4+ T-cell gains after treatment with ART.
- Lymphoid fibrosis, hematopoietic progenitor cell loss, and thymic dysfunction all likely contribute to failure to reinstate normal T-cell homeostasis.
- Chronic inflammation during treated disease has been associated with disease progression.

Combination antiretroviral therapy is highly effective, resulting in complete or near-complete suppression of HIV replication. Consequently, many of the factors that cause progressive immunodeficiency are reversed. Prevention of continued $CD4^+$ T-cell destruction (via both direct and indirect effects) and homeostatic regeneration result in eventual restoration of $CD4^+$ T-cell numbers in blood and tissues in the vast majority of treated PWH. The increase in peripheral $CD4^+$ T-cell counts during therapy appears biphasic (Pakker et al., 1998). A robust increase of approximately 50–100 cells/mm^3 is often observed in the first several weeks following initiation of ART. Because memory cells account for most of the increase, it has long been assumed that the redistribution of cells from tissues to the periphery accounts for this rapid increase. After this early phase, $CD4^+$ T-cell counts increase more slowly (~50 cells/mm^3/year) until they achieve a normal range (Mocroft et al., 2007). The augmented $CD4^+$ T-cell population includes naïve cells and hence is thought to reflect true immune reconstitution. Although less well studied, $CD4^+$ T-cell gains also occur in tissues during effective antiviral therapy.

Although most PWH exhibit some degree of immune reconstitution during therapy, the outcome is variable. Some persons achieving median reference $CD4^+$ T-cell counts nonetheless exhibit a CD4:CD8 ratio below median because of persisting high $CD8^+$ T-cell counts (Gras et al., 2019). A small but clinically important subset of PWH fail to achieve normal peripheral $CD4^+$ T-cell counts, even after many years of therapy. These so-called immunologic nonresponders, or immune-discordant individuals, remain at relatively high risk for cancer, heart disease, liver failure, and other non-AIDS complications, but they usually achieve sufficient restoration of immune function to prevent opportunistic infections. Older persons with HIV and people who start ART during late-stage disease often exhibit suboptimal gains in $CD4^+$ T cells. In one study, approximately 40% of PWH who delayed therapy initiation until their $CD4^+$ T-cell count was less than 200 cells/mm^3 failed to achieve a normal $CD4^+$ T-cell count even after several years of viral suppression (Kelley et al., 2009). Other factors that have been associated with blunted $CD4^+$ T-cell gains include hepatitis C virus coinfection and high levels of T-cell activation.

Given its clinical importance, there is intense interest in determining the pathogenesis of immunologic nonresponsiveness to treatment. In untreated disease, HIV-mediated destruction of hematopoietic stem cells, thymic tissue, lymphoid tissue, and central memory cells contributes to progressive $CD4^+$ T-cell loss. Expression of the immunosuppressive cytokine, IL-10, is induced by SIV infection and is not normalized by ART; indeed, during chronic infection, plasma IL-10 and transcriptomic signatures of IL-10 signaling were correlated with the cell-associated viral DNA content in lymph nodes (Harper et al., 2022). Treatment-mediated suppression of HIV replication only partially restores these factors. Persistent lymph node fibrosis, thymic dysfunction, and loss of cells with stem-like properties have all been associated with $CD4^+$ T-cell regeneration failure and suboptimal gains during therapy (McCune, 2001; Sauce et al., 2011; Schacker et al., 2002; Teixeira et al., 2001). More recently it has been shown that immunologic nonresponders accumulate $CD56^{bright}$ NK cells with cytotoxic activity against autologous, activated $CD4^+$ T cells (Giuliani et al., 2017). Those data suggest that autoreactive NK cells, possibly linked to decreased homeostatic control by a depleted T-reg compartment, contribute to suboptimal immune reconstitution.

Untreated HIV infection is associated with heightened levels of immune activation. Long-term suppression of HIV replication dramatically reduces most measures of immune activation, but this effect is often incomplete, as inflammatory markers typically remain higher in treated PWH than in age-matched uninfected adults (Neuhaus et al., 2010). Persistent inflammation during therapy is associated with excess risk of non-AIDS complications, including heart disease, cancer, liver disease, kidney disease, bone disease, and neurologic complications (Deeks, 2011; Kuller et al., 2008; Phillips et al., 2008). Persistent CMV replication may be an important cause of continued inflammation while on therapy, as higher anti-CMV IgG antibody levels are associated with increased prevalence of carotid artery lesions among women with HIV who achieve HIV suppression on ART, but not among viremic or untreated women (Gómez-Mora et al., 2017; Parrinello et al., 2012).

Persistent and possibly irreversible damage to the infrastructure that supports T-cell homeostasis may account for much of the persistent immunodeficiency and inflammation often observed during therapy. Theoretically, collagen deposition and scarring of the lymphoid system during untreated disease result in a loss of the homeostatic pathways (particularly those involving IL-7 and IL-27) that control T-cell regeneration and global T-cell homeostasis (Ruiz-Riol et al., 2017; Zeng et al., 2012). This disruption can result in persistently low $CD4^+$ T-cell counts and an inability to generate effective memory T cells in response to acute or chronic infections. HIV non-controllers generally harbor cytotoxic $CD8^+$ T cells with lower antigen sensitivity, which means that the cells are less able to kill targets displaying few HIV-derived peptides on their HLA class I molecules (Migueles et al., 2023). The origin of this defect is unproven but seems likely related to poor $CD4^+$ T-cell help and general lymphoid disorganization. Loss of lymphoid structures may additionally result in loss of immune surveillance and development of cancer, as well as a loss of key anti-inflammatory regulatory responses, and, as a result, autoimmune-related clinical syndromes. In a self-perpetuating vicious cycle that persists in absence of any HIV replication, persistent immunodeficiency results in a reduced capacity of host responses to clear pathogens. The resulting burden of these pathogens contributes to more inflammation, which in turn continues to damage the lymphoid tissues. The collective outcome is a combination of low $CD4^+$ T-cell counts and chronic inflammation. Knowledge about these pathways will hopefully lead to novel interventions aimed at preventing or reversing this immunodeficient, pro-inflammatory environment. Such potential treatment options may also help to increase immunological responses to therapeutic vaccines included in HIV cure strategies.

PATHOGENESIS OF IMMUNE RECONSTITUTION INFLAMMATORY SYNDROMES (IRIS)

LEARNING OBJECTIVE

Discuss the leading hypotheses explaining pathogenesis of IRIS syndromes, including antigen persistence and immune dysregulation.

WHAT'S NEW

Presence of a more inflammatory environment in untreated HIV disease is associated with immune reconstitution inflammatory syndrome (IRIS) after treatment initiation. Data on the role of T-regs in IRIS syndromes have been unclear.

KEY POINTS

- Immune reconstitution inflammatory syndromes are seen in most PWH initiating ART with low $CD4^+$ T-cell counts and preexisting opportunistic infections.
- Many IRIS symptoms are localized to sites of previous infection, suggesting the presence of persistent microbial antigens.
- Development of IRIS is associated with increased T-cell activation before initiation of antiretroviral treatment.

A subset of PWH who are immune restored with ART develop inflammatory conditions in the early stages of treatment initiation, known collectively as immune reconstitution inflammatory syndrome (IRIS) (Church, 2017). A large meta-analysis showed that 16% of PWH starting ART therapy developed an IRIS event (Muller et al., 2010). PWH most likely to be affected are those initiating ART with low $CD4^+$ T-cell counts and preexisting opportunistic infections (Muller et al., 2010; Price et al., 2009). The symptoms of IRIS are often localized to sites of previous infection with certain co-pathogens (Lawn et al., 2007), which led to the suggestion that IRIS is caused by adaptive immune responses to persistent co-pathogen-derived antigens (Muller et al., 2010). For example, IRIS in persons with a history of cytomegalovirus retinitis can manifest as inflammation of the posterior uveal tract of the eye (Nussenblatt and Lane, 1998). The most frequent clinical manifestation of cryptococcal IRIS, by contrast, is aseptic meningitis (Boulware et al., 2010).

The hypothesis that IRIS is caused by the host immune response to persistent antigen (in the form of intact organisms, dead organisms, or debris) has the appeal of simplicity, but there are surprisingly few data to support this idea. One study demonstrated that, among PWH with recent cryptococcal meningitis who were placed on ART, those developing cryptococcal IRIS had 4-fold higher titers of cryptococcal antigen in serum (Boulware et al., 2010). However, in a more recent study, low cryptococcal antibody levels were associated with a significantly increased risk of developing C-IRIS (Yoon et al., 2019). Guidelines based on the Cryptococcal Optimal Antiretroviral Timing (COAT) trial (Scriven et al., 2015) recommend initial antifungal treatment, followed by a minimum five-week delayed initiation of ART (Balasko and Keynan, 2019). The approach aims to decrease fungal burden and allow immune balance restoration prior to ART initiation. In cases of *Mycobacterium tuberculosis* or *Mycobacterium avium* complex-associated IRIS, PWH normally convert to skin test positivity, suggesting that at a minimum the disease is mediated by pathogen-specific T cells (French et al., 2004). In the case of CMV immune recovery uveitis, however, the presence of CMV antigens has not been demonstrated in PWH experiencing an IRIS event.

Several studies have suggested that the pre-therapy inflammatory environment predicts IRIS. For example,

Antonelli and colleagues showed that individuals who presented with an IRIS episode had a higher proportion of activated $CD4^+$ T cells before starting ART, compared with those who did not develop IRIS (Antonelli et al., 2010). These activated T cells had a Th1/Th17 skewed cytokine profile before therapy began. Furthermore, PWH with IRIS displayed higher serum IFN-γ levels near the time of their IRIS events. Another study trying to understand the importance of regulatory $CD4^+$ T cells (T-regs) in controlling immune responses to self-antigens suggested that failure to reconstitute these anti-inflammatory cells predisposes to IRIS (Seddiki et al., 2009). However, data on this hypothesis have been inconsistent (Bourgarit et al., 2006; Hartigan-O'Connor et al., 2011). Other groups have argued that poorly regulated innate immune responses may be central to IRIS. Pre-therapy and early treatment-mediated changes in various nonspecific inflammatory biomarkers (including CRP, IL-6, TNF-alpha, and D-dimers) have been associated with increased risk of IRIS and mortality during the first several months of effective ART (Barber, 2012; Boulware et al., 2011). In general, corticosteroids remain the only treatment for paradoxical IRIS whose use is supported by randomized clinical-trial data (Meintjes et al., 2010; Walker et al., 2018).

In summary, the pathogenesis of IRIS seems dependent on the presence of both lymphopenia and antigen-specific $CD4^+$ T cells. These T cells may be responding to persistent pathogen-derived antigens, to self-antigens, or to unrelated foreign antigens. In these latter cases, the opportunistic pathogen may be the trigger rather than the target of the pathogenic T-cell response. The pathogenic response goes hand in hand with marked lymphopenia, which establishes a dysregulated environment in which either the response of the antigen-specific T cells or the effect of that response on the host is exaggerated, and effective control mechanisms of exuberant immune responses have been impaired throughout the period of untreated HIV infection.

MECHANISMS AND CONSEQUENCES OF VIRUS CONTROL IN "ELITE" CONTROLLERS

LEARNING OBJECTIVE

Discuss how some individuals maintain durable control of HIV in the absence of therapy.

KEY POINTS

- HIV-specific $CD8^+$ T cells contribute to durable control of virus in HIV "elite" controllers.
- Despite the lack of readily detectable HIV RNA in plasma, "elite" controllers have higher than normal levels of immune activation, which may contribute to eventual disease progression.
- Neutralizing antibodies are more likely relevant to post-treatment control, than to elite control.

Fewer than 1% of adult PWH who are not taking ART have no readily detectable HIV RNA in plasma. These individuals are generally referred to as "elite" controllers, although other terms have been used to define this or similar groups of individuals who are able to suppress viral replication in absence of ART. The term "long-term non-progressors" refers to a partly overlapping group of PWH who maintain healthy $CD4^+$ T-cell counts despite HIV infection, as well as detectable and sometimes even elevated HIV levels in the blood (Capa et al., 2022). Given that the host mechanisms which might account for virus control in these individuals could inform vaccine and cure research, there has been long-term interest in understanding their mechanisms of viral control, as well as describing the degree to which most elite controllers exhibit any evidence of disease progression.

Researchers interested in determining the mechanisms of virus control in these individuals have assessed specific candidate host factors in controllers and non-controllers. These studies have generally been cross-sectional, making it difficult to determine if a given host response is a cause or consequence of virus control (Deeks and Walker, 2007; Mothe et al., 2009). Some efforts have been made to follow individuals closely during the pre-HIV infection period, both to capture information about the earliest events after infection and to study dynamic changes that may be important for eventual control (Ndhlovu et al., 2015). Confoundingly, there is reason to believe that the immune responses that bring about control of acute HIV infection are distinct from those that maintain long-term viral suppression once control of viremia has been achieved (Goulder and Deeks, 2008).

Although the mechanisms have not been conclusively defined, the collective data support a central role for potent HIV-specific $CD8^+$ T cells (and, to a lesser degree, $CD4^+$ T cells) in maintaining virus control. The importance of these responses is supported by the fact that most genetic predictors of virus control are found on chromosome 6 in the HLA class I region that governs the antigenic specificity of $CD8^+$ T cells (Pereyra et al., 2010). Studies in SIV-infected monkeys further support the importance of virus-specific cytotoxic T-lymphocytes (CTL) responses in virus control, although in the RhCMV-vectored vaccine setting, the responding T cells are MHC class II- and MHC-E-restricted (Hansen et al., 2013a; Hansen et al., 2013b). Similarly, the role of the Th17 cell compartment in sustaining viral replication has been highlighted in monkey and human studies (Hartigan-O'Connor et al., 2012; Ruiz-Riol et al., 2017). Other factors that have been associated with virus control include: (1) strong natural killer (NK) cell responses, including particular NK subsets (Kant et al., 2022; Martin et al., 2007; Rallon et al., 2024; Sips et al., 2012); (2) prevention of apoptosis/cell death in central memory cells (van Grevenynghe et al., 2008); (3) intrinsic intracellular restriction to HIV replication mediated by p21 and other as yet less well characterized factors (Chen et al., 2011; O'Connell et al., 2011; Saez-Cirion et al., 2011); and (4) particular signatures in the antiviral antibody (Kant et al., 2022) or T-cell responses (Romero-Martin et al., 2022). Furthermore, the application of various techniques to samples from HIV controllers and non-controllers has produced an ever-growing list of potentially disease-defining host molecules (De La Torre-Tarazona et al., 2022; Ni et al., 2024). Care must be taken not to confuse causative, functional markers of virus control with simple correlates. For instance, biomarkers such as the proliferative capacity of HIV-specific T cells or specific cytokine profiles may be the consequence of otherwise controlled/uncontrolled HIV infection, rather than its physiological cause (Côrtes et al., 2018; Zhang et al., 2018). Longitudinal studies capturing PWH within days of infection and following them in the absence of treatment may be ethically challenging but could prove highly informative in defining true causes of control in vivo. Significant efforts to establish and study such cohorts have been made in different populations and may yield further insights in the future (Lama et al., 2021; Muema et al., 2020).

At the same time, virologic parameters may also contribute to slow or absent HIV disease progression. Among them, the acquisition of a replication-deficient virus has been studied in a cluster of elite controllers, showing the presence of envelope sequences with a reduced binding affinity to the CD4 receptor (Casado et al., 2018). In addition, the integration site of the proviral DNA in the cellular genome may determine susceptibility of infected cells to antiviral CD8 T cells and influence disease course (Bone and Lichterfeld, 2024; Dragoni et al., 2023). The integration site also appears to influence the level of viral latency and ongoing viral replication, in controllers and even in PWH under ART, and thus directly contributes to a sustained inflammatory environment which in turn might cause end-organ damage including cardiovascular disease (Hatano et al., 2009; Hsue et al., 2009; Hunt et al., 2008; Mens et al., 2010). In addition, potential alterations in the gut microbiota of chronically infected individuals may contribute to controller status, even though the causality remains to be established (Bai et al., 2024).

FUTURE OF IMMUNE-BASED THERAPEUTICS IN HIV DISEASE

LEARNING OBJECTIVE

Discuss experimental approaches to treating chronic inflammation in antiretroviral-treated disease and to boosting immune-based control of HIV replication.

WHAT'S NEW

Many promising immune-based therapeutics are now being tested in advanced human clinical trials.

KEY POINTS

- Proving that HIV-associated inflammation is causally associated with disease progression will ultimately require a clinical endpoint study involving an immune-based therapy that directly affects inflammatory immune mechanisms.
- Promising approaches are now being tested in pathogenesis-oriented studies.
- Recent therapeutic vaccination and combination approaches have shown encouraging clinical signals.

Much of the effort of clinical investigators over the past two decades has focused on the development and optimization of combination ART for treating HIV. Development of several highly effective and well-tolerated regimens has now led to treatment regimens containing long-acting drugs, alleviating the need for daily dosing of ART, helping to increase adherence and reducing stigma (Nachega et al., 2023). With these developments, and since most individuals with access to ART can achieve and maintain undetectable HIV RNA levels for years, it is increasingly apparent that in order to fully restore health, other adjunctive therapies that can control or reverse infection-related comorbidities are needed. Given the consistent observation that inflammation remains elevated despite effective therapy and that the degree of inflammation predicts disease progression, there has been a consistent effort to testing existing drugs for potentially beneficial effects on inflammation in conjunction with suppressed viremia or to developing new approaches that will modify the inflammatory process (Fumaz et al., 2012; Perez-Matute et al., 2015).

Trials of immune-based therapeutics have largely yielded disappointing results. Prednisone, hydroxyurea, cyclosporine, and mycophenolate acid have been studied in numerous trials with minimal or no clinical benefit. Although there was some early promise, all these drugs proved to be either too toxic or to lack any clear efficacy; hence there is limited interest in using nonspecific drugs that globally affect activation and inflammation. The only exceptions to this rule are possibly the HMG-CoA reductase inhibitors (statins). These agents are known to have broad anti-inflammatory effects (though the mechanism for this remains controversial) and are safe and generally well tolerated. Pilot data in adult PWH suggest these drugs might reduce HIV-associated T-cell activation and hence might prove to be beneficial for reasons independent of their lipid-lowering effects (Ganesan et al., 2011). At least one meta-analysis suggests that statins confer moderate mortality benefits in PWH, although they have been consistently under-prescribed for PWH compared to their HIV-uninfected counterparts (De Socio et al., 2016; Ladapo et al., 2017; Uthman et al., 2018; van Zoest et al., 2017). A large clinical study, REPRIEVE, was started in 2015 and has shown effects of statin treatment well beyond their lipid-lowering effects (Grinspoon, 2020; Hoffmann et al., 2019; Looby et al., 2022). Due to this demonstrated potential to improve global health in PWH under suppressive ART (Mehraj et al., 2024), multiple healthcare organizations recommend that all people living with HIV aged 40 and over should take a statin to reduce their risk of heart disease, even if they do not have elevated cholesterol or a high risk of heart disease.

As noted earlier, many factors contribute to persistent immune activation during therapy, including: (1) irreversible breakdown of gut mucosa and subsequent microbial translocation; (2) excess CMV burden and/or enhanced immune responses to CMV (and perhaps other herpes viruses); (3) loss of immunoregulatory cells such as T-regulatory cells; (4) ART toxicity, including generation of pro-inflammatory lipids and development of metabolic syndrome; and (5) lymphoid fibrosis, hematopoietic stem cell dysfunction, and thymic dysfunction. Many, if not all, of these mechanisms can be addressed therapeutically. For example, a number of drugs, including rifaximin (an antibiotic that is not absorbed systemically), sevelamer (which binds LPS/endotoxin in vivo), colostrum-related products (which bind LPS/endotoxin in the gut), chloroquine (which blocks LPS-mediated TLR signaling in myeloid cells), and mesalamine (which is an aspirin-like, anti-inflammatory drug used in ulcerative colitis). have been tested as means to reduce the inflammatory consequences of microbial translocation (Byakwaga et al., 2011; Gori et al., 2011; Murray et al., 2010; Piconi et al., 2011). Interventions that aim to restore certain bacterial species to the gut microbiota are also being studied, although a complete characterization of alterations in gut microbiota and related confounders is still needed before such approaches can be effective (Noguera-Julian et al., 2016; Vujkovic-Cvijin et al., 2020). Valganciclovir-mediated reduction in CMV has been shown to reduce immune activation in HIV disease, and there is new optimism that letermovir may have an even greater effect (Acosta et al., 2020; Hunt et al., 2011). The drug pirfenidone and angiotensin-converting enzyme (ACE) inhibitors, among other drugs, are being studied in nonhuman primates and humans as a means to prevent and/or reverse fibrosis. Interleukin-7 has shown promise as a means to enhance immune function during treated disease (Levy et al., 2009). Treatment with the interleukin-15 "super-agonist" compound N-803 caused increased HIV transcription and proviral DNA initially, but eventually led to a decrease in the frequency of peripheral blood cells with an inducible HIV provirus (Miller et al., 2022). Although these studies will provide important insights into the relationship between immune activation and control, it remains unclear as to how such drugs could eventually be tested in phase III clinical trials.

Immunomodulatory therapies may also have a contribution to make in developing a regimen that could functionally cure HIV infection, permitting durable suppression of viremia in the absence of ART. There has been considerable interest in the potential of antibodies to $\alpha_4\beta_7$ integrin to block homing of lymphocytes to gut tissue and thus eliminate the substrate for viral growth in its most important anatomic site (Guzzo et al., 2017). A first-in-human clinical trial did not confirm early positive signals from SIV models; however, a more recent report demonstrated reduction in both the size and number of lymphoid aggregates in the terminal ileum (Fauci, 2018; Uzzan et al., 2018). This finding is noteworthy because lymphoid aggregates are inductive sites that can support viral replication and possibly contribute to viral reservoirs. Indeed, vedolizumab (an $\alpha_4\beta_7$-blocking monoclonal antibody) showed potential in reducing the viral reservoir in tissue, even though no trial participant achieved undetectable virus levels when ART was stopped (Jimenez-Leon et al., 2024).

Other clinical trials explored or will explore the immunomodulatory effects of interferon-alpha, TLR-7 agonist, TLR-9 agonist, or even vitamin D, some of which have shown promising results in SIV-infected NHP studies (Eckard et al., 2017; Lim et al., 2018; Martinsen et al., 2020; Perreau et al., 2017). However, studies in PWH controllers showed a mixed outcome and pointed toward an important role of microbiota composition on the effectiveness of immune modulation by TLR9 activation (Cai et al., 2024). The TLR9 agonist vesatolimod and others have also been included in combination strategies with therapeutic vaccination.

The most encouraging data were obtained in a recent trial using the HTI immunogen, delivered in a complex vaccination regimen that included DNA, ChAd, and MVA vaccine vectors. In the active arm, 40% of participants remained off ART for 6 or more months after vaccination and ART interruption, compared to only 8% in the placebo arm (Bailón et al., 2022). Subsequent study demonstrated the critical role of HTI-specific T-cell immunity in relative virus control (Mothe Pujades et al., 2023). While neither trial was able to show sustained control of virus replication to undetectable plasma virus levels, further combination strategies with this and other promising vaccine candidates are underway (NCT04357821; NCT06071767). In all of these studies, multiple confounding effects may need to be considered when assessing efficacy, including baseline microbiota composition and epigenetic host gene profiles that have been shown in earlier trials to contribute to the outcome of vaccination and subsequent levels of virus control (Borgognone et al., 2022; Oriol-Tordera et al., 2022).

REFERENCES

Acosta E, Bowlin T, Brooks J, et al. Advances in the development of therapeutics for cytomegalovirus infections. *J Infect Dis.* 2020;221:S32–S44.

Antonelli LR, Mahnke Y, Hodge JN, et al. Elevated frequencies of highly activated CD4+ T cells in HIV+ patients developing immune reconstitution inflammatory syndrome. *Blood.* 2010;116:3818–3827.

Arthos J, Cicala C, Martinelli E, et al. HIV-1 envelope protein binds to and signals through integrin alpha4beta7, the gut mucosal homing receptor for peripheral T cells. *Nat Immunol.* 2008;9:301–309.

Bai X, Sonnerborg A, Nowak P. Elite controllers microbiome: unraveling the mystery of association and causation. *Curr Opin HIV AIDS.* 2024;19(5):261–267. doi:10.1097.

Bailón L, Llano A, Cedeño S, et al. Safety, immunogenicity and effect on viral rebound of HTI vaccines in early treated HIV-1 infection: a randomized, placebo-controlled phase 1 trial. *Nat Med.* 2022;28:2611–2621.

Balasko A, Keynan Y. Shedding light on IRIS: from pathophysiology to treatment of cryptococcal meningitis and immune reconstitution inflammatory syndrome in HIV-infected individuals. *HIV Med.* 2019;20:1–10.

Barber DL, Andrrade BB, Sereti I, Sher A. Immune reconstitution inflammatory syndrome: the trouble with immunity when you had none. *Nat Rev Microbiol.* 2012;10(2):150–156.

Berry NJ, Burns DM, Wannamethee G, et al. Seroepidemiologic studies on the acquisition of antibodies to cytomegalovirus, herpes simplex virus, and human immunodeficiency virus among general hospital patients and those attending a clinic for sexually transmitted diseases. *J Med Virol.* 1988;24:385–393.

Bishop DK, Ferguson RM, Orosz CG. Differential distribution of antigen-specific helper T cells and cytotoxic T cells after antigenic

stimulation in vivo: a functional study using limiting dilution analysis. *J Immunol.* 1990;144:1153–1160.
Bone B, Lichterfeld M. "Block and lock" viral integration sites in persons with drug-free control of HIV-1 infection. *Curr Opin HIV AIDS.* 2024;19:110–115.
Borgognone A, Noguera-Julian M, Oriol B, et al. Gut microbiome signatures linked to HIV-1 reservoir size and viremia control. *Microbiome.* 2022;10:59.
Boulware DR, Hupper Hullsiek K, Puronen CE, et al. Higher levels of CRP, d-dimer, IL-6, and hyaluronic acid before initiation of antiretroviral therapy (ART) are associated with increased risk of AIDS or death. *J Infect Dis.* 2011;203(11):1637–1646.
Boulware DR, Meya DB, Bergemann TL, et al. Clinical features and serum biomarkers in HIV immune reconstitution inflammatory syndrome after cryptococcal meningitis: a prospective cohort study. *PLoS Med.* 2010;7:e1000384.
Bourgarit A, Carcelain G, Martinez V. Explosion of tuberculin-specific Th1-responses induces immune restoration syndrome in tuberculosis and HIV co-infected patients. *AIDS.* 2006;20:F1–F17.
Brenchley JM, Paiardini M, Knox KS, et al. Differential Th17 CD4 T-cell depletion in pathogenic and nonpathogenic lentiviral infections. *Blood.* 2008;112:2826–2835.
Brenchley JM, Price DA, Schacker TW, et al. Microbial translocation is a cause of systemic immune activation in chronic HIV infection. *Nat Med.* 2006;12:1365–1371.
Brodin P, Jojic V, Gao T, et al. Variation in the human immune system is largely driven by non- heritable influences. *Cell.* 2015;160:37–47.
Brust D, Polis M, Davey R, et al. Fluorodeoxyglucose imaging in healthy subjects with HIV infection: impact of disease stage and therapy on pattern of nodal activation. *AIDS.* 2006;20:495–503.
Bujdoso R, Young P, Hopkins J, et al. Non- random migration of CD4 and CD8 T cells: changes in the CD4:CD8 ratio and interleukin 2 responsiveness of efferent lymph cells following in vivo antigen challenge. *Eur J Immunol.* 1989;19:1779–1784.
Byakwaga H, Kelly M, Purcell DF, et al. Intensification of antiretroviral therapy with raltegravir or addition of hyperimmune bovine colostrum in HIV-infected patients with suboptimal CD4+ T-cell response: a randomized controlled trial. *J Infect Dis.* 2011;204:1532–1540.
Cai Y, Podlaha O, Deeks SG, et al. HIV rebound in HIV controllers is associated with a specific fecal microbiome profile. *Eur J Immunol.* 2024;e2350809.
Capa L, Ayala-Suarez R, De La Torre Tarazona HE, et al. Elite controllers long-term non progressors present improved survival and slower disease progression. *Sci Rep.* 2022;12;16356.
Casado C, Marrero-Hernández S, Márquez-Arce D, et al. Viral characteristics associated with the clinical nonprogressor phenotype are inherited by viruses from a cluster of HIV-1 elite controllers. *mBio.* 2018;9:e02338–17.
Chen H, Li C, Huang J, et al. CD4+ T cells from elite controllers resist HIV-1 infection by selective upregulation of p21. *J Clin Invest.* 2011;121:1549–1560.
Cho S, Knox KS, Kohli LM, et al. Impaired cell surface expression of human CD1d by the formation of an HIV-1 Nef/CD1d complex. *Virology.* 2005;337:242–252.
Church LWP, Chopra A, Judson MA. Paradoxical reactions and the immune reconstitution inflammatory syndrome. *Microbiol Spectr.* 2017;5(2), Article 10.1128/microbiolspec.tnmi7-0033-2016. https://doi:10.1128/microbiolspec.TNMI7-0033-2016. PMID: 28303782; PMCID: PMC11687476.
ClinicalTrials.gov. NCT04357821.
ClinicalTrials.gov. NCT06071767.
Coleman CM, Wu L. HIV interactions with monocytes and dendritic cells: viral latency and reservoirs. *Retrovirology.* 2009;6:51.
Côrtes FH, de Paula HHS, Bello G, et al. Plasmatic levels of IL-18, IP-10, and activated CD8(+) T cells are potential biomarkers to identify HIV-1 elite controllers with a true functional cure profile. *Front Immunol.* 2018;9:1576.
Couturier J, Agarwal N, Nehete PN, et al. Infectious SIV resides in adipose tissue and induces metabolic defects in chronically infected rhesus macaques. *Retrovirology.* 2016;13:30.
Couturier J, Suliburk JW, Brown JM. Human adipose tissue as a reservoir for memory CD4+ T cells and HIV. *AIDS.* 2015;29:667–674.
Crakes KR, Santos Rocha C, Grishina I. PPARα-targeted mitochondrial bioenergetics mediate repair of intestinal barriers at the host-microbe intersection during SIV infection. *Proc Natl Acad Sci USA.* 2019;116:24819–24829.
Damouche A, Lazure T, Avettand-Fenoel V, et al. Adipose tissue is a neglected viral reservoir and an inflammatory site during chronic HIV and SIV infection. *PLoS Pathog.* 2015;11:e1005153.
Damouche, A., Pourcher, G., Pourcher, V., et al. High proportion of PD-1-expressing CD4(+) T cells in adipose tissue constitutes an immunomodulatory microenvironment that may support HIV persistence. *Eur J Immunol.* 2017;47:2113–2123.
Decrion AZ, Dichamp I, Varin A, Herbein G. HIV and inflammation. *Curr HIV Res.* 2005;3:243–259.
Deeks SG. HIV infection, inflammation, immunosenescence, and aging. *Annu Rev Med.* 2011;62:141–155.
Deeks SG, Walker BD. Human immunodeficiency virus controllers: mechanisms of durable virus control in the absence of antiretroviral therapy. *Immunity.* 2007;27(3):406–416.
De La Torre-Tarazona E, Ayala-Suarez R, Diez-Fuertes F, Alcami J. Omic technologies in HIV: searching transcriptional signatures involved in long-term non-progressor and HIV controller phenotypes. *Front Immunol.* 2022;1:13:926499.
De Socio GV, Ricci E, Parruti G. Statins and aspirin use in HIV-infected people: gap between European AIDS Clinical Society guidelines and clinical practice: the results from HIV-HY study. *Infection.* 2016;44:589–597.
Dragoni F, Kwaa AK, Traut CC, et al. Proviral location affects cognate peptide-induced virus production and immune recognition of HIV-1-infected T cell clones. *J Clin Invest.* 2023;133(21):e171097.133.
Doisne JM, Urrutia A, Lacabaratz-Porret C, et al. CD8+ T cells specific for EBV, cytomegalovirus, and influenza virus are activated during primary HIV infection. *J Immunol.* 2004;173:2410–2418.
Douek D, Picker LJ, Koup RA. T cell dynamics in HIV-1 infection. *Annu Rev Immunol.* 2003;21:265–304.
Dupin N, Buffet M, Marcelin AG, et al. HIV and antiretroviral drug distribution in plasma and fat tissue of HIV- infected patients with lipodystrophy. *AIDS.* 2002;16:2419–2424.
Eckard AR, O'Riordan MA, Rosebush JC, et al. Vitamin D supplementation decreases immune activation and exhaustion in HIV-1-infected youth. *Antivir Ther.* 2018;23(4):315–324.
Erikstrup C, Kallestrup P, Zinyama-Gutsire RB, et al. Reduced mortality and CD4 cell loss among carriers of the interleukin-10-1082G allele in a Zimbabwean cohort of HIV-1-infected adults. *AIDS.* 2007;21:2283–2291.
Estes JD, Haase AT, Schacker TW. The role of collagen deposition in depleting CD4+ T cells and limiting reconstitution in HIV-1 and SIV infections through damage to the secondary lymphoid organ niche. *Semin Immunol.* 2008;20:181–186.
Fan Y, Gao X, Chen J, et al. HIV Tat impairs neurogenesis through functioning as a notch ligand and activation of notch signaling pathway. *J Neurosci.* 2016;36:11362–11373.
Fauci AS. Durable control of HIV infections in the absence of antiretroviral therapy: opportunities and obstacles. 22nd International AIDS Conference (AIDS 2018), Amsterdam. July 25, 2018.
Favre D, Lederer S, Kanwar B, et al. Critical loss of the balance between Th17 and T regulatory cell populations in pathogenic SIV infection. *PLoS Pathog.* 2009;5:e1000295.
French MA, Price P, Stone SF. Immune restoration disease after antiretroviral therapy. *AIDS.* 2004;18:1615–1627.
Fumaz CR, Gonzalez-Garcia M, Borras X. Psychological stress is associated with high levels of IL-6 in HIV-1 infected individuals on effective combined antiretroviral treatment. *Brain Behav Immun.* 2012;26:568–572.

Ganesan A, Crum-Cianflone N, Higgins J, et al. High dose atorvastatin decreases cellular markers of immune activation without affecting HIV-1 RNA levels: results of a double-blind randomized placebo controlled clinical trial. *J Infect Dis.* 2011;203:756–764.

Giorgi JV, Hultin LE, McKeating JA, et al. Shorter survival in advanced human immunodeficiency virus type 1 infection is more closely associated with T lymphocyte activation than with plasma virus burden or virus chemokine coreceptor usage. *J Infect Dis.* 1999;179:859–870.

Giuliani E, Vassena L, Di Cesare S, et al. NK cells of HIV-1-infected patients with poor CD4(+) T-cell reconstitution despite suppressive HAART show reduced IFN-gamma production and high frequency of autoreactive CD56(bright) cells. *Immunol Lett.* 2017;190:185–193.

Gómez-Mora E, García E, Urrea V, et al. Preserved immune functionality and high CMV-specific T-cell responses in HIV-infected individuals with poor CD4(+) T-cell immune recovery. *Sci Rep.* 2017;7:11711.

Gori A, Rizzardini G, Van't Land B, et al. Specific prebiotics modulate gut microbiota and immune activation in HAART-naive HIV-infected adults: results of the "COPA" pilot randomized trial. *Mucosal Immunol.* 2011;4:554–563.

Goulder P, Deeks SG. HIV control: is getting there the same as staying there? *PLoS Pathog.* 2008;14:e1007222.

Gras L, May M, Ryder LP, et al. Determinants of restoration of CD4 and CD8 cell counts and their ratio in HIV-1-positive individuals with sustained virological suppression on antiretroviral therapy. *J Acquir Immune Defic Syndr.* 2019;80:292–300.

Grinspoon SK, Douglas PS, Hoffman U, Ribaudo HJ. Leveraging a landmark trial of primary cardiovascular disease prevention in human immunodeficiency virus: introduction from the REPRIEVE coprincipal investigators. *J Infect Dis.* 2020;222(Suppl 1):S1–S7.

Grossman Z, Meier- Schellersheim M, Sousa AE. CD4+ T-cell depletion in HIV infection: are we closer to understanding the cause? *Nat Med.* 2002;8:319–323.

Guadalupe M, Reay E, Sankaran S. Severe CD4+ T- cell depletion in gut lymphoid tissue during primary human immunodeficiency virus type 1 infection and substantial delay in restoration following highly active antiretroviral therapy. *J Virol.* 2003;77:11708–11717.

Guillén Y, Noguera-Julian M, Rivera J, et al. Low nadir CD4+ T-cell counts predict gut dysbiosis in HIV-1 infection. *Mucosal Immunol.* 2019;12:232–246.

Guzzo C, Ichikawa D, Park C, et al. Virion incorporation of integrin alpha4beta7 facilitates HIV-1 infection and intestinal homing. *Sci Immunol.* 2017;2(11):eaam7341.

Hage CA, Kohli LL, Cho S, et al. Human immunodeficiency virus gp120 downregulates CD1d cell surface expression. *Immunol Lett.* 2005;98:131–135.

Hammoud DA, Boulougoura A, Papadakis GZ, et al. Increased metabolic activity on 18F-fluorodeoxyglucose positron emission tomography-computed tomography in human immunodeficiency virus-associated immune reconstitution inflammatory syndrome. *Clin Infect Dis.* 2019;68:229–238.

Hansen SG, Piatak M Jr, Ventura AB, et al. Immune clearance of highly pathogenic SIV infection. *Nature.* 2013a;502:100–104.

Hansen SG, Sacha JB, Hughes CM, et al. Cytomegalovirus vectors violate CD8+ T cell epitope recognition paradigms. *Science.* 2013b;340:1237874.

Harper J, Ribeiro SP, Chan CN, et al. Interleukin-10 contributes to reservoir establishment and persistence in SIV-infected macaques treated with antiretroviral therapy. *J Clin Invest.* 2022;15;132(8):e155251.

Hartigan-O'Connor DJ, Abel K, Van Rompay KK, et al. SIV replication in the infected rhesus macaque is limited by the size of the preexisting TH17 cell compartment. *Sci Transl Med.* 2012;4:136ra169.

Hartigan-O'Connor DJ, Jacobson MA, Tan QX. Sinclair E development of cytomegalovirus (CMV) immune recovery uveitis is associated with Th17 cell depletion and poor systemic CMV-specific T cell responses. *Clin Infect Dis.* 2011;52:409–417.

Hatano H, Delwart EL, Norris PJ, et al. Evidence for persistent low-level viremia in individuals who control human immunodeficiency virus in the absence of antiretroviral therapy. *J Virol.* 2009;83:329–335.

He X, Aid M, Ventura JD, et al. Rapid loss of CD4 T cells by pyroptosis during acute SIV infection in rhesus macaques. *J Virol.* 2022;96:e0080822.

Heise C, Miller CJ, Lackner A, Dandekar S. Primary acute simian immunodeficiency virus infection of intestinal lymphoid tissue is associated with gastrointestinal dysfunction. *J Infect Dis.* 1994;169:1116–1120.

Hellerstein M, Hanley MB, Cesar D. Directly measured kinetics of circulating T lymphocytes in normal and HIV-1-infected humans. *Nat Med.* 1999;5:83–89.

Hirao LA, Grishina I, Bourry O. Early mucosal sensing of SIV infection by paneth cells induces IL-1beta production and initiates gut epithelial disruption. *PLoS Pathog.* 2014;10:e1004311.

Hrecka K, Hao C, Gierszewska M, et al. Vpx relieves inhibition of HIV-1 infection of macrophages mediated by the SAMHD1 protein. *Nature.* 2011;474:658–661.

Hsu DC, Wegner MD, Sunyakumthorn P, et al. CD4+ cell infiltration into subcutaneous adipose tissue is not indicative of productively infected cells during acute SHIV infection. *J Med Primatol.* 2017;46:154–157.

Hsue PY, Hunt PW, Schnell A, et al. Role of viral replication, antiretroviral therapy, and immunodeficiency in HIV-associated atherosclerosis. *AIDS.* 2009;23:1059–1067.

Hunt PW, Brenchley J, Sinclair E, et al. Relationship between T cell activation and CD4+ T cell count in HIV-seropositive individuals with undetectable plasma HIV RNA levels in the absence of therapy. *J Infect Dis.* 2008;197:126–133.

Hunt PW, Martin JN, Sinclair E. Valganciclovir reduces T cell activation in HIV-infected individuals with incomplete CD4+ T cell recovery on antiretroviral therapy. *J Infect Dis.* 2011;203:1474–1483.

Hwang I, Zhang T, Scott JM, et al. Identification of human NK cells that are deficient for signaling adaptor FcRgamma and specialized for antibody-dependent immune functions. *Int Immunol.* 2012;24:793–802.

Jimenez-Leon MR, Gasca-Capote C, Roca-Oporto C, et al. Vedolizumab and ART in recent HIV-1 infection unveil the role of alpha4beta7 in reservoir size. *JCI Insight.* 2024;9:e182312.

Jones JL, Phuah CL, Cox AL, et al. TIL-21 drives secondary autoimmunity in patients with multiple sclerosis, following therapeutic lymphocyte depletion with alemtuzumab (Campath-1H). *J Clin Invest.* 2009;119:2052–2061.

Kant S, Dupuy FP, Kiani Z, et al. Contribution of natural killer cells to HIV control in elite controllers. *Virologie (Montrouge).* 2022;26(1):34–49.

Ke R, Cong ME, Li D, et al. On the death rate of abortively infected cells: estimation from simian-human immunodeficiency virus infection. *J Virol.* 2017;91(18):e00352-17.

Kelley CF, Kitchen CM, Hunt PW, et al. Incomplete peripheral CD4(+) cell count restoration in HIV-infected patients receiving long-term antiretroviral treatment. *Clin Infect Dis.* 2009;48:787–794.

King C, Ilic A, Koelsch K, Sarvetnick N. Homeostatic expansion of T cells during immune insufficiency generates autoimmunity. *Cell.* 2004;117:265–277.

Koethe JR, McDonnell W, Kennedy A, et al. Adipose tissue is enriched for activated and late- differentiated CD8+ T cells and shows distinct CD8+ receptor usage, compared with blood in HIV-infected persons. *J Acquir Immune Defic Syndr.* 2018;77:e14–e21.

Kuller LH, Tracy R, Belloso W, et al. Inflammatory and coagulation biomarkers and mortality in patients with HIV infection. *PLoS Med.* 2008;5:e203.

Ladapo JA, Richards AK, DeWitt CM, et al. Disparities in the quality of cardiovascular care between HIV-infected versus HIV-uninfected adults in the United States: a cross-sectional study. *J Am Heart Assoc.* 2017;6(11):e007107.

Laguette MJ, Abrahams Y, Prince S, et al. Sequence variants within the 3′-UTR of the COL5A1 gene alters mRNA stability: implications for musculoskeletal soft tissue injuries. *Matrix Biol.* 2011;30(5–6):338–345.

Lang DJ, Kovacs AA, Zaia JA, et al. Seroepidemiologic studies of cytomegalovirus and Epstein- Barr virus infections in relation to human immunodeficiency virus type 1 infection in selected recipient populations. Transfusion Safety Study Group. *J Acquir Immune Defic Syndr.* 1989;2:540–549.

Lawn SD, Myer L, Bekker LG, Wood R. Tuberculosis-associated immune reconstitution disease: incidence, risk factors and impact in an antiretroviral treatment service in South Africa. *AIDS.* 2007;21:335–341.

Lee J, Zhang T, Hwang I, et al. Epigenetic modification and antibody-dependent expansion of memory-like NK cells in human cytomegalovirus-infected individuals. *Immunity.* 2015;42:431–442.

Lenardo MJ, Angleman SB, Bounkeua C, et al. Cytopathic killing of peripheral blood CD4(+) T lymphocytes by human immunodeficiency virus type 1 appears necrotic rather than apoptotic and does not require env. *J Virol.* 2002;76:5082–5093.

Lenkei R, Andersson B. High correlations of anti-CMV titers with lymphocyte activation status and CD57 antibody-binding capacity as estimated with three-color, quantitative flow cytometry in blood donors. *Clin Immunol Immunopathol.* 1995;77:131–138.

Levy Y, Lacabaratz C, Weiss L, et al. Enhanced T cell recovery in HIV-1-infected adults through IL-7 treatment. *J Clin Invest.* 2009;119:997–1007.

Li D, Xu XN. NKT cells in HIV-1 infection. *Cell Res.* 2008;18:817–822.

Lim SY, Osuna CE, Hraber PT, et al. TLR7 agonists induce transient viremia and reduce the viral reservoir in SIV-infected rhesus macaques on antiretroviral therapy. *Sci Transl Med.* 2018;10(439):eaao4521.

Link A, Vogt TK, Favre S, et al. Fibroblastic reticular cells in lymph nodes regulate the homeostasis of naive T cells. *Nat Immunol.* 2007;8:1255–1265.

Lopez-Verges S, Milush JM, Schwartz BS, et al. Expansion of a unique CD57(+)NKG2Chi natural killer cell subset during acute human cytomegalovirus infection. *Proc Natl Acad Sci USA.* 2011;108:14725–14732.

Maidji E, Somsouk M, Rivera JM, et al. Replication of CMV in the gut of HIV-infected individuals and epithelial barrier dysfunction. *PLoS Pathog.* 2017;13:e1006202.

Manel N, Hogstad B, Wang Y, et al. A cryptic sensor for HIV-1 activates antiviral innate immunity in dendritic cells. *Nature.* 2010;467:214–217.

Margolick JB, Bream JH. Nilles TL, et al. Relationship between T-cell responses to CMV, markers of inflammation, and frailty in HIV-uninfected and HIV-infected men in the Multicenter AIDS Cohort Study. *J Infect Dis.* 2018;218:249–258.

Martin MP, Qi Y, Gao X, et al. Innate partnership of HLA-B and KIR3DL1 subtypes against HIV-1. *Nat Genet.* 2007;39;733–740.

Martinsen JT, Gunst JD, Højen JF, et al. The use of toll-like receptor agonists in HIV-1 cure strategies. *FrontImmunol.* 2020;11:1112.

McCune JM. The dynamics of CD4+ T-cell depletion in HIV disease. *Nature.* 2001;410: 974–979

Meintjes G, Wilkinson RJ, Morroni C, et al. Randomized placebo-controlled trial of prednisone for paradoxical tuberculosis-associated immune reconstitution inflammatory syndrome. *AIDS.* 2010;24: 2381–2390.

Mens H, Kearney M, Wiegand A, et al. HIV-1 Continues to replicate and evolve in patients with natural control of HIV infection. *J Virol.* 2010;84(24):12971–12981.

Migueles SA, Nettere DM, Gavil NV, et al. HIV vaccines induce CD8(+) T cells with low antigen receptor sensitivity. *Science.* 2023;382:1270–1276.

Miller JS, Davis ZB, Helgeson E, et al. Safety and virologic impact of the IL-15 superagonist N-803 in people living with HIV: a phase 1 trial. *Nat Med.* 2022;28:392–400.

Mocroft A, Phillips AN, Gatell J. Normalisation of CD4 counts in patients with HIV-1 infection and maximum virological suppression who are taking combination antiretroviral therapy: an observational cohort study. *Lancet.* 2007;370:407–413.

Mothe B, Ibarrondo J, Llano A, Brander C. Virological, immune and host genetic markers in the control of HIV infection. *Dis Markers.* 2009;27:105–120.

Mothe Pujades B, Curran A, López C, et al. A placebo-controlled randomized trial of the HTI immunogen vaccine and Vesatolimod. Conference on Retroviruses and Opportunistic Infections (Seattle), February 19–23, 2023. Abstract number 443.

Muema DM, Akilimali NA, Ndumnego OC, et al. Association between the cytokine storm, immune cell dynamics, and viral replicative capacity in hyperacute HIV infection. *BMC Med.* 2020;18:81

Muller M, Wandel S, Colebunders R, et al. Immune reconstitution inflammatory syndrome in patients starting antiretroviral therapy for HIV infection: a systematic review and meta-analysis. *Lancet Infect Dis.* 2010;10:251–261.

Murray SM, Down CM, Boulware DR, et al. Reduction of immune activation with chloroquine therapy during chronic HIV infection. *J Virol.* 2010.84:12082–12086.

Ndhlovu ZM, Kamya P, Mewalal N, et al. Magnitude and kinetics of CD8+ T cell activation during hyperacute HIV infection impact viral set point. *Immunity.* 2015;43:591–604.

Neuhaus J, Jacobs DR Jr, Baker JV, et al. Markers of inflammation, coagulation, and renal function are elevated in adults with HIV infection. *J Infect Dis.* 2010;201:1788–1795.

Ni W, Ren L, Liao L, et al. Plasma proteomics analysis of Chinese HIV-1 infected individuals focusing on the immune and inflammatory factors afford insight into the viral control mechanism. *Front Immunol.* 2024;15:1378048.

Noguera-Julian M, Rocafort M, Guillén Y, et al. Gut microbiota linked to sexual preference and HIV infection. *EBioMedicine.* 2016;5:135–146.

Nussenblatt RB, Lane HC. Human immunodeficiency virus disease: changing patterns of intraocular inflammation. *Am J Ophthalmol.* 1998;125:374–382.

O'Connell KA, Rabi SA, Siliciano RF, Blankson JN. CD4+ T cells from elite suppressors are more susceptible to HIV-1 but produce fewer virions than cells from chronic progressors. *Proc Natl Acad Sci USA.* 2011;108:E689–E698.

Oriol-Tordera B, Esteve-Codina A, Berdasco M, et al. Epigenetic landscape in the kick-and-kill therapeutic vaccine BCN02 clinical trial is associated with antiretroviral treatment interruption (ATI) outcome. *EBioMed.* 2022;78:103956.

Pakker NG, Notermans DW, de Boer RJ, et al. Biphasic kinetics of peripheral blood T cells after triple combination therapy in HIV-1 infection: a composite of redistribution and proliferation. *Nat Med.* 1998;4:208–214.

Pandiyan P, Younes SA, Ribeiro SP, et al. Mucosal regulatory T cells and T helper 17 cells in HIV-associated immune activation. *Front Immunol.* 2016;7:228.

Papagno L, Spina CA, Marchant A, et al. Immune activation and CD8(+) T-cell differentiation towards senescence in HIV-1 infection. *PLoS Biol.* 2005;2:E20.

Paquin-Proulx D, Lal KG, Phuang-Ngern Y, et al. Preferential and persistent impact of acute HIV-1 infection on CD4(+) iNKT cells in colonic mucosa. *Proc Natl Acad Sci USA.* 2021;118(46):e2104721118.

Parrinello CM, Sinclair E, Landay AL, et al. Cytomegalovirus immunoglobulin G antibody is associated with subclinical carotid artery disease among HIV-infected women. *J Infect Dis.* 2012;205:1788–1796.

Pereyra F, Jia X, McLaren PJ, et al. The major genetic determinants of HIV-1 control affect HLA class I peptide presentation. *Science.* 2010;330:1551–1557.

Perez-Matute P, Perez-Martinez L, Aguilera-Lizarraga J, et al. Maraviroc modifies gut microbiota composition in a mouse model of obesity: a plausible therapeutic option to prevent metabolic disorders in HIV-infected patients. *Rev Esp Quimioter.* 2015;28:200–206.

Perreau M, Banga R, Pantaleo G. Targeted immune interventions for an HIV-1 cure. *Trends Mol Med.* 2017;23:945–961.

Phillips AN, Neaton J, Lundgren JD. The role of HIV in serious diseases other than AIDS. *AIDS.* 2008;22:2409–2418.

Piconi S, Parisotto S, Rizzardini G, et al. Hydroxychloroquine drastically reduces immune activation in HIV-infected, antiretroviral therapy-treated immunologic nonresponders. *Blood.* 2011;118:3263–3272.

Price P, Murdoch DM, Agarwal U, et al. Immune restoration diseases reflect diverse immunopathological mechanisms. *Clin Microbiol Rev.* 2009;22:651–663.

Raffatellu M, Santos RL, Verhoeven DE, et al. Simian immunodeficiency virus-induced mucosal interleukin-17 deficiency promotes Salmonella dissemination from the gut. *Nat Med.* 2008;14:421–428.

Reeves RK, Li H, Jost S, et al. Antigen-specific NK cell memory in rhesus macaques. *Nat Immunol.* 2015;16:927–932.

Roederer M, Dubs JG, Anderson MT, et al. CD8 naive T cell counts decrease progressively in HIV-infected adults. *J Clin Invest.* 1995;95:2061–2066.

Romero-Martin L, Tarres-Freixas F, Pedreno-Lopez N, et al. T-follicular-like CD8(+) T cell responses in chronic HIV infection are associated with virus control and antibody isotype switching to IgG. *Front Immunol.* 2022;13:92803913.

Ruffin N, Hani L, Seddiki N. From dendritic cells to B cells dysfunctions during HIV-1 infection: T follicular helper cells at the crossroads. *Immunology.* 2017;151:137–145.

Ruiz-Riol M, Berdnik D, Llano A, et al. Identification of interleukin-27 (IL-27)/IL-27 receptor subunit alpha as a critical immune axis for in vivo HIV control. *J Virol.* 2017;91(16):e00441–17.

Ruiz-Riol M, Brander C. Can we just kick-and-kill HIV: possible challenges posed by the epigenetically controlled interplay between HIV and host immunity. *Immunother.* 2019;11:931–935.

Saez-Cirion A, Hamimi C, Bergamaschi A, et al. Restriction of HIV-1 replication in macrophages and CD4+ T cells from HIV controllers. *Blood.* 2011;118:955–964.

Sáez-Cirión A, Sereti I. Immunometabolism and HIV-1 pathogenesis: food for thought. *Nat Rev Immunol.* 2021;21(1):5–19.

Samal J, Kelly S, Na-Shatal A, et al. Human immunodeficiency virus infection induces lymphoid fibrosis in the BM-liver-thymus-spleen humanized mouse model. *JCI Insight.* 2018;3(18):e120430.

Sandberg JK, Fast NM, Palacios EH, et al. Selective loss of innate CD4(+) V alpha 24 natural killer T cells in human immunodeficiency virus infection. *J Virol.* 2002;76:7528–7534.

Sauce D, Larsen M, Fastenackels S, et al. HIV disease progression despite suppression of viral replication is associated with exhaustion of lymphopoiesis. *Blood.* 2011;117(19):5142–5151.

Schacker TW, Nguyen PL, Beilman GJ, et al. Collagen deposition in HIV-1 infected lymphatic tissues and T cell homeostasis. *J Clin Invest.* 2002;110:1133–1139.

Scriven JE, Rhein J, Hullsiek KH, et al. Early ART after cryptococcal meningitis is associated with cerebrospinal fluid pleocytosis and macrophage activation in a multisite randomized trial. *J Infect Dis.* 2015;212:769–778.

Seddiki N, Sasson SC, Santner-Nanan B, et al. Proliferation of weakly suppressive regulatory CD4+ T cells is associated with over-active CD4+ T-cell responses in HIV-positive patients with mycobacterial immune restoration disease. *Eur J Immunol.* 2009;39:391–403.

Silvestri G, Sodora DL, Koup RA, et al. Nonpathogenic SIV infection of sooty mangabeys is characterized by limited bystander immunopathology despite chronic high-level viremia. *Immunity.* 2003;18:441–452.

Sips M, Sciaranghella G, Diefenbach T, et al. Altered distribution of mucosal NK cells during HIV infection. *Mucosal Immunol.* 2012;5:30–40.

Sivro A, Schuetz A, Sheward D, et al. Integrin α(4)β(7) expression on peripheral blood CD4(+) T cells predicts HIV acquisition and disease progression outcomes. *Sci Transl Med.* 2018;10(425):eaam6354.

Srinivasula S, Lempicki RA, Adelsberger JW, et al. Differential effects of HIV viral load and CD4 count on proliferation of naive and memory CD4 and CD8 T lymphocytes. *Blood.* 2011;118:262–270.

Stacey AR, Norris PJ, Qin L, et al. Induction of a striking systemic cytokine cascade prior to peak viremia in acute human immunodeficiency virus type 1 infection, in contrast to more modest and delayed responses in acute hepatitis B and C virus infections. *J Virol.* 2009;83:3719–3733.

Sun JC, Beilke JN, Lanier LL. Adaptive immune features of natural killer cells. *Nature.* 2009;457:557–561.

Surh CD, Sprent J. Homeostasis of naive and memory T cells. *Immunity.* 2008;29:848–862.

Sylwester AW, Mitchell BL, Edgar JB. Broadly targeted human cytomegalovirus-specific CD4+ and CD8+ T cells dominate the memory compartments of exposed subjects. *J Exp Med.* 2005;202:673–685.

Teixeira L, Valdez H, McCune JM, et al. Poor CD4 T cell restoration after suppression of HIV-1 replication may reflect lower thymic function. *AIDS.* 2001;15:1749–1756.

Uthman OA, Nduka C, Watson SI, et al. Statin use and all-cause mortality in people living with HIV: a systematic review and meta-analysis. *BMC Infect Dis.* 2018;18:258.

Uzzan M, Tokuyama M, Rosenstein AK, et al. Anti-α4β7 therapy targets lymphoid aggregates in the gastrointestinal tract of HIV-1-infected individuals. *Sci Transl Med.* 2018;10(461):eaau4711.

van der Vliet HJ, von Blomberg BM, Hazenberg MD, et al. Selective decrease in circulating V alpha 24+V beta 11+ NKT cells during HIV type 1 infection. *J Immunol.* 2002;168:1490–1495.

van Grevenynghe J, Procopio FA, He Z, et al. Transcription factor FOXO3a controls the persistence of memory CD4(+) T cells during HIV infection. *Nat Med.* 2008;14:266–274.

van Zoest RA, van der Valk M, Wit FW, et al. Suboptimal primary and secondary cardiovascular disease prevention in HIV-positive individuals on antiretroviral therapy. *Eur J Prev Cardiol.* 2017;24:1297–1307.

Veazey RS, DeMaria M, Chalifoux LV, et al. Gastrointestinal tract as a major site of CD4+ T cell depletion and viral replication in SIV infection. *Science.* 1998;280:427–431.

Vujkovic-Cvijin I, Dunham RM, Iwai S, et al. Dysbiosis of the gut microbiota is associated with HIV disease progression and tryptophan catabolism. *Sci Transl Med.* 2013;5:193ra191.

Vujkovic-Cvijin I, Sortino O, Verheij E, et al. HIV-associated gut dysbiosis is independent of sexual practice and correlates with noncommunicable diseases. *Nat Commun.* 2020;11:2448.

Walker NF, Stek C, Wasserman S, et al. The tuberculosis-associated immune reconstitution inflammatory syndrome: recent advances in clinical and pathogenesis research. *Curr Opin HIV AIDS.* 2018;13:512–521.

Yoon HA, Nakouzi A, Chang CC, et al. Association between plasma antibody responses and risk for cryptococcus-associated immune reconstitution inflammatory syndrome. *J Infect Dis.* 2019;219:420–428.

Zeng M, Southern PJ, Reilly CS, et al. Lymphoid tissue damage in HIV-1 infection depletes naive T cells and limits T cell reconstitution after antiretroviral therapy. *PLoS Pathog.* 2012;8:e1002437.

Zhang T, Scott JM, Hwang I. Cutting edge: antibody-dependent memory-like NK cells distinguished by FcRgamma deficiency. *J Immunol.* 2013;190:1402–1406.

Zhang W, Ambikan AT, Sperk M, et al. Transcriptomics and targeted proteomics analysis to gain insights into the immune-control mechanisms of HIV-1 infected elite controllers. *EBioMedicine.* 2018;27:40–50.

Zhou J, Amran FS, Kramski M, et al. An NK cell population lacking FcRgamma is expanded in chronically infected HIV patients. *J Immunol.* 2015;194:4688–4697.

6.

HIV TESTING AND COUNSELING

M. Elle Saine and Kyle G. Rodino

CHAPTER GOALS

Upon completion of this chapter, the reader should be able to:

- Discuss the Centers for Disease Control and Prevention's (CDC's) recommendations for both routine HIV testing and HIV testing in special populations, including pregnant women and newborns.
- Describe the types of available tests for screening and diagnoses of HIV and explain the steps of the CDC HIV testing algorithm.
- Present an overview of HIV counseling, including counseling before and after an HIV test is performed.

KEY POINTS

- The CDC recommends that all people aged 13–65 receive an HIV test at least once as part of routine health care. Testing in younger and older persons, as well as repeat testing, should be offered when special circumstances deem this appropriate. Persons identified as at "high risk" for HIV infection should be retested at least annually.
- All persons screened for HIV should be counseled regarding risk-reduction strategies including pre-exposure prophylaxis (PrEP) and other prevention methods depending on test results.
- For routine HIV testing, the CDC algorithm recommends using the most sensitive immunoassay ("fourth-generation" EIA) as a screening test and following any repeatedly reactive/positive results with a different immunoassay that can discriminate between HIV-1 and HIV-2. Samples with a positive screening assay but negative confirmation assay should be tested using a virologic assay (nucleic acid amplification test).
- Post-test counseling for a positive HIV test result should include prompt linkage to care and treatment initiation, discussion of partner notification and transmission-reduction strategies, as well as efforts to address misconceptions and stigma.
- Post-test counseling for a negative HIV test provides an opportunity to engage individuals in information-sharing on HIV/STI prevention interventions including PrEP.

WHAT'S NEW?

- In March 2023, the CDC announced the launch of Together TakeMeHome (TTMH), a project with a goal of distributing up to 1 million HIV self-tests over the next five years.
- The CDC has updated the recommended HIV testing algorithm to recently incorporate FDA-approved HIV nucleic acid amplification tests (NATs) with a diagnostic claim at the third step in situations when the differentiation assay is negative or indeterminate for HIV-1 or HIV-2 antibodies.
- When acute HIV is suspected during pregnancy or the intrapartum period, or while breastfeeding, a plasma HIV RNA assay should be performed in combination with an antigen/antibody immunoassay.

HIV TESTING: HISTORY AND EVOLUTION

An estimated 1.2 million people in the United States have HIV, about 13% of whom are unaware of their status (CDC, 2024a). Persistent disparities in access to prevention and treatment services have limited the population health effectiveness of HIV transmission-reduction strategies (Pitasi et al., 2021). Diagnosis and engagement in care are critical to reducing HIV transmission, with more than 90% of new HIV infections transmitted by people who are either not diagnosed (23%) or are diagnosed but not retained in care (69%) (Frieden et al., 2015). HIV screening and early detection are central to the Ending the HIV Epidemic in the United States (EHE) initiative, which aims to reduce the number of new HIV infections by at least 90% by the year 2030 (DHHS, 2021).

The role of HIV testing as a public health strategy has evolved alongside the development of assays and treatments. In 1985, when HIV testing first became available, the main goal of testing was for blood banks to screen the U.S. blood supply. When it was discovered that people who wanted to learn their HIV status were using blood-donation testing sites for this service, alternative testing sites were implemented. At that time, the value of HIV screening was controversial, as no treatments were available and routes of transmission were still being investigated. By 1987, the public health implications of a positive HIV serology were clear, and the U.S. Public

Health Service and the CDC issued the first set of guidelines for HIV testing and counseling (CDC, 1987).

Early guidelines targeted those in "high-risk groups," but experience has subsequently indicated that a more productive approach, focused on behaviors rather than membership in a particular population, is important. A study in South Carolina found that among 1,784 persons identified as "late-testers" (persons who received an AIDS diagnosis within 1 year of HIV diagnosis), although approximately three-fourths had visited a healthcare facility prior to their HIV diagnosis, the majority of diagnoses for these previous visits probably would not have prompted HIV testing under a risk-based testing strategy (CDC, 2006). Selectively offering HIV screening based on risk assessment alone misses many individuals with HIV (Chen et al., 1998). Compared to risk-based approaches, routine universal screening captures many people who may have been missed and decreases the stigma associated with HIV testing (Branson et al., 2006). Moreover, early diagnosis has the potential to decrease HIV transmission: one meta-analysis showed that the prevalence of high-risk sexual behavior is reduced substantially after people become aware they have HIV, while estimated transmission is 3.5 times higher among persons unaware of their status (Marks et al., 2006). Taken together, the overall magnitude of the benefit of routine screening for HIV infection is substantial.

Beginning in 2006, guidelines recommended that all persons aged 13–64 (regardless of risk factors) be screened for HIV at least once in their lifetime as part of routine health screening (Branson et al., 2006), with more frequent screening for individuals with ongoing risk factors (DiNenno et al., 2017). The U.S. Preventive Services Task Force (USPSTF) Recommendation Summary found convincing evidence that identification of HIV infection and initiation of early treatment with antiretroviral therapy (ART) is of substantial benefit in reducing the risk of AIDS-related events or death and in decreasing the risk of HIV transmission to uninfected sex partners. The USPSTF also found convincing evidence that identification and treatment of pregnant women living with HIV infection is of significant benefit in reducing the rate of mother-to-child transmission (USPTF, 2019).

WHO SHOULD BE TESTED?

The CDC recommends that every individual between the ages of 13 and 64 years should be offered testing at least once in their lifetime, with repeat testing based on specific clinical scenarios and risk factors (Branson et al., 2006). The USPTF similarly recommends screening all adults aged 15–65 years, as well as younger adolescents and older adults at increased risk of infection (grade A recommendation) (USPTF, 2019). The CDC recommends that HIV screening should be offered in the following scenarios:

- Routine screening for all individuals aged 13–64 years in all healthcare settings unless declined (opt-out screening)
- Individuals with signs and symptoms of acute or chronic HIV infection, or an opportunistic infection associated with advanced HIV
- People initiating treatment for tuberculosis (TB)
- Individuals being evaluated for sexually transmitted infections (STIs)
- As part of routine prenatal screening for all pregnant women early in pregnancy. Repeat screening in the third trimester is recommended in certain jurisdictions with elevated rates of HIV among pregnant women.
- Any person whose blood or body fluid is the source of occupational exposure for a healthcare provider should be informed of the incident and tested for HIV infection at the time the exposure occurs, unless recent HIV test results are immediately available.
- Persons at high risk for HIV should be screened for HIV at least annually.

For higher-risk groups, repeat testing may be indicated. Healthcare providers should offer repeat testing, at least annually, to individuals likely to be at increased risk of HIV, such as people who inject drugs; people who engage in sex with partners living with HIV; people who exchange money for sex; gay, bisexual, and other men who have sex with men (GBMSM), or heterosexual persons who had one more sex partner since their last HIV test (Branson et al., 2006). For individuals receiving pre-exposure prophylaxis (PrEP), HIV testing every 2–3 months and immediate testing whenever signs and symptoms of acute HIV infection are reported is indicated (CDC, 2021).

HIV testing should be voluntary, and individuals should be informed verbally that HIV testing will be performed unless they decline (opt-out screening). Separate written consent for HIV testing should not be required; general consent for medical care should be considered sufficient to encompass consent for HIV testing. If a person chooses to decline an HIV test, this decision should be documented in the medical record. While prevention counseling is strongly encouraged for persons at high risk of HIV, and screening provides an opportunity to discuss preventive counseling, this should *not* be required as part of HIV diagnostic testing or HIV screening programs in healthcare settings (Branson et al., 2006).

BLOOD SUPPLY SCREENING

Since 1990, all persons desiring to donate blood or plasma are required to undergo testing, as are those donating sperm for artificial insemination or tissue or organs for transplantation. The donor is notified only if the specimen tests positive. The laboratory assays used for testing blood, blood products, tissues, and organs have evolved along with those used to screen individuals (and often are the same). However, because the volume of testing is larger, pooled testing using nucleic acid tests is commonly done to improve testing and possibly detect blood or blood products from acutely infected persons. Additional details are available in Chapter 14, "HIV Prevention: Pharmacotherapy and Non-Pharmacotherapy-Based Strategies."

GAY, BISEXUAL, AND OTHER MEN WHO HAVE SEX WITH MEN (GBMSM)

GBMSM have been identified as a population at high risk for HIV and other STIs. Male-to-male sexual contact accounts for two-thirds of all new HIV infections (CDC, 2024a). Clinicians can also consider the potential benefits of more frequent HIV screening (e.g., every 3 or 6 months) for some asymptomatic sexually active GBMSM based on individual exposure history, local HIV epidemiology, and local policies (DiNenno et al., 2017).

PERINATAL SCREENING

The USPSTF recommended in 2019 that clinicians screen for HIV infection in all pregnant persons, including those who present in labor or at delivery whose HIV status is unknown (grade A recommendation). HIV screening should be a routine component of prenatal testing and should be performed during the first trimester or at entry into care. Retesting in the third trimester (preferably <36 weeks of gestation) is recommended for women at high risk for HIV exposure, who receive health care in high-incidence areas, and who have signs or symptoms consistent with acute HIV infection (USPSTF, 2019). Repeat HIV testing is also recommended for pregnant people diagnosed with an STI (DHHS, 2024). When acute HIV is suspected during pregnancy, the intrapartum period, or while breastfeeding, a plasma RNA ("viral load") assay should be performed in addition to an HIV antigen/antibody (Ag/Ab) immunoassay (DHHS, 2024).

Women with undocumented HIV status at the time of labor or delivery should be screened with a point-of-care (POC) HIV test unless they opt out. If a mother's HIV status is unknown postpartum, newborn POC testing using an expedited antibody test is recommended (and may be legally mandated in some states) as soon as possible so that antiretroviral prophylaxis can be offered to HIV-exposed infants (DHHS, 2024). The mother should be informed that the identification of HIV antibodies in the newborn is a strong indicator of maternal HIV infection (Branson et al., 2006).

NEWBORNS

Perinatal HIV transmission can occur *in utero*, at the time of labor and delivery, and through breastfeeding (Kourtis et al., 2001). Virologic assays should be used in infants <18 months with perinatal or postnatal exposure to HIV. Children >24 months and children 18–24 months with non-perinatal HIV exposure only should undergo HIV antibody or HIV Ag/Ab testing (DHHS, 2024).

Virologic assays should be performed at birth on infants born to mothers with HIV who meet the following criteria: did not receive prenatal care; did not receive antepartum or intrapartum antiretroviral (ARV) drugs; received intrapartum ARV drugs only; initiated antiretroviral therapy late in pregnancy; were diagnosed with acute HIV during pregnancy; had detectable HIV viral load close to delivery; or received ARV combination drugs but did not have viral suppression (DHHS, 2024; Momplaisir et al., 2015). Infants born to mothers with HIV-2–infection should be tested with HIV-2-specific virologic assays at time points similar to those used for HIV-1 testing. HIV-2 virologic assays are not widely commercially available, but the National Perinatal HIV Hotline (1-888-448-8765) can assist with identification of laboratory resources to pursue this testing (DHHS, 2024).

Additionally, all infants with perinatal HIV exposure should undergo virologic testing at 14–21 days, at 1 or 2 months of age, and at 4–6 months of age. Testing should also be performed for infants with higher risk of perinatal infection 2–4 weeks after cessation of ARV prophylaxis. Some experts also recommend serologic testing to confirm the absence of infection between 12 and 18 months (DHHS, 2024). If any tests are positive, repeat testing is recommended, and the diagnosis of HIV infection can be made based on two separate positive results.

While women living with HIV in the United States have historically been discouraged from breastfeeding, the Department of Health and Human Services (DHHS) recently changed its guidance to now recommend that mothers receive evidence-based counseling to support individualized, shared decision-making about breastfeeding (DHHS, 2024). Additionally, breastfeeding may be recommended for children born in resource-limited settings through the age of 12 months, provided the mother and/or child is receiving ARV prophylaxis, so clinical and laboratory monitoring for HIV transmission should take into consideration ongoing breastfeeding exposures (WHO, 2010). Breastfed infants should have standard virologic testing, as well as testing every 3 months throughout breastfeeding (DHHS, 2024; WHO, 2010). Many experts also recommend monitoring at 4–6 weeks, 3 months, and 6 months after breastfeeding has stopped (DHHS, 2024). Maternal antibody is present at birth and begins to fade with time, but infant antibody production begins after infant infection occurs (Ciaranello et al., 2011). If an infant is initially HIV-negative at birth but later acquires infection through breastfeeding, HIV RNA typically becomes detectable within the first few weeks after infection.

STRATEGIES TO IMPROVE UPTAKE OF HIV TESTING

HIV screening should be voluntary and undertaken only with the person's knowledge and understanding. Testing is optimally undertaken to prevent newly acquired infection in those found to be negative and to provide linkage to care in those found to be positive (Fauci et al., 2019).

Challenges in implementing routine HIV testing include time, cost of testing, follow-up notification of positive results in acute/episodic care settings (e.g., emergency departments, hospital units), and adoption of rapid testing. Provider-initiated HIV testing as part of routine healthcare maintenance in ambulatory settings provides an important opportunity for increasing HIV testing. However, between 2009 and 2017, HIV testing occurred at <1% of visits to physician offices and <3% of visits to community health centers (Hoover et al., 2020). A prior analysis of National HIV Behavioral Surveillance data found that among 333 healthcare-seeking, heterosexual adults at increased risk for acquiring HIV, over half (n = 194 [58%]) reported not receiving an HIV test offer at a recent medical visit, and men were less likely than women to be offered an HIV test (32% vs. 48%). Moreover, compared to people who were offered an HIV test by their provider, those individuals who were not offered an HIV test were less likely to ever have an HIV test (96% vs. 62%) or undergo HIV testing in the past 12 months (71% vs. 16%), emphasizing the significant impact of provider-initiated testing (Diepstra et al., 2018).

The COVID-19 pandemic also likely impacted routine HIV testing. From 2019 to 2020, new HIV diagnoses reported to the CDC decreased by 17% (DiNenno et al., 2022). Targeted home HIV testing programs among GBMSM demonstrated the benefits of increasing access to HIV testing, including reaching individuals who may be hesitant or unable to access clinic-based testing (Hecht et al., 2021).

Importantly, significant health disparities still exist at all stages of the HIV care cascade. Adopting a status-neutral approach to screening and addressing the impacts of systemic racism, stigma toward gender-minority individuals, and structural barriers to health care (e.g., housing and food insecurity) are essential to the population-level effectiveness of HIV-prevention strategies including testing. Coupling stigma-reduction efforts with cultural humility training for healthcare providers has the potential to positively impact patient care experiences and ultimately increase health service uptake and engagement among marginalized and underserved populations (Bagchi and Davis, 2020). Transgender women, for example, who are disproportionally affected by HIV, were more likely to be tested if they had a usual source of health care and comfort with a healthcare provider (Lee et al., 2022).

Features of successful and scalable HIV screening programs include institutional commitment to screening, incorporation of screening into existing clinic workflows, staff education on HIV screening and outcomes, integrated stigma-reduction efforts, use of electronic health record (EHR) prompts and automated laboratory orders, and access to laboratory testing (Bagchi and Davis, 2020; Goetz et al., 2013; Lin et al., 2014). A community-led HIV self-testing study in Malawi showed higher testing rates among adolescents in the community-led testing arm (84.6%) when compared to the standard-of-care arm (67.1%) (Indravudh et al., 2021), demonstrating that community-based interventions may also increase routine testing and HIV identification.

PRETEST COUNSELING

According to the CDC's 2006 recommendations for HIV testing in the healthcare setting, written consent and prevention counseling are not required. However, laws governing consent for HIV testing are state-specific. Although all states require opt-out consent for an HIV test (Halpern, 2005), most states that had required explicit written consent prior to the 2006 CDC recommendations have changed their laws (Neff and Goldschmidt, 2011). In some unique cases, HIV testing without consent may be standard practice. For example, in New York, newborn infants are tested without parental consent if their mother did not consent to HIV testing during pregnancy. There is also variability across state laws regarding explicit exceptions for consent for HIV testing in emergency medical situations (Halpern, 2005), as well as testing of source patients when there has been a potential occupational exposure (e.g., healthcare setting, public safety officer) to HIV. While all states now have laws that explicitly allow minors of a particular age (as defined by each state) to give informed consent to receive sexually transmitted disease (STD) diagnosis and treatment services, the extent to which these laws include provisions for HIV testing is variable. Because laws and regulations vary by state, the clinician is responsible for knowing the appropriate rules in the state in which they practice. Consultation with the local public health officer is advised whenever HIV testing without consent is believed to be necessary. Current state HIV testing laws are compiled by the CDC at https://www.cdc.gov/hiv/policies/law/states/index.html.

The elements of informed consent include some of the information communicated during pretest counseling. The CDC (2006) recommendations define informed consent as follows (Branson et al., 2006, pp. 1–17):

> A process of communication between patient and provider through which, an informed patient can choose whether to undergo HIV testing or decline to do so. Elements of informed consent typically include providing oral or written information regarding HIV, the risks and benefits of testing, the implications of HIV test results, how test results will be communicated, and the opportunity to ask questions.

Effective pretest counseling is an interactive process of assessing risk, recognizing specific risk-inducing behaviors and reviewing risk-reduction strategies. This may be done in various ways—through written material, films, or verbally by trained staff. Of greatest importance is setting a nonjudgmental atmosphere, imparting accurate information in a useful format, offering an opportunity for questions, and maintaining strict confidentiality of personal information. Randomized controlled studies suggest that the quality and delivery of the counseling affects its efficacy on primary prevention (Kamb et al., 1998; Koblin et al., 2004). As such, HIV testing can offer the opportunity to refer people for prevention counseling, especially for people with ongoing exposures.

If deemed to be appropriate, elements of pretest counseling should include the following:

- A functional assessment of the person's decision-making capacity
- The meaning, sensitivity, and specificity of the test
- The potential ramifications of a positive test result

- A discussion about confidentiality and disclosure of test results by the healthcare providers to public health authorities and by the person to sexual and/or drug partners
- A frank discussion of risk-reduction behaviors
- Specific instructions about accessing treatment in the event of a positive result.

HIV TESTING TERMINOLOGY, TYPES, AND ALGORITHM

The first enzyme immunoassay (EIA) was licensed in 1985 (CDC, 1990). The first western blot assay was approved in 1987; thereafter, it was recommended as a confirmatory assay for positive immunoassays (CDC, 1988). Initially, the CDC guidelines focused on the diagnosis of HIV-1 using a sensitive antibody immunoassay with validation of those results by a more specific test such as the western blot or indirect immunofluorescence assay. By 1992, the guidelines also included testing recommendations for the diagnosis of HIV-2. In 2004, protocols for rapid antibody test results were issued with recommendations that all rapid testing be confirmed with either western blot or immunofluorescence assay. With the advent of improved immunoassays and tests, recommendations regarding HIV diagnostic testing have undergone changes.

LABORATORY MARKERS FOR HIV

Following HIV infection there is a brief time frame where no diagnostic markers of infection are present. This time frame between infection and detectable HIV RNA in plasma is referred to as the "eclipse period" and lasts about 5–10 days. The next diagnostic marker to appear is the HIV-1 p24 antigen, present in detectable levels 14–20 days after infection (4–10 days after the appearance of HIV RNA). The period from infection to p24 antigen detection is referred to as the *antigen seroconversion window period*. Although there is no accepted laboratory definition for acute HIV infection, a current operational definition is the detection of HIV RNA or p24 antigen in the blood before antibodies have formed (Cohen et al., 2010). As antibodies develop, the p24 antigens form immune complexes with antibodies and are no longer detectable. Immunoglobulin M antibodies are the first to form, and are expressed about 3–5 days after p24 antigen detection. This is followed by immunoglobulin G antibodies, which persist throughout the course of chronic infection (Branson et al., 2006). The time frame from infection to detectable HIV antibody is considered the antibody seroconversion window period. Figure 6.1 shows the temporal changes expected for laboratory markers after infection. In addition, it is important to understand that viral kinetics and serologic markers may not always be as accurate with non–clade B subtype infections (Hackett, 2012; Swenson et al., 2014). They may also be affected by the presence of antiretroviral medications taken as prophylaxis.

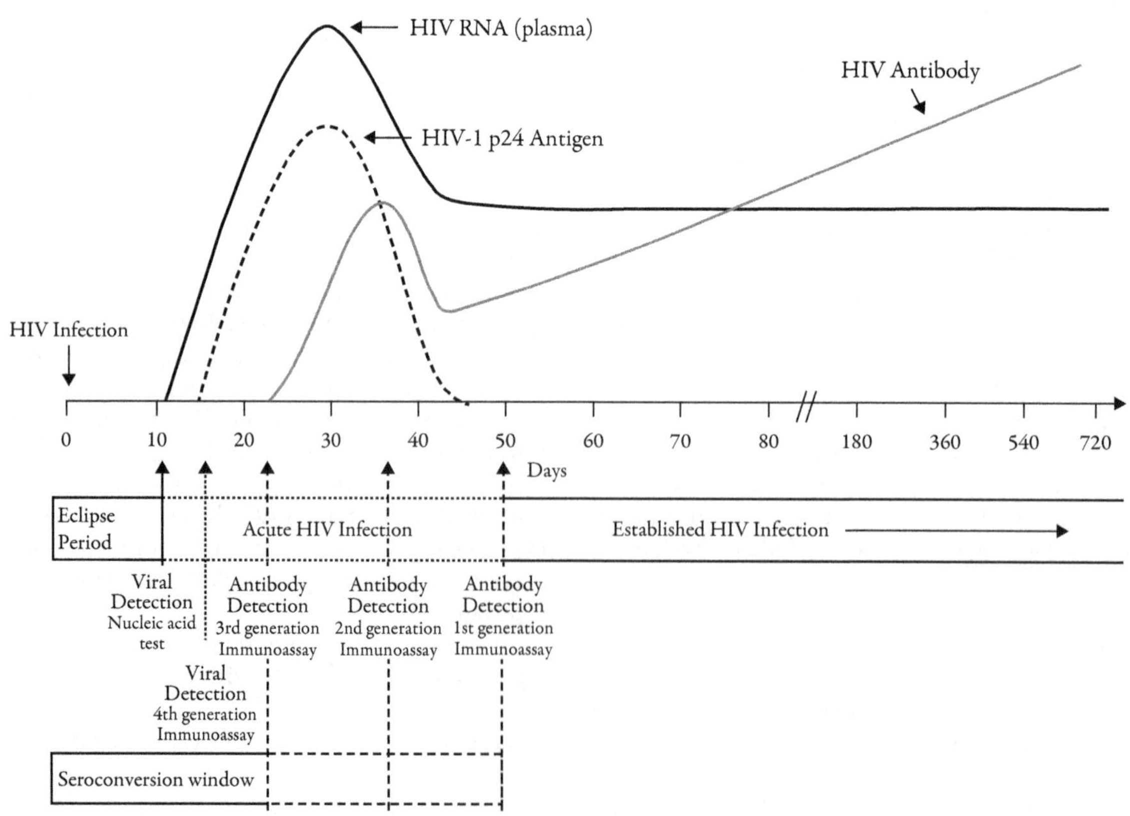

Figure 6.1 Timeline of HIV-1 laboratory markers. SOURCE: Centers for Disease Control and Prevention and Association of Public Health Laboratories. Laboratory Testing for the Diagnosis of HIV Infection: Updated Recommendations. Available at http://dx.doi.org/10.15620/cdc.23447. Published June 27, 2014. Accessed August 22, 2024.

ENZYME IMMUNOASSAYS

Enzyme immunoassays (EIAs) are currently the most reliable and cost-effective screening method for most individuals in the United States. EIAs test blood or other body fluids for the presence of antibodies. However, EIAs are not completely reliable for screening and diagnostic testing for individuals with acute HIV infections (see the section "Virologic Assays"), for self-testing kits (see the section "HIV Self-Testing"), or for screening and diagnosing infants and newborns (see the section "Who Should Be Tested? Newborns").

HIV EIAs are typically described as being from particular "generations," which helps to classify them based on technological advancements throughout the years. These advancements have shortened the detection window significantly. The first-generation EIAs used whole HIV lysate as an antigen to capture antibodies in a blood sample but could only detect HIV-1. These had a significant number of false positives because of cellular protein contamination (Houn et al., 1987; Louie et al., 2006). Second-generation EIAs used recombinant viral proteins or peptides, which limited cellular protein contamination (Chappel et al., 2009). This generation was used to screen blood donations in the 1980s. Third-generation EIAs in the 1990s used a technique that could bind both immunoglobulin G (IgG) and IgM antibodies, further reducing the window period.

Fourth-generation EIAs are antigen/antibody combination assays that detect HIV-1 p24 antigen via a capture immunoassay, in addition to the IgG and IgM antibodies detected by third-generation tests (Kabir et al., 2020). Thus, fourth-generation EIAs reduce the window period further to the time of antigen seroconversion, while maintaining the third-generation test's accuracy (Pandori et al., 2009; Rosenberg et al., 2015; Sickinger et al., 2004). Fifth-generation tests detect HIV-1 p24 antigen and HIV-1 and HIV-2 antibodies, but these are multiplex screening tests that differentiate results for HIV-1 p24 antigen, HIV-1 antibody, and HIV-2 antibody.

In 2014, an updated testing algorithm was issued by the CDC and Association of Public Health Laboratories (APHL) recommending use of the most sensitive immunoassays for primary screening, along with a confirmatory test that discriminates HIV-1 from HIV-2 after a repeatedly positive screening test (Wesolowski et al., 2017). Initial testing should be done with an antigen/antibody combination immunoassay that detects both HIV-1 and HIV-2 antibodies and HIV-1 p24 antigen. If a positive/reactive result is obtained, the specimen should be tested with an antibody immunoassay that differentiates HIV-1 and HIV-2 antibodies. In the event of a reactive antigen/antibody combination immunoassay with a nonreactive or indeterminate HIV-1/HIV-2 antibody differentiation immunoassay, the specimen should be further tested with an HIV-1 nucleic acid test. If the nucleic acid test is reactive, then it indicates acute HIV infection even if the antibody differentiation immunoassay was negative. If the antibody differentiation immunoassay was indeterminate and the nucleic acid test is reactive, this indicates confirmed infection. A negative nucleic acid test indicates a false-positive result of the initial immunoassay. The newly updated HIV diagnostic algorithm includes a third pathway, where recently FDA-approved NATs with a diagnostic claim are incorporated as a third step in the testing algorithm when the differentiation assay is indeterminate. The CDC's guidelines for laboratory testing for HIV are outlined in an algorithm (Figure 6.2).

Table 6.1 enumerates the various types of HIV testing.

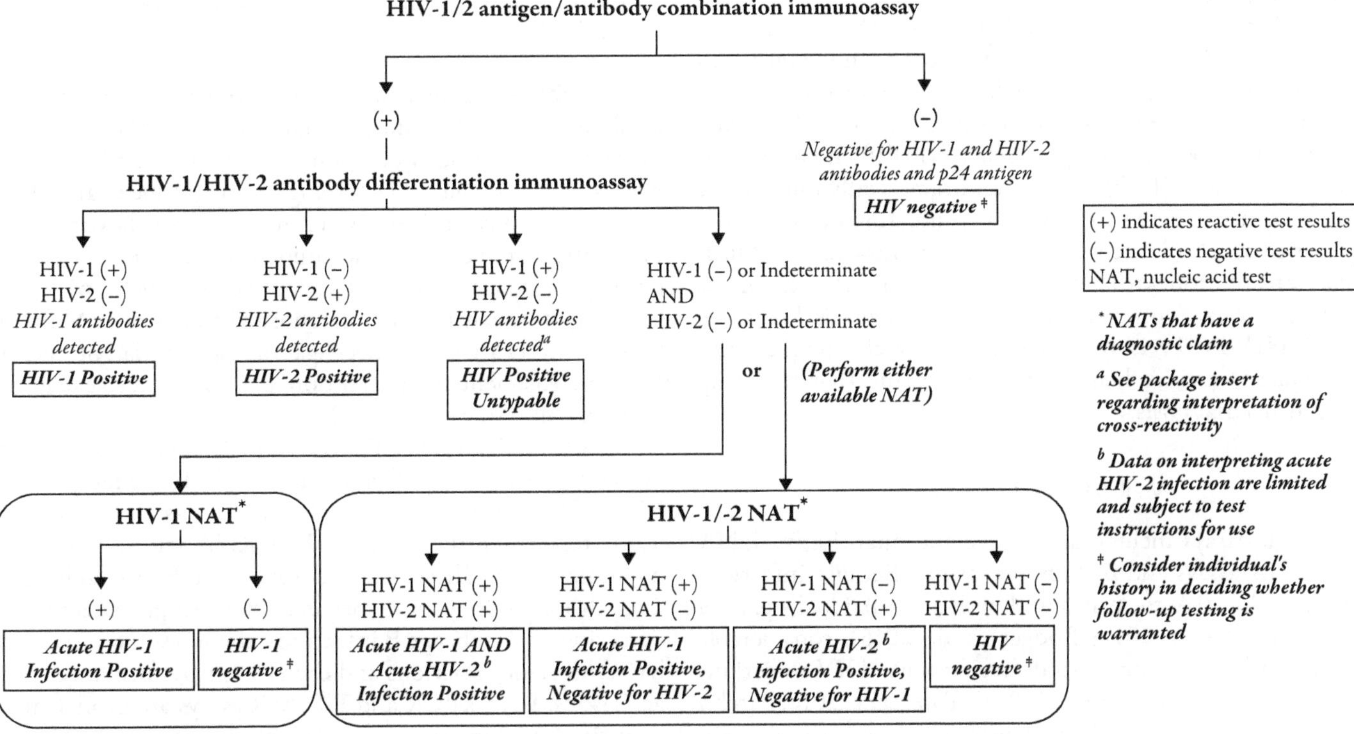

Figure 6.2 CDC recommended laboratory HIV testing algorithm (2023) for serum or plasma specimens. SOURCE: Centers for Disease Control and Prevention and Association of Public Health Laboratories. Technical Update for HIV Nucleic Acid Tests Approved for Diagnostic Purposes. Available at https://www.cdc.gov/hiv/guidelines/recommendations/technical-update-for-hiv.html. Published May 16, 2023. Accessed July 9, 2024.

Table 6.1 HIV TESTING TERMINOLOGY

TEST TYPE	DESCRIPTION
Anonymous testing	No identifying information links the individual to the test sample. At the time of testing, the person is handed a code number, and a matching code number is affixed to the sample. No institutional record of the code is kept. Results are given only verbally because no medical record is created. Treatment cannot be instituted based on this form of testing. Useful for personal informational purposes.
Confidential testing	Test is linked to personal identifiers, and access to results is available for review only by those identified within "need to know" medical standards, including local, state, and national (e.g., CDC) public health agencies.
Screening	Performing an HIV test for all persons in a defined population. For individuals, screening is most cost-effective through an antibody-based test, the most common of which is the enzyme-linked immunosorbent assay (ELISA).
Opt-in screening	The individual approaches the provider and requests HIV testing.
Opt-out screening	Healthcare provider offers routine HIV testing to all individuals unless declined.
Point-of-care or rapid testing	Simplified antibody- or antibody- and antigen-based testing procedure that can give a screening-level result in approximately 20 minutes or less and that can be implemented by a trained non-healthcare individual.
Diagnostic testing	Testing prompted by the presence of clinical signs or symptoms. The term may also refer to the antigen-based confirmation of a positive ELISA. In the United States, the validation test formerly used most often was the western blot analysis. New CDC guidelines now recommend using a fourth-generation HIV Ag/Ab enzyme immunoassay test or HIV RNA test for diagnostic confirmation. The validation testing may also be referred to as *confirmatory testing*.
Targeted testing	Performing an HIV test on persons perceived to be at higher risk, as defined by behavioral, clinical, or demographic characteristics. Formerly the main strategy for HIV testing, it has been supplanted by the recommendation to consider HIV screening as a routine part of medical care.

WESTERN BLOTS

A western blot is another test that detects antibodies by separating the individual proteins of HIV lysate into bands that allow for capturing antibodies specific to selected HIV antigens in an individual's blood or urine (Healey et al., 1992). Assays are reported positive if the bands present meet an established criterion; assays are reported as indeterminate if bands are detected but do not meet the criteria for a positive test (CDC, 1989). Western blots are no longer used in national testing strategies, which evolved to favor more sensitive and less expensive assays (CDC, 2014). However, in the era of pre-exposure prophylaxis (PrEP) and postexposure prophylaxis (PEP) (which can dramatically impact test performance in rare instances when infection occurs in the presence of ART), the western blot may show renewed utility. Consultation with local HIV experts or other resources (e.g., National Clinician Consultation Center's PrEPline, (855) HIV-PrEP) is recommended in such complex and infrequent cases to help coordinate testing that will help establish a diagnosis.

VIROLOGIC ASSAYS

Virologic assays include qualitative and quantitative DNA and RNA assays and p24 antigen assays. Because infection-transmission risk correlates well with an individual's plasma viral load (Chan, 2012; Rodger et al., 2016), considerable attention has been given to detecting acute HIV infections (Cohen et al., 2010; Henn et al., 2017; Patel et al., 2010; Parekh et al., 2018). Individuals experiencing acute infection will typically have relatively high viral loads before seroconverting (Henn et al., 2017). Virologic assays should be considered for the following:

- Diagnosing HIV infection in newborns and infants younger than age 18 months
- Diagnosing acute HIV infections in cases in which individuals would likely not yet have detectable antibodies.

HIV-1 p24 antigen: Fourth- and fifth-generation antigen/antibody combination immunoassays use the HIV-1 p24 core protein as the antigen component and thus can be considered both a serologic and a virologic assay (Stone et al., 2018). Stand-alone p24 antigen assays are available; however, the p24 antigen rapidly becomes undetectable after antibodies develop, thereby limiting the period during which a p24 antigen assay uniquely provides diagnostic information. Multiple p24-only tests are under investigation for a myriad of roles in HIV management and prevention, but no conclusive data are available yet (Gray et al., 2018).

Quantitative HIV-1 RNA assays: Several commercially available nucleic amplification tests (NATs) reliably quantify HIV-1 RNA in plasma, also known as the viral load. These tests quantify plasma HIV-1 RNA within a variable dynamic range. These assays detect most HIV-1 subtypes, and although they have become increasingly effective at detecting non–subtype B infections, there is some variability based on clade variations and each assay's performance characteristics. Both kPCR and RT-PCR assays are proficient at quantitation of many non–clade B strains of HIV-1 (Alvarez et al., 2015; Karasi et al., 2011; Parekh et al., 2018). Because of the rate of false positives, these quantitative assays must be used with caution as a diagnostic test, and most quantitative NATs are not approved by the FDA for diagnosis unless the test has a dual claim allowing it to be used for both HIV-1 diagnosis and clinical management (CDC, 2023b). In acute HIV infection, plasma HIV-1 RNA levels are typically very high, whereas levels of false positives tend to be very low (Henn et al., 2017).

Quantitative HIV-2 RNA assays: Despite increasing use of the HIV-1/HIV-2 differentiation test, few HIV-2 infections are diagnosed in the United States. The CDC continues to recommend that laboratories follow the laboratory-based algorithm with the HIV-1/HIV-2 differentiation test as the second step (Peruski et al., 2020). Moreover, HIV-2 assays are essential in certain locations outside of the United States (Hackett, 2012; Swenson et al., 2014). An FDA-approved quantitative HIV-2 virologic assay is not currently commercially available in the United States. Although some assays may detect a viral load, caution should be exercised when utilizing these results to monitor response to treatment because under-quantification is common when viremia is detected, and not all people with HIV-2 infection will have a detectable viral load (Campbell-Yesufu and Gandhi, 2011). A number of international laboratories use in-house (or laboratory-developed) HIV-2 viral load assays. There are two current labs in the United States with HIV-2 quantitative viral loads available (New York State Department of Health and University of Washington, 2020). Reference laboratory resources are available through the CDC for public health laboratories evaluating HIV-2–reactive specimens.

Qualitative HIV RNA assays: Currently, there are three qualitative virologic assays, frequently referred to as NAAT, which are approved for use by the FDA, as an aid in the diagnosis of HIV. One of these assays (cobas® [Roche Molecular Systems Inc., Branchburg NJ]) detects both HIV-1 and HIV-2 RNA (CDC, 2023b). The other two assays (Aptima® [Hologic Inc., San Diego, CA] and Alinity m [Abbott Molecular, Inc., Des Plaines, IL]) detect HIV-1 RNA only, but these provide both quantitative and qualitative HIV-1 RNA results. The updated CDC HIV testing algorithm incorporating FDA-approved HIV NATs with a diagnostic claim are included in the third step (CDC, 2023b). These assays can be used to assist with diagnosing an acute HIV infection and as an additional test to confirm an HIV-1 infection. Qualitative assays are less commonly available in most clinical laboratories, as viral load monitoring with quantitative assays is the more common application. However, some labs have internally validated the performance of quantitative assays for the application of HIV diagnosis. The qualitative assays' role in point-of-care HIV management, especially in resource-limited settings, is under investigation. Point-of-care HIV viral load testing shows potential due to its ease of use, quick turnaround time for results, and cost-effectiveness (Ochodo et al., 2022). Despite showing acceptable clinical accuracy, more data are required to assess its clinical utility, quality assurance, and its role in future diagnostic algorithms (Agutu et al., 2019).

RAPID HIV TESTS

Rapid HIV tests detect HIV antibodies present in oral fluid, finger-stick (capillary) blood, or venipuncture whole blood/plasma sample. Fourth- and fifth-generation EIAs have shorter detection windows compared to the currently available rapid tests, but rapid tests are as accurate, and test results are available in less than 30 minutes (Kabir et al., 2020). However, there are data that describe lower sensitivity of HIV rapid tests in high-income countries compared to low-income countries, likely because of the larger proportion of acute infections in targeted populations (Tan et al., 2016). They show maximum potential utility in resource-limited settings or to aid timely decision-making processes by avoiding turn-around times (Haleyur Giri Setty and Hewlett, 2014). Individuals with potential exposure and those with ongoing high risk for HIV infection who have negative rapid test results should be counseled to be retested or considered for testing that is more sensitive for detecting acute HIV infections. There are currently more than 15 rapid HIV tests approved by the FDA. Several of these rapid tests have received Clinical Laboratory Improvement Amendment waivers, making them available for point-of-care testing and screening in settings where transporting specimens to a laboratory is either not possible or not practical.

When determining whether to use an approved rapid HIV test or EIA testing for screening and/or diagnosing HIV infections, one should consider the setting in which testing will occur, the cost, and the population being tested. Rapid tests generally cost more than EIA assays, especially if large numbers of tests are being performed. Rapid testing can be beneficial for public health testing programs outside of clinical settings, such as during health fairs or at social venues. Testing on labor and delivery units is another situation in which rapid HIV testing may be a more suitable choice (Haleyur Giri Setty and Hewlett, 2014). Rapid testing platforms for point-of-care HIV RNA testing are also under development (Agutu et al., 2019; Curtis et al., 2016).

TESTING SETTINGS

There are two primary models of HIV testing as per the CDC: routine testing in a standard medical setting and targeted testing in nonclinical settings. Nonclinical settings are sites where medical services are not routinely provided, but select diagnostic services are offered, such as HIV testing. Examples of nonclinical settings include mobile testing units, churches, shelters, syringe service programs, and homes. The essential elements of HIV testing are the same for both a standard medical setting and a nonclinical setting. Facility-based testing uses more sensitive assays, can provide on-site counseling, and accelerates linkage to care. While the goal of HIV testing in a nonclinical setting is to expand access to testing for everyone, it should also focus on linking any persons living with HIV to medical care.

HOME TESTING

HIV self-testing (HIVST) is gaining popularity as a new tool in HIV screening/diagnosis and prevention, with updated guidelines recommending it be offered as an additional approach to traditional HIV testing services (WHO, 2019). Currently, there are only two home HIV tests: the Home Access HIV-1 Test System and the OraQuick In-Home HIV Test. While these seek to empower people and allow them to seek testing outside of healthcare settings, the limitations of oral swab testing are especially worthy of emphasis. HIVST has been shown to have high acceptability in multiple populations (Figueroa et al., 2015; Krause et al., 2013; Stephenson et al., 2017), and could be very promising in low- to middle-income countries (Moshoeu et al., 2019). The processes of dissemination, adoption, and implementation continue to remain significant hurdles, mainly because of challenges with cost, testing performance variability, risk of social harm, and linkage to care (Hurt and Powers, 2014; Johnson et al., 2014; Pant Pai et al., 2013; Ruzagira et al., 2017; WHO, 2019).

The Home Access HIV-1 Test System is a home-collection kit that involves pricking the finger to collect a blood sample, sending the sample to a licensed laboratory, and then calling in for results as early as the next business day. This test is anonymous. If the test is positive, a follow-up test is performed by the lab right away, and the results include the follow-up test. The manufacturer provides confidential counseling and referrals for treatment. The tests conducted on the blood sample collected at home find infection later after exposure than most lab-based tests using blood from a vein but earlier than tests conducted on oral fluid.

The OraQuick In-Home HIV Test is the only HIV test approved by the FDA for home use and self-testing in the United States. OraQuick was approved in 2012 for sale in stores and online to anyone aged 17 years and older. The testing procedure involves swabbing the gums or mucosal surface for an oral fluid sample and using a kit to test it. It tests for HIV-1/2 antibodies in the oral fluid using a swab and delivers results in 20–40 minutes.

If the home test is positive, a follow-up laboratory test will need to be done to confirm the results. The manufacturer provides confidential counseling and referral to follow-up testing sites. Main limitations are lower sensitivity and an extended negative window of at least 3 months after exposure. Because the level of antibody in oral fluid is lower than it is in blood, oral fluid tests detect infection later after exposure compared to blood tests. PrEP or PEP may affect results given their effects on HIV antibody development (Kabir et al., 2020). Up to 1 in 12 people with HIV may falsely test negative.

Data from the eSTAMP trial, a randomized clinical trial evaluating the effectiveness of mailing HIV self-test kits to MSM, showed that compared to control arms, MSM were more likely to test themselves frequently and they identified more HIV infections, did not increase sexually risky behavior, and shared their results with their social network (MacGowan et al., 2020). Despite the lower sensitivity in detecting recent HIV infection, owing to the COVID-19 pandemic, CDC guidelines have added HIVST as options for PrEP monitoring when other options are not available or feasible (home specimen collection kits or self-testing via an oral swab-based test) (CDC, 2024b). In March, 2023, the CDC launched the Together TakeMeHome (TTMH) project, which aims to distribute up to 1 million free HIV self-tests over the next five years. Individuals who are age 17 or older, and regardless of insurance or immigration status, can order up to two free HIV self-tests every 90 days through an online portal (CDC, 2023a).

TESTING IN RESOURCE-LIMITED SETTINGS

Access to early diagnosis of HIV infection is improving in resource-limited settings (Ciaranello et al., 2011), but key barriers continue to exist. Virologic assays are generally more expensive than immunoassays, and additional barriers, such as accurate specimen collection, transport, and laboratory processing, can limit their use in these settings. However, multiple RNA and DNA PCR assays are currently being used, and the use of dried blood spots has decreased the phlebotomy requirements. Dried blood spots may be obtained through a finger or heel stick, are heat stable, noninfectious, and can be shipped via mail or courier (Ciaranello et al., 2011).

POST-TEST COUNSELING

People who undergo HIV testing should be provided post-test counseling, regardless of whether the test is positive or negative. HIV-positive individuals should be informed of their options for treatment and linkage to care.

POSITIVE HIV TEST

Positive HIV results are ideally disclosed during face-to-face meetings in order to optimize opportunities to address individuals' questions and concerns and provide prompt linkage to care. Post-test counseling should, at minimum:

- Review treatments and care options available to individuals, including a discussion of the high effectiveness of antiretroviral therapies
- Provide education about the importance of ongoing medical care
- Provide counseling on transmission-reduction behaviors
- Address disclosure to sexual partner(s) and/or drug-using partners, as well as information on partner services and availability of pre- and post-exposure prophylaxis (PrEP and PEP, respectively) for partners
- Provide counseling targeting stigma reduction (both internalized and perceived stigma), including discussion of U = U and treatment as prevention (TasP)
- Acknowledge individuals' emotions and assess for any intent to harm oneself or others

- Assess for any additional testing needs, including additional STI testing
- Provide referral to additional services, as needed, to address medical and psychosocial needs, including behavioral health counseling, substance use counseling and treatment, reproductive counseling, and case management.

Individuals should be linked to care and initiated on ART as soon as possible, regardless of CD4 count. In settings where comprehensive HIV treatment and care services may not be available, providers should provide prompt linkage to healthcare providers or facilities with specialty expertise in HIV care.

NEGATIVE HIV TEST

Post-test counseling should also be provided for those individuals with a negative HIV test. Depending on the indication for testing (routine testing vs. high-risk exposure or concern for acute infection) and the timing relative to exposure, the validity of a negative test result and the timing of retesting should be assessed. Post-test counseling also provides an opportunity to educate patients on ways to reduce transmission risk, as well as preventive health strategies, such as PrEP, barrier protection use, and safe sex practices. Individuals should also be counseled on and offered comprehensive STI screening. For people with a history of injection drug use, post-test counseling can include education on safe injection practices and syringe services.

PARTNER-NOTIFICATION LEGAL REQUIREMENTS

Many states and some cities have partner-notification laws that require healthcare providers to discuss notification options for sexual or drug injection partners with individuals who test positive for HIV. In some states, violation of partner-notification laws can result in possible civil and/or legal sanctions. States can be categorized into three groups based on their rules and regulations for partner-notification programs: (1) states that require healthcare providers to give the contact's name to the local health officer, and the public health official then notifies the contact; (2) states that give the healthcare provider the choice of notifying either the local health officer or the contacts named by the source patient directly; and (3) states that make such disclosures to a state agency discretionary or optional (Lin and Liang, 2005). Healthcare providers should seek guidance from local public health departments and legal resources as necessary.

In general, PWH should be given the option of directly informing their sexual or needle-sharing contacts. Healthcare providers should be aware of challenges/barriers to HIV disclosure, including fear of being threatened, harmed, or abandoned. When individuals are reluctant to directly disclose their HIV status to partners, partner-notification programs may be helpful (CDC, 2008). For PWH who opt not to inform their partners themselves, these programs typically provide counselors who will inform the at-risk persons of possible HIV exposure without revealing the identity of the person with HIV who may have exposed them. Partner notification may prevent an at-risk individual from acquiring HIV or, if they already have HIV, facilitate linkage to care and treatment initiation. A 2013 Cochrane review of partner-notification strategies in people with an STI/HIV was not able to identify a single optimal method of partner notification (Ferreira et al., 2013). A recent analysis of partner service data submitted to the CDC from 2013 to 2017 found that 97.2% of partners were notified of their potential HIV exposure (Song et al., 2022). However, only 52.3% of partners were tested for HIV, and 23.8% of tested partners were diagnosed with HIV. Additional information can be obtained in Chapter 38, "Legal Issues."

ACKNOWLEDGMENTS

The authors would like to acknowledge the contributions to previous editions of this chapter by Alejandro Delgado, MD.

RECOMMENDED READING

CDC. Technical update for HIV nucleic acid tests approved for diagnostic purposes [Online]. Centers for Disease Control and Prevention and Association of Public Health Laboratories. 2023. https://www.cdc.gov/hiv/guidelines/recommendations/technical-update-for-hiv.html. Accessed July 9, 2024.

Department of Health and Human Services (DHHS). HIV national strategic plan for the United States: a roadmap to end the epidemic 2021–2025 [Online]. Washington, DC: U.S. Department of Health and Human Services; 2021. Accessed July 7, 2024.

DHHS. Recommendations for the use of antiretroviral drugs during pregnancy and interventions to reduce perinatal HIV transmission in the United States [Online]. Department of Health and Human Services. 2024. https://clinicalinfo.hiv.gov/en/guidelines/perinatal. Accessed July 7, 2024.

DiNenno EA, Delaney KP, Pitasi MA, et al. HIV testing before and during the COVID-19 pandemic—United States, 2019–2020. *MMWR*. 2022;71:820–824.

DiNenno EA, Prejean J, Irwin K, et al. Recommendations for HIV screening of gay, bisexual, and other men who have sex with men—United States, 2017. *MMWR*. 2017;66(31):830–832.

Hecht J, Sanchez T, Sullivan PS, et al. Increasing access to HIV testing through direct-to-consumer HIV self-test distribution—United States, March 31, 2020–March 30, 2021. *MMWR*. 2021;70:1322–1325.

Wejnert P. Prevalence of missed opportunities for HIV testing among persons unaware of their infection. *JAMA*. 2018;319(24):2555.

REFERENCES

Agutu CA. Ngetsa CJ, Price MA, et al. Systematic review of the performance and clinical utility of point of care HIV-1 RNA testing for diagnosis and care. *PLoS One*. 2019;14:e0218369.

Alvarez P, Martín L, Prieto L, et al. HIV-1 variability and viral load technique could lead to false positive HIV-1 detection and to erroneous viral quantification in infected specimens. *J Infect*. 2015;71:368–376.

Bagchi AD, Davis T. Clinician barriers and facilitators to routine HIV testing: a systematic review of the literature. *J Int Assoc Provid AIDS Care*. 2020;19:1–17.

Branson BM, Hansfield HH, Lampe MA, et al. Revised recommendations for HIV testing of adults, adolescents, and pregnant women in health-care settings. *MMWR Recomm Rep*. 2006;55:1–17.

Campbell-Yesufu OT, Gandhi RT. 2011. Update on human immunodeficiency virus (HIV)-2 infection. *Clin Infect Dis*. 2011;52:780–787.

Centers for Disease Control and Prevention (CDC). Dear colleague: announcing the launch of Together TakeMeHome. Centers for Disease Control and Prevention. https://www.cdc.gov/nchhstp/director-letters/launch-of-together-takemehome.html. Published March 21, 2023a. Accessed July 9, 2024.

CDC. Estimated HIV incidence and prevalence in the United States, 2018–2022. HIV Surveillance Supplemental Report 2024. [Online]. Centers for Disease Control and Prevention. Available: https://www.cdc.gov/hiv-data/nhss/estimated-hiv-incidence-and-prevalence.html. Published May 21, 2024a. Accessed July 9, 2024.

CDC. Interpretation and use of the western blot assay for serodiagnosis of human immunodeficiency virus type 1 infections. *MMWR Suppl*. 1989;38(7):1–7.

CDC. Issue brief: the role of HIV self-testing in ending the HIV epidemic. [Online]. Centers for Disease Control and Prevention (CDC). https://www.cdc.gov/hiv/policies/data/self-testing-issue-brief.html. Published May 16, 2024b. Accessed July 9, 2024.

CDC. Laboratory testing for the diagnosis of HIV infection: updated recommendations. http://dx.doi.org/10.15620/cdc.23447. Published June 27, 2014. Accessed August 22, 2024.

CDC. Missed opportunities for earlier diagnosis of HIV infection—South Carolina, 1997–2005. *MMWR*. 2006;55:1269–1272.

CDC. Perspectives in disease prevention and health promotion public health service guidelines for counseling and antibody testing to prevent HIV infection and AIDS. *MMWR*. 1987;36:509–515.

CDC. Recommendations for partner services programs for HIV infection, syphilis, gonorrhea, and chlamydial infection. *MMWR Recomm Rep*. 2008;57:1–83.

CDC. Technical update for HIV nucleic acid tests approved for diagnostic purposes. Centers for Disease Control and Prevention and Association of Public Health Laboratories. https://www.cdc.gov/hiv/guidelines/recommendations/technical-update-for-hiv.html. Published May 16, 2023b. Accessed July 9, 2024.

CDC. Update: serologic testing for antibody to human immunodeficiency virus. *MMWR*. 1988;36:833–840, 845.

CDC. Update: serologic testing for HIV-1 antibody—United States, 1988 and 1989. *MMWR*. 1990;39:380–383.

CDC. US Public Health Service: Preexposure prophylaxis for the prevention of HIV infection in the United States—2021 update: a clinical practice guideline. Centers for Disease Control and Prevention. https://www.cdc.gov/hiv/pdf/risk/prep/cdc-hiv-prep-guidelines-2021.pdf. Published 2021. Accessed August 22, 2024.

Chan DJ. Can HIV-1 incidence be estimated from plasma viral load and sexual behaviour? *Int J STD AIDS*. 2012;23:724–728.

Chappel RJ, Wilson KM, Dax EM. Immunoassays for the diagnosis of HIV: meeting future needs by enhancing the quality of testing. *Future Microbiol*. 2009;4:963–982.

Chen Z, Branson B, Ballenger A Peterman TA. Risk assessment to improve targeting of HIV counseling and testing services for STD clinic patients. *Sex Transm Dis*. 1998;25:539–43.

Ciaranello AL, Park JE, Ramirez-Avila L, et al. Early infant HIV-1 diagnosis programs in resource-limited settings: opportunities for improved outcomes and more cost-effective interventions. *BMC Med*. 2011;9:59.

Cohen MS, Gay CL, Busch MP, Hecht FM. The detection of acute HIV infection. *J Infect Dis*. 2010;202 Suppl 2:S270–S277.

Curtis KA, Rudolph DL, Morrison D, et al. Single-use, electricity-free amplification device for detection of HIV-1. *J Virol Methods*. 2016;237:132–137.

Department of Health and Human Services (DHHS). *HIV National Strategic Plan for the United States: A Roadmap to End the Epidemic 2021–2025*. Washington, DC: U.S. Department of Health and Human Services; 2021. https://files.hiv.gov/s3fs-public/HIV-National-Strategic-Plan-2021-2025.pdf. Accessed July 7, 2024.

DHHS. *Recommendations for the Use of Antiretroviral Drugs During Pregnancy and Interventions to Reduce Perinatal HIV Transmission in the United States*. Washington, DC: U.S. Department of Health and Human Services; 2024. https://clinicalinfo.hiv.gov/en/guidelines/perinatal. Accessed July 7, 2024.

Diepstra KL, Cunningham T, Rhodes AG, et al. Prevalence and predictors of provider-initiated HIV test offers among heterosexual persons at increased risk for acquiring HIV infection—Virginia, 2016. *MMWR*. 2018;67:714–717.

DiNenno EA, Delaney KP, Pitasi MA, et al. HIV testing before and during the COVID-19 pandemic—United States, 2019–2020. *MMWR*. 2022;71:820–824.

DiNenno EA, Prejean J, Irwin K, et al. Recommendations for HIV screening of gay, bisexual, and other men who have sex with men—United States, 2017. *MMWR*. 2017;66(31):830–832.

Fauci AS, Redfield RR, Sigounas G, et al. Ending the HIV Epidemic: a plan for the United States. *JAMA*. 2019:321:844–845.

Ferreira A, Young T, Mathews C, et al. Strategies for partner notification for sexually transmitted infections, including HIV. *Cochrane Database Syst Rev*. 2013(10):CD002843.

Figueroa C, Johnson C, Verster A, Baggaley R. Attitudes and acceptability on HIV self-testing among key populations: a literature review. *AIDS Behav*. 2015;19:1949–1965.

Frieden TR, Foti KE, Mermin J. Applying public health principles to the HIV epidemic—how are we doing? *N Engl J Med*. 2015;373:2281–2287.

Goetz MB, Hoang T, Knapp H, et al. Central implementation strategies outperform local ones in improving HIV testing in Veterans Healthcare Administration facilities. *J Gen Intern Med*. 2013;28:1311–1317.

Gray ER, Bain R, Varsaneux O, et al. p24 revisited: a landscape review of antigen detection for early HIV diagnosis. *AIDS*. 2018;32:2089–2102.

Hackett J Jr. Meeting the challenge of HIV diversity: strategies to mitigate the impact of HIV-1 genetic heterogeneity on performance of nucleic acid testing assays. *Clin Lab*. 2012;58:199–202.

Haleyur Giri Setty MK, Hewlett IK. Point of care technologies for HIV. *AIDS Res Treat*. 2014:2014:497046. doi:10.1155/2014/497042014, 497046.

Halpern SD. HIV testing without consent in critically ill patients. *JAMA*. 2005;294:734–737.

Healey DS, Maskill WJ, Howard TS, et al. HIV-1 western blot: development and assessment of testing to resolve indeterminate reactivity. *AIDS*. 1992;6:629–633.

Hecht J, Sanchez T, Sullivan PS, et al. Increasing access to HIV testing through direct-to-consumer HIV self-test distribution—United States, March 31, 2020–March 30, 2021. *MMWR*. 2021;70:1322–1325.

Henn A, Flateau C, Gallien S. Primary HIV infection: clinical presentation, testing, and treatment. *Curr Infect Dis Rep*. 2017;19(10):37.

Hoover KW, Huang YA, Tanner ML, et al. HIV testing trends at visits to physician offices, community health centers, and emergency departments—United States, 2009–2017. *MMWR*. 2020;69:776–780.

Houn HY, Pappas AA, Walker EM Jr. Status of current clinical tests for human immunodeficiency virus (HIV): applications and limitations. *Ann Clin Lab Sci*. 1987;17:279–285.

Hurt CB, Powers KA. 2014. Self-testing for HIV and its impact on public health. *Sex Transm Dis*. 2014;41:10–12.

Indravudh PP, Fielding K, Kumwenda MK, et al. Effect of community-led delivery of HIV self-testing on HIV testing and antiretroviral therapy initiation in Malawi: A cluster-randomised trial. *PLoS Med*. 2021;18: e1003608.

Johnson C, Baggaley R, Forsythe S, et al. Realizing the potential for HIV self-testing. *AIDS Behav*. 2014;18:Suppl 4:S391–S395.

Kabir MA, Zilouchian H, Caputi M, Asghar W. Advances in HIV diagnosis and monitoring. *Crit Rev Biotechnol*. 2020;40:623–638.

Kamb ML, Fishbein M, Douglas JM Jr, et al. Efficacy of risk-reduction counseling to prevent human immunodeficiency virus and sexually transmitted diseases: a randomized controlled trial. Project RESPECT Study Group. *JAMA*. 1998;280: 1161–1167.
Karasi JC, Dziezuk F, Quennery L, et al. High correlation between the Roche COBAS® AmpliPrep/COBAS® TaqMan® HIV-1, v2.0 and the Abbott m2000 RealTime HIV-1 assays for quantification of viral load in HIV-1 B and non-B subtypes. *J Clin Virol*. 2011;52:181–186.
Koblin B, Chesney M, Coates T. Effects of a behavioural intervention to reduce acquisition of HIV infection among men who have sex with men: the EXPLORE randomised controlled study. *Lancet*. 2004;364:41–50.
Kourtis AP, Bulterys M, Nesheim SR, Lee FK. Understanding the timing of HIV transmission from mother to infant. *JAMA*. 2001;285:709–712.
Krause J, Subklew-Sehume F, Kenyon C, Colebunders R. Acceptability of HIV self-testing: a systematic literature review. *BMC Public Health*. 2013;13:735.
Lee K, Trujillo L, Olansky E, et al. Factors associated with use of HIV prevention and health care among transgender women—seven urban areas, 2019–2020. *MMWR*. 2022;71:673–679.
Lin L, Liang BA. HIV and health law: striking the balance between legal mandates and medical ethics. *Virtual Mentor*. 2005;7(10):virtualmentor.2005.7.10.hlaw1-0510. Published 2005 Oct 1. https://doi:10.1001/virtualmentor.2005.7.10.hlaw1-0510.
Lin X, Dietz PM, Rodriguez V, et al. 2014. Routine HIV screening in two health-care settings—New York City and New Orleans, 2011–2013. *MMWR*. 2014;63:537–541.
Louie B, Pandori MW, Wong E, et al. Use of an acute seroconversion panel to evaluate a third-generation enzyme-linked immunoassay for detection of human immunodeficiency virus-specific antibodies relative to multiple other assays. *J Clin Microbiol*. 2006;44:1856–1858.
MacGowan RJ, Chavez PR, Borkowf CB, et al. Effect of internet-distributed HIV self-tests on HIV diagnosis and behavioral outcomes in men who have sex with men: a randomized clinical trial. *JAMA Intern Med*. 2020;180:117–125.
Marks G, Crepaz N, Janssen RS. Estimating sexual transmission of HIV from persons aware and unaware that they are infected with the virus in the USA. *AIDS*. 2006;20:1447–1450.
Momplaisir FM, Brady KA, Fekete T, et al. Time of HIV diagnosis and engagement in prenatal care impact virologic outcomes of pregnant women with HIV. *PLoS One*. 2015;10:e0132262.
Moshoeu MP, Kuupiel D, Gwala N, Mashamba-Thompson TP. The use of home-based HIV testing and counseling in low-and-middle income countries: a scoping review. *BMC Public Health*. 2019;19:132.
Neff S, Goldschmidt R. Centers for Disease Control and Prevention 2006 human immunodeficiency virus testing recommendations and state testing laws. *JAMA*. 2011;305:1767–1768.
Ochodo EA, Olwanda EE, Deeks JJ, Mallett S. Point-of-care viral load tests to detect high HIV viral load in people living with HIV/AIDS attending health facilities. *Cochrane Database Syst Rev*. 2022; 3(3):CD013208.
Pandori MW, Hackett J Jr, Louie B, et al. Assessment of the ability of a fourth-generation immunoassay for human immunodeficiency virus (HIV) antibody and p24 antigen to detect both acute and recent HIV infections in a high-risk setting. *J Clin Microbiol*. 2009;47:2639–2642.
Pant Pai N, Sharma J, Shivkumar S, et al. Supervised and unsupervised self-testing for HIV in high- and low-risk populations: a systematic review. *PLoS Med*. 2013;10:e1001414.
Parekh BS, Ou CY, Fonjungo PN, et al. Diagnosis of human immunodeficiency virus infection. *Clin Microbiol Rev*. 2018;32(1):e00064–18.
Patel P, Mackellar D, Simmons P, et al. Detecting acute human immunodeficiency virus infection using 3 different screening immunoassays and nucleic acid amplification testing for human immunodeficiency virus RNA, 2006–2008. *Arch Intern Med*. 2010;170(1):66–74.
Peruski AH, Wesolowski LG, Delaney KP, et al. Trends in HIV-2 diagnoses and use of the HIV-1/HIV-2 differentiation test—United States, 2010–2017. *MMWR*. 2020;69:63–66.
Pitasi MA, Beer L, Cha S, et al. Vital signs: HIV infection, diagnosis, treatment, and prevention among gay, bisexual, and other men who have sex with men—United States, 2010–2019. *MMWR*. 2021;70:1669–1675.
Rodger AJ, Cambiano V, Bruun T, et al. Sexual activity without condoms and risk of HIV transmission in serodifferent couples when the HIV-positive partner is using suppressive antiretroviral therapy. *JAMA*. 2016;316:171–181.
Rosenberg NE, Pilcher CD, Busch MP, Cohen,MS. How can we better identify early HIV infections? *Curr Opin HIV AIDS*. 2015;10:61–68.
Ruzagira E, Baisley K, Kamali A, et al. Linkage to HIV care after home-based HIV counselling and testing in sub-Saharan Africa: a systematic review. *Trop Med Int Health*. 2017;22(7):807–882.
Sickinger E, Stieler M, Kaufman B, et al. Multicenter evaluation of a new, automated enzyme-linked immunoassay for detection of human immunodeficiency virus-specific antibodies and antigen. *J Clin Microbiol*. 2004;42:21–29.
Song W, Mulatu MS, Rao S, et al. Factors associated with partner notification, testing, and positivity in HIV partner services programs in the United States, 2013 to 2017. *Sex Transm Dis*. 2022;49: 197–203.
Stephenson R, Freeland R, Sullivan SP, et al. Home-based HIV testing and counseling for male couples (Project Nexus): a protocol for a randomized controlled trial. *JMIR Res Protoc*. 2017;6:e101.
Stone M, Bainbridge J, Sanchez AM, et al. Comparison of detection limits of fourth- and fifth-generation combination HIV antigen-antibody, p24 antigen, and viral load assays on diverse HIV isolates. *J Clin Microbiol*. 2018; 56(8):e02045–17.
Swenson LC, Cobb B, Geretti AM, et al. Comparative performances of HIV-1 RNA load assays at low viral load levels: results of an international collaboration. *J Clin Microbiol*. 2014;52:517–523.
Tan WS, Chow EP, Fairley CK, et al. Sensitivity of HIV rapid tests compared with fourth-generation enzyme immunoassays or HIV RNA tests. *AIDS*. 2016;30:1951–1960.
United States Preventive Services Task Force (USPSTF). Screening for HIV infection: US Preventive Services Task Force recommendation statement. *JAMA*. 2019;321:2326–2336.
Wesolowski LG, Parker MM, Delaney KP, Owen SM. Highlights from the 2016 HIV diagnostics conference: the new landscape of HIV testing in laboratories, public health programs and clinical practice. *J Clin Virol*. 2017;91:63–68.
WHO. Consolidated guidelines on HIV testing services for a changing epidemic [Online]. World Health Organization (WHO). https://www.who.int/publications/i/item/consolidated-guidelines-on-hiv-testing-services-for-a-changing-epidemic. Published 2019. Accessed September 26, 2022.
World Health Organization (WHO). *Guidelines on HIV and Infant Feeding 2010: Principles and Recommendations for Infant Feeding in the Context of HIV and a Summary of Evidence*. Geneva: World Health Organization; 2010.

7.

INITIAL EVALUATION OF THE PATIENT WITH HIV

HISTORY, PHYSICAL EXAMINATION, AND LABORATORY EVALUATION

Esteban DelPilar Morales

LEARNING OBJECTIVES

Describe key details of the history and physical examination and appropriate laboratory evaluation for the initial clinical evaluation of a person with HIV (PWH). List unique considerations for the initial evaluation of PWH for some key populations.

WHAT'S NEW?

Gender identity and cultural challenges remain important considerations for the care of some PWH. Given the increasing use of integrase inhibitors (for both HIV prevention and treatment) in resource-rich and resource-limited settings, HIV providers should be familiar with indications for integrase inhibitor resistance testing.

Telehealth continues to be an acceptable and highly utilized care delivery model, including for PWH.

KEY POINTS

- A comprehensive history, including a complete sexual and social history, is key to helping assess an individual's health-associated behaviors and goals, motivations, and potential challenges.
- A comprehensive baseline physical examination and laboratory evaluation are important to help identify any abnormal findings at the time of initial engagement in care which may require prompt intervention, and to provide a baseline and comparison for future examinations.
- Awareness of a person's gender identity and cultural background will allow the healthcare provider to better understand the person's lived experience and is fundamental in caring for PWH.
- PWH presenting for their initial clinic visit may have early infection, asymptomatic chronic infection, or advanced HIV. Recognition of the clinical stage of infection is important so that appropriate prophylactic medications can be prescribed and counseling appropriate to the stage of infection can be provided.

THE HIV-ORIENTED MEDICAL HISTORY

There are several objectives for an initial office/clinic visit with a PWH (either newly diagnosed or with chronic infection). The most obvious purpose is to obtain the necessary information essential for current and future clinical management. Healthcare providers should be cognizant of the fact that some PWH may not feel comfortable disclosing all relevant medical and social history at the first visit. In most cases, as the patient-provider relationship develops over time, people may feel more comfortable sharing information at subsequent visits. The initial visit also represents an opportunity to establish a trust-based relationship between patient and provider. It is important that the provider uses a nonjudgmental tone and provides a safe and supportive environment, as this is more likely to result in a trusting relationship. The patient-provider relationship can affect how a patient views the information and advice received from a provider, including beliefs about the effectiveness of prescribed medications (Berghoff et al., 2018). A strong patient-provider relationship has also been shown to result in improved engagement and retention in care and medication adherence and is predictive of future therapeutic success (Doshi et al., 2015; Flickinger et al., 2013).

If the PWH is accompanied by another person (e.g., friend, spouse, partner, family member), the provider should not assume the accompanying person is aware of the patient's HIV diagnosis or other medical history. Prior to proceeding, the provider should determine if the accompanying person is aware of the patient's HIV status without disclosing the diagnosis. Our practice is to first ask the patient if they prefer the accompanying person to be present during the evaluation or to leave the room. If the patient indicates they want the person to stay, the provider should then ask whether it is okay to discuss "everything" and/or to ask the accompanying person, "Do you know why (patient name) is here today?" In some cases, the accompanying person will indicate that the patient is here for HIV care; however, if it is still not clear that the person is aware of the patient's HIV diagnosis, the provider should ask the person to leave the room so they can ask the patient in private, without disclosing the HIV diagnosis.

A comprehensive history and physical examination, as well as past medical history, social and family history, review of systems, and review of all current and prior medications

Table 7.1 RECOMMENDED PHYSICAL EXAM OF PERSONS WITH HIV (PWH)

BODY ORGAN/ SYSTEM	BE ESPECIALLY ATTENTIVE TO:
Vital signs	Weight loss, body mass index, fat distribution, blood pressure, pulse, respiration rate, temperature
General	Body habitus, nutritional status, pain/tenderness, obvious disabilities
Skin	Rash, seborrheic dermatitis, folliculitis, melanocytic nevi (moles), psoriasis, lichen planus, Kaposi's sarcoma lesions Warts, vesicular lesions, dermatophytes, molluscum contagiosum Needle marks
Head, eyes, ears, nose, and throat (HEENT)	Visual acuity Retinal hemorrhages and exudates (suggestive of CMV) HIV retinopathy (cotton-wool spots) Oral exam: thrush, oral hairy leukoplakia, Kaposi's lesions, gingivitis, aphthous ulcers, chancres, dentition, herpetic lesions, angular cheilitis Thyroid exam
Hemolymphatic	Regional versus generalized lymphadenopathy Splenomegaly
Cardiac	Heart sounds, murmurs, gallop
Pulmonary	Focal or generalized abnormalities
Gastrointestinal	Jaundice, hepatomegaly Abdominal masses Anorectal exam (ulcers, vesicles, chancres, masses, hemorrhoids, warts)
Genitourinary	Ulcers, warts, chancres, herpetic vesicles Gender-specific exam: For people assigned female at birth: pelvic exam, cervical exam For people assigned male at birth: testicular exam
Neurologic	Mental status, cognitive function—consider baseline HIV cognitive assessment (e.g., Montreal Cognitive Assessment test or Mini Mental Status Exam) Cranial nerves, motor strength, sensation, gait, vibratory/proprioceptive exam
Psychiatric	Depression screen should be done at baseline (PHQ-2 or other validated tools) Evidence of self-injury or self-mutilation Evidence of abuse/trauma

and medication allergies, should be performed at the initial visit (Table 7.1, Box 7.1, and Table 7.2). In addition to being aware of possible risk factors for the rapid progression of HIV-related illness and potential complications, the provider should determine the emotional status of the PWH and if they have any issues that may adversely affect adherence, clinical appointment attendance, ability to pay for medications (if necessary), and whether there is sufficient social support.

In addition to the standard history, the following specific items should be addressed:

- Try to determine the emotional status of the patient: What is the level of anxiety regarding their HIV diagnosis? How are they adjusting to the diagnosis? Do they have an established social support network?
- Has the patient disclosed their HIV status to anyone (e.g., partner, family member[s], or friend[s])?
- Have sexual partners (or needle-sharing partners) been exposed to infectious body fluids, which may put them at risk for acquiring HIV? Have they been notified and tested? If not, would the patient be interested in receiving assistance to contact past or recent sexual or needle-sharing partners to discuss HIV screening/testing as well as postexposure prophylaxis (PEP) and/or pre-exposure prophylaxis (PrEP)?

An important aspect of the initial clinic encounter is to determine how the PWH is adjusting to their HIV diagnosis (particularly if newly diagnosed) and their emotional status. It is appropriate to ask if they have shared their diagnosis with anyone (e.g., friends, partner[s], family member[s], or close contacts) (Yu et al., 2018). Non- disclosure of HIV status may be associated with lower medication adherence and increased anxiety. While some PWHs are fearful of the reaction of others to whom they disclose, we generally encourage people to consider disclosing to close, trusted friends and/or family members who may be able to provide support. In our experience, disclosure to close family members or friends often leads to more emotional support, less anxiety, and improved patient well-being. The provider should also ask the patient, "What concerns and fears do you have?" Often, asking and answering

Box 7.1 KEY ELEMENTS IN THE HISTORY/ CURRENT HEALTH STATUS AND REVIEW OF SYSTEMS

- *CONSTITUTIONAL*: INTENTIONAL/ UNINTENTIONAL WEIGHT CHANGE, FEVER, CHILLS, NIGHT SWEATS, FATIGUE, MALAISE
- ***Head, eyes, ears, nose, and throat (HEENT)***: Hearing changes, ear pain, nasal congestion, sinus pain, hoarseness, sore throat, rhinorrhea, swallowing difficulty, oral lesion, eye pain, swelling, redness, foreign body, discharge, vision changes (floaters or blurred vision)
- ***Cardiovascular***: Chest pain, dyspnea, orthopnea, claudication, edema, palpitations
- ***Respiratory***: Cough, sputum, bloody sputum, wheezing, shortness of breath
- ***Gastrointestinal***: Nausea, vomiting, diarrhea, constipation, pain, heartburn, anorexia, dysphagia, hematochezia, melena, flatulence, jaundice
- ***Genitourinary***: Dysmenorrhea, bleeding, dyspareunia, dysuria, urinary frequency, hematuria, urinary incontinence, urgency, flank pain, urinary flow changes, hesitancy, genital lesion
- ***Musculoskeletal***: Arthralgias, myalgias, joint swelling, joint stiffness, back pain, neck pain, injury history
- ***Skin***: Skin lesion, pruritus, hair changes, breast/skin changes, nipple discharge, rash
- ***Neurologic***: Weakness, numbness, paresthesia, loss of consciousness, syncope, dizziness, headache, coordination changes, recent falls
- ***Psychiatric***: Anxiety/panic, depression, insomnia, personality changes, delusions, rumination, suicidal ideation, homicidal ideation, hallucinations, social issues, memory changes, violence/abuse history, eating concerns
- ***Hematologic***: Bruising, bleeding, transfusion history, lymphadenopathy
- ***Endocrine***: Polyuria, polydipsia, heat or cold intolerance

this question can reduce patient anxiety by dispelling myths or misinformation the patient may have heard or read about (Ruffell 2017).

THE MORE A PATIENT KNOWS, THE BETTER THEY CAN CARE FOR THEMSELF

Assessing the PWH's level of understanding of the disease process and the importance of antiretroviral and other medications is important in comprehensive HIV care. Studies have demonstrated that PWH with more knowledge of their disease status do better over time. Incomplete medication knowledge has been associated with lower adherence (Miller et al., 2003; Molla et al., 2018). Levels of sophistication and understanding may differ depending on a person's background, education, health literacy, years of infection, and other factors. Lower educational level does not correlate with lower adherence (Kim et al., 2018). Any opportunity to emphasize education, understanding, and knowledge of the disease state should be fully embraced.

Providers should not assume that patients have a thorough understanding of HIV, even for people with long-standing infections. Open-ended questions such as the following may be helpful: "What do you know about HIV?"; "What do you think you can do to maintain your health long term?"; and "Do you understand the significance of the HIV viral load and T-cell count?"

The provider (or another care team member) should explain, using terms and language appropriate to the patient's health literacy, the significance and meaning of CD4/T cells, HIV viral load, opportunistic infections, and risks and behaviors associated with possible HIV transmission. The "teach back" method is useful to demonstrate the patient's level of understanding and improve treatment adherence in people with chronic diseases (Ha Dinh et al., 2016).

THE PATIENT-PROVIDER RELATIONSHIP

Medical care for PWH should be patient centered, with the primary focus on the person's needs and preferences. Care should be sensitive to the individual's educational, cultural, and socioeconomic background. Understanding each person in their unique circumstances not only helps establish trust, it has also been shown to increase adherence to treatment (Ciechanowski et al., 2001). Previous studies have shown that PWH who feel that their HIV provider is providing personalized, patient-centered care are more likely to be adherent to treatment and to achieve an undetectable viral load (Beach et al., 2006). Ideally the patient-provider relationship will be strengthened with each encounter as the PWH gains more confidence and comfort with the provider.

More recent studies have indicated that motivational interviewing is an effective, evidence-based, and patient-centered communication strategy that enhances readiness for behavioral changes. It can help patients improve their motivation and treatment adherence. Motivational interviewing typically involves empathic listening, shared decision-making, and a change-focused talk, which should elicit personal motivation for behavioral changes (Sued et al., 2022).

SENSITIVE, RESPECTFUL, AND NONJUDGMENTAL

HIV providers frequently care for people with a wide variety of sexual practices, people who have been victims of abuse, people who are/have been commercial sex workers, people who have used intravenous drugs, and individuals in the lesbian/

Table 7.2 KEY CLINICAL HISTORY ELEMENTS TO OBTAIN AT THE INITIAL HIV VISIT

ELEMENT	DETAILS	COMMENTS
HIV-specific history	• Date of seroconversion (if known) • Risk factors for transmission • CD4 count: nadir and pretreatment (if already on treatment) • Detailed history of previous antiretroviral treatment regimens as well as related adverse effects (if any) • Prior HIV drug resistance testing (if any) and HLA-B*5701 (if done)	Patients previously treated might not recall all past treatments. Medical records from previous providers should be obtained.
Past medical history	• Viral hepatitis: Coinfection with hepatitis B or hepatitis C is common, and can progress faster in PWH • Cardiovascular risk/disease: Hypertension, diabetes mellitus, dyslipidemia can affect choice of ART • Other comorbidities: Chronic kidney disease (CKD), endocrine disorders, cerebrovascular disease, etc. • Malignancies: Increased incidence in PWH, some might be indicative of AIDS • OB/GYN: Prior pregnancies, present contraceptives (if any), previous cervical Pap smears and mammography results, potential plans for future pregnancies • Tuberculosis: Risk factors and potential exposures • Previous hospitalizations • Surgeries (including complications, if any) • Childhood infections	Should focus on presence of common comorbidities, particularly those that might affect choice of ART or response to it
Sexual history	• Gender identity and sexual orientation • Sexual partners: Number and gender of partners • Type of sexual activities: Oral, vaginal, anal, use of inanimate objects/sexual toys • Use of condoms: Type and frequency • Activities associated with sex: Alcohol/drug consumption, exchange for favors (money, goods, etc.) • STIs: Any previous diagnosis and treatments • Partners: HIV status and other STIs	Risk of STIs varies greatly if patients are identified by gender identity and sexual orientation rather than just sex (male or female). Can identify PWH who might be candidates for cervical/anal cytology (Pap smears) Can help identify potential sites of testing (example: oral testing for chlamydia in patient that performs oral sex)
Psychiatric history	• Diagnosis and treatments • Sleep patterns: could indicate underlying depression or adverse effects of ART	Depression is frequent in PWH: if not adequately managed can significantly decrease adherence
Medications and allergies	• List all medications presently taken (including over-the-counter and supplements) • Allergies and reactions	Some over-the-counter medications and supplements may interact with ART. Note allergic reaction and severity as well as date of first/last occurrence (if known)
Social history	• Employment and travel: Provides insight into potential exposures and risk factors/behaviors • Alcohol and tobacco use • Substance use: Obtain details of what type, frequency, and method of administration • Domestic/intimate partner violence: Does the patient feel safe at home? • Hobbies and pastimes • Animal/pet exposure	Will provide insight into the patient's safety net and social/home support Can identify potential barriers to treatment
Family history	• First-degree family members • Any family member known to have HIV	May identify potential risk factor for cardiovascular disease, cancers Can provide information regarding support in the family if other members have HIV
Immunizations	• All vaccines with dates (if possible)	Will help determine which vaccines the patient may still require
Healthcare maintenance	• Per guidelines, based on age and other risk factors	Preventive interventions vary by age, gender, and exposures.
Healthcare system information	• Other healthcare providers caring for the patient • Primary contact information (including emergency contacts) • Healthcare proxy and anyone authorized to access patient information • Advance directives • Disclosure information	Patient might want restricted access to their information (including spouse/partner occasionally) Important to reinforce the confidential nature of the information provided

gay/bisexual/transgender/queer (LGBTQ+) communities. Issues of privacy and cultural sensitivity are especially relevant in these encounters. Fostering trust—encouraging truthfulness and openness in the patient-provider relationship—requires special and careful attention to cultivating a nonjudgmental, approachable demeanor. It is important to be sensitive to the individual's priorities, to be respectful of their individuality, and to be aware of their self-perception. When engaging LGBTQ+ individuals it is also important to understand their specific needs and challenges, particularly when obtaining a sexual history (Bass and Nagy, 2024). It is important to understand the terms they prefer to use to describe their sexuality and their sex roles. Providers should be aware that everyone does not feel comfortable with all terms related to the LGBTQ+ community, and that it will be part of the discussion to determine which ones the individual prefers. This is important not only for providers, but for all staff members who interact with the patient.

CULTURAL COMPETENCY AND HUMILITY

It is important for clinicians to be aware of the unique cultural background of each PWH, as theirs may be quite different from that of the clinician providing care. PWH are ethnically and culturally diverse, spanning the spectrum of socioeconomic status. Cultural awareness can identify substantial economic disadvantages, pervasive childhood adversity, limited education, and limited resources that jointly put members of a particular community at risk for the acquisition of HIV, development of depression, and substance use disorders (Le et al., 2016). The effects of cultural competency in the care of PWH were identified early in the HIV epidemic, and its impacts were notable (O'Connor, 1996). Evidence shows that the non-inclusion of cultural norms and values of target populations can act as stumbling blocks in effective communication (Uwah, 2013).

Cultural competency involves not only racial identity but also sexual orientation and gender identity. Cultural humility is an ongoing process of self-reflection and willingness to learn from others, which helps providers better understand and respect cultural differences, if present. At times, specific groups of people can feel disenfranchised if they feel their cultural identity is not being taken into consideration (Shover et al., 2018). By practicing cultural competency and humility in medicine, providers can shape and support patient care and strengthen the patient-provider relationship, leading to increased treatment adherence and improved health outcomes and health literacy. Provider awareness of the cultures surrounding each person can enhance the patient-provider relationship and may result in minimizing barriers to effective treatment. As an example, some communities incorporate their religious beliefs into healthcare (Nyashanu et al., 2022). Being aware of these concepts can help use that faith-based practice to promote health literacy and adherence. Identifying potential gaps in cultural competency as well as ongoing training sessions has been shown to significantly improve knowledge, attitudes, self-efficacy, and intentions among providers (Rhoten et al., 2022). Additional information can be found in Chapter 9, "Diversity and Health Disparities."

LANGUAGE

PWH in the United States and elsewhere originate from many regions of the world. For many patients, English is not their primary language. Thus, an important issue is ensuring effective communication between the patient and healthcare team members. Language-concordant care can provide reassurance that the patient and provider understand each other; it also optimizes health outcomes, advances health equity for diverse populations, and enhances trust between patient and provider (Molina and Kasper, 2019). At times, out of convenience, providers may be tempted to use family members or friends to provide language assistance. These strategies may be associated with a number of problems, including the interpreter not directly translating the provider or patient's intent, leaving out key details, and so on, and it may also result in breaches of confidentiality (Bischoff and Hudelson, 2010). Providing medically trained interpreter services is vital to promoting equitable health care and overcoming misinterpretation and patient-perceived prejudice that can be associated with being a patient who does not speak the local language (Bischoff and Hudelson, 2010; Ngo-Metzger et al., 2009).

THE HIV-ORIENTED PHYSICAL EXAMINATION

Sir William Osler is credited with the saying, "He who knows syphilis knows medicine." The modern-day equivalent of the adage is "He who knows HIV knows medicine," because indeed HIV infection and its sequelae can affect every organ system and can present in every clinical way possible. The HIV-oriented exam, therefore, needs to be especially comprehensive, both for the assessment of current concerns and for establishing a baseline to compare with future findings. At times the physical exam can provide clues to the patient's immunological status. As an example, erythematous candidiasis is often present at $CD4^+$ cell counts between 200 and 500 cells/μL, while pseudomembranous candidiasis often indicates more advanced immunosuppression (CD4 counts ≤ 200 cells/μL), and oral hairy leukoplakia is usually associated with CD4 counts <400 cells/μL (Levy and Jacobson, 2012; Nokta, 2008). The physical exam can also provide insight to any substance use issues (including scars at injection sites or abnormal nasal mucosa associated with frequent inhalation of abrasive substances), personal hygiene patterns, or significant weight loss/gain (Mertens et al., 2008). Other findings should be sought on physical exam that might suggest opportunistic infections, such as skin lesions suggestive of Kaposi's sarcoma or cryptococcemia, or spider angiomata suggestive of chronic liver disease (perhaps from cirrhosis due to viral hepatitis) (Srivastava et al., 2015; Tappero et al., 1995).

RECOGNITION OF ACUTE AND ADVANCED HIV INFECTION

As the trend toward earlier HIV diagnosis continues (prior to any significant immune dysfunction), the majority of PWH presenting to the clinic for initial visits will be asymptomatic or have minor nonspecific symptoms (Robb et al., 2016). Some newly diagnosed PWH may still have signs or symptoms of acute infection, a mononucleosis or flu-like syndrome characterized by fever, lymphadenopathy, sore throat, rash, muscle aches, diarrhea, abdominal pain, and headache (Hoenigl et al., 2016; Niu et al., 1993) (Table 7.3). Symptoms of acute HIV usually resolve within 2 weeks but may persist. The presence of prolonged symptomatic illness appears to correlate with more rapid progression to AIDS (Pedersen et al., 1989; Vanhems et al., 2000). Although usually associated with later stages of HIV disease, opportunistic infections can rarely occur during transient CD4 lymphopenia and early HIV infection (Braun et al., 2015).

Conditions for which HIV screening should be performed or considered:

- Any sexually transmitted infection
- Oral ulcers/aphthous stomatitis
- Oral hairy leukoplakia
- Oral candidiasis in the absence of triggers/risk factors (i.e., inhaled steroids)
- Unexplained weight loss
- Unexplained chronic fatigue
- Unexplained/persistent fevers
- Chronic diarrhea
- Persistent night sweats
- Persistent generalized lymphadenopathy
- Persistent or difficult-to-control seborrheic dermatitis
- Severe or difficult-to-control psoriasis
- Persistent or difficult-to-control vaginal candidiasis
- Herpes zoster/shingles (especially if more than one dermatome or recurrent, especially in young people)
- Chronic or persistent herpes simplex infection of the genital tract or perianal region
- Any sexually transmitted infection
- Chronic thrombocytopenia
- Leukopenia
- Anemia of chronic inflammation, especially without an alternative explanation
- Low lipid levels (low cholesterol, high-density lipoprotein [HDL], and low-density lipoprotein [LDL]), with elevated triglycerides. This has been attributed to chronic inflammatory cytokines (Grunfeld et al., 1992).
- Elevated globulin: albumin ratio, indicating polyclonal gammopathy
- Persistent or intermittent unexplained transaminitis
- Low albumin or prealbumin, especially if wasting is present
- Decreased renal function with proteinuria (could be due to HIV nephropathy)
- Active tuberculosis
- Non-Hodgkin lymphoma or Hodgkin's disease
- Cervical carcinoma in situ
- Listeriosis in an otherwise non-immunosuppressed or pregnant patient
- Extra-intestinal salmonellosis
- Recurrent bacterial pneumonia
- Bacteremic pneumococcal pneumonia
- Pelvic inflammatory disease
- Anal cancer

Table 7.3 **SIGNS AND SYMPTOMS OF ACUTE HIV INFECTION**

SIGNS AND SYMPTOMS	APPROXIMATE INCIDENCE (%)
Fever	48–88
Pharyngitis/sore throat	21–51
Lymphadenopathy	36–45
Rash	12–47
Oral ulcers	12–17
Myalgia/arthralgia	28–46
Diarrhea	17–35
Headache	34–44
Hepatosplenomegaly	10–15
Oral/oropharyngeal or vaginal candidiasis	10
Weight loss	21–39
Neurologic syndromes (e.g., aseptic meningitis, peripheral neuropathy, Guillain–Barré syndrome)	~10

Source: Adapted from Hoenigl et al. *Emerg Infect Dis.* 2016;22(3):532–534.

INITIAL LABORATORY EVALUATION

A comprehensive initial laboratory evaluation should be performed at or before the first clinic visit to establish a baseline CD4 count, HIV viral load, hepatic and renal function, and other markers (see Table 7.4). Laboratory data should ideally be available prior to the initial interaction, but at times people will present for the initial evaluation without any previous records or workup aside from their positive HIV test (Aberg et al., 2014). Laboratory testing can be divided into HIV-specific testing, assessment of risk factors, and routine medical care labs.

Integrase inhibitors have become the backbone of most HIV treatment regimens since their introduction. Due to their high barrier to resistance, routine genotypic testing is usually not recommended in current guidelines. However, there has been an increasing trend in mutations that give minor resistance to integrase inhibitors (Koullias et al., 2017), raising concern. If there is a suspicion for potential resistance,

Table 7.4 INITIAL LABORATORY EVALUATION FOR PWH

CATEGORY	TEST	FREQUENCY	COMMENTS
HIV-specific testing	HIV serology (4th generation Ag/Ab test)	At baseline if not available in records	If no prior results available and viral load is expected to be undetectable (patient on treatment), needed to establish diagnosis
	CD4 count (absolute and percentage)	• At baseline • Monitor every 3 to 6 months initially • If viral load <20 copies/mL and CD4 count more than 300–500 cells/mm^3 for 2 years, repeat only every 12 months • If CD4 >500 cells/mm^3, CD4 monitoring is optional	• Establishes clinical stage of HIV • Establishes risk of opportunistic complications and the need for initiation and discontinuation of opportunistic infection prophylaxis • CD4 percentage, should be noted (less variable than absolute CD4 cell count and may better reflect immune function)
	HIV viral load (RNA)	• At baseline • Repeat 2–8 weeks after starting ART, and every 4–8 weeks until undetectable • Subsequently, every 3–4 months • Every 6 months in adherent patients with consistent viral suppression	• May affect selection of ART (some antiretroviral agents should not be used if viral load is more than 100,000 copies/mL) • Follow-up viral load testing determines response to antiviral therapy.
	Resistance testing	• Initially • Repeat if treatment failure	• Prevalence of HIV drug resistance is 5%–15% in resource-rich settings • Genotypic testing is preferred; phenotypic testing can be helpful in highly treatment-experienced PWH with history of multiple resistance mutations • Integrase resistance testing generally not recommended initially, given low rates of baseline resistance. Consider if failing integrase inhibitor-based regimens or if previously exposed.
	HLA-B*5701	At baseline if considering abacavir	Establishes risk of abacavir hypersensitivity (if positive, abacavir contraindicated)
	Tropism testing	If CCR5 antagonist being considered	Only use maraviroc if virus is CCR5 tropic.
	G6PD screen	Baseline or when appropriate	Deficiency increases risk of hemolytic anemia, particularly with the use of primaquine and dapsone.
General testing	CBC with differential	Baseline; as needed thereafter	• Screen for anemia, leukopenia, lymphopenia, thrombocytopenia (incidence 30%–40% in patients with advanced HIV disease) • Neutropenia could represent bone marrow suppression due to HIV or other infiltrative infections (e.g., *Mycobacterium avium*) • Anemia could indicate medication toxicity (e.g., zidovudine), or viral infection (Parvovirus B19), or nutritional deficiencies (iron, B_{12}, folate) • Eosinophilia may be an indication of parasitic infection, allergy or atopy, eosinophilic folliculitis or drug reaction.

Table 7.4 CONTINUED

CATEGORY	TEST	FREQUENCY	COMMENTS
	Complete metabolic panel	• Baseline • Every 3–6 months thereafter	• Decreased renal function may affect selection of ART and may require renal dosing. • Elevated BUN/creatinine (and proteinuria) may be a sign of HIV-associated nephropathy. • Elevated transaminases and bilirubin levels may suggest possible liver pathology (e.g., viral hepatitis, drug-induced liver injury, steatohepatitis).
	Glucose and lipid profile	• Baseline • Every 6–12 months thereafter or as indicated by cardiovascular risk profile	• Will help identify any baseline metabolic abnormalities and estimate cardiovascular risk • May influence ART choice
	Vitamin D level	• Baseline • As appropriate thereafter	Consider especially if at risk for osteopenia or osteoporosis
	Urinalysis	Baseline	• Assess effect of ART on kidney function (especially tenofovir). • Proteinuria may be a sign of HIV nephropathy.
	Pregnancy test	Baseline and as appropriate thereafter	For people of childbearing capacity/age
Coinfection/ comorbidity testing	Viral hepatitis serologies	• Baseline • Repeat as indicated depending on risk	• If hepatitis A or hepatitis B non-immune, vaccinate • Identifies PWH requiring further evaluation for hepatitis C coinfection • May influence ART selection (particularly hepatitis B)
	Tuberculosis	Baseline and yearly thereafter	• Baseline tuberculin skin test (PPD) or IGRA is indicated in all PWH, unless there is a history of prior positive test or treatment for latent TB. • A PPD result ≥5 mm induration is considered reactive in PWH. • If positive, a chest X-ray should be obtained to rule out active disease, along with a careful history and exam to rule out extrapulmonary TB.
	STIs: Syphilis Chlamydia Gonorrhea	• Baseline • Annually if sexually active • More frequent testing depending on other risk factors	• Screening for trichomonas indicated in women • Test for latent syphilis • Testing for chlamydia/gonorrhea should include pharyngeal, urine, and rectal samples, depending on sexual practices • If positive testing, treatment and counseling on preventing STIs are indicated.
	Toxoplasma (serum IgG)	Baseline	• If seronegative, counseling on avoidance of new infection • If seropositive, prescribe prophylaxis if CD4 count ≤100 cells/mm^3.
	Varicella	Baseline	To identify PWH who may require primary immunization against varicella or against herpes zoster
	CMV	Generally not indicated as seroprevalence >90% in some populations	

(continued)

Table 7.4 CONTINUED

CATEGORY	TEST	FREQUENCY	COMMENTS
Other screening	Cervical Pap test and HPV co-testing	• Baseline • Repeat every 6–12 months (co-testing as indicated by age, history)	Determines if there is dysplasia and HPV infection to help inform risk for neoplastic transformation
	Anal cytology	Baseline	• Consider if there is a history of receptive anal intercourse or a history of genital warts (or abnormal cervical Pap smear in women). • Optimal follow-up not yet established
	Bone density scan		• Baseline screening for osteoporosis in postmenopausal women and men age 50 years or older. • Could be considered in PWH at risk (on tenofovir-based regimens)
	Age-appropriate healthcare maintenance		• Breast and colon cancer screening should follow age-appropriate guidelines • ASCVD score should be considered to evaluate need for statin therapy. • Depression screening with PHQ-2 should be considered. • Cognitive screening with HIV MMSE should be considered. • Dental care is an important component of routine healthcare maintenance. • Other risk-appropriate screening as per U.S. Preventive Service Task Force Recommendations

particularly in patients with previous exposure to this drug class (treatment-experienced, use in long-acting injectable PrEP), testing should be obtained. Additional information on HIV drug resistance can be found in Chapter 17, "HIV Drug Resistance: Evaluation and Clinical Management."

DISCUSSING INITIATION OF THERAPY

In the last several years, some communities have successfully initiated "rapid initiation of ART" programs, in which antiretroviral therapy is started immediately following diagnosis, which represents a significant shift from previous recommendations. In the early years of the HIV epidemic, limited resources and concerns about suboptimal adherence led to a cautious approach in which PWH underwent multiple counseling sessions before starting ART (WHO, 2017). More recent data support earlier ART initiation (within 1 week and at times even the same day) (Ford et al., 2018b). This appears to improve outcomes across the HIV treatment cascade in low- and middle-income settings, including reducing loss to care. However, there is also some evidence that indicates that in certain circumstances, this approach could lead to an increase in loss to follow-up, because of insufficient time to accept and disclose HIV status and to prepare for lifelong treatment (Boyd et al., 2019; Ford et al., 2018a). We agree that, when possible, HIV therapy should be started promptly, taking into consideration social and psychological aspects of committing to lifelong therapy. Certain PWH may have conditions in which rapid starts are contraindicated (concurrent CNS infection with tuberculosis or cryptococcus) since early ART prior to treatment of certain opportunistic infections may increase the likelihood of developing immune reconstitution syndrome and potentially increasing morbidity and mortality (Lawn et al., 2011). Before initiating therapy, a complete and thorough list of all the patient's present medications, as well as any alternative medications or natural supplements, should be sought due to the potential for drug-drug interactions (El Moussaoui et al., 2020). Identifying and managing potential interactions may lead to fewer side effects, less virologic failure, and improved adherence (Castro-Granell et al., 2021).

TELEHEALTH IN HIV

The U.S. Health Resources and Services Administration defines telehealth as the use of electronic information and telecommunications technologies to support long-distance clinical healthcare, patient and professional health-related education, public health, and health administration. Many studies have demonstrated that the use of telehealth can increase convenience for patients by decreasing travel time, improve patient satisfaction, diminish healthcare disparities, and reduce cost, which may lead to improvement in clinical outcomes and quality of care (Kruse et al., 2017). Guaranteeing confidentiality, educating patients and providers, and obtaining insurance reimbursement are some of the challenges that have prevented more widespread implementation of telehealth programs (Dandachi et al., 2019). In the setting of the recent COVID-19 pandemic, the use of telemedicine increased and allowed providers the ability to assess and evaluate patients without exposing patients or healthcare professionals to COVID-19 (Smith et al., 2020).

Recent literature seems to indicate that telehealth programs are viewed positively by most patients. Telehealth for PWH can improve retention in care by decreasing travel time (especially helpful for PWH who live in rural areas) and offer more convenience for the patient's schedule; however, some PWH worry about effective communication and have expressed concerns about the safety and confidentiality of their personal information (Dandachi et al., 2020b). HIV provider-identified benefits of telemedicine include the ability to re-engage patients into care, flexibility, opportunity to engage family members as well as other providers, and enhanced telemedicine efficiency. Providers' concerns with the use of telehealth are usually centered on not being able to perform a physical exam, longer visit times, and inability to connect with the patient. However, in general, providers feel that with the use of telehealth they are able to communicate well with patients, especially with established patients whom the provider knows well and with whom they have previously established a good rapport (Dandachi et al., 2020a). Another concern about routine use of telehealth visits is the lack of interaction between the PWH and case managers, nursing staff, and others.

Barriers to telehealth include lack of access to high-speed internet, which is common in remote areas. Technical challenges such as being comfortable with computers and computer software and new telehealth platforms can also be challenging (Cole et al., 2019). A recent study showed that HIV care delivery in the United States has been quite successful with telehealth adaptations (Labisi et al., 2022). However, despite this success, there are ongoing disparities affecting racial minority groups, older adults, and individuals with low technology literacy, resulting in poor health outcomes compared to other groups. Lack of broadband internet access, as well as compatible devices, also creates significant limitations. In general, when used appropriately, telehealth can be a useful tool for offering HIV care.

RECOMMENDED READING

Feinberg J, Keeshin S. Prevention and initial management of HIV infection. *Ann Int Medi.* 2022;175. 10.7326/AITC202206210.

Thompson MA, Horberg MA, Agwu AL, et al. Primary care guidance for persons infected with Human Immundeficiency Virus: 2020 update by the HIV Medicine Association of the Infectious Disease Society of America. *Clin Infect Dis.* 2021;73:e3572–605.

REFERENCES

Aberg JA, Gallant JE, Ghanem KG, et al.; Infectious Diseases Society of America. Primary care guidelines for the management of persons infected with HIV: 2013 update by the HIV Medicine Association of the Infectious Diseases Society of America. *Clin Infect Dis.* 2014;58(1):1–10.

Bass B, Nagy H. Cultural competence in the care of LGBTQ patients. In: *StatPearls* [Internet]. Treasure Island, FL: StatPearls Publishing; 2023 Nov 13. 2024 Jan–. PMID: 33085323.

Beach MC, Keruly J, Moore RD. Is the quality of the patient-provider relationship associated with better adherence and health outcomes for patients with HIV? *J Gen Intern Med.* 2006;21(6):661–665.

Berghoff CR, Gratz KL, Portz KJ, et al. The role of emotional avoidance, the patient-provider relationship, and other social support in ART adherence for HIV+ individuals. *AIDS Behav.* 2018;22(3):929–938.

Bischoff A, Hudelson P. Communicating with foreign language-speaking patients: is access to professional interpreters enough? *J Travel Med.* 2010;17(1):15–20.

Boyd MA, Boffito M, Castagna A, Estrada V. Rapid initiation of antiretroviral therapy at HIV diagnosis: definition, process, knowledge gaps. *HIV Med.* 2019;20 Suppl 1:3–11.

Braun DL, Kouyos RD, Balmer B, et al. Frequency and spectrum of unexpected clinical manifestations of primary HIV-1 infection. *Clin Infect Dis.* 2015;61(6):1013–1021.

Castro-Granell V, Garin N, Jaén Á, et al. Prevalence, beliefs and impact of drug-drug interactions between antiretroviral therapy and illicit drugs among people living with HIV in Spain. *PLoS One.* 2021;16(11):e0260334.

Ciechanowski PS, Katon WJ, Russo JE, Walker EA. The patient-provider relationship: attachment theory and adherence to treatment in diabetes. *Am J Psychiatry.* 2001;158(1):29–35.

Cole B, Pickard K, Stredler-Brown A. Report on the use of telehealth in early intervention in Colorado: strengths and challenges with telehealth as a service delivery method. *Int J Telerehabil.* 2019;11(1):33–40.

Dandachi D, Dang BN, Lucari B, et al. Exploring the attitude of patients with HIV about using telehealth for HIV care. *AIDS Patient Care STDs.* 2020b;34(4):166–172.

Dandachi D, Freytag J, Giordano TP, Dang BN. It is time to include telehealth in our measure of patient retention in HIV Care. *AIDS Behav.* 2020a;24(9):2463–2465.

Dandachi D, Lee C, Morgan RO, et al. Integration of telehealth services in the healthcare system: with emphasis on the experience of patients living with HIV. *J Investig Med.* 2019;67(5):815–820.

Doshi RK, Milberg J, Isenberg D, et al. High rates of retention and viral suppression in the US HIV safety net system: HIV care continuum in the Ryan White HIV/AIDS Program, 2011. *Clin Infect Dis.* 2015;60(1):117–125.

El Moussaoui M, Lambert I, Maes N, et al. Evolution of drug interactions with antiretroviral medication in people with HIV. *Open Forum Infect Dis.* 2020;7(11):ofaa416. doi:10.1093/ofid/ofaa416.

Flickinger TE, Saha S, Moore RD, Beach MC. Higher quality communication and relationships are associated with improved patient engagement in HIV care. *J Acquir Immune Defic Syndr.* 2013;63(3):362–366.

Ford N, Meintjes G, Calmy A, et al.; Guideline Development Group for Managing Advanced HIV Disease and Rapid Initiation of Antiretroviral Therapy. Managing advanced HIV disease in a public health approach. *Clin Infect Dis.* 2018a;66(Suppl 2):S106–S110.

Ford N, Migone C, Calmy A, et al. Benefits and risks of rapid initiation of antiretroviral therapy. *AIDS.* 2018b;32(1):17–23.

Grunfeld C, Pang M, Doerrler W, et al. Lipids, lipoproteins, triglyceride clearance, and cytokines in human immunodeficiency virus infection and the acquired immunodeficiency syndrome. *J Clin Endocrinol Metab.* 1992;74(5):1045–1052.

Ha Dinh TT, Bonner A, Clark R, et al. The effectiveness of the teach-back method on adherence and self-management in health education for people with chronic disease: a systematic review. *JBI Database System Rev Implement Rep.* 2016 Jan;14(1):210–247.

Hoenigl M, Green N, Camacho M, et al. Signs or symptoms of acute HIV infection in a cohort undergoing community-based screening. *Emerg Infect Dis.* 2016;22(3):532–534.

Kim J, Lee E, Park BJ, et al. Adherence to antiretroviral therapy and factors affecting low medication adherence among incident HIV-infected individuals during 2009–2016: A nationwide study. *Sci Rep.* 2018;8(1):3133.

Koullias Y, Sax PE, Fields NF, et al. Should we be testing for baseline integrase resistance in patients newly diagnosed with human immunodeficiency virus? *Clin Infect Dis.* 2017;65(8):1274–1281.

Kruse CS, Krowski N, Rodriguez B, et al. Telehealth and patient satisfaction: a systematic review and narrative analysis. *BMJ Open*. 2017;7(8):e016242. doi:10.1136/bmjopen-2017-016242.

Labisi T, Regan N, Davis P, Fadul N. HIV care meets telehealth: a review of successes, disparities, and unresolved challenges. *Curr HIV/AIDS Rep*. 2022;19(5):446–453.

Lawn SD, Torok ME, Wood R. Optimum time to start antiretroviral therapy during HIV-associated opportunistic infections. *Curr Opin Infect Dis*. 2011;24(1):34–42.

Le HN, Hipolito MM, Lambert S, et al. Culturally sensitive approaches to identification and treatment of depression among HIV infected African American adults: a qualitative study of primary care providers' perspectives. *J Depress Anxiety*. 2016;5(2):223.

Levy TH, Jacobson DF. (2012), Dermatologic manifestations as indicators of immune status in HIV/AIDS. *J Gen Intern Med*. 2012;27(1):124. doi:10.1007/s11606-011-1743-4.

Mertens JR, Flisher AJ, Satre DD, Weisner CM. The role of medical conditions and primary care services in 5-year substance use outcomes among chemical dependency treatment patients. *Drug Alcohol Depend*. 2008;98(1–2):45–53.

Miller LG, Liu H, Hays RD, et al. Knowledge of antiretroviral regimen dosing and adherence: a longitudinal study. *Clin Infect Dis*. 2003;36(4):514–518.

Molina RL, Kasper J. The power of language-concordant care: a call to action for medical schools. *BMC Med Educ*. 2019;19(1):378. doi:10.1186/s12909-019-1807-4.

Molla AA, Gelagay AA, Mekonnen HS, Teshome DF. Adherence to antiretroviral therapy and associated factors among HIV positive adults attending care and treatment in University of Gondar Referral Hospital, Northwest Ethiopia. *BMC Infect Dis*. 2018;18(1):266.

Ngo-Metzger Q, Sorkin DH, Phillips RS. Healthcare experiences of limited English-proficient Asian American patients: a cross-sectional mail survey. *Patient*. 2009;2(2):113–120.

Niu MT, Stein DS, Schnittman SM. Primary human immunodeficiency virus type 1 infection: review of pathogenesis and early treatment intervention in humans and animal retrovirus infections. *J Infect Dis*. 1993;168(6):1490–501.

Nokta M. Oral manifestations associated with HIV infection. *Curr HIV/AIDS Rep*. 2008;5(1):5–12.

Nyashanu M, Ganga G, Chenneville T. Exploring the impact of religion, superstition, and professional cultural competence on access to HIV and mental health treatment among Black sub-Sahara African communities in the English city of Birmingham. *J Relig Health*. 2022;61(1):252–268.

O'Connor, BB Promoting cultural competence in HIV/AIDS care. *J Assoc Nurses AIDS Care*. 1996;7 Suppl 1:41–53.

Pedersen C, Lindhardt BO, Jensen BL, et al. Clinical course of primary HIV infection: consequences for subsequent course of infection. *BMJ*. 1989;299(6692):154–157.

Rhoten B, Burkhalter JE, Joo R, et al. Impact of an LGBTQ cultural competence training program for providers on knowledge, attitudes, self-efficacy, and intensions. *J Homosex*. 2022;69(6):1030–1041.

Robb ML, Eller LA, Kibuuka H; RV 217 Study Team. Prospective Study of Acute HIV-1 Infection in Adults in East Africa and Thailand. *N Engl J Med*. 2016;374(22):2120–2130.

Ruffell S. Stigma kills! The psychological effects of emotional abuse and discrimination towards a patient with HIV in Uganda. *BMJ Case Rep*. 2017;2017:bcr2016218024. doi:10.1136/bcr-2016-218024

Shover CL, DeVost MA, Beymer MR, et al. Using sexual orientation and gender identity to monitor disparities in HIV, sexually transmitted infections, and viral hepatitis. *Am J Public Health*. 2018;108(S4):S277–S283.

Smith AC, Thomas E, Snoswell CL, et al. Telehealth for global emergencies: implications for coronavirus disease 2019 (COVID-19). *J Telemed Telecare*. 2020;26(5):309–313.

Srivastava GN, Tilak R, Yadav J, Bansal M. Cutaneous cryptococcus: marker for disseminated infection. *BMJ Case Rep*. 2015;2015:bcr2015210898. doi:10.1136/bcr-2015-210898

Sued O, Cecchini D, Rolón MJ, et al. A small cluster randomised clinical trial to improve health outcomes among Argentine patients disengaged from HIV care. *Lancet Reg Health Am*. 2022;13:100307.

Tappero JW, Perkins BA, Wenger JD, Berger TG. Cutaneous manifestations of opportunistic infections in patients infected with human immunodeficiency virus. *Clin Microbiol Rev*. 1995;8(3):440–450.

Uwah C. The role of culture in effective HIV/AIDS communication by theatre in South Africa. *SAHARA J*. 2013;10(3-4):140–149.

Vanhems P, Hirschel B, Phillips AN, et al. Incubation time of acute human immunodeficiency virus (HIV) infection and duration of acute HIV infection are independent prognostic factors of progression to AIDS. *J Infect Dis*. 2000;182(1):334–337.

World Health Organization (WHO). *Guidelines for Managing Advanced HIV Disease and Rapid Initiation of Antiretroviral Therapy*. Geneva: World Health Organization; 2017. License: CC BY-NC-SA 3.0 IGO.

Yu Y, Luo D, Chen X, et al. Medication adherence to antiretroviral therapy among newly treated people living with HIV. *BMC Public Health*. 2018;18(1):825.

8.

HEALTH MAINTENANCE

SELECT TOPICS

Ramiz Kseri

LEARNING OBJECTIVES

Upon completion of this chapter, the reader should be able to:

- Describe tuberculosis (TB) screening indications (including exposure history) and assessment methods (including selection, interpretation, and limitations of screening tests in people with HIV [PWH]).
- Discuss the importance of routine dental care for PWH and essential information to be included in the treating clinician's referral.
- Discuss the immunization schedule for PWH.

HIV HEALTHCARE FLOW SHEETS FOR PRIMARY CARE

Many electronic health record (EHR) systems have the capacity to feature disease-specific flow sheets or "care gap" reminders. For PWH, flow sheets should include HIV-specific information such as $CD4^+$ T-cell counts, HIV-1 viral loads, immunization records, and healthcare maintenance reports (at minimum). Ideally, the EHR flow sheet is designed to prompt clinical reminders regarding the need for opportunistic infection prophylaxis and vaccinations or health maintenance screening based on patients' current $CD4^+$ T-cell counts, serologies, age, sex, and other indicators.

TB SCREENING AND ASSESSMENT

LEARNING OBJECTIVE

Describe TB screening indications (including exposure history) and assessment methods (including selection, interpretation, and limitations of screening tests in PWH).

WHAT'S NEW?

Tuberculosis (TB) screening remains an important component of preventive health care for PWH, both at time of initial HIV diagnosis and routinely thereafter as indicated. New short-course regimens are available for latent TB infection. Given the prevalence of tuberculosis among PWH and unique considerations for interpretation of screening results, HIV providers should be aware of when to screen for TB and how to accurately assess TB status.

KEY POINTS

- Because of immunodeficiency, some PWH are at increased risk for developing active TB disease and should thus be routinely screened.
- PWH also frequently have other indications for TB screening, including contact with persons from areas of the world where there is a high TB incidence and high-risk exposures in correctional and residential facilities.
- In PWH, tuberculin skin testing (TST) or interferon gamma release assays (IGRAs) should be performed at the time of initial HIV diagnosis. For persons whose CD4+ T cells were $<200/mm^3$ who were initially TST (tuberculin skin test) or IGRA (interferon gamma release assay) negative, screening should be repeated when people experience antiretroviral therapy (ART)–associated immune function improvement. Annual testing may be considered in persons with ongoing or repeated exposure to TB.
- TST responses of *5 mm or larger induration* are considered positive in PWH. However, even negative TST or IGRA results may warrant preventive therapy in the setting of high-risk exposures.
- Chest radiography is indicated regardless of TST or IGRA results in PWH with recent exposure to patients with active TB or with a history of symptoms consistent with TB, as well as in any PWH with a positive screening test result.

HIV-associated immune compromise is associated with an increased incidence of TB among PWH, with a relative risk of 10 times that of HIV-negative persons (Horsburgh and Rubin, 2011). As with other opportunistic infections, there has been a substantial decrease in TB incidence among persons receiving consistent ART. However, untreated TB is one of the few opportunistic infections transmissible to others and thus has additional public health implications for prevention and control.

PWH are at increased risk for developing active disease by reactivation of untreated latent TB infection (LTBI), at an estimated rate of 3%–16% *per year* compared to 5%–10%

lifetime risk in HIV-negative persons with no other risk factors. Once infection with *M. tuberculosis* occurs, there can be rapid progression of newly acquired infection to overt clinical disease—for example, within the first month following exposure to an infectious person. Similarly, reactivation disease may also progress rapidly, particularly in highly immunocompromised individuals. The majority of individuals without HIV and infected with TB who develop active disease in the United States were born, previously lived, or traveled for extended periods in TB endemic areas. Currently, 8% of individuals with active TB have underlying HIV disease. However, prior to the advent of ART, in the United States, the proportion of individuals with TB who had underlying HIV was nearly 50%. TB outbreaks were identified among PWH in U.S. institutional settings, including healthcare facilities, correctional facilities, and homeless shelters. Although transmission in institutional settings in the United States is now rare, there is substantial risk in resource-limited settings in which TB is endemic in the general population. PWH who are employees or volunteers in settings identified as high risk by local health authorities should be advised of their risk of exposure to TB and offered alternate sites of work. HIV-positive healthcare workers who intermittently work or volunteer in TB-endemic countries should be similarly advised about their risk. Healthcare providers should seek assistance with assessing the level of risk by evaluating factors such as the community TB prevalence, transmission precautions that are in place, and the healthcare provider's specific duties in those settings.

Compared to HIV-negative persons, PWH (especially individuals with CD4$^+$ T-cell counts less than 200/cells/mm^3) are more likely to present with extrapulmonary TB, miliary pulmonary disease, and disseminated TB. PWH may have active pulmonary TB with normal chest radiographs. Similarly, PWH and TB may present with negative acid-fast bacilli (AFB) sputum in up to 70% of cases (Getahun et al., 2007). In a high-incidence setting and active case-finding study of patients with culture-positive TB, up to 32% had normal chest radiographs; of those who were AFB smear-negative and had normal chest radiographs, 8% had TB, 5% had CD4$^+$ T-cell counts of 350/µL or greater, and 10% had CD4$^+$ T-cell counts of less than 350/µL (Cain et al., 2010). Nucleic acid amplification tests such as Gene Xpert MTB/RIF are more sensitive than AFB smear, and they may identify up to 70% of smear-negative, culture-positive cases (Boehme et al., 2010).

INDICATIONS FOR LTBI SCREENING

Many indications for LTBI screening may be present concurrently in PWH, which represent conditions with higher risk of development of TB than without these conditions, or in situations that pose high risk of exposure or recent infection with *M. tuberculosis*. Indications for screening include the following:

- People who are foreign-born, or in close contact with recent immigrants or refugees, from regions with high rates of TB (i.e., Africa, Asia, Latin America, Russia, and countries of the former Soviet Union)
- Other medical conditions, such as diabetes mellitus, silicosis, chronic renal failure, being underweight (greater than 10% below normal body weight), gastrectomy, injection drug use, malignancies (lymphoma, leukemia, and head and neck cancer), cardiac and renal transplantation, or use of immunosuppressive therapies (especially tumor necrosis factor-α inhibitors)
- Persons in situations with a high risk for person-to-person transmission, such as those working or residing in correctional facilities (3% of TB cases in the United States), homeless shelters (6% of TB cases in the United States), and other congregate settings (Lewinsohn et al., 2017; WHO, 2021)
- Close contacts of persons with active TB, 30%–40% of whom will be found to have LTBI and 1% or 2% of whom will have active disease
- Children born to mothers with HIV-TB coinfection or mothers with HIV who are at high risk for possible LTBI (e.g., close contacts of persons with active disease)
- Persons previously treated for latent or active TB who are re-exposed to someone with active TB can become reinfected, particularly in hyperendemic settings.

SCREENING TESTS FOR *M. TUBERCULOSIS* INFECTION

TUBERCULIN SKIN TESTING

The time-honored method for diagnosis of *M. tuberculosis* infection is the tuberculin skin test (TST), which measures a polycellular delayed-type hypersensitivity response at the site of injection following the administration of purified protein derivative (PPD), an admixture of mycobacterial antigens. The preferred skin test is the intradermal, or Mantoux, method. It is administered by injecting 0.1 mL of 5 tuberculin units (TU) PPD intradermally into the dorsal or volar surface of the forearm. Tests should be read 48–72 hours after test administration, and the diameter of induration transverse to the long axis of the arm should be recorded in millimeters. Multiple puncture tests (i.e., tine test, Heaf test) and PPD strengths of 1 and 250 TU are not sufficiently accurate and should not be used (American Thoracic Society/Centers for Disease Control and Prevention, 2000). Induration of 5 mm or greater in PWH indicates a positive TST. TSTs require two visits to perform and confirm the results of the test, as well as experience in intradermal placement of the test. There is some subjectivity in its interpretation, and false-positive results may occur from exposure to nontuberculous mycobacteria or prior vaccination with *M. bovis* BCG. A positive TST has been shown to be predictive of progression to active TB in PWH, who benefit from preventive therapy with a reduction in TB incidence.

IGRAS

IGRAs are blood tests that measure interferon-γ (IFN-γ) secreted by sensitized T lymphocytes after exposure to TB-specific antigens ESAT-6 and CFP-10. Two tests are currently approved by the U.S. Food and Drug Administration (FDA) and in use for *M. tuberculosis* infection detection: QuantiFERON-TB Gold In-Tube (QFT-GIT) and T-SPOT TB test (T-Spot). QFT measures IFN-γ concentration using an enzyme-linked immunosorbent assay (ELISA), whereas the T-Spot enumerates T cells releasing IFN-γ using an ELISPOT assay. QFT requires fresh blood to be incubated for 18–24 hours with plasma separation, ELISA testing, and comparison to negative and positive mitogen control antigens (phytohemagglutinin). T-Spot assays must be done on fresh blood specimens, processed within 12 hours, and incubated overnight. IGRAs require a single visit, are less subjective in interpretation than TSTs, and are more specific for detection of *M. tuberculosis* infection—that is, less cross-reactivity to nontuberculous mycobacteria (except *M. kansasii*, *M. szulgai*, and *M. marinum*) and BCG (CDC, 2010).

Current evidence suggests that IGRAs have higher specificity (92%–97%) compared to TSTs (56%–95%) (DHHS, 2024). TSTs are more likely to identify persons with long-standing cellular immune responses to TB antigens, and IGRAs are more likely to be positive in persons with recent *M. tuberculosis* infection (Horsburgh and Rubin, 2011). For diagnosis of LTBI, the correlation between TSTs and IGRAs is poor to moderate among PWH (Cattamanchi et al., 2011). For PWH with active TB, in one study, sensitivity was low for both QFT-GIT and TST (63% and 55%, respectively) and was inversely correlated with low $CD4^+$ T-cell counts (Raby et al., 2008). In PWH at low risk of TB exposure, false-positive tests with QFT have also been reported, suggesting the need to repeat testing after an initial positive QFT result to confirm the diagnosis of LTBI when patients are at low risk of exposure (Gray et al., 2012). There have been no definitive comparisons of TSTs and IGRAs for LTBI screening of PWH infection in low-incidence settings.

Either TSTs or IGRAs are appropriate for TB screening among PWH in the United States. Some experts have suggested using both the TST and an IGRA to screen for LTBI, but the predictive value of this approach is not clear, and use of this strategy would be more expensive and more difficult to implement. The routine use of both TSTs and IGRAs to screen for LTBI in the same patient is not recommended in the United States (DHHS, 2024).

TESTING FREQUENCY

PWH should receive a test for LTBI at the time of initial HIV diagnosis, with repeat testing considered for those who are TST or IGRA negative initially with advanced HIV infection ($CD4^+$ T-cell counts <200/μL) and who have improvement in immune function due to ART (CD^+ T-cell counts ≥200/μL). Annual testing may also be considered in PWH who have ongoing or repeated exposure to TB, such as individuals who travel for extended periods of time to hyperendemic TB settings. Intercurrent testing should be done based on recent exposure to a case of active TB, including repeat testing 8–12 weeks after the initial negative test because of how long it may take for the TST or IGRA to become positive following infection.

ANERGY TESTING

Some PWH are at increased risk of impaired delayed-type hypersensitivity responses to skin test antigens because of decreased $CD4^+$ T-cell counts and, therefore, have a compromised ability to react to tuberculin skin testing (i.e., cutaneous anergy). Anergy testing has not been helpful in attempting to distinguish false-negative TST results owing to anergy from true-negative results. Anergy testing is not recommended for routine use in PWH because of problems with test standardization and reproducibility, the variable risk for TB in the setting of anergy, and a lack of demonstrated benefit of preventive therapy in anergic PWH.

CHEST RADIOGRAPHY AND SYMPTOM SCREENING IN PWH

In asymptomatic persons with positive tests for LTBI, chest radiography should be done to exclude active TB. Persons with symptoms of TB, such as cough, fever, and night sweats, should be evaluated for TB regardless of IGRA or skin test results. The absence of these symptoms has a high negative predictive value for excluding active TB (Cain et al., 2010). Chest radiography should also be considered following recent exposure to a person with active TB regardless of skin test or IGRA results. PWH with pulmonary TB are more likely to exhibit atypical radiological presentations, especially individuals with low $CD4^+$ T-cell counts and, in some cases, normal chest radiographs (Palmieri et al., 2002).

PREVENTIVE THERAPY

Preventive therapy is recommended following exposure to persons with active TB, regardless of initial screening, and who have not been treated for active or latent TB and have no clinical evidence of active TB. Preventive therapy should be considered in persons with a history of potential exposure in high-risk settings (as listed previously) regardless of the results of testing for LTBI. Randomized controlled clinical trials have demonstrated that treatment with isoniazid for 6 or 9 months for LTBI in people with HIV reduces the risk of active TB, especially in those with a positive tuberculin skin test (Akolo et al., 2010).

For further information on evaluation and treatment of active TB disease, see Chapter 19, "Opportunistic Infections."

RECOMMENDED READING

Centers for Disease Control and Prevention. Deciding when to treat latent TB. Published March 13, 2018. https://www.cdc.gov/tb/topic/treatment/decideltbi.htm. Accessed August 31, 2024.

Panel on Guidelines for the Prevention and Treatment of Opportunistic Infections in Adults and Adolescents with HIV. Guidelines for the prevention and treatment of opportunistic infections in adults and adolescents with HIV. National Institutes of Health, Centers for Disease Control and Prevention, HIV Medicine Association, and Infectious Diseases Society of America. https://clinicalinfo.hiv.gov/en/guidelines/adult-and-adolescent-opportunistic-infection. Published August 15, 2024. Accessed August 31, 2024.Sterling TR, Njie G, Zenner D, et al. Guidelines for the treatment of latent tuberculosis infection: recommendations from the National Tuberculosis Controllers Association and CDC. *MMWR Recomm Rep.* 2020;69(1):1–11.

DENTAL CARE

LEARNING OBJECTIVE

Discuss the importance of routine dental care for PWH and essential information to be included in the treating clinician's referral.

WHAT'S NEW?

A large proportion of PWH do not receive regular dental and oral health care despite a high burden of need. Referrals for dental care should include information about the patient's risk for secondary infection and bleeding, infectious status, and current medications.

KEY POINTS

- PWH are at increased risk for oral and dental problems because of immunodeficiency, salivary gland dysfunction, substance (including tobacco) use, poor oral hygiene, and limited access to dental care.
- Oral cavity problems can undermine the success of ART by exacerbating existing medical, nutritional, and psychosocial problems; compromise adherence to treatment; and diminish quality of life.
- HIV medical providers should include basic oral screening in routine clinic visits and advocate for regular dental care for patients.
- Referrals for dental care should include information about the patient's risk for secondary infection and bleeding, infectious status, and current medications.

Oral health care is an important part of the medical management of PWH. Oral cavity problems can undermine the success of ART by exacerbating existing medical, nutritional, and psychosocial problems; compromise adherence to treatment; and diminish quality of life (New York State Department of Health AIDS Institute [NYSDOH], 2020).

Oral disease disproportionately affects the same populations that are most affected by HIV and social determinants of health—this includes people with limited health care access/utilization, people who use drugs, and other groups (NYSDOH, 2020). Many PWH do not receive the comprehensive dental care they need. In the HIV Cost and Services Utilization Study, which examined a nationally representative sample of PWH engaged in medical care, 35% of patients had no regular source of dental care; 22% had not received dental care in more than 2 years; 25% had not received needed dental care; and 48% had no dental insurance coverage (Freed et al., 2005).

Significant proportions of PWH have HIV-related oral problems such as untreated caries (39%), gum problems (47%), missing teeth (47%), and xerostomia (dry mouth) (37%) (Freed et al., 2005). PWH with advanced immunosuppression are also at risk for serious systemic opportunistic infections and neoplasms, many of which can manifest in the oral cavity. Examples include candidiasis, hairy leukoplakia, Kaposi's sarcoma, and aphthous ulcerations (Bonito, 2001). The presence of oral candidiasis without medical explanation (e.g., recent antibiotics) is most often related to a low $CD4^+$ T-cell number and is considered a marker for cell-mediated immunodeficiency. Deterioration of oral immunologic functions and changes in salivary flow rate and composition also aid in the development of caries and periodontal diseases, including gingivitis, which can progress to serious necrotizing gingivitis and compromise masticatory functions and nutrition (Bonito, 2001). The presence of necrotizing ulcerative periodontitis, a more aggressive form of periodontal disease, should also be considered a sign of severe immune deterioration. It is a rapidly progressive disease, and treatment should be initiated as early as possible.

Thus, oral health care should be an integral component of primary health care for PWH (NYSDOH, 2020). Providers must become familiar with oral conditions that affect PWH and include basic oral screening in routine clinic visit exams. Providers also must be aware of and advocate for oral health care and dental services in their communities. Finally, providers must counsel patients about the importance of good oral hygiene practices and regular dental care (at least twice annually) (NYSDOH, 2020).

When considering referral to a dental specialist, the main issues of concern are the patient's risk for bleeding, risk for infection, and infectiousness. Accordingly, the following information should be provided in dental referrals:

- *Bleeding risk*: Platelet count (platelet count $<60,000/mm^3$ may require platelet transfusion or steroids prior to dental treatment), liver biochemical tests, history of coagulation or other bleeding disorders, history of liver disease, and current hemoglobin (to ascertain risk of anemia should significant bleeding occur)
- *Infection risk*: Total white blood cell count, absolute neutrophil count, $CD4^+$ T-cell count, history of valvular or congenital heart disease, and other medical risks for infection (e.g., active intravenous drug use posing a risk for endocarditis)

- *Antibiotic prophylaxis*: Based on the individual need of each patient, antibiotic prophylaxis may be indicated prior to dental care. The need for antibiotic prophylaxis is not based on $CD4^+$ T-counts, viral load, or AIDS diagnosis. Patients with severe neutropenia (neutrophil count <500/mm^3) should be premedicated with antibiotics prior to dental treatment. Otherwise, antibiotic prophylaxis is recommended based on the standard guidelines set forth by the American Heart Association (http://www.aha.org) for the prevention of bacterial endocarditis
- *Concurrent infections*: Recent HIV viral load, chronic hepatitis B or hepatitis C coinfection, and contagious respiratory diseases such as active/untreated TB.

Additionally, all medications should be detailed to avoid drug interactions or adverse effects if medications will be used or prescribed as part of the dental care.

RECOMMENDED READING

Integrating HIV Innovating Practices. Implementing oral healthcare into HIV primary care settings curriculum. https://careacttarget.org/library/implementing-oral-health-care-hiv-primary-care-settings-curriculum-0. Published December 2013. Accessed August 30, 2024.

Parish C, Siegel K, Pereyra M, Liguori T. Barriers and facilitators to dental care among HIV-infected adults. *Spec Care Dentist.* 2015;35(6):294–302.

IMMUNIZATIONS

LEARNING OBJECTIVE

Discuss the immunization schedule for PWH.

WHAT'S NEW?

Information in this section is based on the recommendations from the Advisory Committee on Immunization Practices (CDC, 2024b).

KEY POINTS

- Response to vaccinations is based on the $CD4^+$ T-cell count.
- Response to vaccinations is most favorable early after HIV acquisition or soon after immune reconstitution with ART.
- Vaccinations may need to be readministered when immune reconstitution occurs with ART, as immunosuppression can cause a suboptimal response initially in PWH with advanced HIV disease.
- Live-virus vaccinations are not safe in PWH with a $CD4^+$ T-cell count <200 cells/mm^3.

CONCERN WITH IMMUNIZATIONS

Prior to ART in the 1980s, the concern was that immunizations could inadvertently upregulate the immune system and cause elevations in HIV replication, ultimately accelerating infection progression. However, it was determined that increases in HIV RNA were only transient. Also, in PWH on ART, immunizations generally do not cause detectable elevations in HIV RNA levels. The only contraindication to immunizations is low $CD4^+$ T-cell count (less than 200 cells/mm^3) for live vaccinations, as they can cause life-threatening disseminated infections.

CORONAVIRUS (SARS-COV-2 OR COVID-19)

In the general population, individuals who are at highest risk of severe COVID-19 include those aged >60 years; pregnant people; solid organ transplant recipients; and people with certain comorbidities such as cancer, obesity, diabetes mellitus, cardiovascular disease, pulmonary disease, a history of smoking, chronic kidney disease, or chronic liver disease. Many PWH have one or more comorbidities that increase their risk for a more severe course of COVID-19. Three COVID-19 vaccines are authorized or approved for use in the United States. For primary vaccinations, the mRNA vaccines (i.e., BNT162b2 [Pfizer-BioNTech] or mRNA-1273 [Moderna]) as well as protein subunit vaccine NVX-CoV2373 (Novavax) are used. The Ad26.COV2.S (Johnson & Johnson/Janssen) vaccine, because of its risk of serious adverse events and limited efficacy, is no longer recommended. The Advisory Committee on Immunization Practices (ACIP) recommends that people with advanced or untreated HIV receive a three-dose series of the mRNA vaccines, or a two-dose series of the protein subunit vaccine. Advanced HIV is defined as $CD4^+$ T-cell count <200 cells/mm^3, history of an AIDS-defining illness without immune reconstitution, or clinical manifestations of symptomatic HIV.

- Bottom line:
  - Primary vaccine series (2023–2024 updated formula)
    - Three-dose series at 0, 3, 7 weeks for BNT162b2 (Pfizer-BioNTech). This can be given as early as 6 months of age. For patients aged 18 or younger, recommendations are based on age.
    - Three-dose series at 0, 4, 8 weeks for mRNA-1273 (Moderna); can be given 28 days apart in high-risk populations. This can be given as early as 6 months of age. For patients aged 18 or younger, recommendations are based on age.
    - Two-dose series at 0, 3 weeks for NVX-CoV2373 (Novavax). Approved for patients ≥12 years of age.
    - One dose of Ad26.COV2.S (Johnson & Johnson/Janssen) is no longer recommended.

  - Boosters are recommended for most people, preferably either Pfizer-BioNTech or Moderna; these should be administered after the final dose in the primary series. Providers should refer to local guidelines for seasonal booster recommendations.

- For adults aged 50 years and older, a second booster of either Pfizer-BioNTech or Moderna COVID-19 vaccine at least 4 months after the first booster.
- ACIP published booster recommendations in 2024, specifying that "all persons aged ≥65 years receive one additional dose of any updated COVID-19 vaccine (i.e., Moderna, Novavax, or Pfizer-BioNTech). This additional dose should be administered ≥4 months after the previous dose of updated COVID-19 vaccine. For initial vaccination with Novavax COVID-19 vaccine, the two-dose series should be completed before administration of the additional dose. Because Novavax COVID-19 vaccine was initially introduced (and is currently authorized) under Emergency Use Authorization, the recommendation for the updated Novavax COVID-19 vaccine is an interim recommendation. ACIP further recommended that persons aged ≥65 years who are moderately or severely immunocompromised, have completed an initial series, and have received ≥1 updated COVID-19 vaccine dose should receive one additional updated COVID-19 vaccine dose ≥2 months after the last dose of updated vaccine (Panagiotakopoulos et al., 2024).

HAEMOPHILUS INFLUENZA TYPE B (HIB)

Infection caused by *Haemophilus influenzae* is more common in PWH, although the annual incidence remains relatively low. In addition, only about 33% of cases involve *H. influenzae* type b. Therefore, HIB is not recommended for routine administration to adults with HIV.

- Bottom line: Administer one dose only if there is an indication (e.g., sickle cell disease, leukemia, or anatomic or functional asplenia).

HEPATITIS A VIRUS (HAV)

HAV rates in general have declined with introduction of routine vaccination practice in the 1990s. However, rates have increased in people experiencing homelessness, people who inject drugs, and men who have sex with men (MSM). It is recommended to administer hepatitis A vaccine to all non-immune PWH regardless of CD4$^+$ T-cell count.

- Bottom line: For persons without hepatitis A immunity, administer two doses at least 6 months apart. A three-dose series can be administered with combined hep A–hep B vaccine; minimum intervals are 4 weeks between the first and second dose and 5 months between the second and third dose.

HEPATITIS B VIRUS (HBV)

There is an increased risk for PWH of acquiring HBV from injection drug use and/or condomless sex. It is recommended to administer hepatitis B vaccine to all PWH who do not have HBV immunity regardless of CD4$^+$ T-cell count. Screening labs are done pre- and postvaccination to assess baseline status and adequacy of response if vaccines are given.

- Simplified triple screening interpretation (CDC, 2024c):
  - Reactive hepatitis surface antigen (HBsAg), regardless of core antibody (HBcAb) status: acute or chronic infection, no indication for vaccination
  - Reactive hepatitis surface antibody (HBsAb) and reactive core antibody (HBcAb): resolved infection, no need for vaccination
  - Reactive hepatitis surface antibody (HBsAb), negative surface antigen (HBsAg), negative core antibody (HBcAb): receipt of prior vaccination (obtain prior documentation to confirm)
- Bottom line: For PWH without immunity, administer two- or three-dose HBV series. The two-dose series (Heplisav-B) is given 1 month apart. The three-dose series (PreHevbrio or Engerix-B) is given at 0, 1, and 6 months. If screening reveals vaccine nonresponse, re-vaccinate with a second double-dose, three-dose series of recombinant hepatitis B vaccine at 0, 1, 2, and 6 months or re-vaccinate with the two-dose series of HepBCpG (Heplisav-B) (DHHS, 2024). Vaccines containing both hepatitis A and B vaccines are available (Twinrix). If CD4$^+$ T-cell count was below 200 cell/mm^3 with the initial series, waiting until immune reconstitution occurs before doing the second series is an option.

HUMAN PAPILLOMAVIRUS VIRUS (HPV)

For PWH there is a higher incidence of HPV-associated disease. Vaccination is recommended for PWH who are 9 through 26 years of age; some guidelines have recommended extending the age of vaccination up to 45 years.

- Bottom line: Administer three-dose series at 0, 1–2, and 6 months. The two-dose series should NOT be used with PWH. Vaccination should not be given during pregnancy given the lack of clinical trial data. However, a pregnancy test is not required before administration. Series can be continued once people are no longer pregnant.

INFLUENZA

There is a higher risk of adverse outcomes with influenza infection in PWH than in the general population. Recommended influenza vaccines include inactivated influenza vaccine (IIV) or recombinant influenza vaccine (RIV). Live attenuated vaccine is contraindicated in PWH.

- Bottom line: Administer one dose annually of IIV or RIV.

MEASLES MUMPS RUBELLA (MMR)

As with influenza, PWH are at a higher risk of adverse infection outcomes than the general population. It is important to remember that the MMR vaccine is a live-virus vaccine.

- Bottom line: Administer two-dose series if $CD4^+$ T-cell count is 200 cells/mm^3 or greater (for at least 6 months) if born in 1957 or later. Doses should be administered at least 4 weeks apart. Combination vaccination with varicella is NOT recommended. If $CD4^+$ T-cell count is less than 200 cells/mm^3, both MMR and MMRV are contraindicated. The vaccine is also contraindicated in pregnancy, which should be avoided for 28 days after vaccination.

VARICELLA VIRUS (VAR)

For PWH, primary varicella zoster virus infection is uncommon because of immunity from childhood infection. The varicella vaccine is a live-virus vaccine.

- Bottom line: Administer two doses 3 months apart for PWH with no evidence of immunity and a $CD4^+$ T-cell count of 200 cells/mm^3 or greater. The vaccination is contraindicated with low $CD4^+$ T-cell count (<200 cells/mm^3).

ZOSTER

For PWH, the incidence of zoster is 15-fold higher than among age-matched immunocompetent adults, with the highest risk when the $CD4^+$ T-cell count is less than 200 cells/mm^3. Vaccination is intended to prevent zoster and reduce the severity of zoster if it does occur.

- Bottom line:
  - **Recombinant zoster vaccine (RZV)**: Administer two doses, given 2–6 months apart, to persons aged 50 years and older regardless of $CD4^+$ T-cell count. RZV is preferred over zoster vaccine live (ZVL) by the ACIP.
  - **ZVL**: This option is no longer available. Persons who have previously been vaccinated with this product should be vaccinated with two doses of RZV.

MENINGOCOCCUS

PWH are at increased risk of developing meningococcal disease (relative risk is estimated to be 5- to 13-fold higher than in persons without HIV); the risk in PWH appears to be higher with low $CD4^+$ T-cell counts and high HIV RNA levels. Men who have sex with men are at particular risk for meningococcal meningitis. Recent outbreaks of meningococcal meningitis have been reported in networks of MSM.

- Bottom line: For serogroups (A, C, W, Y), administer two doses (8–12 weeks apart) with a booster in 5 years.

  Meningococcal B vaccine is recommended only for PWH aged 18 years or older with an indication for receiving meningococcal B vaccine, such as functional or anatomic asplenia, persistent complement component deficiency, or receiving complement inhibitor. If given, the two-dose serogroup B series is given 1 month apart. If the three-dose series is given, it is at 0, 1–2, and 6 months.

MPOX

In June 2022, clusters of MSM with monkeypox (now referred to as Mpox) began to emerge in the United States (Kumar et al, 2022). The U.S. strategy was announced on June 28, 2022. One vaccine is currently available to adults ages ≥18 years of age based on CDC priority recommendations, the smallpox and Mpox live, non-replicating vaccine (JYNNEOS) (CDC, 2024a). The smallpox (vaccinia) live vaccine (ACAM2000) is not recommended. Vaccination should be given to any at-risk person, which includes:

- Persons who are gay, bisexual, and other MSM, transgender, or nonbinary people who, in the past 6 months, have had:
  - A new diagnosis of at least one sexually transmitted infection
  - More than one sex partner
  - Sex at a commercial sex venue
  - Sex in association with a large public event in a geographic area where Mpox transmission is occurring
- Persons who are sexual partners of the persons described above
- Persons who anticipate experiencing any of the situations described above
  - Bottom line:
    - ACAM2000 is not recommended for PWH regardless of CD4 count.
    - JYNNEOS is a two-dose intradermal series administered 4 weeks apart for at-risk individuals.

PNEUMOCOCCUS

PWH are at increased risk of developing pneumococcal disease, with the relative risk estimated at 7-fold higher than persons without HIV. The ACIP regularly updates its pneumococcal vaccination recommendations. The PCV13 is no longer available (CDC, 2024d).

- Bottom line:
  - **Pneumococcal vaccine-naive**: One dose of PCV20 or PCV15. If PCV15 is used, this should be followed by a dose of PPSV23 given at least 1 year after the PCV15 dose.

A minimum interval of 8 weeks between PCV15 and PPSV23 can be considered for immunocompromised adults to minimize the risk of invasive pneumococcal disease caused by serotypes unique to PPSV23 in these vulnerable groups

RESPIRATORY SYNCYTIAL VIRUS (RSV)

RSV vaccination is recommended for adults age 60 years or older who are at increased risk for severe RSV disease, including those with moderate or severe immune compromise (either attributable to a medical condition or receipt of immunosuppressive medications or treatment).

- Bottom line: Vaccination (single lifetime dose) is recommended for adults 75 years or older, and adults 60–74 who are at increased risk of severe RSV disease.

TETANUS, DIPHTHERIA, AND PERTUSSIS (TDAP)

PWH typically mount an adequate immune response against the toxins produced from these organisms. Therefore, the recommendation for vaccination in PWH does not differ from the general population.

- Bottom line: Administer one dose of Tdap, followed by a Td or Tdap booster every 10 years. If previously received Td only, give one dose of Tdap. Tdap should be given in every pregnancy regardless of immunization history.

RECOMMENDED READING

Thompson MA, Horberg MA, Agwu AL, et al. Primary care guidance for persons with human immunodeficiency virus: 2020 update by the HIV Medicine Association of the Infectious Diseases Society of America. *Clin Infect Dis.* 2021;73(11):E3572–E3605. https://Doi.Org/10.1093/Cid/Ciaa1391

REFERENCES

Akolo C, Adetifa I, Shepperd S, Volmink J. Treatment of latent tuberculosis infection in HIV infected persons. *Cochrane Database Syst Rev.* 2010(1):CD000171. http://www.ncbi.nlm.nih.gov/pubmed/20091503

American Thoracic Society/Centers for Disease Control and Prevention. Targeted tuberculin testing and treatment of latent tuberculosis infection: joint statement of the American Thoracic Society and the Centers for Disease Control and Prevention. *Am J Respir Crit Care Med.* 2000;161:S221–S247.

Boehme CC, Nabeta P, Hillemann D, et al. Rapid molecular detection of tuberculosis and rifampin resistance. *N Engl J Med.* 2010 Sep 9;363(11):1005–1015.

Bonito AJ. *Management of Dental Patients Who Are HIV Positive.* Summary, evidence report/technology assessment: number 37. AHRQ Publication No. 01-E041. Rockville, MD: Agency for Healthcare Research and Quality. http://www.ncbi.nlm.nih.gov/books/NBK11965. Published March 2001. Accessed November 15, 2015.

Cain KP, McCarthy KD, Heilg CM, et al. An algorithm for tuberculosis screening and diagnosis in people with HIV. *N Engl J Med.* 2010;362:707–716.

Cattamanchi A, Smith R, Steingart KR, et al. Interferon-gamma release assays for the diagnosis of latent tuberculosis infection in HIV-infected individuals: a systematic review and meta-analysis. *J AIDS.* 2011;56:230–238.

Centers for Disease Control and Prevention (CDC). Clinical considerations for treatment and prophylaxis of mpox in people who are immunocompromised. https:// www.cdc.gov/poxvirus/mpox/clinicians/people-with-HIV.html. Published June 13, 2024a. Accessed August 18, 2024.

CDC. Clinical testing and diagnosis for hepatitis B. https://www.cdc.gov/hepatitis-b/hcp/diagnosis-testing/index.html. Published March 6, 2024c. Accessed August 31, 2024.

CDC. COVID-19 information for specific groups of people. cdc.gov. https://stacks.cdc.gov/view/cdc/114895. Published Feb 25, 2022. Accessed February 1, 2025.

CDC. Pneumococcal vaccine recommendations. https:// ww.cdc.gov/pneumococcal/hcp/vaccine-recommendations/index.html. Published June 26, 2024d. Accessed August 31, 2024.

CDC. Updated guidelines for using interferon gamma release assays to detect *Mycobacterium tuberculosis* infection—United States, 2010. *MMWR.* 2010;59(RR-5):1–26.

CDC. Vaccine recommendations and guidelines of the ACIP. https://www.cdc.gov/vaccines/hcp/acip-recs/index.html. Published June 2024b. Accessed July 22, 2024d.

Department for Health and Human Services. Panel on Guidelines for the Prevention and Treatment of Opportunistic Infections in Adults and Adolescents with HIV. Guidelines for the prevention and treatment of opportunistic infections in adults and adolescents with HIV. National Institutes of Health, Centers for Disease Control and Prevention, HIV Medicine Association, and Infectious Diseases Society of America. https://clinicalinfo.hiv.gov/en/guidelines/adult-and-adolescent-opportunistic-infection. Published August 15, 2024. Accessed August 18, 2024.

Freed JR, Marcus M, Freed BA, et al. Oral health findings for HIV-infected adult medical patients from the HIV Cost and Services Utilization study. *J Am Dental Assoc.* 2005;136:1396–1405.

Getahun H, Harrington M, O'Brien R, et al. Diagnosis of smear-negative pulmonary tuberculosis in people with HIV infection or AIDS in resource-constrained settings: informing urgent policy changes. *Lancet.* 2007;369(9578):2042–2049.

Gray J, Reves R, Johnson S, et al. Identification of false-positive QuantiFERON-TB Gold In-Tube assays by repeat testing in PLWH at low risk of tuberculosis. *Clin Infect Dis.* 2012;54:e20–e23.

Horsburgh CR, Rubin EJ. Latent tuberculosis infection in the United States. *N Engl J Med.* 2011;364:1441–1448.

Kumar N, Acharya A, Gendelman HE, Byrareddy SN. The 2022 outbreak and pathobiology of the monkeypox virus. *J Autoimmun.* 2022;131:1022855.

Lewinsohn DM, Leonard MK, LoBue PA, et al. Official American Thoracic Society/Infectious Diseases Society of America/Centers for Disease Control and Prevention clinical practice guidelines: diagnosis of tuberculosis in adults and children. *Clin Infect Dis.* 2017;64(2):111–115.

New York State Department of Health AIDS Institute (NYSDOH). HIV and oral health: general principles. http://www.hivguidelines.org/clinical-guidelines/hiv-and-oral-health/general-principles. Published 2020. Accessed July 15, 2020.

Palmieri F, Girardi E, Pellicelli AM, et al. Pulmonary tuberculosis in HIV-infected patients presenting with normal chest radiograph and negative sputum smear. *Infection.* 2002;30(2):68–74.

Panagiotakopoulos L, Godfrey M, Moulia DL, et al. Use of an additional updated 2023–2024 COVID-19 vaccine dose for adults aged ≥65 years: recommendations of the Advisory Committee on Immunization Practices—United States, 2024, April 25. *MMWR.* 2024;73(16):377–381.

Raby E, Moyo M, Devendra A, et al. The effects of HIV on the sensitivity of a whole blood IFN-gamma release assay in Zambian adults with active tuberculosis. *PLoS One.* 2008 Jun 18;3(6):e2489.

World Health Organization (WHO). WHO consolidated guidelines on tuberculosis: module 2: screening: systematic screening for tuberculosis disease. https://www.who.int/publications/i/item/9789240022676. Published March 22, 2021. Accessed August 31, 2024.

9.

DIVERSITY AND HEALTH DISPARITIES

Gary F. Spinner

LEARNING OBJECTIVES

- Provide an understanding of the diversity of PWH, the complexity of unique cultures shaped by a multitude of factors, and the importance of developing a respectful, trusting clinician–patient relationship across cultural differences.
- Discuss the concepts of social determinants of health and racial/ethnic disparities, and how failure to address them leads to health inequity in HIV and other health conditions.
- Discuss the meaning of systemic racism, and how it has contributed to, or failed to rectify, health disparities among many people living with HIV (PWH).
- Explain how clinical trials have generally failed to recruit adequate numbers of women and racial and ethnic minority participants, and the potential clinical implications from failing to do so.
- Discuss how a patient's values, beliefs, and judgments may create barriers to successful treatment if HIV providers are not able to capably navigate cultural differences between patients and healthcare providers.
- Recognize the challenges in addressing racial and ethnic disparities in health care and in HIV.
- Analyze one's personal attitudes, beliefs, and (implicit) biases regarding race, ethnicity, sexual and gender diversity, and cultural practices and understand how these can hinder development of an effective patient–clinician relationship.
- Discuss the impact that culture, ethnicity, immigration status, sexual orientation, gender identity, religion, gender, and behavioral health problems may have on the care of PWH.

WHAT'S NEW?

The COVID-19 pandemic highlighted how Black and Brown communities continue to be more adversely impacted by health disparities. Previous progress to address differences in healthcare access and close gaps on population health outcomes has been disrupted by the pandemic's ongoing effects throughout the United States. Although the CDC is no longer updating its COVID-19 surveillance data, recent trends of declining COVID-19-associated mortality showed more significant declines in Black/African American and Latino/Hispanic people than in White people—possibly due to differences in vaccination uptake (CDC, 2023). During early years of the pandemic, Black and Hispanic people were less likely to receive vaccinations, but these differences diminished over time (CDC, 2023). Despite efforts to develop comprehensive national strategies and implement new funding and policy initiatives which cohesively respond to evolving public health priorities, core structural and societal issues continue to exacerbate HIV-associated inequities among communities of color (Lewis et al., 2024).

Lack of diversity in clinical trials continues to emerge as a key driver in ongoing health inequities. By restricting the demographics of certain populations included in clinical studies, this potentially limits their therapeutic use, undermines trust and relationship-building between health systems and certain communities, and ultimately impedes access to these interventions for populations who may benefit from it.

KEY POINTS

- Patients with HIV come from diverse backgrounds, and some may be mistrustful of healthcare providers and systems.
- Social determinants of health significantly impact persons living with HIV.
- Racism and discrimination have been core drivers of HIV-related inequities; beyond cultural competence, providers should practice cultural humility. It is important for HIV providers to recognize how biases, whether conscious or unconscious, can have a profound impact on patient health outcomes.

INTRODUCTION

HIV providers will encounter thousands of scientific facts, evidence-based guidelines, and various clinical resources aiming to build a compendium of knowledge necessary to provide optimal care to people with HIV (PWH). However, even the most expert healthcare provider, if lacking adequate understanding of how health outcomes are affected by race, ethnicity, gender, and sexual orientation, will not be able to fully support patients in attaining optimal health. This chapter on caring for diverse patient populations aims to provide insight into how varied living conditions, housing, economic factors, geography, neighborhood environment, access to health care, employment, education, and economic factors can be as important to the life of someone living with HIV as effective antiretroviral therapy (ART). It will also provide insight on how clinical trials, which aim to determine whether medications and other therapeutics are safe and effective, have been limited by underrepresentation of women and racial and ethnic minorities. This subsequently leads to profound impacts on diverse populations that might ultimately benefit from those interventions.

In this fifth year of the COVID-19 pandemic and 42nd year of the HIV pandemic, the concept of syndemic theory (first articulated by Singer in 1996) suggests that structural inequalities can interact synergistically to undermine the health of vulnerable populations (Singer, 1996). Syndemic theory helps explain how the interaction of a multitude of social factors impacts the pandemics of HIV and COVID-19, and why populations affected by one pandemic are concurrently and disproportionately impacted by others. A systematic review and meta-analysis of 44 studies of PWH with COVID-19 coinfection observed an increased risk of hospital admission, and two studies demonstrated an increased risk of mortality (Danwang et al., 2022). This chapter will explore the intersectionality of HIV, COVID-19, and systemic racism, and how they synergistically impact each other, and underscore how ending the HIV epidemic will likely require addressing the mutually reinforcing social systems that precipitate the conditions of inequality.

THE IMPORTANCE OF DIVERSITY IN CLINICAL TRIALS

In 2019, emtricitabine plus tenofovir alafenamide (FTC/TAF) was approved by the Food and Drug Administration (FDA) for the prevention of HIV in cisgender men who have sex with men (MSM) and transgender women. The phase 3 DISCOVER trial was a noninferiority trial comparing emtricitabine plus tenofovir disoproxil fumarate (FTC/TDF) to emtricitabine plus tenofovir alafenamide (FTC/TAF) as pre-exposure prophylaxis (PrEP) in approximately 5,300 MSM and transgender women at high risk of acquiring HIV (Mayer et al., 2020a; Mayer et al., 2020b). When the trial demonstrated noninferiority of FTC/TAF as PrEP, the manufacturer requested FDA approval for FTC/TAF to be used in cisgender men, transgender women, as well as cisgender women, even though the study did not include any cisgender women. When the FDA only approved its use in cisgender men and transgender women, citing the fact that no cisgender women were included in the study to prove noninferiority to FTC/TDF, the manufacturer responded that they did not find it feasible to evaluate FTC/TAF in cisgender women because the proposed methodology would require too large a clinical study population of women to prove noninferiority. However, several years later, the manufacturer subsequently began the PURPOSE 1 clinical trial to evaluate long-acting injectable lenacapavir (LEN) as PrEP and included cisgender women as a study group. In addition, PURPOSE 1 included a comparator arm of emtricitabine and tenofovir alafenamide fumarate (FTC/TAF)–subgroup efficacy results could therefore potentially also help determine the effectiveness of FTC/TAF in specific trial populations (Gilead, 2024). While this study found that LEN was highly effective in preventing HIV, it also found no difference in HIV incidence between women randomized to take FTC/TAF compared to the background population of women not on PrEP (Bekker et al., 2024). Although early analyses suggest this may be due to low adherence, it nevertheless underscores the importance of including diverse populations in clinical trials. Without appropriate representation, biomedical research findings will be of limited quality and generalizability, and ultimately impede equitable access to effective medical interventions.

The exclusion of women in clinical trials, despite biological differences between men and women, is not unusual. Women absorb, metabolize, distribute, and eliminate drugs differently compared to men (Ravindran, 2020). The exclusion of women in trials dates back to the 1970s: in 1977, the FDA recommended the exclusion of women of childbearing years from phase 1 and phase 2 studies (Samaei et al., 2022). For many years, this caused clinical trials to almost exclusively recruit white men. However, in 1993, the National Institutes of Health established guidelines for including women and minority populations in all government-funded research (U.S. Congress, 1993). There has been some improvement since then, and the FDA Drug Trials Snapshots of 2015 to 2019 data showed that women represented 51% of clinical trial participants globally and 56% of trial participants in the United States (FDA, 2020). Exclusion of pregnant women has historically been based on concern for the fetus, and while well-intentioned, it results in more than 80% of pregnant patients being prescribed medications that have not been studied in pregnancy (Heyrana et al., 2018). For women with HIV who become pregnant, HIV specialists can help contribute to knowledge on ART safety by reporting all cases to the antiretroviral pregnancy registry (Antiretroviral Pregnancy Registry, 2024).

The FDA underscores the importance of testing drugs and medical products in the people they are meant to help (FDA, 2020). This means that people of different ages, genders, races, and ethnic groups should be included in clinical trials (FDA, 2018). Section 907 of the FDA Safety and Innovation Act directed the FDA to investigate how well demographic subgroups (age, sex, and race and ethnicity) are included in clinical trials and to analyze subgroup-specific safety and effectiveness data (FDA, 2018). It is important to understand that while there are no biologic differences between races and that genetic differences are more common within races than between them, there is a possibility that missed genetic variants in certain populations excluded from clinical trials can potentially lead to differences in efficacy, adverse effects, or incorrect dosing, all of which may lead to patient harm.

In addition to women, racial and ethnic minority groups are significantly underrepresented in clinical research. One review of oncology trials found that over the past 14 years, there has been a decrease in recruitment, with Black and Latino/Hispanic persons and women less likely to be enrolled in cancer trials compared with white men (Duma et al., 2018). There is a significant racial disparity in cancer outcomes, yet clinical trials for cancer treatments are overrepresented by white male participants (Guerrero et al., 2018). For example, prostate cancer–associated incidence and mortality are significantly higher in Black men compared with white men, yet Black men participate significantly less in trials of prostate cancer treatments. In one large trial that *did* include a larger percentage of Black participants, investigators found that the study intervention led to better survival outcomes for Black participants compared to white participants (Sartor et al., 2020). A Pro-Publica analysis found that Black and Native American people are underrepresented in clinical trials for many drugs, even when those groups suffer disproportionately from the condition for which the drug is intended (Chen and Wong, 2018). Bhatnagar and colleagues found that despite Black persons having 2–3 times higher rates of multiple myeloma, pivotal trials for multiple myeloma therapeutics enrolled only 1.8% Black participants (Bhatnagar et al., 2017). In 2021, the FDA published the Drug Trials Snapshots documenting the imbalance of study participants: in studies that included almost 5,000 enrollees which led to approval of 18 new cancer treatments, 73% of participants were white; half were male; 6% were Latino/Hispanic; and only 5% were Black (FDA, 2021).

Given the increasing prevalence of chronic comorbidities among PWH, it's also important for HIV providers to be aware of disparities in chronic noncommunicable disease research. For example, cardiovascular disease (CVD) is the number one cause of death in the United States, and although there are significant racial and ethnic disparities in outcomes from CVD, women, Black persons, and Latino/Hispanic persons are underrepresented in CVD clinical trials (Michos et al., 2021).

WHY ARE THERE INSUFFICIENT NUMBERS OF WOMEN AND RACIAL AND ETHNIC MINORITY PARTICIPANTS IN CLINICAL TRIALS?

There are multiple reasons that racial and ethnic minority populations and women do not participate in clinical trials (FDA, 2018). Mistrust of the healthcare system (discussed elsewhere in this chapter), and of clinical research in particular, has consistently been cited as a long-standing reason for low interest in research participation. This mistrust is based on a multitude of historical examples of experimentation on people of color, and on women, including not being informed of needed treatment, and the withholding of treatment (for example, to enable the study of untreated syphilis) (CDC, 2021). There is also a history of forced sterilization of women without consent in the 1970s (Patel, 2017; Torpy, 2007).

Another significant reason for underrepresentation of racial and ethnic minority groups in clinical trials is lack of access to health care. An FDA draft guidance on Diversity in Clinical Trials (FDA, 2022) cites language and cultural differences, health literacy, lack of transportation, and time and resource constraints, among other reasons, for low rates of minority participation. Lack of access to healthcare centers that conduct clinical research programs for new therapies (Riner et al., 2022) and lack of awareness of clinical trials conducted at those programs may also limit participation. Another access-related barrier is that many U.S. clinicians are not affiliated with large academic medical centers and may be unaware of trials being conducted in their communities to which to refer eligible patients, or they do not have the time to discuss and refer patients to trials. In 2019, of the nearly 30 million patients receiving primary care at Federally Qualified Health Centers (FQHCs), 62% were racial and ethnic minorities (National Institutes of Health, 2020). Many FQHCs lack the resources or time to conduct clinical research, and often, the mission-driven need to provide care to vulnerable patient populations supersedes clinical research involvement. Furthermore, eligibility criteria in some trials can perpetuate disparities. For example, many studies exclude individuals who are unable to read, speak, and/or understand English, or who are not native English speakers (Muthukumar et al., 2021). Other eligibility criteria, such as exclusion for renal dysfunction, are more likely to exclude Black persons (Riner et al., 2022).

THE POTENTIAL FOR CHANGE

The Medicaid program, in which about 20% of the U.S. population overall receive health insurance, has not covered the cost of recipient participation in clinical trials, which thus passes costs to low-income people least able to afford it. At the same time, private insurers are required to provide reimbursement for research participation. The Clinical Treatment Act, passed by the U.S. Congress, went into effect on January 1, 2022, and requires Medicaid to pay the cost of routine care for recipients enrolled in clinical trials who have life-threatening conditions (Raths, 2022). Woodcock and colleagues (2021) argue that it is time for the biomedical industry, policymakers, government agencies, contract research organizations, and patient advocates to support the development and long-term sustainability of an infrastructure that unites clinical research with clinical care. Academic-community-government partnerships in a community engagement model can help address the lack of diversity in clinical trials, with partnerships between community members, clinicians, scientists, governmental officials, and industry (Woodcock et al., 2021).

This chapter explores in more depth the relationship between social determinants of health (SDOH) and health inequity, along with the impact of systemic racism and its impact on health. To further understand the role that SDOH play in clinical outcomes, collecting a uniform data set of demographic and socioeconomic data in clinical trials can facilitate the measurement of care, quality, utilization, and outcomes in highly impacted populations (Kahn et al., 2022). To alleviate the discrepancy between who participates in clinical trials and the real-world experience of patients who ultimately are prescribed the treatments studied, more robust efforts are needed to eliminate barriers of gender, race, and ethnicity in clinical trial participation.

HIV AND COVID-19: TWO PANDEMICS—SAME RACIAL AND ETHNIC DISPARITIES

The dual pandemics of HIV and COVID-19 share much in common beyond their viral etiologies. Both HIV and COVID-19 disproportionately affect Black and Latino/Hispanic populations, yet the health disparities in these two pandemics have nothing to do with any biological differences or virus pathology. These disparities are directly related to SDOH, racial and ethnic health inequities, and societal policies that have either created or failed to address these unequal conditions. To understand the similarities of these two pandemics is to recognize how SDOH create health inequity among people of color, leading to worse outcomes among those with HIV, COVID-19, or many other health conditions.

According to the World Health Organization, "SDOH (SDH) are the conditions in which people are born, grow, work, live, and age, and the wider set of forces and systems shaping the conditions of daily life. These forces and systems include economic policies and systems, development agendas, social norms, social policies, and political systems" (World Health Organization, 2024).

Black people, Latino/Hispanics, and Native Americans all experience significant health disparities in the United States. A *health disparity* is "a particular type of health difference that is closely linked with social, economic, and/or environmental disadvantage." Health disparities adversely affect groups of people who have systematically experienced greater obstacles to health care based on their racial or ethnic group identity; religion; socioeconomic status; gender; age; mental health status; cognitive, sensory, or physical disability; sexual orientation or gender identity; geographic location; or other characteristics historically linked to discrimination or exclusion (DHHS, 2011). While unequal access to health care can be one determinant of less-than-equal health outcomes, disparities go far beyond access to care. For example, even with equal access to services in the Veterans Health Administration, mortality disparities for Black veterans with stage 4 chronic kidney disease, colon cancer, diabetes, HIV, rectal cancer, and stroke have been described, as well as for Native American and Alaska Native veterans undergoing noncardiac major surgery; and for Hispanic/Latino veterans with HIV (Peterson et al., 2018).

HIV: RACIAL AND ETHNIC DISPARITIES

Black and Latino/Hispanic populations account for a vastly disproportionate percentage of PWH. According to CDC data (2022b), while Black persons account for only 12% of the U.S. population, they comprised 37% of all newly diagnosed PWH in 2019. Latino/Hispanic persons comprise 18.5% of the U.S. population but accounted for 42% of HIV incidence in 2019. Black men and women have higher rates of some sexually transmitted infections than other racial/ethnic groups, increasing risk for HIV acquisition and transmission (CDC, 2022b). The lifetime risk of acquiring HIV for Black men is 1 in 27, 1 in 50 for Latino men, compared with 1 in 76 for white men. Black women have a 10 times higher lifetime risk of HIV compared with white women (Singh et al., 2022). Among MSM, 1 of every 2 Black MSM has a lifetime risk of HIV acquisition, compared with 1 in 6 Latino MSM and 1 in 11 white MSM (Hess et al., 2017).

Disparities persist further along the HIV care continuum. White PWH are more likely to be virally suppressed then Black PWH (Crepaz et al., 2018; CDC, 2024): while 56% of white PWH were suppressed, only 41% of Black PWH were suppressed, and this held true by gender, by age, among MSM, and people who inject drugs.

Although Black and Latino/Hispanic MSM have the highest likelihood of acquiring HIV, white MSM are far more likely to be offered key HIV prevention interventions (i.e., PrEP) (Kanny et al., 2019). This disparity persists even among people with health insurance and a usual source of care. Analyses of PrEP prescribing have shown that while PrEP prescriptions increased significantly in all regions of the United States, more PrEP prescriptions were written for white people, and least for Black people (Sullivan et al., 2022). While Black people account for 37% of all new HIV infections, they account for only 14% of PrEP users. Similarly, while Hispanic/Latino people account for 42% of all new HIV diagnoses, they account for only 18% of PrEP users (AIDSVu, 2024).

COVID-19: RACIAL AND ETHNIC DISPARITIES

Like HIV, COVID-19 disproportionately affects people of color. An early analysis of county data found that 97% of predominantly Black counties had at least one COVID-19 case (compared to 80% of other counties), and that counties with a majority of Black residents experienced differences in mortality (Millett et al., 2020b). These counties tended to have lower rates of insurance coverage, higher rates of unemployment, crowded housing, poor air quality, and reduced ability to practice social distancing. In addition, employed persons in predominantly Black counties were more likely to be classified as essential workers, to use public transportation, and to have jobs that did not allow for remote work. Using the same methodology to examine Latino/Hispanic majority counties, a similar outcome of disproportionately high COVID-19 cases and deaths was found. Other surveillance data revealed that severe infection and hospitalization rates were higher for Black and Latino/Hispanic populations as well as Native American/Alaska Native persons (CDC, 2022a).

Key social factors most likely contributing to the increased morbidity and mortality of COVID-19 in racial and ethnic minority populations include poverty, high-density and crowded housing, and differing employment status/remote work flexibility. Other factors include reliance on public transportation; overrepresentation in jails, prisons, homeless shelters, and detention centers where social distancing is not possible; living in multigenerational households where it is difficult to protect older family members; not having sick leave (which increases the likelihood that someone keeps working while ill); lack of health insurance; and distrust of the healthcare system, along with racism, stigma, and systemic inequities (CDC, 2022a).

COVID-19, HIV, AND THEIR LINK TO SYSTEMIC RACISM

Health equity, as defined by the U.S. Department of Health and Human Services, is the attainment of the highest level of health for all people. It requires valuing everyone equally with focused and ongoing societal efforts to address avoidable inequalities, historical and contemporary injustices, and the elimination of health and healthcare disparities (DHHS, 2011).

Significant health disparities experienced by communities of color are examples of health inequity. The unequal adverse health impacts of HIV and COVID-19 hold true for other health conditions, such as certain cancers, respiratory diseases, diabetes, hypertension, and other comorbidities, along with worse clinical outcomes for most of these conditions. Infant mortality for Black infants is 2.5 times higher than for white infants (CDC, 2022d). Black men have a nearly 5-year shorter life expectancy than white men: they are 30% more likely to die from heart disease, twice as likely to be diagnosed with diabetes, twice as likely to have a stroke, and 40% more likely to have hypertension but 10% less likely to have it under control (Graham, 2015). The Black Lives Matter movement, which originated in 2013, gained international attention in the early years of COVID-19 and highlighted other systemic racial injustices: namely, Black persons are over 2.5 times as likely to be killed while in police custody (Roper, 2020) and are incarcerated at 5.1 times the rate for white persons (Nellis, 2016).

To truly understand the racial and ethnic disparities of the HIV and COVID-19 pandemics, one must recognize the pandemic of racism. According to Ibram Kendi (2019), a scholar of race and discriminatory policy in America, "Racism is a marriage of racist policies and racist ideas that produces and normalizes racial inequities, and . . . racial inequity is when two or more racial groups are not standing on approximately equal footing. A racist policy is any measure that produces or sustains racial inequity between racial groups." Social conditions leading to adverse health, including poverty, lack of healthcare access, lower wage employment, segregated and overcrowded housing, and educational disadvantages, are systemic problems related to either policies that have created these disadvantages or a lack of appropriate policies to address and eliminate these disadvantages.

Systemic racism, also known as *institutional racism*, is a form of racism that is embedded as normal practice within society or an organization that can lead to such issues as discrimination in employment, housing, health care, political power, criminal justice, and education, among other issues. It must be recognized for causing many of the social inequities that people of color experience. There are a multitude of programs and policies that can be traced back to racial and ethnic discrimination. For example, the practice of banks denying housing loans to Black people or charging them higher rates of interest with stricter repayment terms has led to fewer Black people owning homes. Historically, the Federal Housing Administration's refusal to insure mortgages in Black neighborhoods and their requirement of developers receiving subsidized loans to build subdivisions that specifically exclude Black people are systemically racist policies that created segregated and more densely populated housing and denied Black people of one of the most common ways to build personal wealth: home ownership (Rothstein, 2017).

Another example of systemic racism relates to unemployment benefits. Almost a quarter of Black workers live in the South, where over half of all new HIV infections occur, and where racism has long played a role in limiting safety net program. During the COVID-19 pandemic, the U.S. unemployment rate skyrocketed. Because unemployment insurance programs are state controlled, and several Southern states have excluded many jobs that are more likely to employ Black and Latino/Hispanic persons, people of color have not received the same degree of unemployment relief from these programs. Indeed, the average high school–educated white person is twice as likely to receive unemployment benefits as the average high school–educated Black person (Nichols, and Simms 2012), and Black persons receive lower rates of compensation than white persons (Badger et al., 2020).

The current U.S. federal initiative to end the HIV epidemic attempts to address some of the geography-based HIV disparities, by directing resources to highly impacted jurisdictions (HRSA, 2020). However, SDOH faced by people of color in these areas threaten to undermine the plan's intended progress. A modeling study of HIV incidence suggests that the goal of ending the HIV epidemic is unlikely to be met because of many barriers, including lack of access to health care, proposed cutbacks to and/or outright elimination of the Affordable Care Act, and failure to expand Medicaid in many of the Southern states (Nosyk et al., 2020). Other researchers have pointed out that income inequality, poverty, the degree of Black/white segregation, housing instability, and homelessness are associated with HIV in certain communities where poverty, vacant housing, unemployment, and isolation are most prevalent (Millett, 2020a).

WHAT NEEDS TO BE DONE?

The Ryan White Program, which serves over half a million PWH in the United States, has been a hugely successful program with significantly better viral suppression outcomes in Ryan White–funded clinics compared with other HIV clinics. Almost three-quarters of PWH served are racial and ethnic minorities, and the majority live below the federal poverty level (Cheever, 2021; CDC, 2022c). Ryan White clinics are funded to address common barriers experienced by patients, such as transportation, primary medical care, food bank services, housing, linguistic services, childcare, emergency financial relief, substance use treatment, case management, and a host of other "wrap around" services. Ryan White–funded clinics attempt to address gaps in health inequities, and much of the program's success can be attributed to its intent to specifically address the racial and ethnic disparities impacting people of color, as well as other marginalized groups. The high degree of success of the Ryan White Program, in which SDOH are actively addressed, can serve as a model of healthcare delivery to all patients.

PROVIDING CULTURALLY COMPETENT CARE

It is not uncommon for healthcare providers to harbor false beliefs about biological differences between people based on race. One study of medical students and residents found that half of survey respondents believed one or more false statements about biological differences between Black and white persons, including the belief that Black persons do not feel pain the same way that whites persons do, or that Black skin is thicker than white skin (Hoffman et al., 2016). These prejudices alienate patients who rightfully perceive the racism and implicit bias that some healthcare providers harbor.

Provider bias, and sometimes overt racism, can lead to longer waiting times for people of color, taking patient concerns less seriously, doing a less thorough workup of health concerns, recommending different treatment options based on a perceived lack of adherence, along with many other differences in the treatment. A systematic review of implicit racial and ethnic bias among healthcare providers found that in the majority of studies, most healthcare providers demonstrated implicit bias through more favorable attitudes toward white patients and negative attitudes toward Black and Latino/Hispanic patients (Hall et al., 2015). Four studies found that healthcare providers saw Black persons as less cooperative, less compliant, and less responsive to medical advice. Several studies found healthcare providers associating poor adherence and noncompliance with Latino/Hispanic patients, and two studies found moderate amounts of bias against darker-skinned patients than lighter-skinned patients.

Even healthcare providers who see themselves as providing equitable care may unknowingly be interacting with patients of color differently and less effectively than with white patients. Clinical education programs need to address issues of race and ethnicity more actively in the training of physicians, nurses, and other healthcare workers. Unless healthcare providers acknowledge and change individual racist and ethnic biases, and work to implement health and social policies that eliminate racism and bias, health systems will continue to perpetuate the disparities witnessed with the HIV and COVID-19 pandemics, and a multitude of other health conditions. Further examples of the importance of diversity are outlined below, so that HIV providers can elevate their awareness and appreciation for the various populations which entrust clinicians with their health care.

RETENTION IN CARE

Retaining patients in care requires culturally competent staff at all levels of an organization. HIV providers may often focus solely on medical aspects of HIV medicine out of habit, and view issues of diversity, cultural competence, and cultural humility as "soft areas" of lesser importance than learning about HIV drug resistance or the latest ART. However, doing so runs the risk of failing to adequately comprehend how patients' behaviors, beliefs, and the characteristics of their unique social, ethnic, racial, religious, gender identity, sexual orientation, or country of origin may affect their engagement with the healthcare system. Failing to understand the important cultural context within which a patient interacts with health systems and providers often leads to poor patient adherence with treatment, misunderstandings about care plans, or worse, disengagement. To successfully provide care to patients and help people achieve their health goals, providers should endeavor to understand the unique context of each patient and provide care that acknowledges specific cultural values that may impact acceptance of treatment.

Research has suggested that PWH who were out of care account for 61% of new HIV infections in the United States (Skarbinski et al., 2015). One North Carolina study that analyzed patients with acute HIV infection found that most transmission events (77%) were attributable to partners with previously diagnosed infection, of whom only 23% were reportedly in care and taking ART within the time that transmission likely occurred (Cope et al., 2015). This is compelling evidence that United States healthcare systems are failing to treat and retain many PWH. This may be due to multiple reasons, including patient disengagement from care, but it underscores the crucial need to improve how healthcare providers interact with patients to successfully retain people in care and adherent to treatment. Failure to develop cultural competence and cultural humility increases the likelihood that PWH will lose contact with care. Therefore, all healthcare providers must develop an awareness of their own values, beliefs, and attitudes, and what biases may be inherent in the providers' own culture.

DIVERSITY OF PATIENTS

Many providers caring for PWH may be serving patients from racial or ethnic groups different from their own. In the United States, PWH are disproportionately Black and Latino/Hispanic, and, regardless of race or ethnicity, are often affected by poverty, substance use and behavioral health conditions, unemployment, housing instability, incarceration, limited education/training, and may also identify as sexual and gender minority. Some patients may be immigrants or refugees whose language and cultural differences may influence acceptance of healthcare services from a system of care culturally different from their own. Understanding how patients' spiritual and religious values may impact their healthcare decision-making is important when caring for diverse groups of patients. However, it is critical to avoid stereotyping people, which also creates barriers to relationship-building. The values, beliefs, and judgments of PWH may differ from those of their healthcare provider, and unless healthcare providers are able to withhold their own judgment of patients' circumstances, trusting relationships may never develop.

THE IMPORTANCE OF TRUST

Trust is a critically important component of an effective patient–clinician relationship. Without trust, a patient is less likely to adhere to a treatment plan. Patients who do not trust their healthcare provider or the healthcare system may be less likely to take prescribed medications, attend appointments, or accept the advice of their clinician.

Mistrust by racial and ethnic minority populations in the United States is common. A Kaiser Family Foundation survey found that one-third of Black and one-third of Latino/Hispanic persons reported experiencing unfair treatment by the healthcare system compared to less than half those numbers of white persons (James, 1999). Black persons were used without providing informed consent in medical experimentation by the U.S. Public Health Service from 1932 to 1972 in the notorious Tuskegee syphilis study (CDC, 2021), which created a legacy of mistrust (Skarbinski et al., 2015). Mistrust has also led to conspiracy theories about the origins of HIV. In 2005, a national telephone survey of 500 Black persons found that 53% agreed that "there is a cure for AIDS, but it is being withheld from the poor"; 27% agreed that "AIDS was produced in a government laboratory"; and 16% agreed that "AIDS was created by the government to control the Black population" (Bogart et al., 2005).

DISPARITIES IN HEALTH CARE

The HIV epidemic in the United States continues to be characterized by significant racial and ethnic disparities and disproportionately affects Hispanic/Latino, Black, Asian, Native Americans/Alaskan Natives, and Native Hawaiian/Other Pacific Islander people in various ways (CDC, 2022c). For many patients, the route of HIV transmission carries significant stigma. Among Black men, of whom 80% acquired HIV by male-to-male sexual contact, being gay or bisexual carries a stigma that is prevalent both in the general population and within the Black community. Stigma creates barriers that keep many men from being tested for HIV or connecting to care once an HIV diagnosis is established. Understanding the effects of stigma and developing nonjudgmental ways to communicate effectively with patients requires that care teams first acknowledge that patients may enter the relationship assuming that providers harbor the same biases as the general population. Becoming culturally competent requires clinicians to thoughtfully develop approaches with each person to allay their fear of disapproval by healthcare providers and provide reassurance that the patient's personal health information will be protected and kept confidential.

The need to provide culturally appropriate HIV care is evident. Failing to adequately understand a patient's culture—best defined as the unique set of beliefs, characteristics, and behaviors formed by the communities in which a patient resides—can create barriers between patients and providers. Lack of trust by the patient hampers successful treatment, and this mistrust may occur especially if patients believe they will receive unequal treatment. Studies examining multiple health conditions have documented the unequal treatment provided to Black and Latino/Hispanic persons. According to the Institute of Medicine (2003), racial and ethnic minorities often receive a lower quality of healthcare services even when insurance status and income are the same as those for non-minorities. Black and Latino/Hispanic patients have higher risk of acute myocardial infarction, re-hospitalization, and death from acute coronary syndrome, yet are less likely than white patients to receive angiography or other coronary interventions (Graham, 2015).

Clinicians need to understand what concerns a patient may have to recommended therapy to better collaborate and share information on potential consequences that may occur without treatment. Asking open-ended questions such as, "What are your concerns about taking this medication?" may allow patients to express their concerns more fully and thus give providers an opportunity to address them.

BIAS IN HEALTHCARE

Cultural *competence* requires taking time to learn what cultural barriers might exist. Cultural *humility* is an ongoing process of self-reflection and self-critique combined with a willingness to learn from others, which helps providers better understand and respect cultural differences, if present. Ethnocentric healthcare providers who only view a patient's culture from the perspective of their own culture risk losing patient trust. Healthcare providers are not immune to the biases that exist in the general population: prior research has found that white males were twice as likely as Black males to be prescribed analgesics for pain, whereas female physicians prescribed higher doses for Black than for white patients (Weisse et al., 2001). A study examining how patient race affects physician perceptions found that physicians rated Black patients as less intelligent, less educated, more likely to abuse drugs and alcohol, and less likely to adhere to treatment even when considering the patient's income and education (van Ryn and Burke, 2000). A systematic review of 15 studies examining racial and ethnic biases found that in all but one study, racial and ethnic bias by healthcare providers existed (Hall et al., 2015). These studies show how racism and personal bias can lead to unequal care provision.

Bias can be either overt (explicit) or covert (implicit). Derogatory comments made by providers or clinic staff about particular "types" of patients are an example of bias. Judgmental comments about how frequently certain patients develop sexually transmitted infections, use the emergency room, request or seek pain medications, and have too many uncared-for children are examples of overt bias and stereotyping. Such comments, in addition to being highly unprofessional and judgmental, may reinforce among other health professionals/staff that bias and judgment are acceptable professional conduct. Negative comments about a patient, especially if overheard by other patients, can impress on patients that they may be the topic of unwanted conversation. Healthcare organizations need to ensure that all staff, regardless of their role, become culturally competent and demonstrate humility. Recognizing the cultural differences that might exist between a patient and healthcare provider is an essential step to welcoming each patient with acceptance and understanding. Only by attempting to recognize and understand these differences can a healthcare provider begin to comprehend what may be needed to best inspire trust in providers, healthcare institutions, and medical therapies.

WOMEN AND HIV

There are 21 million women worldwide living with HIV, and in the United States, 19% of people with HIV are women (UNAIDS, 2024). Most women diagnosed with HIV (84%) acquire the virus through heterosexual sex (CDC, 2024). Black women are disproportionately affected, with 54% of U.S. women living with HIV being Black (CDC, 2024). Women living with HIV experience intimate partner violence at twice the national average (Gruskin et al., 2014). One meta-analysis showed that 55% of women with HIV in the United States have experienced trauma and violence (Gruskin et al., 2014). Cis- and transgender women living with HIV who have experienced trauma and violence have a 4-fold higher likelihood of ART nonadherence. HIV providers should inquire, with sensitivity, about interpersonal violence and refer people to appropriate crisis and intimate partner violence services as needed. Healthcare providers should understand that many survivors of domestic abuse feel powerless and trapped because of factors such as economic dependency, caregiving/childcare responsibilities, and fear of housing instability. Many women may be hesitant to seek timely help. A careful mental health screening should be done, and referral to appropriate behavioral health services should be made when indicated.

SEXUAL AND GENDER MINORITY PATIENTS

Many lesbian, gay, bisexual, transgender, and queer (LGBTQ+) patients do not feel welcome by healthcare providers and organizations, and prior bad experiences may then impact healthcare-seeking behaviors and motivations (National LGBT Health Education Center, 2015). One study of Black MSM found that 29% experienced racial and sexual stigma from their healthcare providers, and 48% reported mistrust of the healthcare system (Eaton et al., 2015). If patients feel uncomfortable speaking about their sexual orientation, they are far more likely not to share important information. Approaches to help LGBTQ+ patients feel more welcome include using gender-neutral pronouns, encouraging the use of preferred names (even if someone's legal name may be different), and training staff to have a nonjudgmental attitude. Learning and using terms and language that patients prefer may also help create a more welcoming, comfortable care environment. For example, patients may use the terms "top" or "bottom" to describe insertive or receptive anal sex. Healthcare providers should inquire about partner(s) without making assumptions about gender identities or sexual preferences, and use more inclusive language (for example, "Do you have a partner?" or "Are you in a relationship?" are more appropriate questions than "Do you have a husband or wife?"). A patient who feels accepted by their care team is more likely to stay engaged in care. Conversely, a patient who perceives disapproval of their lifestyle, sexual orientation, or practices will feel uncomfortable and is much less likely to remain connected.

BEHAVIORAL HEALTH PROBLEMS

The HIV Costs and Services Utilization Study found that nearly 50% of adults treated for HIV have symptoms of a psychiatric disorder—a 4–8 times higher prevalence than the general population (Bing et al., 2001). In the general population, there is a 10- to 20-year reduction in life expectancy in people with severe mental health disorders (Chang et al., 2011) such that psychiatric disorders carry a risk of mortality even greater than that of smoking (Chesney et al., 2014).

Identifying PWH with psychiatric conditions or substance use disorders is crucial, as people with behavioral health conditions may sometimes also experience treatment adherence challenges (Paterson and Swindells, 2000). Providers should carefully collect information on each person's mental health history and refer to additional services as needed and if acceptable to patients. Stigma about mental health may keep many people from accessing services, and on-site behavioral health increases the likelihood that patients will connect to treatment. Many people with substance use disorders may experience a sense of rejection when they reveal their histories and may be fearful that mentioning pain will be perceived as "drug-seeking" (a common stereotype) by a healthcare provider. Cultural competence and humility involve communicating with patients openly and without judgment and require efforts to develop trust and help reduce the stigma associated with substance use.

LANGUAGE AND COMMUNICATION

Language comprehension and effective communication are essential, as barriers can interfere with successful treatment and positive health outcomes. Prior research on people who received emergency room care demonstrated that Spanish-speaking patients were less likely to understand their discharge instructions or carry out follow-up plans (Crane, 1997). Another survey found that 1 in 5 Spanish-speaking patients delayed or declined medical treatment because of language barriers; given the diversity of languages spoken by many PWH, this underscores the need to provide linguistically appropriate services (DHHS, 2011).

Hiring multilingual and multicultural staff is important for advancing organizational infrastructure and cultural competency across healthcare settings. Clinics should utilize high-quality, professional interpreter services (on-site/in-person or telephone-based) as appropriate. Patients who used the interpreter services received significantly more recommended preventive services, made more office visits, and had more prescriptions written and filled (Jacobs et al., 2004). Use of family members or friends as "proxy" interpreters may limit full information-sharing if patients are not comfortable discussing sensitive information in front of family/friends. Language concordance may be especially important for immigrant populations who often experience linguistic barriers, compounding cultural differences which then impede appropriate healthcare service delivery.

RELIGION AND SPIRITUALITY

A 2014 Gallup survey found that 81% of Americans identify with a particular religion (Newport, 2014), and research has also demonstrated that many PWH have strong religious affiliations (Cotton, 2006). People often turn to religion and spirituality in times of illness, and this often influences the way a person perceives and copes with their health situation and decision-making. A patient's faith may sometimes conflict with medical advice, which can impact treatment adherence. It is important that providers ask people about their faith and spiritual beliefs, and how those beliefs may affect perception of illness and acceptance of (and comfort with) recommended treatment.

CREATING A PATIENT-CENTERED HIV PRACTICE

Racial and ethnic diversity in healthcare leadership and staff is necessary to build person-centered healthcare organizations. Including community members and patient/client representatives on governing boards (as is done at FQHCs) can help hold an organization accountable for providing appropriate and respectful care to diverse populations. Patients want empathetic, compassionate healthcare providers who communicate effectively. Clinic materials should be developed with diverse linguistic needs and varying degrees of health literacy in mind. Better healthcare outcomes have been associated with providers with whom patients can share their feelings and thoughts, and patients who have empathic and communicative healthcare providers are more likely to adhere to treatment plans (Sitapati et al., 2012).

Changing the model of care from traditional physician-centered practices to a model that places the patient in the center of the relationship—that is, the patient-centered medical home (PCMH) model—improves quality of care. The PCMH model relies on reorganizing care to ensure that it is comprehensive and responsive to patient-identified needs, with integrated physical and mental health services. Care that is patient-centered also supports patients' efforts to manage their own care to whatever degree they may choose. Services are coordinated so there are smooth transitions across levels of care involving primary care clinics, hospitals, and specialty programs. Services should also be accessible and flexible, with after-hours healthcare provider availability, open access scheduling, and tele-health options as appropriate. Last, focus should be placed on quality and safety, using evidence-based standards and relevant data to recognize opportunities for performance improvement (Agency for Healthcare Research and Quality, 2015). One study demonstrated that the PCMH model improved retention in care for PWH (Sitapati et al., 2012).

Ultimately, a patient-centered approach incorporates interventions to better address the racial, ethnic, and cultural differences between providers and patients, and trains all staff accordingly. Perhaps most importantly, aspiring and established healthcare providers must raise self-awareness of their individual cultural beliefs, values, and attitudes and any biases that may be inherent in them. Increasing mindfulness of one's own biases and engaging in honest attempts to transcend them will allow HIV providers to communicate effectively, with empathy, and without prejudgment—thereby facilitating improved and supportive relationships with patients.

RECOMMENDED READING

National Academies of Sciences, Engineering, and Medicine (NASEM); Policy and Global Affairs; Committee on Women in Science, Engineering, and Medicine; Committee on Improving the Representation of Women and Underrepresented Minorities in Clinical Trials and Research; Bibbins-Domingo K, Helman A, eds. *Improving Representation in Clinical Trials and Research: Building Research Equity for Women and Underrepresented Groups.* Washington, DC: National Academies Press; May 17, 2022.

Why Diverse Representation in Clinical Research Matters and the Current State of Representation Within the Clinical Research Ecosystem. https://www.ncbi.nlm.nih.gov/books/NBK584396/. Accessed August 31, 2024.

REFERENCES

Agency for Healthcare Research and Quality. Defining the PCMH. https://www.pcmh.ahrq.gov/page/defining-pcmh. Published 2015. Accessed. July 23, 2024.

AIDSVu. Deeper look: PrEP. https://aidsvu.org/resources/deeper-look-prep/?gad_source=1&gclid=CjwKCAjwzIK1BhAuEiwAHQmU3ijeQiKYglD3B2-EDSB6R6CNcBHiVA6nF62epxHHLOTqhdPuYtbFiBoCSqwQAvD_BwE. Published 2024. Accessed July 24, 2024.

Antiretroviral Pregnancy Registry. www.apregistry.com. Updated June 2024. Accessed July 23, 2024.

Badger, E, Parlapiano A, Bui Q. Black workers will hurt the most if Congress doesn't extend jobless benefits. *New York Times*, August 7, 2020. https://www.nytimes.com/2020/08/07/upshot/unemployment-benefits-racial-disparity.html

Bekker LG, Das M, Karim QA, et al. Twice-yearly lenacapavir or daily F/TAF for HIV prevention in cisgender women. *NEJM.* 2024;391(13):1179–1192. doi:10.1056/NEJMoa2407001.

Bhatnagar V, Gormley N, Kazandjian D, et al. FDA analysis of racial demographics in multiple myeloma trials. *Blood.* 2017;130(Suppl 1):4352–4352. http://doi: 10.1182/blood.V130.Suppl_1.4352.4352

Bing EG, Burnam A, Longshore D, et al. Psychiatric disorders and drug use among HIV-infected adults in the US. *Arch Gen Psychiatry.* 2001;58:721–728.

Bogart LM, Thorburn S. Are HIV/AIDS conspiracy beliefs a barrier to HIV prevention among African Americans? *J AIDS.* 2005;38(2):213–218.

Centers for Disease Control and Prevention (CDC). Health equity considerations & racial & ethnic minority groups. cdc.gov. https:// www.cdc.gov/coronavirus/2019-ncov/community/health-equity/vaccine-equity.html. Published March 29, 2022a. Accessed August 30, 2022.

CDC. HIV and African American people, 2020. cdc.gov. https://www.cdc.gov/hiv/group/racialethnic/africanamericans/index.html. Published June 28, 2022b. Accessed July 26, 2020.

CDC. HIV by age: viral suppression. cdc.gov. https://www.cdc.gov/hiv/group/age/viral-suppression.html. Published July 1, 2022c. Accessed July 22, 2022.

CDC. HIV fast facts: HIV in the US by race and ethnicity. cdc.gov. https://www.cdc.gov/hiv/data-research/facts-stats/race-ethnicity.html. Published May 21, 2024. Accessed July 24, 2024.
CDC. Reproductive health: infant mortality. https://www.cdc.gov/reproductivehealth/maternalinfanthealth/infantmortality.htm#:~:text=Infant%20Mortality%20Rates%20by%20Race%20and%20Ethnicity%2C%202016,-*Source%3A%20p.&text=Native%20Hawaiian%20or%20other%20Pacific,Asian%3A%203.6. Published June 22, 2022d. Accessed August 18, 2024.
CDC. Risk for COVID-19 infection, hospitalization, and death by race/ethnicity. cdc.gov. Published May 25, 2023. https:// archive.cdc.gov/www_cdc_gov/coronavirus/2019-ncov/covid-data/investigations-discovery/hospitalization-death-by-race-ethnicity.html. Accessed August 18, 2024.
CDC. The US Public Health Service Syphilis Study at Tuskegee: timeline. cdc.gov. http://cdc.gov/Tuskegee/timeline.htm. Published April 21, 2021. Accessed July 24, 2022.
Chang CK, Hayes RD, Perera G, et al. Life expectancy at birth for people with serious mental illness and other major disorders from a secondary mental healthcare case register in London. *PLoS One.* 2011;10:1371.
Chen C, Wong R. Black patients miss out on promising cancer drugs. propublica.org. https://www.propublica.org/article/black-patients-miss-out-on-promising-cancer-drugs. Published September 19, 2018. Accessed August 19, 2024.
Cheever L. HRSA announces increase in HIV viral suppression rate in new 2020 Ryan White HIV/AIDS program client-level data report. https://www.hiv.gov/blog/hrsa-announces-increase-hiv-viral-suppression-rate-new-2020-ryan-white-hivaids-program-client. Published 2021. Accessed July 22, 2022.
Chesney E, Goodwin GM, Fazel S. Risks all-cause and suicide mortality in mental disorders: a meta-review. *World Psychiatry.* June 2014;13(2):153–160.
Cope AB, Power KA, Kuruc JD, et al. Ongoing HIV transmission and the HIV care continuum in North Carolina. *PLoS One.* 2015;10(6):e0127950.
Cotton S. Spirituality and religion in patients with HIV/AIDS. *Gen Intern Med.* 2006;12;21(Suppl 5):S5–S13.
Crane JA. Patient comprehension of doctor–patient communication on discharge from the emergency department. *Emerg Med.* 1997 Jan–Feb;15(1):1–7.
Crepaz N, Dong X, Wang X, et al. Racial and ethnic disparities in sustained viral suppression and transmission risk potential among persons receiving HIV care—United States, 2014. *MMWR.* 2018 Feb 2;67(4):113–118.
Duma N, Vera Aguilera J, Paludo J, et al. Representation of minorities and women in oncology clinical trials: review of the past 14 years. *JCO.* 2018;14(1):e1–e10. http://doi:10.1200/JOP.2017.025288
Danwang C, Noubiap JJ, Robert A, et al. Outcomes of patients with HIV and COVID-19 co-infection: a systematic review and meta-analysis. *AIDS Res Ther.* 2022;19(1):3. doi:10.1186/s12981-021-00427-y
Eaton LA, Driffin DD, Kegler C, et al. The role of stigma and medical mistrust in the routine healthcare engagement of black men who have sex with men. *Am J Public Health.* 2015;105(2):75–82.
US Food & Drug Administration (FDA). 2015–2019 drug trials snapshots summary report: five-year summary and analysis of clinical trial participation and demographics. https://www.fda.gov/media/143592/download?attachment. Published November 2020. Accessed August 18, 2024.
FDA. Diversity plans to improve enrollment of participants from underrepresented racial and ethnic populations in clinical trials guidance for industry. fda.gov. www.fda.gov/media/157635/download. Published April 2022. Accessed August 18, 2024.
FDA. Drug trials snapshots summary report 2020. fda.gov. www.fda.gov/media/145718/download. Published February 2021. Accessed August 2024.
FDA. US Food & Drug Administration Food and Drug Safety and Innovation ACT (FDASIA). https://www.fda.gov/regulatory-information/food-and-drug-administration-safety-and-innovation-act-fdasia/fdasia-title-vii-overview, 2018. Published March 28, 2018. Accessed August 18, 2024.
Gilead.com. Gilead's twice-yearly lenacapavir demonstrated 100% efficacy and superiority to daily Truvada® for HIV prevention. https://www.gilead.com/news-and-press/press-room/press-releases/2024/6/gileads-twiceyearly-lenacapavir-demonstrated-100-efficacy-and-superiority-to-daily-truvada-for-hiv-prevention. June 2024.
Graham G. Disparities in cardiovascular disease risk in the United States. *Curr Cardiol Rev.* 2015;11(3):238–245.
Gruskin S, Safreed-Harmon K, Moore CL, et al. HIV and gender-based violence: welcome policies and programmes, but is the research keeping up? *Reprod Health Matters.* 2014;22(44):174–184.
Guerrero S, López-Cortés A, Indacochea A, et al. Analysis of racial/ethnic representation in select basic and applied cancer research studies. *Sci Rep.* 2018;8(1):1–8. http://doi:10.1038/s41598-018-32264-x
Hall WJ, Chapman MV, Lee KM, et al. Implicit racial/ethnic bias among health care professionals and its influence on health care outcomes: a systematic review. *Am J Public Health.* 2015 Dec;105(12):e60–e76. Accessed July 23, 2024.
Health Resources and Services Administration. Ending the HIV epidemic: a plan for America. https://www.hrsa.gov/ending-hiv-epidemic. Published February 2020. Accessed July 26, 2020.
Hess K, Hu X, Lansky A, et al. Lifetime risk of a diagnosis of HIV infection in the United States. *Ann Epidemiol.* 2017;27(4):238–243.
Heyrana K, Byers HM, Stratton P. Increasing the participation of pregnant women in clinical trials. *JAMA.* 2018;320(20):2077–2078. http://doi:10.1001/jama.2018.17716
Hoffman KM, Trawalter S, Axt JR, Oliver MN. Racial bias in pain assessment and treatment recommendations, and false beliefs about biological differences between Blacks and whites. *Proc Natl Acad Sci USA.* 2016;113(16):4296–301.
Institute of Medicine (US) Committee on Understanding and Eliminating Racial and Ethnic Disparities in Health Care. *Unequal Treatment: Confronting Racial and Ethnic Disparities in Health Care.* Smedley BD, Stith AY, Nelson AR, eds. Washington, DC: National Academies Press; 2003. PMID: 25032386.
Jacobs EA, Shepard D, Suaya JA, et al. Overcoming language barriers in healthcare: costs and benefits of interpreter services. *Am J Public Health.* 2004;94(5):866–869.
James C. *Race Ethnicity and Medical Care: A Survey of Public Perceptions and Experiences.* Kaiser Family Foundation; Washington, DC. September 1999.
Kahn JM, Gray DM, Oliveri JM, Washington CM, DeGraffinreid CR, Paskett ED. Strategies to improve diversity, equity, and inclusion in clinical trials. *Cancer.* 2022;128(2):216–221. http://doi:10.1002/cncr.33905.
Kanny D, Jeffries 4th WL, Chapin-Bardales J, et al. Racial/ethnic disparities in HIV preexposure prophylaxis among men who have sex with men—3 urban areas, 2017. *MMWR.* 2019 Sep 20;68(37):801–806.
Kendi IX. *How to Be Antiracist.* New York: Penguin Random House; 2019.
Lewis TJ, Herring RP, Chinnock RE, Nelson A. Ending the HIV epidemic in Black America: qualitative insights following COVID-19. *J Racial Ethn Health Disparities.* 2024. doi:10.1007/s40615-024-01925-1
Mayer KH, Agwu A, Malebranche D. Barriers to the wider use of pre-exposure prophylaxis in the United States: a narrative review. *Adv Ther.* 2020a;37(5):1778–1811. http://doi:10.1007/s12325-020-01295-0
Mayer KH, Molina J, Thompson MA, et al. Emtricitabine and tenofovir alafenamide vs emtricitabine and tenofovir disoproxil fumarate for HIV pre-exposure prophylaxis (DISCOVER): primary results from a randomized, double-blind, multicenter, active-controlled, phase 3, non-inferiority trial. *Lancet.* 2020b;396(10246):239–254. http://doi:10.1016/S0140-6736(20)31065-5
Michos ED, Reddy TK, Gulati M, et al. Improving the enrollment of women and racially/ethnically diverse populations in cardiovascular clinical trials: an ASPC practice statement. *Am J Prev Cardiol.* 2021;8:100250. https://doi.org/10.1016/j.ajpc.2021.100250
Millett G. Casualties on the road to ending HIV: context matters in addressing HIV disparities. Prime session 1. 40 Year HIV pandemic,

July 7, 2020a. AIDS2020.org. Virtual IAS Conference; July 4–10, 2020a.

Millett G, Jones AT, Benkeser D, et al. Assessing differential impacts of COVID-19 on Black communities. *Ann Epidemiol.* 2020b. PMID: 32419766. Accessed July 23, 2024.

Muthukumar AV, Morrell W, Bierer BE. Evaluating the frequency of English language requirements in clinical trial eligibility criteria: a systematic analysis using ClinicalTrials.gov. *PLOS Med.* 2021;18(9):e1003758. http://doi:10.1371/journal.pmed.1003758

National Institutes of Health. National Health Center Program Uniform Data System, Awardee. https://data.hrsa.gov/tools/data-reporting/program-daata/national. Published 2020.

National LGBT Health Education Center. Providing welcoming services and care for LGBT people. http://www.lgbthealtheducation.org/wp-content/uploads/Learning-Guide.pdf. Published 2015. Accessed December 1, 2015.

Nellis A. The color of justice: racial and ethnic disparity in state prisons. The Sentencing Project. https://sentencingproject.org/staff/ashley-nellis/. Published June 14, 2016. Accessed July 26, 2020.

Newport F. Three-quarters of Americans identify as Christian. Gallup.com. http://www.gallup.com/poll/180347/three-quarters-americans-identify-christian.aspx. Published December 2014. Accessed December 1, 2015.

Nichols A, Simms M. Racial and ethnic differences in receipt of unemployment insurance benefits during the great recession. Urban Institute. https://www.urban.org/sites/default/files/publication/25541/412596-Racial-and-Ethnic-Differences-in-Receipt-of-Unemployment-Insurance-Benefits-During-the-Great-Recession.PDF. Published June 2012. Accessed July 26, 2020.

Nosyk B, Zang X, Krebs E, et al. Ending the HIV epidemic in the USA: an economic modeling study in six cities. *Lancet HIV.* July 2020;7(7):e491–e503.

Patel P. Forced sterilization of women as discrimination. *Pub Health Rev.* 2017;38:7. http:// publichealthreviews.biomedcentral.com/articles/10.1186/s40985-017-0060-9

Paterson DL, Swindells S. Adherence to protease inhibitor therapy and outcomes in patients with HIV infection. *Ann Intern Med.* 2000;133:21–30.

Peterson K, Anderson J, Boundy E, et al. Mortality disparities in racial/ethnic minority groups in the Veterans Health Administration: an evidence review and map. *Am J P Public Health.* 2018;108(3):e1–e10.

Raths D. New law requires Medicaid coverage of clinical trial participation. /policy-value-based-care/medicare-medicaid/news/21251951/new-law-requires-medicaid-coverage-of-clinical-trial-participation. Published 2022. Accessed July 24, 2024.

Ravindran TK. Making pharmaceutical research and regulation work for women. *BMJ.* 2020;371. https://doi.org/101136/bjm.m3808

Riner AN, Girma S, Vudatha V, et al. Eligibility criteria perpetuate disparities in enrollment and participation of Black patients in pancreatic cancer clinical trials. *Journal of Clinical Oncology.* 2022;40(20):2193–2202. http://doi:10.1200/JCO.21.02492

Roper W. Black Americans 2.5 x more likely than whites to be killed by police. Stasta.com. https://www.statista.com/chart/21872/map-of-police-violence-against-black-americans/. Published June 2, 2020. Accessed July 26, 2020.

Ross J, Cunningham CO, Hanna DJ. HIV outcomes among migrants from low- and middle-income countries living in high-income countries: a review of recent evidence. *Curr Opin Infect Dis.* 2018 Feb;31(1):25–32. http://doi:10.1097/QCO.0000000000000415

Samaei M, McGregor AJ, Jenkins MR. Inclusion of women in FDA-regulated premarket clinical trials: a call for innovative and recommended action. *Contemp Clin Trials.* 2022;116:106708. http://doi:10.1016/j.cct.2022.106708

Sartor O, Armstrong AJ, Ahaghotu C, et al. Survival of African-American and Caucasian men after sipuleucel-T immunotherapy: outcomes from the PROCEED registry. *Prostate Cancer Prostatic Dis.* 2020;23(3):517–526. http://doi:10.1038/s41391-020-0213-7

Singer M. A dose of drugs, a touch of violence, a case of AIDS: a conceptualizing of the SAVA syndemic. *Creative Sociol.* 1996;24(2): 99–110.

Singh S, Hu X, Hess K. Estimating the lifetime risk of a diagnosis of HIV infection in the United States. CROI Abstract 43, February 12, 2022. https://www.croiconference.org/abstract/estimating-the-lifetime-risk-of-a-diagnosis-of-hiv-infection-in-the-united-states/. Accessed August 19, 2024.

Sitapati AM, Limneos J, Bonet-Vázquez M, et al. Retention: building a patient-centered medical home in HIV primary care through PUFF (patients unable to follow-up found). *J Health Care Poor Underserved.* 2012;23(3 Suppl):81–95.

Skarbinski J, Rosenberg E, Paz-Bailey G, et al. Human immunodeficiency virus transmission at each step of the care continuum in the United States. *JAMA Intern Med.* 2015;175(4):596–597.

Sullivan PS, DuBose SN, Castel AD, et al. Equity of PrEP uptake by race, ethnicity, sex and region in the United States in the first decade of PrEP: a population-based analysis. *Lancet Reg Health Am.* 2024;33:100738. https://doi:10.1016/j.lana.2024.100738

Sullivan PS. Trends in PrEP inequity by race and census region, United States, 2012–2021. AIDS 2022, Abstract 12943. https://programme.aids2022.org/Abstract/Abstract/?abstractid=12943. Published Accessed.

Torpy SJ. Native American women and coerced sterilization: on the trail of tears in the 1970s. *Am Indian Cul Res J.* 2007;24(2):1–22. http://doi:10.17953/aicr.24.2.7646013460646042

UNAIDS. Fact sheet 2024: global HIV statistics. https:// www.unaids.org/sites/default/files/media_asset/UNAIDS_FactSheet_en.pdf. Published 2024. Accessed August 18, 2024.

U.S. Congress. United States Congress National Institutes of Health Revitalization Act of 1993: Subtitle B: clinical research equity regarding women and minorities. Public Law 103-43.Congress.gov/bill/103rd-congress/senate-bill/1. Accessed July 24, 2022.

U.S. Department of Health and Human Services (DHHS). Office of Minority Health. HHS action plan to reduce racial and ethnic health disparities: a nation free of disparities in health and health care. https:// minorityhealth.hhs.gov/news/title-hhs-announces-plan-reduce-health-disparities-hhs-announces-plan-reduce-health. Published 2011. Accessed August 31, 2024.

van Ryn M, Burke J. The effect of patient race and socioeconomic status on physicians' perceptions of patients. *Social Sci Med.* 2000;50:813–828.

Weisse CS, Sorum PC, Sanders KN, et al. Do gender and race affect decisions about pain management? *J Gen Intern Med.* 2001;16(4): 211–217.

Woodcock J, Araojo R, Thompson T, Puckrein GA. Integrating research into community practice: toward increased diversity in clinical trials. *N Engl J Med.* 2021;385(15):1351–1353. http://doi:10.1056/NEJMp2107331

10.

HIV CARE AND PREVENTION

SPECIAL POPULATIONS

Catherine Silva, Renata Arrington-Sanders, Zil G. Goldstein, Elizabeth Imbert, Matthew D. Hickey, Olabimpe Asupoto, Alysse G. Wurcel, Abby Davids, Ashley Carvalho, Deliana Garcia, Claire M. Hutkins Seda, and Laszlo Madaras

ADOLESCENTS AND HIV

Catherine Silva and Renata Arrington-Sanders

LEARNING OBJECTIVES

- Describe the developmental, cognitive, social, and environmental factors affecting treatment adherence and prevention in adolescents.
- Identify special adolescent populations who are at increased risk of acquiring HIV.
- Discuss HIV pre-exposure prophylaxis (PrEP) options that can be considered for sexually active adolescents.

WHAT'S NEW?

- In the United States, young men of color who have sex with men (MSM) have higher rates of HIV infection compared to white MSM youth.
- Transgender adults and adolescents, especially transgender women of color, have had an increase in HIV infection.
- The COVID-19 pandemic led to a substantial decrease in HIV testing and surveillance activities.
- PrEP should be discussed with all sexually active adolescents.
- In addition to oral formulations of antiretroviral therapy (ART) and PrEP, long-acting injectable options are approved for use in adolescents who are 12 years of age or older or weigh 35 kg or more.

KEY POINTS

- Adolescents are at risk for HIV through sexual behaviors; most adolescents acquire HIV through condomless sex.
- Adolescents in late puberty per Sexual Maturity Rating (SMR) staging (Stages 4–5) can be managed according to adult/adolescent guidelines; prepubescent and early pubescent adolescents (SMR Stages 1–3) can be managed according to pediatric guidelines.
- Psychosocial factors that could affect adherence should be addressed before initiating treatment.
- Sexual risk behaviors in adolescents living with HIV should be given special attention.

The period of adolescence (defined as ages 12–24 years) is a critical time of physical, social, emotional, and cognitive growth and development (Sanders, 2013). In the United States, the average age at first sexual intercourse for males and females is 17 years (Abma et al., 2017). The American Academy of Pediatrics and other professional medical organizations recommend eliciting a thorough sexual history from adolescents to provide appropriate anticipatory guidance, screening, and treatment of sexually transmitted infections including HIV. However, there are multifactorial challenges that adolescents face when accessing appropriate medical care and other services, resulting in a heightened risk for HIV acquisition. Among adolescents, there are significant disparities in HIV infection rates among gender and sexual minority youth, individuals who identify as gay, lesbian, bisexual, or transgender; racial and ethnic minority youth; youth with unstable housing; youth who use injection drugs; individuals who have a mental illness; those who have been sexually or physically abused; and those who are incarcerated or are in foster care.

Health disparities occur as a result of an individual's interaction with socio-environmental factors at the interpersonal (e.g., family and social/sexual networks), intermediate structural (e.g., community, social institutions, culture, social norms, and values), and macrostructural (e.g., socioeconomic conditions) levels that contribute to high rates of HIV. For example, despite the overall drop in new HIV infections, young Black and Hispanic/Latino MSM continue to be disproportionately impacted by HIV in the United States and account for most new HIV transmissions in their age group (CDC, 2024c). Worldwide, adolescent females disproportionately account for new HIV transmissions (UNAIDS, 2024). Such high rates do not result from increased

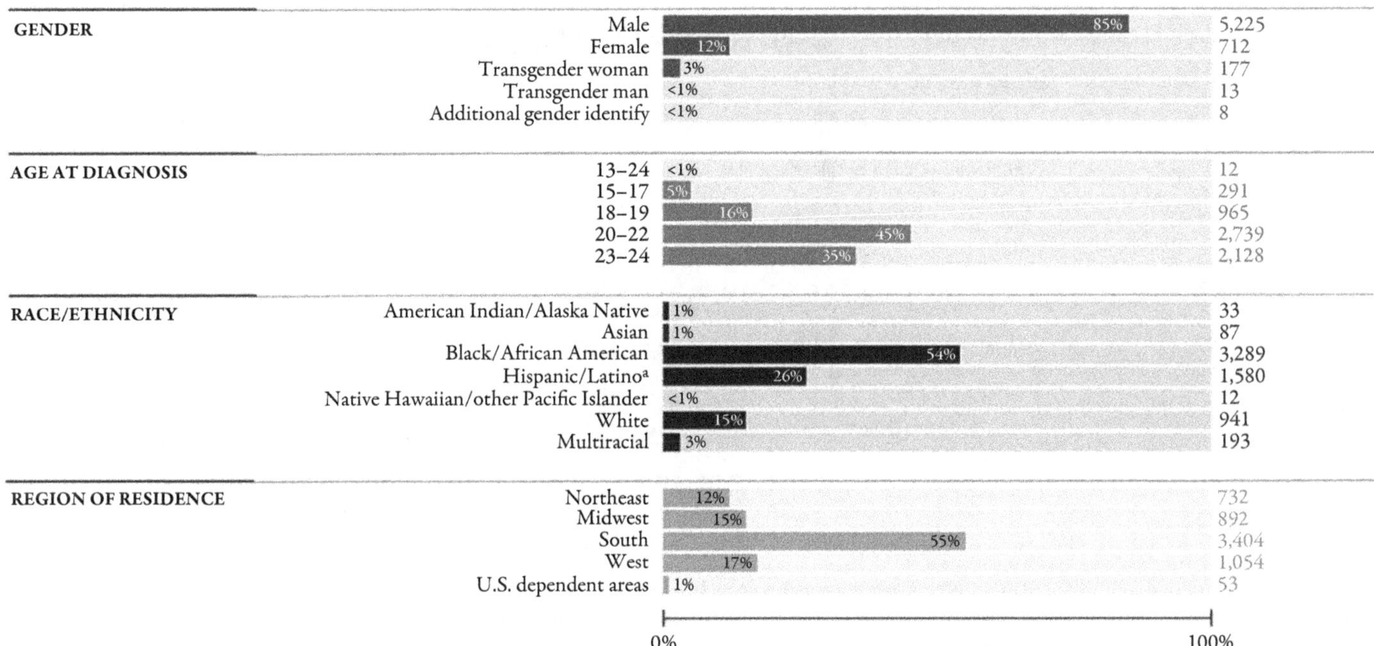

Figure 10.1 Percentage of diagnoses of HIV infection among persons aged 13–24 years, by selected characteristics, 2020, United States and six dependent areas SOURCE: https://www.cdc.gov/hiv/pdf/library/reports/surveillance/cdc-hiv-surveillance-report-2020-updated-vol-33.pdf.

individual behavior but rather from the complex interrelationship of multiple social identities—such as race, ethnicity, gender, socioeconomic status, and sexual orientation—that intersect at the individual's experience, existence within high HIV-prevalent sexual networks, and larger social-structural inequities experienced at the macro level (Raj and Bowleg, 2012). In the United States, approximately 1 million adults and 300,000 youth aged 13–17 years identify as transgender (i.e., a person who has a gender identity that differs from the sex they were assigned at birth) (Herman et al., 2022). In 2019, 2% of new HIV diagnoses in the United States were among transgender or additional gender identity people, with most occurring among African Americans (CDC, 2024c). One meta-analysis estimates that 14% of transgender women in the United States are living with HIV (Becasen et al., 2019). More than one-third (36.3%) of these women were adolescents and young adults less than 24 years old (Becasen et al., 2019). This represents a 34-fold increased odds of HIV infection compared to that of all reproductive-age adults (Baral et al., 2013) (see Figures 10.1 and 10.2).

Transwomen of color are particularly affected. Some have suggested that rates of HIV among Black transgender women are as high as 44% (Becasen et al., 2019). The CDC's National HIV Behavioral Surveillance system, which collects biobehavioral surveillance data every 3 years among individuals at high risk for HIV infection, found that 62% of Black transgender women and 35% of Hispanic transgender women interviewed with living with HIV (CDC, 2020a). Higher rates of HIV are attributed to experiences of stigma, discrimination, negative healthcare encounters, lack of familial support, limited healthcare and housing access, and prevlance of mental health diagnoses (Eaton et al., 2015). These factors contribute to increased drug and alcohol use, sex work, incarceration, homelessness, and attempted suicide.

Adolescents with HIV (AWH) from perinatal transmission are another group of adolescents and young adults living with HIV. Given near universal maternal HIV screening and treatment in most high-income countries, this population is relatively small. The same cannot be said for low-resource countries, however, in which perinatal transmission continues to be an ongoing concern. AWH from perinatal transmission share many common issues with AWH acquired behaviorally—namely, concerns related to stigma, sexuality, disclosure, unplanned pregnancy, nonadherence, and substance misuse. However, this population generally is on more complicated ART regimens based on prior development of HIV drug-resistance mutations during childhood.

The same socioecologic factors (e.g., discrimination, isolation, microaggressions, and minority stress) that contribute to HIV risk predispose youth to comorbidities (e.g., high rates of mental health and substance use disorders) and medical nonadherence in their HIV treatment and management. Differences in the treatment cascade of care by age have been hypothesized as an explanation for the increase in HIV infections by at-risk youth nationally (Zanoni and Mayer, 2014). Less than half (40%) of those aged 13–29 years are aware of their HIV status, and best estimates suggest that only 62% of those are connected to care within their first year of diagnosis (Zanoni and Mayer, 2014). Other studies have suggested that adolescents have much lower linkage rates, ranging from 29% to 73% successfully linked within the first year of diagnosis (Craw et al., 2008). The CDC and the U.S. Preventive Services Task Force recommend routine HIV screening for all youth (Branson et al., 2006; Moyer, 2013). People at ongoing

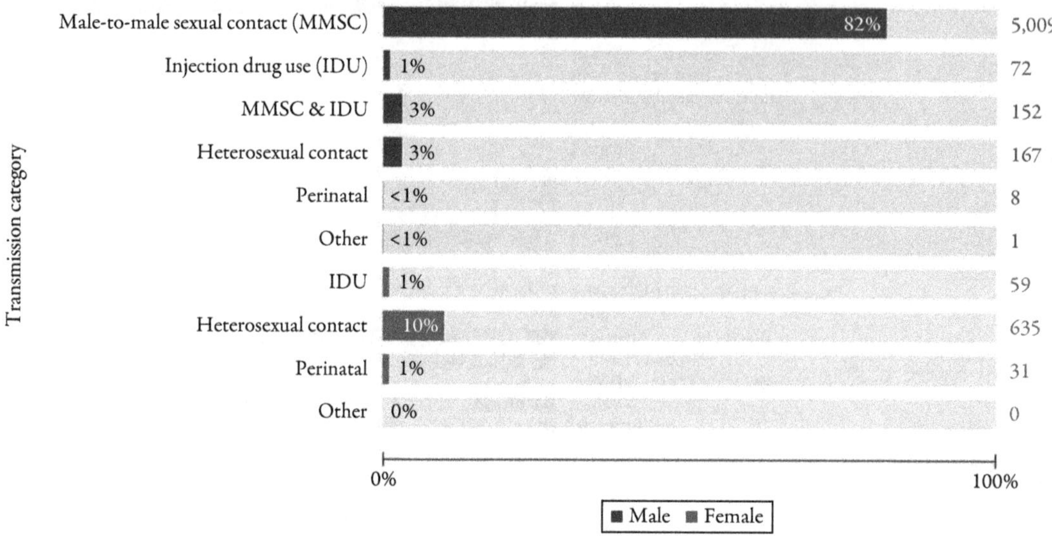

Figure 10.2 Percentage of diagnoses of HIV infection among persons aged 13–24 years, by sex assigned at birth and transmission category, 2020, United States and six dependent areas. SOURCE: https://www.cdc.gov/hiv/pdf/library/reports/surveillance/cdc-hiv-surveillance-report-2020-updated-vol-33.pdf.

risk of HIV acquisition should be screened at least annually. Healthcare providers should increase the frequency of screening every 3–6 months based on sexual risk behavior (e.g., condomless sex) and other groups (e.g., cisgender young men who report sex with other men, transgender or gender-diverse adolescents) who may be at increased risk of HIV infection (Workowski et al., 2021). Venue-based and social networking testing is another effective strategy to reach high-risk youth and increase the identification and linkage of youth into care (Barnes et al., 2010; Boyer et al., 2013; Straub and Tanner, 2018). Once diagnosed with HIV, special efforts to improve engagement in care are often necessary to maximize youth accessing and receiving consistent care.

DEVELOPMENTAL ISSUES

Adolescents face the same barriers to treatment adherence as adults, but they have additional challenges owing to their developmental stage and legal circumstances. Social stigma, fear of alienation from peer groups, medication side effects, lack of transportation, dependence on parents or other caregivers, growing autonomy, and "feeling fine" are major contributors to nonadherence (Ingerski et al., 2021).

MEDICAL MANAGEMENT

U.S. guidelines recommend ART for all individuals with HIV, regardless of $CD4^+$ T- lymphocyte cell count and age (Department of Health and Human Services [DHHS], 2024). Therapy should be initiated as soon as possible, and treatment deferral should be determined on a case-by-case basis. Recent guidelines for adolescents and young adults include data on the efficacy and feasibility of immediate ART and recommendations for certain populations. Earlier initiation of ART has been associated with reduced morbidity and mortality associated with HIV. Data extrapolated from the START and TEMPRANO trials favor initiating ART in all individuals who are able and willing to commit to treatment, understand the benefits and risks of therapy, and understand the importance of adherence (DHHS, 2024). The course of disease in youth is similar to that in adults, and they generally should be treated according to the same guidelines (DHHS, 2024).

Rapid ART initiation has the potential to improve overall health outcomes and reduce the time during which people with newly diagnosed HIV can transmit HIV to others. Two randomized controlled trials in South Africa and in Haiti have demonstrated that rapid ART initiation resulted in higher sustained viral suppression and retention in care (Koenig et al., 2017; Labhardt et al., 2018; Rosen et al., 2016). There have been no randomized trials in the United States; however, data from a city-wide implementation of the San Francisco RAPID program in the United States suggests that either immediate initiation of ART (on the day of diagnosis) or rapid ART initiation (within days or weeks of diagnosis) was associated with 92% virological suppression at one year (Coffey et al., 2019). This study also highlights the intense support required for ART initiation on the same day of HIV diagnosis, clinical evaluation, counseling, laboratory testing, and assessment of insurance coverage (Coffey et al., 2019). Adolescents may also present with high viral loads and multiclass resistance at time of diagnosis (Koay et al., 2021). Guidelines provide details on how to determine the best ART class as guided by the initial viral load level, which is critical.

Concerns have been raised about use of some of antiretroviral agents in certain populations of AWH. Most recently, initial data from the Tsepamo study raised concerns about dolutegravir (DTG)-based regimens predisposing newborns of women on this medication to neural tube defects (NTDs). However, subsequent data involving review of 39,200 births surveyed from March 2019 to April 2020 found that newborns of mothers on DTG at the time of conception were not significantly more likely to have NTDs compared with newborns of mothers taking non-dolutegravir ART (Davey et al., 2020). In the ADVANCE trial, weight gain was more common among study participants receiving DTG-based regimens compared to the EFV-based regimen (Zash et al., 2021).

Prevention is a key component of HIV treatment and current public health efforts. Most adolescents acquire HIV through sexual transmission and are unaware of their diagnosis, making them excellent candidates for prevention counseling, linkage to and engagement in care, and initiation of ART (DHHS, 2024). All adolescents with HIV should be informed that maintaining a plasma HIV RNA (viral load) of <200 copies/mL prevents sexual transmission to their partners ("Undetectable = Untransmittable"). This has been established in a randomized clinical trial and several large observational cohort studies (Cohen et al., 2016). Promoting HIV treatment as prevention can also promote disclosure of one's HIV status by normalizing HIV and removing some of the stigma, fear, and rejection associated with disclosing to partners and publicly (Bavinton et al., 2018; Rodger et al., 2016, 2019).

SEXUAL RISK

High rates of HIV in adolescents are multifactorial. Data suggest that many adolescents do not experience greater numbers of sexual partners. Instead, sexual risk results from multiple psychosocial factors that predispose youth to HIV. Sexual networks with a partner who is living with HIV are more common among adolescents living in higher-density, lower-income areas that are characterized by violence and limited access to care. AWH exist in communities with high rates of unintended pregnancy (Nachman et al., 2009), STIs (Trent et al., 2007), and condomless sex (Clum et al., 2009; Weiner et al., 2007). This, combined with low rates of screening for STIs in HIV clinics that lag rates of non-HIV clinics, can promote high rates of STIs and transmission of HIV (Berry et al., 2015). Additionally, condom negotiation is often not always a simple task for some AWH. In one sample, females with HIV had lower self-efficacy overall ($B = -0.15, p = 0.01$), to discuss safe sex with one's partner ($B = -0.14, p = 0.01$), and to refuse sex without a condom ($B = -0.21, p = 0.01$), and self-efficacy was related to condomless vaginal and anal intercourse episodes (Boone et al., 2015). In young men, some have suggested that age-discordant partnerships, limited condom negotiation, alcohol, and other substances may be key contributors to condomless sex with HIV-negative or unknown status partners (Arrington-Sanders et al., 2013; Bruce et al., 2012; Mustanski and Newcomb, 2013). Other studies suggest a complicated relationship between psychological stress, substance use, and mental health that contributes to condomless sex (Arrington-Sanders et al., 2022). Young transgender women and sexual minority men may also exist within social contexts that predispose them to exchange sex (sex for money or a place to stay), substance use, and violence, which put them at risk for HIV. For some youth with HIV, there is a need to regularly address the risk of pregnancy, acquiring additional STIs, and secondary transmission of HIV to sexual partners.

The CDC recommends screening for STIs in women younger than age 25 years because of the high rates of STIs in this age range. In young MSM, screening for STIs is recommended from extragenital body sites because oropharyngeal, rectal, and urethral infections are commonly present in this population (Workowski et al., 2021). The CDC provides complete screening guidelines for youth living with HIV. Clinic-based motivational interviewing can improve condom use (Xu et al., 2017). The CDC also recommends PrEP for persons at risk for HIV acquisition. PrEP is recommended for sexually active adolescents who had anal or vaginal sex in the past 6 months and any of the following: having a partner living with HIV (partner with unknown or detectable viral load), a bacterial STI in the past 6 months, history of inconsistent or no condom use with sexual partners, and using injection drugs with a partner living with HIV or sharing injection equipment (Workowski et al., 2021). As of 2021, the CDC PrEP Clinical Practice Guidelines were updated to recommend that healthcare providers offer PrEP to all sexually active adolescents even if they do not report high-risk behaviors for HIV infection (CDC, 2021). Normalizing discussions of PrEP with sexually active adolescents may help increase knowledge about PrEP among youth. The oral preparation of PrEP is approved for use in adolescents and young adults weighing 35 kg or more. In 2021, the U.S. Food and Drug Administration (FDA) approved the use of extended-release cabotegravir, a long-acting injectable PrEP option, for use by at-risk adolescents who weighed 35 kg or more (FDA, 2021). The long-acting injectable is given first as two injections 1 month apart, and then every 2 months.

A client-centered approach that includes culturally grounded risk reduction and addresses not only the client's individual risk, but also the complicated contextual factors that impact risk, is most helpful. For example, to be effective, providers will also need to identify and address key social factors that may contribute to risk, including discrimination, housing, employment, food insecurity, mental health, and substance use. Personalized cognitive counseling (PCC) and Many Men, Many Voices (MMMV) are two evidence-based interventions that have been suggested to address the needs of some vulnerable, at-risk communities. PCC uses an individual approach focusing on past sexual risk behavior, while MMMV attempts to address the intersecting factors and identities impacting adolescents (CDC, 2023, 2022d).

SUBSTANCE USE

According to the 2019 National Youth Risk Behavior Survey, approximately 38% of youth described ever having sex, with 27% of high school students reporting that they were currently sexually active. Among youth who described being currently sexually active, 21% drank alcohol or used drugs prior to their most recent sexual intercourse (CDC, 2020b). Substance use predisposes adolescents to other high-risk sexual behaviors like inconsistent or improper condom use, and, for AWH, substance use can interfere with clinical care.

In a large AIDS Treatment Network (ATN) study of 1,712 youth, 61% of males and 45% of females scored 2 or higher on the CRAFFT screening tool, indicating a higher level of risk for substance use disorder (Gamarel et al., 2017). Daily or weekly use of cannabis was 33% for males and 19% for females. Daily or weekly use of alcohol was reported for 27% of males and 12% of females. Substance use prior to and during sex was commonly described. The regular assessment of substance use with appropriate counseling and referral is a key requirement in care.

MENTAL HEALTH

In an ATN study of 1,712 youth, 21% had a positive screen for depression and 15% for anxiety. Further, 15% had reported seriously considering suicide, and 14% were prescribed psychotropics; 70% of the cohort recalled seeing a mental health provider while in care, and 38% of men and 42% of women reported currently wanting to receive mental health services (data presented at the October 2011 ATN meeting). These data suggest that regular screening and referral for mental health disorders is crucial. Stigma is another common concern for youth living with and at risk for HIV (Arrington-Sanders et al., 2020; Dowshen et al., 2009) and can relate to HIV status, sexual identity, or racial/ethnic minority. Stigma can lead to feelings of marginalization, mistrust, and engagement in risky behaviors, including condomless sex, nonadherence to medications, and delays in HIV testing and care. Providers will need to approach AWH from an intersectionality lens to be effective—acknowledging all identities (e.g., race/ethnicity, gender identity, and socioeconomic status).

MEDICATION ADHERENCE

Youth living with HIV are at risk for nonadherence because of psychosocial, developmental, and cognitive factors. Several studies have documented nonadherence in youth living with HIV, with one analysis describing rates of ART adherence during the past 30 days between 28% and 70% (Reisner et al., 2009). Barriers include medical, psychological, and logistical issues. Medical barriers include an AIDS diagnosis (Johnson et al., 2015), difficult ART regimen (Buchanan et al., 2012), absence of symptoms, and an unwelcoming medical environment (Philbin et al., 2014). Psychological barriers include depression, anxiety (Tanney et al., 2012), stigma associated with the diagnosis or transmission history (Rao et al., 2007), and lack of social support (Williams et al., 2022). Positive self-efficacy and outcome expectancy were associated with better adherence, and logistical barriers such as lack of housing, insurance, and transportation were associated with poorer adherence (MacDonell et al., 2016). A comprehensive, multidisciplinary healthcare team is required to serve the medical, logistical, and psychosocial needs of AWH. Individually tailored interventions that address social and psychological factors (e.g., substance use, lack of insurance, access to care, and lack of social support) and structural barriers (e.g., housing and insurance instability) will need to be developed in order to better meet the needs of youth living with HIV. Attention to potential barriers to adherence prior to treatment initiation is likely to improve outcomes.

Long-acting regimens may simultaneously address the psychosocial needs of HIV stigma experienced by adolescents and medication nonadherence. In January 2021, the FDA approved the use of coformulated, extended-release cabotegravir and rilpivirine, a long-acting injectable treatment ART option, for use by adolescents who were 12 years or older or weighed 35 kg or more (US FDA, 2021). In February 2022, the FDA approved an every 2-month maintenance dosing option, and the oral lead-in was made optional in March 2022. This long-acting combination regimen is approved to replace the current oral ART regimen in adolescents who are virologically suppressed (HIV-1 RNA <50 copies/mL), on a stable ART regimen, and have no history of treatment failure or known suspected resistance to either cabotegravir or rilpivirine.

COVID-19 AND OTHER EMERGING CONDITIONS

AWH should continue to follow COVID-19 prevention, testing, treatment, and vaccination guidelines from the Centers for Disease Control and Prevention (CDC). Although there are relatively limited data specific to children and adolescents living with HIV, COVID-19 vaccinations are safe for people with HIV and do not interact or interfere with ART or PrEP regimens. The number of doses for the COVID-19 vaccine will depend on the type of vaccine received; overall, AWH should receive the primary series, followed by boosters. In addition, providers should ensure that adolescents are up to date on all other recommended immunizations, including pneumococcal and influenza immunizations, and are provided with the necessary care for potentially worsening manifestations of mental health and substance use issues that may have increased during the COVID-19 pandemic. These additional comorbidities are prevalent in AWH, so it is vital that providers address these topics and refer them to appropriate mental health and substance use providers when necessary and continue to use a multidisciplinary team to support AWH.

AWH should maintain an adequate supply of medications (i.e., 30 days or longer) to prevent barriers to medication access, especially during disruptions of care that may occur during public health emergencies. Telemedicine may be utilized to help accomodate the schedules of AWH; however, providers should communicate when in-person visits may be especially beneficial (i.e., to facilitate laboratory testing for monitoring and closer assessment of clinical status and needs) (Armbruster et al., 2020). Care models informed by the psychosocial considerations described previously and developmentally based care models that use multidisciplinary care teams are preferable. When a multidisciplinary model is not available, it becomes imperative that the management of complex youth with behavioral problems be facilitated by close communication among HIV primary care providers, nurses, social workers or case managers, and behavioral health providers. Avoiding potentially catastrophic health outcomes, including rapid HIV progression, multiclass HIV drug resistance, depression and suicide, chronic homelessness, prolonged incarceration, substance use disorder, and secondary transmission of HIV, will likely require intensive attention to psychosocial issues. At times, a temporary approach of delaying early ART initiation may improve outcomes by allowing time to focus on developmental and social barriers.

Thus far, reported cases of mpox in children and adolescents (including AWH) are relatively infrequent, and clinical disease is generally not severe. However, providers should counsel AWH on interventions that can effectively prevent mpox. Adolescents with close contact with people with suspected, probable, or confirmed mpox may be eligible for postexposure prophylaxis (PEP) with vaccination, immune globulin, or antiviral medication.

TRANSITION TO ADULT CARE

Finally, clinicians must plan for the transition of AWH into adult care. In a joint statement, the American Academy of Pediatrics, the American Academy of Family Physicians, the American College of Physicians, and the American Society of Internal Medicine affirmed that all adults, including those with special medical needs, benefit from care by clinicians who are trained in adult medicine (Cohen et al., 2002). They recommend that an identified healthcare provider be responsible for the transition, that a portable medical summary be maintained, and that a written transition plan be developed with the AWH and family/caregivers by age 14 years. In addition to these recommendations, Valenzuela and colleagues (2011) recommend the following:

- Optimizing provider communication between adolescent and adult clinics
- Identifying adult care providers willing to care for adolescents and young adults
- Addressing patient and family discomfort or hesitancy regarding the care transition caused by lack of information, concerns about stigma or risk of disclosure, and differences in practice styles
- Helping youth develop life skills, including counseling them on the importance of appropriate use of a primary care provider, managing appointments, symptom recognition and reporting, and self-efficacy
- Identifying an optimal clinic model based on specific needs
- Implementing ongoing evaluation to measure the success of a selected model
- Engaging adult and adolescent care providers in regular multidisciplinary case conferences
- Implementing interventions that may improve outcomes, such as support groups and mental health consultation
- Incorporating a family-planning component into clinical care
- Educating HIV care teams and staff about transitions of care.

The National Health Alliance also has resources that organize transition into the Six Core Elements (http://www.gottransition.org/providers/index.cfm) which can be applied in any clinical setting. Guidance from Straub and Tanner (2018) identifies additional key components of care transitions, including: having formal, written transition policies; staff training in adolescent development; life skills and self-care plans for AWH; tailored programs that target resources for AWH; and integrated panels/registries which allow for information sharing across pediatric and adult clinics.

ADOLESCENT HIV CARE: SUMMARY

Adolescents or youth living with HIV may have multiple developmental, cognitive, social, contextual, and environmental challenges that impact their identification, linkage, and engagement with care. Careful and ongoing attention to the factors described here will likely improve the care, treatment, and adherence of youth living with HIV, and potentially prevent them from "falling through the cracks."

TRANSGENDER POPULATIONS AND HIV

Zil G. Goldstein

LEARNING OBJECTIVE

Equip providers with knowledge and skills to develop and provide gender-affirming primary care, HIV care, and HIV prevention.

WHAT'S NEW

- Transgender people experience disparities in HIV infection, viral load suppression, and pre-exposure prophylaxis (PrEP) utilization and persistence. Biomedical factors are not responsible for these disparities; rather, emerging research connects these observations with experiences of trauma and discrimination because of transgender status.
- Interactions between antiretrovirals (ARVs) and hormone therapy are rare. New modalities of PrEP medications have shown efficacy in transgender populations.

KEY POINTS

- Transgender people have a range of identities and sexual orientations, as well as transition-related goals; each transgender patient should be approached as an individual.

- Special considerations with transgender populations should focus on minimizing transphobia during the healthcare experience, with special attention paid to documentation and use of the correct (patient's preferred) name and pronouns.
- Transgender people and programs should not be aggregated with MSM; programs and materials should be developed specifically for transgender populations using a culturally grounded approach.
- Gender-affirming hormone therapy with estrogens and androgen blockers is generally safe and compatible with ART regimens.
- Hormone therapy and other gender-affirming interventions improve HIV outcomes and reduce risk.
- Gender-affirming surgeries are generally safe among transgender people with HIV (PWH), but should not be considered unless the HIV viral load is suppressed.
- Transgender patients require ongoing primary and preventive care, as do cisgender patients; it is important to tailor transgender primary care based on the hormonal status and individual organ assessment/inventory of each patient.
- Providers should maintain a high index of suspicion for injected silicone and other fillers and be aware of their association with related morbidity.

EPIDEMIOLOGY, DEMOGRAPHICS, AND TERMINOLOGY

Transgender is an umbrella term used to describe persons whose gender identity and/or expression of gender is different from the sex they were assigned at birth. Transgender individuals may identify as men, women, nonbinary, or something else. It is important to ask, record, and use the correct pronouns (such as *he*, *she*, or *they*) and the correct name (which may be different from the legal name and/or the name on insurance documentation) to engage and retain transgender patients. It is also important to recognize that there is no set path for transition. Some transgender people may seek only gender-affirming hormone therapy (HT), whereas others may seek surgical interventions such as genital reassignment surgery or other procedures on the face, breast, or body, with or without concurrent HT. Still other transgender persons may present with a more complex gender identity; some may choose to seek HT or surgical treatments but continue to live part- or full-time in their birth gender, whereas others may assume a fluid gender expression that is not categorizable in either polar gender (Deutsch et al., 2015a). Some transgender people may choose to not pursue any gender-affirming medical or surgical treatments. A 2015 national survey of transgender people found that 30% of respondents identified as genderqueer or nonbinary; that is, neither male nor female (James et al., 2016). Table 10.1 presents a description of selected terminology and identities.

The sexual orientations of transgender persons also vary across a spectrum, with the same 2015 survey responses indicating that 15% identified as heterosexual; 16% as gay or lesbian; 21% as queer; and 32% as bi/pansexual. In most cases, transgender persons define their sexual orientation based on their affirmed gender. For example, a transgender MSM would identify as gay. However, this also varies across cultural and linguistic lines, with many transgender women who have sex with men sometimes also identifying as gay. Instead of focusing on identity, the most effective approach for assessing the sexual history and health of a patient is to ask, "What are the gender(s) of people you have sex with? Are any of them transgender people? What kind of genitals do they have?" or "What kind of genitals are involved in the sex you have?" (Deutsch, 2018). Using the terms *penis* and *vagina* may be alienating to transgender patients who have other words they use to describe their body. Allowing transgender persons to define their own body, identity, and experience will enhance the patient–provider relationship and may serve to improve adherence with ART and other elements of care (Melendez et al., 2009).

The World Professional Association for Transgender Health's *Standards of Care for the Health of Transgender and Gender Diverse People, Version 8* (SOCv8; Coleman et al., 2022) states:

- The expression of gender characteristics, including identities that are not stereotypically associated with one's sex assigned at birth, is a common and culturally diverse human phenomenon that should not be seen as inherently negative or pathological.
- In order to access covered medical and surgical procedures, transgender people are generally given a billable diagnosis. The DSM-V and ICD-10 use "Gender Dysphoria," a state of distress caused by mismatch between gender identity and birth-assigned sex, as the primary diagnosis. The need for a diagnosis to access care, including ongoing routine care when dysphoria is absent after gender transition has occurred has historically forced all transgender people to carry a mental health diagnosis.
- ICD-11 changed this diagnosis to "gender incongruence" and categorizes this term as a condition rather than a disorder, but slow uptake of ICD-11 in the United States hinders progress in de-pathologizing transgender health. (WHO, 2019)

Epidemiologic surveillance in transgender populations has been limited because of inconsistencies in the collection of gender-identity data. Incomplete or inconsistent identification of transgender populations represents a significant structural determinant of the health disparities seen in transgender populations. Best practice for the measurement of gender identity data involves the use of at least two questions, such as gender identity and birth-assigned sex (Cahill and Makadon, 2013, 2014; Deutsch et al., 2013), or some other combination of questions that allow differentiation of all transgender and gender nonbinary people, including those who identify

Table 10.1 DESCRIPTION OF SELECTED TERMINOLOGY AND IDENTITIES

TERM	DESCRIPTION
Transgender	Umbrella term for gender-nonconforming persons; more "modern" and inclusive term, preferred by many
Transsexual	Older, more clinical term, some use to identify those seeking medical or surgical treatment
Trans	Colloquial term increasingly used in place of *transgender*, especially among younger populations
Nonbinary	Describes a range of gender identities that are neither male nor female
Travestí	Term used by some Latina/Spanish speaking transgender women
Gay	Term used by some Latina/Spanish speaking transgender women with complex gender/sexual identities
Transgender woman/ transfeminine person	Person with a female or feminine-spectrum nonbinary gender identity who was assigned male birth sex
Transgender man/ transmasculine person	Person with a male or masculine-spectrum gender identity who was assigned female birth sex
Gender identity	The internal gendered sense of oneself as a man, woman, or something else
Gender expression	Signals that people use to communicate their gender to the outside world, including body modification, the way people dress, talk, or walk; there are numerous ways to alter one's expression with and without medical/surgical intervention

Note: People may use pronouns and/or names that differ from those listed on legal identity documents. Some may use *they/them* or other gender-neutral pronouns.

as "male" or "female," from cisgender people, which records both the current gender identity and the birth-assigned sex (Cahill and Makadon, 2013, 2014; Deutsch et al., 2013). This method has been found to identify twice as many transgender people as a "one-step" method in which a single "sex/gender" question is asked (Tate et al., 2012). The current estimate of the proportion of the transgender population by the UCLA Williams Institute recently doubled, from 0.3% to 0.6% of the U.S. population (Flores et al., 2016).

A 2019 meta-analysis found an HIV prevalence of 14.3% among transgender women living in the United States (Becasen et al., 2019). This striking rate is driven by interactions between structural, personal, behavioral, and biological risks unique to transgender women. Structural factors include a lack of legal recognition or protections that often result in survival sex work. Personal factors include the higher rates of mood disorders seen in transgender populations as a result of ongoing discrimination, as well as drive for gender affirmation; the model of gender affirmation describes the relationship between denial of gender affirmation (through lack of access to medical interventions or legal rights such as the ability to change one's name and gender on identity documents) and high-risk sexual behavior (Sevelius, 2013). Increasing gender affirmation through hormone treatment and surgery has been shown to have a positive effect on viral load suppression (Sevelius et al., 2021). Other behavioral factors include increased rates of condomless sex with primary male partners and anecdotes of increased earnings from sex work when no condom is used. Biological factors have not been explored in depth, but they could include changes to the anal epithelium in the presence of feminizing hormones, reduced erectile function resulting in impaired condom effectiveness, and unknowns such as HIV transmission through receptive vaginal sex in those who have undergone vaginoplasty (Poteat et al., 2015).

Transgender women have lower rates of virologic suppression (84% vs. 89% among cisgender women, and 90% among cisgender men) in 2020 Ryan White HIV/AIDS Program monitoring data (HRSA, 2021). A study of HIV indicators comparing transgender women to cisgender male and female controls found significant differences between transgender women and cisgender men in rates of ART adherence (78.4% vs. 87.4%, $p = 0.014$) for 100% last 3-day adherence and virologic suppression (50.8% vs. 61.4%, $p = 0.013$), but no difference in these measures when compared to cisgender women (Mizuno et al., 2015). Another study found that a high rate of adherence to hormone regimens was associated with a positive odds ratio of 34.5 ($p = 0.002$) for reported high ART adherence, though there was no effect on the rate of undetectable viral load. Satisfaction with current gender expression was also associated with higher reported adherence (OR 2.56, $p = 0.03$) but not with undetectable viral load (Sevelius et al., 2014). Other factors associated with viral load suppression are having a primary care provider who manages both HT and HIV, stable housing, employment, longer time since HIV diagnosis, and achieving gender affirmation as desired (Bukowski et al., 2018; Jin et al., 2019; Sevelius et al., 2021).

Few data exist on HIV risks and prevalence among transgender men, although some data suggest an increased risk (Green et al., 2015). A 2010 San Francisco study found that 61% of transgender men engaged in sex with other men, with 51% participating in vaginal receptive sex, and 39%

participating in anal receptive sex. Transgender men have reported feeling that HIV testing was less accessible to them than to cisgender male controls (43.5% vs. 56.9%, $p = 0.04$) (Sevelius et al., 2014a).

INITIATING HORMONE THERAPY

Gender-affirming HT has been found to have a number of benefits on quality of life and on symptoms of depression, anxiety, and poor social functioning (Colton et al., 2011; Gómez-Gil et al., 2012). SOCv8 defines hormonal and surgical treatment as medically necessary and states that it is unethical to deny surgical care solely on the basis of HIV or hepatitis B or C serostatus. SOCv8 endorses initiating HT with an assessment from a medical provider. There are no minimums with regard to time spent in psychotherapy prior to HT. This "informed consent" pathway destigmatizes and depathologizes transgender identities, and it overcomes several perceived or actual barriers to accessing HT. While some patients may benefit from additional mental health support to address ambivalence around and social barriers to gender-affirming hormone therapy (GAHT), or other issues that come up before and during hormone initiation, a rigorous mental health screening process may be neither available (lack of resources or lack of trained/willing providers) nor culturally applicable (language barriers and cultural differences between Western-oriented psychotherapy and persons of Latinx, African, Aboriginal, or Asian background) (Deutsch et al., 2013). It is also appropriate to offer physician-supervised HT to those patients who may otherwise turn to unprescribed sources of hormones (internet and street purchase) or who have already fully adjusted and socially transitioned to the affirmed (new) gender. A 2009 study of transgender women in New York City found that 10% receiving physician-supervised HT were also obtaining hormones from other sources and that patients were frequently taking two or three concomitant hormone regimens. This same study reported several barriers to accessing physician-supervised HT, including a lack of a knowledgeable provider (32%), lack of a transgender-friendly provider (30%), cost (29%), location (18%), and language (13%) (Sanchez et al., 2009). It is important that transgender persons have reasonable and realistic expectations about what HT and other treatments can and cannot do. Once gender-affirming hormones have begun, there should be continued monitoring for underlying psychosocial factors or mental health conditions, with interventions as indicated.

FEMINIZING HORMONE REGIMENS

Feminizing HT involves testosterone blockade in combination with estrogen replacement and the possible use of a progestogen. The most commonly used testosterone blocker in the United States is spironolactone, a potassium-sparing diuretic taken in divided doses of 50–300 mg twice daily. SOCv8 recommends the use of GNRH agonists and progestogens to achieve testosterone blockade as well (Coleman et al., 2022). In the U.S. context, it is most reasonable to start testosterone blockade with spironolactone because of its cost, efficacy, and common inclusion in drug formularies before progressing to other methods. Caution must be used with patients on angiotensin-converting enzyme (or ACE) inhibitors (because of the potential for increases in serum potassium) or those with impaired renal function. Concomitant use of ART medications that may affect renal function, such as tenofovir, is a theoretical risk; however, no case reports exist of spironolactone causing or worsening renal function in people on tenofovir. If spironolactone, GNRH agonists, and progestogens are unavailable, failed, or contraindicated, it is reasonable to consider 5-alpha reductase inhibitors, which will lower serum dihydrotestosterone levels, but raise total testosterone. Fosamprenavir and amprenavir are the only ARVs known to have interactions with estrogens that result in lower ARV drug levels, but these ARVs are now rarely used. Side effects of spironolactone are mainly orthostatic hypotension and polyuria, both of which tend to resolve after several weeks. Routine monitoring of potassium and renal function (baseline, every 3 months for the first year, and then every 6–12 months) is reasonable. A 2022 systematic review found a nonsignificant drop in serum creatinine (CI: −0.16 to 0.05 mg/dL) among transgender people on feminizing hormone therapy. While interpretation is still under investigation, it is reasonable to consider the amount of time on GAHT as well as muscle mass changes resulting from GAHT in interpreting serum creatinine. Some transgender women, especially those whose only opportunity for income is sustenance (survival) sex work, prefer to retain erectile function and may choose to avoid or use lower doses of testosterone blockers (Hembree et al., 2017).

Estrogen treatment may be via an oral, transdermal, or injectable route. SOCv8 recommends changing to transdermal estrogens at the age of 45 and above because of the lower risk of vascular thrombotic events (VTEs). Transdermal routes of estradiol (50- to 200-μg patch changed 1 or 2 times per week) has been studied extensively and is very safe with respect to risk of thromboembolic disease: a 2008 meta-analysis of VTEs in postmenopausal hormone therapy found a relative risk of VTEs in users of transdermal estradiol of 1.1 versus nonuser controls. This same review found a 2- to 3-fold increased risk of VTEs among users of any type of oral estrogen in the first year of treatment only; however, this increase translates to only an additional 1.5 VTEs per 1,000 woman-years (Canonico et al., 2008). A subsequent 2019 review found the incidence of VTE to be 2.3 events per 1,000 patient-years (Khan et al., 2019). The transdermal route also delivers fairly constant and physiologic serum estradiol levels, which helps minimize common estrogenic symptoms such as migraine, weight gain, or mood swings; however, transdermal preparations tend to be expensive, may irritate the skin, and are not always included in HIV care formularies. Oral 17β-estradiol in divided doses of 2–4 mg twice daily also delivers a constant and physiologic dose and is well tolerated. Some providers recommend administering oral estradiol sublingually to minimize first-pass metabolism and effects on clotting factors. Prior studies reporting 20- to 40-fold increases in VTE risk in transgender women involved the use of high-dose, highly thrombogenic synthetic ethinyl estradiol, which is no longer used in cross-sex treatment, and did not control for tobacco use (Asscheman et al., 1989; van Kesteren et al., 1997). More recent outcome studies of patients using 17β-estradiol have mixed findings, with one cohort of Dutch transgender women using only transdermal estradiol showing no increased risk of VTE, and a U.S. cohort of transgender enrollees in a managed healthcare plan using estrogen therapy showing a 3.2-fold increased risk (Asscheman et al., 2011; Nash et al., 2018).

Many patients may arrive at clinic requesting, or even insisting on, injectable estrogens. Although estradiol valerate 5–30 mg intramuscular every 2 weeks or estradiol cypionate 2.5–10 mg weekly are included in SOCv8, these routes may deliver supraphysiologic estrogen levels that can vary widely over the injection cycle. Almost no data exist on the short- or long-term effects of this route, although anecdotally it is well tolerated. This route may be useful in a harm-reduction setting in which there is concern that a patient may turn to unprescribed hormone sources if an injected medication is not prescribed, or in settings where transdermal estrogens are not available, and drug-drug interactions make avoiding first-pass metabolism a priority. This route may also be useful in people who have a limited level of psychosocial functioning, poor medication adherence, or high pill burden, or to provide an opportunity to "bundle" HIV-related and other care with frequent hormone-injection visits (Ickovics, 2008). Fluctuation of levels may be minimized by dividing the dose into weekly injections and, if needed, titrating peak and trough serum estradiol levels to manage any estrogenic side effects. Further, changes in the hormonal milieu can lead to changes in the balance of Th1–Th2 T lymphocyte function and theoretical alterations in cellular immunity, furthering the argument in favor of constant and physiologic dosing of estrogen.

Data describing interactions between estrogen HT and ART medications are complex and inconsistent. Three small studies have investigated possible drug-drug interactions between HIV pre-exposure prophylaxis (PrEP) and feminizing HT. Tenofovir disoproxil fumarate/emtricitabine (TDF/FTC) does not affect the levels of feminizing HT, and both masculinizing and feminizing HT reduce serum and target tissue TDF concentrations (Hiransuthikul et al., 2018). While a subanalysis of the iPrEx study showed that there was no significant increase in risk for HIV transmission among transgender women with serum levels equivalent to taking TDF/FTC 5 or more times per week, subsequent data suggest that achieving this concentration of serum TDF may require better adherence than was previously thought (Deutsch et al., 2015b). These data also suggest that "on-demand" dosing of oral PrEP requires further study in transgender populations on HT before it can be recommended as an effective prevention strategy.

Results from contraceptive studies are mixed with regard to findings that protease inhibitor (PI) and non-nucleoside reversetranscriptase inhibitor (NNRTI) medications may cause changes in serum estrogen and progesterone levels (Kearney and Mathias, 2009; Marrazzo et al., 2015). However, it is important to monitor serum estradiol levels in all transgender patients, particularly before and after concurrent PI or NNRTI use. In addition to the previously mentioned tests, monitoring of transgender women using HT should include baseline fasting glucose and lipid profiles, with subsequent monitoring as clinically indicated.

Many community members report experience with progestogens helping with breast development; however, a single small (n = 23) study found no effects of progesterone on mood or Tanner stage (Nolan et al., 2022). Clinical practice suggests two main uses for progesterone: as an additional anti-androgen with failure of spironolactone alone, or as a first step to increase energy and libido before trying low-dose testosterone after gonadectomy. It is reasonable to attempt a trial of oral micronized progesterone 100–200 mg every night at bedtime or, if unavailable, medroxyprogesterone acetate 5–10 mg orally at bedtime. However, regardless of the estrogens used, there is an increase in thrombogenicity with the addition of medroxyprogesterone acetate and a lesser increase with the use of other progestogens (Scarabin, 2018).

MASCULINIZING HORMONE REGIMENS

Masculinizing HT primarily involves testosterone administration. The primary goal of therapy is to maintain total testosterone levels in the normal cismale range. Routes include intramuscular or subcutaneous testosterone cypionate or enanthate at 25–100 mg once a week or transdermal routes such as patches (2–8 mg/day) or gels and creams (20–100 mg/day). Testosterone cypionate and enanthate can also be administered in 100–200 mg every 2 weeks, but this dosing may increase peak/trough effects and lead to low energy at trough, often days 10–14 of a 2-week injection cycle. Testosterone undecanoate is available in both an intramuscular (IM) injection formulation that is given every 10 weeks after 2 monthly loading doses or as a twice daily oral regimen. Intranasal testosterone cypionate is also available but must be administered 3 times daily. Long-acting implantable testosterone pellets are also available: insertion involves a minor in-office procedure, and maintaining cisgender male range testosterone levels often requires placement of new pellets every 2–4 months. Oral testosterone undecanoate preparation requires a dosing up-titration and is administered twice daily; an FDA "black box" warning has been placed on this medication regarding a risk of hypertension; notably, the effect size of the increase in blood pressure when observed is small (Swerdloff et al., 2020).

Many providers have begun using the subcutaneous route with testosterone cypionate and enanthate, which is less painful and traumatic and has been found to be noninferior (Olson et al., 2014). This treatment is well tolerated, with a minimum of side effects in most cases. The dose is titrated to the cessation of menses and progression of virilization while keeping total testosterone levels in the normal cismale range. Prior concerns about hepatic injury are currently unfounded with the use of nonoral, nonsynthetic androgens. Monitoring should include baseline and periodic (every 6–12 months) fasting serum lipids, glucose, and hematocrit. Because of the lack of menstruation and the hematopoietic influence of testosterone, hematocrit should be compared to cismale normal ranges. Because testosterone administration alone is not a reliable contraceptive, even in the setting of prolonged amenorrhea, transgender men who are sexually active with a partner who has any detectable sperm in their semen should be counseled on contraceptive use and the teratogenic risks of unplanned pregnancy while using testosterone. While some transgender men may be averse to taking estrogen-containing contraceptives, others may prefer it over more invasive methods. It is important to have an individualized discussion with each person over their contraceptive preferences and consider nonhormonal and progestin-only options (Krempasky et al., 2020). The effects of testosterone on the vagino-cervical mucosa with regards to HIV transmission risk are unknown, though transgender men using testosterone do tend to have higher rates of atrophic vaginitis and inadequate specimens on cervical Pap sampling (Peitzmeier et al., 2014).

Primary human papillomavirus (HPV) screening via self-swab is a viable alternative for transmasculine patients who are uncomfortable with a pelvic exam, and it has been shown to dramatically increase cervical cancer screening rates in this population (Goldstein et al., 2020). This method of screening is preferred by transmasculine people and increases cervical cancer screening rates in the clinical setting, but is less sensitive than traditional provider-collected specimens (Reisner et al., 2017). However, increases in screening rates lead to the detection of more high-risk HPV infection than screening fewer individuals with a more sensitive test (Goldstein et al., 2020). Conversely, since many high-risk HPV infections do not result in cervical dysplasia requiring intervention, high-risk HPV-only screening may result in over-detection and unnecessary subsequent testing such as colposcopy, which can be of particular concern in transgender men and transmasculine people for whom pelvic examinations are traumatic (Deutsch et al., 2020).

SOCv8 requires assessment by a licensed professional prior to any gender-affirming surgery. Common surgical procedures and recommendations from SOCv8 for referral to surgery are listed in Table 10.2. While SOCv8 suggests that the focus of this assessment should be on verifying the patient's gender identity, it is also important to assess for surgical readiness and psychosocial factors that may influence the course of surgery. Expanded insurance coverage for gender-affirming surgeries is available under the Affordable Care Act. Medicaid coverage is on a state-by-state basis and, where available, has made such procedures available to patients with limited levels of psychosocial functioning and health literacy. Providers should consider additional and ongoing assessments of perioperative essentials, such as housing, social support, transportation, and the ability for postoperative care and self-care, and they should provide resources and support to address identified needs or gaps (Deutsch, 2016). Patients may also present with a history of any number of surgical procedures. In some cases, the surgery may have been performed in another state or country; as such, local primary care providers may be called upon to provide postoperative care. Most surgeons are willing to work with local physicians and, when contacted, may ask for photographs to be transmitted by email. For patients with a complex wound care issue and

Table 10.2 COMMON SURGICAL PROCEDURES

PROCEDURE	DESCRIPTION
FEMINIZING	
Vaginoplasty	Creation of a vagina between the urethra and rectum; vaginal lining may vary based on surgical technique
Orchiectomy	Removal of the testes; commonly referred to as castration
Augmentation mammoplasty	Using implants and/or fat grafting to increase the size of the breasts
Facial feminization	Can involve a variety of procedures, including forehead reconstruction, jaw reconstruction, rhinoplasty, tracheal shave, and others to create a more feminine face
Body contouring	Liposuction and fat grafting to create a more feminine figure
MASCULINIZING	
Reduction mammoplasty/ mastectomy	A variety of surgical techniques to create a flat, male-appearing chest and remove mammary and ductal tissue
Hysterectomy ± oophorectomy	Removal of the uterus with or without removing the ovaries
Metoidioplasty	Creation of a small phallus out of the clitoris; can be done with or without vaginectomy and/or urethral reconstruction
Phalloplasty	Creation of a phallus using a skin flap from a variety of techniques varying by donor site
Body contouring	Liposuction and fat grafting to create a more masculine figure

remote surgeon, referral to a local wound care center may be a reasonable alternative approach.

Most vaginoplasties are performed using a penile-inversion technique resulting in a vagina lined by skin. However, it is important to ask each patient if they know how their vagina was created, as different vaginal linings may lead to different bacterial STI susceptibility (Radix et al., 2019). The erectile tissue is removed, and a "neovagina" is created by inverting the penile skin into a pocket created in the pelvis in the very narrow space between the urethra and the rectum. A clitoris is created using the glans penis. The creation of labia minora and majora varies based on the surgeon's technique, with some using skin in the pelvis, and some using scrotal skin if it was not used to line the neovagina. The neovagina requires lifelong periodic dilation and/or sexual activity to maintain depth and girth, and an artificial lubricant is required for penetration.

Health conditions affecting the neovagina usually result from remaining or recurrent granulation tissue or mixed-skin flora or sebum and debris conditions resulting from a deep inverted pocket of keratinized skin. Granulation tissue can be treated with moderate-strength topical steroids applied to a dilator and inserted into the vagina. Cauterization with silver nitrate is also an option but is painful and can lead to rectovaginal fistulae if applied to the posterior vaginal wall. Candida infections are uncommon, and the pH would not be expected to be acidic as in a natal vagina (Weyers et al., 2009). There is no squamocolumnar junction in a neovagina, eliminating the need for Pap testing, but providers should maintain a reasonable index of suspicion for occult penile conditions such as Bowen's disease or other internal skin conditions including skin dysplasia. A small minority of transgender patients receive a vaginoplasty in which a self-lubricating vagina is created using a segment of sigmoid colon. These patients must be monitored for possible malignancy or inflammatory bowel disease of the neovagina. The prostate is not removed during the vaginoplasty procedure; examination of the prostate in a patient who has undergone vaginoplasty may be more effective when performed endovaginally, as the vagina is most often posterior to the prostate. The risk of transmission of HIV via penile-neovaginal receptive sex in transgender women is unknown. Care of transgender women with a history of silicone or saline implant breast augmentation is identical to that of nontransgender persons.

PRIMARY CARE

Transgender persons require the same general primary and preventive care considerations as do nontransgender persons. However, it is important to assess the presence of organs on a patient-by-patient basis. For example, transgender women will retain their prostate after vaginoplasty, and some transgender men may have a hysterectomy but retain their ovaries or cervix. Additionally, chest exams may still be warranted if there is any remaining mammary or ductal tissue after transmasculine patients undergo removal of their breasts. This surgery is not a radical mastectomy; rather, it is an aesthetic surgery most often completed by plastic surgery to create a male-appearing chest, and some mammary or ductal tissue may be left behind. All organ screening should be based on a combination of age and risk factors, maintaining sensitivity to the patient's anxiety, which may be provoked due to examinations and studies on organs related to the birth sex. Screening for breast cancer in transgender women has not been studied; case series exist showing a possible increased risk above that of nontransgender men but lower risk than that of nontransgender women (Brown and Jones, 2015; Gooren et al., 2013). Some experts recommend that after 5–10 years of HT, patients should be considered for breast cancer screening, as are their age-matched nontransgender peers.

Overall, providers should attribute HT as the etiology of any new health condition only after other more common causes have been excluded. Solid, long-term health outcome data are lacking. The largest population-based study on mortality outcomes to date is a retrospective series in the Netherlands of more than 2,000 transgender men and women. In this study, overall mortality among transgender women was increased by 51% in comparison to that of the general Dutch population; however, besides a 64% increase in– risk of death as a result of cardiovascular disease, most of this increase was due to HIV, suicide, and substance abuse, and the study did not control for tobacco use. Transgender men did not have an increased overall mortality compared to the general population, but they had a 25-fold increased mortality relating to substance abuse (Asscheman et al., 2011).

HIV CARE AND PREVENTION CONSIDERATIONS

HIV prevention, care, and research programs have historically grouped transgender women with MSM. This linkage fails to recognize the significant behavioral and social differences between these two groups, not the least of which is that transgender women are not men (Poteat et al., 2015). Other than the possible negative impact of estrogens on amprenavir and fosamprenavir, and theoretical renal function interaction between tenofovir and spironolactone, there are no clear biomedical differences in the prevention or management of HIV in transgender persons (El-Ibiary et al., 2008). The most important considerations are ensuring that programs and clinic settings are culturally appropriate; electronic medical record systems should have the capacity to record and display the correct name and pronoun; social marketing/outreach and recruitment materials should include imaging and messaging appropriate for transgender populations; waiting rooms should have transgender-oriented pamphlets and wall art; and clinic bathroom policies should allow all patients agency in choosing which bathroom to use without being stopped or harassed by clinic staff. Providers and clinic staff should have adequate cultural fluency and sensitivity (Sevelius et al., 2014a).

HIV PrEP in transgender women has not been studied in depth. To date, the only published clinical trial data of PrEP in transgender women is a subgroup analysis of the iPrEx study that found no efficacy on an intention-to-treat basis. However, none of the transgender women who seroconverted had detectible PrEP drug levels at the time of HIV detection. Hormone use was associated with lower drug levels overall, as well as a lower likelihood of having therapeutic drug levels, but the relationship between specific drug levels and HIV risk was identical between MSM and transgender women. It remains to be determined if reduced drug levels in transgender women using hormones are due to a direct interaction or to other confounders, such as increased pill burden or personal fear of interaction between hormones and ARVs (Deutsch et al., 2015b). Trials for long-acting injectable cabotegravir and oral tenofovir alafenamide/emtricitabine as PrEP both included transgender women (Mayer et al., 2020; Landovitz et al., 2021). While no subanalyses have yet been published on these studies specific to transgender participants, inclusion was significant enough in these studies to show efficacy among transgender participants for both regimens. No PrEP studies have included transgender men, and only methods approved for cisgender women should be used in this population. Specifically, tenofovir alafenamide/emtricitabine is not currently recommended for use in transgender men, as neither transgender men nor cisgender women were included in initial clinical trials.

SILICONE

The use of injected silicone and other soft tissue fillers (pumping) has become an increasingly prevalent practice, particularly among transgender women of color and sex workers. Procedures are sought because of a variety of factors; in addition to peer pressure and a lack of understanding of the risks, more complex factors of survival are at play. Patients engaging in survival sex work may believe that they need to obtain a hyperfeminine figure to pay for food and rent. Others may place a priority on erectile function and avoid HT, using silicone as their sole method of body feminization. Still others may live in neighborhoods in which they do not feel safe being identified as a transgender person, and they believe that silicone will assist them in blending in as a nontransgender person (Clark et al., 2008). For many, injected silicone is the only accessible option for body modification beyond hormone therapy.

Numerous acute and chronic health complications may arise with the use of silicone and fillers. Most patients are unaware of exactly what is being injected, and the colloquial "silicone" may refer to any one of a number of injected fillers. Unscrupulous practitioners, medical assistants, or laypersons will inject up to 1 liter or more of medical- or industrial-grade silicone, lubricant oil, insulating caulk, tire sealant, and other chemicals with the intent of bringing drastic and rapid changes to the physique (Silva-Santisteban et al., 2013). In addition to risks associated with exposure to the injected material, risks of acute bacterial infections and sepsis, as well as transmission of HIV and hepatitis, are high under uncontrolled procedural conditions. Thromboembolic events such as deep vein thrombosis (DVT) and pulmonary embolism (PE) have been observed acutely post-silicone injection; patients should be monitored closely if they disclose plans for getting silicone injections. Some patients may have a sterile systemic inflammatory response mimicking sepsis or may suffer embolization syndromes. The free filler substances could serve as an immunoadjuvant that precipitates an immune reconstitution inflammatory syndrome (IRIS) (Alvarez et al., 2016). These episodes are often treated with antibiotics as they can mimic cellulitis; however, particularly painful flares should be treated with systemic steroids. Long-term risks include chronic pain and disfigurement as the injected material migrates and calcifies.

Treatment of silicone-related morbidities is limited and mostly supportive. Two case reports describe improved symptoms with subcutaneous etanercept 25 mg twice weekly; however, the applicability of etanercept when chemicals other than silicone are used, as well as its safety in PWH, is unclear (Desai et al., 2006; Pasternack et al., 2005; Rapaport, 2005). An additional concern is subcutaneous or intramuscular administration of needed medications, such as penicillin or ceftriaxone, and how these injections may be affected by or complicate preexisting soft tissue fillers. One case report described the safe and successful use of subcutaneous enfuvirtide in a patient with extensive migratory silicone material under ultrasound guidance (Gabrielli et al., 2010). It is particularly important to assess for injected fillers when using parenteral hormone regimens or long-acting injectable ARVs, as the location of fillers may affect available injection sites, and the effects of fillers on transdermal estrogens are unknown.

HIV AND TRANSGENDER POPULATIONS SUMMARY

Most of the special considerations in the care of transgender people living with HIV relate to provider and staff cultural competency and respect, tone and content of messaging, using the correct name and pronoun, and avoiding categorizing transgender women together with MSM. Gender affirmation through hormone and surgical treatment improves quality of life and, when bundled with HIV care or prevention efforts, may have synergistic benefits. More study is needed to evaluate the role of PrEP in transgender communities.

CARE OF PWH WHO EXPERIENCE HOMELESSNESS OR UNSTABLE HOUSING

Elizabeth Imbert and Matthew D. Hickey

LEARNING OBJECTIVE

Describe special considerations affecting the clinical management of people experiencing homelessness or unstable housing.

WHAT'S NEW?

- Long-acting injectable ART and innovative, low-barrier models of care improve care engagement and viral suppression.

KEY POINTS

- Establishing mutual trust is paramount.
- Linkage to care and retention in care require enhanced multidisciplinary teamwork.
- Long-acting injectable antipsychotics are important treatment options for individuals with psychosis who face challenges with adherence.
- Long-acting injectable ART is a new innovative tool that is promising for individuals who face challenges with daily adherence.

INTRODUCTION

PWH who experience homelessness or unstable housing have lower rates of viral suppression and higher mortality than their housed counterparts. While housing and other basic needs are ultimately needed to adequately address disparities in HIV outcomes, navigation and linkage to low-barrier clinic-based and mobile care services are promising interventions. Successful linkage to and retention in care are best met through the establishment of a trusting relationship with care teams who can partner with PWH to both treat HIV and simultaneously address housing, mental health, and substance use.

EPIDEMIOLOGY OF HOMELESSNESS AND HIV

Homelessness and unstable housing exist on a spectrum, ranging from unsheltered to living in severely inadequate or insecure accommodations. In the United States, an estimated 580,000 people were unsheltered or in temporary/emergency shelter on a single night in 2020 in the United States (Housing and Urban Development [HUD] Continuum of Care Homeless Assistance Program, 2021). These estimates are based on point-in-time counts of individuals living on the street, in emergency shelters, or in transitional housing and likely significantly underestimate the number of people experiencing homelessness over the course of any given year or experiencing other forms of housing instability.

PWH face a high burden of homelessness and unstable housing. In a representative sample of PWH accessing care at outpatient HIV clinics during 2020–2021, 17% reported homelessness or unstable housing, and 8% reported homelessness in the prior year (CDC, 2022a). People experiencing homelessness also face a disproportionate burden of new HIV diagnoses. In San Francisco, 18% of new HIV diagnoses occurred in people experiencing homelessness, despite representing less than 1% of the total population (Colfax et al., 2021). Once diagnosed with HIV, people experiencing homelessness experience disparities in treatment outcomes throughout the cascade of HIV care. Greater degree of housing instability is associated with lower rates of HIV viral suppression, even among those engaged in care (Clemenzi-Allen et al., 2018; Griffin et al., 2020); further, homelessness at the time of HIV diagnosis is associated with 27-fold greater odds of mortality (Spinelli et al., 2019). In a large study analyzing the differences in causes of death among housed and unhoused individuals diagnosed with HIV in San Francisco between 2002 and 2016, decedents who were homeless were more likely to be younger, Black, female, or transgender, and living below the poverty level; have a history of injection drug use; and were less likely to have been prescribed ART. Compared to those who were housed, those who were homeless were more likely to die of causes related to mental health or substance use disorders (Hessol et al., 2019).

PWH who experience homelessness also face a disproportionate burden of violence, stigma, mental illness, and substance use and may benefit from a syndemic approach to these related conditions (Jones et al., 2020; Tsai et al., 2015; Tsai et al., 2017). Worsening housing instability is associated with more severe mental health symptoms and diagnoses, which are, in turn, associated with worse HIV treatment outcomes (Aidala et al., 2016). Globally, people who inject drugs have an 18% prevalence of HIV (Degenhardt et al., 2017), and concurrent homelessness further increases HIV prevalence and risk of new infection (Stone et al., 2022). Mental health diagnoses and substance use disorders are both associated with lower rates of retention in HIV care (Rooks-Peck et al., 2018). In an analysis in a Ryan White clinic in Miami, Florida, individuals experiencing a combination of homelessness, mental health symptoms, and substance use disorders had lower rates of viral suppression than those with any single isolated condition (Dawit et al., 2021), highlighting the importance of a treatment approach that provides integrated care for HIV, substance use, mental health, and social services to support housing needs.

CARE MODELS FOR PEOPLE EXPERIENCING HOMELESSNESS

Traditional HIV primary care models based on scheduled appointments may be difficult to access for people experiencing homelessness, resulting in higher utilization of urgent and emergency department care (Clemenzi-Allen et al., 2019). Other barriers to care engagement may include competing sustenance needs, lack of secure location to store medications and belongings, insurance challenges, lack of phone availability to receive appointment reminders, and comorbidities such as substance use and mental health diagnoses (Dombrowski et al., 2015; Holtzman et al., 2015; Yehia et al., 2015). Ultimately, supportive housing is the most needed and effective intervention to address homelessness and unstable housing (Wiewel et al., 2020). Housing assistance has an independent effect on improving outcomes for inadequately housed PWH (Aidala et al., 2016).

While simultaneously advocating for greater access to permanent supportive housing, a local partnership between community-based organizations, departments of public health, health systems, and advocacy groups is essential for addressing the current medical and psychosocial needs of PWH and experiencing homelessness. Driven by the UNAIDS "Getting to Zero" campaign and the U.S. Ending the HIV Epidemic initiative, many local jurisdictions have developed forums for collaboration between local organizations that can be invaluable for identifying local resources such as legal aid, showers, and harm-reduction services (Buchbinder and Havlir, 2019; Fauci et al., 2019; UNAIDS, 2010). Engagement with "Getting to Zero" coalitions can facilitate both greater local advocacy and important referral networks for community-based services of which clinicians may not otherwise be aware.

For people experiencing homelessness who are not currently engaged in care, navigation services can provide an important link back into clinical care (Mizuno et al., 2015). Navigators are often peers who can meet patients in the community and accompany them to medical appointments. Navigators often develop close relationships with clients that are critical for both ensuring successful linkage to medical care and building client self-efficacy for active participation in their care (Roland et al., 2020). Because of the intensely personal nature of navigator–client relationships, it is important for navigation programs to provide support for boundary setting and burnout prevention (Roland et al., 2022). Navigation is often most successful when eligible patients are identified by a medical or social service provider, and may be less successful when patients are only identified by public health surveillance reports of patients who are out of care (Dombrowski et al., 2018a; Sachdev et al., 2020). Navigation services also help improve linkage to care and prevent declines in viral suppression post-incarceration (Cunningham et al., 2018; Myers et al., 2018). Clinic-based programs such as the PHAST team in San Francisco are designed to help ensure that recently diagnosed or newly re-engaged patients are immediately started on ART and effectively navigated into routine HIV primary care (Coffey et al., 2019; Bacon et al., 2021a; Bacon et al., 2021b). Other peer navigation interventions have not been successful in improving care engagement for people experiencing homelessness, highlighting the challenges of relinking patients to systems that can provide adequate support for them to remain engaged (Cabral et al., 2018).

Multidisciplinary healthcare teams, clinics, and health systems also play an important role in designing HIV and primary care services in a manner that minimizes barriers for people experiencing homelessness. Research among PWH experiencing homelessness demonstrates that this population has strong preferences for a care team that knows them as a person (as opposed to an urgent care model with an unknown provider) and the ability to drop in for care (vs. a scheduled appointment), with a willingness to trade $32.79 (95% CI: 14.75 to 50.81) and $11.45 (95% CI: 2.95 to 19.95) in gift cards/visit, respectively (Conte et al., 2020). Integration of substance use disorder treatment and mental health services into routine HIV care is also essential for clinics providing care to people experiencing homelessness who face a disproportionate burden of these comorbidities (Garcia and Kushel, 2022; Haldane et al., 2022). The POP-UP low-barrier care model in San Francisco is integrated within the Ward 86 county HIV clinic and provides drop-in comprehensive HIV primary care and social work services for people experiencing homelessness (Hickey et al., 2022; Imbert et al., 2021). The POP-UP model also includes integrated psychiatric and substance use treatment, providing a one-stop-shop for many common patient medical needs. The MAX clinic in Seattle provides similar drop-in services for people experiencing homelessness or other barriers to engagement with routine HIV primary care (Dombrowski et al., 2018b; Dombrowski et al., 2019). Such care models address a key barrier to care by eliminating appointments and providing on-demand access to care, while also routinely reviewing patients who have fallen out of care to conduct outreach when needed.

Mobile care offers another approach to provide care for people whose psychosocial barriers prevent engagement with clinic-based care. Street medicine programs have a long history of providing medical care to people experiencing homelessness outside of traditional clinic settings (Lynch et al., 2022). Street medicine services have successfully delivered mental health services, substance use disorder treatment with low-barrier buprenorphine, and hepatitis C treatment to people living on the streets or in shelters (Carter et al., 2019; Khalili et al. 2022; Lo et al., 2021; Rosecrans et al., 2022). Mobile HIV care programs integrated with medical care and housing navigation services can also improve both health outcomes and successful transition to stable housing (Rajabiun et al., 2020). Other mobile services focus on veterinary care for pets of people experiencing homelessness; this approach can be helpful for engaging patients and for addressing medical needs of their pets that may serve as a barrier to accessing needed healthcare (Geller, 2022). For patients requiring hospitalization but who have a pet, coordination with the local animal care and control to provide temporary boarding for pets can be critical for ensuring the patient can comfortably remain in the hospital to receive needed treatment.

CLINICAL CARE

Clinical care of PWH who experience homelessness and unstable housing should address individual and structural barriers to care. Drop-in access (i.e., no appointments required) to comprehensive primary care with a multidisciplinary care team who can address HIV, mental health diagnoses, substance use disorders, other comorbidities, and housing access is key. Pharmacists and pharmacy technicians can assist with prior authorizations for medications, support clinicians, work with pharmacies, and assist with in-clinic medication distribution. Eligibility workers can assist with insurance issues. Clinics should consider providing gift cards to address immediate sustenance needs, clothing, and hygiene kits; opportunities to pick up medications directly from the clinic; and outreach and navigation, including transportation assistance, for patients who have lapses in care engagement (Imbert et al., 2021). Regular case conferences with the multidisciplinary team are helpful to discuss complex cases, review care gaps, and come up with shared care plans (Hickey et al., 2022). The care team should also work closely with emergency rooms, hospitals, psychiatric services, jails, and community-based organizations, including case managers and navigators, to coordinate care for patients.

Developing a trusting relationship with patients to partner on their care is key (Conte et al., 2020). The care team should elicit PWH's concerns and priorities, share their concerns, and develop a joint care plan with specific next steps. It is important to listen to PWH in a nonjudgmental way and try to understand the challenges they are facing and to elicit ways in which the clinical team might be able to partner with them to address these challenges, recognizing that it may take time to build trust. The care team should address immediate needs (i.e., reason patient came to the visit) and partner with patients on long-term goals. Care teams should be trained in crisis de-escalation, and support for frontline staff should be provided (Audain et al., 2013).

Obtaining information about housing status and stability should be a routine part of obtaining a psychosocial history for PWH. Providers should seek to understand an individual's history of homelessness, exploring factors that precipitated homelessness, psychosocial factors that may impact housing, and patient preferences regarding housing. At each visit, it is important to collect living situation and contact information, including location where the patient is staying and a phone number or email address, or additional contact persons (e.g., family members, friends, case managers) (Audain et al., 2013). For each person, meeting with a social worker to assess source of income, conduct housing assessments, and refer to temporary and long-term housing is important. Compared with unplaced persons not achieving stable housing quickly, persons quickly achieving stable housing were more likely to engage in care, and to be virally suppressed (Wiewel et al., 2020).

In addition to collecting HIV history (diagnosis date, $CD4^{+}$ nadir, history of opportunistic infections, prior ART regimens and side effects, and prior genotypes), it is important to explore adherence, including pattern and duration of nonadherence as well as individual-identified challenges to adherence. When selecting an ART regimen, it is important to elicit personal preferences, including oral (one or more pills) or injectable, side-effects concerns, and medication delivery options (i.e., clinic storage/pick-up, pharmacy, deliver to location, etc.). Having medications in a clinic where PWH can pick up frequently and engage with a medical team and have frequent adherence counseling can be helpful (Imbert et al., 2021). For people receiving methadone at an opioid treatment program or engaging in outpatient psychiatric day programs, consider partnering with these programs to deliver oral ART as directly observed therapy. For individuals who have faced challenges to engagement in care or medication adherence, consider choosing high "genetic barrier to resistance" regimens, including bictegravir/tenofovir alfenamide/emtricitabine or dolutegravir plus tenofovir/emtricitabine. Darunavir-based regimens (particularly fixed-dose darunavir, cobisistat, tenofovir alfenamide, and emtricitabine) have a very high barrier to resistance and may be a good ART option for PWH with inconsistent adherence to oral medications (DHHS, 2024; Lathouwers et al., 2021).

An exciting recent development is the advent of long-acting ART (LA-ART), which is a promising tool for people experiencing homelessness or unstable housing who face barriers to daily oral medication adherence. Because of its extended dosing interval, LA-ART has the potential to mitigate many barriers to daily oral ART adherence, including lack of safe storage for pills, pills getting lost or stolen, pill fatigue, pills as a reminder of living with HIV, fear of inadvertent disclosure from possessing pills, and inability to take a daily medication (Kanazawa et al., 2021; Scarsi and Swindells, 2021). A demonstration project of LA-ART in a diverse group of patients with high levels of substance use and marginal housing in San Francisco demonstrated promising early treatment outcomes, including in PWH with detectable viremia because of adherence challenges. LA-ART was started via a structured process of provider referral, multidisciplinary review by a doctor, nurse, and pharmacist, and monitoring for on-time injections. Inclusion criteria were willingness to receive monthly injections and a reliable contact method; patients with any history of rilpivirine-associated resistance mutations were not considered for LAI-ART; however, the program allowed up to one integrase-associated resistance mutation. The program also allowed patients with hepatitis B coinfection to enter if they are willing to continue or initiate hepatitis B–directed treatment (Christopoulos et al., 2023).

Addressing severe mental illness and substance use disorders is imperative. Integrated psychiatry consultation in primary care can increase access to needed mental health services and support primary care clinicians to meet the psychiatric needs of PWH (Zeidler Schreiter et al., 2013). When treating psychosis, it is important to consider starting an oral antipsychotic that, if tolerated, can be switched to a long-acting injectable antipsychotic (i.e., risperidone or aripiprazole). Long-acting antipsychotics have demonstrated significant benefit as compared to oral antipsychotics in preventing hospitalization or relapse in schizophrenia (Kishimoto et al., 2021). Methamphetamine-induced psychosis can also be treated with antipsychotics (Glasner-Edwards and Mooney, 2014; Verachai et al., 2014); in patients with adherence challenges, long-acting injectable antipsychotics should be considered. Contingency management is an evidence-based intervention to reduce methamphetamine use and should be implemented in outpatient clinics that treat patients with methamphetamine use disorder (Brown and DeFulio, 2020). Assessment for and treatment of opioid use disorder is important during routine HIV care visits, including low-threshold buprenorphine treatment (Jakubowski and Fox, 2020), referral to opioid treatment programs/methadone clinics when indicated, and naloxone distribution (see, e.g., Life-saving naloxone from pharmacies, CDC, 2019). It is also important to offer harm-reduction services, safe education kits, and education during clinic encounters (Peckham and Young, 2020). Given the high prevalence of tobacco use among people experiencing homelessness and its impact on life expectancy for PWH, smoking cessation should also be addressed (Baggett et al., 2013; Reddy et al., 2016). Alcohol use disorder is also high among PWH, and screening and appropriate management are key (Duko et al., 2019).

In addition to partnering with patients on their health goals, it is important to offer standard healthcare maintenance per United States Preventive Services Task Force (USPSTF) guidelines, including routine vaccinations and age-appropriate cancer screening when patients present for care. Specific attention should be given to test and treat for sexually transmitted infections and hepatitis C and ensure vaccination against hepatitis A and hepatitis B, COVID-19, meningitis, and pneumococcus. Tuberculosis screening should be offered, and latent tuberculosis infection treated as indicated (see Chapter 8, "Health Maintenance").

HOMELESSNESS OR UNSTABLE HOUSING CONCLUSION

PWH who experience homelessness or unstable housing face individual and structural barriers that interfere with achieving viral suppression and increase morbidity and mortality. While housing is ultimately needed to address disparities in HIV outcomes, innovative programs that assist with navigation and linkage to low-barrier multidisciplinary care teams who can develop trusting relationships with patients to partner on their care are key.

HIV IN CRIMINAL-LEGAL-INVOLVED PEOPLE

Olabimpe Asupoto and Alysse G. Wurcel

LEARNING OBJECTIVE

Describe the current state of HIV care delivery to people who are criminal-legal involved, with a focus on opportunities for improving care.

WHAT'S NEW?

There is increasing evidence for the feasibility, acceptability, and efficacy of treatment for substance use disorder in PWH. This treatment has been shown to improve rates of retention in HIV care and HIV viral suppression. Although there are challenges to implementation, there are increasing data supporting strategies aimed at broadening access to medication for the prevention of HIV (i.e., PrEP) to people who are incarcerated.

KEY POINTS

- Criminal-legal-involved people are at increased risk for HIV compared to people who have never been incarcerated or detained.
- Rates of HIV in state and federal carceral facilities are decreasing.
- Similar to healthcare standards in the community, all people who are incarcerated and detained should receive HIV medications with the goal of HIV viral suppression.
- HIV viral suppression is suboptimal in people who are released from jail and prison, signaling the need for intensified linkage to care programs upon release.
- Assessment for and treatment of substance use disorder are necessary to provide quality care to PWH who are incarcerated.
- Implementation of programs supporting the provision of PrEP to people at risk for HIV should occur in jails and prisons.

INTRODUCTION

As a result of the intersection of criminalization of drug use disorder, poverty, and racism, HIV prevalence in criminal-legal-involved populations (CLIP) is higher than in people who have never been incarcerated or detained (Bowleg et al., 2022; Brinkley-Rubinstein et al., 2018; Schneider, 1998). The spectrum of criminal-legal involvement is broad and includes the experience of being arrested, being incarcerated in jail or prison, and community supervision, including parole and probation. In 2020, 1 in every 47 adults in the United States were under some form of carceral supervision across this spectrum, and about 75% of CLIP were under community supervision (Kluckow and Zeng, 2022). People who are marginalized, including but not limited to Black, Hispanic/Latino, and Native American people, are more likely than white people to be incarcerated (Dauria et al., 2021). Similarly, PWH who are impacted by criminal justice system are more likely to be Black, Hispanic/Latino, or Native American than white (Bovell-Ammon et al., 2021).

Although there are several commonalities across the criminal-legal spectrum for HIV care, there are setting-specific barriers to the operationalization of HIV care. Here, we focus on four broad carceral settings: (1) prisons and jails, (2) detention centers, (3) resource-limited international carceral settings, and (4) community carceral control and re-entry. We also discuss the importance of testing and treatment for infectious and noninfectious illnesses that co-occur with HIV, HIV transmission in carceral settings, and best practices for HIV-related care and prevention in carceral settings.

Of note, as the language describing people who are incarcerated has shifted away from the use of words like *offender* or *inmate* toward person-first language, we will refer to people with criminal-legal involvement as CLIP, and criminal-legal-involved individuals as CLII. The terms *CLIP* and *CLII* include people who are incarcerated as well as people with a history of previous incarceration.

HIV TREATMENT IN PRISONS AND JAILS

It is important to understand the distinction between prisons and jails. Although the terms *prison* and *jail* are often used interchangeably, there are distinct differences between these facilities, and these differences impact healthcare delivery. Prisons are run at the federal and state level, and incarcerate people for longer periods of time, typically >2 years. Jails are run at the county or city level and typically have shorter periods of incarceration (the average length of jail incarceration in 2020 was 28 days) (Minton and Zhen, 2021).

HIV infection is 3 times more prevalent in state and federal prisons than in the general population (CDC, 2022b). Recently, there has been a decrease (14,180 in 2019 to 11,940 in 2020) in the number of people in state prisons with HIV (Maruschak, 2022). There are no nationally available estimates of people in jails with HIV; however, a 1%–9% range of HIV prevalence has been reported (Javanbakht et al., 2014; Parvez et al., 2013). Approximately 22% of individuals living with HIV who were incarcerated were unaware of their HIV status when they entered prison and jail, and approximately 69% of new infections are transmitted by PWH who are diagnosed with HIV infection but not receiving treatment (Dauria et al., 2022; Iroh et al., 2015).

Most of the research on HIV treatment for people who are in jail and prison is about barriers to receiving HIV medications. One notable study conducted with CLIP in jails demonstrated that while most individuals received ART and met with healthcare providers during incarceration, access to their medication in a timely manner was inadequate (Blue et al., 2022). In this study, participants reported missing medication for extended periods of time because of delays in obtaining correct medications, unpredictable length of stay, jail staff refusing to provide medication because of the financial burden, and lack of communication between correctional officers. Many CLIP were forced to rely on family members to bring their ART to jail, but correctional officers can often prevent this by citing jail policies (Blue et al., 2022). Despite these challenges, one benefit of this study was that CLIP individuals were able to consult with HIV clinicians (Blue et al., 2022). Individuals involved in the study felt well treated, and clinicians tried to improve their care by utilizing local resources (Blue et al., 2022).

Even after barriers to receiving ART are overcome, the methods by which the medications are distributed also pose unique challenges to CLIP living with HIV. The most-common method of ART distribution in carceral settings is direct-observation therapy (DOT), rather than "keep on person" (KOP). Many jails and prisons prefer DOT to keep track of medication adherence. However, for the CLIP with HIV, DOT poses a threat to confidentiality because medical staff may state the medication's name or other CLIP may see the medication during distribution (White et al., 2015a). Other issues with DOT distribution of ART include the inability to take the medication with food and prevention of CLIP with HIV to independently establish their own medication regimen (White et al., 2015a). Prior to release, facilities that use DOT may need to consider introducing a more practical KOP system to help individuals manage their medications.

It is imperative that PWH have consistent access to their medications and their HIV provider. Unfortunately, qualitative research has revealed major gaps in HIV care delivery in jails and prisons. Justice-involved women in Alabama carceral facilities reported barriers to continuous HIV care owing to unfair limitations, including forced isolation, food rationing, refusal to provide counseling after an initial HIV diagnosis, and outright denial of treatment. Disruptions in treatment can also result from transferring between facilities, being segregated, and being in "lockdown," which is when officials restrict individuals from leaving their cells for a period of time (Culbert, 2014).

HIV CARE IN DETENTION SETTINGS

There are over 200 Immigration and Customs Enforcement (ICE) detention facilities in the United States, housing 300,000 people (Terp et al., 2021). Individuals detained in detention settings are subjected to a detention process that is unorganized and complex, which results in gaps in access to appropriate medical care and medications. According to Human Rights Watch, the U.S. immigration detention systems have poor medical care, slow responses to care requests, and inexperienced medical staff, which all contribute to avoidable deaths, including HIV-related deaths (Blunt, 2017). In addition to the poor care offered in detention centers, many people are discouraged from disclosing their HIV status for fear of how it will affect their case or their ability to leave the detention facility (Page et al., 2018). Another barrier for people who are detained in ICE facilities is medication choice because HIV medications vary between countries. Patients with HIV drug resistance may not benefit from first-line treatment because drug resistance patterns in the United States may differ from those in the patient's home country (Beyrer and Pozniak, 2017).

If persons who are detained are able to overcome all the above barriers to receiving care while in a detention facility, they still face significant barriers to high-quality HIV care once they are deported. When they are deported, a 30-day supply of HIV treatment may be prescribed, but only if they receive treatment while in the detention facility (Page et al., 2018). When PWH return to their home countries, returning to the United States often takes precedence over finding HIV clinics for treatment (Grimes et al., 2016). There have been reports of programs aimed at increasing linkage to care for PWH detained in ICE facilities, such as increasing detainee access to specialist consultation during detention (Mishreki et al., 2021). Although some progress has been made in linkage to care, there is still room for improvement in order to encourage ongoing HIV treatment and viral suppression after deportation.

HIV TREATMENT IN RESOURCE-LIMITED INTERNATIONAL CARCERAL SETTINGS

Although the United States has the highest rates of incarceration, jails and prisons exist globally, including in countries that are considered resource-limited settings where HIV prevalence rates are higher. The HIV prevalence in jails and prisons in resource-limited settings is often unknown but is estimated to be quite high, with some countries reporting that 25% of CLIP are living with HIV (Dolan et al., 2016). Prisons in Kyrgyzstan found the prevalence of HIV to be 10.3%, making it the third most common infectious disease they face. More than half of the CLIP living with HIV in these facilities were unaware of their status (Azbel et al., 2016). Twelve of the 15 people who knew their HIV status were taking ART (Azbel et al., 2016). According to a Malaysian study, less than half of CLIP who qualified for ART received it, and a quarter later developed AIDS (Fuge et al., 2020). Similarly, a cross-sectional retrospective study in South African prisons reported that only half of PWH who were eligible for ART initiation were able to do so. Frequently, CLIP were unable to receive HIV care because of a shortage of healthcare workers, disorganized health systems, and facility transfers (Stevenson et al., 2020). An investigation of HIV care access in Malawi's prisons revealed that there is more access to HIV services at entry and throughout incarceration in urban facilities compared to rural ones because of on-site clinics (Gondwe et al., 2021). In contrast, ART was not routinely provided in rural prisons; instead, individuals had to travel to a nearby hospital to receive treatment (Gondwe et al., 2021). Further, many CLII reported significant delays in medical staff providing care for seriously ill patients in urban facilities (Gondwe et al., 2021). Additional barriers that emerged in resource-limited settings include stigma, unequal access to HIV care for women, shortage of healthcare staff, and insufficient diet (Telisinghe et al., 2016).

Structural interventions that address discrimination, HIV stigma, and human rights violations and make health care more accessible are needed in jails and prisons. There is evidence that sub-Saharan African carceral facilities were more aware of HIV risk after employing structural interventions to reduce HIV-related stigma and create safer work environments (Lyons et al., 2020). Further, integrating HIV care with gender-affirming care (Maiorana et al., 2021), mental health services (Collins et al., 2021), and harm reduction (Chang et al., 2021) helps to meet population health and wellness needs. In Kenya, the establishment of community clinics and drop-in centers run by key populations resulted in an immediate improvement in HIV care engagement and a significant increase in individuals initiating ART (DiCarlo et al., 2022). PWH from South African carceral facilities were linked to care within 90 days of release and were interviewed by phone or in person to evaluate medication adherence. The study found that there were no lapses in ART medication (Mabuto et al., 2020).

HIV TRANSMISSION IN CARCERAL SETTINGS

The actual transmission of HIV within jails and prisons is thought to be relatively low, and it is believed to be lower than the transmission rates in the general public (Valera et al., 2017). Especially with increased access to well-tolerated, highly efficacious HIV treatment, transmission in jails and prisons is likely a rare occurrence. However, it is challenging to track HIV transmission in carceral settings because CLIP might be reluctant to report potential exposures for fear of punishment. These exposures include tattooing, injection drug use, and consensual and nonconsensual sexual activity. Despite the need for condoms, only a few carceral facilities provide them. Jails with condoms include Los Angeles, San Francisco, New York City, Philadelphia, and Washington, DC. State prisons in Mississippi and men's prisons in Vermont and California provide condoms (Lucas et al., 2020). Increasing testing, access to HIV-prevention medications, and access to harm-reduction tools, like substance use disorder treatment, are strategies to decrease HIV transmission in jails and prisons (Reddon et al., 2019). These measures should be universally implemented in carceral settings globally to prevent HIV transmission.

RELEASE PLANNING: TRANSITION TO COMMUNITY

Release from jail and prison is a time when people may experience barriers to getting HIV care (Masyukova et al., 2018). The majority (3.9 million) of the 5.5 million people who are CLII in the United States are under some sort of community carceral control. HIV infection rates in community supervision programs in New York are 13% in men and 17% in women, which is significantly higher than the rates in carceral facilities (El-Bassel et al., 2019).

Barriers to care for PWH post-release include interruptions in health insurance, untreated substance use disorders, and mental health conditions (Campbell et al., 2018). One study in Connecticut found that the rates of HIV suppression following release from incarceration were 67% at 1 year and 43% at 3 years (Loeliger et al., 2018b). A study in Illinois compared ART rates between CLII who are incarcerated and CLII who are reincarcerated, and found that the proportion of people on ART decreased from 73% at the time of release to 50% at the time of reincarceration (Badowski and Patel, 2022). Increased linkage to care upon release from prison is critical to maintaining viral suppression. A study conducted in Rhode Island and North Carolina carceral facilities examined the retention of HIV care in CLII post-release and in those already receiving care in the community. HIV care retention in PWH following release was 20% lower than in those already in the community (Costa et al., 2018). Within the first 30 days following release from jail in Connecticut, <20% of people filled their HIV medications or went to an HIV clinic. Less than 50% of those who were released saw an HIV provider within 90 days, and 33% had detectable viremia at the initial appointment (Loeliger et al., 2018a). Conversely, in a study conducted in a Massachusetts jail to evaluate the transition of care back to the community, 70% of participants met with an HIV care provider in a timely manner (within 30 days) (Dong et al., 2021; Sprague et al., 2017). These findings suggest that linkages to care differ by state.

There have been several studies examining the role of a navigator to assist in linkage to care following incarceration (Iryawan et al., 2022; Monroe et al., 2017; Taylor et al., 2018). A case management intervention study was conducted in Baltimore, where justice-involved PWH met with a clinical social worker and an outreach worker to develop treatment plans and attend follow-up visits to assess treatment adherence (Crable et al., 2021). As a result of this intervention, justice-involved PWH were 5.6 times more likely to receive linkage to HIV clinical services, 5.8 times more likely to be prescribed ART, and 4 times more likely to report medication adherence at follow-up visits (Crable et al., 2021). Data to Care (D2C) is a public health strategy that uses available data from HIV surveillance and other sources to re-engage PWH who have fallen out of care to improve health outcomes (Villanueva et al., 2022). A recent qualitative review found that applying the D2C strategy to county jails had both potential benefits for public health and risks for PWH (Buchbinder et al., 2020). Implementing D2C had the advantages of increased public trust in state health services, decreased HIV transmission, improved access to HIV care, and continuity of care following release from jail. However, potential drawbacks include invasions of privacy, unintentional or intentional disclosure of HIV status, threats of violence, and coerced HIV treatment (Buchbinder et al., 2020). Implementating a peer navigator intervention, instead of a D2C intervention, builds trust, reduces stigma, and lessens other discrimination-related barriers to healthcare engagement (Dauria et al., 2022). Once the CLII is released, navigators accompany them to appointments and aid in patient–provider interactions (Woznica et al., 2021). Prior to release, this intervention should be started, and support can be provided to assist individuals in setting goals to overcome barriers to HIV care engagement and medication adherence (Taylor et al., 2018).

Untreated substance use disorder is a major reason that people do not engage in HIV care in the community (Dong et al., 2021; Korthuis and Edelman, 2018). Substance use disorder affects 85% of CLII incarcerated in jail (Rubenstein et al., 2016). There is a strong correlation between mental health conditions and substance use disorders (Baranyi et al., 2019; Baranyi et al., 2022). The presence of a substance use disorder is linked to poor treatment compliance and medication nonadherence (Hunt et al., 2020). Three treatments for opioid use disorder are buprenorphine, naltrexone, and methadone. A study of 21 state carceral facilities found that all three medications were available in 62% of these facilities. Unfortunately, only 7% of the 538 prisons in these 21 carceral facilities offered all three medications (Scott et al., 2021). A study conducted in Rhode Island carceral facilities found that the use of extended-release buprenorphine, a monthly injectable medication, resulted in minimal side effects and was used for longer than other drugs/formulations postrelease. With prolonged use, buprenorphine also prevents return to substance use for a longer duration of time (Martin et al., 2022). Another study conducted with CLII found extended-release naltrexone reduced opioid use relapse (Lier et al., 2022). Internationally, there are also data demonstrating that the initiation of substance use disorder treatment improves linkage to HIV care (Azbel et al., 2018; Mjaland, 2015; Polonsky et al., 2016). Treatment for substance use disorder is an evidence-based intervention that decreases substance use and, therefore, increases linkage to and adherence to HIV care upon release from jails and prisons.

TESTING AND MANAGEMENT OF COMORBID CONDITIONS WITH HIV IN CARCERAL SETTINGS

Any discussion about the optimal treatment of HIV in carceral settings needs to highlight the treatment of noninfectious and infectious illnesses that are prevalent in PWH. HIV medications are highly effective and well tolerated, so morbidity and mortality from HIV and opportunistic infections have decreased (Justiz Vaillant and Naik, 2022). Screening for other infections, including hepatitis B and hepatitis C (HBV, HCV) and sexually transmitted infections like syphilis, is necessary to provide the best care for PWH (Workowski et al., 2021). PWH involved in the justice system who have a history of drug injection have a 78% chance of HIV/HCV coinfection and a 15% chance of HIV/HBV coinfection (Ahmadi et al., 2021). Direct-acting antiviral drugs are the current standard of treatment for HCV and should be offered to all people who are incarcerated and detained. HIV has been linked to premature aging (Aberg, 2020), increased cardiovascular disease (Aberg, 2020), and increased risk of cancer (Castilho et al., 2022). Thus, the treatment of PWH should follow national guidelines for preventive care, including cancer screening and blood pressure control (Lakshmi et al., 2018).

HIV TESTING AND PREVENTION

The Centers for Disease Control and Prevention (CDC) recommend that CLII in carceral facilities be routinely screened for HIV through opt-out HIV testing, offered antiretroviral medication, and evaluated by clinicians with experience treating HIV (CDC, 2022). Opt-out testing is not widely employed in U.S. carceral facilities, according to the most recent research (Solomon et al., 2014). Routine opt-out testing is specifically mentioned at 5% of surveyed jail facilities, and 7% of surveyed jails offered HIV testing for all CLII at intake (Maner et al., 2022). While this is not surprising, routine opt-out testing strategies yield greater numbers of screenings and subsequent HIV diagnoses and, therefore, should be universally employed. Jails, as opposed to prisons, typically have short lengths of stay, high turnover rates, and poor communication with healthcare providers, making routine or opt-out HIV screening and follow-up difficult to implement. The majority of the jails in the nation do not regularly conduct HIV screenings (Hutchinson et al., 2021). Results from studies conducted with individuals who have been incarcerated demonstrated that being African American, having higher education, having been previously incarcerated, and having more HIV knowledge all increased the likelihood of ever receiving HIV screening (Farel et al., 2019). It is critical to promptly diagnose individuals living with HIV to overcome the obstacles preventing effective HIV therapy. The U.S. initiative End the HIV Epidemic encourages state and local health departments to strengthen their existing programs to increase access to HIV testing (Fauci et al., 2019).

People who inject drugs and people who are incarcerated are not routinely offered PrEP, and this is an area where jails and prisons should focus more resources. Medications that prevent HIV transmission have been available as a daily pill since 2012 (Bolland and Grey, 2013; Mayer and Krakower, 2012). PrEP is approved to prevent HIV infection through sexual contact and intravenous drug use (Choopanya et al., 2013; Grant et al., 2010; Murnane et al., 2013). Recently, injectable forms of PrEP have been approved (Garrison and Haberer, 2021). A study on the continuum of PrEP care for men who are incarcerated and at high risk for HIV was conducted in Rhode Island's carceral facilities. The study found that increased PrEP awareness, support from carceral and medical leadership, and linkage to care post-release contributed to the successful use of PrEP in carceral settings (Murphy et al., 2022). In a comparable study conducted in Thailand, where PrEP was administered through directly observed therapy in prison facilities, 94% of CLIP missed fewer than eight doses of oral medication (Colby et al., 2015). With injectable PrEP, frequency of missed doses may be significantly reduced. More research is being conducted about successful implementation of PrEP in carceral settings and during re-entry (Brinkley-Rubinstein et al., 2018; Marcus et al., 2016; Murphy et al., 2022).

RURAL POPULATIONS AND HIV

Abby Davids and Ashley Carvalho

LEARNING OBJECTIVE

Describe obstacles to and best practices for optimal HIV care for PWH in rural settings.

WHAT'S NEW?

PWH in rural areas face unique challenges, including the need for expanded HIV prevention, testing, and care services.

KEY POINTS

- The HIV epidemic in the United States has begun to shift to more rural areas.
- Rural residence creates barriers to HIV care and is a risk factor for lower HIV testing overall, later HIV diagnosis, and increased HIV-related mortality.
- The increasing rurality of the U.S. opioid epidemic highlights additional challenges and needs for both HIV and HCV care in rural areas.

Although the HIV epidemic in the United States began in large cities, it has since moved to more rural areas (Schafer et al., 2017). The Southern United States currently has the highest incidence and prevalence of HIV in the country; accounting for approximately 46% of all HIV transmissions and 49% of new transmissions, while only 37% of the U.S. population lives in the South (CDC, 2024a). Some nonurban counties in the Southern United States now have higher HIV prevalence than many large U.S. cities (Rural Health Information Took Kit, 2022). Racial disparities in the burden of HIV transmissions, particularly among Black populations, are amplified in the South as well (CDC, 2024a).

Rural/nonurban residence creates several barriers to engagement in the HIV care continuum. HIV testing rates are lower in rural areas; in one study, the rate of lifetime HIV testing was 66% for nonurban participants versus 88% for urban participants (Wallace et al., 2011). MSM in rural areas are less likely to be tested for HIV than those in urban areas, as are undocumented migrant and seasonal farmworkers in rural areas (Fernandez et al., 2005; Goldenberg et al., 2014). Rural providers may not offer HIV testing routinely as well; in one study, primary care providers in North Carolina were only 10% adherent to CDC HIV testing guidelines, despite being aware of the recommendations (White et al., 2015b).

Access to care also remains a challenge for PWH in rural areas. Many rural residents travel to urban areas for their medical care, citing a lack of local provider expertise as one reason for this. In 2013, 95% of nonurban counties in the United States lacked a Ryan White HIV medical provider, compared to 69% of urban counties (Vyavaharkar, 2013). In 2017, of the 2,000 organizations funded by the Ryan White program, only 6% were located in rural areas (Klein et al., 2020). Additionally, PWH in rural areas were less likely to have regular outpatient visits with their HIV care provider than PWH in urban areas, and they were less likely to take ART. PWH in rural areas were also less likely to be prescribed newer antiretroviral agents than those living in urban areas (Schafer et al., 2017). In one study from the U.S. Veterans Administration, PWH in rural areas had more advanced HIV infection at diagnosis than those in urban areas, and the mortality hazard ratio for rural PWH versus urban PWH was 1.34 (Ohl et al., 2012). Additional barriers to care for PWH in rural areas include stigma, lack of support services, and transportation difficulties.

Rural areas are also less likely than urban areas to have harm-reduction programs in place. The 2014 outbreak of HIV in rural Scott County, Indiana, underscores the potential for rapid progression of HIV and hepatitis C through communities affected by the opioid epidemic. Currently, in the United States, new opioid injectors reside primarily in nonurban areas, and people using opioids who switch from oral formulations to injection use engage in injection practices with a greater risk of HIV and hepatitis C transmission. The CDC estimates that counties at greatest risk for an injection drug use (IDU)-associated HIV outbreak are mostly rural; this, combined with high rates of poverty and lower educational attainment, makes rural areas particularly vulnerable (CDC, 202b). Hepatitis C similarly affects nonurban populations disproportionately, and many of the areas with the highest rates of acute HCV in the United States are in rural Appalachian states (Schranz et al., 2018).

To provide state-of-the-art health care to the large rural population of PWH, programs are needed to address barriers to care and the stigma that PWH in rural areas face. Strategies that center on the social determinants of health and recognize the importance of involving local community members have proven to be most successful (Schafer et al., 2017; WHO, 2024). These include:

- Community engagement: involving community members in research and programming, such as lay health adviser interventions
- Leveraging existing data sources: agreement on a universal definition of "rurality" in order to study and understand populations in rural areas more fully
- Human resource capacity development: addressing the HIV care provider shortage in rural areas and conducting

needs assessments of rural primary care providers to better understand knowledge gaps and training needs

- Innovative service delivery: consideration of non-clinic-based locations to deliver HIV prevention and testing, such as emergency departments or pharmacies, use of telehealth to reach remote patients, use of teleconferencing to connect specialists in urban areas with primary care providers in rural areas, and optimizing the use of technology including text messaging and app-based services.

Resources for rural HIV care are available through the National Rural Health Association and the Rural Health Information Hub. The Rural Health Information Hub includes an "HIV/AIDS Prevention and Treatment Toolkit" (available at: https://www.ruralhealthinfo.org/toolkits/hiv-aids). A web resource is available to locate nearby federally funded community health centers (U.S. Department of Health and Human Resources; available at: http://findahealthcenter.hrsa.gov/Search_HCC.aspx).

CARE OF MIGRANT AND IMMIGRANT PERSONS WITH HIV

Deliana Garcia, Claire M. Hutkins Seda, and Laszlo Madaras

LEARNING OBJECTIVE

- Discuss the important distinction between "migrants" and "immigrants."
- Discuss the differences in HIV risk, presentation, and comorbidities among immigrants from different regions of the world.
- Discuss the impact of stigma on healthcare-seeking behavior, treatment adherence, and safe practices.

WHAT'S NEW?

- The associations between HIV and migrant health continue to be very dynamic, reflecting long-standing structural and social determinants of health as well as ever-evolving geopolitical environments driving displacement and emerging infections of public health importance.

KEY POINTS

- The complex combination of population characteristics and barriers to care requires careful consideration of each person's circumstances when considering HIV risk, testing, treatment adherence, and perceived or experienced stigma.
- Research in these populations is challenging because of a myriad of factors, including the absence of accommodations in the study structure, recruitment issues, ethical challenges, and subgroup differentiation.
- A distinction in premigration transmission and intra/post-migration transmission appears when considering migrants from the Americas versus those from the African continent and Eastern Europe.
- The prevalence and incidence of HIV in Black and Indigenous people of color in the United States are higher than those of white people, and these populations have less access to care and treatment than do white populations.
- Among immigrant PWH, the prevalence and presentation of opportunistic infections (OIs) or coinfections differ from those of U.S.-born PWH.

Migrants, people in the United States for a time-limited stay, usually engage in remunerated activity like farm work, and newly arrived immigrants, those who wish to resettle permanently in the United States, have largely arrived from Mexico and Central and South America. A smaller percentage are from Africa and Asia (Radford, 2019). Some migrants and recent immigrants live and work in the United States without authorization, although it is unclear how many. A crucial characteristic of these populations is geographic instability and high mobility. Migrants, by definition, move frequently for work purposes, family reunification, or pursuit of safe haven, contributing to an unstable and stressful lifestyle (IOM, 2020).

A natural consequence of such mobility is that migrants face many barriers to accessing care. Migration and immigration—and the federally defined immigration status that migrants and immigrants hold as a result—prevent the acquisition and/or continuation of health insurance. Most people without authorization to live in the United States are not eligible for health insurance or are eligible only for private coverage that is prohibitively expensive. Those with authorization who are migrating within the United States may find it unfeasible to sign up for care after each move as health coverage is geographically fragmented. Mobility is just one negative social determinant of health (SDH), a condition in which people are born, raised, and work. Some SDHs include employment and working conditions, income and social status, social support and connectedness, environment and housing, access to health care and literacy, and gender issues (O'Laughlin, 2018). The discrepancies attributable to these categories shape individual health status and outcomes through their impact on intermediary determinants such as living conditions, psychosocial circumstances, behavioral and/or biological factors, and the health system itself (WHO, 2019). In addition to mobility, migrants and new immigrants face numerous negative SDHs that overlap and amplify each other. They frequently work in labor-based occupations with a high risk for injury and illness (Levy et al., 2007). Low-income status, lack of strong networks in the receiving communities, considerable social and cultural isolation (which frequently result from language barriers, economic limitations, and cultural differences), and fear over immigration status are common SDHs among migrants and new immigrants. In turn, these SDHs limit migrants' and new immigrants' access to HIV health education, testing, and treatment. They also reduce migrants' and new immigrants' participation in data and surveys.

As a result, developing an accurate picture of the HIV epidemic among migrants and immigrants to the United States has been hampered by a lack of national data. The CDC only recently began tracking the country of origin for PWH, and currently, there are few national publications on the topic. Most published reports on HIV and immigrant populations are based on studies at the county, city, and state levels. An example is a report from a study conducted through the San Mateo County Health Department in California. Immigrants within the study population who presented with lower $CD4^+$ T-cell counts were more likely to have an OI and be hospitalized at the time of HIV diagnosis. Immigration status was significantly associated with delayed presentation, although the study did not separate newly arrived immigrants and long-term immigrants (Levy et al., 2007). A cross-sectional population-based survey conducted in Tijuana, Mexico, found that repeat male migrants returning from their home communities were more likely to have sex with men, not use a condom, and use substances before sex (Zhang et al., 2017). Historically, such local epidemiologic studies have been the predominant method for assessing the need and planning services for immigrant populations. A 2018 review of published literature since 2015 on known HIV outcomes among migrants from low- and middle-income countries living in high-income countries suggests that a high proportion of migrants acquire HIV after migration and are disproportionally affected by HIV (Ross et al., 2018). Migrants from Latin America and the Caribbean have the highest rates of post-migration infection, and migrants from Africa have the lowest.

Research in these populations is challenging, as migrants living with HIV may be challenging to identify and follow. The combination of factors such as stigma, along with increased risk behaviors and reluctance to use condoms or seek testing, increases the risk of migrants acquiring HIV infection (Ross et al., 2018). High levels of mobility are predictive of poor engagement in HIV care and ART disruption (Ross et al., 2018). Reliance on the community for daily survival may negatively affect care seeking and adherence if the migrant living with HIV fears ostracism from the social group. Studies of sexual practices among male migrants note riskier behaviors, such as sex with casual female partners and sex workers, condomless anal and vaginal intercourse, and substance use, likely while transiting or in the receiving country. For example, in Mexico, after MSM, the greatest risk for HIV transmission is among those who have migrated to the United States or had a partner who migrated (Hirsch et al., 2002; Hirsch et al., 2007). Poor HIV outcomes are primarily driven by stigma and limited access to care (Ross et al., 2018). Additionally, there is limited evidence on appropriate interventions for migrants living with HIV.

Among immigrants, the picture is slightly clearer, although the available data do not segment newly arrived immigrants from those who may have lived in the United States for many years. HIV was diagnosed in 191,697 persons in the United States between 2007 and 2010, with 16.2% among those born outside the United States. Nearly half of those diagnosed with HIV for whom a specific country or region of birth outside of the United States was known were from Central America and Mexico. A little more than 20% were from the Caribbean, and approximately 15% were from Africa. California, Florida, New York, and Texas reported the highest numbers of persons born outside the United States diagnosed with HIV. They are also the states with the highest overall case rates. Slightly more than 73% of persons born outside the United States living with HIV were male. The racial breakdown for PWH born outside of the United States was 3.3% white, 10% Black, 42.2% Hispanic, and 64.3% Asian. Thirty-nine percent of persons born outside of the United States were infected through heterosexual contact versus 27.2% for U.S.-born persons (Prosser et al., 2012).

The COVID-19 pandemic widened preexisting health disparities. PWH experienced a reduction of access to HIV services as health systems shifted focus to COVID-related care. Disrupted treatment regimens, stalled or discontinued preventive services and educational opportunities, and overwhelmed healthcare facilities contributed to an estimated 10 years' loss of advances in HIV/TB care. Additionally, those with the worst outcomes hospitalized with serious COVID-19 infection were often patients with compromised immune systems from poorly controlled HIV or complicated by chemotherapy for cancer, immunosuppressive medications after organ transplant, and taking medications to suppress chronic autoimmune diseases (Trajman et al., 2022).

In 2022 the emergence of mpox on a global scale presented new challenges for healthcare workers treating HIV. While mpox thus far has not been as lethal to immunocompetent individuals as historical smallpox, those with poor immune systems, especially in places where HIV medication is not readily available, have increased morbidity and mortality. The U.S. public health system is insufficiently comprehensive to be able to respond to emerging health concerns or crises without diverting resources from HIV care, which compromises the gains that have been achieved over years of HIV focus (CDC, 2024b). Additionally, the recent 2024 mpox outbreak has been linked to transmission by people who regularly cross borders for occupational purposes, highlighting the need for attention on mpox as it specifically relates to migrant and immigrant populations.

Migrants and newly arrived immigrants living with HIV are vulnerable to numerous comorbidities and coinfections. Tuberculosis (TB) is the most common presenting comorbidity among migrant and immigrant PWH. In regions of the world where TB is endemic, the *Mycobacterium tuberculosis* (MTB) can persist for years in a person who has been exposed yet has not developed active disease. TB can progress from infection to active disease if the PWH has a suppressed $CD4^+$ count, and it can involve every organ system. Some of the typical medications used in treating MTB must be used with caution in patients also being treated for HIV. For example, when coadministered with the MTB medication rifampin, concentrations of many protease inhibitors are severely diminished, compromising HIV treatment efficacy, yet simultaneous treatment of HIV and MTB can greatly improve global survival in vulnerable populations.

ART may be more toxic in persons with chronic hepatitis, and the prevalence of HBV infection in Asian immigrants may complicate attempts to treat HIV. OIs not usually seen in U.S.-born persons may present in immigrant PWH, reflecting the epidemiology of their country of origin. Examples include *Penicillium marnefii* in persons of Southeast Asian origin, and a variety of parasitic diseases in persons of African descent.

Immigrants and migrants face significant barriers to access medical care, including for diagnosis and treatment of HIV and comorbidities. Efforts to reduce these barriers should include legislation that will support and enhance the public health system, improved access to HIV services, better epidemiologic data on immigrants living with HIV, and enhanced training and support for healthcare providers who serve immigrant populations. Crucial to success in working with migrant and immigrant populations is the utilization of a team approach involving interpreters, social workers, and case managers, including virtual case management to support immigrants between care sites; hiring of culturally appropriate staff; inclusion of peer navigators and community health workers; networking with local community-based organizations working with the impacted populations; Ryan White Program and 340B pharmacy access; and legal services. The CDC has a useful website dedicated to immigrant and refugee health issues (http://www.cdc.gov/immigrantrefugeehealth).

REFERENCES

Aberg JA. Aging and HIV infection: focus on cardiovascular disease risk. *Top Antivir Med*. 2020;27(4):102–105. https://www.ncbi.nlm.nih.gov/pubmed/32224501

Abma JC, Martinez GM. *Sexual Activity and Contraceptive Use Among Teenagers in the United States, 2011–2015*. Hyattsville, MD: National Health Statistics Reports; 2017.

Ahmadi GH, Fararouei M, Mirzazadeh A, et al. The global and regional prevalence of hepatitis C and B co-infections among prisoners living with HIV: a systematic review and meta-analysis. *Infect Dis Poverty*. 2021;10(1):93. https://doi.org/10.1186/s40249-021-00876-7

Aidala AA, Wilson MH, Shubert V, et al. Housing status, medical care, and health outcomes among people living with HIV/AIDS: a systematic review. *Am J Pub Health*. 2016;106(1):e1–e23. https://doi.org/10.2105/AJPH.2015.302905

Alvarez H, Marino A, Garcia-Rodriguez JF, et al. Immune reconstitution in inflammatory syndrome in an HIV-infected patient using subcutaneous silicone fillers. *AIDS*. 2016;30(16):2561–2563.

Armbruster M, Fields EL, Campbell N, et al. Addressing health inequities exacerbated by COVID-19 among youth with HIV: expanding our toolkit. *J Adolesc Health*. 2020;67(2):290–295. http://doi:10.1016/j.jadohealth.2020.05.021

Arrington-Sanders R, Alvarenga A, Galai N, et al. Social determinants of transactional sex in a sample of young black and Latinx sexual minority cisgender men and transgender women. *J Adolesc Health*. 2022;70(2):275–281. http://doi:10.1016/j.jadohealth.2021.08.002

Arrington-Sanders R, Hailey-Fair K, Wirtz AL, et al. Role of structural marginalization, HIV stigma, and mistrust on HIV prevention and treatment among young black latinx men who have sex with men and transgender women: perspectives from youth service providers. *AIDS Patient Care STDS*. 2020;34(1):7–15. https://doi:10.1089/apc.2019.0165

Arrington-Sanders R, Leonard L, Brooks D, et al. Older partner selection in young African-American men who have sex with men. *J Adolesc Health*. 2013;52(6):682–688. http://doi:10.1016/j.jadohealth.2012.12.011

Asscheman H, Giltay EJ, Megens JAJ, et al. A long-term follow-up study of mortality in transsexuals receiving treatment with cross-sex hormones. *Eur J Endocrinol*. 2011;164(4):635–642.

Asscheman H, Gooren LJ, Eklund PL. Mortality and morbidity in transsexual patients with cross-gender hormone treatment. *Metabolism*. 1989;38(9):869–873.

Audain G, Bookhardt-Murray LJ, Fogg CJ, et al. (eds.). *Adapting Your Practice: Treatment and Recommendations for Unstably Housed Patients with HIV/AIDS*. Nashville, TN: Health Care for the Homeless Clinicians' Network, National Health Care for the Homeless Council; 2013.

Azbel L, Polonsky M, Wegman M, et al. Intersecting epidemics of HIV, HCV, and syphilis among soon-to-be released prisoners in Kyrgyzstan: implications for prevention and treatment. *Int J Drug Policy*. 2016;37:9–20. https://doi.org/10.1016/j.drugpo.2016.06.007

Azbel L, Wegman MP, Polonsky M, et al. Drug injection within prison in Kyrgyzstan: elevated HIV risk and implications for scaling up opioid agonist treatments. *Int J Prison Health*. 2018;14(3):175–187. https://doi.org/10.1108/IJPH-03-2017-0016

Bacon O, Chin J, Cohen SE, et al. Decreased time from HIV diagnosis to care, ART initiation, and virologic suppression during the citywide RAPID initiative in San Francisco. *Clin Infect Dis*. 2021a;73(1):e122–e128. http://doi.10.1093/cid/ciaa620

Bacon OML, Coffey SC, Hsu LC, et al. Development of a citywide rapid antiretroviral therapy initiative in San Francisco. *Am J Prev Med*. 2021b;61(5 Suppl 1):S47–S54. https://doi.org/10.1016/j.amepre.2021.06.001

Badowski ME, Patel M. Evaluation of immunologic and virologic function in reincarcerated patients living with HIV or AIDS. *J Correct Health Care*. 2022;28(3):203–206. https://doi.org/10.1089/jchc.20.07.0055

Baggett TP, Lebrun-Harris LA, Rigotti NA. Homelessness, cigarette smoking and desire to quit: results from a US national study. *Addiction*. 2013;108(11):2009–2018. http://doi. 10.1111/add.12292

Baral SD, Poteat T, Strömdahl S, et al. Worldwide burden of HIV in transgender women: a systematic review and meta-analysis. *Lancet Infect Dis*. 2013;13(3):214–222. https://doi:10.1016/S1473-3099(12)70315-8

Baranyi G, Fazel S, Langerfeldt SD, Mundt AP. The prevalence of comorbid serious mental illnesses and substance use disorders in prison populations: a systematic review and meta-analysis. *Lancet Public Health*. 2022;7(6):e557–e568. https://doi.org/10.1016/S2468-2667(22)00093-7

Baranyi G, Scholl C, Fazel S, et al. Severe mental illness and substance use disorders in prisoners in low-income and middle-income countries: a systematic review and meta-analysis of prevalence studies. *Lancet Glob Health*. 2019;7(4):e461–e471. https://doi.org/10.1016/S2214-109X(18)30539-4

Barnes W, D'Angelo L, Yamazaki M, et al. Identification of HIV-infected 12–24-year-old men and women in 15 cities through venue-based testing. *Arch Pediatr Adolesc Med*. 2010;164:273–276.

Bavinton BR, Pinto AN, Phanuphak N, et al. Viral suppression and HIV transmission in serodiscordant male couples: an international, prospective, observational, cohort study. *Lancet HIV*. 2018;5(8):e438–e447. http://doi:10.1016/S2352-3018(18)30132-2

Becasen JS, Denard CL, Mullins MM, et al. Estimating the prevalence of HIV and sexual behaviors among the US transgender population: a systematic review and meta-analysis, 2006–2017. *Am J Public Health*. 2019;109(1):e1–e8. http://doi:10.2105/AJPH.2018.304727

Berry SA, Ghanem KG, Mathews WC, et al. Brief report: gonorrhea and chlamydia testing increasing but still lagging in HIV clinics in the United States. *J AIDS*. 2015;70(3):275–279. http://doi:10.1097/QAI.0000000000000711

Beyrer C, Pozniak A. HIV drug resistance: an emerging threat to epidemic control. *N Engl J Med*. 2017;377(17):1605–1607. https://doi.org/10.1056/NEJMp1710608

Blue C, Buchbinder M, Brown ME, et al. Access to HIV care in jails: perspectives from people living with HIV in North Carolina. *PLoS One*. 2022;17(1):e0262882. https://doi.org/10.1371/journal.pone.0262882

Blunt M. US: detention hazardous to immigrants' health. *Humans Rights Watch*. https://www.hrw.org/report/2017/05/08/systemic-indifference/dangerous-substandard-medical-care-us-immigration-detention. Published 2017. Accessed September 4, 2024.

Bolland MJ, Grey A. Antiretroviral preexposure prophylaxis for HIV prevention. *N Engl J Med*. 2013;368:82.

Boone MR, Cherenack EM, Wilson PA, et al. Self-efficacy for sexual risk reduction and partner HIV status as correlates of sexual beliefs about biological differences between blacks and whites. *AIDS Patient Care STDs*. 2015;29(6):346–353.

Bovell-Ammon BJ, Xuan Z, Paasche-Orlow MK, LaRochelle MR. Association of incarceration with mortality by race from a national longitudinal cohort study. *JAMA Netw Open*. 2021;4(12):e2133083. https://doi.org/10.1001/jamanetworkopen.2021.33083

Bowleg L, Malekzadeh AN, Mbaba M, Boon CA. Ending the HIV epidemic for all, not just some: structural racism as a fundamental but overlooked social-structural determinant of the US HIV epidemic. *Curr Opin HIV AIDS*. 2022;17(2):40–45.

Boyer CB, Hightow-Weidman L, Bether J, et al. An assessment of the feasibility and acceptability of a friendship-based social network recruitment strategy to screen at-risk African American and Hispanic/Latina young women for HIV infection. *JAMA Pediatr*. 2013;3:289–296. http://doi:10.1001/2013.jamapediatrics.398

Branson BM, Handsfield H, Lampe M, et al. Revised recommendations for HIV testing of adults, adolescents, and pregnant women in healthcare settings. *MMWR*. 2006;55(RR-14):1–17.

Brinkley-Rubinstein L, Dauria E, Tolou-Shams M, et al. The path to implementation of HIV pre-exposure prophylaxis for people involved in criminal justice systems. *Curr HIV/AIDS Rep*. 2018;15(2):93–95. https://doi.org/10.1007/s11904-018-0389-9

Brown HD, DeFulio A. Contingency management for the treatment of methamphetamine use disorder: a systematic review. *Drug Alcohol Depend*. 2020;216:108307. http://doi: 10.1016/j.drugalcdep.2020.108307

Brown GR, Jones KT. Incidence of breast cancer in a cohort of 5,135 transgender veterans. *Breast Cancer Res Treat*. 2015;149(1):191–198. http://doi.org/10.1007/ s10549-014-3213-2

Bruce D, Harper GW, Fernandez IM, et al. Age-concordant and age-discordant sexual behavior among gay and bisexual male adolescents. *Arch Sex Behav*. 2012;41(2):441–448. http://doi:10.1007/s10508-011-9730-8

Buchanan A, Montepiedra G, Sirois PA, et al. Barriers to medication adherence in HIV-infected children and youth based on self- and caregiver report. *Pediatrics*. 2012;129(5):e1244–e1251. http://doi:10.1542/peds.2011-1740

Buchbinder M, Blue C, Juengst E, et al. Expert stakeholders' perspectives on a Data-to-Care strategy for improving care among HIV-positive individuals incarcerated in jails. *AIDS Care*. 2020;32(9):1155–1161. https://doi.org/10.1080/09540121.2020.1737641

Buchbinder SP, Havlir DV. Getting to zero San Francisco: a collective impact approach. *J Acquir Immune Defic Syndr*. 2019;82(Suppl 3):S176–S182. https://doi.org/10.1097/QAI.0000000000002200

Bukowski LA, Chandler CJ, Creasy SL, et al. Identifying barriers and facilitators to HIV diagnosis and viral suppression among Black transgender women in the United States. *J Acquir Immune Defic Syndr*. 2018;79(4):413–420.

Cabral HJ, Davis-Plourde K, Sarango M, et al. Peer support and the HIV continuum of care: results from a multi-site randomized clinical trial in three urban clinics in the United States. *AIDS Behav*. 2018;22(8):2627–2639. http://doi:org/10.1007/s10461-017-1999-8

Cahill S, Makadon H. Sexual orientation and gender identity data collection in clinical settings and in electronic health records: a key to ending LGBT health disparities. *LGBT Health*. 2014;1(1):34–41. http:// online.liebertpub.com/doi/abs/10.1089/lgbt.2013.0001.

Cahill S, Makadon HJ. Sexual orientation and gender identity data collection update: US government takes steps to promote sexual orientation and gender identity data collection through meaningful use guidelines. *LGBT Health*. 2014;1(3):157–160. http:// doi.org/10.1089/lgbt.2014.0033.

Campbell ANC, Wolff M, Weaver L, et al. "It's never just about the HIV": HIV primary care providers' perception of substance use in the era of "universal" antiretroviral medication treatment. *AIDS Behav*. 2018;22(3):1006–1017. https://doi.org/10.1007/s10461-017-2007-z. Accessed September 4, 2024.

Canonico M, Plu-Bureau G, Lowe GD, Scarabin PY. Hormone replacement therapy and risk of venous thromboembolism in postmenopausal women: systematic review and meta-analysis. *BMJ*. 2008;336(7655):1227–1231.

Carter J, Zevin B, Lum PJ. 2019. Low barrier buprenorphine treatment for persons experiencing homelessness and injecting heroin in San Francisco. *Addict Sci Clin Pract*. 2019;14(1):20. http://doi:org/10.1186/s13722-019-0149-1

Castilho JL, Bian A, Jenkins CA, et al. CD4/CD8 ratio and cancer risk among adults with HIV. *J Natl Cancer Inst*. 2022;114(6):854–862. https://doi.org/10.1093/jnci/djac053

Centers for Disease Control and Prevention (CDC). Behavioral and clinical characteristics of persons with diagnosed HIV infection: medical monitoring project, United States, 2020 cycle (June 2020–May 2021). HIV Surveillance Special Report 29. cdc.gov. https:// stacks.cdc.gov/view/cdc/149117. Published 2022a. Accessed September 7, 2024.

CDC. CDC recommendations for correctional and detention settings. cdc.gov. https:// www.cdc.gov/nchhstp/director-letters/correctional-settings-recommendations.html?CDC_AAref_Val=https://www.cdc.gov/nchhstp/dear_colleague/2022/dcl-041822-correctional-health.html. Published August 18, 2022b. Accessed September 4, 2024.

CDC. Counties and jurisdictions experiencing or at-risk of outbreaks. https://www.cdc.gov/persons-who-inject-drugs/vulnerable/counties.html. Published 2024b. Accessed July 3, 2024.

CDC. Fast facts: HIV in the US by race and ethnicity. https://www.cdc.gov/hiv/data-research/facts-stats/race-ethnicity.html. Published 2024a. Accessed July 3, 2024.

CDC. HIV surveillance supplemental report: monitoring selected national HIV prevention and care objectives by using HIV surveillance data United States and 6 territories and freely associated states, 2022. https://stacks.cdc.gov/view/cdc/156511. Published May 21, 2024c. Accessed September 5, 2024.

CDC. HIV surveillance report, 2018 (Updated); vol. 31. cdc.gov. https://stacks.cdc.gov/view/cdc/149035. Published May 2020a. Accessed July 26, 2020

CDC. HIV surveillance report, 2020; vol. 33. cdc.gov. https://www.cdc.gov/hiv/library/reports/hiv-surveillance.html. Published May 2022c. Accessed October 22, 2022.

CDC. Life-saving naloxone from pharmacies. cdc.gov. https:// www.cdc.gov/vitalsigns/naloxone/index.html#:~:text=Naloxone%20is%20a%20life-saving%20medication%20that%20can%20reverse,standing%20orders%29%2C%20which%20have%20contributed%20to%20lowering%20deaths. Published 2019. Accessed October 19, 2022.

CDC. Many Men Many Voices. https:// www.cdc.gov/hiv/pdf/research/interventionresearch/compendium/rr/cdc-hiv-intervention-rr-best-3mv.pdf. Published October 20, 2022d. Accessed September 15, 2024.

CDC. Personalized cognitive counseling. cdc.gov. https:// www.cdc.gov/hiv/effective-interventions/diagnose/personalized-cognitive-counseling/index.html. Published April 10, 2023. Accessed September 15, 2024.

CDC. Youth risk behaviour survey data summary and trends report 2009–2019. https:// www.cdc.gov/healthyyouth/data/yrbs/pdf/YRBSDataSummaryTrendsReport2019-508.pdf. Published 2020b. Accessed September 15, 2024.

CDC and US Public Health Service. Preexposure prophylaxis for the prevention of HIV infection in the United States—2021 update: a clinical practice guideline. https://www.cdc.gov/hiv/pdf/risk/prep/

cdc-hiv-prep-guidelines-2021.pdf. Published 2021. Accessed January 24, 2023.
Chang J, Shelly S, Busz M, et al. Peer driven or driven peers? A rapid review of peer involvement of people who use drugs in HIV and harm reduction services in low- and middle-income countries. *Harm Reduct J*. 2021;18(1):15. https://doi.org/10.1186/s12954-021-00461-z
Choopanya K, Martin M, Suntharasamai P, et al. Antiretroviral prophylaxis for HIV infection in injecting drug users in Bangkok, Thailand (the Bangkok Tenofovir Study): a randomised, double-blind, placebo-controlled phase 3 trial. *Lancet*. 2013;381(9883):2083–2090. https://doi.org/10.1016/s0140-6736(13)61127-7
Christopoulos KA, Grochowski J, Mayorga-Munoz F, et al. First demonstration project of long-acting injectable antiretroviral therapy for persons with and without detectable HIV viremia in an urban HIV clinic. *Clin Infect Dis*. 2023;76(3):e645–e651.
Clark RF, Cantrell FL, Pacal A, et al. Subcutaneous silicone injection leading to multi-system organ failure. *Clin Toxicol*. 2008;46(9):834–837. http://doi.org/10.1080/15563650701850025
Clemenzi-Allen A, Geng E, Christopoulos K, et al. Degree of housing instability shows independent "dose-response" with virologic suppression rates among people living with human immunodeficiency virus. *Open Forum Infect Dis*. 2018;5(3):ofy035. http://doi:org/10.1093/ofid/ofy035
Clemenzi-Allen A, Neuhaus J, Geng E, et al. Housing instability results in increased acute care utilization in an urban HIV clinic cohort. *Open Forum Infect Dis*. 2019;6(5):ofz148. http://doi:org/10.1093/ofid/ofz148
Clum G, Chung SE, Ellen JM. Mediators of HIV-related stigma and risk behavior in HIV infected young women. *AIDS Care*. 2009;2(11):1455–1462.
Coffey S, Bacchetti P, Sachdev D, et al. RAPID antiretroviral therapy: high virologic suppression rates with immediate antiretroviral therapy initiation in a vulnerable urban clinic population. *AIDS*. 2019;33(5):825–832. http://doi:10.1097/QAD.0000000000002124
Cohen D, Farley T, Taylor S, et al. When and where do youths have sex? The potential role of adult supervision. *Pediatrics*. 2002;110:1–6.
Cohen MS, Chen YQ, McCauley M, et al. Antiretroviral therapy for the prevention of HIV-1 transmission. *N Engl J Med*. 2016;375(9):830–839. http://doi:10.1056/NEJMoa1600693
Colby D, Srithanaviboonchai K, Vanichseni S, et al. HIV pre-exposure prophylaxis and health and community systems in the Global South: Thailand case study. *J Int AIDS Soc*. 2015;18(4 Suppl 3):19953. https://doi.org/10.7448/IAS.18.4.19953
Coleman E, Bockting W, Botzer M, et al. Standards of care for the health of transsexual, transgender, and gender-nonconforming people, version 7. *Intl J Transgenderism*. 2012;13(4):165–232.
Colfax G, Philip S, Enanoria W, et al. *HIV Epidemiology: Annual Report, 2020*. San Francisco: San Francisco Department of Public Health; 2021.
Collins PY, Velloza J, Concepcion T, et al. Intervening for HIV prevention and mental health: a review of global literature. *J Int AIDS Soc*. 2021;24S2:e25710. https://doi.org/10.1002/jia2.25710
Colton Meier SL, Fitzgerald KM, Pardo ST, et al. The effects of hormonal gender affirmation treatment on mental health in female-to-male transsexuals. *J Gay Lesbian Mental Health*. 2011;15(3):281–299.
Conte M, Eshun-Wilson I, Geng E, et al. Understanding preferences for HIV care among patients experiencing homelessness or unstable housing: a discrete choice experiment. *J Acquir Immune Defic Syndr*. 2020;85(4):444–49. http://doi: 10.1097/QAI.0000000000002476
Costa M, Montague BT, Solomon L, et al. Assessing the effect of recent incarceration in prison on HIV care retention and viral suppression in two states. *J Urban Health*. 2018;95(4):499–507. https://doi.org/10.1007/s11524-018-0255-5
Crable EL, Blue TR, McKenzie M, et al. Effect of case management on HIV outcomes for community corrections population: results of an 18-month randomized controlled trial. *J Acquir Immune Defic Syndr*. 2021;87(1):755–762. https://doi.org/10.1097/QAI.0000000000002624
Craw JA, Gardner LI, Marks G, et al. Brief strengths-based case management promotes entry into HIV medical care: results of the antiretroviral treatment access study-II. *J Acquir Immune Defic Syndr*. 2008;47(5):597–606.
Culbert GJ. Violence and the perceived risks of taking antiretroviral therapy in US jails and prisons. *Int J Prison Health*. 2014;10(2):94–110. https://doi.org/10.1108/IJPH-05-2013-0020
Cunningham WE, Weiss RE, Nakazono T, et al. Effectiveness of a peer navigation intervention to sustain viral suppression among HIV-positive men and transgender women released from jail: the LINK LA randomized clinical trial. *JAMA Intern Med*. 2018;178(4):542–553. http://doi:10.1001/jamainternmed.2018.0150
Dauria EF, Kulkarni P, Clemenzi-Allen A, et al. Interventions designed to improve HIV continuum of care outcomes for persons with HIV in contact with the carceral system in the USA. *Curr HIV/AIDS Rep*. 2022;19(4):281–291. https://doi.org/10.1007/s11904-022-00609-x
Dauria EF, Levine A, Hill SV, et al. Multilevel factors shaping awareness of and attitudes toward pre-exposure prophylaxis for HIV prevention among criminal justice-involved women. *Arch Sex Behav*. 2021;50(4):1743–1754. https://doi.org/10.1007/s10508-020-01834-4
Davey S, Ajibola G, Maswabi K, et al. Mother-to-child HIV transmission with in utero dolutegravir vs. efavirenz in Botswana. *J Acquir Immune Defic Syndr*. 2020;84(3):235–241.
Dawit R, Trepka MJ, Gbadamosi SO, et al. Latent class analysis of syndemic factors associated with sustained viral suppression among Ryan White HIV/AIDS program clients in Miami, 2017. *AIDS Behav*. 2021;25(7):2252–2258. http://doi:10.1007/s10461-020-03153-0
Degenhardt L, Peacock A, Colledge S, et al. Global prevalence of injecting drug use and sociodemographic characteristics and prevalence of HIV, HBV, and HCV in people who inject drugs: a multistage systematic review. *Lancet Glob Health*. 2017;5(12):e1192–e1207. https://doi.org/10.1016/S2214-109X(17)30375-3
Department of Health and Human Services (DHHS). Panel on Antiretroviral Guidelines for Adults and Adolescents: guidelines for the use of antiretroviral agents in adults and adolescents with HIV. Department of Health and Human Services. https://clinicalinfo.hiv.gov/en/guidelines/adult-and-adolescent-arv. Published September 12, 2024. Accessed September 15, 2024.
Desai AM, Browning J, Rosen T. Etanercept therapy for silicone granuloma. *J Drugs Dermatol*. 2006;5(9):894–896.
Deutsch MB. Gender-affirming surgeries in the era of insurance coverage: developing a framework for psychosocial support and care navigation in the perioperative period. *J Health Care Poor Underserved*. 2016;27(2):386–391. doi:10.1353/hpu.2016.0092
Deutsch MB. Pre-exposure prophylaxis in trans populations: providing gender-affirming prevention for trans people at high risk of acquiring HIV. *LGBT Health*. 2018 Oct;5(7):387–390.
Deutsch MB, Bhakri V, Kubicek K. Effects of cross-sex hormone treatment on transgender women and men. *Obstet Gynecol*. 2015a;125(3):605–610.
Deutsch MB, Glidden DV, Sevelius J, et al. HIV pre-exposure prophylaxis in transgender women: a subgroup analysis of the iPrEx trial. *Lancet HIV*. 2015;2(12):e512–9.
Deutsch MB, Green J, Keatley J, et al. Electronic medical records and the transgender patient: Recommendations from the World Professional Association for Transgender Health EMR Working Group. *J Am Med Informat Assoc*. 2013;20(4):700–3.
Deutsch MB, Reisner SL, Peitzmeier S, et al. Recent penile sexual contact is associated with an increased odds of high-risk cervical human papillomavirus infection in transgender men. *Sex Transm Dis*. 2020;47(1):48–53.
DiCarlo MC, Dallabetta GA, Akolo C, et al. Adequate funding of comprehensive community-based programs for key populations needed now more than ever to reach and sustain HIV targets. *J Int AIDS Soc*. 2022;25(7):e25967. https://doi.org/10.1002/jia2.25967
Dolan K, Wirtz AL, Moazen B, Ndeffo-Mbah M, et al. Global burden of HIV, viral hepatitis, and tuberculosis in prisoners and detainees.

Lancet. 2016;388(10049):1089–1102. https://doi.org/10.1016/S0140-6736(16)30466-4
Dong KR, Daudelin DH, Koutoujian PJ, et al. Lessons learned from the Pathways to Community Health Study to evaluate the transition of care from jail to community for men with HIV. *AIDS Patient Care STDs.* 2021;35(9):360–369. https://doi.org/10.1089/apc.2021.0060
Dombrowski JC, Galagan SR, Ramchandani M, et al. HIV care for patients with complex needs: a controlled evaluation of a walk-in, incentivized care model. *Open Forum Infect Dis.* 2019;6(7):ofz294. http://doi:10.1093/ofid/ofz294
Dombrowski JC, Hughes JP, Buskin SE, et al. A cluster randomized evaluation of a health department data to care intervention designed to increase engagement in HIV Care and antiretroviral use. *Sex Transm Dis.* 2018a;45 (6):361–367. https://doi.org/10.1097/OLQ.0000000000000760
Dombrowski JC, Ramchandani M, Dhanireddy S, et al. The Max Clinic: medical care designed to engage the hardest-to-reach persons living with HIV in Seattle and King County, Washington. *AIDS Patient Care STDs.* 2018b;32 (4):149–156. https://doi.org/10.1089/apc.2017.031
Dombrowski JC, Simoni JM, Katz DA, et al. Barriers to HIV care and treatment among participants in a public health HIV care relinkage program. *AIDS Patient Care STDs.* 2015;29(5):279–287. http://doi:10.1089/apc.2014.0346
Dowshen N, Binns HJ, Garofalo R. Experiences of HIV-related stigma among young men who have sex with men. *AIDS Patient Care STDs.* 2009;23(5):371–376. http://doi:10.1089/apc.2008.0256
Duko B, Ayalew M, Ayano G. The prevalence of alcohol use disorders among people living with HIV/AIDS: a systematic review and meta-analysis. *Subst Abuse Treat Prev Policy.* 2019;14(1):52. http://doi:10.1186/s13011-019-0240-3
Eaton LA, Driffin DD, Kegler C, et al. The role of stigma and medical mistrust in the routine healthcare engagement of black men who have sex with men. *Am J Public Health.* 2015;105(2):75–82.
El-Bassel N, Gilbert L, Goddard-Eckrich D, et al. Effectiveness of a couple-based HIV and sexually transmitted infection prevention intervention for men in community supervision programs and their female sexual partners: a randomized clinical trial. *JAMA Netw Open.* 2019;2(3):e191139. https://doi.org/10.1001/jamanetworkopen.2019.1139
El-Ibiary SY, Cocohoba JM. Effects of HIV antiretrovirals on the pharmacokinetics of hormonal contraceptives. *Eur J Contraception Reproduc Health Care.* 2008;13(2):123–132. http:// doi.org/10.1080/13625180701829952
Farel CE, Golin CE, Ochtera RD, et al. Underutilization of HIV testing among men with incarceration histories. *AIDS Behav.* 2019;23(4):883–892. https://doi.org/10.1007/s10461-018-02381-9
Fauci AS, Redfield RR, Sigounas G, et al. Ending the HIV epidemic: a plan for the United States. *JAMA.* 2019;321(9):844–845. http://doi:10.1001/jama.2019.1343
Fernandez M, Collazo JB, Bowen GS et al. Predictors of HIV testing and intention to test among Hispanic farmworkers in South Florida. *J Rural Health.* 2005;21(1):56–64.
Flores AR, Herman JL, Gates GJ, et al. How many adults identify as transgender in the United States? The Williams Institute. https://williamsinstitute.law.ucla.edu/wp-content/ uploads/How-Many-Adults-Identify-as-Transgender-in-the United-States.pdf. Published June 2016. Accessed January 25, 2023.
Fuge TG, Tsourtos G, Miller ER. A systematic review and meta-analyses on initiation, adherence and outcomes of antiretroviral therapy in incarcerated people. *PLoS One.* 2020;15(5):e0233355. https://doi.org/10.1371/journal.pone.0233355
Gabrielli E, Ferraioli G, Ferraris L, et al. Enfuvirtide administration in HIV-positive transgender patient with soft tissue augmentation: US evaluation. *New Microbiologica.* 2010;33:263–265.
Gamarel KE, Nelson KM, Brown L, et al. The usefulness of the CRAFFT in screening for problematic drug and alcohol use among youth living with HIV. *AIDS Behav.* 2017;21(7):1868–1877. http://doi:10.1007/s10461-016-1640-2
Garcia CM, Kushel MB. Integrating mental health and substance use treatment with HIV care for people experiencing homelessness. *Lancet Psych.* 2022;9(8):606–608. http://doi: 10.1016/S2215-0366(22)00228-0
Garrison LE, Haberer JE. Pre-exposure prophylaxis uptake, adherence, and persistence: a narrative review of interventions in the U.S. *Am J Prev Med.* 2021;61(5 Suppl 1): S73–S86. https://doi.org/10.1016/j.amepre.2021.04.036
Geller JM. Street medicine: caring for the pets of the homeless. *J Am Vet Med Assoc.* 2022;260(2):181–185. http://doi:10.2460/javma.21.05.0249
Glasner-Edwards S, Mooney LJ. Methamphetamine psychosis: epidemiology and management. *CNS Drugs.* 2014;28(12):1115–1126. http://doi: 10.1007/s40263-014-0209-8
Goldenberg T, McDougal S, Sullivan P, et al. Preferences for a mobile HIV prevention app for men who have sex with men. *JMIR mHealth uHealth.* 2014;2(4):e47. http://doi: 10.2196/mhealth.3745
Goldstein Z, Martinson T, Ramachandran S, et al. Improved rates of cervical cancer screening among transmasculine patients through self-collected swabs for high-risk human papillomavirus DNA testing. *Transgend Health.* 2020;5(1):10–17. https://doi:10.1089/trgh.2019.0019
Gómez-Gil E, Zubiaurre-Elorza L, Esteva I, et al. Hormone-treated transsexuals report less social distress, anxiety and depression. *Psychoneuroendocrinology.* 2012;37(5):662–670.
Gondwe A, Amberbir A, Singogo E, et al. Prisoners' access to HIV services in southern Malawi: a cross-sectional mixed methods study. *BMC Public Health.* 2021;21(1):813. https://doi.org/10.1186/s12889-021-10870-1
Gooren LJ, van Trotsenburg MAA, Giltay EJ, et al. Breast cancer development in transsexual subjects receiving cross-sex hormone treatment. *J Sexual Med.* 2013;10(12):3129–3134. http:// doi.org/10.1111/ jsm.12319
Grant RM, Lama JR, Anderson PL, et al. Preexposure chemoprophylaxis for HIV prevention in men who have sex with men. *N Eng J Med.* 2010;363(27):2587–2599.
Green N, Hoenigl M, Morris S, et al. Risk behavior and sexually transmitted infections among transgender women and men undergoing community-based screening for acute and early HIV infection in San Diego. *Medicine.* 2015;94(41):e1830.
Griffin A, Dempsey A, Cousino W, et al. Addressing disparities in the health of persons with HIV attributable to unstable housing in the United States: the role of the Ryan White HIV/AIDS program. *PLoS Med.* 2020;17(3) e1003057. http://doi: 10.1371/journal.pmed.1003057
Grimes RM, Hallmark CJ, Watkins KL, et al. Re-engagement in HIV care: a clinical and public health priority. *J AIDS Clin Res.* 2016;7(2):543. doi:10.4172/2155-6113.1000543.
Haldane V, Jung AS, De Foo C, et al. Integrating HIV and substance misuse services: a person-centred approach grounded in human rights. *Lancet Psych.* 2022;9(8):676–688. http://doi:10.1016/S2215-0366(22)00159-6
Health Resources and Services Administration. Ryan White HIV/AIDS program annual client-level data report 2020. www.hab.hrsa.gove/data/data-reports. Published December 2021. Accessed January 25, 2023.
Hembree WC, Cohen-Kettenis P, Gooren L, et al. Endocrine treatment of gender-dysphoric/ gender-incongruent persons: an endocrine society clinical practice guideline. *Endocr Pract.* 2017;23(12):1437.
Herman J, Flores AR, O'Neill KK. How many adults and youth identify as transgender in the US? The Williams Institute. https:// williamsinstitute.law.ucla.edu/wp-content/uploads/Trans-Pop-Update-Jun-2022.pdf. Published 2022. Accessed September 27, 2022.
Hessol NA, Eng M, Vu A, et al. A longitudinal study assessing differences in causes of death among housed and homeless people diagnosed with HIV in San Francisco. *BMC Pub Health.* 2019;19(1):1440. https://doi.org/10.1186/s12889-019-7817-7
Hickey MD, Imbert E, Appa A, et al. HIV treatment outcomes in POP-UP: drop-in HIV primary care model for people experiencing

homelessness. *J Infect Dis*. 2022;jiac267. http://doi: 10.1093/infdis/jiac267
Hiransuthikul A, Himmad K, Kerr S, et al. Drug-drug interactions between the use of feminizing hormone therapy and pre-exposure prophylaxis among transgender women: the iFACT study. TUPDX0107LB. Abstract/13177. http:// programme.aids2018.org/ Abstract/ 13177. Published 2018. Accessed September 8, 2024.
Hirsch J, Higgins J, Bentley M, Nathanson V. The social constructions of sexuality: marital infidelity and sexually transmitted disease–HIV risk in a Mexican migrant community. *Am J Public Health*. 2002;92(8):1227–1237.
Hirsch J, Meneses S, Thompson B, et al. The inevitability of infidelity: sexual reputation, social geographies, and marital HIV risk in rural Mexico. *Am J Public Health*. 2007;97(6):986–996.
Holtzman CW, Shea JA, Glanz K, et al. Mapping patient-identified barriers and facilitators to retention in HIV care and antiretroviral therapy adherence to Andersen's behavioral model. *AIDS Care*. 2015;27(7):817–828. https://doi.org/10.1080/09540121.2015.1009362
Housing and Urban Development (HUD). Continuum of Care Homeless Assistance Program homeless populations and subpopulations reports. HUD Exchange. https:// files.hudexchange.info/reports/published/CoC_PopSub_NatlTerrDC_2021.pdf. Published 2021. Accessed September 8, 2024.
Hunt GE, Malhi GS, Lai HMX, Cleary M. Prevalence of comorbid substance use in major depressive disorder in community and clinical settings, 1990–2019: systematic review and meta-analysis. *J Affect Disord*. 2020;266:288–304. https://doi.org/10.1016/j.jad.2020.01.141
Hutchinson AB, MacGowan RJ, Margolis AD, et al. Costs and consequences of eliminating a routine, point-of-care HIV screening program in a high-prevalence jail. *Am J Prev Med*. 2021;61(5 Suppl 1):S32–S38. https://doi.org/10.1016/j.amepre.2021.06.006
Ickovics JR. "Bundling" HIV prevention: integrating services to promote synergistic gain. *Prevent Med*. 2008;46(3):222–225. http:// doi.org/ 10.1016/ j.ypmed.2007.09.006
Imbert E, Hickey MD, Clemenzi-Allen A, et al. Evaluation of the POP-UP Programme: a multicomponent model of care for people living with HIV with homelessness or unstable housing. *AIDS*. 2021;35(8):1241–1246. http://doi:10.1097/QAD.0000000000002843
Ingerski LM, Means B, Wang F, et al. Preventing medication nonadherence of youth (13–24 years) with HIV initiating antiretroviral therapy. *J Adolesc Health*. 2021;69(4):644–652. http://doi:10.1016/j.jadohealth.2021.04.006
International Organization for Migration. Key migration terms 2020. https://www.iom.int/key-migration-terms. Published 2020. Accessed September 8, 2024.
Iroh PA, Mayo H, Nijhawan AE. The HIV care cascade before, during, and after incarceration: a systematic review and data synthesis. *Am J Public Health*. 2015;105(7):e5–e16. https://doi.org/10.2105/AJPH.2015.302635
Iryawan AR, Stoicescu C, Sjahrial F, et al. The impact of peer support on testing, linkage to and engagement in HIV care for people who inject drugs in Indonesia: qualitative perspectives from a community-led study. *Harm Reduct J*. 2022;19(1):16. https://doi.org/10.1186/s12954-022-00595-8
Jakubowski A, Fox A. Defining low-threshold buprenorphine treatment. *Journal of Addict Med*. 2020;14(2):95–98. http://doi:10.1097/ADM.0000000000000555
James SE, Herman, JL, Rankin, S, et al. *The Report of the 2015 U.S. Transgender Survey*. Washington, DC: National Center for Transgender Equality; 2016.
Javanbakht M, Boudov M, Anderson LJ, et al. Sexually transmitted infections among incarcerated women: findings from a decade of screening in a Los Angeles County jail, 2002–2012. *Am J Public Health*. 2014;104(11):e103–e109.
Jin H, Restar A, Biello K, et al. Burden of HIV among young transgender women: factors associated with HIV infection and HIV treatment engagement. *AIDS Care*. 2019;31(1):125–130.
Johnson M, Samarina A, Xi H, et al. Barriers to access to care reported by women living with HIV across 27 countries. *AIDS Care*. 2015;27(10):1220–1230. http://doi:10.1080/09540121.2015.1046416
Jones AA, Gicas KM, Seyedin S, et al. Associations of substance use, psychosis, and mortality among people living in precarious housing or homelessness: a longitudinal, community-based study in Vancouver, Canada. *PLoS Med*. 2020;17(7):e1003172. http://doi: 10.1371/journal.pmed.1003172
Justiz Vaillant AA, Naik R. HIV-1 associated opportunistic infections. *StatPearls*. https://www.ncbi.nlm.nih.gov/pubmed/30969609. Published 2022. Accessed September 8, 2024.
Kanazawa JT, Saberi P, Sauceda JA, et al. The LAIs are coming! implementation science considerations for long-acting injectable antiretroviral Therapy in the United States: a scoping review. *AIDS Res Human Retrovir*. 2021;37(2):75–88. http://doi: 10.1089/AID.2020.0126
Kearney BP, Mathias A. Lack of effect of tenofovir disoproxil fumarate on pharmacokinetics of hormonal contraceptives. *Pharmacotherapy*. 2009;29(8):924–929. http:// doi.org/10.1592/ phco.29.8.924
Khalili M, Powell J, Park HH, Bush D, et al. Shelter-based integrated model is effective in scaling up hepatitis C testing and treatment in persons experiencing homelessness. *Hepatol Comm*. 2022;6(1):50–64. http://doi:10.1002/hep4.1791
Khan J, Schmidt RL, Spittal MJ, et al. Venous thrombotic risk in transgender women undergoing estrogen therapy: a systematic review and meta-analysis. *Clin Chem*. 2019;65(1):57–66.
Kishimoto T, Hagi K, Kurokawa S, et al. Long-acting injectable versus oral antipsychotics for the maintenance treatment of schizophrenia: a systematic review and comparative meta-analysis of randomised, cohort, and pre–post studies. *Lancet Psychiatry*. 2021;8(5):387–404. http://doi:10.1016/S2215-0366(21)00039-0
Klein PW, Psihopaidas D, Xavier J, Cohen SM. HIV-related outcome disparities between transgender women living with HIV and cisgender people living with HIV served by the Health Resources and Services Administration's Ryan White HIV/AIDS program: a retrospective study. *PLoS Med*. 2020:17(5): e1003125. https://doi.org/10.1371/journal.pmed.1003125
Kluckow R, Zeng Z. Correctional populations in the United States, 2020—statistical tables. https://bjs.ojp.gov/library/publications/correctional-populations-united-states-2020-statistical-tables. Published 2022. Accessed September 15, 2024.
Koay WL, Kose-Otieno J, Rakhmanina N. HIV drug resistance in children and adolescents: always a challenge? *Curr Epidemiol Rep*. 2021;8(3):97–107. http://doi:10.1007/s40471-021-00268-3
Koenig SP, Dorvil N, Devieux JG, et al. Same-day HIV testing with initiation of antiretroviral therapy versus standard care for persons living with HIV: a randomized unblinded trial. *PLoS Med*. 2017;14(7):e1002357. http://doi:10.1371/journal.pmed.1002357
Korthuis PT, Edelman EJ. Substance use and the HIV care continuum: important advances. *Addict Sci Clin Pract*. 2018;13(1):13. https://doi.org/10.1186/s13722-018-0114-4
Krempasky C, Harris M, Abern L, Grimstad F. Contraception across the transmasculine spectrum. *Am J Obstet Gynecol*. 2020;222(2):134–143. https://doi:10.1016/j.ajog.2019.07.043
Labhardt ND, Ringera I, Lejone TI, et al. Effect of offering same-day ART vs usual health facility referral during home-based HIV testing on linkage to care and viral suppression among adults with HIV in Lesotho: the CASCADE randomized clinical trial. *JAMA*. 2018;319(11):1103–1112.
Lakshmi S, Beekmann SE, Polgreen PM, et al. HIV primary care by the infectious disease physician in the United States: extending the continuum of care. *AIDS Care*. 2018;30(5):569–577. https://doi.org/10.1080/09540121.2017.1385720
Landovitz RJ, Donnell D, Clement ME, et al. Cabotegravir for HIV prevention in cisgender men and transgender women. *N Engl J Med*. 2021;385(7):595–608. http://doi:10.1056/NEJMoa2101016
Lathouwers E, Weinsteiger S, Baugh B, et al. Week 96 resistance analyses of the once-daily, single-tablet regimen (STR) darunavir/cobicistat/emtricitabine/tenofovir alafenamide (D/C/F/TAF) in adults living

with HIV-1 from the phase 3 randomized AMBER and EMERALD trials. *J Med Virol.* 2021;93(6):3985–3990. https://doi.org/10.1002/jmv.26721

Levy V, Prentiss D, Balmas G, et.al. Factors in the delayed HIV presentation of immigrants in Northern California: implications for voluntary counseling and testing programs. *J Immigrant Minority Health.* 2007;9:49–54. https://doi.org/10.1007/s10903-006-9015-9

Lier AJ, Seval N, Vander Wyk B, et al. Maintenance on extended-release naltrexone is associated with reduced injection opioid use among justice-involved persons with opioid use disorder. *J Subst Abuse Treat.* 2022;142:108852. https://doi.org/10.1016/j.jsat.2022.108852

Lo E, L'ifland B, Buelt EC, et al. Implementing the street psychiatry model in New Haven, CT: community-based care for people experiencing unsheltered homelessness. *Community Ment Health J.* 2021;57(8):1427–1434. http://doi:10.1007/s10597-021-00846-1

Loeliger KB, Altice FL, Desai MM, et al. Predictors of linkage to HIV care and viral suppression after release from jails and prisons: a retrospective cohort study. *Lancet HIV.* 2018a;5(2):e96–e106. https://doi.org/10.1016/S2352-3018(17)30209-6

Loeliger KB, Meyer JP, Desai MM, et al. Retention in HIV care during the 3 years following release from incarceration: a cohort study. *PLoS Med.* 2018b:15(10):e1002667. https://doi.org/10.1371/journal.pmed.1002667

Lucas KD, Bick J, Mohle-Boetani JC. California's Prisoner Protections for Family and Community Health Act: implementing a mandated condom access program in state prisons, 2015–2016. *Public Health Rep.* 2020;135(Suppl 1):50S–56S. https://doi.org/10.1177/0033354920920629

Lynch KA, Harris T, Jain SH, et al. The case for mobile "street medicine" for patients experiencing homelessness. *J Gen Intern Med.* 2022 Jun 9;37:3999–4001. http://doi: 10.1007/s11606-022-07689-w

Lyons CE, Schwartz SR, Murray SM, et al. The role of sex work laws and stigmas in increasing HIV risks among sex workers. *Nat Commun.* 2020;11(1):773. https://doi.org/10.1038/s41467-020-14593-6

Mabuto T, Woznica DM, Lekubu G, et al. Observational study of continuity of HIV care following release from correctional facilities in South Africa. *BMC Public Health.* 2020;20(1):324. https://doi.org/10.1186/s12889-020-8417-2

Maiorana A, Sevelius J, Keatley J, Rebchook G. "She is like a sister to me": gender-affirming services and relationships are key to the implementation of HIV care engagement interventions with transgender women of color. *AIDS Behav.* 2021;25(Suppl 1):72–83. https://doi.org/10.1007/s10461-020-02777-6

Maner M, Omori M, Brinkley-Rubinstein L, et al. Infectious disease surveillance in U.S. jails: findings from a national survey. *PLoS One.* 2022;17(8):e0272374. https://doi.org/10.1371/journal.pone.0272374

Marcus JL, Volk JE, Pinder J, et al. Successful implementation of HIV preexposure prophylaxis: lessons learned from three clinical settings. *Curr HIV/AIDS Rep.* 2016;13(2):116–124. https://doi.org/10.1007/s11904-016-0308-x

Marrazzo JM, Ramjee G, Richardson BA, et al. Tenofovir-based preexposure prophylaxis for HIV infection among African women. *N Engl J Med.* 2015;372(6):509–518. http:// doi.org/ 10.1056/NEJMoa1402269

Martin RA, Berk J, Rich JD, et al. Use of long-acting injectable buprenorphine in the correctional setting. *J Subst Abuse Treat.* 2022;142:108851. https://doi.org/10.1016/j.jsat.2022.108851

Maruschak LM. HIV in prisons, 2020—statistical tables. ojp.gov. https://www.ojp.gov/library/publications/hiv-prisons-2020-statistical-tables. Published 2022. Accessed September 15, 2024.

Masyukova MI, Hanna DB, Fox AD. HIV treatment outcomes among formerly incarcerated transitions clinic patients in a high prevalence setting. *Health Justice.* 2018;6(1):16. https://doi.org/10.1186/s40352-018-0074-5

Mayer KH, Krakower D. Antiretroviral medication and HIV prevention: new steps forward and new questions. *Am Coll Physicians.* 2012;156:312–314.

Mayer KH, Molina JM, Thompson MA, et al. Emtricitabine and tenofovir alafenamide vs emtricitabine and tenofovir disoproxil fumarate for HIV pre-exposure prophylaxis (DISCOVER): primary results from a randomised, double-blind, multicentre, active-controlled, phase 3, non-inferiority trial. *Lancet.* 2020;396(10246):239–254. http://doi:10.1016/S0140-6736(20)31065-5

Melendez RM, Pinto RM. HIV prevention and primary care for transgender women in a community-based clinic. *J Assoc Nurses AIDS Care.* 2009;20(5):387–397.

Minton DT, Zhen Z. Jail inmates in 2020: statistical tables. bjs.ojp.gov. https://bjs.ojp.gov/library/publications/jail-inmates-2020-statistical-tables. Published 2021. Accessed September 8, 2024.

Mishreki AM, Boardman NJ, Brodine SK, et al. Predictive factors of facilitating linkage to care for HIV-positive detainees in ICE Health Service Corps-staffed facilities. *J Public Health.* 2021;43(3):611–617. https://doi.org/10.1093/pubmed/fdaa003

Mizuno Y, Frazier EL, Huang P, et al. Characteristics of transgender women living with HIV receiving medical care in the United States. *LGBT Health.* 2015;2(3):228034.

Mjaland K. The paradox of control: an ethnographic analysis of opiate maintenance treatment in a Norwegian prison. *Int J Drug Policy.* 2015;26(8):781–789. https://doi.org/10.1016/j.drugpo.2015.04.020

Monroe A, Nakigozi G, Ddaaki W, et al. Qualitative insights into implementation, processes, and outcomes of a randomized trial on peer support and HIV care engagement in Rakai, Uganda. *BMC Infect Dis.* 2017;17(1):54. https://doi.org/10.1186/s12879-016-2156-0

Moyer VA; US Preventive Services Task Force. Screening for HIV: U.S. Preventive Services Task Force recommendation statement. *Ann Intern Med.* 2013;159(1):51–60. http://doi:10.7326/0003-4819-159-1-201307020-00645

Murnane PM, Celum C, Nelly M, et al. Efficacy of pre-exposure prophylaxis for HIV-1 prevention among high risk heterosexuals: subgroup analyses from the Partners PrEP Study. *AIDS.* 2013;27(13):2155–2160.

Murphy M, Sosnowy C, Rogers B, et al. Defining the pre-exposure prophylaxis care continuum among recently incarcerated men at high risk for HIV infection: protocol for a prospective cohort study. *JMIR Res Protoc.* 2022;11(2):e31928. https://doi.org/10.2196/31928

Mustanski B, Newcomb ME. Older sexual partners may contribute to racial disparities in HIV among young men who have sex with men. *J Adolesc Health.* 2013;52(6):666–667. http://doi:10.1016/j.jadohealth.2013.03.019

Myers JJ, Dufour MK, Koester KA, et al. The effect of patient navigation on the likelihood of engagement in clinical care for HIV-infected individuals leaving jail. *Am J Pub Health.* 2018;108(3):385–392. http://doi:10.2105/AJPH.2017.304250

Nachman SA, Cheroff M, Gona P, et al. Incidence of noninfectious conditions in perinatally HIV-infected children and adolescents in the HAART era. *Arch Pediatr Adolesc Med.* 2009;163:164–171.

Nash GD, Flanders WD, Baird TC, et al. Cross-sex hormones and acute cardiovascular events in transgender persons: a cohort study. *Ann Intern Med.* 2018 Aug 21;169(4):205–213. http://doi:10.7326/M17-2785.

Nolan BJ, Frydman AS, Leemaqz SY, et al. Effects of low-dose oral micronised progesterone on sleep, psychological distress, and breast development in transgender individuals undergoing feminising hormone therapy: a prospective controlled study. *Endocr Connect.* 2022;11(5):e220170. http://doi:10.1530/EC-22-0170

Ohl M, Perencevich E, McInnes DK, et al. *Antiretroviral Adherence Among Rural Compared to Urban Veterans with HIV Infection in the United States [issue brief]. Veterans Rural Health Resource Center—Central Region.* Washington, DC: VHA Office of Rural Health; 2012:W(1). https://www.ruralhealth.va.gov/docs/issue-briefs/antiretroviral-adherence-121812.pdf. Accessed September 15, 2024.

O'Laughlin B. Structural reform and the politics of inequality in global public health. *Dev Change.* 2018;47(4):686–711. http://doi:10.1111/dech.12251

Olson J, Schrager SM, Clark LF, et al. Subcutaneous testosterone: an effective delivery mechanism for masculinizing young transgender men. *LGBT Health.* 2014;1(3):165–167. doi:10.1089/lgbt.2014.0018.

Page KR, Grieb SD, Nieves-Lugo K, et al. Enhanced immigration enforcement in the USA and the transnational continuity of HIV care for Latin American immigrants in deportation proceedings. *Lancet HIV.* 2018;5(10):e597–e604. https://doi.org/10.1016/S2352-3018(18)30074-2

Parvez F, Katyal M, Alper H, et al. Female sex workers incarcerated in New York City jails: prevalence of sexually transmitted infections and associated risk behaviors. *Sex Transm Inf.* 2013;89(4):280–284.

Pasternack FR, Fox LP, Engler DE. Silicone granulomas treated with etanercept. *Arch Dermatol.* 2005;141(1):13.

Peckham AM, Young EH. Opportunities to offer harm reduction to people who inject drugs during infectious disease encounters: narrative review. *Open Forum Infect Dis.* 2020;7(11):ofaa503. https://doi.org/10.1093/ofid/ofaa503

Peitzmeier SM, Reisner SL, Harigopal P, et al. Female-to-male patients have high prevalence of unsatisfactory Paps compared to non-transgender females: implications for cervical cancer screening. *J Gen Intern Med.* May 2014;29(5):778–784.

Philbin MM, Tanner AE, Duval A, et al. Linking HIV-positive adolescents to care in 15 different clinics across the United States: creating solutions to address structural barriers for linkage to care. *AIDS Care.* 2014;26(1):12–19. http://doi:10.1080/09540121.2013.808730

Polonsky M, Azbel L, Wickersham JA, et al. Accessing methadone within Moldovan prisons: prejudice and myths amplified by peers. *Int J Drug Policy.* 2016;29:91–95. https://doi.org/10.1016/j.drugpo.2015.12.016

Poteat T, Wirtz AL, Radix A, et al. HIV risk and preventive interventions in transgender women sex workers. *Lancet.* 2015;385(9964):274–286. http:// doi.org/10.1016/ S0140-6736(14)60833-3

Prosser AT, Tang T, Hall HI. HIV in persons born outside the United States 2007–2010. *JAMA.* 2012:308:(6):601–607.

Radford J. Key findings about U.S. immigrants. Pew Research Center. https://www.pewresearch.org/fact-tank/2019/06/17/key-findings-about-u-s-immigrants/. Published 2019. Accessed January 25, 2023.

Radix AE, Harris AB, Belkind U, Ting J, Goldstein ZG. Chlamydia trachomatis infection of the neovagina in transgender women. *Open Forum Infect Dis.* 2019 Nov 11;6(11):ofz470. doi:10.1093/ofid/ofz470.

Raj A, Bowleg L. Heterosexual risk for HIV among Black men in the United States: a call to action against a neglected crisis in Black communities. *Am J Men's Health.* 2012;6(3):178–181. http://doi:10.1177/1557988311416496

Rajabiun S, Davis-Plourde K, Tinsley M, et al. Pathways to housing stability and viral suppression for people living with HIV/AIDS: findings from the building a medical home for multiply diagnosed HIV-positive homeless populations initiative. *PloS One.* 2020;15(10):e0239190. http://doi: 10.1371/journal.pone.0239190

Rao D, Kekwaletswe TC, Hosek S, et al. Stigma and social barriers to medication adherence with urban youth living with HIV. *AIDS Care.* 2007;19(1):28–33. http://doi:10.1080/09540120600652303

Rapaport MJ. Silicone granulomas treated with etanercept. *Arch Dermatol.* 2005;141(9):1171. http:// doi.org/ 10.1001/ archderm.141.9.1171-a

Reddon H, Marshall BDL, Milloy MJ. Elimination of HIV transmission through novel and established prevention strategies among people who inject drugs. *Lancet HIV.* 2019;6(2):e128–e136. https://doi.org/10.1016/S2352-3018(18)30292-3

Reddy KP, Parker RA, Losina E, et al. Impact of cigarette smoking and smoking cessation on life expectancy among people with HIV: a US-based modeling study. *J Infect Dis.* 2016;214(11):1672–1681. http://doi:10.1093/infdis/jiw430

Reisner SL, Deutsch MB, Peitzmeier SM, et al. Comparing self- and provider-collected swabbing for HPV DNA testing in female-to-male transgender adult patients: a mixed-methods biobehavioral study protocol. *BMC Infect Dis.* 2017;17(1):444.

Reisner SL, Mimiaga MJ, Skeer M, et al. A review of HIV antiretroviral adherence and intervention studies among HIV-infected youth. *Top HIV Med.* 2009;17(1):14–25.

Rodger AJ, Cambiano V, Brunn T, et al. Risk of HIV transmission through condomless sex in serodifferent gay couples with the HIV-positive partner taking suppressive antiretroviral therapy (PARTNER): final results of a multicentre, prospective, observational study. *Lancet.* 2019;393(10189):2428–2438. http://doi:10.1016/S0140-6736(19)30418-0

Rodger AJ, Cambiano V, Bruun T, et al. Sexual activity without condoms and risk of HIV transmission in serodifferent couples when the HIV-positive partner is using suppressive antiretroviral therapy. *JAMA.* 2016;316(2):171–181. http://doi:10.1001/jama.2016.5148

Roland KB, Higa DH, Leighton CA, et al. Client perspectives and experiences with HIV patient navigation in the United States: a qualitative meta-synthesis. *Health Promot Pract.* 2020;21(1):25–36. https://doi.org/10.1177/1524839919875727

Roland KB, Higa DH, Leighton CA, et al. HIV patient navigation in the United States: a qualitative meta-synthesis of navigators' experiences. *Health Promot Pract.* 2022;23 (1):74–85. http://doi:10.1177/1524839920982603

Rooks-Peck CR, Adegbite AH, Wichser ME, et al. Mental health and retention in HIV care: a systematic review and meta-analysis. *Health Psychol.* 2018;37(6):574–585. http://doi: 10.1037/hea0000606

Rosecrans A, Harris R, Saxton RE, et al. Mobile low-threshold buprenorphine integrated with infectious disease services. *J Subst Abuse Treat.* 2022;133:108553. http://doi: 10.1016/j.jsat.2021.108553

Rosen S, Maskew M, Fox MP, et al. Initiating antiretroviral therapy for HIV at a patient's first clinic visit: the RapIT randomized controlled trial. *PLoS Med.* 2016;13(5):e1002015. http://doi:10.1371/journal.pmed.1002015

Ross J, Cunningham CO, Hanna DJ. HIV outcomes among migrants from low- and middle-income countries living in high-income countries: a review of recent evidence. *Curr Opin Infect Dis.* 2018;31(1):25–32. http://doi:10.1097/QCO.0000000000000415

Rubenstein LS, Amon JJ, McLemore M, et al. HIV, prisoners, and human rights. *Lancet.* 2016;388(10050):1202–1214. https://doi.org/10.1016/S0140-6736(16)30663-8

Rural Health Information Hub. RHI Hub tool kit. https://ww.ruralhealthinfo.org/toolkits/hiv-aids. Published April 8, 2022. Accessed September 8, 2024.

Sachdev DD, Mara E, Hughes AJ, et al. "Is a bird in the hand worth 5 in the bush?": a comparison of 3 data-to-care referral strategies on HIV care continuum outcomes in San Francisco. *Open Forum Infect Dis.* 2020;7(9):ofaa369. http://doi: 10.1093/ofid/ofaa369

Sanchez NF, Sanchez JP, Danoff A. Health care utilization, barriers to care, and hormone usage among male-to-female transgender persons in New York City. *Am J Public Health.* 2009;99(4):713.

Sanders RA. Adolescent psychosocial, social, and cognitive development. *Pediatr Rev.* 2013 Aug;34(8):354–358.

Scarabin PY. Progestogens and venous thromboembolism in menopausal women: an updated oral versus transdermal estrogen meta-analysis. *Climacteric.* 2018;21(4):341–345.

Scarsi KK, Swindells S. The promise of improved adherence with long-acting antiretroviral therapy: what are the data? *J Int Assoc Provid AIDS Care.* 2021;20:23259582211009011. https://doi.org/10.1177/23259582211009011

Schafer KR, Albrecht H, Dillingham R, et al. The continuum of HIV Care in rural communities in the United States and Canada: what is known and future research directions. *J Acquir Immune Defic Syndr.* 2017;75(1):35–44. http://doi:10.1097/QAI.0000000000001329. PMID: 28225437; PMCID: PMC6169533.

Schneider, CL. Racism, drug policy, and AIDS. *Polit Sc Q.* 1998;113(3):427–446.

Schranz AJ, Barrett J, Hurt CB, et al. Challenges facing a rural opioid epidemic: treatment and prevention of HIV and hepatitis C. *Curr HIV/AIDS Rep.* 2018;15(3):245–254. http://doi:10.1007/s11904-018-0393-0

Scott CK, Dennis ML, Grella CE, et al. The impact of the opioid crisis on U.S. state prison systems. *Health Justice.* 2021;9(1):17. https://doi.org/10.1186/s40352-021-00143-9

Sevelius JM. Gender affirmation: a framework for conceptualizing risk behavior among transgender women of color. *Sex Roles.* 2013;68(11–12):675–689.

Sevelius J, Chakravarty D, Neilands TB, et al. Evidence for the model of gender affirmation: the role of gender affirmation and healthcare

empowerment in viral suppression among transgender women of color living with HIV. HRSA SPNS Transgender Women of Color Study Group. *AIDS Behav.* 2021;25(Suppl 1):64–71. doi:10.1007/s10461-019-02544-2.
Sevelius JM, Patouhas E, Keatley JG, et al. Barriers and facilitators to engagement and retention-in-care among transgender women living with human immunodeficiency virus. *Ann Behav Med.* 2014a;47(1):5–16.
Sevelius JM, Saberi P, Johnson MO. Correlates of antiretroviral adherence and viral load among transgender women living with HIV. *AIDS Care.* August 2014b;26(8):976–982.
Silva-Santisteban A, Segura ER, Sandoval C, et al. Determinants of unequal HIV care access among people living with HIV in Peru. *Global Health.* 2013;9(1):22.
Solomon L, Montague BT, Beckwith CG, et al. Survey finds that many prisons and jails have room to improve HIV testing and coordination of postrelease treatment. *Health Aff.* 2104;33(3):434–442.
Spinelli MA, Hessol NA, Schwarcz S, et al. Homelessness at diagnosis is associated with death among people with HIV in a population-based study of a US city. *AIDS.* 2019;33(11):1789–1794. http://doi:10.1097/QAD.0000000000002287
Sprague C, Scanlon ML, Radhakrishnan B, Pantalone DW. The HIV prison paradox: agency and HIV-positive women's experiences in jail and prison in Alabama. *Qual Health Res.* 2017;27(10):1427–1444. https://doi.org/10.1177/1049732316672640
Stevenson KA, Podewils LJ, Zishiri VK, et al. HIV prevalence and the cascade of care in five South African correctional facilities. *PLoS One.* 2020;15(7):e0235178. https://doi.org/10.1371/journal.pone.0235178
Stone J, Artenie A, Hickman M, et al. The contribution of unstable housing to HIV and hepatitis C virus transmission among people who inject drugs globally, regionally, and at country level: a modelling study. *Lancet Public Health.* 2022;7(2):e136–e145. http://doi:10.1016/S2468-2667(21)00258-9
Straub DM, Tanner AE. Health-care transition from adolescent to adult services for young people with HIV. *Lancet Child Adolesc Health.* 2018;3:214–222. http://doi:10.1016/S2352-4642(18)30005-1
Swerdloff RS, Wang C, White WB, et al. A new oral testosterone undecanoate formulation restores testosterone to normal concentrations in hypogonadal men. *J Clin Endocrinol Metab.* 2020;105(8):2515–2531.
Tanney MR, Naar-King S, MacDonnel K. Depression and stigma in high-risk youth living with HIV: a multi-site study. *J Pediatr Health Care.* 2012;26(4):300–305. http://doi:10.1016/j.pedhc.2011.02.014
Tate CC, Ledbetter JN, Youssef CP. A two-question method for assessing gender categories in the social and medical sciences. *J Sex Research.* 2012;50:1–10.
Taylor BS, Fornos L, Tarbutton J, et al. Improving HIV care engagement in the South from the patient and provider perspective: the role of stigma, social support, and shared decision-making. *AIDS Patient Care STDs.* 2018;32(9):368–378. https://doi.org/10.1089/apc.2018.0039
Telisinghe L, Charalambous S, Topp SM, et al. HIV and tuberculosis in prisons in sub-Saharan Africa. *Lancet.* 2016;388(10050):1215–1227. https://doi.org/10.1016/S0140-6736(16)30578-5
Terp S, Ahmed S, Burner E, et al. Deaths in Immigration and Customs Enforcement (ICE) detention: FY2018–2020. *AIMS Public Health.* 2021;8(1):81–89. https://doi.org/10.3934/publichealth.2021006
Trajman A, Felker I, Alves LC, et al. The COVID-19 and TB syndemic: the way forward. *Int J Tuberc Lung Dis.* 2022;26(8):710–719. https://doi:10.5588/ijtld.22.0006
Trent M, Chung SE, Ellen JM, et al. New sexually transmitted infections among adolescent girls infected with HIV. *Sex Transmitted Infect.* 2007;83:468–469.
Tsai AC, Mendenhall E, Trostle JA, et al. Co-occurring epidemics, syndemics, and population health. *Lancet.* 2017;389(10072):978–982. http://doi:10.1016/S0140-6736(17)30403-8
Tsai AC, Weiser SD, Dilworth SE, et al. Violent victimization, mental health, and service utilization outcomes in a cohort of homeless and unstably housed women living with or at risk of becoming infected with HIV *Am J Epidemiol.* 2015;181(10):817–826. http://doi:10.1093/aje/kwu350.
UNAIDS. *Getting to Zero: 2011–2015 Strategy.* Geneva: Joint United Nations Programme on HIV/AIDS; 2010.
UNAIDS. UNAIDS fact sheet 2024. unaids.org. https: www.unaids.org/en/resources/fact-sheet Published 2024. Accessed September 15, 2024.
U.S. Food and Drug Administration (FDA). FDA approves first injectable treatment for HIV pre-exposure prevention. fda.gov. https://www.fda.gov/news-events/press-announcements/fda-approves-first-injectable-treatment-hiv-pre-exposure-prevention. Published 2021. Accessed September 15, 2024.
Valenzuela JM, Buchanan CL, Radcliffe J, et al. Transition to adult services among behaviorally infected adolescents with HIV: a qualitative study. *J Pediatr Psychol.* 2011;36(2):134–140. http://doi:10.1093/jpepsy/jsp051
Valera P, Chang Y, Lian Z. HIV risk inside U.S. prisons: a systematic review of risk reduction interventions conducted in U.S. prisons. *AIDS Care.* 2017;29(8):943–952. https://doi.org/10.1080/09540121.2016.1271102
van Kesteren PJ, Asscheman H, Megens JA, et al. Mortality and morbidity in transsexual subjects treated with cross-sex hormones. *Clin Endocrinol.* 1997;47(3):337–42.
Verachai V, Rukngan W, Chawanakrasaesin K, et al. Treatment of methamphetamine-induced psychosis: a double-blind randomized controlled trial comparing haloperidol and quetiapine. *Psychopharmacology.* 2014;231(16):3099–3108. http://doi: 10.1007/s00213-014-3485-6
Villanueva M, Miceli J, Speers S, et al. Advancing data to care strategies for persons with HIV using an innovative reconciliation process. *PLoS One.* 2022;17(5):e0267903. https://doi.org/10.1371/journal.pone.0267903
Vyavaharkar M, Glover S, Leonhirth D, et al. *HIV in Rural America: Prevalence and Service Availability: A Technical Report by the South Carolina Rural Health Research Cente*r. South Carolina Rural Health Research Center; University of South Carolina, Columbia, South Carolina, USA; 2013.
Wallace SA, McLellan-Lemal E, Harris MJ, et al. Why take an HIV test? Concerns, benefits, and strategies to promote HIV testing among low-income heterosexual African American young adults. *Health Educ Behav.* 2011;38(5):462–470. http://doi:10.1177/1090198110382501
Weiner LS, Battles HR, Wood LV. A longitudinal study of adolescents with perinatally or transfusion acquired HIV infection: sexual knowledge, risk reduction self-efficacy and sexual behavior. *AIDS Behav.* 2007;11:471–478.
Weyers S, Verstraelen H, Gerris J, et al. Microflora of the penile skin-lined neovagina of transsexual women. *BMC Microbiol.* 2009;9(1):102. http://doi.org/10.1186/1471-2180-9-102
White BL, Golin CE, Grodensky CA, et al. Effect of directly observed antiretroviral therapy compared to self-administered antiretroviral therapy on adherence and virological outcomes among HIV-infected prisoners: a randomized controlled pilot study. *AIDS Behav.* 2015a;19(1):128–136. https://doi.org/10.1007/s10461-014-0850-8
White BL, Walsh J, Rayasam S, et al. What makes me screen for HIV? Perceived barriers and facilitators to conducting recommended routine HIV testing among primary care physicians in the Southeastern United States. *J Int Assoc Provid AIDS Care.* 2015b;14(2):127–135. http://doi:10.1177/2325957414524025
Wiewel EW, Singh TP, Zhong Y, et al. Housing subsidies and housing stability are associated with better HIV medical outcomes among persons who experienced homelessness and live with HIV and mental illness or substance use disorder. *AIDS Behav.* 2020;24(11):3252–3263. http://doi:10.1007/s10461-020-02810-8
Williams RS, Stetten NE, Cook C, et al. The meaning and perceptions of HIV-related stigma in African American women living with HIV in rural Florida: a qualitative study. *J Assoc Nurses AIDS Care.* 2022;33(2):118–131. http://doi:10.1097/JNC.0000000000000252

Workowski K, Bachmann L, Chan P, et al. Sexually transmitted infections treatment guidelines, 2021. *MMWR Recomm Rep.* 2021;70(4):13–26.

World Health Organization (WHO). International classification of diseases, eleventh revision (ICD-11). 2019/2021. WHO. https://icd.who.int/browse11. Published 2024. Accessed September 8, 2024.

WHO. Social determinants of health. WHO. https://www.who.int/social_determinants/en/. Updated 2024. Accessed September 8, 2024.

Woznica DM, Fernando NB, Bonomo EJ, et al. Interventions to improve HIV care continuum outcomes among individuals released from prison or jail: systematic literature review. *J Acquir Immune Defic Syndr.* 2021;86(3):271–285. https://doi.org/10.1097/QAI.0000000000002523

Xu Y, Chen X, Yu B, et al. The effects of self-efficacy in bifurcating the relationship of perceived benefit and cost with condom use among adolescents: a cusp catastrophe modeling analysis. *J Adolesc.* 2017;61:31–39. http://doi:10.1016/j.adolescence.2017.09.004

Yehia BR, Stewart L, Momplaisir F, et al. Barriers and facilitators to patient retention in HIV care. *BMC Infect Dis.* 2015;15:246. http://doi:10.1186/s12879-015-0990-0

Zanoni BC, Mayer KH. The adolescent and young adult HIV cascade of care in the United States: exaggerated health disparities. *AIDS Patient Care STDs.* 2014 Mar;28(3):128–135. http://doi:10.1089/apc.2013.0345. PMID: 24601734; PMCID: PMC3948479.

Zash R, Caniglia EC, Diseko M, et al. Maternal weight and birth outcomes among women on antiretroviral treatment from conception in a birth surveillance study in Botswana. *J Int AIDS Soc.* 2021;24(6):e25763.

Zeidler Schreiter EA, Pandhi N, Fondow MDM, et al. Consulting psychiatry within an integrated primary care model. *J Health Care Poor Underserved.* 2013;24(4):1522–1530. https://doi.org/10.1353/hpu.2013.0178

Zhang X, Rhoads N, Rangel MG, et al. Understanding the impact of migration on HIV risk: an analysis of Mexican migrants' sexual practices, partners, and contexts by migration phase. *AIDS Behav.* 2017;21(3):935–948.

11.

HIV CARE COORDINATION

Margret O. Nelson

LEARNING OBJECTIVE

Describe the importance of an interdisciplinary team approach to the optimal management of people with HIV (PWH).

KEY POINTS

- As PWH are surviving longer, there is an increased prevalence of other comorbidities, resulting in an increasing need for chronic disease management.
- Coordination of care with a patient-centered interdisciplinary care model can be an effective strategy to increase engagement in care and reduce barriers, especially for patients with many comorbidities and/or few resources.
- Care goals should be addressed regularly with PWH as the complexity of their needs evolves over time. Discussions should include the patient's goals, quality of life, palliative care and hospice care (as indicated), and offer emotional and spiritual support.

IMPORTANCE OF AN INTERDISCIPLINARY APPROACH TO HIV CARE

Currently available antiretroviral therapies (ART) have higher efficacy and favorable side effect profiles, such that newer and simpler ART regimens are associated with improved medication adherence compared to older ART options from previous decades. This has led to prolonged survival in PWH, approaching that of the general population (Samji et al., 2014; Wada et al., 2014). Increasing longevity, coupled with the fact that the U.S. incidence of HIV has decreased only moderately over the past decade (Centers for Disease Control and Prevention [CDC], 2024), has resulted in an expanded population of PWH overall, including many who need complex medical care and support.

In 2022, 54% of PWH were aged 50 years or older (CDC, 2024), and this population of PWH is growing. HIV accentuates the complications of aging, manifested by the earlier onset of cardiovascular and renal disease, cognitive impairment, and certain types of cancer and diabetes in PWH relative to their HIV-negative peers (Condo et al., 2023). With longer survival and increased comorbidities, PWH often require chronic disease management in addition to the treatment of HIV infection (Chu and Selwyn, 2011; Guaraldi et al., 2018). Thus, optimal care for PWH is provided by clinicians with expertise in general medicine, behavioral health, and substance use treatment, in addition to HIV medicine and infectious diseases. In this setting, an interdisciplinary approach is thought to be the best management strategy and has been shown to increase rates of viral suppression (Elgalib et al., 2018). The Agency for Healthcare Research and Quality (AHRQ, 2018) suggests that care coordination involves deliberately organizing patient care activities and sharing information among all participants concerned with a patient's care to achieve safer and more effective care. Quality interdisciplinary care requires highly organized systematic sharing of knowledge and treatment plans between multiple care providers and facilities.

A recent study identified six major barriers to HIV care: HIV-related stigma, mental health disorders, substance abuse and misuse, insurance issues, food insecurity, and homelessness (Tarfa et al., 2023). The social determinants of health (SDOH) play an important role in caring for PWH, who may also experience more challenges navigating the increasingly complicated U.S. healthcare system, resulting in fragmented care or disengagement. If not addressed, these issues may result in lower levels of viral suppression and poorer health outcomes. Social workers/case managers, financial counselors, nurses, community health workers, and integrated behavioral health staff can contribute to reducing barriers to care.

THE HIV CONTINUUM OF CARE

The goals of HIV clinical care are to suppress viral replication, decrease HIV-related morbidities, improve immune status, prolong survival, improve quality of life, and decrease HIV transmission (HIV.gov, 2022; U.S. Department of Health and Human Services [USDHHS], 2024). The key steps needed to achieve these goals have been described as the HIV continuum of care, and include timely diagnosis, linkage to and subsequent retention in care, and initiation and continuation of ART (HIV.gov, 2022). These steps in the HIV continuum are the basis of the U.S. "Ending the HIV Epidemic: A Plan for America" initiative, which includes the goal of decreasing HIV incidence by 90% by 2030 (USDHHS, 2023).

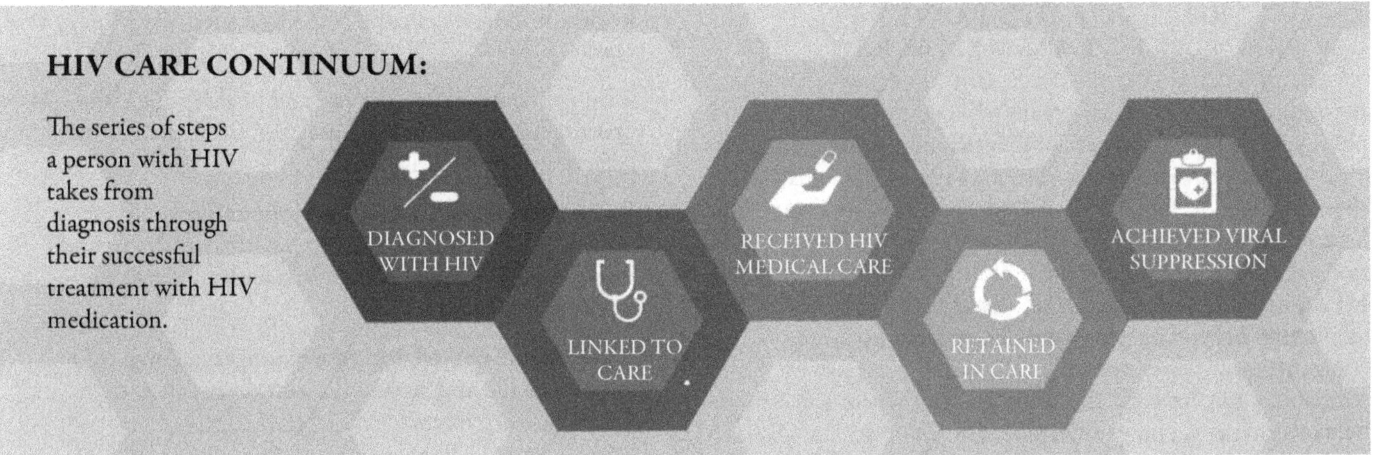

Figure 11.1 The HIV care continuum. SOURCE: Centers for Disease Control and Prevention. HIV.Care.Continuum/HIV.gov. https://www.hiv.gov/federal-response/policies-issues/hiv-aids-care-continuum.

The U.S. national HIV/AIDS strategy also recognizes the need to focus prevention, care, and treatment efforts to end the HIV epidemic on populations bearing the greatest burden. These higher risk and underserved populations include men who have sex with men (MSM), especially Black, Hispanic/Latino, and American Indian/Alaska Native men; Black women; transgender women; youth 13–24 years old; and people who inject drugs (HIV.gov, 2023). Black MSM have the highest rates of new infection (CDC, 2024). Ongoing stigma discourages HIV testing and may result in later presentations to care with more advanced disease. There may be real or perceived personal, cultural, or system-based barriers to care (Bauman et al., 2013; Irvine et al., 2014; Scanlon and Vreeman, 2013), which in some individuals can result in lower levels of ongoing engagement in care and result in suboptimal viral suppression (Gardner et al., 2011; White House Office of National AIDS Policy, 2014) (Figure 11.1).

The first step in the HIV continuum of care is the timely diagnosis of HIV infection. This requires a combination of targeted community outreach to increase testing in high-risk populations as well as routine HIV screening in the general population (USPSTF, 2019). The next step is prompt linkage to care, followed by engagement in care, and retention of the patient in care while ART is initiated. A growing body of literature supports the prolonged benefits of increased likelihood of viral suppression and retention in care with same-day or rapid (within 14 days of diagnosis) ART initiation (Ford et al., 2018). Once ART is initiated—and for decades to follow—the patient needs to be effectively followed and supported in care to ensure durable virologic suppression. There are obstacles to success at each step in the continuum, which need to be identified, anticipated, and addressed by the care team. The goals in the HIV continuum can be challenging and often require input and expertise from members of an interdisciplinary team working together to identify and address potential barriers, including depression, substance use, lack of housing, and lack of medical insurance (Dombrowski et al., 2015). Social support plays a significant role in determining health-related quality of life, which has been shown to be associated with positive clinical outcomes across the entire HIV care cascade (Han et al., 2024).

INTERDISCIPLINARY TEAM CARE

Because of the complexities of caring for some PWH, including the often concomitant diagnoses of substance use and psychiatric disorders, coordinated, patient-centered care is optimally delivered in an ambulatory, chronic disease model by an interdisciplinary team (Gallant et al., 2011; Mugavero et al., 2011; Ojikutu et al., 2014). In this integrated HIV care model, HIV primary care is combined with mental health and substance use services into a single coordinated program. The integrated HIV care model, which has been used effectively to meet the medical and social needs of PWH for decades (largely via Ryan White funding; see later discussion), is essentially a patient-centered medical home. In fact, it has been suggested that the HIV integrated care model can be used as a template for primary care clinic medical homes (Beane et al., 2014). In the integrated or coordinated care model, the goal is to treat the *patient* rather than the *disease*. Team members work together with the patient to clarify goals of care. This leads to improved outcomes by engaging various healthcare workers to work together to help the patient navigate various processes in a complex healthcare system (Bauman et al., 2013; Boyd and Lucas, 2014; Chu and Selwyn, 2011).

Studies have demonstrated that shared and coordinated patient care among different disciplines can increase the efficiency of care without duplication of services among multiple healthcare service providers (Gallant et al., 2011; Horberg et al., 2012). A recent study of Medicaid-enrolled PWH who had co-occurring chronic health conditions (e.g., asthma, chronic obstructive pulmonary disease, diabetes, and congestive heart failure) and psychiatric illness and/or substance use disorders found that patients in a medical home model of care had more efficient care, which resulted in substantial cost savings compared to patients not cared for in a medical home model (Crits-Christoph et al., 2018).

ROLES OF HIV PATIENT CARE TEAM MEMBERS

A comprehensive HIV care team will typically have at least a physician and/or an advanced practitioner, a nurse, a behavioral health provider, and a case manager. Other disciplines that enhance a care team include social work, nutrition, health education, clinical pharmacy, substance use/addiction medicine, and financial counseling (Gallant et al., 2011; HIV.gov, 2023; Horberg et al., 2012). The makeup of any particular HIV care team will be specific to needs of the community/patients served and available resources. Some teams may not have all the listed positions, and some members of a care team may undertake tasks not traditionally part of their job description. In many cases, the roles may overlap (see Table 11.1).

- Public health workers, nurses, and health educators offer initial HIV screening, provide HIV-prevention education, including information on pre- and postexposure prophylaxis (PrEP and PEP) if HIV negative, and link PWH to an HIV provider.
- Physicians and advanced practice providers diagnose, prescribe/treat, refer to other specialists (including oral health professionals), and often lead interdisciplinary care teams.
- Clinical pharmacists, nurses, and health educators provide assistance with medication information and adherence counseling.
- Psychiatrists, therapist/counselors, and substance use counselors provide mental health assessment and treatment, psychosocial support, and substance use disorder treatment.
- Administrative staff and case managers arrange appointments and serve as liaisons between patients and healthcare providers.
- Social workers and financial advisors link patients to available community resources (e.g., housing, disability, and food assistance) and assist with applications for healthcare insurance, including ADAP.
- Nutritionists provide education on nutrition, adherence, and healthy lifestyles.

The designated team leader, most often a physician or advanced practice provider, should facilitate communication among team members to support the goal of quality care. Ongoing

Table 11.1 HIV CONTINUUM AND HIV CARE TEAM ROLES

STAGE	GOALS	INTERVENTIONS	EXAMPLES OF TEAM MEMBERS WHO HELP SUPPORT OPTIMAL OUTCOMES AT EACH STAGE
Diagnosed	Identify patients with HIV Reduce transmission Educate, normalize testing and prevention	Accessible testing events and sites Timely linkage to PCP HIV screening Pre- and postexposure prophylaxis (PrEP and PEP)	Public health worker Nurse Health educator
Receipt of care	Connect with PCP Address barriers to care Educate and navigate	Arrange and accompany individuals to appointments Address insurance, child care, transportation, schedule conflicts (e.g., work duties) Link to community resources	Administrative staff Community health worker Nurse Case manager
Retained in care	Connect/engage with the care team Regularly attend follow-up visits Engage in health maintenance/ preventive health Educate and connect to resources	Offer PCP care team services: BH, SW, SUD TX Offer community resources for support Outreach to out-of-care patients	Behavioral health Social worker Case manager Substance use counselor
Viral suppression	Achieve and maintain undetectable viral load	Educate on the importance of medication adherence and "U = U" Address medication side effects	PCP or HIV specialist Nurse Pharmacist Health educator
Linked to care	Engage in health maintenance with ongoing care and continued viral suppression	Regular follow-up visits Lab monitoring Patient-centered primary care	PCP and/or HIV specialist Nurse Behavioral health Case manager Pharmacists

BH = behavioral health; PCP = primary care physician; SW = social work; SUD TX = substance use disorder treatment.

communication between the interdisciplinary team and the patient is essential to ensure collaborative and patient-centered care (Gallant et al., 2011; Nancarrow et al., 2013). The patient's preference for mode of communication should be clearly described/visible in the electronic health record (EHR).

Regular meetings to discuss the needs of patients and to reassess team member roles are important. The complexity of the patient's medical and psychosocial needs can often be overwhelming. Learning the patient's priorities and making partnered decisions with the patient can improve outcomes and help coordination of care among the healthcare team and the patient (Gallant et al., 2011; Mugavero et al., 2011). There are limited data on standardized ways of measuring interdisciplinary team care (Boyd and Lucas, 2014). However, the periodic internal review of the interdisciplinary member responsibilities and infrastructure can help improve and consolidate responsibilities, avoid duplication of tasks, and augment the efficiency and effectiveness of the team. One survey indicated that patients who received care in an interdisciplinary HIV care model had high levels of satisfaction (Vachirasudlekha et al., 2014).

Numerous factors, including high rates of homelessness/unstable housing, substance use, and mental illness, often result in the need for more resources to support PWH. Providing comprehensive care often requires referrals to other healthcare providers, financial counselors, social workers, and ancillary services. Depending on the model and scope of HIV care, referrals may occur within the same interdisciplinary HIV team, to another provider in the same institution, or to an external provider/organization. Effective referrals can be initiated and tracked through a structured referral process utilizing established referral sources. Making one team member responsible for tracking the status of referrals helps ensure their completion.

While there is no single approach that will work for all HIV providers or delivery models with regard to appropriate referrals, certain practices may be widely applicable. Initially, an assessment of the patient's referral needs should be performed, and objectives for those referrals should be clearly defined. Ideally, providers from different disciplines should collaborate to meet the identified patient healthcare needs. With an interdisciplinary team-based approach, decisions regarding referrals and patient care are shared. In collaborative arrangements, decision-making responsibilities are shared, and ownership of changes in care may shift depending on the level of expertise required at a given time. It is important to communicate changes to the interdisciplinary team and document them clearly.

It is often helpful for team members to become familiar with various agencies/resources in their community, especially organizations that maintain a core group of professionals committed to the care of PWH. This encourages further support and involvement in the patient's progress. Referral of patients to on-site providers is preferred, but referrals off-site may occasionally be necessary or desired. This can present its own set of challenges, especially regarding transportation, communication, and reimbursement. In some cases, if resources allow, case managers or community health workers may accompany patients to ensure that they attend external appointments and that any recommendations are understood by the patient and are carried out.

Transitions from the hospital back to the community carry a high level of risk for missed medication changes and treatment plans. Recently, one analysis found that nurse-led hospital-to-community transitional care programs had better outcomes than a hospital-only program (Moen et al., 2023). Clear two-way communication between the HIV provider and specialist is important for goals of care to be met. Referring providers should clearly identify the specific questions and requests being asked of specialists. After the consult, specialists should communicate the plan of care to referring providers and patients. A shared EHR can help to improve communication. However, direct communication between the referring provider and specialist, as well as with other team members, is optimal.

Responsibility for the implementation and follow-up of recommended changes in the plan of care should be well outlined. Frequent and timely communication between the referring organization and the referral providers can decrease gaps in care and ensure continuity of quality care.

COMPLEXITY OF PWH CARE NEEDS

The following are illustrative case examples of the types of complex comorbidities and chronic conditions that characterize the care of PWH:

1. An obese 55-year-old woman has a history of major depression and prior inconsistent medication adherence, which led to virologic failure; she is currently taking ART and has an undetectable viral load.

This patient stopped seeing her therapist and psychiatrist one year ago because she felt she no longer required mental health treatment. However, she was recently divorced, lost her job (and thus her health insurance), and has found it challenging to accept her new diagnosis of type 2 diabetes mellitus. Although the patient's HIV is currently controlled, the HIV provider is concerned about recent major life events leading to a depressive episode, which may eventually impact medication adherence (this happened in the past and contributed to prior inconsistent medication adherence, with resultant decreased efficacy of the patient's initial HIV regimen). This patient will need several issues addressed simultaneously, including treatment of her depression, applying for Medicaid and the AIDS Drug Assistance Program (ADAP), and treatment of her obesity and diabetes. She would benefit from prompt referrals to behavioral health (both a therapist and psychiatrist), a case manager and financial counselor for Medicaid and ADAP assistance, and a nutritionist and endocrinologist for treatment of coexisting medical problems.

2. A 61-year-old man with a history of anxiety, depression, uncontrolled hypertension, and cirrhosis is currently suppressed on ART (CD4 = 352 cells/mm^3, VL<20 copies/mL). Much of his anxiety is based in fear of disclosure of

his HIV status. To this end, he drives over an hour to see an HIV specialist. His few episodes of missed medication doses were prompted by risk of disclosure. He presents for his follow-up appointment requesting a change to long-acting injectable ART. He has Medicare and Medicaid insurance.

The HIV provider had some concerns about this patient's availability/capacity to return to clinic reliably for each dose of long-acting ART. They discussed this at great length, including the risk of developing resistance if doses were missed and the logistics of traveling so far for each appointment. The patient is hesitant to see other providers/nurses and have his diagnosis known more widely to other providers, especially those closer to home. Because of this, he declined an option to see a provider nearer to him. He reassures his HIV specialist that he can travel to frequent injection appointments reliably. The clinical pharmacy team reviewed the patient's insurance coverage and reported that he is covered 100% and will have access to long-acting injectable HIV therapy without a copay. Nursing staff will need to meet with the patient to again review details of large-volume injections, the importance of visit adherence to avoid development of HIV drug resistance, and ongoing plans for monitoring labs. After consultation and feedback to the HIV specialist, prescriptions will be sent to the pharmacy and the patient can switch to his new regimen. Nursing will follow for adherence, lab monitoring, and injection side effects.

3. A 58-year-old man with multiple comorbidities, including large granular lymphocytic leukemia, is currently suppressed on ART (CD4 >650 cells/mm^3, VL<20 copies/mL). He also has metabolic dysfunction-associated steatotic liver disease (MASLD), type 2 diabetes mellitus, coronary artery disease, seizure disorder, anxiety, post-traumatic stress disorder, and chronic back pain. He presents to the Emergency Department with new pancytopenia and concern for myelodysplastic syndrome.

Despite having the benefit of stable housing and good insurance coverage, this patient has many needs that may challenge his team's ability to communicate between institutions. He was admitted to the hospital to work up his pancytopenia, address chronic back pain, and monitor and treat his escalating anxiety related to being hospitalized. His hospital-based oncology team can guide aspects of the medical workup without introducing unfamiliar clinicians and aggravating his anxiety. His primary care team can provide detailed historical and psychosocial information for the hospitalist team. Care coordination between sites will be very important for discharge planning and post-hospitalization follow-up. The patient and his caregivers will need support through the stress of any new diagnosis. If a serious illness/complication is present, a palliative care consult could provide guidance and continuity across primary care and specialists, ensuring that the patient's treatment plan is based in shared decision-making, accurately reflects the patient's preferences, and addresses the patient's complex needs.

PALLIATIVE CARE AND HOSPICE CARE

In the setting of advancements in ART and life expectancy for PWH, advance care planning should be addressed as it would with any patient. Discussions about advanced care planning should be prioritized with all people diagnosed with a serious illness to help lay the groundwork for choices later in care. These discussions should include intervention preferences, favored care settings, feelings about palliative/hospice care, and the documented selection of a healthcare proxy. Studies have shown that patients who have participated in advance care planning are more likely to be satisfied with their care (Steel and Owen, 2020; Yuen, 2021).

The terms *palliative care* and *hospice care* are often used interchangeably. While both use an interdisciplinary approach and include a focus on comfort and symptom management and the inclusion of the person and their caregivers in decision-making, there are important differences.

Palliative care is the broader term and *hospice care* is a component. Palliative care is designed to address treatment choices for serious illnesses or chronic conditions, manage symptoms and treatment side effects, and improve quality of life at any stage of illness, from diagnosis to recovery or death. This whole-person approach is most effective when engaged well before end-of-life care is needed. Symptom management interventions can be delivered while treatment for serious illness continues. Palliative care is meant to enhance a person's current care by focusing on quality of life (NIA, 2017). This level of care can be provided in hospitals, nursing homes, outpatient palliative care clinics, or at home.

Hospice care is a specialized form of palliative care that is delivered in the final months or weeks of life. Hospice care is focused on comfort and quality of life when curative treatment options are no longer effective and life expectancy is limited (typically 6 months or less). Like palliative care, hospice care provides comprehensive comfort care and support for caregivers. When hospice care is delivered at home, a member of the hospice team visits regularly, and they are available by phone around the clock, with individuals close to the patient often serving as primary caregivers. Dedicated hospice facilities, whether in hospitals or free-standing hospice homes, are staffed by licensed and unlicensed caregivers. Unfortunately, many patients are enrolled in hospice care very late in their treatment course, missing the opportunity to benefit from longer durations of hospice care. Beginning hospice care earlier can provide months of meaningful care and quality time with loved ones. Early enrollment in palliative and hospice care services can improve quality of life, reduce use of ineffective aggressive treatments, lower costs, and extend survival (Temel et al., 2010).

FUNDING FOR HIV CARE

RYAN WHITE HIV/AIDS PROGRAM

The Ryan White HIV/AIDS Program (RWHAP) is an essential component of HIV patient care in the United States

(Health Resources and Service Administration [HRSA] HIV/AIDS, 2022; Sood et al., 2014). This federal program, which began in 1991, funds health care and services to PWH. Program funding is distributed among Parts A–F. Part A provides emergency assistance to eligible areas that are most severely affected by HIV/AIDS, often through large municipal departments of public health. Part B, which funds the AIDS Drug Assistance Program (ADAP), provides grants to all 50 states and U.S. territories or associated jurisdictions to help cover the costs of HIV medications. Part C funds are granted directly to clinics providing outpatient-based comprehensive primary healthcare for PWH, supporting the multidisciplinary care teams discussed in the section above. Part D provides family-centered care for women, infants, children, and youth. Part F covers dental programs, the Minority AIDS Initiative, as well as the educational arm of the RWHAP, which includes a variety of programs, such as the AIDS Education and Training Centers Regional offices, National Clinician Consultation Center, National Coordinating Resource Center/National AETC Support Center, and special projects of national significance.

The RWHAP funds cities, states, and local community-based organizations to provide HIV care and treatment services and "wrap-around" support to more than half a million people each year and assists approximately 52% of all people diagnosed with HIV in the United States. However, coverage and requirements of RWHAP-funded programs may vary from state to state, and grantee renewal requirements may vary from year to year (this includes required data collection and conformance with standards of care) (HRSA, 2022). The RWHAP is always the "payer of last resort," as it is meant to fill gaps where other programs such as Medicaid, Medicare, private insurances, and medical education fall short in addressing the complex care needs of varied HIV communities.

A critical component of the RWHAP, the Part B AIDS Drug Assistance Program (ADAP, also known in some states as the HIV Drug Assistance Program), provides medication support to low-income PWH who have limited or no medication health coverage from private insurance, Medicaid, or Medicare. ADAP funds may also be used to purchase health insurance for eligible clients and for services that enhance access to, adherence to, and monitoring of drug treatments. States have varied eligibility criteria and renewal processes, including documentation of income status (15 states established income eligibility at 200% or less of the federal poverty level); diagnosis of HIV, opportunistic infections, and chronic medical conditions; and/or other service needs (HRSA, 2022).

Several studies have demonstrated better clinical outcomes for patients receiving care at RWHAP-funded clinics versus nonfunded clinics. Wrap-around clinical and case management services provided by the RWHAP result in increased retention in care and consequently in increased viral suppression (Kay et al., 2018). Assistance with necessities such as food and transportation (utilized by 1 in 3 patients served by the RWHAP) and housing (utilized by 1 in 5 patients) are key components to supporting people with HIV with incomes at or below the poverty level. In a study of 8,000 PWH, nearly 75% of patients receiving care at RWHAP-funded facilities achieved viral suppression despite a greater likelihood of poverty and unstable housing. Further, patients with incomes at or below the poverty level were more likely to achieve viral suppression if they received care at a RWHAP-funded facility (Weiser et al., 2015).

The RWHAP ensures access to ART among un- and underinsured PWH and is thus associated with increased viral suppression among those populations. In an analysis of over 18,000 patients in which 41% of patients had RWHAP assistance, patients whose private or Medicaid coverage was supplemented by the RWHAP were both more likely to be prescribed ART and sustain viral suppression than those without such supplementation (Bradley et al., 2016). A recent study of over 3,000 MSM enrolled in the Miami-Dade County RWHAP demonstrated that nearly 85% of the men achieved sustained viral suppression (Sheehan et al., 2020). In this study, one of the factors associated with increased sustained viral suppression was having an HIV clinician who serves a larger volume of RWHAP clients. The central role of the medical case manager as part of the multidisciplinary RWHAP team was identified as one reason the rate of viral suppression was higher than expected.

QUALITY IMPROVEMENT

The primary goals of HIV care are to optimize patient health, decrease HIV transmission, and end the HIV epidemic. A clear vision with focused efforts to improve clinical outcomes and quality can help to develop, improve, and sustain effective patient care practices (Gallant et al., 2011; Mugavero et al., 2011). An up-to-date and available patient registry with relevant clinical and care engagement/retention data can help monitor and measure patient care outcomes. Examples of relevant clinical and engagement/retention data include adherence, missed appointments, recent contact information and outreach, detectable viral load, ART status, and evidence of failing or failed care (e.g., development of HIV drug resistance, new opportunistic infections, onset or worsening of comorbid conditions, or overall clinical decline).

In a resource-limited setting, targeted data collection may be beneficial instead of attempting to obtain all data continuously. For example, it may be beneficial to prioritize and focus resources on high-risk and vulnerable patients, such as those who have been out of care for over 6 months or have a detectable viral load. A patient registry with clinical and laboratory data can also support the measurement of the quality of care delivered and improve patient outcomes by strategizing on select quality-improvement projects. Examples include annual influenza vaccination among patients with HIV and appropriate sexually transmitted disease screening.

ACKNOWLEDGMENTS

Special thanks to Amanda A. Westlake, Sally Spencer-Long, Daniel J. Skiest, and Christian Ramers, who authored portions of this chapter in prior editions.

RECOMMENDED READING

Gardner LI, Giordano TP, Marks G, et al. Enhanced personal contact with HIV patients improves retention in primary care: a randomized trial in six US HIV clinics. *Clin Infect Dis*. 2014;59(5):725–734.

Newhouse RP, Spring B. Interdisciplinary evidence-based practice: moving from silos to synergy. *Nurs Outlook*. 2010;58(6):309–317.

Shah M, Risher K, Berry SA, et al. The epidemiologic and economic impact of improving HIV testing, linkage, and retention in care in the United States. *Clin Infect Dis*. 2016;62(2):220–229.

REFERENCES

Agency for Healthcare Research and Quality (AHRQ). Care coordination. https://www.ahrq.gov/ncepcr/care/coordination.html. Content last reviewed August 2018. Accessed July 15, 2024.

Bauman LJ, Braunstein S, Calderon Y, et al. Barriers and facilitators of linkage to HIV primary care in New York City. *J AIDS*. 2013;64(1):S20–S26.

Beane SN, Culyba RJ, DeMayo M, Armstrong W. Exploring the medical home in Ryan White HIV care settings: a pilot study. *J Assoc Nurses AIDS Care*. 2014 May–Jun;25(3):191–202.

Boyd CM, Lucas GM. Patient-centered care for people living with multimorbidity. *Curr Opin HIV AIDS*. 2014;9(4):419–427.

Bradley H, Viall AH, Wortley PM, et al. Ryan White HIV/AIDS program assistance and HIV treatment outcomes. *Clin Infect Dis*. 2016 Jan 1;62(1):90–98.

Centers for Disease Control and Prevention (CDC). HIV surveillance report: diagnoses, deaths, and prevalence of HIV in the United States and 6 territories and freely associated states, 2022. https://www.cdc.gov/hiv-data/nhss/hiv-diagnoses-deaths-prevalence.html. Published May 21, 2024, Accessed July 15, 2024.

Chu C, Selwyn PA. An epidemic in evolution: the need for new models of HIV care in the chronic disease era. *J Urban Health*. 2011;88(3):556–566.

Condo A, Baim-Lance A, Golstein N. Bringing geriatric care into the HIV primary care clinic: A combined HIV/Geriatric multidisciplinary clinic model. *Innov Aging*. 2023;7(Suppl 1):117–118.

Crits-Christoph P, Gallop R, Noll E, et al. Impact of a medical home model on costs and utilization among comorbid HIV-positive Medicaid patients. *Am J Manag Care*. 2018;24:368–375.

Dombrowski JC, Simoni JM, Katz DA, et al. Barriers to HIV care and treatment among participants in a public health HIV care relinkage program. *AIDS Patient Care STDs*. 2015;29:279–287.

Elgalib A, Al-Sawafi H, Kamble B, et al. Multidisciplinary care model for HIV improves treatment outcome: a single-centre experience from the Middle East. *AIDS Care*. 2018;*30*(9):1114–1119.

Ford N, Migone C, Calmy A, et al. Benefits and risks of rapid initiation of antiretroviral therapy. *AIDS*. 2018;32(1):17–23.

Gallant JE, Adimora AA, Carmichael JK, et al. Essential components of effective HIV care: a policy paper of the HIV Medicine Association of the Infectious Diseases Society of America and the Ryan White Medical Providers Coalition. *Clin Infect Dis*. 2011;53:1043–1050.

Gardner EM, McLees MP, Steiner JF, et al. The spectrum of engagement in HIV care and its relevance to test-and-treat strategies for prevention of HIV infection. *Clin Infect Dis*. 2011;52(6):793–800.

Guaraldi G, Malagoli A, Calcagno A, et al. The increasing burden and complexity of multi-morbidity and polypharmacy in geriatric HIV patients: a cross sectional study of people aged 65–74 years and more than 75 years. *BMC Geriatr*. 2018;18(1):99.

Han S, Wang X, Hu Y, et al. Defining HIV-related social support: what types of social support do people with HIV need? *J Assoc Nurses AIDS Care*. 2024;35(4):367–371.

HIV.gov. HIV care continuum. https://www.hiv.gov/federal-response/policies-issues/hiv-aids-care-continuum. Updated October 28, 2022. Accessed July 15, 2024.

HIV.gov. Types of providers. https://www.hiv.gov/hiv-basics/starting-hiv-care/find-a-provider/types-of-providers. Updated October 27, 2023. Accessed July 15, 2024.

Horberg MA, Hurley LB, Towner WJ, et al. Determination of optimized multidisciplinary care team for maximal antiretroviral therapy adherence. *J AIDS*. 2012;60(2):183–190.

Irvine MK, Chamberlin SA, Robbins RS, et al. Improvements in HIV care engagement and viral load suppression following enrollment in a comprehensive HIV care coordination program. *Clin Infect Dis*. 2014;60:298–310.

Kay ES, Batey DS, Mugavero MJ. The Ryan White HIV/AIDS Program: supplementary service provision post–Affordable Care Act [published correction appears in *AIDS Patient Care STDs*. 2019 Aug;33(8):379–380]. *AIDS Patient Care STDs*. 2018;32(7):265–271. doi:10.1089/apc.2018.0032

Moen M, Doede M, Johantgen M, et al. Nurse-led hospital-to-community care, clinical outcomes for people living with HIV and health-related social needs. *J Adv Nurs*. 2023;79(5):1949–1958.

Mugavero MJ, Norton WE, Saag MS. Health care system and policy factors influencing engagement in HIV medical care: piecing together the fragments of a fractured health care delivery system. *Clin Infect Dis*. 2011;52(Suppl 2):S238–S246.

Nancarrow SA, Booth A, Ariss S, et al. Ten principles of good interdisciplinary team work. *Hum Resour Health*. 2013;11:19.

National Institutes on Aging (NIA). What are palliative care and hospice care? National Institute on Aging. https://www.nia.nih.gov/health/what-are-palliative-care-and-hospice-care. Published May 17, 2017. Accessed January 25, 2023.

Ojikutu B, Holman J, Kunches L, et al. Interdisciplinary HIV care in a changing healthcare environment in the USA. *AIDS Care*. 2014;26(6):731–735.

Samji H, Cescon A, Hogg RS, et al. Closing the gap: increases in life expectancy among treated HIV-positive individuals in the United States and Canada. *PLoS One*. 2014;8(12):e81355.

Scanlon ML, Vreeman RC. Current strategies for improving access and adherence to antiretroviral therapies in resource-limited settings. *HIV AIDS (Auckl)*. 2013;5:1–17.

Sheehan DM, Dawit R, Gbadamosi SO, et al. Sustained HIV viral suppression among men who have sex with men in the Miami-Dade County Ryan White program: the effect of demographic, psychosocial, provider and neighborhood factors. *BMC Public Health*. 2020;20(1)326. doi:10.1186/s12889-020-8442-1

Sood N, Juday T, Vanderpuye-Orgle J, et al. HIV care providers emphasize the importance of the Ryan White program for access to quality of care. *Health Aff*. 2014;33(3):394–400.

Steel AJ, Owen LH. Advance care planning: the who, what, when, where and why. *Br J Hosp Med*. 2020;81(2):1–6. doi: 10.12968/hmed.2019.0396. Epub 2020 Feb 25.

Tarfa A, Pecanac K, Olayinka O, et al. A qualitative inquiry into the patient-related barriers to linkage and retention in HIV care within the community setting. *Explor Res Clin Soc Pharm*. 2023;9:100207.

Temel JS, Greeg JA, Muzikansky A, et al. Early palliative care for patients with metastatic non-small-cell lung cancer. *N Engl J Med*. 2010;363(8):733–742.

U.S. Department of Health and Human Services Administration (USDHHS). EHE overview. https://www.hiv.gov/federal-response/ending-the-hiv-epidemic/overview. Published December 4, 2023. Accessed July 15, 2024.

USDHHS. Panel on Antiretroviral Guidelines for Adults and Adolescents. Guidelines for the use of antiretroviral agents in adults and adolescents with HIV. Department of Health and Human Services. https://clinicalinfo.hiv.gov/en/guidelines/adult-and-adolescent-arv. Published February 27, 2024. Accessed July 15, 2024.

U.S. Department of Health Resources and Human Services. HIV/AIDS Bureau. Published December, 2022. Accessed July 15, 2024.

U.S. Preventive Services Task Force, Owens DK, Davidson KW, Krist AH, et al. Screening for HIV infection: US Preventive Services Task Force recommendation statement. *JAMA*. June 18, 2019;321(23):2326–2336.

Wada N, Jacobson LP, Cohen M, et al. Cause-specific mortality among HIV-infected individuals, by CD4+ cell count at HAART initiation, compared with HIV-uninfected individuals. *AIDS*. 2014;28:257–265.

Weiser J, Beer L, Frazier E, et al. Service delivery and patient outcomes in Ryan White HIV/AIDS program-funded and—nonfunded health care facilities in the United States. *JAMA Intern Med.* 2015;175(10):1650–1659.

White House Office of National AIDS Policy. *National HIV/AIDS Strategy: Update of 2014 Federal Actions to Achieve National Goals and Improve Outcomes Along the HIV Care Continuum*. Washington, DC: The White House Office of National AIDS Policy; 2014.

Vachirasudlekha B, Cha A, Berkowitz L, et al. Interdisciplinary HIV care: patient perceptions. *Int J Health Care Qual Assur.* 2014;27(5): 405–413.

Yeun YR. The effects of advance care planning on decision conflict and psychological distress: a systematic review and meta-analysis of randomized controlled trials. *J Hosp Palliat Care*. 2021;24(3):144–153. doi:10.14475/jhpc.2021.24.3.144

12.

THE PHARMACIST'S ROLE IN HIV CARE

Jennifer Cocohoba

INTRODUCTION

Medications are essential tools used for prevention, treatment, and management of co-occurring conditions in persons with HIV (PWH) and for persons who may acquire HIV. A multidisciplinary approach to HIV care should include a pharmacist because of pharmacists' broad expertise in medication therapy. Pharmacists play an important role across the spectrum of HIV care: they facilitate access to medications, ensure accurate dispensing, and provide patients with education on their medications. Pharmacist specialists have also become essential members of the HIV healthcare team because their expertise extends beyond dispensing to providing expert consultation, facilitating patient adherence, and co-managing antiretroviral therapy (ART) and HIV prevention services. When incorporated into the healthcare team, HIV pharmacists' expertise can improve the selection, safety, efficacy, and overall quality of medication therapy.

LEARNING OBJECTIVES

- Describe common settings in which HIV pharmacists practice.
- List three potential ways in which pharmacists can contribute to HIV care.

WHAT'S NEW

- Data and experience continue to accumulate on the innovative and meaningful ways in which pharmacists contribute to improved health outcomes in persons with HIV. Pharmacists are increasingly being recognized as an important resource for advancing HIV prevention efforts through testing and furnishing of pre-exposure prophylaxis (PrEP) or postexposure prophylaxis (PEP). Pharmacists are also emerging as essential team members for long-acting injectable antiretroviral programs.

KEY POINTS

- HIV pharmacists are a diverse group of healthcare providers who work to improve the health of persons with HIV via medication therapy management, quality-assurance practices, research, and other avenues.
- HIV pharmacists are skilled at managing complex antiretroviral drug-drug interactions, recommending therapies for people with complex ART resistance patterns, and providing patient education and adherence support.
- If practicing with a physician under a collaborative drug therapy management agreement, an HIV pharmacist may be able to provide disease state management (e.g., furnishing and adjusting medications and ordering lab tests) for PrEP, HIV treatment, and medications for associated chronic conditions.

THE HIV PHARMACIST SPECIALIST

Medications for HIV have become more convenient but not less complex. Approximately half of people with HIV in the United States are over the age of 50 years, and a large proportion take five or more medications (Okoli et al., 2020). For this reason, having an HIV pharmacist on the healthcare team can greatly enhance HIV care. HIV-specialized clinical pharmacists typically receive advanced HIV training during postdoctoral residencies, infectious diseases fellowship programs, or through HIV-specific fellowships. Completion of programs such as the American Academy of HIV Medicine's HIV Pharmacist (AAHIVP) certification, the HIV Pharmacotherapy Continuing Education Program offered through the University of Buffalo, or the AIDS Education and Training Centers' National HIV Curriculum can distinguish pharmacists who are well versed in many aspects of HIV pharmacotherapy (McLaughlin et al., 2018). Many HIV pharmacists also pursue Board of Pharmacy Specialties certification in infectious diseases (BCIDP) or ambulatory care (BCACP) owing to the wide knowledge base, roles, and responsibilities that can be associated with caring for people with HIV. Although pathways exist for formal training or certification, some HIV pharmacists have simply acquired their knowledge and expertise through extensive practice-based experience and self-study.

EXPANDED PATIENT CARE ROLES

Some HIV pharmacists hold an expanded scope of practice beyond traditional dispensing. The mechanisms for this include collaborative practice agreements (CPA), autonomous prescribing, and credentialing and privileging (American Pharmacists Association, 2024). A CPA is a formal relationship which allows a prescriber to designate certain functions that a specific pharmacist may perform. CPAs may allow HIV pharmacists to select and initiate ART or opportunistic infection prophylaxis, order and interpret pertinent labs, simplify regimens using fixed-dose combination tablets, and manage common antiretroviral-related side effects such as nausea and diarrhea. Knowledgeable pharmacists may order, interpret, and change a patient's ART based on resistance tests. For example, in one cohort, 1,255 persons with HIV referred to a clinical pharmacist for treatment initiation were significantly more likely (HR = 1.37) to achieve viral suppression during the first 2 years of therapy as compared to people who received standard initiation by a primary care provider (Nevo et al., 2015). All 50 states within the United States have legislation or regulatory authority allowing pharmacists to engage in collaborative practice with prescribers; however, the requirements and regulations vary from state to state (Howell et. al, 2023).

Some states authorize pharmacists to independently prescribe medications or specific categories of medications. This advanced scope of practice can be achieved through issuance of statewide protocols or standing orders, or through state-designated medication categories for prescribing. At the facility level, healthcare institutions can expand pharmacists' scope of practice through a process of vetting their credentials and granting them additional patient care privileges. Elevating the role of pharmacists enhances HIV interdisciplinary care and extends the practitioner's ability to reach the greatest number of patients. Responsibilities of HIV pharmacists in clinical practice are likely to expand in the future as the profession continues to advocate for pharmacists to be recognized as healthcare providers under U.S. federal law.

SETTINGS IN WHICH HIV PHARMACISTS PROVIDE PATIENT CARE

Pharmacists contribute to HIV care across the spectrum of disease and medical visits. When a patient is acutely ill, they may interact with an HIV-specialized pharmacist in the hospital. In many health systems, infectious diseases (ID) experts oversee consultative care for PWH, and HIV/ID-specialized pharmacists on these multidisciplinary teams contribute their skills and knowledge to improve outcomes. For example, patients taking antiretrovirals who are admitted to the intensive care unit may require evaluation for complex drug-drug interactions or need close monitoring to dose adjust medications for renal insufficiency or hepatic dysfunction (Walker et al., 2022). Inpatient HIV pharmacists assist teams in selecting appropriate ART and opportunistic infection regimens, screen for drug interactions, may order and interpret resistance testing or therapeutic drug monitoring assays (if indicated), provide discharge counseling for patients initiating new ART, and may help coordinate transitions of care for persons with HIV who are entering or leaving the hospital (Durham et al., 2017).

Patients may interact with HIV-specialized pharmacists who work as part of an interdisciplinary ambulatory care team in a clinic. These HIV pharmacists have a wide range of duties commensurate with their experience and level of expertise. Responsibilities can include dispensing medications in a clinic-associated pharmacy; acting as a liaison between the clinic and community dispensing pharmacy to improve medication access; performing medication-use evaluations to ensure optimal pharmacotherapy in a population; providing patient education; consulting with patients and medical providers regarding medication-related problems, adherence, or resistance testing results; initiating and managing ART or PrEP; administering vaccinations, ordering lab tests; and initiating, adjusting, or discontinuing medications for opportunistic infections and other concomitant disease states.

ART is typically dispensed by a community pharmacist. Nearly all people with HIV will interact with community pharmacists at some point; in fact, the community pharmacist may be the healthcare provider with whom a healthy patient interacts most frequently. The act of picking up medication refills might seem simple, yet personal, intrapersonal, and system-related barriers may complicate the process for some patients (Johnson et al., 2020). Larger metropolitan areas may have pharmacies that specialize in HIV care. These HIV-focused pharmacies may be part of large retail chains, independently owned, or integrated within a larger health system, or may assist patients through mail-order services. Pharmacies can elect to undergo an accreditation process to be officially recognized as a specialty pharmacy, although this designation typically indicates expertise in multiple disease states and not just HIV alone. Patient education and counseling, provision of reminder devices and adherence aids, managing the practical aspects of synchronizing and coordinating medication refills, facilitating procurement of antiretrovirals, and working with patients to address medication-related financial barriers (e.g., enrolling patients in manufacturer assistance programs) are just a few of the activities conducted by HIV community pharmacists. As a testament to some of the less tangible but positive impact of community pharmacies, a large Centers for Disease Control and Prevention (CDC) demonstration project found a 12.9% improvement in retention in care when medical clinics partnered with community pharmacies in a patient-centered medical home model (Byrd et al., 2019).

PHARMACIST CONTRIBUTIONS TO HIV CARE: A SAMPLE OF SPECIFIC SKILLS AND IMPACT

Pharmacists' contributions to care for persons with HIV are diverse, and it can be challenging to define or list all the skills and patient-related activities that an HIV pharmacist can engage in. The American Society of Health Systems Pharmacists publishes a statement that attempts to summarize the scope of practice for pharmacist involvement in HIV care (Schafer et al., 2016). This statement is currently under revision given that the last version was published in 2016, and pharmacist roles have evolved since then. The

Infectious Disease Society of America, in partnership with the HIV Medicine Association, also published a statement on Team-Based Care, which included a brief description of the roles of clinical pharmacists (Infectious Diseases Society of America, 2024).

Pharmacists make ideal treatment facilitators because of their extensive training in comprehensive medication therapy management (MTM). The goal of MTM is for a pharmacist to optimize a patient's treatment through the identification, resolution, and prevention of medication-related problems (American Pharmacists Association and the National Association of Chain Drug Stores Foundation, 2008). This definition of MTM is intentionally broad so that it may accommodate the wide variety of activities a pharmacist may perform to optimize a patient's therapy. This section presents a sample of some of the evidence supporting the positive impact that pharmacists have when caring for people with HIV.

ENHANCING TREATMENT EFFICACY AND REDUCING ANTIRETROVIRAL THERAPY ERRORS

HIV pharmacists have a strong impact on ART efficacy. A systematic review found that pharmacist care significantly improved antiretroviral adherence (OR = 2.70), viral load suppression (OR = 4.13), and CD4+ cell count (median +66.83 cells/mm^3) when compared to usual care strategies (Ahmed et al., 2022). A pharmacist-led comprehensive pharmacogenomic testing program that was implemented in persons with HIV resulted in 39% of enrolled patients receiving a new recommendation for ART dose adjustment or monitoring (Zeuli et al., 2023). Pharmacist influence on treatment efficacy is not limited to ART; some collaborative practice agreements allow them to assess and adjust medication therapy for other HIV-related conditions and comorbidities such as depression, diabetes, hypertension, hepatitis C, and dyslipidemia. A retrospective cohort study found that an interdisciplinary primary care team that included an HIV pharmacist produced significantly improved outcomes in lipid management and smoking cessation for patients with HIV and diabetes, hypertension, or hyperlipidemia when compared to a control group that was managed by an individual healthcare provider (Cope et al., 2015). The interdisciplinary team achieved cost savings of approximately $3,000 per patient.

Published literature suggests that people with HIV are at high risk of medication errors when hospitalized. These errors may occur at various points during the hospital stay and include incorrect antiretroviral regimens, incorrect dosing strategies or scheduling, or unresolved drug-drug interactions. Pharmacist-led antiretroviral stewardship programs have resulted in reduced ART medication errors in hospitalized persons with HIV. A joint statement endorsed by the American Academy of HIV Medicine, HIV Medicine Association, and Infectious Disease Society of America recommends inclusion of a clinical pharmacist on interdisciplinary antiretroviral stewardship teams and highlights the contributions of pharmacists in improving antiretroviral use in hospitalized patients (Koren et al., 2020). An ARV stewardship program in Philadelphia found that out of 567 hospital admissions involving persons with HIV, 43% required at least one intervention, and the cost savings associated with the stewardship program was estimated at $263,428 over a 1-year period (DePuy et al., 2019). Successful pharmacist-led stewardship programs may have greater impact beyond the immediate correction of medication errors. An ARV stewardship program in Chicago found statistically significant reductions in ARV error rates (17% to 6%), reductions in 30-day hospital readmissions (27% to 12%), and increases in linkage to care for patients served (Brizzi et al., 2020). Similarly, a hospital system in North Carolina found significantly reduced ARV error rates and increased linkage to care with a pharmacist-led ARV stewardship program (Roshdy et al., 2021).

MANAGING DRUG-DRUG INTERACTIONS AND POLYPHARMACY

People with HIV take increasingly more medications as they age. The proportion of persons with HIV and polypharmacy (typically defined as taking 5 or more medications) has ranged from 36% to 94% when observed in various cohorts of older persons with HIV in the United States (Back and Catia, 2020). In a single-center study, 248 persons with HIV were referred to a clinical pharmacist for medication review (McNicholl et al., 2017). The pharmacist identified medications that were potentially inappropriate (as defined by BEERS criteria) in 63% of the cohort, uncovered contraindicated drug interaction pairs in 20 patients, and was able to de-prescribe at least one medication for 69% of patients. Some antiretroviral agents strongly induce or inhibit the cytochrome P450 system, particularly the 3A4 isoform. Because approximately 60% of the most commonly prescribed drugs are also metabolized via cytochrome P450 3A4, pharmacists are trained to carefully review a patient's medication list to identify adverse drug interactions that may result in excess toxicity or subtherapeutic levels of the object drug, or that may result in alterations in the HIV drug concentrations. Pharmacists provide management strategies for known interactions. For important theoretical interactions, pharmacists may suggest using therapeutic drug monitoring and can help interpret the levels garnered from these tests.

SUPPORTING MEDICATION ADHERENCE, ACCESS, AND EDUCATION

In every setting, HIV pharmacists strive to support patient adherence to antiretroviral medications by addressing system-related and patient-related barriers to taking medications (Kibicho and Owczarzak, 2011). One very basic barrier is the inability to afford medications, resulting in suboptimal adherence. Pharmacists can provide patients with information and resources regarding manufacturer-supported patient assistance programs, or state-run AIDS drug assistance programs (ADAPs), and PrEP assistance programs to help reduce costs. Navigating insurance and pharmacy benefit management systems can be challenging for clinicians and patients. Pharmacists and technicians can play a critical role in selecting antiretroviral regimens that adhere to insurance formulary guidelines, provide clinical justification for prior authorizations, and manage those submissions so that patients do not have lapses in therapy.

Pharmacists can encourage the use of reminder devices and other tools to improve antiretroviral adherence (Hubbard-Mcree et al., 2020). Some community pharmacies offer specialized dose packaging in medication cards ("bubble packs" or "blister packs") to help patients synchronize and organize their pills and remember to take them. Pharmacists can also guide patients on how to set up and use weekly medication boxes. Some community and clinic pharmacists offer text messaging medication reminders or may work with patients to set up cell phone alarms to encourage timely medication taking. Pharmacies may offer a variety of other adherence-enhancing services, such as online management of medications, automatic prescription refills, telephone refill reminders, and home mailing or courier medication delivery.

An important adherence service that pharmacists provide is tailored patient counseling. They offer personalized education regarding HIV as a chronic disease, HIV treatment and opportunistic infection prophylaxis, and management of adverse effects. Using evidence-based counseling techniques such as motivational interviewing, pharmacists may help assess a patient's readiness to initiate ART and can help motivate the patient toward that goal (D'Antonio, 2010; Krummenacher et al., 2011). Although these topics may be discussed during the treating clinician's visit rather than during a pharmacist visit, this type of assessment and information sharing often takes up more time than allowed in a brief clinic visit that is typically focused on acute medical problems. A visit with a pharmacist provides additional time for complementary education and serves as an extension of the provider's care.

Pharmacists may package their services into structured adherence programs that span the range of patient assessment, education, and counseling, offering reminder devices, dispensing medications, and providing continuity in the refill process. These highly heterogeneous programs have been situated within community clinics, hospital clinics, and academic medical center clinics, and have found improvements in $CD4^+$ counts, increased rates of viral suppression, fewer acute medical visits, and increased adherence for patients who interact with an HIV clinical pharmacist. Although no two pharmacist-managed adherence programs are exactly alike, various studies have illustrated their benefits with regard to patient outcomes. Two early seminal studies conducted within Kaiser Permanente found that teams composed of a clinical pharmacist, social worker/benefits coordinator, and primary care provider were the most effective at increasing antiretroviral adherence (8.1% increase in mean adherence) and that patients who had been seen by an HIV clinical pharmacist had significantly improved refill adherence at 24 months compared to those who did not (Horberg et al., 2007; Horberg et al., 2012). Evidence supporting the benefits of pharmacist-led HIV adherence programs continues to grow (Ahmed et al., 2022). Future research should focus on cost savings associated with pharmacist adherence support. One small study provided a cost-avoidance estimate of $49,702 for 16 PWH who completed a 6-month, pharmacist-led adherence program (Dilworth et al., 2018). Adherence programs situated within community pharmacies may also have an important impact on antiretroviral adherence and patient outcomes. A specialty pharmacy which offered medication access and financial assistance, delivery, and patient outreach calls found ART adherence to be significantly higher in their intervention group as compared to the group that opted out of services (100% vs. 94%) (Barnes et al., 2020). While ART adherence did not substantially change for a group of 765 persons with HIV who were cared for in a community pharmacy-medical clinic patient-centered medical home, rates of viral suppression improved significantly from 75% pre-implementation to 86% post-implementation (Byrd et al., 2020). The estimated incremental cost per virally suppressed patient was $5,039 (Shrestha et al., 2020). These studies suggest potential for improvements in adherence and HIV viral suppression when patients use HIV-knowledgeable community pharmacies.

PHARMACIST ROLES IN THE IMPLEMENTATION OF LONG-ACTING INJECTABLE ANTIRETROVIRAL THERAPY

Long-acting injectable antiretroviral therapies (LA-ART) are revolutionizing HIV care. Currently available LA-ART must be administered by a healthcare provider and is typically administered in clinic settings. Given high costs, complex insurance coverage, and limited distribution, HIV pharmacists have increasingly served on clinic implementation and leadership teams for these specialty medications. In early implementation studies, HIV pharmacist expertise was leveraged to review patient insurance eligibility, assess their clinical eligibility, and provide patient education on LA-ART (Christopoulos et al., 2023; Hill et al., 2023). In one health center, an HIV pharmacist worked closely with health information technology services to establish work queues, create tracking databases, and facilitate billing and reimbursements (Collins et al., 2022). In four New York clinics, a pharmacist-led program to transition patients onto long-acting injectable cabotegravir with rilpivirine resulted in a 43% initiation rate and 84% treatment retention at the end of the 2-year study period (Nguyen et al., 2024). Including HIV pharmacists on LA-ART implementation teams will be critical for expanding access to these novel therapies.

HIV TESTING

HIV testing is a service that is emerging predominantly in community pharmacies. These models of care typically employ point-of-care "rapid" HIV tests, counseling, and linkage to confirmatory testing and/or care. The CDC notes that HIV testing in retail pharmacies is an effective intervention for enhancing diagnosis of HIV. This was supported by a 2011 demonstration project where 1,540 point-of-care HIV tests were administered across 21 retail pharmacy sites, with pre- and post-test counseling requiring 3–4 minutes, and patient wait time averaging 23 minutes for test results (Weidle et al., 2014). The cost per person tested ranged from $32.17 to $47.21 (Lecher et al., 2015). A statewide HIV testing program implemented in pharmacies in Virginia also found that HIV testing in pharmacies was a successful way to connect with "hard-to-reach" populations (Collins et al., 2018). Of 3,630 tests conducted over a 2-year period, 46% of clients reported that they had either never been tested before or were unsure whether they had received an HIV test. Collectively, these studies, as well as others, demonstrate the importance of pharmacies serving as HIV testing sites and pharmacists as key personnel identifying new HIV infections.

ENHANCING PREVENTION EFFORTS WITH PREP

PrEP utilization has grown impressively over the past 6 years, but large gaps in utilization remain (CDC, 2024). Some of these gaps may be due to lack of clinician familiarity with PrEP, or lack of time to discuss or manage PrEP, or certain populations who might benefit from PrEP lacking general health care. Pharmacists may offer unique access to some of these patient populations. In the southeastern United States, one study noted uneven distribution of PrEP prescribing locations across Ending the HIV Epidemic (EHE) focus areas, whereas pharmacies were evenly distributed within those EHE areas (Harrington et al., 2023).

HIV pharmacists can screen for clinical appropriateness, prescribe PrEP under protocol, order and review monitoring labs, assess and support adherence, and refill as appropriate. Various studies have confirmed patients' acceptability of pharmacists screening them for PrEP indications and for pharmacy-run PrEP programs (Crawford et al., 2020; Lutz et al., 2021; Zhu et al., 2020). The One-Step-PrEP program in Seattle, Washington, is an example of a pharmacy-run PrEP program operating under a collaborative drug therapy agreement (CDTA) (Tung et al., 2018). From 2015 to 2018, 714 patients sought out this pharmacy-based PrEP service. Of those seeking PrEP, 695 initiated PrEP and most of these patients (98%) did not have to pay for their PrEP medication. An impressive retention rate of 75% was achieved over the first 3 years of operations. This study demonstrates that pharmacy-based PrEP services are feasible and desired, and remain a promising avenue for pharmacists to contribute to the public health goal of preventing new infections. As additional biomedical options for PrEP are approved and become more widely available (i.e., long-acting injectable cabotegravir), the role of pharmacists in expanding PrEP access may develop even further.

The critical need to expand access to HIV prevention therapies has led to several states passing laws to grant pharmacists direct prescribing authority for PrEP and postexposure prophylaxis (PEP). One of the first states to pass this type of legislation was California; after initial legislation was passed, a follow-up study conducted 3 years later involving 919 pharmacists and pharmacy students indicated that only 11% of pharmacists initiate PrEP at their pharmacy and 13% initiate PEP (Hunter et al., 2023). Cited barriers to implementation included: inadequate pharmacy staffing, lack of ease with performing recommended testing, and reimbursement for time and services rendered. Some states who subsequently passed similar laws incorporated provisions for pharmacist reimbursement or laboratory testing, but further studies will be needed to understand how to make these important pharmacy-based HIV prevention initiatives as successful as possible.

A novel avenue for pharmacists to enhance prevention efforts is to facilitate rapid ART and PrEP initiation. A pharmacist was the first point of contact for persons newly diagnosed with HIV for a pharmacist-driven rapid ART program at a Ryan White–funded clinic in Rhode Island in 2019 (Brotherton et al., 2020). During the visit, the pharmacist assessed ART readiness, provided education, screened for drug interactions, facilitated ART access, recommended patient-specific ART to the triage physician for initiation, and called the client 2 weeks after initiation. A retrospective analysis of the program found significantly reduced time from intake to ART start (16 vs. 0 days) and reduced time to viral suppression (81 vs. 34 days). A pharmacist-led program at an HIV testing center in Mississippi facilitated PrEP initiation for 69 patients, 89% of whom received their prescriptions within the same day (Khosropour et al., 2020). Programs such as this hold great potential to rapidly reduce viral loads and potentially impact HIV transmissions.

PHARMACISTS: UNLIMITED POTENTIAL

The benefit of having an HIV clinical pharmacist extends beyond direct patient services. Pharmacists are becoming increasingly essential members of HIV hospital and clinic quality-improvement teams. Performance measures often involve chart abstraction and generation of reports to benchmark rates of ART, viral suppression, opportunistic infection prophylaxis, and adherence. HIV pharmacists have the clinical background and skills to assess these and other key indicators quickly, accurately, and thoroughly. Pharmacists can also offer valuable insight for "plan–do–study–act" projects designed to improve any below-target performance measures.

Finally, an increasing number of trained HIV clinical pharmacist scientists are making a strong impact on HIV-related research. A solid understanding of study design, drug therapy monitoring, and pharmacotherapy makes HIV clinical pharmacists ideal study coordinators or project managers for research studies being conducted within clinical settings. Advanced training through master's degree programs and complementary PhD programs also places HIV clinical pharmacists in an optimal position to serve as principal investigators on research studies regarding pharmacokinetics, pharmacodynamics, investigational drugs, adherence, drug resistance, or provision of health services. As more pharmacists gain training in clinical research methods, they will continue to contribute valuable information to the body of HIV care knowledge.

CONCLUSION

HIV clinical pharmacists are a diverse group of healthcare practitioners with specialized skills and knowledge. Whether they are engaged in direct patient care, quality assurance, research, or a combination of these, they strive to benefit people with HIV through their efforts. Although not all clinics or hospitals have available resources or funding to house an HIV-specialized pharmacist, collaborations with HIV-focused community retail pharmacists can ensure that patients have access to this valuable healthcare team member and that they receive the highest-quality medication-management care possible.

RECOMMENDED READING

Durham SH, Badowski ME, Liedtke MD, Rathbun RC, Fulco PP. Acute care management of the HIV-infected patient: a report from the HIV Practice and Research Network of the American College of Clinical Pharmacy. *Pharmacotherapy*. 2017;37:611–629.

Hill LA, Ballard C, Cachay ER. The role of the clinical pharmacist in the management of people living with HIV in the modern antiretroviral era. *AIDS Rev*. 2019;21(4):195–210.

Koren DE, Scarsi KK, Farmer EK, et al. A call to action: the role of antiretroviral stewardship in inpatient practice, a joint policy paper of the Infectious Diseases Society of America, HIV Medicine Association, and American Academy of HIV Medicine. *Clin Infect Dis*. 2020 May 23;70(11):2241–2246.

Schafer JJ, Cocohoba JM, Sherman EM, Tseng AL (eds.). *HIV Pharmacotherapy: The Pharmacist's Role in Care and Treatment*. Bethesda, MD: American Society of Health-System Pharmacists; 2018.

REFERENCES

Ahmed A, Dujaili JA, Rehman IU, et al. Effect of pharmacist care on clinical outcomes among people living with HIV/AIDS: a systematic review and meta-analysis. *Res Soc Admin Pharm*. 2022;18:2962–2980.

American Pharmacist Association. Scope of practice. https://www.pharmacist.com/Practice/Practice-Resources/Scope-of-Practice/. Accessed July 10, 2024.

American Pharmacists Association and National Association of Chain Drug Stores Foundation. Medication therapy management in pharmacy practice: core elements of an MTM service model (version 2.0). *J Am Pharm Assoc (2003)*. 2008;48(3):341–353.

Back D, Catia M. The challenge of HIV treatment in an era of polypharmacy. *J Int AIDS Soc*. 2020;23(2):e25449.

Barnes E, Zhao J, Giumenta A, Johnson M. The effect of an integrated health system specialty pharmacy on HIV antiretroviral therapy adherence, viral suppression, and CD4 count in an outpatient infectious disease clinic. *JMCP*. 2020;26(2):95–102.

Brizzi MB, Burgos RM, Chiampas TD, et al. Impact of pharmacist-driven antiretroviral stewardship and transitions of care interventions on persons with human immunodeficiency virus. *Open Forum Infect Dis*. 2020:24;7(8):ofaa073.

Brotherton AL, Shah RB, Garland J, et al. Pharmacist-driven rapid ART reduces time to virologic suppression in Rhode Island. Abstract #498. Conference on Retroviruses and Opportunistic Infections. Boston, MA; March 8–11, 2020.

Byrd KK, Hardnett F, Clay PG, et al. Retention in HIV care among participants in the patient-centered HIV care model: a collaboration between community-based pharmacists and primary medical providers. *AIDS Patient Care STDs*. 2019 Feb;33(2):58–66.

Byrd KK, Hou JG, Bush T, et al. Adherence and viral suppression among participants of the patient-centered human immunodeficiency virus (HIV) care model project: a collaboration between community-based pharmacists and HIV clinical providers. *Clin Infect Dis*. 2020 Feb 14;70(5):789–797.

Centers for Disease Control and Prevention (CDC). Core indicators for monitoring the Ending the HIV Epidemic initiative: National HIV Surveillance System data reported through December 2023. HIV Surveillance Data Tables 2024;5(1). https://www.cdc.gov/hiv-data/initiatives/index.html. Published May 2024. Accessed July 2, 2024.

Christopoulos KA, Grochowski J, Mayorga-Munoz F, et al. First demonstration project of long-acting injectable antiretroviral therapy for persons with and without detectable human immunodeficiency virus (HIV) viremia in an urban HIV clinic. *Clin Inf Dis*. 2023;76(3):e645–e651.

Collins B, Bronson H, Elamin F, Yerkes L, Martin E. The "no wrong door" approach to HIV testing: results from a statewide retail pharmacy-based HIV testing program in Virginia, 2014–2016. *Public Health Rep*. 2018 Nov–Dec;133(Suppl 2):34S–42S.

Collins LF, Corbin-Johnson D, Asrat M, et al. Early experience implementing long-acting injectable cabotegravir/rilpivirine for human immunodeficiency virus-1 treatment at a Ryan White-funded clinic in the US South. *Open Forum Infect Dis*. 2022;9(9):ofac455.

Cope R, Berkowitz L, Arcebido R, et al. Evaluating the effects of an interdisciplinary practice model with pharmacist collaboration on HIV patient co-morbidities. *AIDS Patient Care STDs*. 2015;29(8):445–453.

Crawford ND, Albarran T, Chamberlain A, et al. Willingness to discuss and screen for pre-exposure prophylaxis in pharmacies among men who have sex with men. *J Pharm Pract*. February 18, 2020:897190020904590.

D'Antonio N. Including motivational interviewing skills in the PharmD curriculum. *Am J Pharm Educ*. 2010;74(8):152d.

DePuy AM, Samuel R, Mohrien KM, Clayton EB, Koren DE. Impact of an antiretroviral stewardship team on the care of patients with human immunodeficiency virus infection admitted to an academic medical center. *Open Forum Infect Dis*. 2019 Jul;6(7):ofz290.

Dilworth TJ, Klein PW, Mercier RC, et al. Clinical and economic effects of a pharmacist-administered antiretroviral therapy adherence clinic for patients living with HIV. *JMCP*. 2018;24(2):165–172.

Harrington KRV, Chandra C, Alohan DI, et al. Examination of HIV preexposure prophylaxis need, availability, and potential pharmacy integration in the southeastern US. *JAMA Network Open*. 2023;6(7):e2326028.

Hill LA, Abulhosn KK, Yin JF, Bamford LP. Single-center experience evaluating and initiating people with HIV on long-acting cabotegravir/rilpivirine. *AIDS*. 2023;37(4):605–609.

Horberg MA, Bartemeier Hurley L, James Towner W, et al. Determination of optimized multidisciplinary care team for maximal antiretroviral therapy adherence. *J Acquir Immune Defic Syndr*. 2012;60(2):183–190.

Horberg MA, Hurley LB, Silverberg MJ, et al. Effect of clinical pharmacists on utilization of and clinical response to antiretroviral therapy. *J AIDS*. 2007;44(5):531–539.

Howell L. Collaborative practice now allowed in all 50 states. *Pharmacy Today*. 2023;29(12). https://www.pharmacist.com/CEO-Blog/collaborative-practice-now-allowed-in-all-50-states. Accessed July 10, 2024.

Hubbard-McCree D, Byrd KK, Johnston M, Gaines M, Weidle PJ. Roles for pharmacists in the "Ending the HIV Epidemic: A Plan for America" initiative. *Public Health Reports®*. 2020;135(5):547–554. https://doi:10.1177/0033354920941184

Hunter LA, Packel LJ, Chitle P, et al. Opportunities to increase access to HIV prevention: evaluating the implementation of pharmacist-initiated pre-exposure prophylaxis in California. *Open Forum Infect Dis*. 2023;10(11):ofad549.

Infectious Diseases Society of America. Position of the Infectious Diseases Society of America and the HIV Medicine Association on team-based infectious diseases care and the roles of advanced practice providers and clinical pharmacists. *Clin Infect Dis*. 2024;79(4):807–809. doi:10.1093/cid/ciae265

Johnson SR, Giordano TP, Markham C, et al. Patients' experiences with refilling their HIV medicines: facilitators and barriers to on-time refills. *Perm J*. 2020;24:1–3.

Khosropour CM, Backus KV, Means AR, et al. A pharmacist-led, same-day, HIV pre-exposure prophylaxis initiation program to increase PrEP uptake and decrease time to PrEP initiation. *AIDS Patient Care STDs*. 2020 Jan;34(1):1–6.

Kibicho J, Owczarzak J. Pharmacists' strategies for promoting medication adherence amongst patients with HIV. *J Am Pharm Assoc (2003)*. 2011;51(6):746–755.

Koren DE, Scarsi KK, Farmer EK, et al. A call to action: the role of antiretroviral stewardship in inpatient practice, a joint policy paper of the Infectious Diseases Society of America, HIV Medicine Association, and American Academy of HIV Medicine. *Clin Infect Dis*. 2020 May 23;70(11):2241–2246.

Krummenacher I, Cavassini M, Bugnon O, et al. An interdisciplinary HIV-adherence program combining motivational interviewing and electronic antiretroviral drug monitoring. *AIDS Care*. 2011;23(5):550–561.

Lecher SL, Shrestha RK, Botts LW, et al. Cost analysis of a novel HIV testing strategy in community pharmacies and retail clinics. *J Am Pharm Assoc (2003)*. 2015;55(5):488–492.

Lutz S, Heberling, M, Goodlet KJ. Patient perspectives of pharmacists prescribing HIV pre-exposure prophylaxis: a survey of patients receiving antiretroviral therapy. *J Am Pharm Assoc (2003)*. 2021;61(2):e75–e79.

McLaughlin M, Gordon LA, Kleyn TJ, Lamsen M, Scott J. Assessment of the benefits of and barriers to HIV pharmacist credentialing. *J Am Pharm Assoc (2003)*. 2018 Mar–Apr;58(2):168–173.

McNicholl IR, Gandhi M, Hare CB, Greene M, Pierluissi E. A pharmacist-led program to evaluate and reduce polypharmacy and potentially inappropriate prescribing in older HIV-positive patients. *Pharmacotherapy*. December 2017;37(12):1498–1506.

Nevo ON, Lesko CR, Colwell B, et al. Outcomes of pharmacist-assisted management of antiretroviral therapy in patients with HIV infection: a risk-adjusted analysis. *Am J Health Syst Pharm*. 2015;72:1463–1470.

Nguyen NM, Kavanagh R, Gozar M, et al. Implementation of a pharmacist-led, long-acting, injectable cabotegravir/rilpivirine program for HIV-1 at health system-based clinics in the New York Metropolitan Area. *AIDS Patient Care STDs*. 2024;38(3):115–122.

Okoli C, de los Rios P, Eremin A, Brough G, Young B, Short D. Relationship between polypharmacy and quality of life among people in 24 countries living with HIV. *Prev Chronic Dis*. 2020;17:190359.

Roshdy D, McCarter M, Meredith J, et al. Implementation of a comprehensive intervention focused on hospitalized patients with HIV by an existing stewardship program: successes and lessons learned. *Ther Adv Infect Dis*. 2021;19(8):20499361211010590.

Schafer JJ, Gill TK, Sherman EM, McNicholl IR. ASHP guidelines on pharmacist involvement in HIV care. *Am J Health-Syst Pharm*. 2016;73:468–494. http://www.ajhp.org/content/73/7/468. Accessed August 31, 2024.

Shrestha RK, Schommer JC, Taitel MS, et al. Costs and cost-effectiveness of the patient-centered HIV care model: a collaboration between community-based pharmacists and primary medical providers. *J Acquir Immune Defic Syndr*. 2020;85(3):e48–e54.

Tung EL, Thomas A, Eichner A, Shalit P. Implementation of a community pharmacy-based pre-exposure prophylaxis service: a novel model for pre-exposure prophylaxis care. *Sex Health*. 2018 Nov;15(6):556–561.

Walker CK, Shaw CM, Moss Perry MV, Claborn MK. Antiretroviral therapy management in adults with HIV during ICU admission. *J Pharm Practice*. 2022;35(6):952–962.

Weidle PJ, Lecher S, Botts LW, et al. HIV testing in community pharmacies and retail clinics: a model to expand access to screening for HIV infection. *J Am Pharm Assoc (2003)*. 2014 Sep–Oct;54(5):486–492.

Zeuli JD, Rivera CG, Wright JA, et al. Pharmacogenomic panel testing provides insight and enhances medication management in people with HIV. *AIDS*. 2023;37(10):1525–1533.

Zhu V, Tran D, Banjo O, Onuegbu R, Seung H, Layson-Wolf C. Patient perception of community pharmacists prescribing pre-exposure prophylaxis for HIV prevention. *J Am Pharm Assoc (2003)*. 2020 Apr 15:S1544–S3191(20):30128.

13.

PRINCIPLES AND SCIENTIFIC BASIS OF HIV THERAPY

Neha Sheth Pandit, David E. Koren, and Emily Heil

LEARNING OBJECTIVES

Upon completion of this chapter, the reader should be able to:

- Describe the classes of antiretroviral (ARV) agents and their mechanisms of action.
- Discuss the clinical trials underpinning new trends in antiretroviral therapy (ART).
- Explain the basic principles of applied pharmacokinetics, pharmacodynamics, and pharmacogenomics of ARV agents.
- Recognize the benefits of co-formulated ART regimens versus the need for tailored ARV dosing.
- Enumerate key principles of clinical trial design and expanded-access programs.

CLASSES AND MECHANISMS OF ANTIRETROVIRAL AGENTS

LEARNING OBJECTIVE

- Describe the mechanisms of action of all ARV classes.

WHAT'S NEW?

The long-acting injectable (LAI) combination of cabotegravir and rilpivirine is a newer two-drug regimen containing an integrase strand transfer inhibitor (INSTI) and non-nucleoside reverse transcriptase inhibitor (NNRTI), respectively, approved for use in people with HIV (PWH) who are virologically suppressed on an oral ARV regimen. The combination of these LAI ARVs is approved to be administered every month or every 2 months. In addition, a novel injectable capsid inhibitor, lenacapavir, has been approved for PWH with multidrug-resistant HIV and is administered every 6 months.

KEY POINTS

- There are six major categories of antiretroviral agents: entry inhibitors, non-nucleoside and nucleoside reverse transcriptase inhibitors, protease inhibitors, integrase inhibitors, and capsid inhibitors.
- Combination ART is recommended for all people living with HIV (PWH).

INTRODUCTION

Conventional terminology refers to individual antiretroviral agents as ARVs, whereas a combination of ARVs taken together to treat HIV infection effectively is known as antiretroviral therapy, or ART. As recommended by the U.S. Department of Health and Human Services (DHHS) since 2012 (DHHS, 2024) and as further validated by the START (INSIGHT START GROUP, 2015) and TEMPRANO (TEMPRANO ANRS 12136 STUDY GROUP, 2015) trials, ART is indicated for all persons living with HIV without regard to CD4 cell count. There have been 68 U.S. Food and Drug Administration (FDA)–approved agents to treat HIV, including combinations of individual agents and reformulations of existing ones, not all of which are currently available. These medications target the five major steps in the HIV replication cycle (Figure 13.1) as well as capsid formation (not shown in the figure). Classes of ARVs can be divided into nucleoside/nucleotide reverse transcriptase inhibitors (NRTIs), non-nucleoside reverse transcriptase inhibitors (NNRTIs), protease inhibitors (PIs), integrase strand transfer inhibitors (INSTIs), entry inhibitors (comprising an attachment inhibitor [AI]), a fusion inhibitor (FI), a C-C chemokine receptor type 5 coreceptor antagonist (CCR5A), and a post-attachment inhibitor (PAI) and capsid inhibitors. The primary goal of ART is to achieve and maintain viral suppression (DHHS, 2024).

NUCLEOSIDE/NUCLEOTIDE REVERSE TRANSCRIPTASE INHIBITORS

NRTIs inhibit the HIV-encoded reverse transcriptase enzyme in the host cell. This blocks the conversion of single-stranded viral RNA to double-stranded viral DNA, ultimately preventing incorporation of HIV genetic material into the host double-stranded DNA. NRTIs are nucleoside and nucleotide analogs; when reverse transcriptase incorporates them into the growing DNA, chain elongation is terminated. NRTIs must first be activated in the cell through three phosphorylation steps before they can become active chain terminators; nucleotide reverse transcriptase inhibitors only require two phosphorylation steps. NRTIs are poor substrates for human nuclear DNA polymerase alpha, but some NRTIs can be utilized by human mitochondrial DNA polymerase gamma and thus can cause mitochondrial toxicity. This class of antiretrovirals include the nucleosides abacavir (ABC), emtricitabine

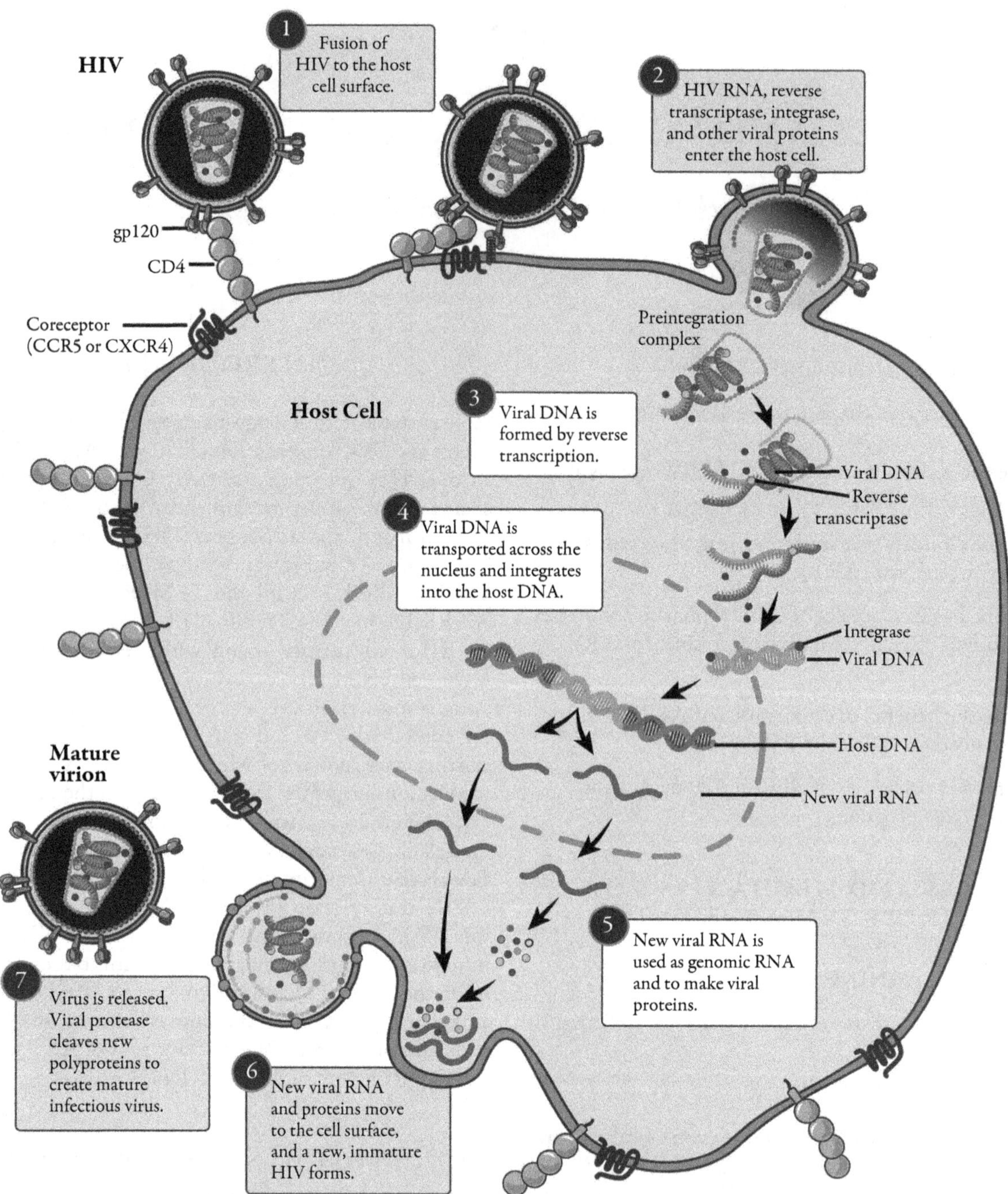

Figure 13.1 HIV viral replication. SOURCE: NIH. https://www.niaid.nih.gov/diseases-conditions/hiv-replication-cycle.

(FTC), lamivudine (3TC), and zidovudine (AZT or ZDV) and nucleotides tenofovir disoproxil fumarate (TDF) and tenofovir alafenamide (TAF). Older NRTIs that are no longer marketed include didanosine (ddI), zalcitabine (ddC), and stavudine (d4T).

NON-NUCLEOSIDE REVERSE TRANSCRIPTASE INHIBITORS

NNRTIs inhibit viral reverse transcriptase in the host cell. They act at the same point in the HIV-1 replication cycle as do the nucleotide reverse transcriptase inhibitors, but NNRTIs bind to the reverse transcriptase adjacent to the active site, causing structural alterations in the enzyme that sterically prevent it from adding any new nucleosides to the growing DNA chain. As the mechanism of action is different, the viral mutations that encode for resistance to NNRTIs are different from those that encode for resistance to NRTIs. Doravirine (DOR), efavirenz (EFV), etravirine (ETR), and rilpivirine (RPV) make up the clinically relevant, FDA-approved NNRTIs. Older NNRTIs that are no longer available or widely used in adolescents/adults in the United States include nevirapine (NVP) and delavirdine (DLV).

PROTEASE INHIBITORS

PIs act when a nearly mature virion is budding from the surface of the infected host cell. These compounds bind HIV-1 protease, preventing it from cleaving the gag precursor polyproteins, an essential process for HIV core maturation. Thus, the viruses that bud from the cell have immature cores, rendering them defective and unable to infect further host cells. PI regimens administered with pharmacokinetic enhancers (boosted PIs) are associated with no to very low rates of treatment-emergent HIV drug resistance at the time of virologic failure. While there are nine currently FDA-approved PIs, only two, atazanavir (ATV) and darunavir (DRV), are recommended in the DHHS guidelines (DHHS, 2024) in certain clinical situations. The remaining that are not clinically relevant or no longer marketed in the United States include saquinavir (SQV), indinavir (IDV), ritonavir-boosted lopinavir (LPV/r), nelfinavir (NFV), fosamprenavir (FPV), and tipranavir (TPV).

INTEGRASE STRAND TRANSFER INHIBITORS

INSTIs inhibit the viral enzyme integrase, which is responsible for inserting HIV proviral DNA into the host cell's DNA. There are five FDA-approved integrase inhibitors: bictegravir (BIC), cabotegravir (CAB), dolutegravir (DTG), elvitegravir (EVG), and raltegravir (RAL). Regimens that include an INSTI are associated with the most rapid viral load declines of all ARVs and greater CD4 cell increases compared to NNRTI- or PI-based regimens. Due to its high potency, minimal drug-drug interactions, and high tolerability, INSTI-based regimens are considered preferred for initial antiretroviral therapy for most PWH.

ENTRY INHIBITORS

HIV entry inhibitors are a diverse class with different mechanisms of action. Fostemsavir (FTR) is an attachment inhibitor that binds to the HIV envelope protein gp120 and prevents viral attachment to the CD4 cell surface receptor. Enfuvirtide (T-20), a fusion inhibitor, binds the HIV envelope protein gp41, preventing virus envelope–cell membrane fusion. Chemokine coreceptor antagonists act by binding to the CCR5 coreceptor, resulting in allosteric changes that prevent HIV gp120 binding and attachment. The only FDA-approved coreceptor antagonist is maraviroc (MVC), a CCR5 coreceptor antagonist, which requires testing for viral coreceptor tropism prior to utilization. PWH who harbor viruses that partially or fully use the alternative chemokine coreceptor, CXCR4, should not be prescribed MVC, because it will not antagonize this coreceptor. Ibalizumab (IBA), a monoclonal antibody characterized as a post-attachment inhibitor, sterically inhibits post-CD4 receptor binding through attachment to domain 2 of the CD4 receptor of T- cells. Lenacapavir (LEN) is the most recently approved antiretroviral medication, with a novel mechanism involving capsid inhibition. The inhibition of capsid allows for LEN to impact multiple steps in the HIV viral replication cycle. To accomplish this, LEN binds between subunits of capsid hexamers and polymers to prevent nuclear uptake of HIV proviral DNA, viral assembly and release, and capsid core formation.

KEY CHARACTERISTICS AND FINDINGS OF RECENT CLINICAL TRIALS INCLUDED IN UPDATED U.S. DHHS-RECOMMENDED REGIMENS

LONG-ACTING INJECTABLE-BASED REGIMENS FOR SWITCH THERAPY

In March 2020, two studies evaluated the use of cabotegravir/rilpivirine, a combination injectable long-acting CAB (an INSTI) and RPV (an NNRTI), after oral induction with these same agents for initial treatment of HIV-1 (FLAIR) and maintenance of suppression (ATLAS). The common focus of these studies was to evaluate the use of a long-acting, injectable, two-drug ART to improve the overall antiretroviral adverse effects profile, decrease the burden of daily oral regimens, and improve engagement with care.

FLAIR was a phase 3, randomized, open-label trial that enrolled 629 ART-naive PWH (Orkin et al., 2020). All participants were given 20 weeks of daily oral induction therapy with DTG/ABC/3TC, and at 16 weeks (once HIV-1 RNA levels were less than 50 copies/mL) were randomly assigned to continue this regimen or switch to oral cabotegravir plus rilpivirine for 1 month, followed by monthly injections of the same agents. Sixty-three participants withdrew from the trial before randomization, and the remaining 566 were randomly assigned to the two treatment groups. By weeks 48, 96, and 124, an HIV-1 RNA level of 50 copies/mL or more was found in 6 (2.1%), 9 (3%), and 14 (5%) participants, respectively, in the long-acting treatment arm. Comparatively, 7 (2.5%) and 9 (3%) participants were found to have an HIV RNA of ≥50 copies/mL in the oral therapy arm at 48 and 96 weeks, respectively. At 96 weeks, participants assigned to the oral treatment arm were given the option to switch to LAI or withdraw from the study. An additional 232 participants switched to LAI at this time and were assigned to do either an oral lead-in of CAB/RPV prior to injectable therapy or switch directly to injectable CAB/RPV. After 24 weeks of LAI, only 2 participants (2%) had an HIV RNA of ≥50 copies/mL (Orkin et al., 2020; Orkin et al., 2021a; Orkin et al., 2021b). The most common side effect was injection-site reaction (88% of participants). Virologic failure was seen in 4 participants in the long-acting therapy arm, with 1 additional failure seen within 24 weeks in the open-label extension phase. Possible correlations to virologic failure may have been body mass index >30 kg/m^2, integrase polymorphisms, and low drug concentrations. Despite the reported adverse reactions, satisfaction scores were higher in the long- acting therapy group.

ATLAS was a randomized, multicenter, parallel-group, open-label trial of long-acting CAB/RPV switch therapy compared to current oral therapy in virologically suppressed (HIV RNA <50 copies/mL) participants with HIV-1 infection (Swindells et al., 2020). Participants were randomly assigned to continue their current oral therapy or switch to injectable CAB/RPV every 4 weeks. At week 48, an HIV RNA <50 copies/mL was found in 92.5% of participants in the LAI arm and 95.5% in the oral therapy arm, meeting the criteria for noninferiority. At 52 weeks, participants had the opportunity to continue long-acting CAB/RPV monthly (long-acting arm), switch from oral ART to injectable CAB/RPV (switch arm), or transition to ATLAS-2M (to compare different administration schedules of CAB/RPV, i.e., every 2 months). At 96 weeks, 100% in the LAI arm (23/23) and 97% in the switch arm (28/29) achieved an HIV RNA of <50 copies/mL (Swindells et al., 2022). Injection-site reactions occurred in 83% of participants in the LAI group, causing study withdrawal for 4 participants (1%). At week 44, participants in the LAI group reported greater treatment satisfaction. Per the HIV Treatment Satisfaction Questionnaire assessment, 97% of participants in the LAI group selected the injectable regimen over the daily oral therapy as their preferred HIV treatment.

ATLAS-2M was a randomized, multicenter, open-label study evaluating long-acting CAB/RPV administered every 8 weeks (q8wk) versus every 4 weeks (q4wk). The study randomly assigned 1,045 participants, 522 in the q8wk arm and 523 in the q4wk arm. At 48 weeks, 94% of PWH in the q8wk group achieved HIV RNA <50 copies/mL compared to 93% in the q4wk group in the intention-to-treat analysis (Overton et al., 2020). At 96 weeks, 91% and 90% of PWH maintained HIV RNA <50 copies/mL in the q8wk group and q4wk, respectively (Jaeger et al., 2021). At 152 weeks, 87.4% and 85.9% of PWH maintained HIV RNA <50 copies/mL in the q8wk group and q4wk, respectively (Overton et al., 2023). No new safety signals were identified, and toxicities were similar to those in the ATLAS study.

CAB/RPV intramuscular injections were subsequently approved by the U.S. FDA for monthly dosing in December 2021, every 2-month dosing in February 2022, and with the option to defer the oral lead-in in March 2022.

LONG-ACTING INJECTABLE-BASED REGIMENS FOR MULTIDRUG-RESISTANT HIV

In December 2022, LEN was approved by the U.S. FDA for the treatment of HIV-1 in heavily treatment-experienced adults with multidrug-resistant infection. Lenacapavir is the first antiretroviral in a class of medications known as capsid inhibitors. Inhibition of the HIV-1 capsid is a novel mechanism of action that allows for disruption of the HIV life cycle in multiple different stages compared to traditional NRTI, NNRTI, INSTI, and PI medications. This medication is administered every 6 months as subcutaneous injections after an oral lead-in.

The CAPELLA study evaluated two cohorts of PWH, one that was on failing ART (HIV RNA ≥400 copies/mL) for at least 8 weeks with resistance to two ARVs in 3 of 4 classes of antiretroviral medications (NRTI, NNRTI, PI, or INSTI), and one on effective ART (HIV RNA<400 copies/mL). Seventy-two PWH were included in this study, 36 in each cohort.

The first cohort comprised two groups receiving either placebo (n = 12) or oral LEN (600 mg on days 1 and 2, and 300 mg on day 8, n = 24) in addition to their failing regimen (optimized background therapy, or OBT) for 14 days. On day 15, 88% of those in the oral LEN group achieved an HIV RNA 0.5 log decrease compared to 17% in the placebo group. The oral LEN group was then switched to subcutaneous LEN every 6 months (q6mo) and the placebo group was crossed over to an oral LEN lead-in followed by q6mo subcutaneous injections. Both groups in this cohort continued on OBT throughout.

The second cohort of virologically controlled PWH received oral LEN and their OBT for 14 days and then transitioned to subcutaneous q6mo LEN + OBT.

By week 26 it was noted that 81% and 83% of cohorts 1 and 2 had achieved an HIV RNA <50 copies/mL, respectively, demonstrating excellent efficacy of LEN+OBT in both maintaining viral suppression or achieving it against multidrug-resistant virus. Common adverse events noted in this study included injection-site reactions and GI-related toxicities (Segal-Maurer et al., 2022).

As will be discussed in Chapter 14, covering HIV preexposure prophylaxis, LEN was also recently shown to have outstanding efficacy in preventing HIV infection.

WHAT'S ON THE HORIZON?

The landscape of antiretroviral therapies includes advancing new combinations and formulations, allowing for decreased frequency of medication administration and alternatives to oral daily therapies.

Although long-acting CAB/RPV is currently only approved for PWH already stable on oral ART, a demonstration project identified 57 participants who were viremic at the time of LAI CAB/RPV initiation. The mean $\log_{10}$ HIV RNA level was 4.21, and by a median of 33 days, 54/57 (94.7%) patients achieved virologic suppression (Gandhi et al., 2023). In 2024, the IAS-USA HIV treatment guidelines were updated to note that LAI CAB/RPV may be considered in PWH with viremia if no other treatment options are effective (Sax et al., 2024). Further analyses are needed regarding the use of this combination ART in PWH with viremia.

In another study of LAI therapy, a phase 2 study enrolled 182 treatment-naïve PWH to be randomized into one of four groups: (1) subcutaneous LEN plus TAF/FTC for 28 weeks, then subcutaneous LEN plus TAF; (2) subcutaneous LEN plus TAF/FTC for 28 weeks, then subcutaneous LEN plus BIC; (3) oral LEN plus TAF/FTC; or (4) oral BIC/TAF/FTC. At week 28, 94%, 92%, 94%, and 100% achieved HIV RNA <50 copies/mL in each group, respectively. At 54 weeks, 90%, 85%, 85%, and 92% achieved HIV RNA <50 copies/mL in each group, respectively. The most common adverse reactions include erythema, swelling, pain, headaches, and nausea (Gupta et al., 2023). The success of this study is a stepping stone to the development of alternative treatment options, including CAB plus LEN.

RECOMMENDED READING

Orkin C, Gorgolas M, et al. Long-acting cabotegravir and rilpivirine after oral induction for HIV-1 infection. *N Engl J Med.* 2020;382:1124–1135.

Segal-Maurer S, DeJesus E, Stellbrink HJ, et al. Capsid inhibition with lenacapavir in multidrug-resistant HIV-1 infection. *N Engl J Med.* 2022;386(19):1793–1803.

Swindells S, Andrade-Villanueva J, Richmond GJ, et al. Long-acting cabotegravir and rilpivirine for maintenance of HIV-1 suppression, *N Engl J Med.* 2020;382:1112–1123.

PHARMACOKINETICS, PHARMACODYNAMICS, AND PHARMACOGENOMICS

LEARNING OBJECTIVE(S)

- Describe the basic pharmacokinetic properties of classes of ARV agents.
- Explain the benefits and shortcomings of using ritonavir or cobicistat (COBI) for pharmacokinetic enhancement of PIs and/or INSTIs.
- Review the potential role of therapeutic drug monitoring (TDM) for ARV agents.
- Demonstrate how pharmacogenomics is applied in the clinical management of PWH.

KEY POINTS

- Pharmacokinetics and local drug exposure can differ significantly within anatomical sanctuary sites compared with the systemic compartment.
- High variability in interpatient ARV concentrations is common, which makes population ARV pharmacokinetics difficult to interpret.
- Suboptimal ARV concentrations can result in HIV drug resistance and virologic failure.
- TDM can be considered in certain cases.
- Pharmacogenomic testing for the HLA-B*5701 haplotype reduces the risk of abacavir hypersensitivity reaction and is recommended prior to the initiation of abacavir-containing therapy.

INTRODUCTION

The science of *pharmacokinetics* studies the amount of drug in various compartments of the body and attempts to explain the effect that the body has on the drug through the assessment of multiple factors known as **ADME**: (1) **a**bsorption or bioavailability of the drug, (2) **d**istribution of the drug throughout body compartments, (3) **m**etabolism of the drug, and (4) **e**limination or excretion of the drug from the body. Clinical pharmacokinetics is the application of these pharmacokinetic principles to the therapeutic management of a drug in an individual with the goal of enhancing efficacy while minimizing toxicity.

In contrast, *pharmacodynamics* examines the relationship between the drug concentration and response, or the impact that the drug has on the body, which may have both intended and unintended pharmacologic effects. It also attempts to describe how drugs may interact with each other and display synergistic/multiplying or antagonistic effects. An example is the combination of AZT and ganciclovir, causing additive bone marrow toxicity resulting in neutropenia. The combination of FTC and 3TC is antagonistic as both drugs compete for the same site of action on the viral reverse transcriptase target, given similar chemical structures (DHHS, 2024).

Finally, *pharmacogenomics* is the practice of using host or viral genetic variation to individualize therapeutic decisions.

PHARMACOKINETICS

ABSORPTION

Medication absorption highly depends on the route of administration. Oral formulations of ARV medications have varying degrees of bioavailability that affect a PWH's serum ARV concentration. Currently, AZT and IBA are available in an intravenous formulation; enfuvirtide and LEN are available for subcutaneous injection; and CAB and RPV are administered as intramuscular injections. Ibalizumab, a humanized monoclonal antibody, is either an intravenous infusion or push given every 14 days for heavily treatment-experienced PWH (Emu et al., 2017). Long-acting injectable formulations of RPV and CAB are approved for administration every 4 weeks or every 8 weeks. Lencapavir is a capsid inhibitor for heavily treatment-experienced PWH dosed every 26 weeks. For the solid dosage forms, absorption first requires the dissolution of the tablet or capsule, allowing the drug to be absorbed through the gastrointestinal (GI) tract and then into the systemic circulation, from which it will be distributed to its site of action.

Drug absorption is a function of ionization and aqueous solubility, which can be impacted by factors such as gastric pH, gastric mobility (emptying), absorptive capacity, biliary function, GI enzymes, splanchnic blood flow, CYP enzyme expression in the gut, and transporters, such as P-glycoprotein. Absorption can be further affected under different individual conditions, such as the use of nasogastric or percutaneous endoscopic gastrostomy tubes (g-tube) for medication administration, or when liquid formulations of medications are required, such as for pediatric PWH or individuals who have difficulty swallowing solid dosage forms. Many ARVs are available in oral solutions or suspensions to facilitate administration in these circumstances. The bioavailability of many ARV medications can be significantly compromised by manipulation of the dosage form, such as crushing tablets or opening up the contents of capsules (Bastiaans et al., 2014). For example, administration of crushed LPV/r tablets significantly decreased the exposure of both components, with a decrease in area under the plasma drug concentration-time curve (AUC) of 45% and 47%, respectively, compared to swallowing the tablets whole (Best et al., 2011). Additionally, certain medications like RPV are insoluble in water, so crushing for administration via g-tube could compromise drug concentrations (Janssen Pharmaceuticals, 2024).

Food can impact the bioavailability and rates of absorption for certain medications because food increases the pH in the stomach and delays gastric emptying to the small intestine, which serves as the site of absorption for many medications. For example, the exposure of RPV is 40% lower when taken on an empty stomach compared to a food of at least 533 kcals (Janssen Pharmaceuticals, 2024). The solubility of a drug and surface area for absorption can be affected by gastric bypass procedures, which may impact the absorption of ART (Smith et al., 2011). In addition, the AUC and trough concentrations of INSTIs can be significantly reduced when coadministered with polyvalent cation products such as iron and calcium supplements or antacids containing aluminum, magnesium, or calcium. INSTIs should be given at least 2 hours before polyvalent cations under fasting conditions, or at the same time if administered with food (DHHS, 2024).

Some antiretrovirals require an acidic environment for solubility to occur, and acid-reducing agents may impact the dissolution of these drugs. Atazanaivir is a PI whose absorption is dependent on a highly acidic environment. Up to 40 mg by mouth twice daily of famotidine with boosted and unboosted ATV was found to decrease ATV AUC by approximately 20% (Wang et al., 2011). A pharmacokinetic study of boosted ATV and omeprazole 20 mg reported a 42% reduction in ATV AUC and a 46% reduction in ATV trough concentration (C_{trough}) compared with boosted ATV alone (Zhu et al., 2011). Increased gastric pH by acid-reducing agents such as proton pump inhibitors (PPIs) do not cause changes in absorption with other PIs such as DRV/RTV (DHHS, 2024). Increased gastric pH will also decrease RPV absorption, leading to suboptimal concentrations. RPV 150 mg was given with omeprazole 20 mg to 16 HIV-negative participants, which resulted in an AUC and C_{max} decrease of 40%. Based on this study, PPIs are contraindicated with RPV, and H_2 antagonists should be taken 12 hours before or 4 hours after RPV ingestion (Crauwels et al., 2008).

DISTRIBUTION

After ARVs are absorbed into the bloodstream, they distribute into the interstitial and intracellular fluids depending on the individual physiochemical properties (pK, molecular weight/size, and lipophilicity) of each drug (Minuesa et al., 2011). Many of the ARVs circulate in the bloodstream reversibly bound to plasma proteins. Albumin primarily binds acidic drugs, and α_1 acid glycoprotein primarily binds basic drugs. Only if free, or unbound, is the drug pharmacologically active, and the greater the free fraction of the drug, the better it distributes into tissues or compartments. A decrease in plasma protein binding may be seen in people with cirrhosis or cancer (Morse et al., 2006). Unbound drugs can enter cells or tissues primarily through carrier-mediated transport mechanisms, although some drugs can pass through via transcellular diffusion (Griffin et al., 2011).

The individual distribution characteristics of ARV compounds are under extensive investigation because each ARV drug may differ in the ability to penetrate into "sanctuary sites" throughout the body. These are areas where HIV can undergo compartmentalized viral replication with the potential to select resistant viral mutations due to suboptimal ARV drug concentrations within these sites, such as the male and female genital tract and/or the central nervous system (CNS) (Pomerantz, 2002; Tseng et al., 2014). Drug distribution to the male and female genital tracts is influenced by many factors, including hormonal changes, inflammation, concomitant sexually transmitted infections, and drug factors such as protein binding and lipophilicity (Trezza and Kashuba, 2014). Consequently, understanding drug distribution in the genital tract is essential for selecting agents for pre-exposure prophylaxis (PrEP).

METABOLISM

Many ARV drugs, including CCR5 inhibitors, attachment inhibitors, NNRTIs, and PIs, are metabolized by CYP enzymes, which are located in the smooth endoplasmic reticulum in cells throughout the body, primarily the liver and intestines. Inhibition of gut CYP3A4 enzymes leads to increased bioavailability of these agents, whereas inhibition of liver CYP3A4 metabolism results in delayed elimination and a prolonged elimination half-life. RTV, an early protease inhibitor, is a highly potent CYP3A4 inhibitor, and coadministration of a subtherapeutic dose (~100 mg) of ritonavir is sufficient to enhance (or "boost") the pharmacokinetic profile of all but one (NFV) of the currently licensed PIs (Larson et al., 2014). Cobicistat (COBI), a similarly potent inhibitor of CYP3A enzymes, is approved by the FDA to provide pharmacokinetic enhancement to PIs such as DRV and an INSTI, EVG. Because of its selective inhibition of CYP3A enzymes, COBI has less potential for off-target drug interactions compared to RTV. Unlike RTV, COBI has no anti-HIV activity; it is also more soluble than RTV, facilitating the development of coformulated products (Larson et al., 2014; Shah et al., 2013).

Pharmacokinetic enhancement of PI and INSTI concentrations with RTV or COBI, although increasing the risk of interactions with other agents, has several benefits, including:

- Higher C_{trough} levels, reducing the risk of selection for drug-resistant viral quasispecies
- Higher plasma levels throughout the day, minimizing or eliminating:
    - the need for food requirements

- the significance of interactions with other agents that induce the metabolism of PIs and INSTIs
- the effects of interpatient variations in drug levels due to factors such as sex, smoking, alcohol consumption, or liver disease.

- Increased plasma half-life, resulting in reduced dosing frequency and pill burden
- Increased levels of "forgiveness" with missed or late doses, potentially delaying/preventing the development of viral mutations.

P-glycoprotein (P-gp) is a cellular protein pump involved in transporting molecules in and out of the cell. P-gp is found extensively in the intestine, and its action is important in drug exposure and bioavailability. PIs are known to be substrates for P-gp. Overexpression of P-gp by certain individuals may result in lower intracellular concentrations of some PIs and thus decrease overall drug exposure (Sankatsing et al., 2004). RTV is a potent inhibitor of P-gp, whereas COBI is a weak P-gp substrate and inhibitor that does not lead to clinically relevant interactions (Larson et al., 2014; Shah et al., 2013).

EXCRETION

ARVs are eliminated from the body either unchanged by the process of excretion or converted to metabolites that may be more readily excreted. The kidney is the most important organ for eliminating drugs and their metabolites, whereas the liver is the principal organ responsible for drug metabolism and biliary excretion (Verbeeck et al., 2009). Renal and hepatic diseases are progressive illnesses that may occur as comorbidities in PWH. Chronic kidney disease is a condition marked by deteriorating kidney function and subsequent decreases in medication elimination. NRTIs are primarily eliminated via the kidney, with the exception of ABC. If there is a decrease in the glomerular filtration rate (GFR) in chronic kidney disease, it may be necessary to decrease the NRTI dose or increase the dosing frequency interval to prevent high systemic drug concentrations that may lead to adverse drug reactions.

It is important for the clinician to routinely check kidney function at least every 6 months (DHHS, 2024). The National Kidney Foundation Kidney Disease Outcomes Quality Initiative recommends the use of kidney function estimating equations of either Cockroft–Gault or the Modification of Diet in Renal Disease for the routine estimation of GFR. Note that most FDA medication package-insert dosage guidelines for renal impairment are based on only the Cockroft–Gault estimating equation. Guidelines for renal dosage adjustments of ARV agents are provided in all prescribing information, in addition to DHHS guidelines (DHHS, 2024).

PHARMACODYNAMICS AND THERAPEUTIC DRUG MONITORING

The need to maintain adequate drug concentrations that are effective in controlling HIV replication and preventing ARV resistance has resulted in considerable interest in the relationship between ARV drug exposure, virologic response, and drug-related toxicity. The ideal ARV dosing strategy ensures the highest probability of success at maintaining viral suppression with the lowest possible dose. This relationship can be examined through therapeutic drug monitoring (TDM). A retrospective study of 1,807 samples found that most concentrations for ARVs are above the upper therapeutic threshold and could likely benefit from dose optimization using TDM (Cattaneo et al., 2014). Currently, the only ARV approved at the lowest efficacious dose was RPV, but post-approval dose reduction has been seen with ARVs such as AZT, DDI, D4T, and EFV. Other medications shown to be efficacious but not yet approved at lower doses include LPV, ATV, DRV, and RAL (Crawford et al., 2012).

DTG has predictable pharmacokinetics, with minimal inter-subject variability and a defined exposure-response relationship (Cottrell et al., 2013). Early studies showed that DTG toxicities occurred at dosing ranges used for evaluation (Boffito et al., 2020). A study of 43 people over the age of 60 years living with HIV showed a significantly higher C_{min} of DTG compared to control with many PWH presenting with toxicities of DTG (Elliot et al., 2019). Despite this, the use of TDM for routine ART management has not been standard of care in most situations because of a lack of several key elements, including large prospective studies showing improved outcomes, established therapeutic concentration ranges for ARV agents, and laboratories that reliably perform ARV concentrations. These factors, plus intra-person variability in drug concentrations, challenge the use of ARV TDM in clinical practice (DHHS, 2024; Pretorius et al., 2011).

Nevertheless, TDM of ARVs could be considered for people who may have compromised ADME or in populations where pharmacokinetic studies are limited. For example, absorption may be disrupted in PWH with drug interactions or impairment of GI, hepatic, and renal function. TDM of ARVs may be beneficial in pregnant, pediatric, obese, or elderly PWH (Cattaneo et al., 2020; DHHS, 2024). Metabolism may be affected in PWH on concurrent CYP P450-interacting ARVs, and excretion may be compromised, leading to toxicities for individuals with hepatic or renal impairment (Cattaneo et al., 2020; DHHS, 2024). For PWH experiencing virologic rebound, adherence to their treatment regimen should be thoroughly evaluated prior to TDM, as medication nonadherence is the most common cause for treatment failure.

PROTEASE INHIBITORS

All PIs are CYP3A4 substrates, and most are CYP3A inhibitors; thus, there is a risk of drug interactions with commonly used medications that may be substrates of, may induce, or may inhibit the same CYP enzymes. The most common example of this type of interaction is the boosting effect of RTV or COBI on other PIs or the INSTI EVG. However, many medications used for comorbidities common in PWH also have CYP3A4-based interactions. In addition, boosting can potentiate the toxicity of the target drug. A retrospective analysis of 240 PWH on boosted and unboosted ATV found a direct correlation between ATV plasma concentrations and the incidence and severity of hyperbilirubinemia, percentage increase in triglycerides, and incidence of nephrolithiasis. These toxicities and increased plasma concentrations were seen mostly in the boosted ATV group, and the study suggested that concentrations greater than 800 ng/mL were likely the cause (Gervasoni et al., 2015).

NON-NUCLEOSIDE REVERSE TRANSCRIPTASE INHIBITORS

Like PIs, NNRTIs are substrates of the CYP3A4 enzyme. Although most NNRTIs are CYP3A4 inducers, not inhibitors like PIs, NNRTIs are similarly at high risk for drug interactions. Whereas PIs have a high genetic barrier to resistance, single-point mutations such as K103N or Y181C can cause complete virologic resistance to first-generation NNRTIs. Second-generation NNRTIs, such as ETR, RPV, and DOR, largely have a higher genetic barrier to resistance (Usach et al., 2013) and were designed to maintain activity against K103N virus. As one might expect, the risk of virologic failure with EFV-based ART was associated with low EFV plasma levels in one small study (Marzolini et al., 2001). In a larger study, however, trough levels and AUC_{24} of NVP and EFV were not significantly predictive of virologic failure, although for EFV there was an association between these parameters and virologic failure (Van Leth et al., 2006). An analysis of ETR from the DUET trials failed to show any relationship between ETR pharmacokinetics and efficacy or toxicities (Kakuda et al., 2010). These studies suggest that when reliably taken at prescribed doses, NNRTIs retain full activity, with resistance occurring more because of improper adherence than pharmacokinetic issues.

Given intramuscularly, long-acting RPV avoids first-pass metabolism, so gastric pH concerns for oral rilpivirine absorption are not a concern. LAI RPV has been approved to be administered every 4 or 8 weeks. The elimination half-life of LAI RPV is 13 to 28 weeks (ViiV Healthcare, 2023).

EFV-induced CNS toxicities have been correlated with elevated plasma concentrations (Marzolini et al., 2001). Through the use of TDM and dose adjustment, elevated plasma EFV concentrations were reduced to the recommended therapeutic range while maintaining undetectable viral loads (Mello et al., 2011). Although subjects in this trial were stable on long-term EFV, a significant improvement in anxiety scores and a trend toward lower stress scores were noted with the reduction in concentrations. When EFV 400 mg was compared to the standard 600 mg dose, it was found noninferior for virologic suppression and was associated with fewer EFV-related adverse events (ENCORE1 Study Group, 2014). A fixed-dose combination tablet including EFV 400 mg is FDA-approved to help minimize toxicities (Mylan Laboratories, 2019).

INTEGRASE STRAND TRANSFER INHIBITORS

RAL, DTG, BIC and CAB are metabolized by UGT1A1, whereas EVG acts similarly to a PI as a substrate of CYP3A4 requiring pharmacokinetic enhancing, with the attendant potential for drug interactions. BIC is a minor substrate of CYP3A4, so coadministration of potent inducers of CYP3A, P-gp, or UGT1A1 should be avoided.

A study in treatment-naive individuals that evaluated RAL 800 mg once daily compared to 400 mg twice daily, both given with FTC/TDF, found that although PWH in both groups had similar AUCs, a 6-fold decrease was seen in C_{trough} in the 800 mg group (Rizk et al., 2012). Even with the decrease in C_{trough}, similar response rates were seen in both groups with a baseline viral load of 100,000 copies/mL or less. However, the once-daily dosing arm was statistically inferior to the standard twice-daily dosing arm in those persons with a baseline viral load of more than 100,000 copies/mL and a $CD4^+$ T-cell count 200 mm^3 or less (Eron et al., 2011). A different study comparing RAL 1200 mg once daily to 400 mg twice daily, both in combination with TDF/FTC, in ART-naive PWH found that the once-daily option was noninferior to twice-daily dosing. RAL HD 600 mg tablets are available and FDA approved for a total 1,200 mg dosage taken orally once daily (Deeks, 2017).

A final feature seen with INSTIs has been a rapid decline in HIV viral load after initiation. DTG 50 mg daily was shown to achieve a 2.5 log decrease in HIV RNA after 10 days of therapy (Lalezari et al., 2009), and similar results were seen with the use of EVG, which resulted in a greater than 1 log decrease in HIV RNA after once- and twice-daily dosing (DeJesus et al., 2006).

The advent of long-acting ARVs has created alternatives for PWH who are no longer able to maintain daily oral medication adherence. Intramuscular CAB allows for extended interval dosing due to its pharmacokinetic profile. Pharmacokinetic studies have shown that detectable concentration of LAI CAB can be seen up to 18 months after last dosing of intramuscular administration. A study of 177 participants also found that the CAB terminal half-life to be 1.33 times longer in females than in males. Higher body mass indexes also showed a statistically significant increase in terminal half-life (Landovitz et al., 2020). This extended half-life and elimination, also known as the pharmacokinetic tail, has the potential to lead to toxicities, resistance, and drug interactions if medications are not discontinued and monitored appropriately.

CNS EFFECTIVENESS OF ARVS

The CNS is reached by considerable blood flow, but two anatomical barriers, the blood–brain barrier and the blood–cerebrospinal fluid (CSF) barrier, prevent the free passage of drugs into the brain (Calcagno et al., 2014). The CNS HIV Antiretroviral Therapy Effects Research (CHARTER) study group developed the CNS penetration-effectiveness (CPE) ranking scheme of CNS effectiveness of ARVs based partly on the physiochemical properties of the drug, such as lipophilicity, protein binding, and efflux substrate, that affect penetration into the CNS (Letendre et al., 2008). Regimens with higher CPE scores were proposed to have greater effectiveness in controlling HIV replication in the CSF. However, the use of CPE rankings to affect the course and severity of HIV-associated neurocognitive disorder (HAND) has not been demonstrated consistently (Caniglia et al., 2014; Ellis et al., 2014; Mukerji et al., 2018; Santos et al., 2019).

PHARMACOGENOMICS

Pharmacogenomics refers to the concept of using information about genetic variation to identify the most effective or well-tolerated ARV medications for an individual. Pharmacogenomic applications can be broadly categorized into the following areas: (1) ARV susceptibility, (2) explaining pharmacokinetic or pharmacodynamic variability, and (3) predicting adverse drug reactions. An example of the first category is genotypic resistance testing, which uses viral, not host genetic markers to predict susceptibility to ARV medications and is recommended prior to the initiation of treatment and in response to treatment failure. An example of the third category is seen with efavirenz, which is associated with characteristic neuropsychological side effects correlating with plasma levels. Its metabolism is variable, with higher levels associated with genetic polymorphisms of cytochrome CYP2B6 (Rotger et al., 2007). In one clinical trial from Japan, individuals harboring the CYP2B6*6 or -*26 allele successfully maintained plasma efavirenz levels despite dose reduction (Gatanaga et al., 2007).

Perhaps the best example of using pharmacogenomic biomarkers to predict adverse drug reactions is the association between the HLA-B*5701 allele and ABC hypersensitivity. Without genetic screening, approximately 5%–8% of individuals exposed to abacavir develop a hypersensitivity reaction (HSR), which can be fatal upon drug rechallenge. Genetic screening identified the HLA-B*5701 allele as a predictor of HSR; subsequently, the PREDICT study (Mallal et al., 2008) randomized 1,956 predominantly white individuals who were treated with ABC-containing ART. The use of HLA genetic screening dramatically reduced clinically suspected HSR from 7.8% to 3.4%. Skin patch test immunologically confirmed HSR was reduced from 2.7% to 0%. In a large, racially diverse group of North American patients, HLA-B*5701 screening resulted in 0.8% of individuals having clinically suspected HSR and no immunologically confirmed cases (Young et al., 2008). HLA-B*5701 allele screening is now recommended prior to the use of abacavir by multiple national treatment guidelines (DHHS, 2024).

SUMMARY

Understanding the basic principles of applied clinical pharmacokinetics, pharmacodynamics, and pharmacogenomics can help the clinician gain insight into contemporary HIV pharmacotherapy and improve therapeutic responses. This information can be used to improve ART for the individual by gaining a fundamental working knowledge of concepts that contribute to the occurrence of drug-drug interactions, adverse drug reactions, poor adherence, decreased efficacy, and the selection of viral resistance. These factors, alone or in combination, can lead to treatment failure of ART and subsequent progression of HIV disease.

ARV DOSING AND COFORMULATIONS

LEARNING OBJECTIVE(S)

- Describe food requirements, typical dosing, and modified dosing according to weight, renal and hepatic clearance for FDA-approved ARV therapies.
- Identify co-formulations used in HIV therapy.

WHAT'S NEW?

LAI CAB/RPV is now approved for administration every 4 or 8 weeks.

KEY POINTS

- The selection of an ARV dose should take into consideration the drug concentration that inhibits viral replication and the concentration that causes toxicity.
- Current oral ARV agents are dosed either once or twice daily without need for exact 24- or 12-hour dosing.
- Multiple factors affect drug exposures, including renal and/or hepatic insufficiency, ARV food requirements, and drug interactions.
- Co-formulated medications reduce pill burden and improve adherence to ART.

The selection of an appropriate ARV dosage is based on the amount of drug needed to inhibit viral replication and the ability to physiologically obtain these concentrations without causing significant toxicities. Ideally, the maximum concentration should not cause adverse events, and the minimum drug concentrations at the end of a dosing interval should be in excess of the target concentration needed to inhibit viral replication.

Many ARV agents are metabolized by the liver and/or eliminated by the kidney; thus, changes in hepatic or renal function can cause drug accumulation. This increases the potential for adverse drug events and might necessitate dose changes. A single-arm, open-label study by Eron and colleagues dosed EVG/COBI/TAF/FTC daily in PWH with severe renal dysfunction (with estimated creatinine clearances <15 mL/min) and in participants on intermittent hemodialysis; no significant adverse effects were seen (Eron et al., 2019). From these data, the FDA expanded dosing recommendations among several tablets that include these agents. However, in situations in which renal and/or hepatic impairment requires dosage modifications, the use of certain fixed-dose, single-tablet regimens (STRs; e.g., Atripla, Biktarvy, Complera, Delstrigo, Dovato, Genvoya, Odefsey, Stribild, and Triumeq) may not be possible; these situations may require the use of individual agents, when available, with the proper dosage adjustment for each agent. As of 2024, there are 23 co-formulations licensed for use as HIV therapy in the United States (Table 13.1).

Table 13.1 FDA-APPROVED COMBINATION ARV FORMULATIONS

TRADE NAME	COMPONENTS	CLASSES	DOSE
Combivir[a] (1997)	AZT (300 mg) 3TC (150 mg)	2 NRTIs	1 tablet by mouth daily
Trizivir[a] (2000)	AZT (300 mg) 3TC (150 mg) ABC (300 mg)	3 NRTIs	1 tablet by mouth twice daily
Kaletra (2000)	LPV (200 mg) RTV (50 mg)	1 PI + 1 PKE	2 tablets by mouth twice daily For treatment-naive patients only: 4 tablets by mouth daily
Truvada (2004)	FTC (200 mg) TDF (300 mg)	2 NRTIs	1 tablet by mouth daily
Epzicom (2004)	ABC (600 mg) 3TC (300 mg)	2 NRTI	1 tablet by mouth daily
Atripla (2006)	FTC (200 mg) TDF (300 mg) EFV (600 mg)	2 NRTIs + 1 NNRTI	1 tablet by mouth daily
Complera (2011)	FTC (200 mg) TDF (300 mg) RPV (25 mg)	2 NRTIs + 1 NNRTI	1 tablet by mouth daily
Stribild (2012)	EVG (150 mg) COBI (150 mg) FTC (200 mg) TDF (300 mg)	2 NRTIs + 1 INSTI + 1 PKE	1 tablet by mouth daily
Triumeq (2014)	ABC (600 mg) 3TC (300 mg) DTG (50 mg)	2 NRTIs + 1 INSTI	1 tablet by mouth daily
Prezcobix (2015)	DRV (800 mg) COBI (150 mg)	1 PI + 1 PKE	1 tablet by mouth daily
Evotaz (2015)	ATV (300 mg) COBI (150 mg)	1 PI + 1 PKE	1 tablet by mouth daily
Genvoya (2015)	EVG (150 mg) COBI (150mg) FTC (200 mg) TAF (25 mg)	2 NRTIs + INSTITI + 1 PKE	1 tablet by mouth daily
Odefsey (2016)	RPV (25 mg) TAF (25 mg) FTC (200 mg)	2 NRTIs + 1 NNRTI	1 tablet by mouth daily
Descovy (2016)	TAF (25 mg) FTC (200 mg)	2 NRTIs	1 tablet by mouth daily
Juluca (2017)	RPV (25 mg) DTG (50 mg)	1 NNRTI + 1 INSTI	1 tablet by mouth daily
Biktarvy (2018)	TAF (25 mg) FTC (200 mg) BIC (50 mg)	2 NRTIs + 1 INSTI	1 tablet by mouth daily
Cimduo (2018)	TDF (300 mg) 3TC (300 mg)	2 NRTIs	1 tablet by mouth daily
Symfi (2018)	TDF (300 mg) 3TC (300 mg) EFV (600 mg)	2 NRTIs + 1 NNRTI	1 tablet by mouth daily
Symfi Lo (2018)	TDF (300 mg) 3TC (300 mg) EFV (400 mg)	2 NRTIs + 1 NNRTI	1 tablet by mouth daily

Table 13.1 CONTINUED

TRADE NAME	COMPONENTS	CLASSES	DOSE
Symtuza (2018)	TAF (10 mg) FTC (200 mg) DRV (800 mg) COBI (150 mg)	2 NRTIs + 1 PI +1 PKE	1 tablet by mouth daily
Delstrigo (2018)	DOR (100 mg) TDF (300 mg) 3TC (300 mg)	2 NRTIs + 1 NNRTI	1 tablet by mouth daily
Dovato (2019)	3TC (300 mg) DTG (50 mg)	1 NRTI + 1 INSTI	1 tablet by mouth daily
Cabenuva (2021)	Every month: Initial injection at month 1: CAB (600 mg) RPV (900 mg) Monthly maintenance injection starting at month 2: CAB (400 mg) RPV (600 mg) *Every 2 months*: Initial injection at month 1: CAB (600 mg) RPV (900 mg) Every 2-month maintenance injection starting at month 2: CAB (600 mg) RPV (900 mg)	1 NNRTI + 1 INSTI	CAB (600 mg) = 3 mL IM injection RPV (900 mg) = 3 mL IM injection CAB (400 mg) = 2 mL IM injection RPV (600 mg) = 2 mL IM injection

[a] Only generic formulation is available in the United States.

ABC = abacavir; ARV = antiretroviral; ATV = atazanavir; AZT = zidovudine; BIC = bictegravir; BID = twice daily; CAB = cabotegravir; COBI = cobicistat; DOR = doravirine; DRV = darunavir; DTG = dolutegravir; EFV = efavirenz; EVG = elvitegravir; FTC = emtricitabine; INSTI = integrase strand transfer inhibitor; LPV = lopinavir; NRTI = nucleoside reverse transcriptase inhibitor; NNRTI = non-nucleoside reverse transcriptase inhibitor; NtRTI = nucleotide reverse transcriptase inhibitor; PI = protease inhibitor; PKE = pharmacokinetic enhancer; PO = oral; RAL = raltegravir; RPV = rilpivirine; RTV = ritonavir; 3TC = lamivudine; TAF = tenofovir alafenamide; TDF = tenofovir disoproxil fumarate.

Counseling PWH on optimal dosing and adherence is critical to the success of ART. Evidence-based guidelines for improving adherence are available and include recommendations for the routine collection of self-reported adherence data and the use of pharmacy refill data adherence monitoring (International Advisory Panel on HIV Care Continuum Optimization, 2015). Nearly all ARV medications currently prescribed are dosed either once or twice daily. Note that this does not imply, nor require, that PWH take their medications exactly every 24 or 12 hours; rather, they may aim to take their medications within a more generous time window.

Many ARV medications should be taken with food for optimal absorption. Some medications require an acidic stomach environment and may have negative drug interactions with acid-lowering agents such as PPIs (e.g., ATV and RPV). Others require dietary fat for optimal absorption (e.g., RPV). Counseling and adherence to dietary restrictions are important elements for optimal response to ART. The adult and adolescent DHHS guidelines list the standard dose, food requirements, and dosage adjustments in renal and/or hepatic impairment for the FDA-approved ARVs (DHHS, 2024).

Co-formulated ARV medications have been used for the treatment of HIV since 1997. The rationale for co-formulation is to decrease pill burden, thereby facilitating treatment adherence while decreasing risk of selective nonadherence or supply chain gaps. A meta-analysis comparing STRs to multi-tablet ARV regimens (MTRs) concluded that STRs were associated with statistically significantly higher adherence compared to PWH on MTRs of any frequency (odds ratio [OR] 2.37; 95% confidence interval [CI]: 1.68–3.35; p <0.001; four studies), twice-daily MTR (OR 2.53; 95% CI: 1.13–5.66; p = 0.02; two studies), and once-daily MTR (OR 1.81; 95% CI: 1.15–2.84; p = 0.01; two studies) (Clay, 2015). The relative risk (RR) for 48-week viral load suppression was improved with STRs (RR 1.09; 95% CI: 1.04–1.15; p = 0.0003; three studies), whereas RR of grade 3 to 4 laboratory abnormalities was lower among PWH on STRs (RR 0.68; 95% CI: 0.49–0.94; p = 0.02; two studies).

RECOMMENDED READING

Cattaneo D, Baldelli S, Cozzi V, Clementi E, Marriott DJE, Gervasoni C. Impact of therapeutic drug monitoring of antiretroviral drugs in routine clinical management of people living with HIV: a narrative review. *Ther Drug Monit.* 2020;42(1):64–74. http://doi:10.1097/FTD.0000000000000684

Clay PG, Nag S, Graham CM, et al. Meta-analysis of studies comparing single and multi-tablet fixed dose combination HIV treatment regimens. *Medicine.* 2015;94(42):e1677.

CLINICAL RESEARCH AND ACCESS PROGRAMS

Clinical care teams play an important role in sharing information with PWH about the availability of clinical research trials. National resources for ongoing clinical trials such as https://clinicaltrials.gov/ should be made available to all PWH.

LEARNING OBJECTIVE

Describe the differences between phase 1, 2, 3, and 4 research clinical trials and expanded-access programs.

KEY POINTS

- Phase 1 studies are the earliest clinical trials, focusing mainly on safety, pharmacokinetics, and dosing.
- Phase 2 studies further evaluate safety and begin to evaluate efficacy.
- Phase 3 studies focus on safety and efficacy in the target population.
- Phase 4 studies, sometimes referred to as *post-marketing trials*, occur after FDA approval and study the use of the drug in different populations and long-term safety.
- Expanded-access programs make a drug available to all PWH who are in particular need before the drug is commercially available. These programs are generally not established until after phase 3 studies have been fully enrolled.

PHASES OF CLINICAL TRIALS

In general, there are four phases to drug development, which are guided by procedures described in the U.S. Code of Federal Regulations 21 CFR 314.126 (FDA, 2017):

- Phase 1 is the most preliminary clinical work in small numbers of human subjects and helps to determine safety/toxicity (FDA, 2017). Phase 1 studies usually start as single-dose studies and then progress to multiple-dose studies, mainly using healthy volunteers. They evaluate a range of aspects, such as pharmacokinetics (including drug bioavailability), dose and dosing interval, food effects, tolerability, and toxicity to define the maximum tolerated dose, sentinel adverse effects, and target organ toxicity.
- Phase 2 studies further evaluate toxicity and the drug's effectiveness for a particular indication in a larger number of PWH who have the disease or condition under study Although most PWH get the same dose based on phase 1 trials, some phase 2 studies may evaluate different doses (FDA, 2017). This is usually the initial assessment of activity or proof-of-concept study. It includes several doses and a short course of monotherapy or functional monotherapy. It may include randomized dosing and control or dose escalation. Phase 2 studies also collect data on pharmacokinetics, dose response, tolerability, and toxicity. In HIV, these studies are usually divided into phase 2a and phase 2b. Phase 2a trials are generally conducted in a small number of PWH and usually are of short duration. Phase 2b trials usually involve longer-term dosing, are almost always in combination with other agents, and have a control arm. Longer-term tolerability, toxicity, and effectiveness are important outcomes.
- Phase 3 studies are primarily geared toward large cohort efficacy and, along with the accumulated weight of safety and toxicity studies, form the basis for submission to and approval by the FDA (FDA, 2017). Phase 3 studies are typically large, randomized studies that provide the core information for submission and regulatory approval. They frequently include blinded therapy. For ARVs, the endpoint for the most part has traditionally been some measurement of HIV-1 RNA response.
- Phase 4 studies are post-marketing or post-approval trials and may be mandated by the FDA to further determine long-term toxicities or may serve as vehicles for expanded indications or dosing changes (FDA, 2018a).

Expanded-access programs are often created for PWH in particular need, to make a drug available before it is licensed. These programs are an outgrowth of the expedited review process for HIV therapies and are usually limited in the number of individuals enrolled and the duration of availability. Typically, expanded-access programs are established after phase 3 studies have been fully enrolled and before drug approval. They are subject to FDA oversight (FDA, 2024), although considerably less so than are registrational trials. Because of the number of treatment options available today, expanded-access programs are much less common than in the past.

INTERPRETING CLINICAL TRIAL RESULTS

PER-PROTOCOL (PP) VERSUS INTENT-TO-TREAT (ITT) ANALYSIS

In randomized trials, a per-protocol (PP) analysis (also known as as-treated analysis, observed analysis, or on treatment analysis) examines outcomes in only those study participants who remain on their assigned study regimen for the duration of the trial or, in the case of an interim analysis, up to a particular time point. In comparison, an ITT analysis evaluates each participant according to the treatment group to which they were originally randomly assigned, regardless of whether the participant received the treatment or completed the study. Both ITT and PP analyses are valuable in understanding the findings of a clinical trial.

By removing from the analysis those participants who were lost to follow-up, do not complete the study (for any reason), drop out because of side effects, or do not stay on their prescribed study regimen, a PP analysis selects for participants who tolerated study medication(s). This analysis method is, therefore, intrinsically biased toward a best-case scenario and may systematically bias results such that poor outcomes associated with a treatment that is not well tolerated may be hidden. The value of the ITT analysis is that it limits bias by evaluating the entire population of participants randomly assigned to a given study regimen. ITT analyses more completely encompass efficacy, tolerability, adverse events, and the myriad other reasons why participants do not remain on or deviate from the assigned drug regimen; therefore, it accounts for the influence of these factors on outcomes (Lang et al., 1997). The more rigorous ITT approach conveys a truer sense of a treatment's overall effectiveness, is less subject to bias, and reflects "real-world" practice.

Because of the inherent differences in these approaches, the PP analysis will frequently report better outcomes than will the ITT analysis (e.g., a higher proportion of participants achieving an undetectable HIV RNA level). PP analyses exclude participants who are noncompliant with study medications, procedures, and/or study visits and those who drop out because of intolerance of the assigned regimen. If more participants are excluded from one treatment arm than another, the PP analysis may report a clinical difference that is quite different from the actual treatment difference obtained when all subjects are analyzed. Conversely, a PP analysis may find no difference between two treatments, whereas an ITT analysis, which better accounts for tolerability, may find a superior outcome for a treatment because of less study drop out or discontinuation.

PRIMARY EFFICACY ENDPOINT

Achieving an undetectable HIV RNA level (viral load) is the most widely accepted endpoint for antiretroviral clinical trials, as it is the most clinically relevant surrogate marker for outcomes that may take years to occur (e.g., progression to AIDS and death). As such, investigational antiretroviral drug regimens are frequently evaluated by assessing the percentage of participants achieving low (suppressed) plasma levels of HIV RNA. Because assays that detect HIV RNA have different limits of detection, it is important to know which prespecified level of HIV RNA was considered "suppressed" or "undetectable." Often, trials will allow some "forgiveness" in statistical analysis to account for small elevations or "blips" in viral load that likely do not affect ultimate clinical outcome.

In addition to measuring the failure to achieve or maintain HIV RNA suppression that exceeds such blips, the time to loss of virologic response (TLOVR) analysis also considers the introduction of a new antiretroviral drug, death, or loss to follow-up as failures (FDA, 2015). Depending on the study population, the FDA suggests the Snapshot method of analyzing results with the goal of simplifying the evaluation of study results. Snapshot differs from TLOVR in that it primarily focuses on a virologic response at a predetermined endpoint (e.g., 24 or 48 weeks). Specifically, an outcome will be measured only if a participant is a responder with an HIV RNA <50 copies/mL at week 48, +/− a 1- to 2-week window) (Qaqish et al., 2010). Twenty-four weeks of follow-up data are often appropriate for drugs that have some benefit over existing options (i.e., for PWH with multiple ARV drug resistance where it may not be possible to construct a fully suppressive treatment regimen; or improved efficacy, tolerability, or ease of administration), while 48 weeks is recommended for investigational therapies with comparable characteristics to existing options (FDA, 2015). Both analysis methods have value, and clinical trials often report results in both forms, although more recent analyses have favored the Snapshot algorithm.

NONINFERIORITY ANALYSIS

In contrast to statistical analyses used to demonstrate superiority, new drug regimens may be evaluated to demonstrate equivalence or noninferior efficacy relative to a standard drug regimen. The noninferiority trial is used mainly when the added value of a new drug/regimen is related to factors such as improved convenience, better tolerability, simpler dosing schedule, lower toxicity, or lower cost (Wittkop et al., 2010). FDA industry guidance regarding procedures for new drug approval has helped to standardize the statistical methods used in clinical trials of this nature. The proportion of treatment responders at 48 weeks is often used to assess noninferiority, as this provides sufficient time for emergence of loss of tolerability, ARV drug resistance, or other relevant measurable outcomes, using a specific margin of difference that is acceptable between study arms (FDA, 2015). In practical terms, a noninferiority analysis is a statistically rigorous way in which a clinical trial can demonstrate that a new therapy/regimen is at least as good as a currently available option. Often, efficacy results may appear numerically different, with one regimen achieving a slightly higher proportion of participants with undetectable viral loads at week 48, for example. In a noninferiority trial, numerical difference is less important than whether efficacy of both regimens falls within the prespecified "noninferiority margin," which then helps determine clinical equivalence. Trials are often powered differently, with larger numbers of participants if they aim to show superiority of one regimen over another rather than noninferiority. The FDA has tightened this noninferiority margin to ensure that new drugs are truly equivalent to existing therapies before coming to market.

CLINICAL VERSUS STATISTICAL SIGNIFICANCE

When evaluating research findings, clinicians should be aware of the difference between a statistically significant and a clinically significant difference. One of the most common errors in interpreting and reporting clinical trial results is not correctly distinguishing between clinical and statistical significance (Braitman, 1991). A *clinically significant finding* is one that has important implications for patient care. A *statistically significant finding* is a conclusion that there is evidence against the "null hypothesis"; that is, a low probability exists of getting a result as extreme or more extreme than the one observed in the study data by chance alone. *Statistical significance*, when applied to the terms *noninferiority* or *superiority*, indicates that the result of a clinical trial would be unlikely to occur by chance. It does not necessarily mean that the result will be important for treating patients (Braitman, 1991; Lang et al, 1997). Clinically significant findings typically must involve outcomes with particular relevance to clinical medicine and must have an effect size that is large enough to influence clinical decision-making.

MECHANISMS FOR EXPANDED ACCESS

There are three general approaches to expanded access, whether for an individual, intermediate-size participant population, or widespread use (FDA, 2018b, FDA, 2023).

INDIVIDUAL PERSON

For an emergency investigational new drug (E-IND) or protocol, a physician, on behalf of the individual, contacts the FDA and/or pharmaceutical manufacturer. In this type of emergency situation, a telephonic or electronic request/authorization may be used given the time-sensitive nature of the request and will either be submitted as a new IND or under the existing IND by the sponsor (manufacturer) as the situation allows. In such extreme emergency cases, institutional board (IRB) approval may not have been able to be acquired; however, this is expected to be reported to an IRB within 5 working days (FDA, 2018b).

INTERMEDIATE-SIZE PARTICIPANT POPULATION

Access for use by more than one person (but fewer participants than would otherwise be part of a normal IND) would be submitted as either a new IND or as a protocol addendum to the existing IND as the situation allows. Both FDA and IRB approval are required before treatment may begin. A request of this type may be submitted for an already approved medication or related product that would not otherwise normally be available because of extenuating circumstances (e.g., alternative manufacturers of products owing to drug shortages).

WIDESPREAD USE

Access for expanded/emergency widespread use must be submitted under either a new IND, or as a protocol addendum to the existing IND as the situation allows. The FDA must approve the protocol with a subsequent 30-day waiting period before treatment can begin unless the FDA decides that treatment should begin at an earlier time.

ACKNOWLEDGMENTS

The authors acknowledge Christian Ramers and Sarah Rojas, authors of this chapter in previous editions.

RECOMMENDED READING

U.S. Food and Drug Administration (FDA). Expanded access. https://www.fda.gov/news-events/public-health-focus/expanded-access. Published February 2024. Accessed August 26, 2024.

REFERENCES

Bastiaans DET, Cressey TR, Vromans H, Burger DM. The role of formulation on the pharmacokinetics of antiretroviral drugs. *Expert Opin Drug Metab Toxicol*. 2014;10(7):1019–1037.

Boffito M, Waters L, Cahn P, et al. Perspectives on the barrier to resistance for dolutegravir + lamivudine, a two-drug antiretroviral therapy for HIV-1infection. *AIDS Res Human Retroviruses*. 2020;36(1):13–18. http://doi:10.1089/AID.2019.0171

Best BM, Capparelli EV, Rossi SS, et al. Pharmacokinetics of lopinavir/ritonavir crushed versus whole tablets in children. *JAIDS*. 2011;58(4):385–391.

Braitman LE. Confidence intervals assess both clinical significance and statistical significance. *Ann Intern Med*. 1991;114:515–517.

Calcagno A, Di Perri G, Bonora S. Pharmacokinetics and pharmacodynamics of antiretrovirals in the central nervous system. *Clin Pharmacokinet*. 2014;53(10):891–906.

Caniglia EC, Cain LE, Justice A, et al. Antiretroviral penetration into the CNS and incidence of AIDS-defining neurologic conditions. *Neurology*. 2014;83(2):134–141.

Cattaneo D, Baldelli S, Castoldi S, et al. Is it time to revise antiretrovirals dosing? A pharmacokinetic viewpoint. *AIDS*. 2014;28(16):2477–2479.

Cattaneo D, Baldelli S, Cozzi V, et al. Impact of therapeutic drug monitoring of antiretroviral drugs in routine clinical management of people living with HIV: a narrative review. *Ther Drug Monit*. 2020;42(1):64–74.

Cottrell ML, Hadzic T, Kashuba ADM. Clinical pharmacokinetic, pharmacodynamic, and drug interaction profile of the integrase inhibitor dolutegravir. *Clin Pharmacokinet*. 2013;52(11):981–994.

Crauwels HM, van Heeswijk RP, Kestens D, et al. The pharmacokinetic interaction between omeprazole and TMC 278, an investigational NNRTI. Abstract P239. Presented at the 9th International Congress on Drug Therapy in HIV Infection. Glasgow, Scotland; November 2008.

Crawford KW, Ripin DHB, Levin AD, et al. Optimising the manufacture, formulation, and dose of antiretroviral drugs for more cost-effective delivery in resource-limited settings: a consensus statement. *Lancet Infect Dis*. 2012;12(7):550–560.

DeJesus E, Berger D, Markowitz M, et al. Antiviral activity, pharmacokinetics, and dose response of the HIV-1 integrase inhibitor GS-9137 (JTK-303) in treatment-naive and treatment-experienced patients. *J Acquir Immune Defic Syndr*. 2006;43(1):1–5.

Department of Health and Human Services (DHHS), Panel on Antiretroviral Guidelines for Adults and Adolescents. Guidelines for the use of antiretroviral agents in adults and adolescents. https://clinicalinfo.hiv.gov/en/guidelines/adult-and-adolescent-arv/whats-new-guidelines. Published February 2024. Accessed July 29, 2024.

Elliot ER, Wang X, Singh S, et al. Increased dolutegravir peak concentrations in people living with human immunodeficiency virus aged 60 and over, and analysis of sleep quality and cognition. *Clin Infect Dis*. 2019;68(1):87–95.

Ellis RJ, Letendre S, Vaida F, et al. Randomized trial of central nervous system-targeted antiretrovirals for HIV-associated neurocognitive disorder. *Clin Infect Dis*. 2014;58(7):1015–1022.

Emu B, Fessel WJ, Schrader S, et al. Forty-eight-week safety and efficacy on-treatment analysis of ibalizumab in patients with multi-drug resistant HIV-1. *Open Forum Infect Dis*. 2017;4(Suppl 1):S38–S39. http://doi:10.1093/ofid/ofx162.093

ENCORE1 Study Group. Efficacy of 400 mg efavirenz versus standard 600 mg dose in HIV-infected, antiretroviral-naive adults

(ENCORE1): a randomised, double-blind, placebo-controlled, non-inferiority trial [published correction appears in Lancet. 2014 Apr 26;383(9927):1464]. *Lancet*. 2014;383(9927):1474–1482. doi:10.1016/S0140-6736(13)62187-X

Eron JJ, Lelievre JD, Kalayjian R, et al. Safety of elvitegravir, cobicistat, emtricitabine, and tenofovir alafenamide in HIV-1-infected adults with end-stage renal disease on chronic haemodialysis: an open-label, single-arm, multicenter, phase 3b trial. *Lancet HIV*. 2019;6(1):e15–e24. http://doi:10.1016/S2352-3018(18)30296-0

Eron JJ, Rockstroh JK, Reynes J, et al. Raltegravir once daily or twice daily in previously untreated patients with HIV-1: a randomised, active-controlled, phase 3 non-inferiority trial. *Lancet Infect Dis*. 2011;11(12):907–915. http://doi:10.1016/S1473-3099(11)70196-7

Food and Drug Administration (FDA). Expanded access categories for drugs (including biologics). https://www.fda.gov/news-events/expanded-access/expanded-access-categories-drugs-including-biologics. Published 2018b. Accessed July 2024.

FDA. Expanded access | information for physicians. https://www.fda.gov/news-events/expanded-access/expanded-access-information-physicians. Published 2023. Accessed July 2024.

FDA. FDA's drug review process. https://www.fda.gov/drugs/information-consumers-and-patients-drugs/fdas-drug-review-process-ensuring-drugs-are-safe-and-effective. Published 2017. Accessed July 2024.

FDA. FDA post-market drug safety monitoring. https://www.fda.gov/patients/drug-development-process/step-5-fda-post-market-drug-safety-monitoring. Published 2018a. Accessed July 2024.

FDA. *Guidance for Industry Submitting Select Clinical Trial Data Sets for Drugs Intended to Treat Human Immunodeficiency Virus-1 Infection*. Washington, DC: U.S. Department of Health and Human Services; 2015. https://www.fda.gov/media/112667/download. Accessed August 26, 2024.

Gandhi M, Hickey M, Imbert E, et al. Demonstration project of long-acting antiretroviral therapy in a diverse population of people with HIV. *Ann Intern Med*. 2023;176(7):969–974. doi:10.7326/M23-0788

Gatanaga H, Hayashida T, Tsuchiya K, et al. Successful efavirenz dose reduction in HIV type 1-infected individuals with cytochrome P450 2B6*6 and *26. *Clin Infect Dis*. 2007;45(9):1230–1237. http://doi:10.1086/522175

Gervasoni C, Meraviglia P, Minisci D, et al. Metabolic and kidney disorders correlate with high atazanavir concentrations in HIV-infected patients: is it time to revise atazanavir dosage? *PLoS One*. 2015;10(4):1–12. http://doi:10.1371/journal.pone.0123670

Griffin L, Annaert P, Brouwer KL. Influence of drug transport proteins on the pharmacokinetics and drug interactions of HIV protease inhibitors. *J Pharm Sci*. 2011;100(9):3636–3654. http://doi:10.1002/jps.22655

Gupta SK, Berhe M, Crofoot G, et al. Lenacapavir administered every 26 weeks or daily in combination with oral daily antiretroviral therapy for initial treatment of HIV: a randomized open-label, active-controlled, phase 2 trial. *Lancet HIV*. 2023;10(1):e15–e23.

INSIGHT START Study Group. Initiation of antiretroviral therapy in early asymptomatic HIV Infection. *N Engl J Med*. 2015;373(9):795–807. http://doi:10.1056/NEJMoa1506816

International Advisory Panel on HIV Care Continuum Optimization. IAPAC guidelines for optimizing the HIV care continuum for adults and adolescents. *J Int Assoc Provide AIDS Care*. 2015; 14(Suppl. 1):S3–S34. http://doi:10.1177/2325957415613442

Jaeger H, Overton ET, Richmond G, et al. Long-acting cabotegravir and rilpivirine dosed every 2 months in adults with HIV-1 infection (ATLAS-2M), 96-week results: a randomized, multicentre, open-label, phase 3b, non-inferiority study. *Lancet HIV*. 2021;8(11):e679–e689.

Janssen Therapeutics. Endurant package insert. https://www.janssenlabels.com/package-insert/product-monograph/prescribing-information/EDURANT-pi.pdf. Published March 2024. Accessed July 2024.

Kakuda TN, Wade JR, Snoeck E, et al. Pharmacokinetics and pharmacodynamics of the non-nucleoside reverse-transcriptase inhibitor etravirine in treatment-experienced HIV-1-infected patients. *Clin Pharmacol Ther*. 2010;88(5):695–703. http://doi:10.1038/clpt.2010.181

Lalezari J, Sloan L, DeJesus E, et al. Potent antiviral activity of S/GSK1349572, a next generation integrase inhibitor (INI) in INI-naive HIV-1-infected patients: ING111521 protocol. Abstract TUAB105. Presented at the 5th Conference on HIV Pathogenesis, Treatment and Prevention. Cape Town, South Africa; July 19–22, 2009.

Landovitz RJ, Li S, Eron JJ, et al. Tail-phase safety, tolerability, and pharmacokinetics on long-acting injectable cabotegravir in HIV-uninfected adults: a secondary analysis of the HPTN 077 trial. *Lancet HIV*. 2020;7(7):e472–e481.

Lang TA, Secic M. *How to Report Statistics in Medicine: Annotated Guidelines for Authors, Editors, and Reviewers*. Philadelphia, PA: American College of Physicians; 1997.

Larson KB, Wang K, Delille C, et al. Pharmacokinetic enhancers in HIV therapeutics. *Clin Pharmacokinet*. 2014;53(10):865–872. http://doi:10.1007/s40262-014-0167-9

Letendre S, Marquie-Beck J, Capparelli E, et al. Validation of the CNS penetration-effectiveness rank for quantifying antiretroviral penetration into the central nervous system. *Arch Neurol*. 2008;65(1):65–70. http://doi:10.1001/archneurol.2007.31

Mallal S, Phillips E, Carosi G, et al. HLA-B*5701 screening for hypersensitivity to abacavir. *N Engl J Med*. 2008;358(6):568–579. http://doi:10.1056/NEJMoa0706135

Marzolini C, Telenti A, Decosterd LA, et al. Efavirenz plasma levels can predict treatment failure and central nervous system side effects in HIV-1-infected patients. *AIDS*. 2001;15(1):71–75. http://doi:10.1097/00002030-200101050-00011

Mello AF, Buclin T, Decosterd LA, et al. Successful efavirenz dose reduction guided by therapeutic drug monitoring. *Antivir Ther*. 2011;16(2):189–197. http://doi:10.3851/IMP1742

Minuesa G, Huber-Ruano I, Pastor-Anglada M, et al. Drug uptake transporters in antiretroviral therapy. *Pharmacol Ther*. 2011;132(3):268–279. http://doi:10.1016/j.pharmthera.2011.06.007

Morse GD, Catanzaro LM, Acosta EP. Clinical pharmacodynamics of HIV-1 protease inhibitors: use of inhibitory quotients to optimise pharmacotherapy. *Lancet Infect Dis*. 2006;6(4):215–225. http://doi:10.1016/S1473-3099(06)70436-4

Mukerji SS, Misra V, Lorenz DR, et al. Impact of antiretroviral regimens on cerebrospinal fluid viral escape in a prospective multicohort study of antiretroviral therapy-experienced human immunodeficiency virus-1-infected adults in the United States. *Clin Infect Dis*. 2018;67(8):1182–1190. http://doi:10.1093/cid/ciy267

Mylan Laboratories. Symfi Lo package insert. https://dailymed.nlm.nih.gov/dailymed/fda/fdaDrugXsl.cfm?setid=86aad85d-5460-4c38-9761-a225e6bce190&type=display. Published October 2019. Accessed July 2024.

Orkin C, Bernal Morell E, Tan DHS, et al. Initiation of long-acting cabotegravir plus rilpivirine as direct-to-injection or with an oral lead-in in adults with HIV-1 infection: week 124 results of the open-label phase 3 FLAIR study. *Lancet HIV*. 2021b;8(11): e668–e678.

Orkin C, Keikawus A, Górgolas Hernández-Mora M, et al. Long-acting cabotegravir and rilpivirine after oral induction for HIV-1 infection. *N Engl J Med*. 2020;382:1124–1135.

Orkin C, Oka S, Philibert P, et al. Long-acting cabotegravir plus rilpivirine for treatment in adults with HIV-1 infection: 96-week results of the randomized, open-label, phase 3 FLAIR study. *Lancet HIV*. 2021a;8(4):e185–e196.

Overton ET, Richmond G, Rizzardini G, et al. Long-acting cabotegravir and rilpivirine doses every 2 months in adults with HIV-1 infection (ATLAS-2M), 48-week results: a randomized, multicentre, open-label, phase 3b, non-inferiority study. *Lancet*. 2020;396(10267):1994–2005.

Overton ET, Richmond G, Rizzardini G, et al. Long-acting cabotegravir and rilpivirine dose every 2 months in adults with human immunodeficiency virus 1 type 1 infection: 152-week results from ATLAS-2M, a randomized, open-label, phase 3b, noninferiority study. *Clin Infect Dis*. 2023;76(9):1646–1654.

Pomerantz RJ. Reservoirs of human immunodeficiency virus type 1: the main obstacles to viral eradication. *Clin Infect Dis*. 2002;34(1):91–97. http://doi:10.1086/338256

Pretorius E, Klinker H, Rosenkranz B. The role of therapeutic drug monitoring in the management of patients with human immunodeficiency virus infection. *Ther Drug Monit*. 2011;33:265–274.
Qaqish R, van Wyk J, King M. A comparison of the FDA TLOVR and FDA Snapshot algorithms based on studies evaluating once-daily vs. twice daily lopinavir/ritonavir (LPV/r) regimens. *J Intl AIDS Soc*. 2010;13:58.
Rizk ML, Hang Y, Luo WL, et al. Pharmacokinetics and pharmacodynamics of once-daily versus twice-daily raltegravir in treatment-naive HIV-infected patients. *Antimicrob Agents Chemother*. 2012; 56(6):3101–3106. http://doi:10.1128/AAC.06417-11
Rotger M, Tegude H, Colombo S, et al. Predictive value of known and novel alleles of CYP2B6 for efavirenz plasma concentrations in HIV-infected individuals. *Clin Pharmacol Ther*. 2007;81(4):557–566. http://doi:10.1038/sj.clpt.6100072
Sankatsing SUC, Beijnen JH, Schinkel AH, et al. P glycoprotein in human immunodeficiency virus type 1 infection and therapy. *Antimicrob Agents Chemother*. 2004;48(4):1073–1081. http://doi:10.1128/aac.48.4.1073-1081.2004
Santos GMA, Locatelli I, Métral M, et al. Cross-sectional and cumulative longitudinal central nervous system penetration effectiveness scores are not associated with neurocognitive impairment in a well-treated aging human immunodeficiency virus-positive population in Switzerland. *Open Forum Infect Dis*. 2019;6(7):ofz277. doi.org/10.1093/ofid/ofz277
Sax PE, Thompson MA, Saag MS, IAS-USA Treatment Guidelines Panel. Updated treatment recommendation on use of cabotegravir and rilpivirine for people with HIV from the IAS-USA Guidelines Panel. *JAMA*. 2024;331(12):1060–1061.
Segal-Maurer S, DeJesus E, Stellbrink HJ, et al. Capsid inhibition with lenacapavir in multidrug-resistant HIV-1 infection. *N Engl J Med*. 2022;386(19):1793–1803.
Shah BM, Schafer JJ, Priano J, Squires KE. Cobicistat: a new boost for the treatment of human immunodeficiency virus infection. *Pharmacotherapy*. 2013;33(10):1107–1116. http://doi:10.1002/phar.1237
Smith A, Henriksen B, Cohen A. Pharmacokinetic considerations in Roux-en-Y gastric bypass patients [published correction appears in Am J Health Syst Pharm. 2012;69(3):182]. *Am J Health Syst Pharm*. 2011;68(23):2241–2247. doi:10.2146/ajhp100630
Swindells S, Andrade-Villanueva J, Richmond GJ, et al. Long-acting cabotegravir and rilpivirine for maintenance of HIV-1 suppression. *N Engl J Med*. 2020;382(12):1112–1123. http://doi:10.1056/NEJMoa1904398
Swindells S, Lutz T, Van Zyl L, et al. Week 96 extension results of a Phase 3 study evaluating long-acting cabotegravir with rilpivirine for HIV-1 treatment. *AIDS*. 2022;36(2):185–194.
TEMPRANO ANRS 12136 Study Group. A trial of early antiretrovirals and isoniazid preventive therapy in Africa. *N Engl J Med*. 2015;373(9):808–822. http://doi:10.1056/NEJMoa1507198
Trezza CR, Kashuba AD. Pharmacokinetics of antiretrovirals in genital secretions and anatomic sites of HIV transmission: implications for HIV prevention. *Clin Pharmacokinet*. 2014;5(7)3:611–624. http://doi: 10.1007/s40262-014-0148-z
Tseng A, Seet J, Phillips EJ. The evolution of three decades of antiretroviral therapy: challenges, triumphs and the promise of the future. *Br J Clin Pharmacol*. 2014;79(2):182–194. http://doi:10.1111/bcp.12403
Usach I, Melis V, Peris JE. Non-nucleoside reverse transcriptase inhibitors: a review on pharmacokinetics, pharmacodynamics, safety and tolerability. *J Int AIDS Soc*. 2013;16(1):1–14. http://doi:10.7448/IAS.16.1.18567
Van Leth F, Kappelhoff BS, Johnson D, et al. Pharmacokinetic parameters of nevirapine and efavirenz in relation to antiretroviral efficacy. *AIDS Res Hum Retroviruses*. 2006;22(3):232–239. http://doi:10.1089/aid.2006.22.232
Verbeeck RK, Musuamba FT. Pharmacokinetics and dosage adjustment in patients with renal dysfunction. *Eur J Clin Pharmacol*. 2009;65(8):757–773. http://doi:10.1007/s00228-009-0678-8
ViiV Healthcare. Cabenuva package insert. https://viivhcmedinfo.com/search-medical-scientific-information/viiv-document-viewer?cmd=GSKMedicalInformation&token=23108-862a5aad-0610-40a2-95ac-0ef4073ff7be&dns=gsk-medcomms.veevavault.com&medcommid=REF--US-000964&product=Cabotegravir+and+Rilpivirine. Published December 2023. Accessed July 2024.
Wang X, Boffito M, Zhang J, et al. Effects of the H2-receptor antagonist famotidine on the pharmacokinetics of atazanavir-ritonavir with or without tenofovir in HIV-infected patients. *AIDS Patient Care STDS*. 2011;25(9):509–515. doi:10.1089/apc.2011.0113
Wittkop L, Smith C, Fox Z, et al. Methodological issues in the use of composite endpoints in clinical trials: examples from the HIV field. *Clin Trials*. 2010 Feb;7(1):19–35.
Young B, Squires K, Patel P, et al. First large, multicenter, open-label study utilizing HLA-B*5701 screening for abacavir hypersensitivity in North America. *AIDS*. 2008;22(13):1673–1681. http://doi:10.1097/QAD.0b013e32830719aa
Zhu L, Persson A, Mahnke L, et al. Effect of low-dose omeprazole (20 mg daily) on the pharmacokinetics of multiple dose atazanavir with ritonavir in health subjects. *J Clin Pharmacol*. 2011;51(3):368–377. http://doi:10.1177/0091270010367651

14.

HIV PREVENTION

PHARMACOTHERAPY AND NON-PHARMACOTHERAPY-BASED STRATEGIES

Katrina Baumgartner, Christopher M. Bositis, Wyatt Hanft, and Carolyn Chu

INTRODUCTION

HIV prevention encompasses a vast range of approaches and tools across behavioral, social, structural, and biomedical dimensions. Multiple highly efficacious biomedical options, including long-acting pharmacotherapies for HIV pre-exposure prophylaxis (PrEP), are available, although uptake differs across populations. Behavioral and social factors remain key drivers of the HIV epidemic, and inequitable access to and/or support for the utilization of effective interventions among historically marginalized communities remain a concern. Implementation science highlights opportunities to improve the acceptance and application of evidence-based interventions across "real-world" settings.

LEARNING OBJECTIVES

- Discuss behavioral factors and opportunities surrounding HIV prevention, including considerations for unique circumstances and populations.
- Describe safety of the U.S. blood supply and transfusion medicine considerations related to early antiretroviral therapy (ART) initiation for people with HIV and PrEP use among donors.
- Recognize structural and systems-level considerations that influence HIV transmission.

WHAT'S NEW

Behavioral interventions for HIV prevention, developed for use at the individual, dyadic, and organizational levels, continue to be optimized for acceptability, feasibility, and effectiveness. Technology-based strategies remain an active area of investigation—especially for younger populations. Although contemporary testing technologies and successful advocacy have led to blood product donation policy changes in many resource-rich settings, ART use (especially as long-acting injectable PrEP) poses screening and diagnostic challenges for blood supply monitoring. HIV outbreaks continue to affect networks of people who use drugs, particularly in resource-limited areas impacted by a largely unregulated drug supply and without widely accessible harm-reduction interventions and/or substance use disorder treatment.

KEY POINTS

- Providers should elicit comprehensive socio-behavioral histories in a person-centered, respectful manner and engage with patients through collaborative decision-making to identify acceptable and effective HIV prevention opportunities.
- The U.S. blood supply remains extremely safe, and policy changes regarding donor deferral practices among men who have sex with men (MSM) have not been associated with increased incidence of HIV seropositivity among donors.
- Expanded harm-reduction services, increased access to (and use of) medications for substance use disorder treatment, integrated substance use and HIV care, and large-scale public health and policy efforts are necessary to curb the HIV epidemic.

BEHAVIORAL INTERVENTIONS

Behavioral interventions to prevent HIV transmission include general informational campaigns about sexual health, substance use, and mental health, as well as messages tailored for various populations or practices. Some people adopt "sero-adaptive" strategies to utilize knowledge of an individual's HIV and virologic suppression status (self-reported or confirmed) when identifying potential sex partners or engaging in specific practices (Malekinejad et al., 2023; Mann et al., 2022). "PrEP-sorting" has also been described, whereby partners are selected based on current PrEP use (Maloney et al., 2022).

Adolescents, younger adults, and cisgender women remain a focus of global HIV prevention efforts; these populations are particularly impacted by multiple socioeconomic and cultural factors (e.g., trafficking and violence, sexual coercion, economic inequality) and also unique perinatal/postpartum and postmenopausal physiologic considerations (Bhushan et al., 2022; Eastment and McClelland, 2018; Thompson et al., 2018). Behavioral interventions developed especially for younger cisgender women and adolescents often involve delaying sexual debut; condom promotion; reducing partner concurrency and/or changes; increasing HIV/STI-related knowledge and screening, self-efficacy, and resilience;

building social capital and assets/economic social protection; and addressing unmet substance use and mental health needs (Alexander et al., 2023; Chang and Ashcraft, 2020; Fu et al., 2023; Mathur et al., 2023; Opara et al., 2022; Wilkins et al., 2022). Effective modalities include peer educator support models and group-based knowledge transfer/skills training to increase sexual negotiation capacity and healthy relationship building.

For people who use drugs (including people who inject drugs), most behavioral interventions have utilized individual- and/or group-based methods to promote safer sex and drug use practices. Interventions often focus on sharing information/counseling to elicit motivational and behavioral change in addition to cognitive-behavioral strategies, social-cognitive approaches, and strengths-based case management (Elkbuli et al., 2019).

Transgender and gender nonbinary communities continue to experience some of the highest rates of HIV infection globally, and many individuals face social and legal exclusion and marginalization, sexual and physical violence, economic susceptibility, high levels of stigma and bias, and transphobia. Substance use and transactional or exchange sex, as well as low rates of HIV screening, condom use, and pre-/postexposure prophylaxis utilization also drive transmissions (Malone et al., 2021; Phillips et al., 2023; Poteat et al., 2017; Sevelius et al., 2020; Toribio et al., 2023). Studies indicate that welcoming gender-affirming care environments and peer support/navigation resources may improve HIV prevention outcomes such as engagement in care and adherence (Ayala et al., 2021; Lee et al., 2022; Van Gerwen and Blumenthal, 2023).

Broad adoption of virtual/distance-based health programming and widespread availability of mobile devices facilitate ongoing development of web- and mobile health-based strategies. As one study notes, "technology can be used to engage users in novel and innovative ways that are less dependent on existing institutional structures and may use democratizing approaches to promote community engagement and ownership" (Jones et al., 2022, p. 10). Accordingly, technology-based interventions, including social media and other digital platforms, may be particularly acceptable to younger audiences, including younger MSM. Digital health interventions have demonstrated efficacy regarding delaying sexual initiation and reducing other HIV-associated risk behaviors, increasing HIV/STI knowledge and condom self-efficacy, increasing HIV testing and PrEP awareness, and may also help address stigma (Ibitoye et al., 2021; Lee et al., 2023; Maloney et al., 2020; Melendez-Torres et al., 2022; Romero et al., 2021; Veronese et al., 2020).

Regular HIV/STI screening and treatment remain a cornerstone of prevention. A link between sexually transmitted infections (STIs) and HIV transmission/acquisition has been supported by both biologic plausibility (e.g., genital tract inflammation leading to increased viral shedding in persons with HIV and increased access of HIV to subepithelial target cells) and epidemiologic synergy (Cohen et al., 2019b; Mayer and Venkatesh, 2011). Periodic HIV screening/testing is especially important for people using PrEP, people who are or may become pregnant, and people with ongoing regular exposures. Universal HIV screening aims to: (1) ensure that people know their status, (2) reliably identify early infection, and (3) assist with timely linkage to care and treatment. Screening outside of primary care and sexual health/HIV settings, such as through emergency departments, may help increase uptake, especially in populations not regularly engaged with primary and preventive care services (Lyons et al., 2023; Simmons et al., 2023; White and Solnick, 2024). Self-testing also remains an important option, as some individuals prefer testing outside of traditional clinic-based channels (CDC, 2021a). The COVID-19 pandemic helped accelerate and expand home-based HIV/STI testing: for example, opt-out HIV screening coupled with COVID testing led to increased detection of acute HIV for some programs (Spears et al., 2022). In 2023, the Centers for Disease Control and Prevention (CDC) and agency partners launched the most extensive self-testing program in U.S. history, "Together TakeMeHome" (CDC, 2023)

STRUCTURAL AND SYSTEMS-LEVEL INTERVENTIONS

SAFETY OF THE U.S. BLOOD SUPPLY

With the incorporation of nucleic acid testing and global improvements in quality oversight processes, the risk of transfusion-transmitted HIV is approximately 1 infectious unit per 2–10 million transfusions in the United States and other resource-rich settings (Busch, 2022; Faddy et al., 2024). Recently, many regulatory entities have adopted a reduced deferral period for some donor groups. For example, the U.S. Food and Drug Administration (FDA) now recommends a 3-month deferral since last sex for MSM (Bloch, 2022; FDA, 2020). However, early ART initiation and PrEP use both pose challenges for transfusion-related screening and testing practices, since ART used for either treatment or prevention can alter infection biomarker progression and may (in rare cases) result in delayed antibody development or even "seroreversion" (Custer et al., 2020; Leblanc et al., 2023; Nishiya et al., 2021; Seed et al., 2021). In particular, long-acting injectable PrEP may lead to ambiguous testing results and/or delayed HIV diagnoses among potential donors (Donnell et al., 2017; Marzinke et al., 2021).

SUBSTANCE USE, HARM REDUCTION, AND HIV PREVENTION

Injection drug use has long been linked to HIV transmission, with risk estimates ranging from 0.63% to 2.4% per act (Baggaley et al., 2006). Although the connection has been demonstrated most clearly for intravenous drug use, subcutaneous and intramuscular injections involving exposure to virus-containing material can potentially also lead to transmission. Alcohol and sedative/hypnotic use have also been associated with HIV transmission by affecting decision-making and negotiation around condom use and/or other sex or injection practices (Berry and Johnson, 2018; Hoenigl et al., 2016; Ickowicz et al., 2015). *Chemsex* refers to the planned use of one or more psychoactive and/or non-psychoactive substances to enhance sexual experiences; it typically involves drugs such as crystal methamphetamine, ecstasy, and/or GHB. Chemsex among gay, bisexual, and other MSM communities has been associated with behaviors that increase HIV/STI transmission such as condomless anal sex and problematic drinking (Ivey et al., 2023). Rather than viewing participation in chemsex as an either/or phenomenon, an integrated harm-reduction framework can help identify opportunities for behavioral, social, and biomedical HIV prevention interventions along a continuum (Strong et al., 2022).

The intersections between substance use and HIV encompass a broad and complex array of micro- and macro-environmental and structural factors. Ongoing cross-sector responses should be well-coordinated and include: (1) increased access to naloxone and other life-saving harm-reduction interventions, including syringe exchange services and supervised consumption spaces; (2) improved recognition and decreased stigma surrounding substance use, as well as broad HIV/viral hepatitis education and screening, including use of peer-based programming; (3) low-barrier, co-located comprehensive substance use/mental health and HIV services, including pre- and postexposure prophylaxis (PrEP and PEP) and rapid ART initiation; (4) flexible, trauma-informed care which upholds dignity and autonomy and supports health promotion; and (5) policy and structural changes which address racism and discrimination, and decrease disparities in housing and economic opportunities, incarceration, and criminalization of HIV and drug possession/use (Biello et al., 2018; Broz et al., 2021; Perlman and Jordan, 2018; Rich et al., 2018; Touesnard et al., 2022).

ADDITIONAL STRUCTURAL AND SYSTEMS-LEVEL CONSIDERATIONS

Several other structural factors influence HIV risk and delivery of evidence-based HIV prevention services; these represent an extensive landscape of physical, sociocultural, organizational, economic, and policy-related dynamics. Physical factors such as proximity and convenience of HIV services can affect motivation to seek care and testing. Stigma, structural racism, sexism and gender-based violence, and intersectional discrimination often influence decision-making related to accessing health systems, screening/testing and engagement in care, status disclosure (including to healthcare providers), sexual and substance use/mental health, and PrEP uptake (Bowleg et al., 2022; Decker et al., 2022; Harrison et al., 2022; Sutton et al., 2021). Settings that discreetly offer co-located services and expanded access can help facilitate engagement in care and increase uptake. Pharmacy, emergency department, and street medicine/homeless outreach-based HIV screening and PrEP programs have been implemented in some communities (Jackson et al., 2024; Mehtani et al., 2024; Zhao et al., 2022). Inadequate housing, racial segregation, and inequitable housing policies all pose significant barriers to care and have been associated with increased HIV transmission (Aidala et al., 2015; Brawner et al., 2022; Garcia et al., 2015).

Economic factors are closely intertwined with HIV: resource-limited settings are disproportionately affected by high rates of HIV, often related to deindustrialization and unemployment. These disparities involve inequalities in poverty, gender, race, and education; economic instability; labor migration; health insurance status; access to health resources and health literacy; local infrastructure and resources; and other factors (Del Rio, 2020; Zanakis et al., 2007). Cash transfer programs have been associated with fewer STIs, increased HIV testing, and reduced infections among cisgender women (Richterman and Thirumurthy, 2022; Stoner et al., 2021). COVID-19 further exacerbated disparities in HIV prevention among many communities of color, which are also heavily impacted by socioeconomic inequity, such as women, youth, and some sexual and gender minority individuals (DiNenno et al., 2022; Hong et al., 2023; Rimmler et al., 2022; Santos et al., 2022).

The epidemiology of incarceration closely reflects that of HIV and involves a complex interplay between racial and economic disparities in arrest and incarceration rates, substance use, and HIV (Iroh et al., 2015; Wirtz et al., 2018). People in correctional settings often have low rates of HIV awareness, screening/testing, care engagement, and access to PrEP; correctional health programs are highly varied in the comprehensiveness and quality of HIV services offered (Belenko et al., 2017; Murphy et al., 2024; Valera et al., 2017). The post-release period represents a unique, high-impact opportunity for reducing unmet HIV screening and prevention needs (Khan et al., 2019; Stone et al., 2018).

TREATMENT AS PREVENTION: "UNDETECTABLE = UNTRANSMITTABLE"

In 2016, the Prevention Access Campaign launched the "Undetectable = Untransmittable (U = U)" health equity and anti-stigma initiative, based on several multinational trials (e.g., HPTN 052, PARTNER, and PARTNER2, Opposites Attract) demonstrating no cases of linked sexual transmission of HIV when the seropositive partner was durably suppressed on ART. Prior to this, the concept of "treatment as prevention" had been accepted such that most clinical guidelines had removed specific $CD4^+$ thresholds for ART initiation and universally favored early ART for all people with HIV. In 2017, the CDC endorsed the campaign, and in 2022 the U.S. government officially supported "U = U" at the International AIDS Conference.

BIOMEDICAL INTERVENTIONS FOR HIV TRANSMISSION PREVENTION

LEARNING OBJECTIVES

- Describe recommended baseline and follow-up assessments for people receiving oral or injectable PrEP, occupational postexposure prophylaxis (oPEP), and nonoccupational postexposure prophylaxis (nPEP), as well as common side effects and other potential concerns.

- Discuss current PrEP inequities in the United States and review potential strategies to close these gaps.
- Describe new or investigational biomedical interventions for HIV prevention and how they complement existing interventions.

WHAT'S NEW

Long-acting early viral inhibition (LEVI) syndrome is characterized by HIV viral suppression and delayed or diminished HIV antibody expression when HIV acquisition occurs in the setting of long-acting cabotegravir (CAB-LA) used as PrEP and may result in delayed HIV diagnosis. Innovative strategies to deliver low-barrier pre- and postexposure prophylaxis services may increase access and utilization. Parenteral and long-acting prevention therapies continue to be actively investigated.

KEY POINTS

- Both oral and injectable PrEP are safe and highly effective for preventing HIV acquisition.
- Significant inequities in PrEP coverage based on race, gender, geography, and mode of exposure exacerbate existing HIV-related disparities.
- Postexposure prophylaxis (PEP), when taken within 72 hours of exposure, is safe and effective; PEP may be considered as a bridge to PrEP in individuals with anticipated ongoing exposures.
- Continued development and evaluation of novel biomedical prevention approaches are key to an effective and sustainable global reduction in new HIV transmissions.

INTRODUCTION

Biomedical interventions that prevent HIV transmission and acquisition include PrEP, oPEP, and nPEP; voluntary medical male circumcision; and ART-mediated perinatal HIV transmission prevention. The care of pregnant people and infants is discussed elsewhere in this volume; this chapter is focused on options for pre- and post-exposure prophylaxis and other biomedically oriented interventions.

HIV PRE-EXPOSURE PROPHYLAXIS (PREP)

For people who do not have HIV, PrEP involves taking antiretroviral medications before potential exposures to prevent HIV acquisition.

DATA: CLINICAL TRIALS AND REAL-WORLD EFFECTIVENESS

The FDA first approved daily use of tenofovir disoproxil fumarate (TDF) 300 mg plus emtricitabine (FTC) 200 mg (co-formulated as fixed-dose TDF/FTC) to reduce the likelihood of sexually acquired HIV in 2012. This was based on multiple studies demonstrating that, when taken consistently, TDF-based PrEP effectively reduced HIV acquisition in multiple populations, including men who have sex with men (MSM), transgender women who have sex with men, people who inject drugs, and heterosexual women and men (Table 14.1). The CDC estimates PrEP efficacy to be 99% for preventing sexual transmission of HIV with "optimal or consistent use" (CDC, 2022a) based on real-world data from the U.S. Kaiser Cohort and UK PROUD studies, which together showed no incident HIV infections among approximately 5,000 individuals, the majority MSM, who took daily oral PrEP consistently (Marcus et al., 2017; McCormack et al., 2016; Volk et al., 2015).

Data also support the efficacy of "on-demand" or "event-driven" PrEP (often referred to as "2-1-1" dosing): 2 pills of TDF/FTC taken together 2–24 hours prior to sexual exposure, 1 pill 24 hours after the initial 2 pills, and 1 pill again 24 hours after that (or 1 pill daily until 2 sex-free days). The IPERGAY and PRÉVENIR studies showed high efficacy rates among MSM using this strategy (Molina et al., 2015, 2017, and 2022) (Table 14.1), including participants who reported infrequent sex (Antoni et al., 2020). Moreover, PRÉVENIR demonstrated a high level of interest in event-driven PrEP, with almost 50% of participants choosing this option over daily TDF/FTC: discontinuations because of side effects were rare, supporting its tolerability as well (Molina et al., 2022). As with daily PrEP, adherence is key: in HPTN 067/ADAPT, differences in adherence between daily and event-driven PrEP led to an estimated 18% efficacy reduction with the latter (Dimitrov et al., 2020). CDC guidelines include 2-1-1 dosing of TDF/FTC as an option for adult MSM who request it and who report infrequent sex (less than once/week), and who can anticipate or delay sex to ensure the first dose is taken correctly (CDC, 2021b). Guidance from IAS-USA and WHO extrapolate these findings to also support 2-1-1 dosing for cisgender men of any sexual orientation and transgender women who are not on hormonal therapy (Gandhi et al., 2023; WHO, 2022). Some experts advise caution for transgender women on hormonal therapy, as tenofovir rectal tissue levels may be decreased with estrogen (Shieh et al., 2019). Given insufficient data at this time, 2-1-1 dosing is not recommended for receptive vaginal sex. Additionally, although daily adherence to TDF/FTC is optimal for cisgender women, pooled analyses suggest a minimum of 4 doses per week is expected to provide effective protection for most females (Marrazzo et al., 2024).

In 2019, the DISCOVER trial led to FDA approval of tenofovir alafenamide/emtricitabine (TAF/FTC) as an alternative oral PrEP medication (Mayer et al., 2020). DISCOVER showed noninferiority of daily TAF/FTC compared to TDF/FTC among MSM and transgender women who have sex with

Table 14.1 SUMMARY OF SELECT PHASE 3 RANDOMIZED CONTROLLED PREP TRIALS

TRIAL (REFERENCE)	*N*, STUDY POPULATIONS; SETTINGS	INTERVENTION(S)	ESTIMATED RELATIVE REDUCTION IN HIV ACQUISITION
iPrEX (Grant et al., 2010)	2,499 men who have sex with men (MSM) and transgender women (TGW); United States, South America, Thailand, South Africa	Daily TDF/FTC	44%
Partners PrEP (Baeten et al., 2012)	4,747 heterosexual women and men; Kenya and Uganda	Daily TDF Daily TDF/FTC	67% 75%
Bangkok Tenofovir Study (Choopanya et al., 2013)	2,413 people who inject drugs (PWID); Thailand	Daily TDF	49%
FEM-PrEP (Van Damme et al., 2012)	2,120 heterosexual women; Africa	Daily TDF/FTC	No significant risk reduction (hazard ratio 0.94)
IPERGAY (Molina et al., 2015)	414 MSM; France and Canada	2-1-1 TDF/FTC	86%
DISCOVER (Ogbuagu et al., 2021)	5,387 MSM and TGW; Europe and North America	Daily TAF/FTC vs. Daily TDF/FTC	53% fewer infections in TAF/FTC arm
HPTN 083 (Landovitz et al., 2020)	4,566 MSM and TGW; United States, Latin America, Asia, Africa	CAB-LA vs. daily TDF/FTC	66% fewer infections in CAB-LA arm
HPTN 084 (Delany-Moretlwe et al., 2022a)	3,224 cisgender women who have sex with men (WSM); Africa	CAB-LA vs. daily TDF/FTC	89% fewer infections in CAB-LA arm
The RING Study (Nel et al., 2016)	1,959 cisgender WSM; Africa	Monthly DPV ring	31%
ASPIRE/MTN020 (Baeten et al., 2016)	2,629 cisgender WSM; Africa	Monthly DPV ring	27%
PURPOSE 1 (Bekker et al., 2024)	5,345 cisgender adolescent girls and young WSM; South Africa and Uganda	Twice-yearly LEN vs. oral daily TAF/FTC and TDF/FTC	0 incident infections in LEN group (100%)

men (Table 14.1). Multiple ongoing studies are evaluating safety and efficacy of TAF/FTC for prevention in cisgender women, including those who are pregnant and breastfeeding (ClinicalTrials.gov. NCT05140954; ClinicalTrials.gov. NCT04994509; Joseph Davey et al., 2022); at this time, it is not yet recommended by CDC as an HIV prevention option for vaginal exposures. Similarly, TAF/FTC is not currently approved for on-demand dosing, although preliminary data from macaque and *ex vivo* models are promising (Bekerman et al., 2021; Herrera et al., 2023).

Injectable cabotegravir (CAB-LA) is another PrEP option for all sexually active adults and adolescents (CDC, 2021b). Its use is based on safety and efficacy data from HPTN 083 and 084, which found that long-acting cabotegravir (CAB) given via intramuscular injection every 8 weeks was superior to TDF/FTC in reducing incident sexually acquired HIV in MSM, transgender women, and cisgender women (Delany-Moretlwe et al., 2022a; Landovitz, et al., 2021) (Table 14.1). While these findings were driven primarily by lower adherence among participants receiving TDF/FTC, CAB-LA was found to be 66% more effective at preventing HIV in MSM and transgender women, and 88% more effective in cisgender women. There are no data on use of CAB-LA in persons whose primary risk for HIV acquisition is via injection drug use, although CDC guidelines endorse its use in persons who inject drugs based on their sexual risk (CDC, 2021b). At the 2024 International AIDS Conference, interim results from the PURPOSE 1 trial of twice-yearly injectable lenacapavir in cisgender women were announced (see section "New and Investigational Interventions for HIV Prevention" in this chapter).

The FDA controversially decided not to review the dapavirine ring application for U.S. approval, despite evidence demonstrating that cisgender women often prefer this option. WHO guidelines include it as an alternative PrEP option for cisgender women (Ngure et al., 2022; WHO, 2021).

PREP INDICATIONS

Multiple guidelines on PrEP indications and use have been released and are periodically updated; this chapter highlights specific recommendations from the 2021 CDC/USPHS guidelines. Other guidelines of interest include those from the World Health Organization (WHO, 2021); International Antiviral Society–USA (Gandhi et al., 2023); and New York State Department of Health AIDS Institute (New York State

Department of Health, 2022). The U.S. Preventive Services Task Force also recommends PrEP for individuals with risk factors for HIV acquisition (Grade A) (USPSTF, 2023).

PrEP is recommended as a prevention option for adults and adolescents with an increased likelihood of acquiring HIV (CDC, 2021b). Importantly, guidelines recommend that clinicians discuss PrEP with all sexually active adults and adolescents, individuals who inject nonprescription drugs, and individuals with substance use disorders, and also offer it to anyone who requests it, as some people may be hesitant to disclose sexual or substance use behaviors (CDC, 2021b; Gandhi et al., 2023). Stringent eligibility criteria and risk-based calculators may inadvertently exclude individuals who may be at heightened HIV risk based on network or community prevalence, intimate partner violence, criminal justice involvement, or partner characteristics rather than personal behavioral attributes; this has been seen in studies of PrEP eligibility in cisgender women of color and young Black MSM (Adams et al., 2021; Calabrese et al., 2019; Lancki et al., 2018). The IAS-USA guidelines recommend against using specific criteria or screening tools to determine eligibility (Gandhi et al., 2023). One simple, nonstigmatizing and non-judgmental question is: "Are you interested in learning more about medications to prevent HIV?" Table 14.2 summarizes indications and key clinical points for current FDA-approved PrEP medication options.

PRESCRIBING PREP

Initiation of PrEP

At the time of PrEP initiation, clinicians should document the following:

- Absence of acute or chronic HIV
- Assessment of renal function: creatinine clearance (CrCl) should be ≥60 mL/min for TDF/FTC use; or ≥30 mL/min for TAF/FTC use
- Assessment of hepatitis B (HBV) status

To document the absence of acute or chronic HIV, the CDC recommends following algorithms shown in Figure 14.1 or Figure 14.2 (for people without vs. with recent antiretroviral prophylaxis use, respectively), with a negative test result documented within the week prior or day of PrEP initiation. Oral rapid HIV testing should not be used due to lower sensitivity for detecting HIV compared to blood-based tests. For individuals reporting signs or symptoms of acute HIV (or who had an exposure of significant clinical concern) within the previous 4 weeks, both an HIV RNA and HIV antigen/antibody (Ag/Ab) test should be done. HIV RNA and Ag/Ab co-testing is also recommended for anyone who has received PEP or oral PrEP within the previous 3 months, or injectable PrEP within the last 12 months, to most accurately determine baseline HIV status prior to PrEP initiation (CDC, 2021b).

When a person not on PrEP has a possible HIV exposure, U.S. guidelines recommend PEP initiation within 72 hours and continuation for 28 days (see PEP sections below) before transitioning to PrEP ("PEP to PrEP"), after confirming ongoing negative HIV status (CDC, 2021b). If the timing of the last possible exposure was more than 72 hours but less than 2–3 weeks prior (or is uncertain), and HIV cannot yet be confidently ruled out with available testing results, the risks and benefits of same-day PrEP should be weighed carefully. One strategy for individuals in this scenario who are asymptomatic and seeking PrEP is to provide a 30-day supply and close clinical and laboratory follow-up (i.e., repeat HIV Ag/Ab and RNA testing at 1 month); this strategy of same-day prescribing may improve PrEP uptake (Kamis et al., 2019) and is concordant with IAS-USA guidelines which recommend against delaying PrEP for individuals at ongoing risk of HIV (Gandhi et al., 2023).

Extra caution should be taken when considering long-acting injectable PrEP initiation if a person is potentially in the HIV testing "window period," as establishing a laboratory diagnosis of infection may be challenging once a person receives CAB-LA (see LEVI syndrome below). The optimal strategy for initiating PrEP in individuals with frequent, high-risk exposures who are consistently in the window or eclipse period for HIV testing is unclear and may contribute to PrEP underutilization in persons who inject drugs daily (Taylor et al., 2019).

PrEP Medication Options

Providers should consider multiple factors when deciding among different PrEP options with patients, including availability of population-specific safety and efficacy data; co-occurring conditions (e.g., hepatitis B, kidney disease, or osteopenia/osteoporosis) and co-medications; patient preference; availability; and cost. Daily TDF/FTC is the most commonly prescribed option and can be used by most adults and adolescents—further, a generic formulation is available, which makes it the most cost-effective option currently (Marcus et al., 2022). Event-driven TDF/FTC, daily TAF/FTC, and CAB-LA are additional options (CDC, 2021b) (Table 14.2).

PrEP Monitoring

Recommendations for baseline and follow-up laboratory testing and monitoring for various PrEP options are detailed in Table 14.2.

LEVI Syndrome

Regular and sensitive HIV testing has become critical with the advent of long-acting injectable PrEP, given emerging evidence regarding delayed HIV diagnoses with ongoing PrEP administration, concerns for HIV drug resistance development, and the characterization of long-acting early viral inhibition (LEVI) syndrome. First observed in HPTN 083/084, LEVI syndrome refers to altered HIV replication dynamics and immunologic responses seen when HIV is acquired despite on-time CAB-LA injections, or after recent CAB-LA administration (Eshleman et al., 2023 and 2022). In many

Table 14.2 SUMMARY OF FDA-APPROVED HIV PRE-EXPOSURE PROPHYLAXIS (PREP) MEDICATION OPTIONS FOR ADOLESCENTS AND ADULTS $\geq$35 KG

PrEP candidates include: Anyone requesting PrEP, has condomless anal and/or vaginal sex, injects drugs, recent STIs, or has partners with positive or unknown HIV status.

Medication	Tenofovir disoproxil fumarate (TDF) 300 mg *plus* emtricitabine (FTC) 200 mg (Co-formulation available as emtricitabine/tenofovir disoproxil fumarate or generic)	Tenofovir alafenamide (TAF) 25 mg plus emtricitabine (FTC) 200 mg (Co-formulation available as emtricitabine/ tenofovir alafenamide)	Long-acting injectable cabotegravir 600 mg (3 ml) injection (LA-CAB) (Co-formulation available as cabotegravir)
Indication	Preferred oral regimen for most PrEP candidates	Insufficient data for use with receptive vaginal exposures or injection drug use Alternative oral option for people with (or at risk for) kidney disease or osteopenia/osteoporosis who have insertive/ receptive anal sex	Alternative for people who prefer non-oral PrEP option, need to avoid tenofovir (i.e., people with kidney disease), and/or may have challenges adhering to regular oral medication schedule
Dosing and administration	1 tablet by mouth daily *or* 2-1-1 "on-demand" (2 tablets 2–24 hours before insertive or receptive anal sex, then 1 tablet 24 hours after the first 2-pill dose, and then 1 tablet again 24 hours after that)	1 tablet by mouth daily	Initial 2 "loading" doses administered as intramuscular (IM) injections 4 weeks apart, then "maintenance" (continuation) injections every 8 weeks; ventrogluteal site recommended, but dorsogluteal approach acceptable Oral lead-in (oral cabotegravir 30 mg daily) is optional, and may help assess medication tolerability.
Contra-indications	Absolute: Acute, "early" or chronic HIV infection; creatinine clearance less than 60 mL/min for TDF/FTC (or less than 30 mL/min for TAF/FTC) Caution: Hepatitis B with cirrhosis/transaminitis (close monitoring advised when discontinuing TDF/FTC or TAF/FTC due to concern for potential hepatitis flare); people at risk for kidney disease; osteoporosis or history of fragility fracture for TDF/FTC		Absolute: Unknown or positive HIV status; co-use of carbamazepine, oxcarbazepine, phenobarbital, phenytoin, rifampin, or rifapentine Caution: Co-use with certain anticonvulsants and antimycobacterial agents; severe renal impairment/end-stage kidney disease not yet on dialysis; presence of gluteal fillers/implants; taking anticoagulants or bleeding diathesis/ thrombocytopenia
Side effects	*Short-term*: Headache, nausea, diarrhea, and abdominal discomfort (symptoms usually resolve within few weeks with or without supportive measures). If tenofovir-associated renal impairment develops, kidney function often improves after medication discontinuation.		*More common*: Injection site reactions, diarrhea, headache, fever, fatigue, dizziness, nausea, and vomiting *Less common*: Hepatotoxicity, weight gain, depression, hypersensitivity reaction
Other considerations for initiation, missed doses, discontinuation	Limited data on time to efficacy/protection across all populations and types of exposures: refer to clinical trial study protocols, specific guidelines for additional detail. For MSM taking "on-demand" oral PrEP, an initial double-dose (2 pills) of TDF/FTC is thought to confer adequate protection within 24 hours. Continue daily dosing for 2 days after last exposure. For all other populations, protection is likely after 7 daily doses (and can be continued for 7 days after last exposure). Limited data on TAF/FTC: some experts anticipate likely protection after 7 daily doses (and can be continued for 7 days after last exposure).		Limited data on time to efficacy/protection: many experts anticipate likely effective within 7 days after initiation. See package insert for recommendations on missed or late doses, and refer to text on monitoring after discontinuation. Consider oral "bridge" with TDF/FTC or TAF/FTC as indicated.
Initiation visit	Evaluate for potential exposures within the last 72 hours and consider need for postexposure prophylaxis (PEP). *Evaluate readiness for PrEP initiation*: Build rapport; explore interest/motivation(s); offer information on efficacy, side effects, and monitoring; identify factors to support ongoing adherence; troubleshoot insurance coverage; establish plan for communicating refill and other needs, appointments, and general follow-up. *At every follow-up visit*: Assess refill need, support adherence, assess side effects, explore other interests regarding sexual wellness, review exposures (e.g., number of partners, anal/vaginal insertive/receptive exposures, condom use, substance use), affirm interest in continuing PrEP.		

(*continued*)

	Labs: HIV Ag/Ab ("4th generation" test), kidney function assessment (e.g., serum creatinine), site-specific gonorrhea/chlamydia, syphilis screening, HAV IgG, HBsAg, HBcAb (total), HBsAb, HCV Ab (with reflex RNA if available), and pregnancy test if indicated. For people starting FTC/TAF, obtain lipid panel. **Also obtain HIV-1 RNA if:** symptoms of acute HIV infection, history of oral PrEP or PEP within last 3 months, or history of long-acting injectable PrEP within last 12 months. Consider if recent exposure(s) of significant clinical concern. Counsel to return for repeat HIV testing if off PrEP for over 7 days and possible exposure.	**Labs:** HIV Ag/Ab ("4th generation" test) *and* HIV-1 RNA, site-specific gonorrhea/chlamydia, syphilis screening, pregnancy test (if indicated). Viral hepatitis serologies are also recommended to inform additional prevention interventions. Counsel on "tail" phase: once injections are discontinued, CAB-LA concentrations decrease over many months and preventive efficacy is no longer assured. Consider alternative HIV prevention options.
Follow-up visits	*After one month*: HIV Ag/Ab with or without HIV-1 RNA may be repeated if clinically indicated. *Every three months*: HIV Ab/Ag (also HIV-1 RNA if available/clinically indicated), site-specific GC/CT and syphilis screening, pregnancy and kidney function assessment[1] (as indicated) *Yearly*: HCV Ab (with reflex RNA if available) for people who inject drugs and people having receptive anal sex, lipid panel for people taking FTC/TAF *Discontinuation*: HIV Ab/Ag (also HIV-1 RNA if available/clinically indicated), site-specific GC/CT and syphilis screening, kidney function assessment	*After one month*: HIV Ag/Ab *and* HIV-1 RNA *Every two months*: HIV Ag/Ab *and* HIV-1 RNA, pregnancy test (as indicated) *Every four months*: Site-specific GC/CT and syphilis screening *Yearly*: HCV Ab (with reflex RNA if available) for people who inject drugs and people having receptive anal sex *Discontinuation*: HIV Ag/Ab and HIV-1 RNA, site-specific GC/CT and syphilis screening

Note: CDC recommends kidney function assessment every 6 months for people over 50 years of age, people with baseline creatinine clearance less than 90 mL/min, or other risk factors for kidney disease.

Source: Adapted from 2021 CDC/US Public Health Service Guidelines and 2022 IAS-USA Treatment and Prevention Guidelines.

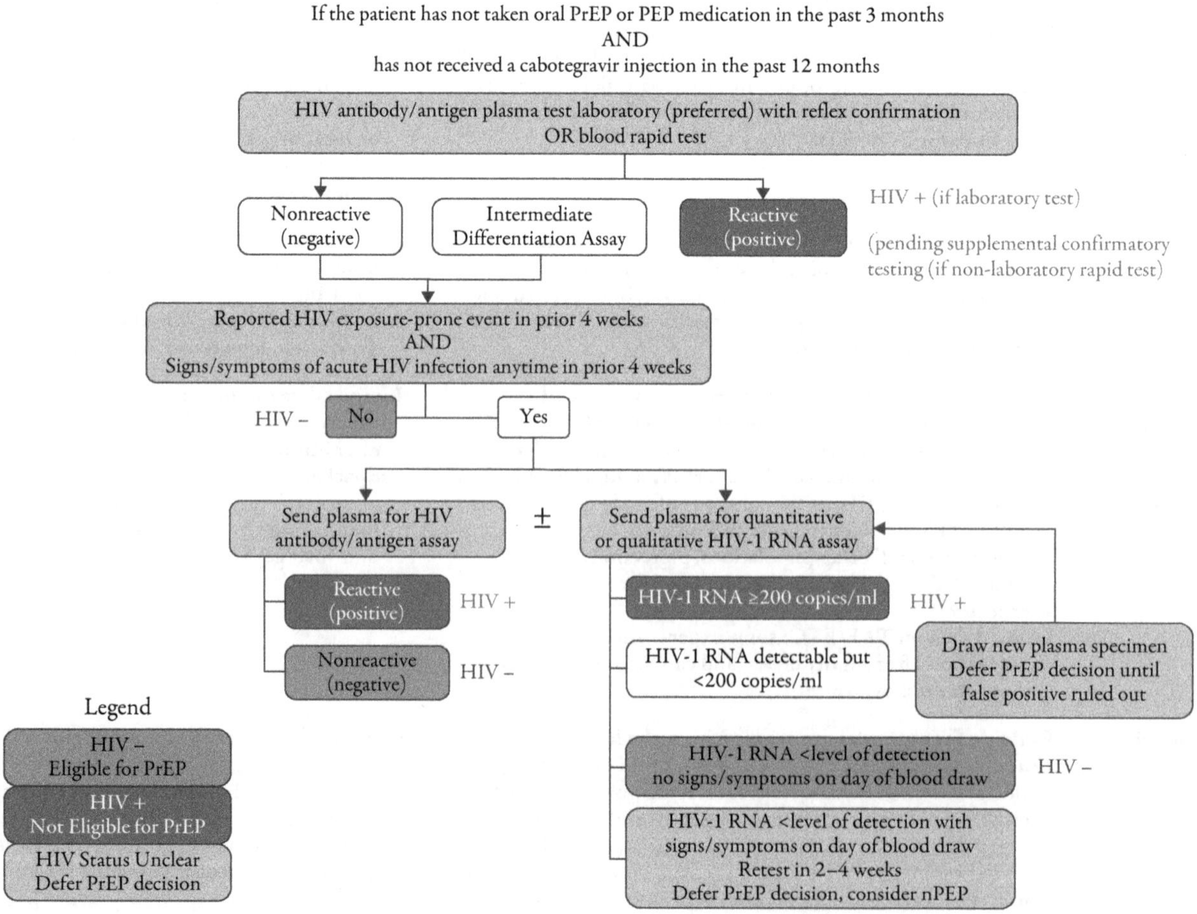

If the patient has not taken oral PrEP or PEP medication in the past 3 months
AND
has not received a cabotegravir injection in the past 12 months

HIV antibody/antigen plasma test laboratory (preferred) with reflex confirmation OR blood rapid test

Nonreactive (negative)
Intermediate Differentiation Assay
Reactive (positive)
HIV + (if laboratory test)
(pending supplemental confirmatory testing (if non-laboratory rapid test)

Reported HIV exposure-prone event in prior 4 weeks AND Signs/symptoms of acute HIV infection anytime in prior 4 weeks

HIV – No
Yes

Send plasma for HIV antibody/antigen assay
±
Send plasma for quantitative or qualitative HIV-1 RNA assay

Reactive (positive) HIV +
Nonreactive (negative) HIV –

HIV-1 RNA ≥200 copies/ml HIV +
HIV-1 RNA detectable but <200 copies/ml
Draw new plasma specimen Defer PrEP decision until false positive ruled out
HIV-1 RNA <level of detection no signs/symptoms on day of blood draw HIV –
HIV-1 RNA <level of detection with signs/symptoms on day of blood draw Retest in 2–4 weeks Defer PrEP decision, consider nPEP

Legend
HIV – Eligible for PrEP
HIV + Not Eligible for PrEP
HIV Status Unclear Defer PrEP decision

Figure 14.1 Assessment of HIV status prior to PrEP initiation: no recent antiretroviral prophylaxis use SOURCE: https://www.cdc.gov/hiv/pdf/risk/prep/cdc-hiv-prep-guidelines-2021.pdf, Figure 4a.

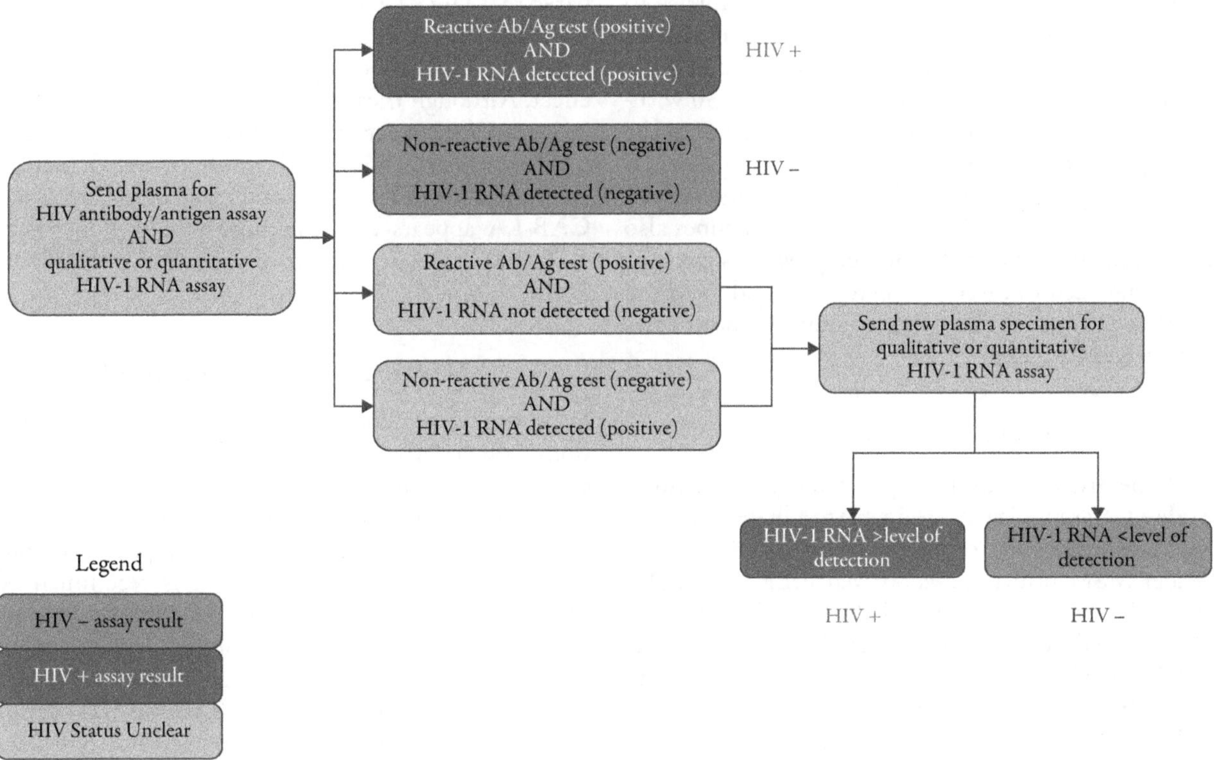

Figure 14.2 Assessment of HIV status prior to PrEP initiation: recent or current antiretroviral prophylaxis use. SOURCE: https://www.cdc.gov/hiv/pdf/risk/prep/cdc-hiv-prep-guidelines-2021.pdf, Figure 4b.

cases, viral replication was suppressed (including low or undetectable HIV DNA), antibody detection was diminished or delayed, and cases involved minimal or no clinical symptoms. This newly described syndrome contrasts starkly with the typical presentation of acute HIV, which generally occurs in the absence of recent/current antiretroviral (ARV) use and involves a classically symptomatic syndrome with high-level viremia and reliable pattern of testing results. In initial trials, previous testing algorithms initially failed to diagnose HIV for the majority of cases of HIV acquisition with recent CAB-LA administration. As a result, CAB-LA was inadvertently continued in many cases, and major integrase strand transfer inhibitor (INSTI) resistance was seen in most of these (Eshleman et al., 2023, 2022).

While indeterminate test results leading to late HIV diagnosis can occur with both oral and injectable PrEP, it seems to be more common with the latter, and has been associated with longer delays (Marzinke et al., 2021; Sivay et al., 2017). Therefore, combined HIV Ag/Ab and HIV viral load testing (e.g., either a qualitative or quantitative RNA) is recommended with every CAB-LA injection; repeat viral load should be strongly considered in the event of a detectable/positive monitoring viral load in order to differentiate true- vs. false-positive cases (CDC, 2021b; Ghandi et al., 2023; Landovitz et al., 2024). While CDC guidelines also recommend quarterly HIV Ag/Ab and HIV RNA for individuals on oral PrEP, it may be reasonable to consider utilizing RNA co-testing only in certain situations (e.g., PrEP discontinuations greater than 1 week in duration, use of on-demand dosing, symptoms of acute HIV infection). One recent study involving thousands of oral PrEP users showed 99.8% concordance between HIV Ag/Ab and RNA testing (Zhu et al., 2024).

PrEP Delivery Strategies

To improve PrEP access and persistence, several effective delivery strategies have been modeled, including same-day PrEP and PrEP via tele-health ("tele-PrEP") (Goedel et al., 2022; Kamis et al., 2019). The CDC guidelines include recommendations for PrEP management utilizing both models. New clusters of HIV among individuals experiencing homelessness and active substance use have also prompted programs to reimagine PrEP care, with a focus on "low-threshold" prescribing. Various strategies have been employed and appear to be successful for historically "harder to reach" populations: approaches include engagement outside of traditional clinic settings (e.g., syringe services programs, mobile outreach, low-barrier bridge programs, street/shelter-based services), intensive team-based PrEP outreach, and tailored prescribing (e.g., short-course PrEP prescriptions, provision of safe med storage, on-site pharmacies/medication delivery, and/or observed dosing) (Bazzi et al., 2023; Braun et al., 2022). Other promising strategies include text messaging/electronic reminders, patient navigation, provider training, and utilization of adjunct rapid/point-of-care HIV testing for PrEP initiation (Kamis et al., 2019; Siegler et al., 2020).

In 2022, the WHO called for PrEP de-medicalization and simplification in low- and middle-income countries to expand access and uptake. Its guidelines also simplified lab testing prior to initiation (e.g., allowing for deferral of baseline renal function testing in individuals under age 30 without comorbidities, and guidance to not withhold PrEP in the absence of hepatitis B and hepatitis C testing) and added HIV self-testing as an option for oral PrEP and dapivirine vaginal ring prescribing (WHO, 2022). International guidelines also support the development of differentiated programs globally, highlighting the need to diversify where, how, and to whom PrEP is delivered and emphasizing community-based and integrated, tailored services.

Discontinuing PrEP

PrEP should be discontinued in people who experience unacceptable side effects or toxicities, are unable to adhere to the prescribed regimen or follow-up care, or elect to discontinue PrEP. For cisgender MSM utilizing event-driven PrEP with TDF/FTC, it should be continued for two daily doses (i.e., 48 hours) after the last sexual exposure (Molina et al., 2017; Molina et al., 2019; WHO, 2019). For other exposure types/indications, various guidelines advise oral TDF/FTC PrEP continuation for 7–28 days after the last possible HIV exposure (USDHHS Perinatal Guidelines, 2024a; Rutstein et al., 2020). Data guiding TAF/FTC discontinuations are limited at this time.

Because CAB-LA levels remain significant for almost 1 year after the last injection, people who discontinue CAB-LA and may have ongoing exposures should be provided with oral PrEP for 12 months to reduce the risk of HIV drug resistance development during this "tail phase." Additionally, regular laboratory monitoring with HIV Ag/Ab and RNA testing is recommended during this time (CDC, 2021b; Landovitz et al., 2020).

OTHER CLINICAL CONCERNS RELATED TO PREP USE

TOLERABILITY AND ADVERSE EFFECTS

Oral PrEP (both TDF/FTC and TAF/FTC) is generally well tolerated, with less than 10% of users experiencing serious adverse events (CDC, 2021b; Ogbuagu et al., 2021). Common "start-up" side effects include nausea, headache, and weight loss. Most symptoms resolve within the first month and can usually be managed supportively. More serious potential oral PrEP toxicities include acute and/or chronic kidney injury and bone demineralization, which often resolve with medication discontinuation (Mulligan et al., 2015; Solomon et al., 2014). Compared to TDF/FTC, TAF/FTC was associated with more favorable and significant differences in bone mineral density and renal marker changes in the DISCOVER trial (Ogbuagu et al., 2021). However, participants receiving TAF/FTC experienced more weight gain and less favorable lipid changes; the long-term significance of these observations is unclear. In one cohort analysis, TAF/FTC was linked to increased hypertension diagnoses and statin initiation compared to TDF/FTC (Rivera et al., 2023).

CAB-LA is generally very well tolerated, with local injection site reactions being the most common reported side effect. Although these occur frequently (over 80% of HPTN 083 participants experienced injection site reactions), symptoms are typically mild, rarely result in CAB-LA discontinuation, and become less significant over time (Landovitz, 2020). CAB-LA appears to cause more weight gain compared to TDF/FTC (Delany-Moretlwe et al., 2022a; Landovitz et al., 2021).

MEDICATION INTERACTIONS

Drug-drug interactions between PrEP and other medications are relatively uncommon. Enzyme-inducing antiepileptic medications such as carbamazepine should not be administered with either TAF/FTC or CAB-LA. Use of the anti-tuberculous agent rifampicin is contraindicated with LA-CAB, and caution is recommended when coadministered with TAF/FTC. Before prescribing PrEP, clinicians should obtain a full list of all prescribed and over-the-counter medications and supplements. Multiple resources (e.g., the University of Liverpool's online HIV drug interaction checker) are available to help assess for possible interactions. Similarly, medications that may be administered during the "tail phase" of CAB-LA (~12 months) should be assessed for drug-drug interactions, given lingering cabotegravir concentrations (Landovitz et al., 2020).

BREAKTHROUGH HIV INFECTION AND HIV RESISTANCE AFTER PREP USE

Breakthrough HIV acquisition and ARV drug resistance with consistent use of oral PrEP is rare but has been reported, primarily because of transmitted drug resistance (Cohen et al., 2018; Colby et al., 2018; Knox et al., 2017; Markowitz et al., 2017; Spinelli et al., 2021; Thaden et al., 2018). Most cases occurred in people with undiagnosed HIV at the time of PrEP initiation, underscoring the importance of accurate baseline HIV testing and clinical assessment.

Incident HIV infections in people receiving CAB-LA remain extremely uncommon; however, a number of breakthrough infections have occurred in individuals receiving on-time injections and with high plasma cabotegravir concentrations (Landovitz et al., 2022; Landovitz et al., 2023). Unlike with oral PrEP, HIV drug resistance development has been observed in most of these cases, raising global concern given the central role that INSTIs play in treatment across both resource-limited and resource-rich settings (Landovitz et al., 2022; Landovitz et al., 2023; Marzinke et al., 2021). HIV acquisition within several months of last CAB-LA dose has been linked to ARV resistance development (Landovitz et al., 2023). Additionally, as with oral PrEP, breakthrough infections without ARV resistance were also observed in HPTN 083/084 in the setting of injectable PrEP initiation or missed/delayed injections (Eshelman et al., 2022; Marzinke et al., 2021). The possibility of breakthrough infections and subsequent risk of acquired HIV drug resistance underscores the need for highly sensitive assays that can identify HIV as early as possible, especially for people initiating and continuing CAB-LA.

Individuals who acquire HIV while taking oral or injectable PrEP should be transitioned to antiretroviral therapy (ART) in accordance with current treatment guidelines. Given the heightened concern for INSTI resistance, if HIV is diagnosed after receiving CAB-LA, darunavir-based ART should be utilized for rapid treatment initiation in this scenario until INSTI resistance can be ruled out (USDHHS, 2024b). Refer to Chapter 17 on "HIV Drug Resistance" for additional detail regarding ARV resistance in the context of PrEP use.

COINFECTIONS

STIs are commonly diagnosed among PrEP users. Care must be taken to ensure that concerns about increased rates of STIs or "risk compensation" are not used to justify withholding PrEP. Rather, the focus should turn toward promoting sexual health using shared decision-making based on individual preferences and priorities, regular STI screening and consideration of other STI prevention interventions, and engagement in care (Marcus et al., 2019). Sex-positive collaboration may include information sharing on doxycycline prophylaxis for STI prevention. For additional detail, refer to the Chapter 37, "Sexually Transmitted Infections."

Because tenofovir has dual antiviral activity against both HIV and HBV, testing for HBV prior to or concurrent with PrEP initiation is important to guide integrated counseling and HBV vaccination or treatment (as indicated) (CDC, 2021b; WHO 2022). Individuals with chronic hepatitis B, as evidenced by a reactive HBV surface antigen (HBsAg) test, should be evaluated by an HBV-treatment experienced clinician (CDC, 2021b). Persons with evidence of current (HBsAg reactive) or prior (HBcAb reactive) hepatitis B may receive oral PrEP but should be counseled on potential hepatic flares, HBV reactivation, and/or need for HBV treatment initiation should tenofovir-containing PrEP be abruptly discontinued without close monitoring. Quarterly laboratory monitoring with HBV DNA and liver function testing should be performed for 12 months after oral PrEP cessation (Mizushima et al., 2023; Mohareb et al., 2022; Solomon et al., 2016). On-demand TDF/FTC is not recommended by the CDC for individuals with chronic hepatitis B, and alternatives should be sought.

In the global context, expanding access to oral PrEP may help curb morbidity and mortality associated with the HBV-HIV syndemic. Contrary to U.S. guidance, the WHO supports use of both daily and event-driven tenofovir-based PrEP in individuals with HBV, in an effort to expand access to effective HIV prevention tools in significantly impacted populations (WHO, 2022). Real-world data support the use of both daily and on-demand oral tenofovir-based PrEP as an effective HBV prevention strategy in individuals without HIV (Mizushima et al., 2023). Cabotegravir does not have intrinsic anti-HBV activity; data are currently lacking on its safety in people with chronic HBV, although HBV is not a contraindication to its use.

PREGNANCY AND LACTATION

Providers should discuss PrEP with all sexually active individuals, including anyone trying to conceive, as well as pregnant, postpartum, or chestfeeding people first. PrEP should be offered to anyone who desires or is otherwise eligible (USDHHS, 2024a; USDHHSb). Currently, daily TDF/FTC is the only FDA-approved option validated for vaginal exposures and has been well-studied in peri-conception, pregnancy, and breastfeeding (in the context of HIV as well as HBV treatment) (USDHHS, 2024a). Completed PrEP efficacy trials to date did not enroll pregnant or breastfeeding individuals, and this evidence gap contributes to ongoing inequities in PrEP accessibility and uptake (Joseph Davey et al., 2022). Data from the Antiviral Pregnancy Registry demonstrate no evidence of harm to fetuses exposed to TDF/FTC (Antiretroviral Pregnancy Registry, 2024), and likewise, the use of TDF/FTC during lactation appears to be safe (USDHHS, 2024a; CDC, 2021b).

Although TAF/FTC is approved for use as part of combination HIV treatment in pregnant people with HIV, limited data exist on its use as PrEP in pregnancy (primarily from analyses of TAF/FTC for preventing HIV through vaginal sex in nonpregnant individuals). Currently, TAF/FTC is not recommended as a PrEP option for cisgender or pregnant women, although studies are ongoing (ClinicalTrials.gov.NCT05140954; ClinicalTrials.gov.NCT04994509 ("PURPOSE 1"); Joseph Davey et al., 2022). Similarly, information is limited on CAB-LA safety and efficacy in people who are pregnant or breastfeeding: data from HPTN 084 including participants in the open-label extension who became (or were) pregnant while receiving CAB-LA suggest that it is generally well-tolerated and safe in pregnancy (Delany-Moretlwe et al., 2022b; Delany-Moretlwe et al., 2024). CDC guidance supports patient-centered discussions around CAB-LA for PrEP in pregnancy, and initiation or continuation when benefits may outweigh risks or unknowns (CDC, 2021b).

PREP INEQUITIES

Since initial FDA approval, the number of individuals taking PrEP in the United States has increased, and this has likely contributed to overall declines in HIV incidence (CDC, 2024b; Sullivan et al., 2024). However, PrEP inequities persist, and populations with heightened HIV incidence (namely BIPOC and people in the Southern United States) are not seeing the utilization increases needed to mitigate disparities in HIV acquisition. While absolute rates of PrEP use in white and Black populations were similar by 2021, the PrEP-to-need ratio for white populations was much higher than for Black populations, with data showing much lower PrEP coverage among Black and African American individuals (Sullivan et al., 2024). Lower PrEP coverage has also been seen for U.S. Hispanic and Latino populations (Sullivan et al., 2024). By geography, PrEP-to-need ratios are highest in the Northeast and lowest in the South, where over half of new HIV diagnoses occurred in 2022 (CDC, 2024b; Sullivan et al., 2024). PrEP use is greatest among MSM and substantially lower among cisgender women and persons who inject drugs (Kuo et al., 2018; Mayer et al., 2018; Streed et al., 2022; Sullivan et al., 2024).

Of particular concern in the United States, inequitable PrEP distribution could worsen as a result of the 340B drug pricing system, which (paradoxically) promotes the use of more expensive and less accessible options over less expensive generic ones (Marcus et al., 2022), the end result being perpetuation of already stark inequities. Efforts to close these gaps must include individual and population-level strategies to address inequity-promoting factors, including internalized biases and structural racism. Increased capacity building (especially for clinicians serving communities of color), community-level education to promote awareness and reduce stigma, and inclusive public health campaigns may have an impact, as would ensuring equitable access to health care, insurance, and medication assistance programs (Kanny et al., 2019; Sullivan et al., 2024).

PREP CONSULTATION

Providers seeking clinical guidance on PrEP should contact local experts, if available. The National Clinician Consultation Center (nccc.ucsf.edu) offers free PrEP teleconsultation to U.S. providers: 1-(855) 448-7737 | 1-(855) HIV-PrEP.

PEP

Post-exposure prophylaxis (PEP) for HIV prevention is a pharmacotherapeutic intervention that takes advantage of the window of time it takes HIV to cross the mucosal barrier, begin viral replication, and establish infection. Ethical considerations have precluded conducting PEP efficacy trials, and data supporting its use are largely derived from animal models, inference from postnatal prophylaxis studies, observational studies, and an early retrospective case-control study showing an 81% reduction in HIV acquisition among healthcare workers who took postexposure zidovudine (Cardo et al., 1997; Lunding et al., 2015; Ogata-Aoki et al., 2018; Otten et al., 2000; Shih et al., 1991; Young et al., 2007). Along with a scientific understanding of HIV viral kinetics, these studies have laid the foundation for the recommendation to initiate PEP urgently after possible exposure, ideally within 24 hours (and at most within 72 hours), and to continue it for 28 days. U.S. occupational and nonoccupational PEP guidelines were updated in 2013 and 2016, respectively, by the CDC/U.S. Public Health Service (Dominguez et al., 2016; Kuhar et al., 2013). Recent guidance for occupational and nonoccupational exposures was published by the New York State Department of Health AIDS Institute (DeHaan et al., 2022), and WHO published guidelines in 2024 (WHO, 2024). See Box 14.1.

Box 14.1 GENERAL PEP PRINCIPLES

- People who experience a potential HIV exposure should seek urgent medical evaluation; when indicated, PEP should be started as soon as possible and within 72 hours from the time of exposure.
- HIV status of the source individual should be determined, when possible, to guide the need for PEP initiation and/or continuation.
- PEP initiation, if indicated, should not be delayed while awaiting HIV or other baseline testing from the exposed or source individual, or while awaiting expert consultation.
- Recommended PEP regimens include three oral antiretroviral medications taken for 28 days; initial provision of a complete 28-day PEP course is recommended to improve completion rates.
- Close follow-up services, including counseling, repeat HIV testing, and medication monitoring, should be provided. HIV follow-up testing should be done at 4–6 weeks and 3–4 months (if using a combination HIV antigen/antibody test).

OCCUPATIONAL EXPOSURES

The use of ART to prevent HIV acquisition for healthcare personnel experiencing significant occupational exposure was first recommended in 1990. Occupational exposures encompass penetrating injuries (predominantly sharps or percutaneous needlesticks) and splash injuries to mucus membranes and/or nonintact skin. The likelihood of HIV acquisition appears to be related to viral inoculum size, which is in turn influenced by clinical status of the source person with HIV and quantity of blood/infectious fluid involved (Kuhar et al., 2013).

For occupational exposures (where the source is more often identified and potentially available), timely source person testing is important to guide decisions around whether to initiate and/or continue PEP. If the source's HIV status is unknown, consent should be obtained for testing; if source HIV status is confirmed negative, PEP should be discontinued. If source HIV Ag/Ab testing is negative, but they had an exposure to HIV in the prior 4 weeks, source HIV RNA should also be obtained and PEP should be continued until the RNA returns negative. It is important to note that there have been no reported cases of occupational HIV transmission due to source persons in the window period (Kuhar et al., 2013).

If the source is known to be a person with HIV, oPEP initiation is generally recommended—if possible, information on the source person's most recent viral load, current and prior ART and resistance history, and prescriber information should be obtained. It is unknown whether oPEP needs to be continued for exposures where the source person's HIV viral load is undetectable. Given the well-established evidence base supporting "U = U" for sexual exposures, some groups (e.g., British HIV Association) do not recommend

Table 14.3 EXPOSURES SCENARIOS TO CONSIDER POSTEXPOSURE PROPHYLAXIS (PEP) INITIATION

Higher likelihood of HIV acquisition—**PEP initiation generally recommended**	**Receptive or insertive vaginal or anal sex with a source person with HIV not known to be virologically suppressed on ART[1]** **Needle sharing with a partner who is a person with HIV.** **Penetrating sharps injury involving blood or other potentially infectious material (e.g., needlestick involving device recently placed in blood vessel, or is visibly bloody) from a source known to be a person with HIV.** **Mucosal contact (mouth, nose, eyes) or nonintact skin (e.g., open wound/abrasion) involving blood, visibly bloody fluid, or other potentially infectious material (e.g., semen, vaginal fluid) from a source known to be a person with HIV.** **Sexual assault involving mucosal-to-mucosal contact, or mucosal or broken-skin contact to potentially infectious body fluid. If history is limited or cannot be obtained during sexual assault evaluation (including pediatric cases), PEP is recommended if any physical evidence of sexual abuse.**
Lower or unknown likelihood of HIV acquisition—**Case-by-case assessment and shared decision-making recommended**	**Exposure of any type where the source person's HIV status is unknown[2]** **Exposure of any type involving exposed persons consistently on PrEP**
No likelihood of HIV acquisition—**PEP initiation not warranted**	**Kissing** **Human bites not involving blood** **Mutual masturbation without skin breakdown or blood exposure** **Oral-to-oral contact without mucosal damage or visible blood (e.g., mouth-to-mouth resuscitation)** **Exposure to solid-bore needles or sharps *not* in recent contact with blood/infectious material[3]**

Notes: [1] Given robust evidence regarding "U = U," if the source is *known* to be virologically suppressed on ART, then PEP is unlikely to confer additional benefit; however, it *may be initiated* while awaiting confirmation of the source person's recent viral load and subsequently discontinued once confirmed.

[2] The NYSDOH guidelines consider exposure to a source person with unknown HIV status as a "higher-risk" scenario; CDC guidelines recommend a case-by-case determination regarding PEP use in this scenario.

[3] HIV is intolerant of environmental exposure to air, and the likelihood of HIV acquisition from community-based needle stick injuries (e.g., discarded or "found" needles) is extremely low. There have been no documented transmissions through community needle sticks and PEP is generally not recommended in these scenarios.

Source: Adapted from 2016 and 2013 CDC/US Public Health Service Guidelines and 2022 New York State Department of Health guidelines.

oPEP when the source person's viral load is confirmed to be undetectable at the time of exposure. Debate remains as to whether oPEP should be initiated when the source person's HIV status is unknown: while New York State DOH guidelines recommend its use in this scenario, U.S. national guidelines recommend expert consultation, and British guidelines generally recommend against it. Given these differing recommendations, we recommend that an informed, shared decision-making framework be employed so that exposed persons can identify the course of action most consistent with their goals and values. Table 14.3 reviews general PEP initiation recommendations for various exposure scenarios.

NONOCCUPATIONAL EXPOSURES

Nonoccupational exposures encompass consensual sex, sexual assault, needle sharing, penetrating injuries (sharps or percutaneous needlesticks), bites with blood exposure, and mucosal/splash injuries. Careful clinical assessment of the exposure is critical, as nPEP initiation is generally only indicated for scenarios where there is higher likelihood for HIV acquisition (Table 14.3); these include when the source is known to be a person with HIV, and on a case-by-case basis when source HIV status is unknown (DeHaan et al., 2022). New York State DOH guidance suggests focusing on the nature of the exposure and recommends PEP for all higher-risk exposures whether the source person's HIV status is unknown or known to be positive; this includes exposures from receptive and insertive vaginal or anal intercourse, needle sharing, penetrating injury, or bites with visible bleeding in the mouth that causes bleeding in the exposed individual (DeHaan et al., 2022).

U.S.-based guidelines recommend against using geography, the residence of the exposed individual, or the perceived or assumed source person's "risk behavior" to guide PEP initiation (DeHaan et al., 2022). British guidelines recommend assessing not only the nature of the exposure, but also the likelihood of the source having HIV with detectable viremia, ART use, and susceptibility of the exposed individual (i.e., presence of ulcerative genital disease in sexual exposures) (Cresswell et al., 2022). British recommendations to initiate PEP are based on a calculated risk of transmission dependent on the known prevalence of HIV viremia in a specific risk group multiplied by the risk of transmission based on the type of exposure—this varies greatly from U.S. guidelines. Of note, British guidelines were developed based on UK-specific population-level data analyzed by risk, gender, race, and location and in the context of a largely diagnosed, treated, and virally suppressed national population, which is not globally generalizable (Cresswell et al., 2022).

While basic principles of PEP initiation and prescribing largely overlap between nonoccupational and occupational exposures, there are several specific considerations for nonoccupational exposures:

- Providers and patients should consider future exposures, with attention to a timely transition to PrEP especially if ongoing HIV exposures are anticipated after PEP completion. Offering a 1-month supply of PrEP to start immediately after PEP completion ("PEP to PrEP") has been shown to be efficacious in increasing subsequent PrEP uptake (Cockbain and Whitlock, 2022).
- For consensual sexual exposures, baseline evaluation should include HIV testing, site-specific gonorrhea and chlamydia testing, syphilis screening, and pregnancy testing (if indicated).
- For sexual assault victims, while baseline HIV testing is indicated, other STI testing can be offered but should not be routinely collected, except in situations of pediatric assault. This is because some victims are at increased risk of repetitive assault, and STI results may subsequently enter bias into court proceedings (DeHaan et al., 2022).
- Other considerations for sexual assault victims include consideration of PEP if there is any mucosal-to-mucosal contact (including oral-penile), or mucosal or broken-skin contact to infectious body fluids, as apparent or occult physical trauma and bleeding are common (DeHaan et al., 2022).
- PEP is not generally indicated for exposed individuals consistently adherent to oral or injectable PrEP; for patients who are only taking PrEP sporadically, particularly if oral PrEP was not taken in the week prior to exposure, nPEP may be indicated (CDC, 2021b).
- For consensual sexual exposures, given the evidence behind "U = U," PEP is not recommended when the source person is known to be living with HIV and is consistently on ART with a confirmed undetectable viral load (Cresswell et al., 2022; DeHaan et al., 2022).

RECOMMENDED PEP REGIMENS

PEP regimens should be convenient, with minimal side effects and drug interactions, to support medication continuation and adherence. For most adults and adolescents, U.S. as well as international guidelines generally prefer TDF/FTC together with an integrase strand transfer inhibitor (INSTI) (Table 14.4). Because INSTI medications act prior to HIV integration with cellular DNA, they provide a theoretical advantage over alternative regimens. Further, a growing body of data from clinical practice support the use of complete single-tablet regimens (STR) for PEP, demonstrating high tolerability, low discontinuation rates, and no HIV seroconversions during the follow-up period (Gan et al., 2024; Gantner et al., 2020; Foster et al., 2015; Malinverni et al., 2021; Mayer et al., 2017; Mayer et al., 2022, Tan et al., 2024). Accordingly, various guidelines now include STR options for PEP (EACS, 2023; Gandhi et al., 2023;). In light of this, we recommend a combination of co-formulated TXF (i.e., TDF or TAF) plus XTC (i.e., FTC or 3TC) with a second-generation INSTI as PEP for most individuals.

Traditional methods of PEP service delivery require that exposed persons present to care within 72 hours after a potential HIV exposure and, depending on the institution, follow up with a different provider to attain a full 28-day supply of medication if this was not provided initially. Such practices create barriers to PEP initiation and completion. PEP in pocket (PIP) is an emerging strategy wherein persons who may have future exposures are given a full, 28-day prescription of PEP to self-initiate after a potential exposure—this approach may be especially useful for people with infrequent and/or unanticipated exposures. People prescribed PIP benefit from low-barrier, immediate access to PEP when needed, and should be advised to seek appropriate follow-up if PIP is initiated. Early studies of PIP have demonstrated high levels of acceptability with high rates of appropriate use (89%) and no cases of inappropriate non-use after high-risk exposures (Rashotte et al., 2024). Additionally, offering PIP may increase both PEP and subsequent PrEP uptake, as observed

Table 14.4 **POSTEXPOSURE PROPHYLAXIS (PEP) REGIMENS FOR MOST ADULT AND ADOLESCENT EXPOSED PERSONS***

DUAL NUCLEOSIDE/NUCLEOTIDE REVERSE TRANSCRIPTASE INHIBITOR (NRTI) "BACKBONE"	ANTIRETROVIRAL (ARV) "ANCHOR"
Tenofovir disoproxil fumarate 300 mg/emtricitabine 200 mg (TDF/FTC) one tablet by mouth once daily *or* **Tenofovir disoproxil fumarate 300 mg/lamivudine 300 mg (TDF/3TC) one tablet by mouth once daily** *or* **Tenofovir alafenamide 25 mg/emtricitabine 200 mg (TAF/FTC) one tablet by mouth once daily** ***PLUS one of the following recommended or alternative "anchor" ARV agents (see next column)***	*Recommended*: **Dolutegravir (DTG) 50 mg one tablet by mouth once daily** *or* **Bictegravir (BIC) 50 mg one tablet by mouth once daily** *Alternative*: **Raltegravir (RAL) 400 mg one tablet by mouth twice daily** *or* **Raltegravir HD (RAL HD) 1200 mg one tablet by mouth once daily** *or* **Elvitegravir/cobicistat (EVG/cobi) available as co-formulation with both FTC/TDF and FTC/TAF**

* Refer to product package inserts for specific age/weight, kidney function, and pregnancy/breastfeeding considerations. The majority of ARVs listed are safe during periconception and in pregnancy unless noted. For people with kidney impairment, NRTI dose adjustment may be advised.

by the SEARCH Dynamic Choice HIV Prevention trials in Kenya and Uganda (Ayieko et al., 2024). To date, no HIV seroconversions have been documented in patients using this method (Alghamdi et al., 2020; Billick et al., 2023; Rashotte et al., 2024). Due to its novelty, PIP has not yet entered most state or national PEP guidelines.

BASELINE TESTING AND MONITORING

For all exposures, recommended baseline testing of the exposed individual includes laboratory-based HIV Ag/Ab testing; hepatitis B and C serologies; and (if indicated) renal and liver function assessment and pregnancy testing. For consensual sexual exposures, additional baseline testing should include syphilis and site-directed STI screening; STI testing can be offered but should not be routinely performed for sexual assault exposures, as results may instill bias in future potential court proceedings (DeHaan et al., 2022).

All hepatitis B–susceptible individuals with possible exposure to hepatitis B (source with confirmed hepatitis B infection or unknown status) should initiate the hepatitis B vaccine series within 24 hours. Individuals without immunity who are exposed to someone with known acute or chronic HBV should also receive hepatitis B immune globulin. Currently, PEP for hepatitis C is not recommended or approved for occupational or nonoccupational exposures (Moorman et al., 2020). In cases of sexual assault, a first dose of HPV vaccine should be administered, and exposed individuals should be offered empiric STI treatment (DeHaan et al., 2022). Emergency contraception should be offered for sexual exposures if the exposed person is of childbearing potential.

Follow-up HIV testing includes HIV Ag/Ab at 4–6 weeks and again at 3–4 months. While laboratory-based testing is preferred because of improved sensitivity, some guidelines indicate that point-of-care HIV Ag/Ab tests may be used for follow-up testing (DeHaan et al., 2022). For people with potential exposure to HCV, newer guidelines emphasize early follow-up with HCV NAT for earlier detection (DeHaan et al., 2022; Moorman et al., 2020). See Table 14.5 for detailed testing and monitoring recommendations.

SPECIAL PEP CONSIDERATIONS

- The combination of DTG or RAL, taken with TDF/FTC (or either TAF/FTC or TDF/3TC), is safe in pregnancy and in persons of childbearing potential. BIC/TAF/FTC is currently considered an alternative option for HIV treatment in pregnant people with HIV; its use as PEP in pregnancy remains limited at this time. Although available data suggest it is safe, providers should engage in shared decision-making before prescribing it as PEP for people who are pregnant or of childbearing potential.
- For exposed individuals who are breastfeeding, person-centered counseling and shared decision-making should be utilized, including discussions of the potential risks and benefits of continued breastfeeding (with or without PEP) and tailored clinical and laboratory follow-up. Limited data preclude the ability to develop standardized recommendations; additional options include temporary interruption of breastfeeding (with pumping and storing or discarding in the interim) until early repeat HIV testing can be completed to facilitate reassessment, or complete weaning. Factors that should be considered include source person HIV status and availability for testing; nature of the exposure; review of breastfeeding-associated transmission (acute infection with high level viremia confers elevated risk); infant age; whether or not breastfeeding is well established; and feasibility/desirability of other infant feeding options.
- If exposed individuals are found to have hepatitis B at the time of baseline exposure assessment, they should be linked to/followed by a provider with HBV management and treatment experience to determine whether anti-HBV therapy should be continued after PEP completion. Until this assessment occurs, TXF/XTC continuation should be considered, as medication discontinuation may inadvertently lead to hepatic flares.
- PEP duration may need to extend beyond 28 days if the exposed person is subsequently found to have an indeterminate HIV test result or experiences symptoms suggestive of acute retroviral syndrome/acute HIV infection during follow-up. If the exposed individual is pregnant or breastfeeding, careful monitoring/testing and ARV management are warranted.
- Expert consultation is recommended in various scenarios (Table 14.6).

VOLUNTARY MEDICAL MALE CIRCUMCISION

The presence of penile foreskin may facilitate sexual HIV acquisition as a result of low-grade inflammation and resultant dysbiosis (Cohen et al., 2019a). Three large, randomized trials in sub-Saharan Africa demonstrated that voluntary circumcision led to an approximate 50% risk reduction for heterosexual HIV acquisition (Auvert et al., 2005; Bailey et al., 2007; Gray et al., 2007; Siegfried et al., 2009). This benefit did not appear to extend to female partners of circumcised men with HIV (Weiss et al., 2009). Based on observational data, circumcision may benefit MSM who practice primarily insertive anal sex, especially in low- and middle-income countries (Yuan et al., 2019). Data for individuals having receptive anal sex is lacking, and there have been no randomized trials examining this: thus, a population-level benefit among MSM has not been proven. Regardless, voluntary medical male circumcision (VMMC) remains a critical evidence-based strategy for adolescent boys and cisgender men engaging in heterosexual sex in areas of high HIV transmission rates (primarily sub-Saharan Africa) as recommended by the WHO and UNAIDS since 2007 (WHO, 2020). The WHO's 2020

Table 14.5 RECOMMENDED SERVICES INCLUDING COUNSELING, LABORATORY MONITORING, AND OTHER CLINICAL MANAGEMENT AFTER EXPOSURE TO SOURCE WITH KNOWN OR UNKNOWN HIV STATUS

TIME FROM EXPOSURE	RECOMMENDED SERVICES	
	COUNSELING	LABORATORY TESTING AND MANAGEMENT
Baseline	Transmission prevention: condom use, avoidance of blood/tissue donation, etc. Sexual assault: ensure close follow-up care including support from crisis counselor or outreach worker Recommended clinical and laboratory monitoring People initiating PEP: potential side effects, adherence, drug interactions	HIV Ag/Ab testing For persons without documented vaccine-induced immunity: hepatitis B surface antigen (HBsAg), hepatitis B total core antibody (HBcAb), and hepatitis B surface Ab (HBsAb). All hepatitis B-susceptible persons with possible exposure to hepatitis B (source with confirmed hepatitis B infection or unknown status) should initiate hepatitis B vaccine series. Individuals without immunity who are exposed to someone with known acute or chronic HBV should also receive hepatitis B immune globulin. Hepatitis C antibody (HCV Ab) with reflex to RNA if available If sexual exposure: site-specific gonorrhea and chlamydia testing, syphilis, pregnancy test (if indicated). In cases of adults presenting after sexual assault, baseline STI screening may be offered but is not routinely required; offer empiric STI treatment, HPV vaccination, and emergency contraception. If initiating PEP: kidney function and pregnancy testing (if indicated)
24–48 hours (may be conducted by telephone)	If available, review additional information about exposure or source person to guide PEP continuation (if initiated) and other follow-up Behavioral support and transmission prevention People taking PEP: side effects, adherence, drug interactions	
2 weeks (may be conducted by telephone)	People taking PEP: side effects, adherence, drug interactions Recommended clinical and early laboratory monitoring Transmission prevention	If taking PEP and baseline testing identified laboratory abnormalities, or person is experiencing adverse effects: repeat laboratory testing as indicated
4–6 weeks	Recommended clinical and final laboratory monitoring Transmission prevention For people with ongoing exposures or interest in PrEP: counsel on PEP to PrEP transition options, testing, and timing	HIV Ag/Ab testing If source person has known HCV infection or unknown status: HCV RNA If sexual exposure: consider repeat STI screening Pregnancy testing (if indicated)
3–4 months	Recommended clinical and final laboratory monitoring Transmission prevention For people with ongoing exposures or interest in PrEP: counsel on PEP to PrEP transition options, testing, and timing	HIV Ag/Ab testing (if negative, HIV acquisition from the initial exposure can be excluded with a high degree of confidence) If exposed person was hepatitis B-susceptible at baseline: repeat HBsAg and HBcAb[1] If source person has known HCV infection or unknown status: HCV Ab at 4–6 months

Note: [1]HBsAb may also be obtained 1–2 months *after* completion of vaccination series, to demonstrate immunity. For persons who received HBIG, defer testing until anti-HBs from HBIG are no longer detectable (i.e., 6 months).

Source: Adapted from 2016 and 2013 CDC/US Public Health Service Guidelines and 2022 New York State Department of Health guidelines.

update on VMMC continues to not recommend circumcision specifically for MSM, given the paucity of high-quality data, but states that MSM should not be excluded in settings where VMMC programs are active for HIV prevention (WHO, 2020). In the United States, VMMC is not recommended broadly as an HIV prevention intervention, and decisions should be based on individualized discussions incorporating population-specific data, individual behaviors, and potential procedural risks (CDC, 2024a).

NEW AND INVESTIGATIONAL INTERVENTIONS FOR HIV PREVENTION

NOVEL PREP ANTIRETROVIRALS AND DELIVERY METHODS

Ongoing active investigation of alternate delivery methods and novel ARVs promises to further expand HIV prevention options. Studies are underway for a once-weekly pill,

Table 14.6 SCENARIOS IN WHICH EXPERT PEP CONSULTATION IS RECOMMENDED*

SCENARIO	CONSIDERATIONS
Delayed (i.e., later than 72 hours) exposure report	If timing of last exposure involving higher likelihood of HIV acquisition occurred over 72 hours ago (or is uncertain), and HIV cannot be confidently ruled out with immediate testing
Unknown identity of source person (e.g., needle in sharps disposal container)	Determine PEP use on a case-by-case basis: consider severity of exposure and other relevant factors. Do not test needles or other sharp instruments for HIV.
Known or possible pregnancy in the exposed individual, or exposed individual is breastfeeding	PEP should not be delayed while awaiting expert consultation; medication selection and care plan may be adjusted (as indicated) after consultation.
Source has known or suspected ARV drug resistant HIV or current/historical ART failure	PEP should not be delayed while awaiting HIV resistance testing results or history; PEP regimen may be adjusted as indicated after consultation.
Significant adverse side effects, toxicity, or drug-drug interactions with PEP medications.	Symptoms (e.g., gastrointestinal symptoms, headache) are often manageable without modifying PEP regimen—providers can offer analgesics, antimotility, and antiemetic agents as indicated. Significant underlying health condition (e.g., kidney disease) or polypharmacy may increase risk of medication-associated toxicity, drug-drug interactions, and need for ARV dose-adjustment or alternative PEP regimen.

* Consultation can be sought with local experts; the National Clinician Consultation Center (nccc.ucsf.edu) offers free postexposure prophylaxis teleconsultation to U.S. providers: 1-(888)-448-4911.

Source: Adapted from 2013 CDC/US Public Health Service Guidelines and 2022 New York State Department of Health guidelines.

additional long-acting injectable options, and sustained-release implants that may provide long-acting coverage.

Lenacapavir (LEN), a capsid inhibitor that acts across multiple stages of the HIV life cycle, is in phase 3 clinical trials as a 6-month subcutaneous injection for PrEP, hoping to expand options to adolescent girls and young women (PURPOSE 1; Clinicaltrials.gov.NCT04994509) as well as men (cisgender, transgender, and nonbinary individuals) who have sex with men and transgender women (PURPOSE 2; Clinicaltrials.gov. NCT04925752). Recent results from an interim analysis of PURPOSE-1 data revealed 100% efficacy, with zero incident infections in participants randomized to receive LEN compared to 16 infections in participants receiving TDF/FTC and 39 in participants receiving TAF/FTC. Importantly, there was no statistically significant difference in HIV incidence between the TDF/FTC and TAF/FTC arms. However, incidence in the TAF/FTC arm was not statistically superior to background incidence (Bekker et al., 2024). Closer analyses of PURPOSE 1 data, including medication adherence details, are needed to determine whether TAF/FTC may be effective for people having receptive vaginal sex. Studies of islatravir (a novel nucleoside reverse transcriptase translocation inhibitor) as PrEP were initially promising but have been discontinued because of safety concerns. Other investigational PrEP options actively being explored include a long-acting, in situ forming implant of CAB (Massud et al., 2022; Young et al., 2023).

MICROBICIDES

Microbicides are products applied locally to the vaginal or rectal mucosa to reduce risk of STI/HIV acquisition and may be especially acceptable as behaviorally congruent alternatives to condom use and/or oral PrEP/PEP (Bauermeister et al., 2023). The use of microbicides or other local drug-delivery devices, such as vaginal rings, have several potential benefits. First, they deliver high concentrations of a drug to the desired tissue with minimal systemic exposure (Hendrix et al., 2013) and can thus potentially provide on-demand protection. Many products are also targeted toward cisgender women, a group disproportionately excluded from many ART and PrEP trials (but who comprise almost half of new HIV transmissions globally) (UNAIDS, 2023). These options may be used discretely, can potentially be co-formulated with other medications such as contraceptives, and importantly, may be highly acceptable to some users. This was particularly well illustrated in the REACH trial: after a period of use of each product, 67% of adolescents and young women chose the once-monthly dapivirine vaginal ring over once-daily oral PrEP, with fewer than 5% of visits during the choice period showing no-low adherence (Ngure et al., 2022).

Tenofovir gel as a vaginal microbicide has been extensively studied with mixed results, with greatest protection seen in women with high adherence (Abdool Karim et al., 2010). Given low rates of adherence to this method across multiple trials, as well as concerns that efficacy may be impacted by vaginal dysbiosis or inflammation, it is no longer under active investigation (Abdool Karim et al., 2022). Rectal tenofovir gel in MSM and transwomen is under investigation, and has been shown to be safe and acceptable in early-stage trials (Cranston et al., 2017). Single-dose tenofovir rectal douche (DREAM-01 trial, Clinicaltrials.gov.NCT02750540) has been shown to achieve colorectal antiviral concentrations exceeding oral TDF (Weld et al., 2024). Pre-clinical trials of on-demand TAF/elvitegravir vaginal (CONRAD-128, Clinicaltrials.gov.NCT03762772) and rectal (MTN-039, Clinicialtrials.gov.NCT04047420) inserts have proven to be safe and efficacious, and display clinical PK/PD profiles compatible with HIV protection (Riddler et al., 2023; Thurman et al., 2023).

MULTIPURPOSE PREVENTION TECHNOLOGIES (MPT)

Options integrating contraception and HIV/STI prevention into single combined agents, or multipurpose prevention technology (MPT), have led to significant optimism for expanded choice in women's sexual and reproductive health. Building on already approved and marketed products, the "Dual Prevention Pill" (DPP, a co-formulated combined oral contraceptive once-daily pill with TDF/FTC) may be the first MPT available in the ensuing years (Friedland et al., 2021). A trial to assess DPP acceptability, adherence, and preference compared to 2-pill regimens is currently underway (Friedland et al., 2024). The 28-day dapivirine (DPV) vaginal ring is already recommended by the WHO as a stand-alone microbicidal option for HIV prevention for cisgender women (WHO, 2021). In phase 1 trials, 90-day combined dapivirine-levonorgestrel (DPV/LNG) rings have been shown to be safe, well tolerated, and capable of achieving cervical and plasma DPV concentrations exceeding that of single-agent rings while also providing LNG plasma concentrations comparable to other efficacious contraceptives (Achilles et al., 2024). Similarly, the phase 2a CONRAD-128 study showed that a 90-day continuous use tenofovir-levonorgestrel (TFV/LNG) ring was safe, with adequate protective levels of both medication components (Mugo et al., 2021). Building upon this work, the phase 2a CONRAD-144 study demonstrated similar safety and tolerability, and that both TFV/LGN and single agent tenofovir rings achieved cervical vaginal tenofovir levels suggesting anti-HSV-2 activity—adding to the multipurpose utility of this intervention (Mugo et al., 2023). Long-acting cabotegravir/levonorgestrel (CAB/LNG) injectables and pellet implants are under preclinical investigation. Many other MPTs for HIV prevention, including intravaginal films, gels, and patches using antiviral, microbicide, and monoclonal antibody platforms, are in varying stages of development (MPT Product Development Database).

VACCINES AND BROADLY NEUTRALIZING ANTIBODIES

Multiple challenges, both biomedical and social, have impeded development of an effective HIV vaccine. These include HIV diversity and pathogenesis, difficulty in generating broadly neutralizing antibodies, identification of appropriate immune correlates of protection, community preparedness and concerns about vaccine-induced positivity, and expanded PrEP use (Hammer, 2015). With the exception of the modestly positive Thai vaccine trial RV 144, which demonstrated a 31% reduction in incident HIV among recipients, clinical trials of HIV vaccines have largely been disappointing.

Nevertheless, the pursuit of an effective vaccine remains relevant. Even with widespread ART availability and pharmacologic HIV prevention methods, an effective vaccine is essential to effectively address the global HIV epidemic (Fauci, 2017). The ability of a vaccine to elicit broadly neutralizing antibodies (bNAbs, antibodies that can protect against multiple pathogenic HIV strains by binding to highly conserved regions of the virus) is crucial but thus far has been elusive. Recent advances in the identification and understanding of bNAbs have injected new hope into HIV prevention research. While two randomized trials of VRC01, a bNAb targeting the HIV-1 CD4 binding site, did not show broad benefit when administered as infusions, there was a reduction in HIV incidence of HRC01-sensitive HIV-1 isolates, supporting a proof-of-concept that bNAbs can be effective tools for HIV prevention (Corey et al., 2021). While there are no current vaccine candidates in clinical trials, contemporary vaccine development efforts are directed toward novel approaches to induce bNAb production, such as B-cell lineage vaccine design, germline-targeting vaccine design, and epitope-focused vaccine design; as well as toward novel vaccine delivery methods (including use of CMV vectors and heterologous viral vector vaccination, both of which appear to promote strong T-cell mediated immune responses) as well as mRNA mediated vaccine delivery similar to that used for COVID-19 (Nkolola, 2024).

RECOMMENDED READING

Bowleg L, Malekzadeh AN, Mbaba M, Boone CA. Ending the HIV epidemic for all, not just some: structural racism as a fundamental but overlooked social-structural determinant of the US HIV epidemic. *Curr Opin HIV AIDS*. 2022;17(2):40–45.

Gamarel KE, King WM, Operario D. Behavioral and social interventions to promote optimal HIV prevention and care continua outcomes in the United States. *Curr Opin HIV AIDS*. 2022;17(2):65–71.

Girometti N, Delpech V, McCormack S, et al. The success of HIV combination prevention: the Dean Street model. *HIV Med*. 2021;22(10):892–897.

Joseph Davey DL, Bekker LG, Bukusi EA, et al. Where are the pregnant and breastfeeding women in new pre-exposure prophylaxis trials? The imperative to overcome the evidence gap. *Lancet HIV*. 2022 Mar;9(3):e214–e222.

Krakower DS, Daskalakis DC, Feinberg J, Marcus JL. Tenofovir alafenamide for HIV preexposure prophylaxis: what can we DISCOVER about its true value? *Ann Intern Med*. 2020;172(4):281–282. http://doi:10.7326/M19-3337

Marcus JL, Killelea A, Krakower DS. Perverse incentives: HIV prevention and the 340B drug pricing program. *N Engl J Med*. June 2022;386(22):2064–2066.

Perlman D, Jordan AE. The syndemic of opioid misuse, overdose, HCV, and HIV: structural-level causes and interventions. *Current HIV/AIDS Reports*. 2018;15:96–112.

Sullivan PS, DuBose SN, Castel AD, et al. Equity of PrEP uptake by race, ethnicity, sex and region in the United States in the first decade of PrEP: a population-based analysis. *Lancet Reg Health Am*. 2024;33:100738.

CONCLUSION

Tremendous strides continue to be made in the vast field of HIV prevention. Although much attention has focused on ART-based interventions such as treatment as prevention and PrEP, implementation in real-world practice and population health program experiences continue to raise important questions for clinical care delivery across varied resource landscapes, many of which remain unanswered. Ongoing disparities in access, uptake, and persistence of many prevention interventions threaten to exacerbate existing disparities in HIV outcomes. HIV providers are important champions in addressing bias and structural factors driving inequities. Ultimately, a multifaceted approach including behavioral, structural, and established biomedical interventions is necessary to end the global HIV epidemic.

REFERENCES

Abdool Karim Q, Abdool Karim SS, Frohlich JA, et al. Effectiveness and safety of tenofovir gel, an antiretroviral microbicide, for the prevention of HIV infection in women. *Science*. 2010;329(5996):1168–1174.

Abdool Karim SS, Baxter C, Abdool Karim Q. Advancing HIV prevention using tenofovir-based pre-exposure prophylaxis. *Antiviral Therapy*. 2022;27(2):13596535211067589. doi:10.1177/13596535211067589

Achilles SL, Kelly CW, Hoesley CJ, et al.; MTN-030/IPM 041 and MTN-044/IPM 053/CCN019 Protocol Teams for the Microbicide Trials Network and the Contraceptive Clinical Trials Network. Phase 1 randomized trials to assess safety, pharmacokinetics, and vaginal bleeding associated with use of extended duration dapivirine and levonorgestrel vaginal rings. *PLoS One*. 2024;19(6):e0304552.

Adams JW, Khan MR, Bessey SE, et al. Preexposure prophylaxis strategies for African-American women affected by mass incarceration. *AIDS*. 2021;35(3):453-462.

Aidala AA, Wilson MG, Shubert V, et al. Housing status, medical care, and health outcomes among people living with HIV/AIDS: a systematic review. *Am J Public Health*. 2015;106:e1–e23.

Alexander KA, Mpundu G, Duroseau B, et al. Intervention approaches to address intimate partner violence and HIV: a scoping review of recent research. *Curr HIV/AIDS Rep*. 2023;20(5):296–311.

Alghamdi A, Hempel A, Heendeniya A, Clifford-Rashotte M, Tan DHS, Bogoch II. HIV postexposure prophylaxis-in-pocket: long-term follow-up of individuals with low-frequency, high-risk HIV exposures. *AIDS*. 2020;34(3):433–437.

Antiretroviral Pregnancy Registry Steering Committee. *Antiretroviral Pregnancy Registry Interim Report for January 1, 1989 Through January 31, 2024*. Wilmington, NC: Registry Coordinating Center; 2024. www.APRegistry.com. Accessed July 13, 2024.

Antoni G, Tremblay C, Delaugerre C, et al. On-demand pre-exposure prophylaxis with tenofovir disoproxil fumarate plus emtricitabine among men who have sex with men with less frequent sexual intercourse: a post-hoc analysis of the ANRS IPERGAY trial. *Lancet HIV*. 2020;7(2):e113–e120.

Auvert B, Taljaard D, Lagarde E, et al. Randomized, controlled intervention trial of male circumcision for reduction of HIV infection risk: the ANRS 1265 trial. *PLoS Med*. 2005;2(11):e298.

Ayala G, Sprague L, van der Merwe LL, et al. Peer- and community-led responses to HIV: a scoping review. *PLoS One*. 2021;16(12):e0260555.

Ayieko J, Balzer L, Kakande E, et al. Uptake and predictors of PEP uptake in the SEARCH Dynamic Choice HIV Prevention trials. Abstract 1135. Conference on Retroviruses and Opportunistic Infections, March 3–6, 2024.

Baeten JM, Donnell D, Ndase P, et al. Antiretroviral prophylaxis for HIV prevention in heterosexual men and women. *N Engl J Med*. 2012;367:399–410.

Baeten JM, Palanee-Phillips T, Brown ER; MTN-020–ASPIRE Study Team. Use of a vaginal ring containing dapivirine for HIV-1 prevention in women. *N Engl J Med*. 2016;375(22):2121–2132.

Baggaley R, Boily M-C, White RG, et al. Risk of HIV-1 transmission for parenteral exposure and blood transfusion: a systematic review and meta-analysis. *AIDS*. 2006;20(6):805–812.

Bailey RC, Moses S, Parker CB, et al. Male circumcision for HIV prevention in young men in Kisumu, Kenya: a randomizedd controlled trial. *Lancet*. 2007;369:643.

Bauermeister JA, Dominguez Islas C, Jiao Y, et al; MTN-035 Protocol Team. A randomized trial of safety, acceptability and adherence of three rectal microbicide placebo formulations among young sexual and gender minorities who engage in receptive anal intercourse (MTN-035). *PLoS One*. 2023;18(4):e0284339.

Bazzi AR, Shaw LC, Biello KB, et al. Patient and provider perspectives on a novel, low-threshold HIV PrEP program for people who inject drugs experiencing homelessness. *J Gen Intern Med*. 2023;38(4):913–921.

Bekerman E, Cox S, Babusis D, et al. Two-dose emtricitabine/tenofovir alafenamide plus bictegravir prophylaxis protects macaques against SHIV infection. *J Antimicrob Chemother*. 2021;76(3):692–698.

Bekker L-G, Das M, Abdool Karim Q, et al; PURPOSE 1 Study Team. Twice-yearly lenacapavir or daily F/TAF for HIV prevention in cisgender women. *N Engl J Med*. 2024. doi:10.1056/NEJMoa2407001

Belenko S, Visher C, Pearson F, et al. Efficacy of structured organizational change intervention on HIV testing in correctional facilities. *AIDS Educ Prev*. 2017;29(3):241–255.

Berry MS, Johnson MW. Does being drunk or high cause HIV sexual risk behavior? A systematic review of drug administration studies. *Pharmacol Biochem Behav*. 2018;164:125–138.

Bhushan NL, Stoner MCD, Groves AK, Kahn K, Pettifor AE. Partnership dynamics and HIV-related sexual behaviors among adolescent mothers in South Africa: a longitudinal analysis of HIV Prevention Trials Network 068 data. *J Adolesc Health*. 2022;71(1):63–69.

Biello KM, Bazzi AT, Mimiaga MJ, et al. Perspectives on HIV pre-exposure prophylaxis (PrEP) utilization and related intervention needs among people who inject drugs. *Harm Reduct J*. 2018;15(1):55.

Billick MJ, Fisher KN, Myers S, Tan DHS, Bogoch II. Brief report: outcomes of individuals using HIV postexposure prophylaxis-in-pocket ("PIP") for low-frequency, high-risk exposures in Toronto, Canada. *J Acquir Immune Defic Syndr*. 2023;94(3):211–213.

Bloch EM. Deferral of men who have sex with men from blood donation: policy and change. *Transfus Clin Biol*. 2022;29(3):195–197.

Bowleg L, Malekzadeh AN, Mbaba M, Boone CA. Ending the HIV epidemic for all, not just some: structural racism as a fundamental but overlooked social-structural determinant of the US HIV epidemic. *Curr Opin HIV AIDS*. 2022;17(2):40–45.

Braun HM, Walter C, Farrell N, Biello KB, Taylor JL. HIV exposure prophylaxis delivery in a low-barrier substance use disorder bridge clinic during a local HIV outbreak at the onset of the COVID-19 pandemic. *J Addict Med*. 2022;16(6):678–683.

Brawner BM, Kerr J, Castle BF, et al. A systematic review of neighborhood-level influences on HIV vulnerability. *AIDS Behav*. 2022;26(3):874–934.

Broz D, Carnes N, Chapin-Bardales J, et al. Syringe services programs' role in ending the HIV epidemic in the U.S.: why we cannot do it without them. *Am J Prev Med*. 2021;61(5 Suppl 1):S118–S129.

Busch MP. Four decades of HIV and transfusion safety: much accomplished but ongoing challenges. *Transfusion*. 2022;62(7):1334–1339.

Calabrese SK, Willie TC, Galvao RW, et al. Current US guidelines for prescribing HIV pre-exposure prophylaxis (PrEP) disqualify many women who are at risk and motivated to use PrEP. *J Acquir Immune Defic Syndr*. 2019;81(4):395–405.

Cardo DM, Culver DH, Ciesielski CA, et al.; Centers for Disease Control and Prevention Needlestick Surveillance Group. A case control study of HIV seroconversion in health care workers after percutaneous exposure. *N Engl J Med*. 1997;337(21):1485–1490.

CDC. Announcing the launch of Together TakeMeHome. https://www.cdc.gov/nchhstp/director-letters/launch-of-together-takemehome.html. Published 2023. Accessed July 15, 2024.

CDC. Effectiveness of prevention strategies to reduce the risk of acquiring or transmitting HIV. cdc.gov. https://www.cdc.gov/hiv/risk/

estimates/preventionstrategies.html. June 17, 2022a. Accessed July 10, 2024.
CDC. Male circumcision for HIV prevention fact sheet. cdc.gov. https://www.cdc.gov/nchhstp-newsroom/factsheets/male-circumcision-for-hiv-prevention.html. March 6, 2024a. Accessed July 21, 2024.
CDC. Monitoring selected national HIV prevention and care objectives by using HIV surveillance data—United States and 6 territories and freely associated states, 2022. HIV Surveillance Supplemental Report 2024; 29(No. 2). https://www.cdc.gov/hivdata/nhss/national-hiv-prevention-and-care-outcomes.html. Published May 2024b. Accessed 11 July 2024.
CDC. Self-testing. cdc.gov. https://www.cdc.gov/hiv/effective-interventions/diagnose/hiv-self-testing/index.html. July 31, 2021a (last reviewed June 26, 2023). Accessed July 21, 2024.CDC. US Public Health Service: preexposure prophylaxis for the prevention of HIV infection in the United States—2021 update: a clinical practice guideline. cdc.gov. https://www.cdc.gov/hiv/pdf/risk/prep/cdc-hiv-prep-guidelines-2021.pdf. Published December 2021b. Accessed 11 July 2024.
Chang JJ, Ashcraft AM. Human immunodeficiency virus in adolescents: risk, prevention, screening, and treatment. *Prim Care.* 2020;47(2):351–365.
Choopanya K, Martin M, Suntharasamai P, et al. Antiretroviral prophylaxis for HIV infection in injecting drug users in Bangkok, Thailand (the Bangkok Tenofovir Study): a randomised, double-blind, placebo-controlled phase 3 trial. *Lancet.* 2013;381:2083–2090. https://clinicaltrials.gov/ct2/show/NCT03762772. Accessed August 31, 2024.
Cockbain B, Whitlock G; Dean Street Collaborative Group. Immediate PrEP when accessing PEP: a service evaluation. *HIV Med.* 2022;23(10):1108–1112. doi:10.1111/hiv.13310
Cohen MS, Council OD, Chen, JS. Sexually transmitted infections and HIV in the era of antiretroviral treatment and prevention: the biologic basis for epidemiologic synergy. *J Int AIDS Soc.* 2019a;22(S6):e25355.
Cohen SE, Sachdev D, Lee SA, et al. Acquisition of tenofovir-susceptible, emtricitabine-resistant HIV despite high adherence to daily pre-exposure prophylaxis: a case report [published online ahead of print, 2018 Nov 29]. *Lancet HIV.* 2018;S2352–3018(18)30288–1. doi:10.1016/S2352-3018(18)30288-1
Cohen YZ, Butler AL, Millard K, et al. Safety, pharmacokinetics, and immunogenicity of the combination of the broadly neutralizing anti-HIV-1 antibodies 3BNC117 and 10-1074 in healthy adults: a randomized, phase 1 study. *PLoS One.* 2019;14(8):e0219142.
Colby DJ, Kroon E, Sacdalan C, et al. Acquisition of multidrug-resistant human immunodeficiency virus type 1 infection in a patient taking preexposure prophylaxis. *Clin Infect Dis.* 2018;67(6):962–964.
Corey L, Gilbert P, Juraska M, et al. Two randomized trials of neutralizing antibodies to prevent HIV-1 acquisition. *N Engl J Med.* 2021;18;384(11):1003–1014.
Cranston RD, Lama JR, Richardson BA, et al. MTN-017: a rectal phase 2 extended safety and acceptability study of tenofovir reduced-glycerin 1% gel. *Clin Infect Dis.* 2017;64(5):614–620.
Cresswell F, Asanati K, Bhagani S, et al.; British HIV Association. UK guideline for the use of HIV post-exposure prophylaxis 2021. https://www.bhiva.org/file/6183b6aa93a4e/PEP-guidelines.pdf. Published February 14, 2022; 2023 amendment. Accessed August 31, 2024.
Custer B, Quiner C, Haaland R, et al. HIV antiretroviral therapy and prevention use in US blood donors: a new blood safety concern. *Blood.* 2020;136(11):1351–1358.
Decker MR, Lyons C, Guan K, et al. A systematic review of gender-based violence prevention and response interventions for HIV key populations: female sex workers, men who have sex with men, and people who inject drugs. *Trauma Violence Abuse.* 2022;23(2):676–694.
DeHaan E, McGowan JP, Fine SM, et al.; New York State Department of Health AIDS Institute Medical Care Criteria Committee. *Post-Exposure Prophylaxis (PEP) to Prevent HIV Infection.* Baltimore, MD: Johns Hopkins University; August 11, 2022 (last reviewed/updated April 17, 2023). https://cdn.hivguidelines.org/wp-content/uploads/20230417131815/NYSDOH-AI-PEP-to-Prevent-HIV-Infection_4-17-2023_HG.pdf. Accessed July 21, 2024.
Delany-Moretlwe S, Hughes JP, Bock P, et al. Cabotegravir for the prevention of HIV-1 in women: results from HPTN 084, a phase 3, randomized clinical trial. *Lancet.* 2022a;399(10337):1779–1789.
Delany-Moretlwe S, Hughes JP, Guo X, et al. Evaluation of CAB-LA safety and PK in pregnant women in the blinded phase of HPTN 084. Abstract 700. Conference on Retroviruses and Opportunistic Infections. Virtual; February 12–16, 2022b.
Delany-Moretlwe S, Voldal E, Saidi F, et al. Initial evaluation of injectable cabotegravir (CAB-LA) safety during pregnancy in the HPTN 084 open-label extension. International AIDS Conference. Munich, Germany; July 22–26, 2024.
Del Rio C. How do we stop the band from playing on in the US? Abstract 61. Conference on Retroviruses and Opportunistic Infections. Boston, MA; March 8–11, 2020.
DiNenno EA, Delaney KP, Pitasi MA, et al. HIV testing before and during the COVID-19 pandemic—United States, 2019–2020. *MMWR.* 2022;71(25):820–824.
Dimitrov D, Moore JR, Wood D, et al. Predicted effectiveness of daily and nondaily preexposure prophylaxis for men who have sex with men based on sex and pill-taking patterns from the Human Immuno Virus Prevention Trials Network 067/ADAPT study. *Clin Infect Dis.* 2020;71(2):249–255. http://doi:10.1093/cid/ciz799
Dominguez K, Smith DK, Vasavi T, et al. Updated guidelines for antiretroviral postexposure prophylaxis after sexual, injection drug use, or other non-occupational exposure to HIV—United States, 2016. US Centers for Disease Control and Prevention. http://stacks.cdc.gov/view/cdc/38856. Published May 23, 2018. Accessed August 31, 2024.
Donnell D, Ramos E, Celum C, et al. The effect of oral preexposure prophylaxis on the progression of HIV-1 seroconversion. *AIDS.* 2017;31(14):2007–2016.
EACS Guidelines version 12.0, October 2023. https://www.eacsociety.org/media/guidelines-12.0.pdf. Accessed July 27, 2024.
Eastment MC, McClelland RS. Vaginal microbiota and susceptibility to HIV. *AIDS.* 2018;32(6):687–698.
Elkbuli A, Polcz V, Dowd B, et al. HIV prevention intervention for substance users: a review of the literature. *Subst Abuse Treat Prev Policy.* 2019;14(1):1.
Eshleman SH, Fogel JM, Piwowar-Manning E, et al. Characterization of human immunodeficiency virus (HIV) infections in women who received injectable cabotegravir or tenofovir disoproxil fumarate/emtricitabine for HIV prevention: HPTN 084. *J Infect Dis.* May 16, 2022;225(10):1741–1749.
Eshleman SH, Fogel JM, Piwowar-Manning E, et al. The LEVI Syndrome: characteristics of early HIV infections with cabotegravir for PrEP. Abstract 160. Conference on Retroviruses and Opportunistic Infections. February 19–22, 2023. Seattle, WA.
Faddy HM, Osiowy C, Custer B, et al; Virology and Surveillance; Risk Assessment and Policy subgroups of the ISBT Working Party on Transfusion-Transmitted Infectious Diseases. International review of blood donation nucleic acid amplification testing. *Vox Sang.* 2024;119(4):315–325.
Fauci AS. An HIV vaccine is essential for ending the HIV/AIDS pandemic. *JAMA.* October 24, 2017;318(16):1535–1536. http://doi:10.1001/jama.2017.13505
Foster R, McAllister J, Read TR, et al. Single-tablet emtricitabine-rilpivirine-tenofovir as HIV postexposure prophylaxis in men who have sex with men. *Clin Infect Dis.* 2015 Oct 15;61(8):1336–1341.
Friedland BA, Mathur S, Haddad LB. The promise of the dual prevention pill: a framework for development and introduction. *Front Reprod Health.* 2021;3:682689. http://doi:10.3389/frph.2021.682689
Friedland BA, Mgodi NM, Palanee-Phillips T, et al. Assessing the acceptability of, adherence to and preference for a dual prevention pill (DPP) for HIV and pregnancy prevention compared to oral pre-exposure prophylaxis (PrEP) and oral contraception taken separately: protocols for two randomised, controlled, cross-over studies in South Africa and Zimbabwe. *BMJ Open.* 2024;14(3):e075381.
Fu R, Hou J, Gu Y, Yu NX. Do couple-based interventions show larger effects in promoting HIV preventive behaviors than individualized

interventions in couples? A systematic review and meta-analysis of 11 randomized controlled trials. *AIDS Behav.* 2023;27(1):314–334.

Gan L, Xie X, Fu Y, et al. Safety and adherence of bictegravir/emtricitabine/tenofovir alafenamide for HIV post-exposure prophylaxis among adults in Guiyang China: a prospective cohort study. *BMC Infect Dis.* 2024;24(1):565.

Gandhi RT, Bedimo R, Hoy JF, et al. Antiretroviral drugs for treatment and prevention of HIV infection in adults: 2022 recommendations of the International Antiviral Society-USA Panel. *JAMA.* 2023;329(1):63–84.

Gantner P, Hessamfar M, Souala MF, et al.; E/C/F/TAF PEP Study Group. Elvitegravir-cobicistat-emtricitabine-tenofovir alafenamide single-tablet regimen for human immunodeficiency virus postexposure prophylaxis. *Clin Infect Dis.* 2020 Feb 14;70(5):943–946.

Garcia J, Parker C, Parker RG, et al. "You're really gonna kick us all out?" Sustaining safe spaces for community-based HIV prevention and control among Black men who have sex with men. *PLoS One.* 2015;10(10):e0141326.

Goedel WC, Rogers BG, Li Y, et al. Pre-exposure prophylaxis discontinuation during the COVID-19 pandemic among men who have sex with men in a multisite clinical cohort in the United States. *J Acquir Immune Defic Syndr.* 2022 Oct 1;91(2):151–156.

Grant RM, Lama JR, Anderson PL, et al. Preexposure chemoprophylaxis for HIV prevention in men who have sex with men. *N Engl J Med.* 2010;363:2587–2599.

Gray RH, Kigozi G, Serwadda D, et al. Male circumcision for HIV prevention in men in Rakai, Uganda: a randomised trial. *Lancet.* 2007;369:657–666.

Hammer SM. Advances in preventive HIV vaccines: efficacy trial evolution [Oral session 0021]. ID Week 2015. San Diego, CA; October 7–11, 2015.

Harrison SE, Muessig K, Poteat T, et al. Addressing racism's role in the US HIV epidemic: qualitative findings from three Ending the HIV Epidemic prevention projects. *J Acquir Immune Defic Syndr.* 2022;90(S1):S46–S55.

Hendrix CW, Chen BA, Guddera V, et al. MTN-001: randomized pharmacokinetic cross-over study comparing tenofovir vaginal gel and oral tablets in vaginal tissue and other compartments. *PLoS One.* 2013;8(1):e55013.

Herrera C, Serwanga J, Else L, et al.; CHAPS. Dose finding study for on-demand HIV pre-exposure prophylaxis for insertive sex in sub-Saharan Africa: results from the CHAPS open label randomised controlled trial. EBioMedicine. 2023;93:104648.

Hoenigl M, Chaillon A, Moore DJ, et al. Clear links between starting methamphetamine and increasing sexual risk behavior: a cohort study among men who have sex with men. *J AIDS.* 2016;71(5):551–557.

Hong C, Huh D, Schnall R, et al. Changes in high-risk sexual behavior, HIV and other STI testing, and PrEP use during the COVID-19 pandemic in a longitudinal cohort of adolescent men who have sex with men 13 to 18 years old in the United States. *AIDS Behav.* 2023;27(4):1133–1139.

Ibitoye M, Lappen H, Freeman R, et al. Technology-based interventions to increase point-of-care HIV testing and linkage to care among youth in the US: a systematic review. *AIDS Behav.* 2021;25(6):1829–1838.

Ickowicz S, Hayashi K, Dong H, et al. Benzodiazepine use as an independent risk factor for HIV infection in a Canadian setting. *Drug Alcohol Depend.* 2015;155:190–194.

Iroh PA, Mayo H, Nijhawan AE. The HIV care cascade before, during, and after incarceration: a systematic review and data synthesis. *Am J Public Health.* 2015;105(7):e5–e16.

Ivey K, Bernstein KT, Kirkcaldy RD. Chemsex drug use among a national sample of sexually active men who have sex with men: American Men's Internet Survey, 2017–2020. *Subst Use Misuse.* 2023;58(5):728–734.

Jackson KJ, Chitle P, McCoy SI, White DAE, et al. A systematic review of HIV pre-exposure prophylaxis (PrEP) implementation in US emergency departments: patient screening, prescribing, and linkage to care. *J Community Health.* 2024;49(3):499–513.

Jones J, Knox J, Meanley S, et al. Explorations of the role of digital technology in HIV-related implementation research: case comparisons of five Ending the HIV Epidemic supplement awards. *J Acquir Immune Defic Syndr.* 2022;90(S1):S226–S234.

Joseph Davey DL, Bekker LG, Bukusi EA, et al. Where are the pregnant and breastfeeding women in new pre-exposure prophylaxis trials? The imperative to overcome the evidence gap. *Lancet HIV.* March 2022;9(3):e214–e222.

Kamis KF, Marx GE, Scott KA, et al. Same-day HIV pre-exposure prophylaxis (PrEP) initiation during drop-in sexually transmitted diseases clinic appointments is a highly acceptable, feasible, and safe model that engages individuals at risk for HIV into PrEP care. *Open Forum Infect Dis.* 2019;6(7):ofz310.

Kanny D, Jeffries WL IV, Chapin-Bardales J, et al. Racial/ethnic disparities in HIV preexposure prophylaxis among men who have sex with men—23 urban areas, 2017. *MMWR.* 2019;68:801–806.

Khan MR, McGinnis KA, Grov C, et al. Past year and prior incarceration and HIV transmission risk among HIV-positive men who have sex with men in the US. *AIDS Care.* 2019;31(3):349–356.

Knox DC, Anderson PL, et al. Multidrug-resistant HIV-1 infection despite preexposure prophylaxis. *N Engl J Med.* 2017;376:501–502.

Kuhar DT, Henderson DK, Struble KA, et al. Updated USPHS guidelines for the management of occupational exposures to human immunodeficiency virus and recommendations for post-exposure prophylaxis. *Infect Control Hosp Epidemiol.* 2013;34(9):875–892.

Kuo I, Agopian A, Opoku J, et al. Assessing PrEP needs among heterosexuals and people who inject drugs, Washington, DC. Abstract 1030. Conference on Retroviruses and Opportunistic Infection. Boston, MA; March 4–7, 2018.

Lancki N, Almirol E, Alon L, et al. Preexposure prophylaxis guidelines have low sensitivity for identifying seroconverters in a sample of young Black MSM in Chicago. *AIDS.* 2018;32 (3):383–392.

Landovitz RJ, Donnell D, Clement ME, et al. Cabotegravir for HIV prevention in cisgender men and transgender women. *N Engl J Med.* 2021;385(7):595–608.

Landovitz RJ, Donnell D, Tran H, et al. Updated efficacy, safety, and case studies in HPTN 083: CAB-LA vsTDF/FTC for PrEP. Abstract 96. Conference on Retroviruses and Opportunistic Infections. Virtual; February 12–16, 2022.

Landovitz RJ, Gao F, Fogel JM, et al.; HPTN 083 Study Team. Performance characteristics of HIV RNA screening with long-acting injectable cabotegravir (CAB-LA) pre-exposure prophylaxis (PrEP) in the multicenter global HIV Prevention Trials Network 083 (HPTN 083) Study. International AIDS Conference. Munich, Germany; July 22–26, 2024.

Landovitz RJ, Hanscom B, Clement M, et al. Efficacy and safety of long-acting cabotegravir compared with daily oral tenofovir disoproxil fumarate plus emtricitabine to prevent HIV infection in cisgender men and transgender women who have sex with men 1 year after study unblinding: a secondary analysis of the phase 2b and 3 HPTN 083 randomised controlled trial. *Lancet HIV.* 2023;10:e767–778.

Landovitz RJ, Li S, Eron JJ Jr, et al. Tail-phase safety, tolerability, and pharmacokinetics of long-acting injectable cabotegravir in HIV-uninfected adults: a secondary analysis of the HPTN 077 trial. *Lancet HIV.* 2020 Jul;7(7):e472–e481.

Leblanc J, Custer B, Van de Laar T, et al. HIV pre-exposure prophylaxis, blood donor deferral, occult infection, and risk of HIV transmission by transfusion: a fine balance between evidence-based donor selection criteria and transfusion safety. *Transfus Med Rev.* 2023;37 (3):150754.

Lee JJ, Verdugo JL, Xiao AY, Vo K. Digital interventions to enhance PrEP update and adherence through stigma reduction. *Curr HIV/AIDS Rep.* 2023;20 (6):458–469.

Lee K, Trujillo L, Olansky E, et al. Factors associated with use of HIV prevention and health care among transgender women—seven urban areas, 2019–2020. *MMWR.* 2022;71(20):673–679.

Lunding S, Katzenstein TL, Kronborg G, et al. The Danish PEP Registry: experience with the use of post-exposure prophylaxis following blood exposure to HIV from 1999–2012. *Infect Dis (Lond).* 2016;48(3):195–200. doi:10.3109/23744235.2015.1103896

Lyons MS, Chawarski MC, Rothman R, et al. Missed opportunities for HIV and hepatitis C screening among emergency department patients with untreated opioid use disorder. *J Addict Med.* 2023;17(2):210–214.

Malekinejad M, Jimsheleishvili S, Barker EK, et al. Sexual practice changes post-HIV diagnosis among men who have sex with men in the United States: a systematic review and meta-analysis. *AIDS Behav.* 2023;27(1):257–278.

Malinverni S, Bédoret F, Bartiaux M, et al. Single-tablet regimen of emtricitabine/tenofovir disoproxil fumarate plus cobicistat-boosted elvitegravir increase adherence for HIV postexposure prophylaxis in sexual assault victims. *Sex Transm Infect.* 2021;97(5):329–333. http://doi:10.1136/sextrans-2020-054714

Malone J, Reisner SL, Cooney EE, et al. Perceived HIV acquisition risk and low uptake of PrEP among a cohort of transgender women with PrEP indication in the Eastern and Southern United States. *J Acquir Immune Defic Syndr.* 2021;88(1):10–18.

Maloney KM, Benkeser D, Sullivan PS, et al. Sexual mixing by HIV status and pre-exposure prophylaxis use among men who have sex with men: addressing information bias. *Epidemiology.* 2022;33(6):808–811.

Maloney KM, Bratcher A, Wilkerson R, Sullivan PS, et al. Electronic and other new media technology interventions for HIV care and prevention: a systematic review. *J Int AIDS Soc.* 2020;23(1):e25439.

Mann LM, Kelley CF, Siegler AJ, Stephenson R, Sullivan PS. Seroadaptive strategy patterns of young black gay, bisexual, and other men who have sex with men in Atlanta, Georgia. *J Acquir Immune Defic Syndr.* 2022;89(1):40–48.

Marcus JL, Hurley LB, Nguyen DP, et al. Redefining human immunodeficiency virus (HIV) preexposure prophylaxis failures. *Clin Infect Dis.* 2017;65(10):1768–1769.

Marcus JL, Katz KA, Krakower DS, Calabrese SK. Risk compensation and clinical decision making: the case of HIV preexposure prophylaxis. *N Engl J Med.* 2019;380(6):510–512.

Marcus JL, Killelea A, Krakower DS. Perverse incentives: HIV prevention and the 340B Drug Pricing Program. *N Engl J Med.* 2022;386(22):2064–2066.

Markowitz M, Grossman H, Anderson PL, et al. Newly acquired infection with multidrug-resistant HIV-1 in a patient adherent to preexposure prophylaxis. *J Acquir Immune Defic Syndr.* 2017;76(4):e104–E106.

Marrazzo J, Tao L, Becker M, et al. HIV preexposure prophylaxis with emtricitabine and tenofovir disoproxil fumarate among cisgender women. *JAMA.* 2024;331 (11):930–937.

Marzinke MA, Grinsztejn B, Fogel JM, et al. Characterization of human immunodeficiency virus (HIV) infection in cisgender men and transgender women who have sex with men receiving injectable cabotegravir for HIV prevention: HPTN 083. *J Infect Dis.* 2021;224(9):1581–1592.

Massud I, Kovarova M, Wong-Sam A, et al. In situ forming implants with cabotegravir for ultra long-acting PrEP. Abstract 855. Conference on Retroviruses and Opportunistic Infections; February 12–16, 2022.

Mathur S, Mahapatra B, Mishra R, et al. Which intervention synergies maximize AGYW's HIV outcomes? A classification and regression tree analysis of layered HIV prevention programming. *J Acquir Immune Defic Syndr.* 2023;94(4):317–324.

Mayer KH, Gelman M, Holmes J, et al. Safety and tolerability of once daily coformulated bictegravir, emtricitabine, and tenofovir alafenamide for postexposure prophylaxis after sexual exposure. *J Acquir Immune Defic Syndr.* 2022;90(1):27–32.

Mayer KH, Grasso C, Levine K, et al. Increasing PrEP uptake, persistent disparities in at-risk patients in a Boston Center. Abstract 101. Conference on Retroviruses and Opportunistic Infections. Boston, MA; March 4–7, 2018.

Mayer KH, Jones D, Oldenburg C, et al. Optimal HIV postexposure prophylaxis regimen completion with single tablet daily elvitegravir/cobicistat/tenofovir disoproxil fumarate/emtricitabine compared with more frequent dosing regimens. *J Acquir Immune Defic Syndr.* 2017;75(5):535–539.

Mayer KH, Molina JM, Thompson MA, et al. Emtricitabine and tenofovir alafenamide vs emtricitabine and tenofovir disoproxil fumarate for HIV pre-exposure prophylaxis (DISCOVER): primary results from a randomised, double-blind, multicentre, active-controlled, phase 3, non-inferiority trial. *Lancet.* 2020;396(10246):239–254.

Mayer KH, Venkatesh KK. Interactions of HIV and other sexually transmitted diseases, and genital tract inflammation facilitating local pathogen transmission and acquisition. *Am J Reprod Immunol.* 2011;65:308–316.

McCormack S, Dunn DT, Desai M, et al. Pre-exposure prophylaxis to prevent the acquisition of HIV-1 infection (PROUD): effectiveness results from the pilot phase of a pragmatic open-label randomised trial. *Lancet.* 2016;387(10013):53–60.

Mehtani NJ, Strough A, Strieff S, et al. Feasibility of implementing a low-barrier long-acting injectable antiretroviral program for HIV treatment and prevention for people experiencing homelessness. *J Acquir Immune Defic Syndr.* 2024;96(1):61–67.

Melendez-Torres GJ, Meiksin R, Witzel TC, et al. eHealth interventions to address HIV and other sexually transmitted infections, sexual risk behavior, substance use, and mental ill-health in men who have sex with men: systematic review and meta-analysis. *JMIR Public Health Surveill.* 2022;8(4):e27061.

Mizushima D, Takano M, Aoki T, et al. Effect of tenofovir-based HIV pre-exposure prophylaxis against HBV infection in men who have sex with men. *Hepatology.* 2023;77(6):2084–2092.

Mohareb AM, Larmarange J, Kim AY, et al. Risks and benefits of oral HIV pre-exposure prophylaxis for people with chronic hepatitis B. *Lancet HIV.* August 2022;9(8):e585–e594.

Molina JM, Capitant C, Spire B, et al; ANRS IPERGAY Study Group. On-demand preexposure prophylaxis in men at high risk for HIV-1 infection. *N Engl J Med.* 2015;373(23): 2237–2246.

Molina JM, Charreau I, Spire B, Cotte L, Chas J, Capitant C. Efficacy, safety, and effect on sexual behavior of on-demand pre-exposure prophylaxis for HIV in men who have sex with men: an observational cohort study. *Lancet.* 2017;4(9): E402–E410.

Molina JM, Ghosn J, Algarte-Génin M, et al; ANRS Study Group. Incidence of HIV-infection with daily or on-demand PrEP with TDF/FTC in Paris area. Update from the ANRS Prévenir Study. Abstract TUAC0202. IAS Conference on HIV Science; July 21–24, 2019.

Molina JM, Ghosn J, Assoumou L, et al. Daily and on-demand HIV pre-exposure prophylaxis with emtricitabine and tenofovir disoproxil (ANRS PREVENIR): a prospective observational cohort study. *Lancet HIV.* 2022;9(8):e554–e562.

Moorman AC, de Perio MA, Goldschmidt R, et al. Testing and clinical management of health care personnel potentially exposed to hepatitis C virus—CDC guidance, United States, 2020. *MMWR Recomm Rep.* 2020;69(RR-6):1–8.

MPT Product Development Database. https://mpts101.org/?fwp_indication=hiv. Accessed July 9, 2024.

Mugo N, Mudhune V, Heffron R, et al. Randomized, placebo-controlled trial of safety, pharmacokinetics, and pharmacodynamics of 90-day intravaginal rings (IVRs) releasing tenofovir (TFV) with and without levonorgestrel (LNG) among women in Western Kenya. Abstract OA06.02. HIV Research for Prevention (HIVR4P). Virtual conference; 2021.

Mugo NR, Mudhune V, Heffron R, et al. Randomized controlled phase IIa clinical trial of safety, pharmacokinetics and pharmacodynamics of tenofovir and tenofovir plus levonorgestrel releasing intravaginal rings used by women in Kenya. *Front Reprod Health.* 2023; 5:1118030.

Mulligan K, Glidden DV, Anderson PL, et al. Effects of emtricitabine/tenofovir on bone mineral density in HIV-negative persons in a randomized, double-blind, placebo-controlled trial. *Clin Infect Dis.* 2015;61(4):572–580.

Murphy M, Rogers BG, Ames E, et al. Implementing preexposure prophylaxis for HIV prevention in a statewide correctional system in the United States. *Public Health Rep.* 2024;139(2):174–179.

Nel A, van Niekerk N, Kapiga S, et al; Ring Study Team. Safety and efficacy of a dapivirine vaginal ring for HIV prevention in women. *N Engl J Med*. 2016;375 (22):2133–2143.

New York State Department of Health AIDS Institute. PrEP to prevent HIV and promote sexual health. https://www.hivguidelines.org/guideline/hiv-prep/?mycollection=pep-prep. May 20, 2022. Accessed September 15, 2022.

Ngure K, Nair G, Szydlo D, et al. Choice and adherence to dapivirine ring or oral PrEP by young African women in REACH. Abstract 82. Conference on Retroviruses and Opportunistic Infections. Virtual; February 12–16, 2022.

Nishiya AS, Salles NA, de Almeida-Neto C, et al. Influence of unreported HIV prophylaxis on the kinetics of post-blood donation HIV seroconversion. *Transfusion*. 2021;61(12):3488–3492.

Nkolola JP, Barouch DH. Prophylactic HIV-1 vaccine trials: past, present, and future. *Lancet HIV*. 2024 Feb;11(2):e117–e124.

Ogata-Aoki H, Higashi-Kuwata N, Hattori SI, et al. Raltegravir blocks the infectivity of red-fluorescent-protein (mCherry)-labeled HIV-1JR-FL in the setting of post-exposure prophylaxis in NOD/SCID/Jak3-/- mice transplanted with human PBMCs. *Antiviral Res*. 2018;149:78–88.

Ogbuagu O, Ruane PJ, Podzamczer D, et al. Long-term safety and efficacy of emtricitabine and tenofovir alafenamide vs emtricitabine and tenofovir disoproxil fumarate for HIV-1 pre-exposure prophylaxis: week 96 results from a randomised, double-blind, placebo-controlled, phase 3 trial. *Lancet HIV*. 2021;8(7):e397–e407.

Opara I, Pierre K, Assan MA, et al. A systematic review on sexual health and drug use prevention interventions for black girls. *Int J Environ Res Public Health*. 2022;19(6):3176.

Otten RA, Smith DK, Adams DR, et al. Efficacy of postexposure prophylaxis after intravaginal exposure of pig-tailed macaques to a human-derived retrovirus (human immunodeficiency virus type 2). *J Virol*. 2000;74(20):9771–9775.

Perlman D, Jordan AE. The syndemic of opioid misuse, overdose, HCV, and HIV: structural-level causes and interventions. *Curr HIV/AIDS Rep*. 2018;15:96–112.

Phillips G 2nd, Davoudpour S, Floresca YB, et al. Disparities in HIV testing, condom use, and HIV education between transgender and not transgender high school-aged youth: findings from the 2019 Youth Risk Behavior Survey. *Health Educ Behav*. 2023;50(1):29–40.

Poteat T, Malik M, Scheim A, Elliott A. HIV prevention among transgender populations: knowledge gaps and evidence for action. *Curr HIV/AIDS Rep*. 2017;14(4):141–152.

Rashotte MC, Yoong D, Naccarato M, et al. Appropriate usage of post-exposure prophylaxis-in-pocket for HIV prevention by individuals with low-frequency exposures. *Int J STD AIDS*. 2024;35(6):446–451.

Rich KM, Bia J, Altice FL, et al. Integrated models of care for individuals with opioid use disorder: how do we prevent HIV and HCV? *Curr HIV/AIDS Rep*. 2018;15(3):266–275.

Richterman A, Thirumurthy H. The effects of case transfer programmes on HIV-related outcomes in 42 countries from 1996 to 2019. *Nat Hum Behav*. 2022;6(10):1362–1371.

Riddler SA, Kelly C, Hoesley C, et al. Safety and PK/PD of a tenofovir alafenamide/elvitegravir insert administrated rectally. Abstract 164. Conference on Retroviruses and Opportunistic Infections. February 19–22, 2023. Seattle, WA.

Rimmler S, Golin C, Coleman J, et al. Structural barriers to HIV prevention and services: perspectives of African American women in low-income communities. *Health Educ Behav*. 2022;49(6):1022–1032. doi:10.1177/10901981221109138

Rivera AS, Pak KJ, Mefford MT, et al. Use of tenofovir alafenamide fumarate for HIV pre-exposure prophylaxis and incidence of hypertension and initiation of statins. *JAMA Netw Open*. 2023;6(9):e2332968.

Romero RA, Klausner JD, Marsch LA, Young SD. Technology-delivered intervention strategies to bolster HIV testing. *Curr HIV/AIDS Rep*. 2021;18(4):391–405.

Rutstein SE, Smith DK, Dalal S, et al. Initiation, discontinuation, and restarting HIV pre-exposure prophylaxis: ongoing implementation strategies. *Lancet HIV*. 2020;7(10):e721–e730.

Santos GM, Hong C, Wilson N, et al. Persistent disparities in COVID-19-associated impacts on HIV prevention and care among a global sample of sexual and gender minority individuals. *Glob Public Health*. 2022;17(6):827–842.

Seed CR, Styles CE, Hoad VC, et al. Effect of HIV pre-exposure prophylaxis (PrEP) on detection of early infection and its impact on the appropriate post-PrEP deferral period. *Vox Sang*. 2021;116 (4):379–387.

Sevelius JM, Poteat T, Luhur WE, et al. HIV testing and PrEP use in a national probability sample of sexually active transgender people in the United States. *J Acq Imm Def Syndr*. 2020;84(5):437–442.

Shieh E, Marzinke MA, Fuchs EJ, et al. Transgender women on oral HIV pre-exposure prophylaxis have significantly lower tenofovir and emtricitabine concentrations when also taking oestrogen when compared to cisgender men. *J Int AIDS Soc*. 2019;22(11):e25405.

Shih CC, Kaneshima H, Rabin L, et al. Post exposure prophylaxis with zidovudine suppresses human immunodeficiency virus type 1 infection in SCID-hu mice in a time-dependent manner. *J Infect Dis*. 1991;163(3):625–627.

Siegfried N, Muller M, Deeks JJ, et al. Male circumcision for prevention of heterosexual acquisition of HIV in men. *Cochrane Database Syst Rev*. 2009;2:CD003362.

Simmons R, Plunkett J, Cieply L, et al. Blood-borne virus testing in emergency departments: a systematic review of seroprevalence, feasibility, acceptability and linkage to care. *HIV Med*. 2023;24(1):6–26.

Sivay MV, Li M, Piwowar-Manning E, et al; HPTN 067/ADAPT Study Team. Characterization of HIV seroconverters in a TDF/FTC PrEP Study: HPTN 067/ADAPT. *J Acquir Immune Defic Syndr*. 2017;75(3):271–279.

Solomon MM, Lama JR, Glidden DV, et al. Change in renal function associated with oral FTC/TDF use for HIV pre-exposure prophylaxis. *AIDS*. 2014;28:851–859.

Solomon MM, Schechter M, Liu AY, et al. The safety of tenofovir–emtricitabine for HIV pre-exposure prophylaxis (PrEP) in individuals with active hepatitis B. *J AIDS*. 2016;71(3):281–286.

Spears CE, Taylor BS, Liu AY, Levy SM, Eaton EF. Intersecting epidemics: the impact of COVID-19 on the HIV prevention and care continua in the United States. *AIDS*. 2022;36(13):1749–1759.

Spinelli MA, Lowery B, Shuford JA, et al. Use of drug-level testing and single-genome sequencing to unravel a case of HIV seroconversion on PrEP. *Clin Infect Dis*. 2021;72(11):2025–2028.

Stone J, Fraser H, Lim AG, et al. Incarceration history and risk of HIV and hepatitis C virus acquisition among people who inject drugs: a systematic review and meta-analysis. *Lancet Infect Dis*. 2018;18(12):1397–1409.

Stoner MCD, Kilburn K, Godfrey-Faussett P, Ghys P, Pettifor AE. Cash transfers for HIV prevention: a systematic review. *PLoS Med*. 2021;18(11):e1003866.

Streed CG, Morgan JR, Gai MJ, et al. Prevalence of HIV preexposure prophylaxis prescribing among persons with commercial insurance and likely injection drug use. *JAMA Netw Open*. 2022;5(7):e2221346.

Strong C, Huang P, Li CW, et al. HIV, chemsex, and the need for harm-reduction interventions to support gay, bisexual, and other men who have sex with men. *Lancet HIV*. 2022;9(10):e717–e725. doi:10.1016/S2352-3018(22)00124-2

Sullivan PS, DuBose SN, Castel AD, et al. Equity of PrEP uptake by race, ethnicity, sex and region in the United States in the first decade of PrEP: a population-based analysis. *Lancet Reg Health Am*. 2024 Apr 22;33:100738.

Sutton MY, Martinez O, Brawner BM, et al. Vital voices: HIV prevention and care interventions developed for disproportionately affected communities by historically underrepresented, early-career scientists. *J Racial Ethn Health Disparities*. 2021;8(6)1456–1466.

Tan D, Persaud R, Qamar A, et al. BIC/FTC/TAF as HIV PEP was well-tolerated with high adherence and no seroconversions. Abstract 1134. Conference on Retroviruses and Opportunistic Infections. March 3–6, 2024. Denver, CO.

Taylor JL, Walley AY, Bazzi AR. Stuck in the window with you: HIV exposure prophylaxis in the highest risk people who inject drugs. *Subst Abus*. 2019;40(4):441–443.

Thaden JT, Gandhi M, Okochi H, Hurt CB, McKellar MS. Seroconversion on preexposure prophylaxis: a case report with segmental hair analysis for timed adherence determination. *AIDS.* 2018;32(9):F1–F4.

Thompson KA, Hughes JP, Baeten J, et al. Increased risk of HIV acquisition among women throughout pregnancy and during the postpartum period: a prospective per-coital-act analysis among women with HIV-infected partners. *J Infect Dis.* 2018;218(1):16–25.

Thurman AR, Ouattara LA, Yousefieh N, et al. A phase I study to assess safety, pharmacokinetics, and pharmacodynamics of a vaginal insert containing tenofovir alafenamide and elvitegravir. *Front Cell Infect Microbiol.* 2023;13:1130101.

Toribio M, Cetlin M, Fulda ES, et al. Hormone prescription and HIV screening/preventive practices among clinicians providing care for transgender individuals. *Transgend Health.* 2023;8(1):64–73.

Touesnard N, Brothers TD, Bonn M, Edelman EJ. Overdose deaths and HIV infections among people who use drugs: shared determinants and integrated responses. *Expert Rev Anti Infect Ther.* 2022;20(8):1061–1065.

UNAIDS. 2023 epidemiological estimates. https://www.unaids.org/en/resources/fact-sheet. December 2023. Accessed July 21, 2024.

U.S. Food and Drug Administration (FDA). Coronavirus (COVID-19) update: FDA provides updated guidance to address the urgent need for blood during the pandemic. fda.gov. https://www.fda.gov/news-events/press-announcements/coronavirus-covid-19-update-fda-provides-updated-guidance-address-urgent-need-blood-during-pandemic. Published April 2, 2020. Accessed August 31, 2024.

U.S. Preventive Services Task Force. Preexposure prophylaxis to prevent acquisition of HIV: US Preventive Services Task Force Recommendation Statement. *JAMA.* 2023;330(8):736–745.

U.S. Department of Health and Human Services. Panel on Antiretroviral Guidelines for Adults and Adolescents. Guidelines for the use of antiretroviral agents in adults and adolescents with HIV. Department of Health and Human Services. https://clinicalinfo.hiv.gov/en/guidelines/. Published February 2024b. Accessed July 13, 2024.

USDHHS. Panel on Treatment of Pregnant Women with HIV Infection and Prevention of Perinatal Transmission. Recommendations for use of antiretroviral drugs in pregnant women with HIV infection and interventions to reduce perinatal HIV transmission in the United States. https://clinicalinfo.hiv.gov/en/guidelines/. Published January 2024a. Accessed July 13, 2024.

Valera P, Chang Y, Lian Z. HIV risk inside US prisons: a systematic review of risk reduction interventions conducted in US prisons. *AIDS Care.* 2017;29(8):943–952.

Van Damme L, Corneli A, Ahmed K, et al. Preexposure prophylaxis for HIV infection among African women. *N Engl J Med.* 2012;367:411–422.

Van Gerwen OT, Blumenthal JS. Providing gender-affirming care to transgender and gender-diverse individuals with and at risk for HIV. *Top Antivir Med.* 2023;31(1):3–13.

Veronese V, Ryan KE, Hughes C, et al. Using digital communication technology to increase HIV testing among men who have sex with men and transgender women: systematic review and meta-analysis. *J Med Internet Res.* 2020;22(7):e14230.

Volk JE, Marcus JL, Phengrasamy T, et al. No new HIV infections with increasing use of HIV preexposure prophylaxis in a clinical practice setting. *Clin Infect Dis.* 2015;61(10):1601–1603.

Weiss HA, Hankins CA, Dickson K. Male circumcision and risk of HIV infection in women: a systematic review and meta-analysis. *Lancet Infect Dis.* 2009;9:669–677.

Weld ED, McGowan I, Anton P, et al. Tenofovir douche as HIV preexposure prophylaxis for receptive anal intercourse: safety, acceptability, pharmacokinetics, and pharmacodynamics (DREAM 01). *J Infect Dis.* 2024;229(4):1131–1140.

White DA, Solnick RE. Communicable disease screening and human immunodeficiency virus prevention in the emergency department. *Emerg Med Clin North Am.* 2024;42(2):369–389.

Wilkins NJ, Rasberry C, Liddon N, et al. Addressing HIV/sexually transmitted diseases and pregnancy prevention through schools: an approach for strengthening education, health services, and school environments that promote adolescent sexual health and well-being. *J Adolesc Health.* 2022;70(4):540–549.

Wirtz AL, Yeh PT, Flath N, et al. HIV and viral hepatitis among imprisoned key populations. *Epidemiologic Rev.* 2018;40(1):12–26.

WHO. *Consolidated Guidelines on HIV Prevention, Testing, Treatment, Service Delivery and Monitoring: Recommendations for a Public Health Approach.* Geneva: World Health Organization; 2021. License: CC BY-NC-SA 3.0 IGO.

WHO. *Guidelines for HIV Post-Exposure Prophylaxis.* Geneva: World Health Organization; 2024. License: CC BY-NC-SA 3.0 IGO.

WHO. *Preventing HIV Through Safe Voluntary Medical Male Circumcision for Adolescent Boys and Men in Generalized HIV Epidemics: Recommendations and Key Considerations.* Geneva: World Health Organization; 2020. License: CC BY-NC-SA 3.0 IGO.

WHO. Technical brief: Differentiated and simplified pre-exposure prophylaxis for HIV prevention: update to WHO implementation guidance. https://www.who.int/publications/i/item/9789240053694. Published July 2022. Accessed July 10, 2024.

WHO. Technical brief: What's the 2+1+1? Event-driven oral pre-exposure prophylaxis to prevent HIV for men who have sex with men: update to WHO's recommendation on oral PrEP. https://apps.who.int/iris/bitstream/handle/10665/325955/WHO-CDS-HIV-19.8-eng.pdf?ua=1. Published July 2019. Accessed July 10, 2024.

Young TN, Arens FJ, Kennedy GE, et al. Antiretroviral post-exposure prophylaxis (PEP) for occupational HIV exposure. *Cochrane Database Sys Rev.* 2007;1:CD002835.

Young IC, Massud I, Cottrell ML, et al. Ultra-long-acting in-situ forming implants with cabotegravir protect female macaques against rectal SHIV infection. *Nat Commun.* 2023;14(1):708.

Yuan T, Fitzpatrick T, Ko NY, et al. Circumcision to prevent HIV and other sexually transmitted infections in men who have sex with men: a systematic review and meta-analysis of global data. *Lancet Glob Health.* 2019 Apr;7(4):e436–e447.

Zanakis SH, Alvarez C, Li V. Socio-economic determinants of HIV/AIDS pandemic and nations efficiencies. *Eur J Operational Res.* 2007;176:1811–1838.

Zhao A, Dangerfield DT 2nd, Nunn A, et al. Pharmacy-based interventions to increase use of HIV pre-exposure prophylaxis in the United States: a scoping review. *AIDS Behav.* 2022;26(5):1377–1392.

Zhu W, Huang Y, Delaney K, et al. Few discordant HIV Ag/Ab and RNA test results among persons in a national cohort of PrEP users. Abstract 206. Conference on Retroviruses and Opportunistic Infections. March 3–6, 2024. Denver, CO.

15.

ANTIRETROVIRAL THERAPY SELECTION/DECISION-MAKING

INITIAL AND SUBSEQUENT REGIMENS

Saira Ajmal, Zelalem Temesgen, Poonam Mathur, and David E. Koren

LEARNING OBJECTIVES

Upon completion of this chapter, the reader should be able to:

- Enumerate the goals of antiretroviral treatment (ART) and rationale for treatment as soon as possible of all persons with HIV (PWH).
- List the U.S. Department of Health and Human Services (DHHS) recommended initial HIV treatments.
- Describe important criteria in selecting an initial treatment regimen.
- Identify when ART should be switched and how to do so.

OVERVIEW OF ART

WHAT'S NEW?

- DHHS guidelines recommend starting ART immediately or as soon as possible after the diagnosis of HIV is made.
- HIV integrase inhibitor-based combinations are the standard of care for initial therapy, with additional recommendations for certain clinical situations.
- Bictegravir (BIC), dolutegravir (DTG), or boosted darunavir (DRV/r) paired with emtricitabine/tenofovir (FTC plus either TDF or TAF) can be used for rapid ART initiation before initial lab results are available, including HIV drug resistance testing (i.e., genotype).
- The DHHS ART Guidelines recommend that the DTG + lamivudine (3TC) fixed-dose two-drug regimen may be used for initial treatment except for individuals with HIV RNA >500,000 copies/mL, hepatitis B virus (HBV) coinfection, or in whom ART is to be started before the results of HIV genotypic resistance testing or HBV testing are available.

KEY POINTS

- Uncontrolled HIV replication is associated with inflammation, accelerated aging, and a higher rate of comorbid illnesses, effects which have been shown to be reduced by earlier initiation of ART.
- Studies demonstrate improved clinical outcomes with treatment initiation at $CD4^+$ T-cell counts greater than 500 cells/mm^3, and treatment is now recommended for all PWH regardless of $CD4^+$ T-cell count.
- Timely HIV treatment is highly effective at preventing HIV-1 transmission.
- ART regimen selection considers what is best suited for the patient to support adherence and long-term durability with regard to medication tolerability and toxicities, HIV drug resistance, and patient comorbidities.

INTRODUCTION

Great strides have been made in HIV pharmacotherapy with ART since the introduction of zidovudine in 1987 and combination therapy in 1996. ART has reduced both HIV-associated and non-HIV-associated morbidity and mortality, making HIV a chronic disease that can be managed with potent and simple medication regimens, affording PWH a low risk of AIDS-related complications, few (if any) significant medication side effects, and near-normal life expectancy (ATCC, 2017; Samji et al., 2013). In addition, treatment with ART has been shown to dramatically reduce HIV transmission. However, as of 2021, only 66% of PWH in the United States had suppressed viral loads (HIV.gov, 2023). Of note, in 2021, the number of PWH receiving regular ART had dropped to 54% from 58% in 2018. It is not clear why there has been a drop in the number of PWH retained in care, but access issues during the COVID-19 pandemic may have played a role.

Paramount to the success of ART is the patient's willingness and commitment to adhere to long-term therapy. In the past, acute and long-term adverse effects associated with ART limited adherence to therapy, often leading to treatment failure. However, current combinations are associated with less toxicity, reduced pill burden, and improved potency, allowing many PWH to achieve greater than 95% adherence required for stable, long-term viral suppression. Most patients can start with a single-pill comprising a two- or three-drug regimen, typically based on an "anchor" integrase strand transfer inhibitor (INSTI). For the first time, guidelines also now recommend a long-acting, two-drug combination antiretroviral regimen injected intramuscularly once every 4 or 8 weeks for patients with stable viral suppression. Nevertheless, PWH continue to face several factors which can have a significant impact on ART success, including access to and the cost of long-term ART, particularly in resource-limited areas; drug interactions; comorbid medical conditions such as hepatitis B and C, tuberculosis, cardiovascular and renal disease, diabetes, osteoporosis or osteopenia, psychological disorders and substance use, weight gain, and other social, economic, geographic, racial, and gender-identity factors that disproportionately impact PWH. Recognizing and addressing the individual barriers to adherence for each patient prior to ART initiation, as well as long term, can have a dramatic effect on treatment outcomes.

There are 32 Food and Drug Administration (FDA)–approved individual antiretroviral (ARV) drugs classified based on their mechanism of action, 1 pharmacokinetic enhancer, and 21 fixed-dose combinations to treat PWH. A panel of leading HIV specialists, convened by the DHHS, has been developing and updating recommendations for use of ARV agents in PWH since the early ART era. These guidelines and those published by the International Antiviral Society-USA (IAS-USA) (Gandhi, 2023) are similar and are periodically updated to reflect the release of new medications and HIV treatment in special populations. Guidelines also emphasize patient readiness for therapy, barriers to adherence, and comorbid conditions, and provide information on dosing and drug interactions. At the time of this writing, the most recent DHHS guidelines update, released on September 12, 2024, included key updates regarding the initiation of statin therapy in PWH (DHHS, 2024).

CURRENT TREATMENT GUIDELINES: WHEN TO START

Both DHHS and IAS-USA guidelines recommend starting ART immediately or as soon as possible after the diagnosis of HIV is made, with an intent to improve the uptake of ART and linkage to care, decrease the time to virologic suppression, and reduce HIV transmission (DHHS, 2024; Gandhi, 2023). If possible, ART should be started within 7 days of diagnosis ("Rapid ART"). This guidance has not changed since the last publication, and it reflects data from the START and TEMPRANO trials supporting treatment in all PWH regardless of $CD4^+$ T-cell count to reduce the morbidity and mortality associated with HIV infection (ATCC, 2017; Lundgren et al., 2015). START and HPTN-052 (first in 2011, again in 2020) also demonstrated the power of ART-driven viral suppression to prevent HIV transmission (Cohen et al., 2011; Cohen et al., 2020), a phenomenon known as "treatment as prevention," or TasP. Specifically, prompt ART initiation may prevent sexual or perinatal transmission, especially when viral loads are suppressed to <200 copies/mL (for sexual transmission) and <50 copies/mL (for perinatal transmission) (Bavinton et al., 2018; Cohen et al., 2016; Rodger et al., 2016; Townsend et al., 2008; Tubiana et al., 2010). Lastly, the completeness of $CD4^+$ T-cell count recovery is related to the $CD4^+$ T-cell count at the time of treatment initiation, supporting the notion that ART should be started as soon as possible and not deferred. Many individuals who start treatment with $CD4^+$ T-cell counts <350 cells/mm^3 do not achieve $CD4^+$ T-cell counts >500 cells/mm^3 even after 10 years of ART, and they have a shorter life expectancy than PWH who initiate ART at higher $CD4^+$ T-cell counts (Moore and Keruly, 2007; Palella et al., 2016; Samji et al., 2013).

In some cases, ART initiation may be deferred because of psychosocial factors, but these cases should be the exception, and ART should be started as soon as these issues have stabilized, and the patient is ready for treatment. The following specific scenarios should be considered urgent, and deferral of treatment initiation is generally discouraged: pregnancy; $CD4^+$ T-cell count <200 cells/mm^3; malignancies (both AIDS- and non-AIDS-defining); opportunistic infections and conditions such as HIV-associated dementia, HIV-associated nephropathy, HBV or HCV coinfection, and acute or early HIV infection.

An exception to immediate ART initiation in the setting of opportunistic infections applies to PWH with tuberculosis or cryptococcal meningitis. For patients with tuberculosis *without* meningitis, ART should be started within 2 weeks of tuberculosis therapy initiation if the $CD4^+$ count is <50 cells/mm^3, and within 8 weeks if the $CD4^+$ count is ≥50 cells/mm^3. In cases of tuberculous meningitis, the timing of ART initiation remains controversial: DHHS recommends withholding ART until completion of 8 weeks of tuberculosis treatment, whereas IAS-USA recommends initiating ART within 2 weeks of starting TB meningitis treatment (DHHS 2024; Gandhi, 2023). In cases of cryptococcal meningitis, ART initiation should be deferred for 2–6 weeks after starting anticryptococcal therapy (DHHS, 2024; Gandhi, 2023).

"Rapid ART" refers to the initiation of ART as soon as possible (i.e., within 7 days) after HIV diagnosis. "Immediate ART" and "Same-day ART" refer to starting HIV treatment on the day of diagnosis or during the first clinic visit (DHHS, 2024; Gandhi, 2023). Rapid ART is supported by randomized clinical trials conducted in South Africa (Rosen et al., 2016), Haiti (Koenig et al., 2017), and Lesotho (Labhardt et al., 2018). Additionally, clinic-based observational cohort studies in San Francisco (Rapid ART Program for Individuals with an HIV Diagnosis, or RAPID), Atlanta (Rapid Entry and ART in Clinic for HIV, or REACH), and San Diego demonstrated a significant decrease in time to viral suppression and time to initial provider appointment with immediate ART initiation (Coffey et al., 2019; Colasanti et al., 2018; Hoenigl et al., 2016; Pilcher et al., 2017).

These studies provide evidence that same-day HIV diagnosis and ART initiation are feasible and may be beneficial, whether in a resource-rich setting with a multidisciplinary support system or in more resource-limited settings. Additionally, since persons recently infected with HIV often have very high viral loads during the first several weeks and are therefore at increased risk of transmitting to others, coupling early diagnosis with rapid ART initiation has great potential to reduce HIV transmission. However, data from the CASCADE study in Lesotho (Labhardt et al., 2018) suggested that favorable virologic outcomes with same-day ART are not sustainable after 12 months (Amstutz et al., 2019), a finding that needs further exploration in both resource-limited and resource-rich settings. Other data show that same-day ART in resource-limited settings is challenging, as it requires adequate resources, including staffing, readily available drugs, no payer concerns, and attention to housing and food challenges (Coffey et al., 2019). Although there are no randomized clinical trials demonstrating the success of same-day ART in resource-limited settings, observational studies have shown decreased time to viral suppression and high rates of viral suppression at 1 year compared with standard of care (Coffey et al., 2019; Seybolt et al., 2020). It is unclear, however, if same-day ART leads to improvement in retention in care or sustainable viral suppression after 1 year (Amstutz et al., 2019; Cuzin et al., 2019).

Overall, implementing rapid ART has been shown to reduce barriers to care (Colasanti et al., 2018). The combination of data showing both personal and public health benefits of universal ART for PWH creates a powerful impetus to improve all facets of the HIV care continuum (i.e., to diagnose all PWH and assist them in linkage, engagement, and retention in health care that provides fully suppressive ART and comprehensive medical care). High ART potency and low pill and side-effect/toxicity burdens make this more feasible than ever before.

CURRENT TREATMENT GUIDELINES: WHAT TO START

SELECTION OF AN INITIAL ANTIRETROVIRAL REGIMEN

Currently, there are over 30 different ARV agents comprising different mechanisms of action aimed at providing maximal viral suppression when used in combination (DHHS 2024; Gandhi et al., 2023). The available classes of agents and pharmacokinetic (PK) enhancers are reviewed extensively in Chapter 13. Regimens that do not require boosting are favored in order to reduce the potential for drug interactions (Gandhi et al., 2023). Historically, effective combination ART regimens had been defined as a three-drug combination consisting of two NRTIs (NRTI "backbone") with an "anchor" non-nucleoside reverse transcriptase inhibitor (NNRTI), protease inhibitor (PI), or INSTI. Such regimens have resulted in favorable virologic and immunologic outcomes in most patients in clinical trials, as well as in clinical practice, particularly as pill burdens and toxicities decreased over the years. Additional data now support the use of the two-drug regimen DTG/3TC for initial treatment of some PWH (Cahn et al., 2018, 2020, 2022).

Per the September 2024 DHHS HIV treatment guidelines, three regimens (all INSTI-based) are recommended as initial therapy for most PWH. These recommendations are based on efficacy and toxicity, as evidenced from large randomized clinical trials. Guidelines also specify recommendations for the initial treatment of PWH who previously used long-acting cabotegravir (CAB-LA) for HIV pre-exposure prophylaxis (PrEP). Due to the long half-life of CAB-LA, drug levels may be present for up to 4 years at levels suboptimal to prevent infection (Landovitz et al., 2020). This may select for INSTI resistant virus due to possible cross-resistance of CAB-resistant mutations to other INSTIs (Eshelman et al., 2022; Landovitz et al., 2021).Therefore, the guidelines recommend against initiating an INSTI- based regimen in this population if treatment is begun before results of genotypic testing are available. In this scenario, initiation of therapy with boosted darunavir plus tenofovir plus emtricitabine/lamivudine is recommended. Further details on the topic of genotypic resistance testing can be found in Chapter 17, "HIV Drug Resistance: Evaluation and Clinical Management."

Previous guidelines recommended against the use of DTG during the first trimester of pregnancy and in people of childbearing potential who are trying to conceive or are sexually active and not using effective contraception, because of preliminary data from Botswana suggesting an increased risk of neural tube defects (0.9%) (Zash et al., 2018). Updated results now show that the prevalence of neural tube defects in neonates with maternal exposure to DTG is substantially lower than suggested by preliminary data (Raesima et al., 2019; Zash et al., 2020), and not significantly different compared to that noted with maternal exposure to non-DTG regimens. The DHHS now considers DTG a recommended option for people of childbearing potential, with the provision that risks and benefits should be discussed with patients, allowing them to make an informed decision.

The long-acting injectable combination of CAB and RPV is now recommended for treatment of PWH who have already achieved virologic suppression on oral ART.

When selecting an ART regimen, providers must consider comorbid conditions, past and present resistance test results, patient readiness, and barriers to adherence, such as cost and convenience (e.g., pill burden and dosing frequency); pregnancy state or potential among women of childbearing age; and the potential for drug interactions. A summary of patient- and regimen-specific factors to consider when selecting an ARV regimen is provided in Table 15.1, and the three DHHS-recommended initial HIV regimens are shown in Box 15.1.

Weight gain can occur after initiation of any ART regimen because of ART-induced reversal of HIV-associated inflammation, catabolism, and anorexia (Gandhi et al., 2023). Weight gain can lead to obesity in individuals who are of normal weight or overweight prior to initiation of ART, increasing the risk of comorbidities. There are several risk factors for excess weight

Table 15.1 FACTORS FOR CONSIDERATION IN ART SELECTION

PATIENT CHARACTERISTICS	COMORBIDITIES	REGIMEN-SPECIFIC CONSIDERATIONS
Pretreatment HIV RNA level	Cardiovascular disease, hyperlipidemia, renal disease, osteoporosis, psychiatric illness/ substance use disorders, neurologic disease, co-medications	Regimen's genetic barrier to resistance
Pretreatment CD4$^+$ T-cells	Pregnancy or pregnancy potential	Potential adverse effects of medications
HIV drug resistance	Coinfections: hepatitis C, hepatitis B, tuberculosis	Drug interactions
HLA-B*5701 status	Concern for excess weight gain	Convenience—pill burden, dosing frequency, availability of fixed-dose combination products, food requirement
Anticipated medication adherence	-	Cost
PWH preference	-	Timing of initiation

Source: Adapted from Adult Panel on Antiretroviral Guidelines for Adults and Adolescents. Guidelines for the use of antiretroviral agents in adults and adolescents with HIV. DHHS, 2024. https:// clinicalinfo.hiv.gov/en/guidelines/hiv-clinical-guidelines-adult-and-adolescent-arv/what-start-initial-antiretroviral?view=full.

gain with ART initiation, including low pretreatment CD4$^+$ T-cell count, high pretreatment viral load, Black race, and female sex (Bares et al., 2018; Bhagwat et al., 2018; Sax et al., 2020). Differences in risk of weight gain are also seen among the ART classes (Sax et al., 2020). INSTI-containing regimens induce greater weight gain than comparator regimens (Bhagwat et al., 2018; Kouanfack et al., 2019; Venter et al., 2019). DRV-based regimens have also been implicated with more weight gain than EFV-based regimens when either was combined with FTC and tenofovir alafenamide fumarate (TAF) (Ruderman et al., 2021). Among NRTIs, TAF-containing regimens are associated with greater weight gain than tenofovir disoproxil fumarate (TDF)- or abacavir (ABC)-containing regimens.

The mechanisms underlying increased weight gain for certain ART classes versus others are unclear. For example, it is unknown if the greater weight gain seen with INSTIs is due to a direct effect on appetite or metabolism or because there are fewer adverse effects with INSTIs (Gandhi et al., 2023). In addition, further analysis of the ADVANCE study (Venter et al., 2019) showed that the weight gain observed with DTG- versus EFV-based regimens was primarily dependent on CYP2B6 polymorphisms associated with slow EFV metabolism (and presumably, higher EFV levels). Among those with rapid EFV metabolism genotype, there was no weight gain difference between the participants treated with DTG and EFV (Griesel et al., 2021). A placebo-controlled study of PrEP (Mayer et al., 2020) showed that TDF inhibited weight gain, which may explain why TAF is associated with greater weight gain when compared to TDF. The distribution of weight gain is also different for women with HIV compared to men

Box 15.1 RECOMMENDED INITIAL ART REGIMENS

INSTI-BASED REGIMENS (IN ALPHABETICAL ORDER)

Bictegravir/emtricitabine/tenofovir alafenamide[a] (AI)
Dolutegravir plus tenofovir/emtricitabine (DTG + TDF/FTC or TAF/FTC)[b,c,d] (AI)
Dolutegravir/lamivudine if HIV RNA ≤500,000 copies/mL, no HBV coinfection, able to wait for HIV genotypic resistance and HBV testing results, and no concern for INSTI resistance related to prior use of long-acting cabotegravir (CAB) as pre-exposure prophylaxis (AI)

[a] Single-pill, once-daily regimen.
[b] Lamivudine (3TC) may be interchanged with emtricitabine (FTC) or vice versa.
INSTI, integrase strand transfer inhibitors.
[c] Fixed-dose, co-formulated product for nucleoside backbone.
[d] TAF and TDF are two forms of tenofovir approved by the FDA. TAF is associated with better bone demineralization and kidney toxicity biomarkers than TDF, while TDF is associated with lower lipid levels and lack of weight gain. Safety, cost, and access are among the factors to consider when choosing between these drugs.
SOURCE: Adapted from Adult Panel on Antiretroviral Guidelines for Adults and Adolescents. Guidelines for the use of antiretroviral agents in adults and adolescents with HIV. DHHS 2024. https:// clinicalinfo.hiv.gov/en/guidelines/hiv-clinical-guidelines-adult-and-adolescent-arv/what-start-initial-antiretroviral?view=full.

with HIV on ART, with women gaining more fat than lean body mass compared to men, and more weight concentrated in the limbs and trunk (Kerchberger et al., 2020; Lake et al., 2020; Venter et al., 2020). At present, differences among ART classes and individual drugs in their potential for causing excess weight gain are not fully understood, and therefore are not yet reliable criteria for initial ART regimen selection. Regardless, prior to initiation of ART, PWH should receive information on diet, exercise, and behavior modifications that can mitigate weight gain associated with ART initiation. Further details on weight gain associated with ART can be found in Chapter 32, "Endocrine Disorders and Metabolic Complications in HIV."

CHOOSING BETWEEN RECOMMENDED NRTI BACKBONES

The NRTI combinations of tenofovir disoproxil fumarate or tenofovir alafenamide (TAF/FTC, TDF/3TC, or TDF/FTC) or ABC/3TC comprise the nucleoside backbones in recommended and alternative regimens, with the exception of the two-drug regimens DTG/3TC, DTG/RPV, and CAB/RPV. All these NRTI combinations are available as co-formulated, fixed-dose tablets and as components of co-formulated single-tablet regimens. Choosing between the NRTI pairs or single NRTI is directed mainly by differences between TDF, TAF, and ABC. TDF and TAF are oral prodrugs of tenofovir (TFV) and are available in several co-formulated single-tablet regimen (STR) preparations and as single medications. ABC is available in an STR with DTG and 3TC as DTG/ABC/3TC, in the dual NRTI tablet ABC/3TC, or as a single medication.

Studies comparing the efficacy of ABC/3TC to that of TDF/FTC as components of three-drug regimens have yielded conflicting results. ACTG 5202 compared the efficacy and safety of ABC/3TC to that of TDF/FTC when each was used in combination with either efavirenz (EFV) or ritonavir-boosted atazanavir (ATV/r); significant differences in virologic efficacy favoring TDF/FTC were noted in those with baseline HIV RNA level greater than 100,000 copies/mL, leading to unblinding of this cohort (Sax et al., 2009). The ASSERT study compared ABC/3TC to TDF/FTC, with participants in each group also receiving EFV. The proportion of participants with HIV RNA less than 50 copies/mL was lower among ABC/3TC-treated participants compared to the TDF/FTC group (Post et al., 2010). In contrast to these two trials, other studies have documented virologic equivalence between ABC/3TC and TDF/FTC. The HEAT study compared ABC/3TC to TDF/FTC, each in combination with ritonavir-boosted lopinavir (LPV/r); there was no difference in virologic efficacy, including in patients with baseline HIV RNA greater than 100,000 copies/mL (Smith et al., 2009). Similarly, ABC/3TC has shown comparable virologic efficacy to TDF/FTC when used in combination with DTG (Walmsley et al., 2013).

There are also differences in the safety profile of these NRTI drugs for certain PWH. The serious and potentially fatal ABC hypersensitivity reaction (HSR) was reviewed in Chapter 13, but the importance of testing patients for the HLA-B*5701 allele before starting therapy to predict the risk of the ABC HSR bears repeating, as individuals who test positive should not take ABC (ViiV Healthcare, 2023). ABC has also been associated with myocardial infarction (MI) in some, but not in all, observational studies (Monforte et al., 2013; Palella et al., 2015; Sabin et al., 2014; Worm et al., 2010; Young et al., 2015) and is therefore sometimes avoided in patients with increased cardiac risk profiles.

TDF has been associated with renal impairment and reduced bone mineral density, which may be exacerbated when TDF is used in regimens containing PIs boosted with ritonavir or cobicistat or elvitegravir boosted with cobicistat (McComsey et al., 2011; Mocroft et al., 2015). TAF is an oral prodrug of tenofovir (TFV) that was designed to enhance the pharmacokinetics (absorption from the gut) and pharmacodynamics (intracellular concentration) to achieve higher active metabolite (TFV-DP) concentrations inside peripheral blood $CD4^+$ mononuclear cells; it may therefore be administered at lower doses than TDF with comparable antiviral efficacy but less renal and bone mineral biomarker-based adverse effects. The approval of TAF by itself and as part of two STRs—EVG 150mg/COBI 150mg/FTC 200mg/TAF 10mg (EVG/c/TAF/FTC) and RPV 25mg/TAF 25mg/FTC 200 mg (RPV/TAF/FTC)—was supported by 48-week data from two pivotal phase 3 studies. In the first, EVG/c/TAF/FTC was found to be noninferior to elvitegravir 150 mg/cobicistat 150 mg/FTC 200 mg/TDF 300 mg (EVG/c/TDF/FTC) among treatment-naive adult PWH. The safety and efficacy of TAF/FTC were also demonstrated in one switch study of virologically suppressed PWH randomly assigned to continue TDF/FTC or switch to TAF/FTC (Gallant et al., 2016; Pozniak et al., 2016). Bioequivalence studies (which compare drug levels between approved and investigational drug products in humans without clinical safety or efficacy assessed) also demonstrated that stand-alone TAF/FTC achieved the same drug levels of TFV-DP in target cells as with EVG/c/TDF/FTC. Similar studies also demonstrated that RPV/TAF/FTC achieved similar drug levels of FTC and TFV in the blood as with EVG/c/TAF/FTC, and similar drug levels of RPV as stand-alone RPV. It is important to note that for RPV/TAF/FTC and TAF/FTC, head-to-head comparison to a non-RTV, COBI-boosted regimen in treatment-naive patients has not been accomplished as it was with EVG/c/TAF/FTC vs. EVG/c/TDF/FTC, which included rigorous clinical follow-up. Finally, in a large, randomized, double-blind, multicenter, placebo-controlled, phase 3 study comparing BIC/TAF/FTC to DTG + TAF/FTC in previously untreated adult PWH, the bictegravir regimen was noninferior to the dolutegravir regimen (GS-US-380-1490; Sax).

TAF/FTC is now included as a component of the first-line recommended for most patients, co-formulated with bictegravir and emtricitabine (BIC/TAF/FTC) Two doses of TAF have been FDA-approved: 25 mg and 10 mg, the latter intended for use in combination with ritonavir or cobicistat because of the "boosting" effect that cobicistat has on tenofovir, in order to lessen the risk for renal and bone demineralization toxicity. A recent meta-analysis of 14 clinical trials, involving almost 15,000 PWH on ART, showed TAF to have greater treatment efficacy compared to TDF, but only when used in ART regimens containing pharmacokinetic (PK) boosters (ritonavir or cobicistat). This difference in overall treatment efficacy was attributed to increased proximal renal tubular toxicity from higher levels of TFV when dose-unadjusted TDF was used with a boosting agent. Conversely, there was no difference in overall efficacy or in bone-related or proximal renal toxicity between TAF- and TDF-containing unboosted regimens (Pilkington et al., 2020).

On the HIV prevention side, the DISCOVER trial, a randomized, double-blind, phase 3 trial comparing the efficacy and safety of FTC/TAF to FTC/TDF, was the largest clinical trial to directly compare the adverse effects of these two NRTI pairs in HIV-negative persons at risk for HIV. There was no difference in the incidence of new HIV infections between the two groups. However, FTC + TAF was associated with less bone demineralization and adverse renal biomarkers (hip bone mineral density; spine bone mineral density; urine β2-microglobulin to creatinine ratio; retinol-binding protein to creatinine ratio; distribution of urine protein to creatine ratio above the clinically significant threshold of 22.6 mg/mmol; and change in serum creatinine from baseline). Weight gain was significantly greater in the TAF versus the TDF group. However, there were no statistically significant differences between the two groups in serious adverse events or discontinuation because of adverse events, including renal and bone demineralization toxicities (Mayer et al., 2020).

CHOOSING BETWEEN THIRD DRUG OPTIONS

The choice of the third drug in an initial ARV regimen lies between an INSTI, NNRTI, or PI, and is based on consideration of overall regimen efficacy, genetic barrier to resistance, safety profile, convenience, comorbidities, and potential for drug interactions. Based on these considerations, the following observations have been noted (complementing and reinforcing data presented in Chapter 12):

- The efficacy and safety of DTG-based regimens with either ABC/3TC or TDF/FTC have been evaluated in three clinical trials (SPRING-2, SINGLE, and FLAMINGO), where they were found to be noninferior or superior to other INSTI-, NNRTI-, or PI-based regimens. Thus, DTG/ABC/3TC and DTG + TDF/FTC are among recommended first-line ART regimens (Clotet et al., 2014; Raffi et al., 2013; Walmsley et al., 2013).
- The two-drug regimen of DTG/3TC has been added as a recommended initial regimen for select patients based on 96-week data from the GEMINI-1 and GEMINI-2 trials showing efficacy similar to the three-drug regimen of DTG plus TDF/FTC (Cahn et al., 2020). Extended 144-week analyses of GEMINI-1 and GEMINI-2 provided evidence of the durable efficacy and long-term tolerability of DTG + 3TC (Cahn et al., 2022).
- The efficacy and safety of RAL (with either TDF/FTC or ABC/3TC) have been evaluated in a number of clinical trials, in which it was shown to be superior to EFV-, ATV/r-, and DRV/r-based regimens and noninferior to DTG-based regimens (Lennox et al., 2009; Lennox et al., 2015; Raffi et al., 2013). However, this INSTI is no longer recommended for most people with HIV because of the pill burden and lower barrier to resistance.
- The fixed-dose combination EVG/c/TDF/FTC was evaluated in two randomized clinical trials and found to be noninferior to EFV/TDF/FTC or ATV/r plus TDF/FTC (Rockstroh et al., 2013; Zolopa et al., 2013). Similar to RAL, EVG-based regimens have a lower barrier to resistance than DTG- or BIC-containing regimens. In addition, EVG requires pharmacokinetic boosting with cobicistat (a strong cytochrome P 3A4 inhibitor) and thus has a greater potential for drug interactions.
- BIC is available only as part of a single-tablet, once-daily regimen that includes TAF and FTC (BIC/TAF/FTC). The efficacy of BIC in ART-naive adults was compared to DTG plus two NRTIs in two large phase 3 randomized, double-blind clinical trials (Gallant et al., 2017; Sax et al., 2017). The proportion of participants with plasma HIV RNA less than 50 copies/mL at week 48 in the BIC arms was noninferior to that noted in the DTG arms in both trials (89% vs. 93% and 92.4% vs. 93%, respectively). Longer-term follow-up of these two studies have confirmed these results.
- Clinical studies of DRV/r + TDF/FTC have shown it to be noninferior to RAL and superior to LPV/r. Compared to DTG-based regimens in the FLAMINGO study, DRV/r was inferior to DTG on an intent-to-treat basis, with adverse events being the primary driver for this difference (Clotet et al., 2014).
- Previously, ATV/r + TDF/FTC was among the preferred first-line ARV regimens based on its virologic efficacy, which is equivalent to that of a number of comparator regimens, including EFV/TDF/FTC, EFV + ABC/3TC, LPV/r + TDF/FTC, and EVG/c/TDF/FTC. However, a more recent study, ACTG 5257, compared ATV/r with DRV/r or RAL, each in combination with TDF/FTC. On-treatment virologic efficacy was comparable among the three groups; however, more adverse events and treatment discontinuations were noted among patients on ATV/r compared to the other two groups (Lennox et al., 2015). Thus, ATV/r has been moved to the "Recommended Initial Regimens in Certain Clinical Situations" category.
- Historically, EFV, particularly the STR EFV/TDF/FTC, played a central role in the preferred first-line ARV regimen category. This was based on its demonstrated superiority or noninferiority to all the regimens against which it was compared. However, more recent studies have shown superiority of DTG,

RAL, and RPV (the latter in patients with baseline HIV RNA<100,000 copies/mL and $CD4^+$ cell count >200 cells/mm^3) over EFV; these results were primarily driven by differences in adverse events. Concern regarding EFV-related adverse events was further enhanced by a possible association with suicidality observed in one analysis of four clinical trials (Mollan et al., 2014). Thus, EFV/TDF/FTC was also moved to the alternative "Recommended Initial Regimens in Certain Clinical Situations" category.

- The DRIVE-AHEAD and DRIVE-FORWARD randomized controlled trials showed noninferiority of doravirine (DOR) to both EFV and DRV/r when either of these drugs was taken with two NRTIs (Molina et al., 2018; Orkin et al., 2019). Advantages of DOR include CNS tolerability (vs. EFV), favorable lipid effects (vs. DRV/r, EFV), and fewer drug interactions (vs. EFV, RPV). In addition, in a cross-trial analysis, DOR was not associated with weight gain compared with EFV (600 mg) or boosted DRV (Orkin et al., 2021).

RECOMMENDED INITIAL REGIMENS IN CERTAIN CLINICAL SITUATIONS

The U.S. DHHS guidelines provide an evidence-based menu for selecting an initial ART regimen, and most PWH will be eligible for one of the recommended initial regimens. However, it remains the responsibility of managing clinicians to select the regimen most suited to the clinical scenario at hand. Other ART regimens listed as alternatives in the DHHS guidelines tables are effective but may have some potential disadvantages (e.g., pill burden, dosing, schedule, toxicity profile, and baseline HIV RNA levels or $CD4^+$ T-cell count restrictions) compared to the preferred regimens, or they may have fewer supporting data from randomized clinical trials. Nevertheless, there may be situations in which these agents might be preferred for an individual patient. These alternative regimens are categorized as INSTI-, NNRTI-, and PI-based regimens and regimens when ABC, TAF, and TDF cannot be used. These regimens and clinical scenarios that might prompt their use are shown here in Tables 15.2, 15.3, and 15.4.

Table 15.2 OTHER INITIAL ANTIRETROVIRAL REGIMENS FOR CERTAIN CLINICAL SCENARIOS

INSTI-BASED REGIMENS	NNRTI-BASED REGIMENS	PI-BASED REGIMENS	WHEN ABC, TAF AND TDF CANNOT BE USED
			DTG/3TC[a]—if HIV RNA ≤500,000 copies/mL, no HBV coinfection, able to wait for HIV genotypic resistance testing to determine sensitivity to 3TC, and no concern for INSTI resistance (AI)
	Rilpivirine/tenofovir alafenamide/ emtricitabine (RPV/ TAF/FTC[a])—if pretreatment HIV RNA<100,000 copies/mL and $CD4^+$ T-cell count >200 cells/mm^3 (BII)		
Dolutegravir/abacavir/ lamivudine (DTG/ ABC/3TC [a]) —if HLA-B*5701 negative (BI)	**Doravirine/tenofovir disoproxil fumarate/ lamivudine (BI) or doravirine plus tenofovir alafenamide/emtricitabine (BIII) (DOR/TDF/3TC [a]) or (DOR plus TAF/FTC[b])**	**Cobicistat-boosted darunavir (DRV/c) or ritonavir-boosted darunavir (DRV/r) plus abacavir/lamivudine (ABC/3TC[b])—if HLA-B*5701 negative (BII)**	
		Cobicistat-boosted darunavir (DRV/c) or ritonavir-boosted darunavir (DRV/r) plus tenofovir (TAF or TDF[c]) plus emtricitabine or lamivudine (FTC or 3TC[d]) (BI) **DRV/c/F/TAF available as single-pill once-daily regimen**	-

INSTI = integrase strand inhibitors; NNRTI = nonnucleoside reverse transcriptase inhibitors; PI = protease inhibitor.

[a] Single-pill, once-daily regimen.

[b] Fixed-dose, co-formulated product for nucleoside backbone.

[c] TAF and TDF are two forms of tenofovir approved by the FDA. TAF has fewer bone and kidney toxicities than TDF, while TDF is associated with lower lipid levels. Safety, cost, and access are among the factors to consider when choosing between these drugs.

[d] Lamivudine (3TC) may be interchanged with emtricitabine (FTC) or vice versa.

Table 15.3 BASELINE CONDITIONS

SCENARIO	RECOMMENDED ACTION
Low CD4+ T-cell count (<200 cells/mm^3)	Do not use RPV or DRV/r plus RAL.
Pretreatment HIV RNA >100,000 copies/mL	Do not use RPV, ABC/3TC[a] with EFV or ATV/r, or DRV/r plus RAL.
Pretreatment HIV RNA >500,000 copies/mL	Do not use RPV based regimens, ABC/3TC[a] with ATV/r, DRV/r plus RAL, or DTG/3TC.
ARV to be started before HIV-drug-resistance results are available	Recommended regimens: BIC/TAF/FTC, DTG plus (TAF or TDF) plus (3TC or FTC), or (DRV/r or DRV/c) plus (TAF or TDF) plus (3TC or FTC) Avoid ABC, NNRTI-based regimens, and DTG/3TC.

Source: Adapted from Adult Panel on Antiretroviral Guidelines for Adults and Adolescents. Guidelines for the use of antiretrovirals in adults and adolescents with HIV. DHHS, 2024. https:// clinicalinfo.hiv.gov/en/guidelines/hiv-clinical-guidelines-adult-and-adolescent-arv/what-start-initial-antiretroviral?view=full.

[a] Lamivudine (3TC) may be interchanged with emtricitabine (FTC) or vice versa.

WHEN TO SWITCH OR SIMPLIFY ANTIRETROVIRAL THERAPY

The approach to changing ARV regimens can be considered in one of two broad categories: in the settings of virologic suppression and failure. In PWH with viral suppression, the main goal of switching therapy is typically to simplify treatment or avoid a present or future side effect or toxicity while maintaining virologic control and not jeopardizing future treatment options. Because PWH must take antiretroviral medications for life, side effects and toxicities must be addressed to avoid metabolic complications and adherence problems that can lead to virologic failure. A complete review of the patient's treatment history, resistance testing, treatment tolerance, and drug interactions should be conducted prior to designing a new regimen. According to the IAS-USA and DHHS, the following are some reasons to consider changing therapy (DHHS, 2024; Gandhi et al., 2023):

1. Reduce pill burden or dosing frequency
2. Reduce short- or long-term toxicity and enhance tolerability
3. Changes in food or fluid requirements
4. Minimize drug-drug or drug-food interactions
5. Optimize ART regimen for pregnancy or in case of pregnancy
6. Reduce costs.
7. Change route of administration to meet the individual's health or lifestyle needs.

With the advent of newer agents with improved toxicity profiles, easier dosing schedules, and fewer pills, providers are often confronted with the question of whether to change individual agents or entire regimens. Because some medications are only available in combination tablets, simply changing one agent may not be possible. Switching to a simplified, less adverse effect–laden regimen in PWH with an extensive treatment history can, therefore, be complex. Although the optimal time for changing therapy remains undetermined, most studies have investigated changes in therapy for PWH who have been controlled on an ART regimen for at least 6 months, and in most cases, study participants are tolerating their current ART regimens well.

In general, the two approaches to changing therapy in virally suppressed PWH are changing one agent to another within the same class or to a different class (DHHS, 2024). Within-class simplification can decrease toxicity, dosing frequency, and pill burden, especially when co-formulated agents are used. One example of a within-class change is switching from TDF to TAF for decreased long-term chances of bone and/or proximal renal tubular adverse effects (Gallant et al., 2016). Similar to NRTIs, within-class simplification of NNRTIs can reduce toxicities and adverse side effects. For example, switching efavirenz to rilpivirine (Hagins et al., 2018) or doravirine (Johnson et al., 2019) demonstrated noninferior efficacy for maintaining virologic suppression for 96 weeks and 48 weeks, respectively, and both rilpivirine and doravirine have fewer neuropsychiatric adverse effects when compared to efavirenz (Orkin et al., 2019; van Lunzen et al., 2016).

The majority of studies investigating class switches have evaluated the replacement of a boosted PI with an alternative class, such as an NNRTI or INSTI. This can be done to reduce toxicity or drug interactions or to change to a simpler, once-daily co-formulated combination. Although this is generally successful in PWH without resistance, it can lead to virologic failure in PWH with previous underlying resistance. This was seen in the cases of the SWITCHMRK 1 and 2 studies, where PWH randomly assigned to change from LPV/r to RAL had improved serum lipid concentrations but also had a higher virologic failure rate than those who remained on LPV/r, leading to premature study termination at 24 weeks (Eron et al., 2010). Therefore, DHHS recommends a careful review of the HIV drug-resistance profile and consultation with a clinician who has expertise in drug resistance before modifying ART in persons with a history of treatment failure and drug resistance (DHHS, 2024).

Over the past decade, there has been growing evidence for the use of two-drug ARV therapy for not just treatment-naive, but also for treatment-experienced PWH. Each component's side effects and drug-drug interactions need to be reviewed prior to switching therapy. Patients should have no prior evidence of resistance to either drug in the combination prior to switching. Some of the most thoroughly investigated two-drug regimens have included DTG/3TC, DTG/RPV, and 3TC with a boosted PI. Noninferiority of switching to DTG/3TC through 144 weeks was observed when compared to continuing a three- or four-drug TAF-containing regimen in the TANGO study (van Wyk et al., 2020) and through 48 weeks when compared to continuation

Table 15.4 CONCOMITANT MEDICAL CONDITIONS

SCENARIO	RECOMMENDED ACTION
Cardiac disease	Consider avoiding ABC, LPV/r, and DRV/r.
Chronic kidney disease	Avoid TDF with a PK enhancer, in particular: EVG/cobi/TDF/FTC ATV/cobi with TDF DRV/cobi with TDF. Avoid ATV. TAF may be used if CrCL >30 mL/min or if on chronic hemodialysis.[b] ABC may be used if HLA-B*5701 negative. Option when ABC, TAF, or TDF cannot be used: DTG/3TC (only if HIV RNA ≤500,000 copies/mL, no HBV coinfection, genotype confirms sensitivity to 3TC, and no concern for INSTI resistance)
HIV-associated dementia	Avoid EFV because its psychiatric side effect profile may complicate clinical assessment and management. Favor use of DRV- or DTG-based regimens because of the possibility of increased central nervous system penetration.
Osteoporosis/ osteopenia	Avoid TDF.
Hyperlipidemia	EFV, ABC, PI/r or PI/cobi, and EVG/cobi have been associated with increases in lipids. TDF lowers lipids; therefore switching from TDF to TAF is associated with increased lipids.
Psychiatric illness	Consider avoiding EFV and RPV, which can exacerbate psychiatric symptoms and may be associated with suicidality.
HBV coinfection	Use TDF or TAF plus FTC or 3TC. If TDF or TAF use is contraindicated, recommend use of FTC or 3TC with entecavir.
Tuberculosis	Rifampin is a potent inducer of CYP (mostly 3A and 2C subfamilies) enzyme system, P-gp, and UGT1A1. Check drug-interaction resources; DTG 50 mg may be given twice daily when coadministered with rifampin. If no concern for HIV drug resistance, EFV/TDF/FTC may be used. If a PI/r-based ART regimen is used, rifabutin is the rifamycin of choice in the tuberculosis regimen but requires dose adjustment.
Gastroesophageal reflux disease requiring proton pump inhibitors	Avoid ATV or RPV.
Situations when neither tenofovir nor abacavir can be used	DTG/3TC (no HBV coinfection, no history of resistance, and HIV RNA <500,000 copies/mL) DTG/RPV or CAB/RPV (virally suppressed with no previous virologic failure)

[a] Lamivudine (3TC) may be interchanged with emtricitabine (FTC) or vice versa.

[b] Only studied with EVG/cobi/TAF/FTC and BIC/TAF/FTC.

Adapted from Adult Panel on Antiretroviral Guidelines for Adults and Adolescents. Guidelines for the use of antiretroviral agents in adults and adolescents with HIV. DHHS, 2024. https:// clinicalinfo.hiv.gov/en/guidelines-search?guideline%5B0%5D=title_bookpart%3AHIV%20Clinical%20Guidelines%3A%20 Adult%20and%20Adolescent%20ARV.

of a three- or four-drug ART regimen containing two NRTIs plus an INSTI, NNRTI, or PI-based regimen in the SALSA study (Llibre et al., 2023). This is similar to DTG/RPV in the SWORD-1 and SWORD-2 studies. Noninferiority was demonstrated at week 100, when 89% of the early-switch arm (start of study) and 93% of the late-switch arm (week 52) had maintained HIV RNA <50 copies per mL (Aboud et al., 2019). Lastly, several smaller studies have found combinations of 3TC with a boosted protease inhibitor (PI) to be noninferior to the same boosted PI with two NRTIs. One example is the SALT study (Perez-Molina et al., 2017), which compared virologically controlled participants randomized to receive either ATV/r + 3TC or ATV/r + 2NRTIs, and found similar virologic response with observed rates of viral load <50 copies/mL of 74% for both groups at 96 weeks.

The efficacy of long-acting injectable combination of CAB/RPV was studied in the FLAIR, ATLAS, and ATLAS-2M registrational trials, delivering the medication via gluteal intramuscular injections every 4 or every 8 weeks among persons with existing viral suppression. Participants in the FLAIR Trial (Orkin et al., 2020) were ART-naive at baseline, and initially achieved viral suppression with oral ART prior to initiation of LA CAB/RPV. PWH in the ATLAS Trial (Swindells et al., 2020) were stably virally suppressed for at least 6 months on an oral ART regimen prior to starting LA CAB/RPV. Ultimately, both studies found long-acting, injectable CAB/RPV therapy to be noninferior to oral ARV therapy with regard to HIV viral suppression when administered at 4-week intervals. Further, the ATLAS-2M trial (Overton et al., 2021) found that an 8-week dosing schedule was noninferior to the 4-week dosing regimen in terms of viral suppression and risk of virologic failure. Injection site reactions (including pain in 70% and nodules in 10%–20%) were the most common adverse event, occurring in 75%–86% of patients (Orkin et al., 2020; Swindells et al., 2020). Among these episodes, 99% were reported as mild to moderate, and only about 1% of participants withdrew from the studies because of injection site reactions (Orkin et al., 2020).

Clinicians should consider challenges they may encounter with more frequent patient visits, including changes to clinic infrastructure and operations to ensure successful delivery of long-acting medications on a monthly or every other month basis. The CUSTOMIZE trial (Czarnogorski et al., 2021) noted useful changes to clinic structure, including extending clinic hours, ensuring available rooms, dedicating refrigerator space for storage, and implementing a reminder system for patients.

Switching an ART regimen in a patient who is experiencing virologic failure requires a somewhat different approach than in the setting of virologic suppression. In such cases, one of the primary goals is to design a regimen with sufficient active agents to achieve virologic control, with particular attention to prior resistance testing. In an update to the previously held standard that PWH experiencing virologic failure should be switched to a regimen including three active drugs, the DHHS guidelines now say that a new regimen should strive to use two fully active ARV drugs from two different classes if at least one with a high resistance barrier is included, such as DTG or boosted DRV (DHHS, 2024). If a regimen cannot be crafted that satisfies these criteria, a provider should attempt to create a regimen including three fully active drugs from at least two different classes.

If regimen switching is prompted by virologic failure or suboptimal viral load reduction, HIV drug-resistance testing must be performed to guide the selection of active ARV drugs. For PWH with virologic failure while on an INSTI, genotype testing specifically for INSTI resistance should be performed, in addition to the standard genotyping performed on the protease and reverse transcription regions of the genome. Genotyping should be done while the patient is either on ART or within 4 weeks of discontinuation, as the dominant viral strains may decrease in prevalence so that they become too low to detect. This is commonly referred to as "reversion to wild-type virus." The addition of phenotypic testing to genotypic testing was traditionally recommended for PWH with complex resistance patterns, although over time, the sophistication and reliability of algorithmic genotype interpretations such as the Stanford Drug Resistance Database have largely obviated the need for phenotypic testing. Further details on the topic of HIV drug-resistance testing can be found in Chapter 17, "HIV Drug Resistance: Evaluation and Clinical Management."

Several new medications may potentially be utilized for the treatment of multidrug-resistant HIV-1, though guidance from an HIV specialist is recommended. The attachment inhibitor fostemsavir is an option for patients expected to have incomplete activity from an optimized background regimen, with one study demonstrating that this may help 84% of such patients achieve HIV-1 RNA counts <200 copies/mL by 48 weeks (Kozal et al., 2020). Ibalizumab is a humanized IgG4 monoclonal antibody that blocks entry of HIV-1 by targeting the $CD4^+$ extracellular domain 2. In one study, 50% of 40 patients with multidrug-resistant HIV-1 infection attained viral load <200 copies/mL at 25 weeks (Emu et al., 2018). Lastly, lenacapavir (a new capsid inhibitor), when paired with an optimized background regimen, yielded a viral load <50 copies/mL at week 26 in 81% of PWH with multidrug-resistant virus (Segal-Maurer et al., 2022).

When switching regimens for patients with hepatitis B coinfection, a combination effective for both HIV and HBV should be used. Although 3TC and FTC have anti-HBV activity, resistance to these agents typically develops within 4 years, and thus, they cannot be used alone against HBV. Therefore, most often, either TDF or TAF, both potent and durable against HBV, are included in the ART regimen. If that is not possible, entecavir, another potent anti-HBV agent, should be added to the ART regimen (however, for people with prior exposure to HBV monotherapy with 3TC or FTC, HBV resistance against entecavir must be considered). Notably, none of the two-drug ART regimens have adequate anti-HBV activity and are therefore not recommended by themselves for persons with HBV coinfection or unknown HBV status (DHHS, 2024).

Some PWH may also want to switch regimens due to weight gain. Weight gain can occur with any ART regimen but has been most pronounced with the combination of an INSTI and TAF, particularly when switching off older weight-suppressive agents such as EFV or TDF. Monitoring of weight gain can be done with serial BMIs, waist circumference, and waist-to-hip ratio measurements. There are no recommendations on how much weight gain warrants an ART switch, or which regimen patients should be switched to, but it is recommended that patients receive counseling on lifestyle modification and dietary interventions if they experience weight gain while on ART, since the metabolic concerns associated with INSTIs and TAF do not override the potential benefit of these drugs (DHHS, 2024; Gandhi et al., 2023).

After switching regimens, PWH should be evaluated closely to ensure that no new side effects have emerged, and a repeat viral load 4–8 weeks after a regimen change should be obtained to ensure the patient is virally suppressed. If preexisting laboratory abnormalities were attributed to the prior ART regimen (e.g., hyperlipidemia assumed to be from PIs), these laboratory values should be rechecked 3 months after switching regimens (DHHS 2024).

SUMMARY

The DHHS, IAS-USA, World Health Organization, European AIDS Clinical Society, and British HIV Association guidelines now recommend treatment of all PWH regardless of the $CD4^+$ T-cell count. Currently, the critical issues in antiretroviral treatment are focused on optimizing regimens for the individual patient. Barriers to adherence and addressing those factors remain paramount, and resolution prior to treatment initiation is important to achieve treatment success. Once patients are ready for therapy, an ART regimen must be tailored to their medical comorbidities (with attention to side-effect profiles) and lifestyle. Switching to newer agents must be done prudently, with careful consideration of similar factors and any HIV drug-resistance history. Finally, just as there has been enormous progress in the past, we will continue to witness significant change in the future as we seek to find the optimal treatments for PWH.

RECOMMENDED READING

DHHS. US Department of Health and Human Services guidelines for the use of antiretroviral agents in adults and adolescents with HIV. https://clinicalinfo.hiv.gov/en/guidelines/hiv-clinical-guidelines-adult-and-adolescent-arv/whats-new. Published February 27, 2024. Accessed August 7, 2024.

Gandhi RT, Bedimo R Hoy JF, et al. Antiretroviral drugs for treatment and prevention of HIV infection in adults: 2020 recommendations of the International Antiviral Society-USA panel. *JAMA*. 2023; 329(1):63–84. doi:10.1001/jama.2022.22246.

REFERENCES

Aboud M, Orkin C, Podzamczer D, et al. Efficacy and safety of dolutegravir-rilpivirine for maintenance of virological suppression in adults with HIV-1: 100-week data from the randomised, open-label, phase 3 SWORD-1 and SWORD-2 studies. *Lancet HIV*. 2019;6(9):e576–e587.

Amstutz A, Brown J, Ringera I, et al. Engagement in care, viral suppression, drug resistance, and reasons for nonengagement after home-based, same-day antiretroviral therapy initiation in Lesotho: a two-year follow-up of the CASCADE trial. *Clin Inf Dis*. 2019;71(10):2608–2614.

Antiretroviral Therapy Cohort C (ATCC). Survival of HIV-positive patients starting antiretroviral therapy between 1996 and 2013: a collaborative analysis of cohort studies. *Lancet HIV*. 2017;4(8):e349–e356.

Bares SH, Smeaton LM, Xu A, et al. HIV-infected women gain more weight than HIV-infected men following the initiation of antiretroviral therapy. *J Womens Health (Larchmt)*. 2018;27(9):1162–1169.

Bavinton BR, Pinto AN, Phanuphak N, et al. Viral suppression and HIV transmission in serodiscordant male couples: an international, prospective, observational, cohort study. *Lancet HIV*. 2018;5(8):e438–e447.

Bhagwat P, Ofotokun I, McComsey GA, et al. Changes in waist circumference in HIV-infected individuals initiating a raltegravir or protease inhibitor regimen: effects of sex and race. *Open Forum Infect Dis*. 2018;5(11):ofy201.

Cahn P, Madero JS, Arribas JR, et al. Durable efficacy of dolutegravir plus lamivudine in antiretroviral treatment-naive adults with hiv-1 infection: 96-week results from the GEMINI-1 and GEMINI-2 randomized clinical trials. *J Acquir Immune Defic Syndr*. 2020;83(3):310–318.

Cahn P, Sierra Madero JS, Arribas JR, et al. Dolutegravir plus lamivudine versus dolutegravir plus tenofovir disoproxil fumarate and emtricitabine in antiretroviral-naïve adults with HIV-1 infection (GEMINI-1 and GEMINI-2): week 48 results from two multicenter, double-blind, randomized, non-inferiority, phase 3 trials. *Lancet*. 2018;393(10167):143–155. doi:10.1016/S0140-6736(18)32462-0

Cahn P, Sierra Madero J, Arribas JR, et al. Three-year durable efficacy of dolutegravir plus lamivudine in antiretroviral therapy—naive adults with HIV-1 infection. *AIDS*. 2022;36(1):39–48.

Clotet B, Feinberg J, van Lunzen J, et al. Once-daily dolutegravir versus darunavir plus ritonavir in antiretroviral-naive adults with HIV-1 infection (FLAMINGO): 48 week results from the randomised open-label phase 3b study. *Lancet*. 2014;383(9936):2222–2231.

Coffey S, Bacchetti P, Sachdev D, et al. RAPID antiretroviral therapy: high virologic suppression rates with immediateantiretroviral therapy initiation in a vulnerable urban clinic population. *AIDS*. 2019;33(5):825–832.

Cohen MS, Chen YQ, McCauley M, et al. Prevention of HIV-1 infection with early antiretroviral therapy. *N Engl J Med*. 2011;365:493–505.

Cohen MS, Chen YQ, McCauley M, et al. Antiretroviral therapy for the prevention of HIV-1 transmission. *N Engl J Med*. 2016;375(9):830–839.

Cohen MS, Gamble T, McCauley M. Prevention of HIV transmission and the HPTN 052 study. *Annu Rev Med*. 2020;71:347–360. doi:10.1146/annurev-med-110918-034551. PMID: 31652410.

Colasanti J, Sumitani J, Mehta CC, et al. Implementation of a rapid entry program decreases time to viral suppression among vulnerable persons living with HIV in the Southern United States. *Open Forum Infect Dis*. 2018;28;5(6):ofy104.

Cuzin L, Cotte L, Delpierre C, et al.; Dat'AIDS study group. Too fast to stay on track? Shorter time to first anti-retroviral regimen is not associated with better retention in care in the French Dat'AIDS cohort. *PLoS One*. 2019;14(9):e0222067.

Czarnogorski M, Garris C, D'Amico R, et al. Customize: overall results from a hybrid III implementation-effectiveness study examining implementation of cabotegravir and rilpivirine long-acting injectable for HIV treatment in US Healthcare settings; final patient and provider data. 11th IAS Conference on HIV Science. Virtual; July 18–21, 2021.DHHS. US Department of Health and Human Services guidelines for the prevention and treatment of opportunistic infections in adults and adolescents with HIV. https://clinicalinfo.hiv.gov/en/guidelines/hiv-clinical-guidelines-adult-and-adolescent-opportunistic-infections/whats-new. Published August 15, 2024. Accessed August 26, 2024.

DHHS. US Department of Health and Human Services guidelines for the use of antiretroviral agents in adults and adolescents with HIV. https://clinicalinfo.hiv.gov/en/guidelines/hiv-clinical-guidelines-adult-and-adolescent-arv/whats-new. Published September 12, 2024. Accessed August 7, 2024.

Emu B, Fessel J, Schrader S, et al. Phase 3 study of Ibalizumab for multidrug-resistant HIV-1. *N Engl J Med*. 2018;379(7):645–654.

Eron JJ, Young B, Cooper DA, et al. The SWITCHMRK 1 and 2 investigators. Switch to a raltegravir-based regimen versus continuation of a lopinavir–ritonavir-based regimen in stable HIV-infected patients with suppressed viremia (SWITCHMRK 1 and 2): two multicentre, double-blind, randomized controlled trials. *Lancet*. 2010;375:396–407.

Eshleman SH, Fogel JM, Halvas EK, et al. HIV RNA screening reduces integrase strand transfer inhibitor resistance risk in persons receiving long-acting cabotegravir for HIV prevention. *J Infect Dis*. 2022;226(12):2170–2180. doi:10.1093/infdis/jiac415

Gallant JE, Daar ES, Raffi F, et al. Efficacy and safety of tenofovir alafenamide versus tenofovir disoproxil fumarate given as fixed-dose combinations containing emtricitabine as backbones for treatment of HIV-1 infection in virologically suppressed adults: a randomised, double-blind, active-controlled phase 3 trial. *Lancet HIV*. 2016;3(4):e158–e165.

Gallant J, Lazzarin A, Mills A, et al. Bictegravir, emtricitabine, and tenofovir alafenamide versus dolutegravir, abacavir, and lamivudine for initial treatment of HIV-1 infection (GS-US-380-1489): a double-blind, multicentre, phase 3, randomised controlled non-inferiority trial. *Lancet*. 2017;390(10107):2063–2072.

Gandhi RT, Bedimo R Hoy JF, et al. Antiretroviral drugs for treatment and prevention of HIV infection in adults: 2020 recommendations of the International Antiviral Society-USA panel. *JAMA*. 2023; 329(1):63–84. doi:10.1001/jama.2022.22246

Griesel R, Maartens G, Chirehwa M, et al. CYP2B6 genotype and weight gain differences between dolutegravir and efavirenz. *Clin Infect Dis*. 2021;73(11):e3902–e3909.

Hagins D, Orkin C, Daar ES, et al. Switching to coformulated rilpivirine (RPV), emtricitabine (FTC) and tenofovir alafenamide from either RPV, FTC and tenofovir disoproxil fumarate (TDF) or efavirenz,

FTC and TDF: 96-week results from two randomized clinical trials. *HIV Med*. 2018;19(10):724–733.

HIV.gov. Overview: data and trends: US statistics. https://www.hiv.gov/hiv-basics/overview/data-and-trends/statistics. Published December 7, 2023 Accessed August 7, 2024.

Hoenigl M, Chaillon A, Moore DJ, et al. Rapid HIV viral load suppression in those initiating antiretroviral therapy at first visit after HIV diagnosis. *Sci Rep*. 2016;6:32947.

Johnson M, Kumar P, Molina JM, et al. Switching to doravirine/lamivudine/tenofovir disoproxil fumarate (DOR/3TC/TDF) maintains HIV-1 virologic suppression through 48 weeks: results of the DRIVE-SHIFT trial. *J Acquir Immune Defic Syndr*. 2019;81(4):463–472.

Kerchberger AM, Sheth AN, Angert CD, et al. Weight gain associated with integrase stand transfer inhibitor use in women. *Clin Infect Dis*. 2020;71(3):593–600.

Koenig SP, Dorvil N, Devieux JG, et al. Same-day HIV testing with initiation of antiretroviral therapy versus standard care for persons living with HIV: a randomized unblinded trial. *PLoS Med*. 2017;14(7):e1002357. doi:10.1371/journal.pmed.1002357

Kouanfack C, Mpoudi-Etame M, Omgba Bassega P, et al; NAMSALANRS 12313 study group. Dolutegravir-based or low-dose efavirenz-based regimen for the treatment of HIV-1. *N Engl J Med*. 2019;381(9):816–826.

Kozal M, Aberg, J, Pialoux G, et al. Fostemsavir in adults with multidrug-resistant HIV-1 infection. *N Engl J Med*. March 2020; 382:1232–1243.

Labhardt ND, Ringera I, Lejone TI, et al. Effect of offering same-day ART vs usual health facility referral during home-based HIV testing on linkage to care and viral suppression among adults with HIV in Lesotho: the CASCADE randomized clinical trial. *JAMA*. 2018;319(11):1103–1112.

Lake JE, Wu K, Bares SH, et al. Risk factors for weight gain following switch to integrase inhibitor-based antiretroviral therapy. *Clin Infect Dis*. 2020;71(9):e471–e477.

Landovitz RJ, Donnell D, Clement ME, et al. Cabotegravir for HIV prevention in cisgender men and transgender women. *N Engl J Med*. 2021;385(7):595–608.

Landovitz RJ, Li S, Eron JJ, Jr., et al. Tail-phase safety, tolerability, and pharmacokinetics of long-acting injectable cabotegravir in HIV-uninfected adults: a secondary analysis of the HPTN 077 trial. *Lancet HIV*. 2020;7(7):e472–e481.

Lennox JL, DeJesus E, Lazzarin A, et al. Safety and efficacy of raltegravir-based versus efavirenz-based combination therapy in treatment-naïve patients with HIV-1 infection: a multicentre, double-blind randomised controlled trial. *Lancet*. 2009 Sep 5;374(9692):796–806.

Lennox JL, Landovitz RJ, Ribaudo HJ. Three nonnucleoside reverse transcriptase inhibitor-sparing antiretroviral regimens for treatment-naïve volunteers infected with HIV-1. *Ann Intern Med*. 2015 Mar 17;162(6):461–462.

Llibre JM, Brites C, Cheng CY, Efficacy and safety of switching to the 2-drug regimen dolutegravir/lamivudine versus continuing a 3- or 4-drug regimen for maintaining virologic suppression in adults living with human immunodeficiency virus 1 (HIV-1): week 48 results from the phase 3, noninferiority SALSA randomized trial. *Clin Infect Dis*. 2023;76(4):720–729.

Lundgren J, Babiker A, et al.; INSIGHT START Study Group. Initiation of antiretroviral therapy in early asymptomatic HIV infection. *N Engl J Med*. 2015;373(9):795–807.

Mayer KH, Molina JM, Thompson MA, et al. Emtricitabine and tenofovir alafenamide vs emtricitabine and tenofovir disoproxil fumarate for HIV pre-exposure prophylaxis (DISCOVER): primary results from a randomised, double-blind, multicentre, active-controlled, phase 3, non-inferiority trial. *Lancet*. 2020;396(10246):239–254. doi:10.1016/S0140-6736(20)31065-5

McComsey GA, Kitch D, Daar ES, et al. Bone mineral density and fractures in antiretroviral-naive persons randomized to receive abacavir-lamivudine or tenofovir disoproxil fumarate-emtricitabine along with efavirenz or atazanavir-ritonavir: AIDS Clinical Trials Group A5224s, a substudy of ACTG A5202. *J Infect Dis*. 2011; 203(12):1791–1801.

Mocroft A, Lundgren JD, Ross M, et al. Exposure to antiretrovirals (ARVs) and development of chronic kidney disease (CKD). Abstract 142. Presented at the 2015 Conference on Retroviruses and Opportunistic Infections. Seattle, WA; February 23–24, 2015.

Molina JM, Squires K, Sax PE, et al. Doravirine versus ritonavir-boosted darunavir in antiretroviral-naive adults with HIV-1 (DRIVE-FORWARD): 48-week results of a randomised, double-blind, phase 3, non-inferiority trial. *Lancet HIV*. 2018;5(5):e211–e220.

Mollan KR, Smurzynski M, Eron JJ, et al. Association between efavirenz as initial therapy for HIV-1 infection and increased risk for suicidal ideation or attempted or completed suicide: an analysis of trial data. *Ann Intern Med*. 2014 Jul 1;161(1):1–10.

Monforte AD, Reiss P, Ryom L, et al. Atazanavir is not associated with an increased risk of cardio- or cerebrovascular disease events. *AIDS*. 2013 Jan 28;27(3):407–415.

Moore RD, Keruly JC. CD4+ cell count 6 years after commencement of highly active antiretroviral therapy in persons with sustained virologic suppression. *Clin Infect Dis*. 2007;44(3):441–446.

Orkin C, Arasteh K, Górgolas Hernández-Mora M, et al. Long-acting cabotegravir and rilpivirine after oral induction for HIV-1 infection. *N Engl J Med*. 2020;382(12):1124–1135.

Orkin C, Elion R, Thompson M, et al. Changes in weight and BMI with first-line doravirine based therapy. *AIDS*. 2021;35(1):91–99.

Orkin C, Squires KE, Molina JM, et al. Doravirine/lamivudine/tenofovir disoproxil fumarate is non-inferior to efavirenz/emtricitabine/tenofovir disoproxil fumarate in treatment-naive adults with human immunodeficiency virus-1 infection: week 48 results of the DRIVE-AHEAD trial. *Clin Infect Dis*. 2019;68(4):535–544.

Overton ET, Richmond G, Rizzardini G, et al. Long-acting cabotegravir and rilpivirine dosed every 2 months in adults with HIV-1 infection (ATLAS-2M), 48-week results: a randomised, multicentre, open-label, phase 3b, non-inferiority study. *Lancet*. 2021;396(10267):1994–2005.

Palella F, Althoff KN, Moore R, et al. NA-ACCORD: recent abacavir use and risk of MI. Abstract 749 LB. Presented at the 2015 Conference on Retroviruses and Opportunistic Infections. Seattle, WA; February 23–26, 2015.

Palella FJJ, Armon C, Chmiel JS, et al. CD4 cell count at initiation of ART, long-term likelihood of achieving CD4 >750 cells/mm3 and mortality risk. *J Antimicrob Chemother*. 2016;71(9):2654–2662.

Perez-Molina JA, Rubio R, Rivero A, et al. Simplification to dual therapy (atazanavir/ritonavir + lamivudine) versus standard triple therapy [atazanavir/ritonavir + two nucleos(t)ides] in virologically stable patients on antiretroviral therapy: 96 week results from an open-label, non-inferiority, randomized clinical trial (SALT study). *J Antimicrob Chemother*. 2017;72(1):246–253.

Pilcher CD, Ospina-Norvell C, Dasgupta A, et al. The effect of same-day observed initiation of antiretroviral therapy on HIV viral load and treatment outcomes in a U.S. public health setting. *J Acquir Immune Defic Syndr*. 2017;74(1):44–51.

Pilkington V, Hughes SL, Pepperrell T, et al. Tenofovir alafenamide vs. tenofovir disoproxil fumarate: an updated meta-analysis of 14 894 patients across 14 trials. *AIDS*. 2020;34(15):2259–2268.

Post FA, Moyle GJ, Stellbrink HJ, et al. Randomized comparison of renal effects, efficacy, and safety with once-daily abacavir/lamivudine versus tenofovir/emtricitabine, administered with efavirenz, in antiretroviral-naive, HIV-1-infected adults: 48-week results from the ASSERT study. *J AIDS*. 2010;55(1):49–57. doi:10.1097/QAI.0b013e3181dd911e

Pozniak A, Arribas JR, Gathe J, et al. Switching to tenofovir alafenamide, coformulated with elvitegravir, cobicistat, and emtricitabine, in HIV-infected patients with renal impairment: 48-week results from a single-arm, multicenter, open-label phase 3 study. *J AIDS*. 2016 Apr 15;71(5):530–537.

Raesima MM, Ogbuabo CM, Thomas V, et al. Dolutegravir use at conception: additional surveillance data from Botswana. *N Engl J Med*. 2019;381(9):885–887.

Raffi F, Jaeger H, Quiros-Roldan E, et al. Once-daily dolutegravir versus twice-daily raltegravir in antiretroviral-naive adults with HIV-1 infection (SPRING-2 study): 96 week results from a randomised, double-blind, non-inferiority trial. *Lancet Infect Dis*. 2013;13(11):927–935.

Rockstroh J, DeJesus E, Henry K, et al. A randomized, double-blind comparison of coformulated elvitegravir/cobicistat/emtricitabine/tenofovir DF vs. ritonavir-boosted atazanavir plus coformulated emtricitabine and tenofovir DF for initial treatment of HIV-1 infection: analysis of week 96 results. *J AIDS*. 2013;62(5):483–486.

Rodger AJ, Cambiano V, Bruun T, et al. Sexual activity without condoms and risk of HIV transmission in serodifferent couples when the HIV-positive partner is using suppressive antiretroviral therapy. *JAMA*. 2016;316(2):171–181.

Rosen S, Maskew M, Fox MP, et al. Initiating antiretroviral therapy for HIV at a patient's first clinic visit: the RapIT randomized controlled trial. *PLoS Med*. 2016;13(5):e1002015. doi:10.1371/journal.pmed.1002015. Erratum in: *PLoS Med*. 2016;13(6):e1002050. doi:10.1371/journal.pmed.1002050

Ruderman S, Crane H, Nance, R, et al. Brief report: weight gain following ART initiation in ART-naïve people living with HIV in the current treatment era. *J AIDS*. 2021;86(3):339–343.

Sabin C, Reiss P, Ryom L, et al. Is there continued evidence for an association between abacavir and myocardial infarction risk? Abstract 747. Presented at the 21st Conference on Retroviruses and Opportunistic Infections. Boston, MA; 2014.

Samji H, Cescon A, Hogg RS, et al.; North American AIDS Cohort Collaboration on Research and Design (NA-ACCORD) of IeDEA. Closing the gap: increases in life expectancy among treated HIV-positive individuals in the United States and Canada. *PLoS One*. 2013 Dec 18;8(12):e81355. doi:10.1371/journal.pone.0081355. PMID: 24367482; PMCID: PMC3867319.

Sax PE, Erlandson KM, Lake JE, et al. Weight gain following initiation of antiretroviral therapy: risk factors in randomized comparative clinical trials. *Clin Infect Dis*. 2020;71(6):1379–1389.

Sax PE, Pozniak A, Montes ML, et al. Coformulated bictegravir, emtricitabine, and tenofovir alafenamide versus dolutegravir with emtricitabine and tenofovir alafenamide, for initial treatment of HIV-1 infection (GS-US-380-1490): a randomised, double-blind, multicentre, phase 3, non-inferiority trial. *Lancet*. 2017;390(10107):2073–2082.

Sax P, Tierney C, Collier A, et al. Abacavir–lamivudine versus tenofovir–emtricitabine for initial HIV-1 therapy. *N Engl J Med*. 2009 Dec 3;361(23):2230–2240.

Segal-Maurer S, DeJesus E, Stellbrink HJ, et al. Capsid inhibition with lenacapavir in multidrug-resistant HIV-1 infection. *N Engl J Med*. 2022;386(19):1793–1803.

Seybolt L, Conner K, Butler I, et al. Rapid start lead to sustained viral suppression in young people in the South [Abstract 1073] in special issue: abstracts from the 2020 Conference on Retroviruses and Opportunistic Infections. *Top Antivir Med*. 2020;28(1):407.

Smith KY, Patel P, Fine D, et al. Randomized, double-blind, placebo-matched, multicenter trial of abacavir/lamivudine or tenofovir/emtricitabine with lopinavir/ritonavir for initial HIV treatment. *AIDS*. 2009 Jul 31;23(12):1547–1556.

Swindells S, Andrade-Villanueva JF, Richmond GJ, et al. Long-acting cabotegravir and rilpivirine for maintenance of HIV-1 suppression. *N Engl J Med*. 2020;382(12):1112–1123.

Townsend CL, Cortina-Borja M, Peckham CS, et al. Low rates of mother-to-child transmission of HIV following effective pregnancy interventions in the United Kingdom and Ireland, 2000–2006. *AIDS*. 2008;22(8):973–981.

Tubiana R, Le Chenadec J, Rouzioux C, et al. Factors associated with mother-to-child transmission of HIV-1 despite a maternal viral load <500 copies/ml at delivery: a case-control study nested in the French perinatal cohort (EPF-ANRS CO1). *Clin Infect Dis*. 2010;50(4):585–596.

van Lunzen J, Antinori A, Cohen CJ, et al. Rilpivirine vs. efavirenz-based single-tablet regimens in treatment-naive adults: week 96 efficacy and safety from a randomized phase 3b study. *AIDS*. 2016;30(2):251–259.

van Wyk J, Ajana F, Bisshop F, et al. Efficacy and safety of switching to dolutegravir/lamivudine fixed-dose 2-drug regimen vs continuing a tenofovir alafenamide-based 3- or 4-drug regimen for maintenance of virologic suppression in adults living with human immunodeficiency virus type 1: phase 3, randomized, noninferiority TANGO study. *Clin Infect Dis*. 2020;71(8):1920–1929.

Venter WDF, Moorhouse M, Sokhela S, et al. Dolutegravir plus two different prodrugs of tenofovir to treat HIV. *N Engl J Med*. 2019;381(9):803–815.

Venter WDF, Sokhela S, Simmons B, et al. Dolutegravir with emtricitabine and tenofovir alafenamide or tenofovir disoproxil fumarate versus efavirenz, emtricitabine, and tenofovir disoproxil fumarate for initial treatment of HIV-1 infection (ADVANCE): week 96 results from a randomised, phase 3, non-inferiority trial. *Lancet HIV*. 2020;7(10):e666–e676. doi:10.1016/S2352-3018(20)30241-1

ViiV Healthcare. Ziagen (abacavir) US prescribing information. http://gskpro.com/content/dam/global/hcpportal/en_US/Prescribing_Information/Ziagen/pdf/ZIAGEN-PI-MG.PDF Published July 2023. Accessed August 26, 2024.

Walmsley SL, Antela A, Clumeck N, et al. Dolutegravir plus abacavir–lamivudine for the treatment of HIV-1 infection. *N Engl J Med*. 2013;369(19):1807–1818.

Worm SW, Sabin C, Weber R, et al.; DAD Study Group. Risk of myocardial infarction in patients with HIV infection exposed to specific individual antiretroviral drugs from 3 major drug classes. *J Infect Dis*. 2010;201:318–330.

Young J, Xiao Y, Moodier EE, et al. Effect of cumulating exposure to abacavir on the risk of cardiovascular disease events in patients from the Swiss HIV cohort study. *J AIDS*. 2015;69(4):413–421.

Zash R, Holmes L, Diseko M, et al. Update on neural tube defects with antiretroviral exposure in the Tsepamo study, Botswana. Presented at AIDS 2020, 23rd International AIDS Conference. Virtual; 2020.

Zash R, Makhema J, Shapiro RL. Neural-tube defects with dolutegravir treatment from the time of conception. *N Engl J Med*. 2018;379(10):979–981.

Zolopa A, Sax P, DeJesus E, et al. A randomized double-blind comparison of coformulated elvitegravir/cobicistat/emtricitabine/tenofovir disoproxil fumarate versus favirenz/emtricitabine/tenofovir disoproxil fumarate for initial treatment of HIV-1 infection: analysis of week 96 results. *J AIDS*. 2013;63:96–100.

16.

ANTIRETROVIRAL TREATMENT AND STEWARDSHIP IN HOSPITAL SETTINGS

David E. Koren and Yoseph Aldras

LEARNING OBJECTIVE

Recognize the relative priority of initiating and/or maintaining antiretroviral therapy (ART) for hospitalized people with HIV (PWH) with significant comorbid conditions. Discuss the benefit of antiretroviral stewardship programs. Describe issues regarding continuity of care after discharge from the inpatient setting.

WHAT'S NEW?

- New ART agents (including long-acting formulations) have been approved, and HIV providers should be familiar with clinical indications and their access/availability, especially as it pertains to the care of hospitalized PWH.
- Given the ongoing importance of weight gain for some PWH, renewed attention should be given to changes in antiretroviral (ARV) absorption and pharmacokinetic effects of bariatric surgery.

ANTIRETROVIRAL STEWARDSHIP: HOSPITALIZATION-RELATED CONCERNS

The introduction of highly active antiretroviral therapy has changed hospitalization patterns among PWH. In the pre-ART era, progressive opportunistic infections (OIs) and end-stage AIDS were the main causes of recurrent hospitalizations. These causes (as well as overall hospitalization rates) have dramatically declined with modern ART. Recent drivers for hospitalization have diversified and are now associated with an increased incidence of chronic, noncommunicable health conditions such as diabetes, cardiovascular disease, chronic kidney diseases, and malignancies (Paul et al., 2002). There are many important considerations for ART use and management during hospitalization, encompassing two broad scenarios.

The first scenario involves PWH who are not on ART at the time of hospital admission, which may be due to nonadherence or not having been diagnosed with HIV until the hospitalization itself (possibly owing to initial presentation with an OI). The key question in this scenario is whether to start ART during the hospitalization. Concerns regarding additional pill burden, increased potential for side effects and drug interactions, and possible immune reconstitution inflammatory syndrome must be weighed against faster recovery from severe/opportunistic infections and ultimate morbidity/mortality benefits. An early randomized trial helped inform this issue, concluding that early ART initiation resulted in less progression to AIDS/death with no increase in adverse events or loss of virologic response compared to deferred ART (Zolopa et al., 2009). Current U.S. Department of Health and Human Service (DHHS) guidelines cite the START and TEMPRANO trials in its recommendation to initiate "ART immediately (or as soon as possible) after HIV diagnosis in order to increase the uptake of ART and linkage to care, decrease the time to viral suppression for individual patients, and improve the rate of virologic suppression among persons with HIV." This may occur via a "rapid start" scenario, where ART is initiated prior to having results of all baseline HIV-associated laboratory testing (DHHS, 2024, n.p.). In a multisite cohort of 801 people with HIV and substance use disorders, ART initiation during hospitalization was associated with a shorter time to first HIV care visit (29 days among those who initiated ART while hospitalized compared to 54 days among those who did not) (Jacobs et al., 2020). These data, however, did not reveal an association between inpatient ART initiation and either retention or viral suppression over 12 months, demonstrating that further ongoing interventions may be required.

A critical additional factor in deciding whether to initiate ART during hospitalization is the importance of ensuring that patients will be able to access and continue ART upon discharge to prevent lapses in adherence and potential HIV drug resistance. This necessitates both the immediate availability of ART on discharge (i.e., ensuring that patients have access to outpatient medications via insurance coverage or the Ryan White AIDS Drug Assistance Program [ADAP]) and ensuring that patients are linked to resources that can help support ongoing adherence and engagement in care. Hospital teams should assess housing stability, unmet substance use disorder treatment needs, mental healthcare optimization, and the patient's motivation/willingness to take ART consistently. In all cases, it is essential that PWH have streamlined access to ongoing outpatient HIV specialty care and that strong linkages are made before discharge to prevent lapses in ART adherence.

The second scenario involves PWH who are already diagnosed and on ART at the time of admission. PWH who are stably on oral ART and admitted should continue receiving their regimen while hospitalized, with few exceptions. Issues that impact oral ART continuation include the reason for admission and if it impacts the ability to take oral medications—for example, severe gastrointestinal (GI) disturbances such as intractable vomiting, diarrhea, or bowel obstruction may require ART modification. In such cases, ART use may need to be temporarily suspended until GI symptoms resolve sufficiently and the patient is able to tolerate oral medications again (this approach avoids intermittent absorption and subtherapeutic drug levels predisposing to development of HIV drug resistance). Temporary oral ART discontinuation may additionally need to be considered for persons with severe lactic acidosis, pancreatitis, severe hepatic enzyme elevations, altered mental status/reduced level of alertness or consciousness, or emergent surgical issues. ART dosing should be resumed as soon as safely possible when the patient has clinically improved from these initial severe presentations.

If possible, PWH who are *nihil per os* (NPO) should continue oral ART with water unless there is an acute GI problem rendering them strictly NPO. PWH with nasogastric tubes should be given all ART in liquid form, when available, or crushed/reconstituted if no liquid form is available. An updated reference table, informed by a literature review of ARVs that can be crushed or sprinkled (and also includes information on liquid formulation availability) can be found at: www.hiv-druginteractions.org/prescribing_resources/hiv-guidance-swallowing. Of note, patients receiving fully injectable, long-acting antiretroviral regimens (e.g., cabotegravir-rilpivirine) would not be subject to the same potential for GI tract–related interruptions as described above.

Drug interaction issues need to be considered routinely during hospitalizations for all PWH. Any new medications given should be checked for interactions with patients' current ART regimen, and dose adjustments or medication changes should be made as needed, ideally in concert with an HIV specialty pharmacist. Particular attention should be paid to proton pump inhibitor (PPI) interactions, because PPIs are often started for ulcer prophylaxis or other reasons during hospitalization. Atazanavir and rilpivirine are particularly susceptible to subtherapeutic drug levels because of PPI interaction; therefore, extra care should be taken to mitigate problematic interactions. Additionally, integrase strand inhibitor agents (bictegravir, dolutegravir, elvitegravir, and raltegravir) may have decreased activity in the context of simultaneous administration with medications containing di/polyvalent cations. These examples are only some of many potential pharmacokinetic/dynamic interactions. An updated reference for drug-drug interactions concerning ARVs can be found at: http://www.hiv-druginteractions.org.

Some other ART considerations during hospitalization include formulary availability, especially at smaller hospitals with less HIV experience, and adequate stock of all commonly used ARV agents. It is important to work with hospital pharmacies to ensure that correct ART is available without delay in the correct dosing form and that, if there are any supply problems, appropriate class substitutions are considered in consultation with an HIV expert. Recent approval of long-acting injectable cabotegravir-rilpivirine may lead to unique issues during medication reconciliation, and clinicians not familiar with ART may require further education on the long-acting nature of newer formulations, particularly if a patient is hospitalized during an injection window. If a patent is receiving an investigational medication via a clinical research study, it is imperative that their treating physician and the research team administering the investigational drug are notified of the person's hospital admission because they must make arrangements to bring the drug to the hospital and arrange for its administration.

ANTIRETROVIRAL STEWARDSHIP

Given reported inpatient ART error rates as high as 86%, which may include, but are not limited to, incomplete ARV regimens and drug-drug interactions, the need has arisen for increased safety monitoring of PWH during transitions of care as well as in the hospital setting (Li and Foisy, 2014). To address issues of inpatient HIV management, a joint call to action was published in 2020 by the American Academy of HIV Medicine, HIV Medicine Association, and Infectious Disease Society of America, defining antiretroviral stewardship as, "coordinated interventions designed to improve continuity of care of patients receiving ARVs through the utilization of evidence-based ARV practices including medication reconciliation, dosing, mitigation of drug interactions, and prevention of viral resistance" (Koren et al., 2020). These activities, tailored to the needs of each individual institution, are generally conducted by stakeholders with experience in ART, and may consist of clinical checklists to ensure safe prescribing practices, standardized computerized physician order entry sets to prevent inadvertent errors, and/or prospective review strategies by physician-pharmacist collaborations to maintain patient safety throughout a hospitalization. In doing so, stewardship initiatives may prevent virologic failure, emergent HIV drug resistance, deleterious drug interactions, and adverse drug events. ARV stewardship activities should be routinely monitored for outcomes/efficacy and incorporated into reporting alongside other non-HIV-related stewardship initiatives (Koren et al., 2020).

PERIOPERATIVE CARE, SURGICAL ISSUES, AND BARIATRIC CONSIDERATIONS FOR PWH

KEY POINTS

- Overall, evidence does not suggest worse surgery-associated morbidity and mortality in PWH undergoing procedures.
- Perioperative complications may be more frequent or severe/complex in very immunosuppressed PWH.

- There are some specific anesthesia considerations for PWH.
- Bariatric procedures may affect antiretroviral absorption. Considerations should be made regarding the person's specific ARV regimen and type of procedure during the pre-surgical evaluation.

Overall, data suggest similar postoperative morbidity and mortality outcomes in PWH compared to people without HIV. The number of operations for AIDS-related surgical illnesses has decreased considerably with the advent of highly effective ART (Saltzman et al., 2005). Studies comparing PWH who are virologically suppressed to HIV-negative persons indicate that HIV infection does not significantly change surgical outcomes across a variety of procedures (Dominici and Chello 2020; Gahagan et al., 2016; Sandler et al., 2019). Given the vastly improved survival and longevity of PWH using ART alongside ongoing comorbidities that have increased with an aging PWH population, the need for non-HIV-related surgical operations and anesthesia has become far more commonplace.

POSTOPERATIVE COMPLICATIONS AND HIV INFECTION

Data regarding the influence of HIV infection on postoperative wound healing and complication rates are mixed. Evidence suggests that advanced HIV infection, determined by low $CD4^+$ count or presence/recent history of OIs or certain malignancies, may complicate postoperative wound healing and increase risk of infections such as pneumonia (Cacala et al., 2006; Gahagan et al., 2016; Horberg et al., 2006; Sandler et al., 2019). This may be due to debility and wasting as much as immunosuppression. Recent $CD4^+$ T-cell count and viral load measurements are useful when assessing surgical risks and related prognoses for PWH (Evron et al., 2004; Saltzman et al., 2005). Postoperative $CD4^+$ T-cell counts of 200 cells/mm^3 or less are associated with higher mortality rates irrespective of surgical procedure (Gahagan et al., 2016; Horberg et al., 2006; Sandler et al., 2019). One study noted a 13.3% mortality rate with a $CD4^+$ T-cell count less than 50 cells/mm^3 and 0.8% mortality rate with $CD4^+$ T-cell count greater than 200 cells/mm^3 6 months postoperatively (Evron et al., 2004). Another study noted that viral load >30,000 copies/mL, and not $CD4^+$ count, was associated with increased risk of surgical complications (Horberg et al., 2006).

To reduce operative complications, PWH with a history or signs of cardiac, pulmonary, or other comorbidities should undergo all standard preoperative assessments (e.g., Revised Cardiac Risk Index evaluation) as well as relevant laboratory, radiographic, and other testing when indicated. PWH may have an earlier and more frequent history of coronary artery disease (CAD), malignancy, and venous thromboembolism, which should be considered when assessing operative risk (Evron et al., 2004). Treatment history for malignancy (e.g., cardiotoxic chemotherapy) should also be considered.

ANESTHESIA CONSIDERATIONS AND DRUG INTERACTIONS

Information about the relative general hazards of anesthesia and surgery for PWH is scarce (Evron et al., 2004). Many ARVs may interact directly with anesthetic drugs and can cause side effects that influence which anesthetics are used and how they are administered (Evron et al., 2004; Hughes, 2004). This issue is continually evolving, given interaction profiles of each ARV or anesthetic agent.

Specific considerations when administering general anesthesia to PWH include the possible effects of anesthesia and opioids on the immune system, the cardiopulmonary and neurologic status of the person, and possible interactions with ART medications.

- *Opioids*: although there is laboratory evidence that opioids may detrimentally affect immune function, the clinical significance of short-term opioid administration during general anesthesia is unclear, and not enough clinical data are available to justify its avoidance.
- *Neurologic considerations*: neurologic manifestations, such as overt dementia, may impair the ability of PWH to provide preoperative consent and may increase brain sensitivity to sedative or psychoactive drugs such as opioids, benzodiazepines, and neuroleptics.
- *General central nervous system (CNS)*: increased intracranial pressure (ICP) and CNS infections (i.e., meningitis, encephalopathy, or myelopathy) are contraindications to neuraxial anesthesia.
- *Cerebrospinal fluid analysis and nerve or muscle biopsy* may be required, and radiological studies of the spinal cord should be performed as part of the neurological evaluation to exclude compressive lesions in symptomatic PWH. OIs may be associated with increased ICP, especially in the case of CNS toxoplasmosis or cryptococcal meningitis. Because these infections respond to medical therapy, surgery should be postponed whenever possible if these are present.
- *Pulmonary considerations*: pulmonary complications can occur as a consequence of many OIs, leading to respiratory distress and hypoxemia.

Regional anesthesia has been shown to be associated with reduced morbidity and mortality for a wide range of patients, including PWH having cesarean delivery under spinal anesthesia. However, a high motor block with intercostal muscle paralysis may not be tolerated (Evron et al., 2004). Regional anesthesia is less likely to interfere with immune function or interact with ARV drugs. Sepsis and platelet abnormalities are contraindications to regional anesthesia, and neuropathy may also interfere. Post–dural puncture headache may occur after regional anesthesia and may necessitate epidural blood patch. No increase in neurologic abnormalities in six PWH receiving an epidural blood patch during a follow-up period of 2 years was observed, and there is no evidence to contraindicate the use of blood patch in PWH (Evron et al., 2004; Tom et al., 1992).

Some non-nucleoside reverse transcriptase inhibitors such as efavirenz or etravirine induce the cytochrome P450 enzyme system (CYP3A3/4) and may decrease serum levels of some anesthetic or sedative drugs that use this metabolic pathway, such as midazolam and fentanyl (Evron et al., 2004). Etomidate, atracurium, remifentanil, and desflurane are not dependent on CYP450 hepatic metabolism and may be preferable in persons receiving ART (Evron et al., 2004).

Protease inhibitors (PIs) primarily use the cytochrome P450 system as well (CYP3A4). Because PIs often inhibit and may also induce this enzyme, they may increase or decrease the effects of other drugs using the same metabolic pathway; any anesthetics used concomitantly should be carefully titrated. Ritonavir is the most potent inhibitor of CYP3A4 and CYP2D6. Another CYP3A inhibitor, cobicistat, is commonly used as an ART boosting agent and has similar interactions to ritonavir, with similar need for dosing considerations. Fentanyl is metabolized mainly by CYP3A4 (Evron et al., 2004); ritonavir can reduce fentanyl clearance by up to 67%. This strong interaction suggests that fentanyl (as well as other anesthetics) should be carefully titrated and monitored in PWH on a concomitant boosting agent. These effects may be deleterious, and careful respiratory monitoring should be maintained in the setting of this interaction, as the risk of respiratory depression for an increased duration will likely be higher (Hughes, 2004). Integrase strand inhibitors themselves are neither inductive nor inhibitory to the cytochrome P450 system, though if used in combination with other products, such as elvitegravir with cobicistat, this will have the aforementioned inhibitory effects.

BARIATRIC SURGERY AND ANTIRETROVIRAL THERAPY

Although bariatric surgeries have proven effective in both reducing obesity-related mortality and obesity-related comorbidities, they warrant consideration of pharmacologic complications that may arise depending on the type of surgery performed (e.g., Roux-en-Y gastric bypass or sleeve gastrectomy). Generally, these considerations consist of absorptive and dietary concerns. While the exact site of absorption is only known among a few ARVs, among those that are identified, many are absorbed in the small intestine. Therefore, Roux-en-Y procedures may compromise absorption (Cimino et al., 2018; Zino et al., 2022). Additionally, if an antiretroviral requires a caloric and/or fat requirement, and the stomach volume is reduced significantly because of a procedure, this will inevitably result in subtherapeutic absorption as well. During evaluative workup prior to a procedure, considerations should be made as to available formulations of the patient's ART regimen (including whether the medication can be crushed or is available in liquid form), potential for drug-drug interactions (including acid-suppression and di/polyvalent cations), and the type of bariatric procedure. Minimal systematic data exist on this issue given the broad array of potential bariatric procedures and antiretroviral combinations; however, some recent studies have provided insight. One retrospective cohort analysis showed that virologic failure was rare in PWH following bariatric surgery (Zino et al., 2023). Another retrospective cohort analysis compared the efficacy and safety of bariatric surgery in PWH to people without HIV and showed similarity between the two (Zino et al., 2024). Notably, patients receiving long-acting injectable ART (e.g. cabotegravir-rilpivirine) are not expected to face the same concerns for postoperative drug absorption via the GI tract given parenteral administration.

RECOMMENDED READING

Huesgen E, DeSear KE, Egelund EF, et al. A HAART-breaking review of alternative antiretroviral administration: practical considerations with crushing and enteral tube scenarios. *Pharmacotherapy*. 2016;36(11):1145–1165.

REFERENCES

Cacala SR, Mafana E, Thompson SR, et al. Prevalence of HIV status and CD4 counts in a surgical cohort: their relationship to clinical outcome. *Ann R Coll Surg Engl*. 2006;88(1):46–51.

Cimino C, Binkley A, Swisher R, et al. Antiretroviral considerations in HIV-infected patients undergoing bariatric surgery. *J Clin Pharm Ther*. 2018;43:757–767.

Dominici C, Chello M. Impact of human immunodeficiency virus (HIV) infection in patients undergoing cardiac surgery: a systematic review. *Rev Cardiovasc Med*. 2020 Sep 30;21(3):411–418.

Evron S, Glezerman M, Harow E, et al. Human immunodeficiency virus: anesthetic and obstetric considerations. *Anesth Analg*. 2004;98(2):503–511.

Gahagan JV, Halabi WJ, Nguyen VQ. Colorectal surgery in patients with HIV and AIDS: trends and outcomes over a 10-year period in the USA. *J Gastrointest Surgery*. 2016 Jun;20(6):1239–1246.

Horberg MA, Hurley LB, Klein DB, et al. Surgical outcomes in human immunodeficiency virus-infected patients in the era of highly active antiretroviral therapy. *Arch Surg*. 2006;141(12):1238–1245.

Hughes SC. HIV and anesthesia. *Anesthesiol Clin North Am*. 2004;22(3):379–404.

Jacobs P, Feaster DJ, Pan Y, et al. Initiation of antiretroviral therapy in the hospital is associated with linkage to human immunodeficiency virus (HIV) care for persons living with HIV and substance use disorder. *Clin Infect Dis*. 2020;73(7):e1982–e1990.

Koren DE, Scarsi KK, Farmer EK, et al. A call to action: the role of antiretroviral stewardship in inpatient practice, a joint policy paper of the Infectious Diseases Society of America, HIV Medicine Association, and American Academy of HIV Medicine. *Clin Infect Dis*. 2020;70(11):2241–2246.

Li EH, Foisy MM. Antiretroviral and medication errors in hospitalized HIV-positive patients. *Ann Pharmacother*. 2014;48(8):998–1018.

Paul S, Gilbert HM, Lande L, et al. Impact of antiretroviral therapy on decreasing hospitalization rates of HIV-infected patients in 2001. *AIDS Res Hum Retroviruses*. 2002;18:501–506.

Saltzman DJ, Williams RA, Gelfand DV, et al. The surgeon and AIDS: twenty years later. *Arch Surg*. 2005;140(10):961–967.

Sandler BJ, Davis KA, Schuster KM. 2019. Symptomatic human immunodeficiency virus–infected patients have poorer outcomes following emergency general surgery. *J Trauma Acute Care Surg*. 2019;86(3):479–488.

Tom DJ, Gulevich SJ, Shapiro HM, et al. Epidural blood patch in the HIV-positive patient. Review of clinical experience. San

Diego HIV Neurobehavioral Research Center. *Anesthesiology.* 1992;76(6)943–947.

U.S. Department of Health and Human Services (DHHS). Panel on Antiretroviral Guidelines for Adults and Adolescents. Guidelines for the use of antiretroviral agents in adults and adolescents living with HIV. https://clinicalinfo.hiv.gov/en/guidelines/hiv-clinical-guidelines-adult-and-adolescent-arv/whats-new. Published 2024. Accessed June 14, 2024.

Zino L, Chen QR, Deden L, et al. 2024. Efficacy and safety of bariatric surgery in Dutch people living with HIV: a retrospective matched cohort analysis. *Obes Surg.* 2024;34(5):1584–1589.

Zino L, Kingma JS, Marzolini C, et al. Implications of bariatric surgery on the pharmacokinetics of antiretrovirals in people living with HIV. *Clin Pharmacokinet.* 2022;61(5):619–635.Zino L, Wit F, Rokx C, et al. Outcomes of bariatric surgery in people with human immunodeficiency virus: a retrospective analysis from the ATHENA cohort. *Clin Infect Dis.* 2023;77(11):1561–1568.

Zolopa AR, Anderson J, Powderly W, et al. Early antiretroviral therapy reduces AIDS progression/death in individuals with acute opportunistic infections: a multicenter randomized strategy trial. *PLoS One.* 2009;4(5)e5575. doi:10.1371/journal.pone.0005575

17.

HIV DRUG RESISTANCE

EVALUATION AND CLINICAL MANAGEMENT

Carolyn Chu, Avani Dalal, and Robert W. Shafer

LEARNING OBJECTIVES

- Outline various types of HIV drug resistance (HIVDR) testing assays and clinical considerations for their use and interpretation.
- Define transmitted HIV drug resistance (TDR) and acquired HIV drug resistance (ADR), and general principles/approaches to their management.
- Describe unique considerations regarding HIVDR evaluation and management for select clinical scenarios, including antiretroviral therapy (ART) switches/simplification, rapid ART initiation, pregnancy/breastfeeding, recent pre-exposure prophylaxis (PrEP) use, including long-acting injectable PrEP, and care of persons with HIV (PWH) in low- and middle-income countries.

WHAT'S NEW?

Relatively few countries are on track to meet the UNAIDS "95-95-95" target of 95% of people on ART achieving viral suppression (United Nations Programme on HIV/AIDS [UNAIDS], 2023), underscoring ongoing gaps in HIV care. For some PWH, HIVDR is a factor contributing to ongoing viremia on ART. Current U.S. and international guidelines incorporate specific antiretroviral (ARV) recommendations after first- and second-line treatment failures, which account for prevalent resistance patterns that emerge across different scenarios. Proviral DNA sequencing remains an area of interest, given ongoing attention to regimen simplification/"switch" and nucleoside reverse transcriptase inhibitor (NRTI)-sparing strategies, including long-acting injectable combinations. For people who acquired HIV in the setting of oral or long-acting injectable PrEP use, subsequent ART treatment selection should take potential TDR and/or ADR into account.

KEY POINTS

- Guidelines in the United States and other high-income settings continue to recommend HIVDR testing at initial diagnosis and for people experiencing virologic failure on therapy.
- HIVDR testing is typically conducted with genotypic testing; simultaneous phenotypic testing may be considered if complex drug resistance mutation (DRM) patterns are of concern.
- ADR remains important, especially with increasing use of second-generation INSTIs (in particular, dolutegravir) for multiple clinical scenarios globally; thus providers should continue to emphasize medication adherence and timely virologic monitoring.
- Access to HIVDR testing remains limited for some recently approved ARVs (e.g., ibalizumab, fostemsavir, lenacapavir) which are typically considered only for heavily treatment-experienced individuals; therefore, optimization of the "background" ART regimen for people on these newer agents is critical.
- Proviral DNA resistance testing may be considered for regimen simplifications/switches, particularly when a comprehensive history of prior plasma genotype testing results and ART use is not available. Results should be interpreted and applied carefully.

INTRODUCTION

Before highly active combination treatment, HIVDR was the main obstacle to successful therapy. As newer ARV drugs spanning different therapeutic classes have continued to be developed and approved, it has become possible to overcome HIVDR in many cases such that its management may be less of a challenge in the current treatment era. However, because HIV is a lifelong infection, the cumulative development of DRMs has the potential to limit treatment options for some PWH. HIV drug resistance, therefore, remains an important clinical concern, and providers should be aware of basic prevention and management approaches. Although the overall prevalence of HIVDR has generally declined over time in resource-rich settings due to the use of more robust combination regimens, international surveillance approaches are shifting in response to the widespread roll-out of DTG-based therapy among both treatment naive and experienced populations, as well as scale-up of long-acting cabotegravir as PrEP

Table 17.1 HIVDR-ASSOCIATED TERMS AND DEFINITIONS

Drug resistance mutations (DRMs)	Amino acid changes selected by ARV therapy, reducing ARV susceptibility in vitro, and/or reducing virological response to therapy
Polymorphism	Amino acid changes in the targets of ARV therapy that are often present in ART-naive persons. Although most polymorphisms do not influence ARV susceptibility, some are selected by therapy and contribute to reduced ARV susceptibility, nearly always in combination with nonpolymorphic DRMs.
Transmitted drug resistance (TDR)	Presence of one or more DRMs in an ART-naive person
Pretreatment drug resistance (PDR)	Presence of one or more DRMs in a PWH initiating or re-initiating ART in settings where pre-therapy genotypic resistance testing is not routinely performed. Persons with PDR may include ART-naive persons, as well as pregnant persons who received ART for perinatal transmission prevention, persons receiving PrEP/PEP, and persons who discontinued first-line ART without a documented history of virological failure.
Acquired drug resistance (ADR)	DRMs that are selected during antiretroviral therapy, which can happen when viral replication is not fully suppressed in the presence of drug
Genetic barrier to resistance	A function of the number and type of mutations required to reduce virus susceptibility to an ARV, the likelihood that these mutations will develop upon ARV drug exposure, and the impact of reduced ARV susceptibility on virological outcome. Some mutations rarely occur because they are associated with markedly reduced virus replication. The impact of reduced ARV susceptibility on virological outcome is highly heterogeneous.
Genotyping	Analysis for HIVDR through examination of viral genetic structure, specifically involving the sequencing of molecular targets of therapy to determine the presence of mutations known to confer decreased ARV drug susceptibility
Phenotyping	Analysis for HIVDR which employs the measurement of drug susceptibility of virus by determining the concentration of drug that inhibits viral replication in tissue culture
Sanger sequencing	Sequencing method of choice for commercially available genotypic resistance testing for over 20 years: DNA sequencing method used following reverse transcription of the viral ribonucleic acid genome (based on selective incorporation of chain-terminating dideoxynucleotides by DNA polymerase during in vitro DNA replication)
Next-generation HIVDR testing	High-throughput DNA sequencing technologies, where millions of DNA strands can be sequenced in parallel, yielding substantially more throughput and minimizing need for the fragment-cloning methods often used in Sanger sequencing
Proviral DNA sequencing	Sequencing approach which samples the "archived" HIV viral reservoir found in PBMCs
Wild-type virus	Naturally occurring, non-mutated strain of a virus
Thymidine analogue mutations (TAM)	Non-polymorphic mutations selected by the thymidine analogs AZT and d4T: the accumulation of TAMs leads to progressive decrease in drug susceptibility for all approved NRTIs.

Adapted from Günthard HF, et al. *Clin Infect Dis.* 2019;68(2):177–187.

(World Health Organization [WHO], 2024). Further, resistance to recently approved ARVs continues to be observed in clinical trials and real-world settings; therefore, ongoing monitoring is necessary as more people initiate these agents. Evolving practices for second-line therapy and management of ART-experienced individuals raise important considerations for HIVDR. Table 17.1 includes a list of terms and definitions used in this chapter.

MECHANISMS OF HIV DRUG RESISTANCE

HIV mutates at a high rate during replication, resulting in nearly one nucleotide change per cycle (Abram et al., 2010). Among PWH receiving incompletely suppressive ART, some mutations result in amino acid changes that reduce susceptibility to one or more ARVs an individual is receiving (Coffin, 1995). In PWH on ART who do not maintain sufficiently high levels of medication adherence, viral variants possessing mutations that reduce ARV susceptibility will have a selective replication or "fitness" advantage. When strains harboring such mutations first emerge, they are part of a diverse swarm of viral variants (often referred to as a *quasispecies*) whose complexity is also increased by the high recombination rate occurring whenever more than one viral variant infects the same cell (Eberle and Gutler, 2012b; Levy et al., 2004). With sufficient selective ARV pressure, new variants will merge and become dominant (Figure 17.1). By contrast, if a person maintains virus suppression through consistent ART use, HIV is

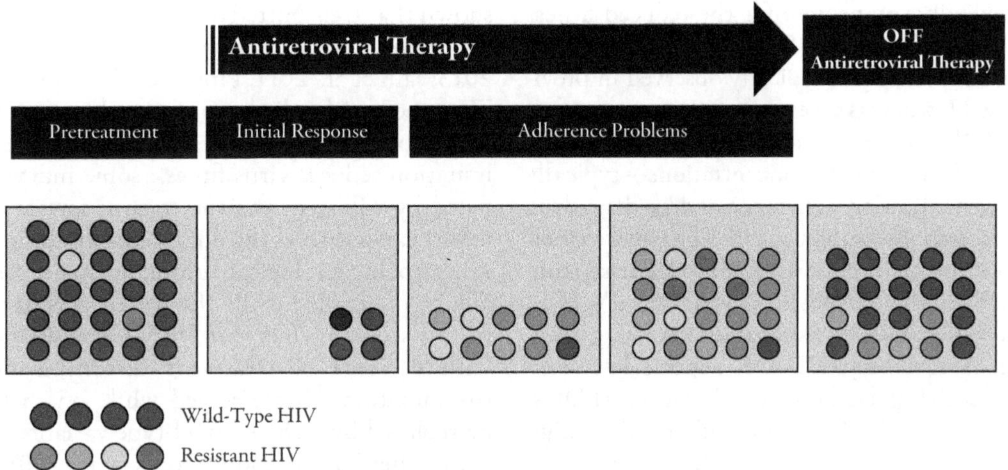

Figure 17.1 Suboptimal ART and poor ART adherence lead to development of ARV-resistant strains. SOURCE: National HIV Curriculum, https://www.hiv.uw.edu/go/antiretroviral-therapy/evaluation-management-virologic-failure/core-concept/all.

unable to replicate to a level high enough to support ongoing evolution and HIVDR development (Siliciano and Siliciano, 2013; van Zyl et al., 2018).

HIVDR is mediated almost entirely by mutations in the molecular targets of ART, including the reverse transcriptase (RT) gene in persons receiving nucleoside RT inhibitors (NRTIs) or non-nucleoside RT inhibitors (NNRTIs), the protease gene in persons receiving protease inhibitors (PIs), the integrase gene in persons receiving integrase strand transfer inhibitors (INSTIs); and the envelope genes (gp120 and gp41) in persons receiving entry inhibitors. Phenotypic resistance to INSTIs may also arise from mutations in the 3′ polypurine tract or through accumulation of multiple *Env* DRMs; the clinical significance of this is unknown (Hikichi et al., 2024; Malet et al., 2019). The "genetic barrier to resistance" to an ARV is a useful concept that indicates that ARVs differ in their vulnerability to HIVDR by virtue of the number and type of mutations required for clinically significant reductions in drug susceptibility and the likelihood that these mutations will develop upon drug exposure (Figure 17.2). Further, some HIVDR-associated mutations occur rarely because they are associated with markedly reduced virus replication.

During its replication cycle, HIV-1 integrates into host chromosomal DNA and is then usually expressed leading to productive infection and cell killing. In resting memory $CD4^+$ T-cells, however, integrated proviral DNA may persist for years, forming a stable reservoir. As a result, proviral DNA levels in peripheral blood mononuclear cells (PBMCs) remain detectable even in PWH on stably suppressive ART such that the DRMs present in proviral DNA will often reflect resistance that emerged prior to the most recent regimen (see section "Proviral DNA Sequencing" below).

HIVDR is usually caused by "major" DRMs that reduce drug susceptibility by themselves, as well as accessory "minor"

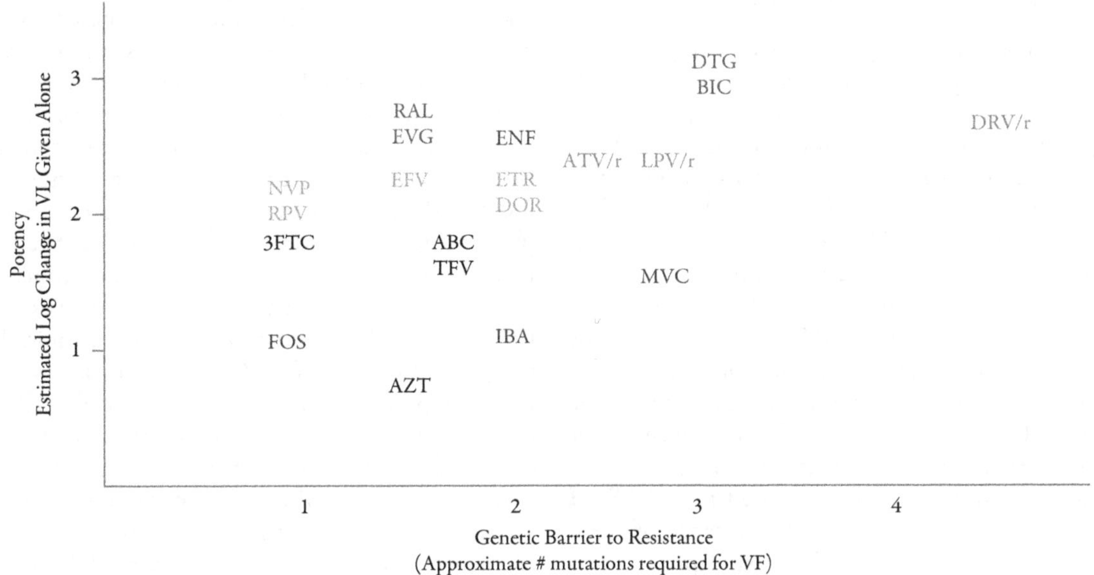

Figure 17.2 Schematic indicating genetic barrier to resistance (estimated) for select, approved ARV agents.

mutations that generally compensate for the reduced fitness associated with many of the major DRMs. With a few notable exceptions, major DRMs are not typically observed in previously untreated PWH, whereas accessory mutations are often polymorphic. HIVDR emerges in viruses from PWH exposed to suboptimal ARV inhibitory concentrations—typically due to low levels of medication adherence and/or drug-drug interactions or occasionally patient-specific pharmacokinetics. Most cases of virologic failure with HIVDR arise from incomplete adherence, which exposes viruses from PWH to incompletely suppressive ARV levels capable of exerting drug-selective pressure. Accordingly, HIVDR appears less commonly in patients receiving fixed-dose combinations (FDCs) containing ARVs with similar half-lives (and, ideally, a high genetic barrier to resistance) because incomplete adherence to these combinations is less likely to expose a virus to selective drug pressure (Llibre et al., 2011; Stella et al., 2022). Lower rates of HIVDR have also been associated with routine viral load monitoring practices in which early detection of rebound prompts careful adherence assessment/counseling, evaluation for drug-drug interactions, and/or ART modification (as necessary prior to the evolution of multiple significant DRMs) (Bachmann et al., 2019).

Group M HIV-1 strains have evolved into many subtypes and circulating recombinant forms (Rambaut et al., 2004). However, none of the subtypes are intrinsically resistant to the main ARV classes. Although viruses belonging to different subtypes occasionally differ in the frequency with which they develop different DRMs, the phenotypic effect of these mutations appear to be subtype- independent; thus, it is not generally necessary to know an individual's virus subtype to select therapy or interpret HIVDR testing results when considering commonly used ARVs (Günthard et al., 2019).

HIV DRUG RESISTANCE TESTING

INDICATIONS AND TIMING

U.S. guidelines recommend drug resistance testing at diagnosis/entry into care, regardless of whether someone initiates ART soon thereafter. It is also recommended for people experiencing virologic failure on therapy and confirmed RNA levels greater than 200 copies/mL, as well as people with suboptimal viral load reduction (DHHS, 2024a; Günthard et al., 2019). For ART-naive PWH, the role of baseline resistance evaluation is to guide initial regimen selection (or early modification in the case of immediate ART initiation prior to results of baseline testing). For ART-experienced persons with virologic failure, resistance testing can help ascertain the cause of failure, as well as determine which ARVs may have been compromised and which agents still retain activity for potential incorporation into subsequent regimens.

Timely resistance testing is recommended for all PWH because resistant variants are less fit in the absence of ARV selection pressure compared to wild-type susceptible virus variants. Retrospective studies involving stored samples have shown that transmitted drug-resistant variants are frequently outcompeted by wild-type revertants over time (Castro et al., 2013; Jain et al., 2011; Pingen et al., 2014; Yanik et al., 2012). The speed with which transmitted mutations are no longer detectable within plasma depends on the extent to which a mutation reduces virus fitness: some mutations are outcompeted by wild-type variants within several months, whereas others can persist as the dominant variant for years. In PWH experiencing virological failure, resistance testing should ideally be performed while the patient is still on ART because in this scenario emergent DRMs may no longer be detected within weeks of treatment discontinuation—specifically, the mutations that emerged while on therapy will rapidly be replaced by archived wild-type variants that were present before therapy initiation (Deeks et al., 2001; Devereux et al., 1999). If resistance testing cannot be performed while a person is on therapy, testing performed within 4 weeks after oral/non-long-acting ART discontinuation may still be informative (DHHS, 2024a). By contrast, given the long half-lives of long-acting injectable ARVs, PWH with virologic failure on long-acting ART should undergo timely resistance testing regardless of when the last dose was received—INSTI resistance testing should be included for people who have received long-acting cabotegravir.

GENOTYPIC AND PHENOTYPIC RESISTANCE TESTING

HIVDR testing can be performed genotypically (by sequencing the molecular targets of therapy) or phenotypically (by determining drug susceptibility in cell culture); both use PCR products directly amplified from cDNA that has been reverse-transcribed from plasma RNA. Genotypic resistance testing involves direct sequencing of the viral genome using conventional population (Sanger) sequencing methodologies to identify mutations in the RT, protease (PR), and INSTI genes of circulating plasma RNA. Although genotypic tests are more complex than typical antimicrobial susceptibility tests, their ability to detect mutations present as mixtures (i.e., co-circulating with wild-type variants), even if the mutation is present at a level too low to affect drug susceptibility in a phenotypic assay, provides insight into the potential for resistance to emerge. Sequencing tests can also detect transitional mutations that do not cause drug resistance by themselves but rather indicate the presence of selective drug pressure. Compared to phenotypic testing, additional advantages of genotypic testing include lower cost and shorter turnaround time.

Phenotypic susceptibility testing involves the identification of ARV drug concentration that inhibits HIV replication by 50% (IC_{50}). The IC_{50} of a clinically sampled virus is then compared to that of a drug-susceptible laboratory reference strain and expressed as a ratio (referred to as *fold change*) of the IC_{50} of the sampled virus relative to the reference control (Figure 17.3). Most phenotypic tests use recombinant viruses created by inserting PCR-amplified clinical virus gene segments (RT/PR, integrase, envelope) into the backbone of a wild-type laboratory clone (Petropoulos et al., 2000).

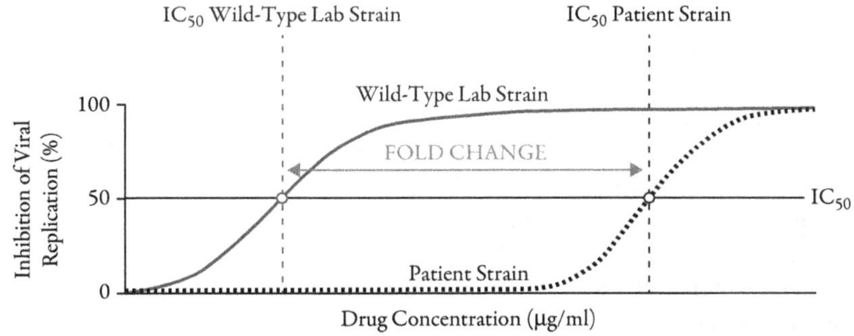

Figure 17.3 Calculating level of phenotypic resistance. This graph shows the method for calculating the level of phenotypic resistance of a single ARV. The ARV is tested on a patient's HIV isolate and a laboratory reference (wild-type strain). The IC_{50} represents the concentration of the ARV required to cause 50% inhibition of HIV replication. The fold change is calculated by dividing the IC_{50} of the patient's isolate by the IC_{50} of the wild-type laboratory strain. As shown, as the curve shifts to the right, a higher concentration of ARV would be required to inhibit HIV replication and thus the strain of HIV would be more resistant. The further the curve shifts to the right (for the patient's HIV strain tested), the greater the level of resistance SOURCE: National HIV Curriculum, https://www.hiv.uw.edu/go/antiretroviral-therapy/evaluation-management-virologic-failure/core-concept/all.

Phenotypic testing is not generally necessary at baseline for newly diagnosed PWH. However, it may be a valuable complement to genotypic testing in persons who have experienced virologic failure on multiple treatment regimens and/or who have complicated DRM patterns (DHHS, 2024a; Günthard et al., 2019). It may also be useful in cases of acquired multiclass resistance. When phenotypic testing is indicated, it should be performed simultaneously with genotypic testing because of the ability of genotypic testing to detect emerging resistance, as indicated previously.

HIV THERAPEUTIC TARGETS FOR RESISTANCE TESTING

Sequencing of protease and the 5′ part of RT usually constitutes one assay, and INSTI sequencing usually constitutes a second, distinct assay. Whereas RT/PR genotypic testing is routinely recommended for all newly diagnosed PWH and in people with virologic failure, INSTI genotypic testing is recommended primarily in persons with virologic failure (or incomplete/delayed virologic response) on an INSTI-containing regimen. Baseline INSTI resistance testing should be considered in select persons with TDR, such as those with reduced NRTI susceptibility or multiclass resistance, and in persons who acquired HIV from a PWH failing an INSTI-containing regimen (Günthard et al., 2019). It is also recommended in persons who acquired HIV after receiving cabotegravir-based PrEP, as emergent INSTI-associated DRMs were detected in some clinical trial participants who were subsequently diagnosed with HIV (see section "ARV Resistance Considerations for Special Circumstances" below) (DHHS, 2024a; Eshleman et al., 2022; Marzinke et al., 2021).

Lenacapavir is the first-in-class HIV capsid inhibitor licensed for use in the United States and other high-income countries. The entry inhibitor class now includes pre- and post-attachment inhibitors, CCR5 antagonists, and fusion inhibitors. Clinical information on HIVDR for some of these newer agents is primarily derived from resistance analyses and outcomes among trial participants who experienced virologic failure (Emu et al., 2018; Gartland et al., 2022; Margot et al., 2022). Currently, there are no commercially available genotypic or phenotypic resistance tests for ibalizumab, fostemsavir, or lenacapavir. Genotypic testing for HIV-1 tropism (to evaluate the activity of the CCR5 antagonist maraviroc) and enfuvirtide susceptibility is available in several U.S.-based reference laboratories; phenotypic testing for these two ARVs is also available. To date, cross-resistance between attachment and entry inhibitors, or between lenacapavir and entry inhibitors, has not been described (Margot et al., 2023; Rose et al., 2022).

HIV-1 RNA THRESHOLDS FOR GENOTYPIC TESTING

Clinical guidelines in the United States and other high-income settings recommend HIVDR testing for PWH with virologic failure and confirmed RNA (i.e., viral load) levels greater than 200 copies/mL (DHHS, 2024a; EACS, 2023; Waters et al., 2023). Standard resistance testing may be unsuccessful in people with viral load greater than 200 copies/mL but less than 500 copies/mL; however, it should still be considered since repeated viral loads from 200 to 500 copies/mL are associated with an increased risk of HIVDR and/or subsequent increased viremia (Delaugerre et al., 2012b; Elvstam et al., 2017; Esber et al., 2019; Fleming et al., 2019; Hermans et al., 2018; Joya et al., 2019; Laprise et al., 2013; Li et al., 2012; Swenson et al., 2014; Vandenhende et al., 2015). Most nested PCR-based genotypic assays are able to yield interpretable results for many PWH with viral loads between 200 and 500 copies/mL (Gonzalez-Serna, 2014; Mackie et al., 2010).

PROVIRAL DNA SEQUENCING

Proviral DNA sequencing is being increasingly employed for PWH with virologic suppression who are considering therapy modification, including transitions to the dual-therapy combination of long-acting cabotegravir plus rilpivirine (Armenia et al., 2018; Cervo et al., 2023; Cutrell et al., 2021; Ellis et al., 2019; Rauschning et al., 2023; Rodriguez et al., 2021; van Wyk et al., 2020). Current U.S. guidelines support consideration of proviral DNA testing for PWH with viral suppression seeking regimen simplification, particularly if complex or semi-complex preexisting HIVDR is suspected (e.g., multiple prior treatment failures) (DHHS, 2024a). There is a strong but imperfect correlation between the DRMs in PBMC proviral DNA and plasma HIV-1 RNA from the same blood samples (Derache et al., 2015; Devereux et al., 2000; Gaitan et al., 2023; Hoffman et al., 2022; Porter et al., 2016; Verhofstede et al., 2004). Specifically, in patients with suppressed plasma viral load, proviral DNA genotyping will detect many but not all DRMs identified via historical plasma genotypic resistance testing (Allavena et al., 2018; Boukli et al., 2018; Delaugerre et al., 2012a; Margot, 2020; Wirden et al., 2011; Zaccarelli et al., 2016). This may occur particularly if previous episodes of virologic failure with emergent HIVDR were either not prolonged or were associated with high-level viremia (Chu et al., 2022). Proviral DNA testing has also been studied in PWH with detectable viremia, including low-level viremia, but its clinical usefulness in this setting is less well characterized (Boukli et al., 2018; Curanovic et al., 2023; Lubke et al., 2015; Lv et al., 2023; Villalobos et al., 2020; Zaccarelli et al., 2016). In general, proviral DNA resistance testing results should be interpreted with caution and accompanied by careful review of prior ART history and plasma RNA genotype results if available.

NEXT-GENERATION SEQUENCING

Newer sequencing technologies—collectively referred to as next-generation sequencing (NGS)—are replacing population-based Sanger sequencing for many applications in diagnostic microbiology laboratories and continue to be used in research settings. The cost of NGS can be considerably lower than that of Sanger sequencing should a sufficient number of samples be tested in the same run (Lapointe et al., 2015; Noguera-Julian et al., 2017). Additionally, the ability of NGS to simultaneously sequence all genetic regions of interest and detect low-abundance DRMs (i.e., present at a prevalence below 15%–20%) has potential advantages for improving individual outcomes among PWH, although clinically relevant thresholds for various drug classes and specific ARVs are not well-defined or standardized at this time (Avila-Rios et al., 2020; Balakrishna et al., 2023; Li et al., 2011; Teo et al., 2022). NGS may also be particularly useful for settings where NNRTI-based and maraviroc-inclusive regimens are still widely used (Avila-Rios et al., 2016a; Boltz et al., 2011; Cozzi-Lepri et al., 2015; Pou et al., 2014; Westby et al., 2006). Given the above, NGS continues to gain popularity for use in individuals as well as for population-level HIVDR evaluation in resource-limited settings (Baxter et al., 2021; Manyana et al., 2021). Nonetheless, Sanger sequencing has been used for over two decades to identify HIVDR and has been shown to be highly reproducible and interpretable in clinical settings, whereas laboratory NGS procedures and approaches to sequence analysis continue to evolve (Avila-Rios et al., 2020; Keys et al., 2015; Mbunkah et al., 2020). Moreover, it has been difficult to translate the theoretical benefits of increased sensitivity for low-abundance variants into a practical clinical benefit, especially as ARV agents have become more potent and as most NGS assays have displayed reduced reproducibility at mutation detection thresholds below 5% (Avila-Rios et al., 2016a; Balakrishna et al., 2023; Huber et al., 2017; Inzaule et al., 2018).

INTERPRETATION OF RESISTANCE TESTING RESULTS

Genotypic resistance testing produces a list of DRMs which is accompanied by a prediction of which ARVs are likely to have reduced activity. As the many known DRMs occur in complex patterns and cause varying levels of reduced drug susceptibility, interpretation algorithms and systems are required to predict which ARVs are likely to retain activity. Three commonly used, publicly available interpretation systems include the Stanford HIVDB interpretation system (Paredes et al., 2017), ANRS system (Eberle and Gurtler, 2012a), and Rega system (Eberle and Gutler, 2012a). The International AIDS Study-USA Antiviral Group also maintains a list of DRMs considered to be the most clinically relevant (Wensing et al., 2022). These are summarized in Tables 17.2 and 17.3.

Genotypic resistance interpretation system rules are usually developed by considering several types of published data, including whether a DRM has been selected by a drug either in vitro or in PWH, whether a DRM reduces drug susceptibility in vitro, and whether there are data showing that a DRM interferes with virological response to an ART regimen containing the relevant drug. Although one might expect that DRMs present at low levels would have a lesser clinical impact than those present at higher levels, there are no interpretation systems that treat low-abundance DRMs

Table 17.2 SELECT RESOURCES ON HIVDR CLINICAL EVALUATION AND MANAGEMENT

U.S. DHHS Guidelines	**https://clinicalinfo.hiv.gov/en/guidelines/adult-and-adolescent-arv/whats-new-guidelines**
IAS-USA: Drug resistance mutations in HIV-1	**https://www.iasusa.org/resources/hiv-drug-resistance-mutations/**
Stanford HIV Database	**https://hivdb.stanford.edu/**
National HIV Curriculum (ART overview)	**https://www.hiv.uw.edu/go/antiretroviral-therapy**
National Clinician Consultation Center	**https://nccc.ucsf.edu/**
HIV-ASSIST	**https://hivassist.com**
Clinical Care Options (HIV portfolio)	**https://clinicaloptions.com/hiv**

Table 17.3 COMMON HIVDR MUTATIONS AND IMPACT ON ARV SUSCEPTIBILITY, BY CLASS AND MEDICATION

ARV DRUGS	DRUG RESISTANCE MUTATIONS (DRMS)
Nucleoside/nucleotide RT inhibitors	
Abacavir (ABC)	K65R/N, L74V/I, Y115F, M184V/I: 1 mutation confers low-level and 2 confer high-level resistance. T215Y/F + 2 additional TAMS: intermediate- to high-level resistance MDR mutations: high-level resistance K70E/Q/N/T: low-level phenotypic resistance
Lamivudine (3TC); Emtricitabine (FTC)	M184V/I confer high-level resistance. K65R, MDR mutations, and 4–5 TAMs confer intermediate levels of resistance.
Tenofovir (TFV) disoproxil fumarate (TDF); Tenofovir alafenamide (TAF)	K65R: confers low-level phenotypic resistance but potentially high-level clinical resistance. T215Y/F + 2 additional TAMS: intermediate- to high-level resistance MDR mutations: intermediate- to high-level resistance depending on the specific mutations K70E/Q/N/T: low-level phenotypic resistance
Zidovudine (AZT)	TAMs: confer intermediate- to high-level resistance. MDR mutations confer high-level resistance.
	TAMs (thymidine analog mutations) are defined as M41L, D67N, K70R, L210W, T215F/Y, K219Q/E. T215F/Y is the most important of these, and the combination of M41L+L210W+T215Y has the greatest phenotypic and virological impact. MDR mutations are defined as (i) Q151M, usually in combination with ≥2 of the following: A62V, V75I, F77L, and F116Y; (ii) an amino acid insertion at position 69, which nearly always occurs with ≥1 TAM. M184V/I increase susceptibility to AZT, TDF, and TAF; K65R increases susceptibility to AZT. TAF and TDF have similar resistance profiles. However, TAF achieves >4-fold higher intracellular levels of the active inhibitor TFV-diphosphate, suggesting that it is likely to be more active than TDF at inhibiting both drug-susceptible and drug-resistant viruses. However, most genotypic resistance interpretation systems do not distinguish between the two TFV prodrugs. T215S/C/D/E/I/V are commonly transmitted mutations consistent with previous thymidine analog selection pressure. These mutations have much less clinical significance than T215Y/F.
Non-nucleoside RT inhibitors	
Efavirenz (EFV)	L100I, K101E/P, K103N/S, V106A/M, Y188L/C/H, G190A/S/E/Q, P225H, F227C, and M230L
Etravirine (ETR)	L100I, K101E/P, Y181C/I/V, G190E/Q, F227C, and M230L
Rilpivirine (RPV)	L100I, K101E/P, E138A/G/K/Q/R, Y181C/I/V, Y188L, G190E/Q, F227C, and M230L.
Doravirine (DOR)	L100I, V106A/M, Y188L, G190E/S, F227C/L, M230L, L234I, Y318F
General comments	Common accessory relatively nonpolymorphic DRMs: A98G, V106I, V108I, V179D/E/F, H221Y, and P225H High-level DOR resistance in persons receiving DOR usually includes one of the following DRMs: V106A, Y188L, F227L/C, M230L, L234I, or Y318F. The common DRMs K103N, Y181C, and G190A are not associated with clinically significant reductions in DOR susceptibility. However, many combinations of ≥2 DRMs that emerge in persons receiving other NNRTIs can be associated with reductions in DOR susceptibility that are likely to be clinically significant. ETR usually requires ≥2 mutations for intermediate- or high-level resistance. Although E138K causes low-level RPV resistance, it is one of the most commonly emerging DRMs in persons developing virologic failure while receiving RPV. E138A, which is polymorphic in certain subtypes, minimally reduces RPV susceptibility but is of uncertain clinical significance.
Protease inhibitors	
Atazanavir (ATV/r)	V32I, M46I/L, I47V, G48V/M, I50L, I54V/T/A/S/L/M, V82A/C/F/M/S/T, I84V/A/C, N88S, and L90M
Darunavir (DRV/r)	V32I, I47V/A, I50V, I54L/M, L76V, V82F, and I84V/A/C
Lopinavir (LPV/r)	L24I, V32I, M46I/L, I47V/A, G48V/M, I50V, I54V/T/A/S/L/M, L76V, V82A/C/F/M/S/T, I84A/C/V, and L90M
General comments	Common accessory nonpolymorphic DRMs: L10F, V11I/L, K20T, L33F, G73/S/T/C/A, T74P, and L89V DRV/r has the highest genetic barrier to resistance, usually requiring 2–3 of the listed mutations and 2–3 of the accessory mutations to develop high-level resistance. LPV/r has a lower genetic barrier to resistance compared with DRV/r but likely a higher genetic barrier to resistance than ATV/r.

(continued)

Table 17.3 CONTINUED

ARV DRUGS	DRUG RESISTANCE MUTATIONS (DRMS)
Integrase strand transfer inhibitors	
Raltegravir (RAL)	T66K, E92Q, G118R, F121Y, Y143C/R/H/A/G/K/S, Q148H/R/K, and N155H
Elvitegravir (EVG)	T66A/I/K, E92Q, G118R, F121Y, P145S, Q146P, S147G, Q148H/R/K, N155H, and R263K
Dolutegravir (DTG)	T66K, E92Q, G118R, Q148H/R/K, N155H, and R263K
Bictegravir (BIC)	T66K, E92Q, G118R, Q148H/R/K, N155H, and R263K
Cabotegravir (CAB)	T66K, E92Q, G118R, Q148H/R/K, N155H, and R263K
Notes	Accessory uncommon nonpolymorphic DRMs: H51Y, Q95K, E138A/K/T, G140S/A/C, G149A, S153Y/F, and S230R Accessory polymorphic DRMs: L74M, T97A, E157Q, G163K/R/E, D232N Many of the EVG and RAL-associated DRMs appear to be DTG and BIC-accessory DRMs. There are 3 somewhat overlapping RAL-resistance mutational pathways: Y143C/R/H vs. Q148H/R/K vs. N155H often in combination with an additional mutation such as E92Q, E138K/A/T, G140S/A/C, and/or an accessory mutation. Persons receiving EVG are less likely to develop Y143 mutations and more likely to develop T66A/I/K, E92Q, and S147G, but there is a high-level of cross-resistance between RAL and EVG. There are somewhat overlapping DTG-resistance mutation pathways: Q148H/K/R + 1–2 additional mutations; N155H + ≥ additional mutations; R263K; and G118R. Although R263K is the most commonly occurring DRM in persons developing DTG-associated virologic failure, it is associated with just a 2-fold reduction in susceptibility. BIC has a nearly identical resistance profile compared with DTG. High-level resistance to RAL and EVG usually requires just 1–2 DRMs, while high-level resistance to DTG and BIC appears to require 2–3 DRMs. Additionally, DRMs emerge less frequently in persons receiving DTG or BIC compared with those receiving RAL or EVG. DRMs associated with reduced DTG or BID susceptibility generally cause a greater reduction in CAB susceptibility.
Entry inhibitors	
Enfuvirtide (fusion inhibitor)	Mutations in gp41 codons 36–45, the region to which enfuvirtide binds. The key mutations are G36D/E/S/V, I37V, V38E/A/G/M, Q40H, N42T, N43D/K/S, L44M, L45M and Q48H. A single mutation usually reduces susceptibility about 10-fold, whereas two mutations usually reduce susceptibility about 100-fold.
Maraviroc (CCR5 inhibitor)	CXCR4-tropic gp120 variants: positively charged residues at positions 11 and 25 of the V3 loop of gp120 and several other combinations of mutations, primarily but not exclusively within the V3 loop, are associated with CXCR4 tropism. The most common mechanism of resistance is the expansion of preexisting CXCR4-tropic variants that were not detected before therapy. Resistance can also emerge as a result of gp120 mutations that allow HIV-1 to bind to an altered CCR5 receptor. There is no consistent pattern of these mutations.
Ibalizumab (post-attachment inhibitor)	Loss of potential N-linked glycosylation sites (PNGS) in the V5 loop of gp120 allows HIV-1 to bind CD4 and enter cells despite the presence of ibalizumab; examples include N460Q, N464Q, and variations at amino acids close to asparagine that disrupt N-linked glycosylation (Blair, 2020).
Fostemsavir	Several gp120 mutations, including M426L and S375M, are considered major fostemsavir-resistance mutations, while M434I and M475I are considered to have a lesser effect on susceptibility. The amino acids that explain why CRF01_AE viruses are usually resistant to fostemsavir map to 375H and 475I (Zhou et al., 2014)
Capsid inhibitor	
Lenacapavir	A number of major and minor (accessory) mutations have been identified, mostly through in vitro studies and initial clinical trials. Major DRMs include: L56I, M66I, Q67H/Y/N/K, K70N/H/R/S, and N74D/S.

Adapted from Shafer RW, et al. *Manual of Clinical Microbiology*, 13th ed. ASM Press; 2023.

differently from those present at higher levels. Further, interpretation systems often differ in the number of levels of resistance assigned. For example, most systems assign three levels: *susceptible*, *low-level/possible resistance*, and *resistance*. The Stanford HIVDB system assigns five levels: *susceptible*, *potential low-level resistance*, *low-level resistance*, *intermediate resistance*, and *high-level resistance*. Overall, the systems are rarely completely discordant (i.e., a virus is rarely scored as being fully susceptible to a drug by one system but fully resistant by another system). Nonetheless, formal comparison of the various interpretation systems has found subtle differences (Rhee et al., 2009).

Phenotypic test results also require interpretation because the clinical significance of fold reductions in susceptibility differ among ARVs (de Meyer et al., 2008; Eron et al., 2013; Vingerhoets et al., 2010; Winters et al., 2009). Whenever possible, phenotypic tests provides three thresholds for fold reductions in drug susceptibility: (i) the reduction in susceptibility that exceeds the uppermost value for wild-type viruses, often referred to as the *biological threshold* (Parkin et al., 2004); (ii) the lowest fold-reduction in susceptibility that indicates a PWH will have a reduced likelihood of response (*lower clinical threshold*); and (iii) the lowest fold-reduction in susceptibility that indicates a drug will likely be completely inactive (*upper clinical threshold*). Upper and lower clinical thresholds have been developed for ARVs that have been used in salvage therapy situations for treatment of PWH with viruses containing DRMs affecting the same ARV class, including tenofovir (Miller et al., 2004), etravirine (Vingerhoets et al., 2010), darunavir (De Meyer et al., 2008), and dolutegravir (Eron et al., 2013).

Importantly, genotypic and phenotypic test interpretations alone do not contain sufficient information to construct a clinically appropriate ART regimen for an individual. In addition to results of recent resistance testing, it is necessary to consider prior treatment history and previous resistance-testing results. Genotypic and phenotypic resistance-interpretation systems also vary in how they take into account differences in ARV potency and thus do not incorporate fundamental principles of how treatment regimens should be constructed. Therefore, clinicians must place the results of drug resistance assays within the context of current treatment guidelines.

TRANSMITTED HIV DRUG RESISTANCE

EPIDEMIOLOGY

TDR is defined as the presence in an ART-naive person of one or more DRMs that are polymorphic in that they do not occur naturally in the absence of selective drug pressure. For practical purposes, polymorphic mutations have been defined as mutations occurring at a prevalence below 0.5% in all major HIV subtypes in ART-naive persons at times and in regions where TDR has been uncommon. The most common list of mutations used for TDR surveillance was published in 2009 and is often referred to as the WHO list (Bennett et al., 2009). The U.S. Centers for Disease Control and Prevention uses a more expansive list (Wheeler et al., 2010), and a subset of major IAS-USA mutations has also been used in various analyses (Wensing et al., 2022). Recent studies have examined the impact of adding new candidate surveillance DRMs to previously established lists, given evolving treatment practices and availability of newer ARVs (Rhee et al., 2021).

Over the past decade, TDR prevalence has been approximately 15% in the United States, 10%–15% in Europe and the Latin America and Caribbean regions, and 5%–15% in sub-Saharan Africa and Asia (Avila-Rios et al., 2016b; Gupta et al., 2018; Kirichenko et al., 2022; McClung et al., 2022; Miranda et al., 2022; Rhee et al., 2015; Rhee et al., 2020b; WHO, 2024). TDR prevalence has been stable in most regions except for sub-Saharan Africa, where rates of transmitted NRTI and NNRTI resistance have increased, particularly among persons with pretreatment resistance (PDR), which includes ARV-naive persons as well as PWH who received prior ARVs to prevent perinatal HIV transmission or who are reinitiating therapy without a documented history of virologic failure; see "Resource-Limited Settings" below. By contrast, samples obtained from PWH in upper-income countries with identified NRTI, NNRTI, and PI-associated TDR generally contain DRMs associated with ARVs that are now used infrequently, such as thymidine analog mutations (TAMs), certain NNRTI-resistance mutations, and mutations associated with older PIs (Drescher et al., 2014; Machnowska et al., 2019; Margot at al., 2017; Pingen et al., 2014; Rhee et al., 2019a; Rhee et al., 2021). Many of these circulating TDR strains are considered most likely to be established among ART-naive persons, rather than reflecting direct transmission from persons experiencing virologic failure.

Given recent international scale-up of dolutegravir-based therapy and introduction of long-acting cabotegravir across various global settings/care models, transmitted INSTI resistance is likely to remain a public health and clinical concern for the foreseeable future. The prevalence of transmitted INSTI resistance has been below 1.0% in most regions, with one review suggesting low prevalence of surveillance DRMs even in regions where INSTIs have been widely used for several years (Bailey et al., 2021; de Salazar et al., 2023; McClung et al., 2022). However, a few U.S. studies have reported slightly higher rates of 1.4%–2.2% (McClung et al., 2020; Poschman and Spencer, 2020).

MANAGEMENT OF TDR

In the United States and other high-income countries, the risk posed by TDR to the success of first-line therapy is low because, as noted previously, most of the currently transmitted DRMs do not compromise currently recommended first-line ART regimens. Moreover, the routine practice of baseline genotypic resistance testing facilitates early identification of transmitted DRMs that would compromise currently recommended first-line ART regimens and consideration of alternatives.

Given the lack of clinical trials comparing treatment approaches for persons in whom baseline resistance testing reveals the presence of TDR, several retrospective studies provide useful insight. First, because there is no cross-resistance between drug classes, persons with transmitted NNRTI resistance are expected to have an undiminished response to treatment using an INSTI- or PI-containing first-line ART regimen. Second, the presence of the most commonly transmitted NRTI-associated DRMs—TAMs other than T215Y/F—do not appear to influence virological response to first-line tenofovir-containing regimens (Margot et al., 2017; Sörstedt et al., 2018). Third, although the presence of baseline TDR-associated DRMs suggests the possible presence of additional undetected mutations (i.e., those that have faded to low levels following competition with wild-type revertants) (Castro et al., 2013; Jain et al., 2011; Mbunkah et al., 2020; Pingen et al., 2014), such additional DRMs have not been detected frequently by sensitive NGS methods (Clutter et al., 2017; Dauwe et al., 2016; Toni et al., 2009; Varghese et al., 2009). Moreover, in retrospective studies, PWH with TDR detected by baseline genotype do not appear to have higher rates of virologic failure when testing results are subsequently used to appropriately guide therapy (Borghetti et al., 2021; Geretti et al., 2019; Knyphausen et al., 2014; Margot et al., 2017; Metzner et al., 2010; Peuchant et al., 2008; Rhee et al., 2020a).

ACQUIRED HIV DRUG RESISTANCE

EPIDEMIOLOGY

Collectively, the increased use of ARVs with a high genetic barrier to resistance (particularly second-generation INSTIs) and use of FDCs, often administered as complete, single-tablet regimens, make it less likely that medication nonadherence will result in a person's virus becoming exposed to an incompletely suppressive regimen. Many clinical trials and several cohort studies in upper-income countries have reported that fewer persons beginning ART have developed virologic failure or acquired HIVDR during the past two decades in general (ATCC, 2017; Carr et al., 2019; Davy-Mendez et al., 2018; Li et al., 2019; Lodi et al., 2018; Lombardi et al., 2021; Miranda et al., 2022; Nance et al., 2018; Rhee et al., 2020a; Scherrer et al., 2016). Additionally, laboratory-based studies have observed a decline in the proportion of submitted viruses with HIVDR and multiclass resistance (Kagan et al., 2019; Paquet et al., 2014), although this trend may primarily reflect an increasing proportion of tests ordered for persons with newly diagnosed HIV rather than virologic failure. There is also a decreasing proportion of heavily treatment-experienced PWH overall (Bajema et al., 2020). Of note, although global data are relatively limited at this time, findings from recent country-level surveillance programs have indicated that the emergence of acquired dolutegravir resistance may be higher than anticipated, particularly in people with extensive treatment experience (CDC, 2024; WHO, 2024).

Nonetheless, lifelong adherence to daily oral therapy is a continuing challenge, particularly in populations facing logistical, social, and financial barriers to obtaining HIV care and accessing treatment (Benson et al., 2020; Rich et al., 2020; Siefried et al., 2017). Moreover, despite increased use of FDCs and ARVs with a high genetic barrier to resistance, such regimens are not available to some PWH, particularly those who have experienced previous virologic failure or who have coexisting medical conditions/co-medications that might preclude use of certain agents. Recent approval of long-acting ARVs has now also ushered in a host of new questions regarding HIVDR management for which limited evidence is available (Rhee et al., 2022); for example, how best to prevent, identify, and manage ADR in PWH receiving long-acting ART.

MANAGEMENT OF ADR

In PWH developing virologic failure on an initial ART regimen, those who develop HIVDR often have predictable patterns of DRMs. For example, persons receiving an NNRTI-containing regimen will usually have both NRTI and NNRTI-associated DRMs, while those receiving a first-generation INSTI-containing regimen will often have both NRTI and INSTI-associated DRMs (DHHS, 2024a; Gregson et al., 2016; Rhee et al., 2020a). In these two scenarios, the most common NRTI-associated DRMs are the 3TC/FTC mutations M184V/I; additionally, approximately 30% of PWH will also develop a tenofovir-associated DRM (usually K65R or K70E/Q). In low- and middle-income countries, the proportion of persons developing a tenofovir-associated DRM on a first-line NRTI/NNRTI-containing regimen is higher and approaches 60% (Gregson et al., 2016). Among PWH receiving an initial boosted PI or second-generation INSTI-containing regimen, those who develop HIVDR will usually just acquire M184V/I (DHHS, 2024a; Dolling et al., 2013; El Bouzidi et al., 2014; Lathouwers et al., 2020; Rhee et al., 2019b, 2020b; Scarsi et al., 2020). As a result of these predictable patterns, the U.S. guidelines incorporate recommendations for first-line treatment failure scenarios: specific recommendations most commonly involve modifying therapy to include at least one fully active NRTI and either a second-generation INSTI or boosted darunavir (Table 17.4).

In PWH who have experienced virologic failure on multiple ART regimens, the patterns of observed HIV-associated DRMs are often less predictable. In this scenario, most guidelines recommend expert consultation and modification of therapy to include at least two fully active drugs from different ARV drug classes, with at least one having a high barrier to resistance (DHHS, 2024a; Gandhi et al., 2023). The vast majority of clinical trials performed in heavily treated PWH have been registration trials designed to study the impact of "salvage therapy" with ART regimens containing either boosted darunavir, dolutegravir, ibalizumab, or fostemsavir (McCluskey et al., 2019).

With the demonstration that both dolutegravir and boosted darunavir plus a single fully active NRTI are fully suppressive ART regimens for many PWH, and the recent approval of several additional ARVs (e.g., doravirine, ibalizumab, fostemsavir, and now lenacapavir), the prospects for constructing a fully suppressive regimen in nearly all treatment-experienced PWH with virologic failure are high (Bajema et al., 2020; Emu et al., 2018; Marcelin et al., 2021; Paton et al., 2022; Puertas et al., 2020; Raymond et al., 2020; Saladini et al., 2023). Among INSTI-naive PWH or among INSTI-experienced persons with viruses retaining susceptibility to dolutegravir, the combination of dolutegravir plus one fully active NRTI and/or fully active NNRTI (e.g., rilpivirine or doravirine) may be sufficient (DHHS, 2024a).

Table 17.4 TREATMENT OPTIONS FOR PWH WITH VIROLOGIC FAILURE ON A FIRST-LINE REGIMEN

CLINICAL SCENARIO	TYPE OF FAILING REGIMEN	HIVDR CONSIDERATIONS	NEW REGIMEN OPTIONS
First regimen failure	NNRTI plus 2 NRTIs	Likely resistance to NNRTI ± XTC (i.e., NNRTI mutations ± M184V/I). Additional NRTI mutations may be present.	Boosted PI (preferably boosted DRV) plus 2 NRTIs (at least 1 fully active); *or* DTG (possibly BIC) plus 2 NRTIs (at least 1 fully active); *or* Boosted PI plus INSTI (preferably boosted DRV plus DTG)
	Boosted PI plus 2 NRTIs	Most likely no resistance, or resistance limited to XTC (i.e., M184V/I without resistance to other NRTIs)	Second-generation INSTI plus 2 NRTIs (at least 1 fully active—if only one of the NRTIs is fully active or if adherence is a concern, DTG is preferred INSTI although BIC might be considered); *or* Continue same regimen; *or* Another boosted PI plus second-generation INSTI; *or* Another boosted PI plus 2 NRTIs (at least 1 fully active)
	INSTI plus 2 NRTIs	No INSTI resistance (can have XTC resistance, i.e., only M184V/I, usually without resistance to other NRTIs)	Boosted PI plus 2 NRTIs (at least 1 fully active); *or* DTG (possibly BIC) plus 2 NRTIs (at least 1 fully active); *or* Boosted PI plus DTG
		RAL or EVG ± XTC resistance. May have XTC resistance. Resistance to first-line BIC or DTG is rare.	Boosted PI plus 2 NRTIs (at least 1 fully active); *or* DTG twice daily or possibly BIC (if virus is sensitive) plus 2 NRTIs (at least 1 fully active); *or* DTG twice daily or possibly BIC (if virus is sensitive) plus boosted PI

DRV = darunavir; BIC = bictegravir; DTG = dolutegravir; EVG = elvitegravir; RAL = raltegravir; XTC: 3TC/FTC.

Source: Panel on Antiretroviral Guidelines for Adults and Adolescents. Guidelines for the use of antiretroviral agents in adults and adolescents with HIV. Department of Health and Human Services. Adapted from Table 11. https://clinicalinfo.hiv.gov/sites/default/files/inline-files/AdultandAdolescentGL.pdf. Last updated January 31, 2024. Accessed September 14, 2024.

For some PWH with INSTI-resistant viruses, susceptibility to dolutegravir may be retained if dosed twice a day (Akil et al., 2015; Castagna et al., 2014; Eron et al., 2013). Although guidelines indicate bictegravir may be considered rather than dolutegravir for treatment-experienced PWH, it has not been studied for salvage therapy (in contrast to dolutegravir), and its dose cannot be doubled/adjusted to compensate for INSTI-related DRMs—therefore, careful consideration of its use in this scenario is warranted. Likewise, for PWH whose viruses retain complete or nearly complete susceptibility to boosted darunavir, the combination of boosted darunavir plus one fully active NRTI and/or fully active NNRTI (e.g., etravirine or doravirine) may be sufficient. Regimens including dolutegravir plus boosted darunavir have been increasingly used among treatment-experienced PWH with viremia (Armenia et al., 2021; Capetti et al., 2018; D²EFT Study Group, 2024; Jablonowska et al., 2019)—this may reflect provider preferences for avoiding NNRTIs when their inclusion is considered to be of questionable benefit.

In the presence of preexisting resistance to dolutegravir *and* boosted darunavir, current options are more complicated. However, even in this scenario, there are several potentially useful treatment approaches, including the use of two or more active drugs from the four main ARV classes and possibly the use of one or more entry inhibitors or other novel agents (Puertas et al., 2020; Raymond et al., 2020). In most PWH, fostemsavir may have a similar degree of antiviral activity as ibalizumab; however, a small subset of persons will harbor intrinsically resistant viruses (Kozal et al., 2020).

ARV RESISTANCE CONSIDERATIONS FOR SPECIAL CIRCUMSTANCES

There are a number of special scenarios where guidelines offer specific recommendations for HIVDR evaluation and management. A few are described below.

ART SWITCH/SIMPLIFICATION (MODIFYING ART IN THE SETTING OF VIROLOGIC SUPPRESSION)

At times, providers and/or PWH may consider changing to a different fully suppressive regimen. This may be due to concerns regarding safety profile, side effects, new drug-drug interactions, pill burden, challenges navigating food or fluid requirements, pregnancy status/intentions, or cost/access. In these situations, providers should consider the person's complete treatment and resistance-testing history to construct a cumulative resistance profile (DHHS, 2024c; Gandhi et al., 2023; McCluskey et al., 2019). The fundamental clinical principle with regimen optimization/simplification is to maintain virologic suppression and not compromise future options. If comprehensive resistance data are not available, clinicians may be able to extrapolate information from the treatment history—for example, a person with prior virologic failure while taking ARVs with relatively low barrier to resistance (most NNRTIs, first-generation INSTIs, lamivudine/emtricitabine) can be assumed to have accumulated resistance to these drugs (DHHS, 2024a). Proviral DNA sequencing may be considered, but results should be interpreted in conjunction with the knowledge of HIVDR that may have emerged during past episodes of virological failure and previous genotypic resistance test results.

U.S. guidelines list several specific optimization strategies that can be considered (Table 17.5), taking into account factors listed above as well as others (e.g., hepatitis B coinfection) (DHHS, 2024a; Gandhi et al., 2023). Individuals with no suspected or documented history of HIVDR generally have multiple options for switching regimens, either between or within classes. However, clinicians should still exercise caution and generally avoid switching to an agent with a lower genetic barrier to resistance, given the risk of virologic failure in the case of TDR or existing ADR from prior failure (DHHS, 2024a; Eron et al., 2010). Of note, a number of two-drug regimens (including cabotegravir plus rilpivirine, both administered as long-acting injections) are currently identified as potential "switch" options—it would be especially prudent to have a high degree of confidence in a patient's full HIVDR profile when considering switching to a dual-therapy regimen, to ensure that both ARVs are fully active.

With increasing use and availability of long-acting cabotegravir plus rilpivirine, several considerations must be made prior to switching to this regimen. Current U.S. guidelines recommend considering this combination for people who are engaged in care, are virologically suppressed for 3–6 months, agree to regular clinic visits for injections, and do not have HBV coinfection (unless the patient is on a specific HBV regimen). When viremia occurs, resistance testing including integrase testing should be performed (DHHS, 2024a). A pooled analysis from the FLAIR, ATLAS, and ATLAS-2M trials demonstrated that virologic failure was rare across studies (approximately 1%); risk factors included presence of baseline proviral rilpivirine-associated mutations, HIV-1 subtype A6/A1, higher BMI (≥30 kg/m^2), and lower week 8 rilpivirine trough concentrations (Cutrell et al., 2021).

For people with a history of limited HIVDR, clinicians can consider a switch from one drug to another within the same class or in a different class, as long as the new drug has a high genetic barrier to resistance and there is no known or suspected resistance to the new agent. Dolutegravir plus two NRTIs (one of which is fully active) should be effective as a switch strategy in PWH without underlying dolutegravir resistance (DHHS, 2024a). Bictegravir/emtricitabine/tenofovir alafenamide has also been examined as a switch option in both trials and real-world settings, including for treatment-experienced PWH (Acosta et al., 2020; Armenia et al., 2022; Rolle et al., 2021; Sax et al., 2022). Expert consultation may be especially helpful when considering regimen switching/simplification for heavily ART-experienced PWH, as individuals who have undergone multiple regimen modifications have often done so because of virologic failure and ADR, and may have multiclass HIVDR (DHHS, 2024a; Gandhi, et al., 2023).

RAPID ART INITIATION AND RAPID ART REINITIATION

U.S. guidelines currently recommend initiating ART at time of diagnosis (when possible) or soon afterward "to increase the uptake of ART, decrease the time required to achieve linkage to care and virologic suppression, and improve the rate of virologic suppression" (DHHS, 2024a, n.p.). This approach has been demonstrated to be feasible and acceptable across different settings (Boyd et al., 2019; Coffey et al., 2019; Colasanti et al., 2018; Martin et al., 2021; Rodriguez et al., 2019). In addition to benefits at the individual patient level, public health benefits include decreased risk of HIV transmission to others (Ford et al., 2018; Mateo-Urdiales, 2019; Pilcher et al., 2017). A randomized study looking at a universal test-and-treat strategy with immediate ART initiation found no evidence of increased HIVDR prevalence with this strategy compared to standard of care (Fogel et al., 2022). One retrospective cohort analysis also found no difference in one-year probability of virologic suppression among people initiating ART with versus without baseline genotype results (Bavaro et al., 2022).

Since regimen selection for rapid ART initiation occurs prior to availability of baseline resistance-testing results, options should have a suitably high likelihood of effectiveness and favorable safety and side-effect profiles; local TDR patterns may also need to be considered. To date, the most commonly used rapid ART combination options in the United States, despite baseline INSTI- and NRTI-associated mutations, for ART-naive individuals are dolutegravir or bictegravir based regimens (Acosta et al., 2021; D'Antoni et al., 2022; Shafran et al., 2023).

Currently, the only specific medication recommendations provided in U.S. guidelines on rapid ART selection are to avoid NNRTI-based regimens, abacavir, and the dual-therapy combination of dolutegravir plus lamivudine. Additionally, INSTI-based regimens should be avoided in people who received long-acting cabotegravir for PrEP prior to HIV acquisition; instead, a regimen containing boosted darunavir should be used until drug resistance testing confirms no INSTI resistance. Given the potential impact of TDR and overall prevalence of hepatitis B among PWH, more experience with rapid ART using dolutegravir plus lamivudine may be beneficial (Kessler et al., 2020; Rolle et al., 2023).

For PWH who have been out of care and/or off ART, "rapid ART re-initiation" decisions may not be straightforward, especially if limited history is available. Depending on the individual's prior treatment history, some providers would consider obtaining resistance testing at the first clinical re-engagement visit; however, as indicated previously, testing performed in the absence of recent ART use may be of limited utility. Although it may provide useful information to guide therapy modification *after* rapid ART re-initiation (in the event that DRMs are identified), historically selected mutations may not be reflected accurately without the presence of

Table 17.5 TREATMENT OPTIONS FOR OPTIMIZING ART IN THE SETTING OF VIROLOGIC SUPPRESSION

CLINICAL SCENARIO	TYPE OF SWITCH	STRATEGIES THAT HAVE EVIDENCE FOR SUCCESS
No suspected or documented HIVDR	Within-class switch	• TDF or ABC to TAF • RAL or EVG/c to DTG or BIC • DTG to BIC or BIC to DTG • EFV to RPV or DOR • RPV to DOR
	Between-class switch	• Boosted PI to second-generation INSTI • Boosted PI to RPV or DOR • NNRTI to second-generation INSTI or boosted PI
	Switch from 3-drug to 2-drug regimen (both drugs should be fully active)	• DTG + RPV • DTG + XTC • 3TC + boosted PI (e.g., DRV/r or DRV/cobi or ATV/r or LPV/r) • Boosted DRV + DTG • Long-acting CAB + RPV[a]
History of limited drug resistance	Within-class switch	• Switch from one drug with a high genetic barrier to resistance to another (i.e., from DTG to BIC) • Switch to a drug with a higher genetic barrier to resistance (i.e., from RAL to DTG or BIC)
	Between-class switch	• Switch from one drug with a high genetic barrier to resistance to another (i.e., from boosted PI to DTG or BIC) • Switch to a drug with a higher genetic barrier to resistance (i.e., from EFV to DTG or BIC or boosted PI)
History of complex underlying resistance	Proceed with caution; follow the same principles outlined under "Management of ADR" and consider expert consultation	

3TC = lamivudine; ABC = abacavir; ATV = atazanavir; ATV/r = ritonavir-boosted atazanavir; BIC = bictegravir; CAB = cabotegravir; DRV = darunavir; DRV/cobi = cobicistat-boosted darunavir; DRV/r = ritonavir-boosted darunavir; DTG = dolutegravir; DOR = doravarine; EFV = efavirenz; EVG/c = elvitegravir/cobicistat; LPV/r = ritonavir-boosted lopinavir; MVC = maraviroc; RAL = raltegravir; RPV = rilpivirine; TAF = tenofovir alafenamide; TDF = tenofovir disoproxil fumarate.

Note: [a] Given limited data and experience, U.S. guidelines recommend that the dual regimen of long-acting CAB + RPV can be used to replace an existing, stable oral ARV regimen in PWH with sustained viral suppression for 3–6 months (optimal duration is not defined), who have good adherence and engagement in care, no known or suspected resistance to either medication, and no prior treatment failures. If the person being considered for long-acting CAB + RVP has active or occult HBV infection, they should be receiving HBV therapy if indicated. Persons being considered for long-acting CAB + RPV should also not be receiving medications with significant drug interactions.

Source: Panel on Antiretroviral Guidelines for Adults and Adolescents. Guidelines for the use of antiretroviral agents in adults and adolescents with HIV. Department of Health and Human Services. Adapted from text. http://www.aidsinfo.nih.gov/ContentFiles/AdultandAdolescentGL.pdf. Last updated January 31, 2024. Accessed September 14, 2024.

selective drug pressure. In other words, the absence of detectable resistance must be viewed cautiously when interpreting results. Expert input is generally recommended for "rapid ART re-initiation" decisions (especially for heavily ART-experienced PWH) since multiple factors should be taken into account, such as prior ART exposure and response, previous resistance-testing results, and concern for potential untreated central nervous system (CNS) opportunistic infections. If the viral load does not decrease as anticipated after re-initiating therapy, providers should have a low threshold to repeat resistance testing to guide further management.

HEAVILY TREATMENT-EXPERIENCED PATIENTS

Assessment and management of highly treatment-experienced patients who are experiencing virologic failure is complex; however, the goal of treatment remains the same: achieving virological suppression. Virological failure can occur for a multitude of factors related to the individual, HIV infection, and/or ART regimen. Evaluation should include assessment of a person's complete treatment and HIVDR history, medication adherence and tolerability patterns, and prior viral load and $CD4^+$ count trends. Resistance testing should be performed while the patient is taking the failing regimen or within 4 weeks of discontinuation of a non-long-acting regimen. If resistance testing is obtained after that time period, it can still provide useful information but may not detect previously selected mutations (DHHS, 2024a). Adding a single ARV drug to an already failing regimen is generally not recommended, as this rarely results in virologic suppression and increases the risk of further HIVDR. When choosing a new regimen in highly treatment-experienced patients, two fully active ARVs can be utilized if at least one has a high barrier to resistance (e.g., DTG or boosted DRV). If no fully active

ARV with a high resistance barrier is available, the new regimen should attempt to include three fully active agents. Fully active ARVs may include drugs in classes without selected drug-resistant virus, newer members of existing classes with higher barriers to resistance, and drugs with novel mechanisms that the patient has not previously received. Examples include lenacapavir, ibalizumab, and fostemsavir (DHHS, 2024a). Clinicians can also consider enrolling patients in clinical trials of investigational agents or expanded access of investigational agents (DHHS, 2024a).

PREGNANCY AND INFANT FEEDING

The fundamental principles of HIVDR testing/evaluation and management for pregnant people are the same as those in people who are not pregnant (i.e., perform drug-resistance testing at diagnosis, at initiation or re-initiation of ART, and in the event of virologic failure) (DHHS, 2024c). However, it is important to achieve virologic suppression as early and as quickly as possible in pregnancy to reduce the likelihood of perinatal transmission. Because resistance testing results may not be available for several weeks, U.S. guidelines recommend immediate ART initiation if HIV is diagnosed during pregnancy (DHHS, 2024c). In ART-experienced pregnant PWH, therapy should be guided by what is known about previous ART regimens, responses to therapy, and available resistance-testing results. In both scenarios, treatment should be modified if necessary once resistance-testing results are available, and ARV safety and dosing should also be considered in pregnancy. In one study, 16% of ART-naive and 33% of treatment-experienced PWH had one or more resistance-associated mutations at the time of pregnancy. The most common finding in both ART-naive (81%) and treatment-experienced (91%) patients was NNRTI resistance (da Silveira Gouvêa et al., 2023). If therapy must be stopped for any reason, all ARV drugs should be stopped simultaneously and re-initiated as soon as possible to minimize HIVDR. Pregnant persons who have documented zidovudine resistance should still receive intravenous zidovudine during labor when indicated (i.e., HIV RNA >1,000 copies/mL near delivery).

Unique pregnancy-associated factors may lead to incomplete viral suppression and HIVDR development, such as nausea and vomiting affecting adherence and pharmacokinetic changes such as increased plasma volume and renal clearance. Some ARVs require dose adjustment during pregnancy; U.S. guidelines provide detailed information (DHHS, 2024c). If perinatal/postnatal HIV transmission does occur in the setting of incomplete maternal viral suppression, maternal HIVDR can be transmitted to the infant, potentially limiting treatment options for the infant (Boyce et al., 2022; Delaugerre et al., 2009; Weyland et al., 2022). Decisions about ARV prophylaxis and/or treatment for infants exposed to drug-resistant virus should therefore be made in consultation with a pediatric HIV specialist.

Updated guidelines, particularly in resource-rich settings, now support evidence-based, person-centered counseling for infant feeding, and therefore more mothers with virologic suppression on ART may opt to breastfeed (DHHS, 2024b). If an infant acquires HIV infection during breastfeeding, resistance testing should be performed on the infant's virus and ART should be adjusted accordingly. The PROMISE (Promoting Maternal and Infant Survival Everywhere) trial included over 2,400 women with CD4 >350 cells/mm^3 and compared the efficacy of extended infant prophylaxis using nevirapine to maternal ART alone in preventing breastfeeding-associated HIV transmission. Investigators found that maternal viral load and HIVDR were independently associated with breastfeeding transmission (Boyce et al., 2022). Furthermore, many ARVs have been detected in breast milk: since the levels of these ARVs are noted to be lower than that in maternal serum plasma, it is generally considered unlikely that infants would experience toxicity from breastmilk ARV exposures. However, infants who acquire HIV through breastfeeding are at risk of developing HIVDR due to subtherapeutic levels of ARVs in breast milk as well as dosing of ARVs given as prophylaxis (Bamford et al., 2024; Bishop et al., 2024; Boyce et al., 2022; DHHS, 2024b; Fogel et al., 2013; Volpe et al., 2022; Waitt et al., 2018).

CHILDREN AND YOUTH

U.S. guidelines include separate, distinct recommendations for ART management of infants, children, and other youth with HIV infection (DHHS, 2024b). Many of the principles are the same as in adults (e.g., obtain genotype testing when HIV viral loads are detectable, and select treatment based on ARV history and resistance-testing results). Changes to ART may occur for a multitude of reasons, including regimen simplification, modification to include agents with a higher resistance barrier, adverse effects, and treatment failure. However, some special considerations are particularly noteworthy for children and youth. Infants with perinatally/postnatally acquired infection can have complex HIVDR patterns given subtherapeutic ARV exposure during pregnancy and breastfeeding. Furthermore, resistance can develop rapidly due to high levels of viral replication (DHHS, 2024). For infants with high pretreatment viral loads, it can often take over 6 months to achieve suppression; however, ongoing non-suppression (especially while on NNRTI-based regimens) increases the risk of developing resistance (Babiker et al., 2011).

Virologic failure in children can occur for many reasons, and the main challenge is often suboptimal adherence. Persistent viremia in the setting of no identifiable ARV resistance is most commonly due to low levels of adherence. However, other factors must be considered, including poor medication absorption, drug-drug interactions, and incorrect dosing. Resistance testing is most optimally assessed while the child is on the failing ARV regimen. As with adults, viral strains may quickly revert back to wild-type virus after ART cessation, and subsequently drug-resistant strains may no longer be detected. Importantly, INSTIs are more frequently being utilized in pediatric treatment regimens (especially for children who have experienced treatment failure on NNRTI- or PI-based regimens) (Briand et al., 2017; DHHS, 2024b;

Viani et al., 2020). Although raltegravir has been most commonly studied thus far, both dolutegravir and bictegravir have the advantage of once daily dosing, smaller pill size, and higher barrier to resistance. They also often retain activity in some people who have experienced virologic failure or are highly treatment experienced.

HIV ACQUISITION IN THE SETTING OF PREP USE

There have been two main concerns regarding PrEP and HIVDR: the first is whether PrEP will remain effective in areas with high TDR prevalence, and the second is whether PrEP will lead to increased cases of HIVDR. Additionally, as more long-acting options become available and PrEP is further implemented globally, new considerations arise (Parikh et al., 2022). Regarding the first concern, studies have shown that transmission of viruses resistant to tenofovir and/or 3TC/FTC is generally uncommon (with M184V/I occurring in 0.8% and K65R in 0.1% of newly diagnosed PWH in the United States), although pretreatment drug resistance may be >10% among sub-populations in various regions (Macdonald et al., 2020; McClung et al., 2020). Approximately 0.5% of newly diagnosed PWH in the United States are predicted to have cabotegravir resistance (McClung et al., 2020); low rates have also been reported from other regions thus far (Charpentier et al., 2021). By contrast, among PWH experiencing virologic failure, approximately 15% have 3TC/FTC and/or tenofovir resistance, and approximately 5% have cabotegravir resistance. Therefore, the risk of PrEP failure may be higher if a person on PrEP acquires HIV from a PWH experiencing virologic failure.

Regarding the second concern of whether global PrEP scale-up will increase HIVDR, data from PrEP clinical trials have indicated that there are two scenarios in which HIVDR can emerge: persons experiencing acute infection at the time of PrEP initiation, and persons who acquire infection at a later time point (usually as a result of subtherapeutic PrEP drug exposure most commonly caused by low medication adherence) but continue to take PrEP. When HIVDR does occur with oral PrEP use, it is nearly always associated with M184V/I and 3TC/FTC resistance and rarely with K65R and tenofovir resistance (Gibas et al., 2019; Girometti et al., 2022; Johnson et al., 2021; Landovitz et al., 2024; Misra et al., 2024; Parikh et al., 2016). One examination of multiple studies found that, out of 310 individuals who acquired HIV while taking tenofovir disoproxil fumarate/emtricitabine in clinical settings, 20% had PrEP-associated HIVDR (WHO, 2024). For people taking "event-driven" (or "on-demand") oral PrEP, low levels of adherence to this dosing strategy appear to increase the likelihood of HIV acquisition and also the potential for development of resistance (Laurent et al., 2023; Raccagni et al., 2022). Nevertheless, despite increased HIVDR risk in people who acquire HIV after recent PrEP exposure, rapid ART initiation can still be feasible and has been shown to achieve virologic suppression (even with known HIVDR including M184V/I) (Girometti et al., 2022).

Since 2021, long-acting options for PrEP have become more widely available and now include the dapivirine vaginal ring (approved in several African countries) and injectable cabotegravir (approved in both resource-rich and resource-limited settings). Among dapivirine trial participants who acquired HIV infection, risk of NNRTI resistance was not significantly higher among those who had received the dapivirine vaginal ring versus placebo (Baeten et al., 2021; Nel et al., 2021; Parikh et al., 2021). Further research is needed regarding its efficacy in preventing HIV acquisition in the setting of drug-resistant virus (WHO, 2024).

Cases of emergent INSTI-associated DRMs were observed among clinical trial participants who received long-acting cabotegravir and were subsequently diagnosed with HIV (Eshelman et al., 2022; Marzinke et al., 2021). To date, 10 of these 16 cases were found to have INSTI resistance, and all 10 had cross-resistance to dolutegravir (Marzinke et al., 2023). The development of INSTI resistance in this scenario is thought to primarily be due to the long pharmacokinetic "tail" of the drug after cessation of injections (creating an extended time frame of subtherapeutic drug exposure) and delayed HIV detection, which collectively increases the risk for selection of virus with INSTI-associated DRMs. Observations from clinical trials indicate that use of a more sensitive HIV RNA assay for screening would have detected infection before INSTI-resistance mutations occurred in most cases, and before the mutations accumulated in other cases (Eshleman et al., 2022; Marzinke et al., 2023). Importantly, one key limitation to widespread adoption of this diagnostic tool for earlier HIV detection is that universal RNA monitoring is neither feasible nor affordable in many settings. Although this and other mitigation strategies have yet to be fully characterized or operationalized, cases of INSTI resistance related to long-acting cabotegravir as PrEP are generally expected to be infrequent given its high overall efficacy. Additionally, because HIV RNA levels were low at time of diagnosis in people who acquired HIV on long-acting cabotegravir, the chance of transmitted drug resistance to others is likely to be reduced in early infection. However, a systematic review demonstrated that dolutegravir resistance was identified in nearly 1 in 4 people who acquired HIV while receiving long-acting cabotegravir (Ahluwalia et al., 2022).

RESOURCE-LIMITED SETTINGS (LOW- AND MIDDLE-INCOME COUNTRIES)

The primary differences regarding evaluation and management of HIVDR between high-income countries and low-/middle-income countries (LMIC) include: (a) absence of universal access to routine genotypic resistance testing; (b) less frequent viral load monitoring; (c) high prevalence of infants and children with perinatally acquired infection whose treatment options are limited because of transmitted or acquired DRMs; and (d) the large proportion of PWH who have failed previously recommended first-line therapy combinations (with resultant development of dual NRTI-NNRTI resistance) or who have failed first- *and* second-line therapy (with subsequent three-class drug resistance).

Pretreatment drug resistance (PDR) refers to DRMs detected in PWH before they start ART. This may arise with either transmission of a drug-resistant strain (i.e., TDR) or DRMs, owing to previous ART exposure, such as with time-limited perinatal/postpartum ART use, PrEP or PEP, or interrupted first-line ART. For LMIC, global surveillance data have indicated a notable rise in pretreatment resistance to NNRTIs after initial ART scale-up, primarily because of use of first-generation NNRTIs with a low genetic barrier to resistance (Bertagnolio et al., 2022). Current WHO guidelines recommend dolutegravir-based ART as preferred first- and second-line treatment, and over 25 million people worldwide are receiving dolutegravir. In these populations, virologic suppression rates exceed 90%; however, as part of increasing dolutegravir utilization, WHO recommends routine HIVDR surveillance. Recent observational and country-specific data have indicated that levels of HIVDR to dolutegravir are higher than those reported from clinical trials. Currently, the WHO does not suggest they are high enough to require country-level action; however, closer national monitoring with widespread information-sharing is essential to guide clinical practice regarding ART management for people who have failed dolutegravir-based ART (WHO, 2024). In a systematic analysis, the prevalence of INSTI-associated DRMs among previously dolutegravir-naive individuals was less than 3%. Data from eight cohorts from high-income countries showed that 4.8% of participants receiving dolutegravir-based ART with ongoing viremia had resistance to dolutegravir. In contrast, data from studies in LMIC demonstrated the prevalence of dolutegravir resistance ranging from 3.9% to 19.6% among individuals on dolutegravir-based therapy experiencing viremia. As of July 2023, 10 countries had implemented surveys to address increasing dolutegravir resistance (3 are ongoing, 24 more are planned). Furthermore, only 6 countries have implemented surveys among children and adolescents (1 is ongoing, and 14 are planned). More data are required regarding risk factors, patterns of emergent drug resistance, and its impact on pregnant people and breastfed infants. The 2024 updated WHO HIV drug-resistance strategy provides an overview of core recommended activities, including country-level monitoring of quality-of-care indicators associated with predicting HIVDR, as well as survey implementation (WHO, 2024).

Importantly, as global scale-up of long-acting cabotegravir as PrEP continues to move forward, ongoing population-level HIVDR (and particularly INSTI resistance) monitoring will be essential in preserving INSTIs as first-line therapy for HIV treatment in resource-limited settings. Programs which have been established to evaluate PrEP-associated HIVDR have been shown to be beneficial and feasible, with the most common limitation being laboratory capacity (Levy et al., 2022). A modeling study from sub-Saharan Africa attempted to predict INSTI resistance in the setting of long-acting cabotegravir implementation. The model predicted that about 20 years after the introduction of long-acting cabotegravir, 13% of people initiating ART would have preexisting INSTI resistance versus 1.7% in the absence of long-acting cabotegravir initiation. Despite the total increase in INSTI resistance, the implementation of long-acting cabotegravir would lead to a 29% decrease in HIV incidence and reduction in the number of people dying of HIV-related causes (Smith et al., 2023).

HIV-2

HIV-2 infection (and HIV-1/-2 coinfection) remains rare in the United States. However, HIV-2 is endemic in many regions experiencing high overall HIV prevalence, such as West Africa. The two types not only have different susceptibility to various ARV agents but also exhibit different pathways to resistance (Moranguinho et al., 2023). HIV-2 has demonstrated intrinsic, high-level resistance to NNRTIs and enfuvirtide. Therefore, NNRTI-containing regimens, including long-acting cabotegravir plus rilpivirine, are not recommended. Protease inhibitors exhibit variable activity against HIV-2; boosted lopinavir and darunavir are believed to have the most clinically useful potency. HIV-2 is susceptible to INSTIs, as well as all NRTIs currently in clinical use; however, data suggest differences in INSTI and NRTI mutation selection and HIVDR mechanisms/pathways between HIV-2 and HIV-1 (Boyer et al., 2012; Gottlieb et al., 2009; Moranguinho et al., 2023; Requena et al., 2017; Tzou et al., 2020). Of note, recent studies continue to find novel INSTI mutations in HIV-2 not previously characterized. One study found a number of DRMs causing extensive cross-resistance between raltegravir and dolutegravir (Smith et al., 2022). Three small, single-arm, open-label trials have assessed the effectiveness of INSTI-based regimens (raltegravir, boosted elvitegravir, or dolutegravir in combination with 2 NRTIs): all demonstrated favorable 48-week clinical outcomes (Ba et al., 2018; Matheron et al., 2018; Pacheco et al., 2023). These studies provide the best evidence to date for HIV-2 treatment recommendations, which now recommend an INSTI plus two NRTIs as the optimal strategy in treating people with HIV-2 mono- or coinfection.

With regard to newer and less commonly used agents, lenacapavir and ibalizumab both demonstrate in vitro potency against HIV-2; in vitro studies suggest that HIV-2 is intrinsically resistant to fostemsavir (Le Hingrat et al., 2022; Nowicka-Sans et al., 2012; Smith et al., 2024;). Maraviroc appears to be active against isolates of HIV-2 in vitro; however, there is no FDA-approved assay that can be used to determine HIV-2 receptor tropism (Moranguinho et al., 2023; Visseaux et al., 2012). In general, there are significant limitations to HIV-2 testing in the United States, including HIV-2 drug-resistance testing, which is not commercially available. Some research laboratories (e.g., the University of Washington) have limited capacity to perform genotype testing under research protocols. Some local, national, and international guidelines include alternative ARV regimens for initial and second-line ART for HIV-2; however, at this time no comparative controlled trial data exist to support the effectiveness of a specific regimen over others (New York State Department of Health, 2012; WHO, 2021; WHOr, 2013).

CONCLUSION

ADR and, to a lesser extent, TDR continue to pose challenges to the successful treatment of PWH. In the absence of selective drug pressure, DRMs can quickly be replaced by wild-type variants, so resistance testing should be performed as close to HIV diagnosis as possible and, ideally, while PWH are still on ART when virologic failure is identified. Identified DRMs should be documented and taken into account when considering ART re-initiation or modification. PBMC DNA sequencing can be useful for ART switch/simplification in PWH who are virologically suppressed, but results should be interpreted with caution. Management of ADR and TDR should take into account HIV-specific factors and other key individual conditions and/or factors to construct a clinically appropriate regimen that includes at least two fully active drugs from different ARV drug classes. Several specific clinical scenarios pose unique considerations for prevention and management of HIVDR.

RECOMMENDED READING

Carr A, Mackie NE, Paredes R, Ruxrungtham K. HIV drug resistance in the era of contemporary antiretroviral therapy: a clinical perspective. *Antivir Ther.* 2023;28(5):13596535231201162. doi:10.1177/13596535231201162

Johnson MM, Jones CE, Clark DN. The effect of treatment-associated mutations on HIV replication and transmission cycles. *Viruses.* 2023;15(1):107.

Temereanca A, Ruta S. Strategies to overcome HIV drug resistance: current and future perspectives perspectives. *Front Microbiol.* 2023;14:1133407.

REFERENCES

Abram ME, Ferris AL, Shao W, et al. Nature, position, and frequency of mutations made in a single cycle of HIV-1 replication. *J Virology.* 2010;84(19):9864–9878.

Acosta RK, Chen GQ, Chang S, et al. Three-year study of pre-existing drug resistance substitutions and efficacy of bictegravir/emtricitabine/tenofovir alafenamide in HIV-1 treatment-naïve participants. *J Antimicrob Chemother.* 2021;76(8):2153–2157.

Acosta RK, Willkom M, Andreatta K, et al. Switching to bictegravir/emtricitabine/tenofovir alafenamide (B/F/TAF) from dolutegravir (DTG) + F/TAF or DTG + F/tenofovir disoproxil fumarate (TDF) in the presence of pre-existing NRTI resistance. *J Acquir Immune Defic Syndr.* 2020;85(3):363–371.

Ahluwalia AK, Inzaule S, Baggaley RC, et al. Characterization of dolutegravir drug resistance in persons diagnosed with HIV after exposure to long-acting injectable cabotegravir for preexposure prophylaxis. *AIDS.* 2022;36(13):1897–1898.

Akil B, Blick G, Hagins DP, et al. Dolutegravir versus placebo in subjects harbouring HIV-1 with integrase inhibitor resistance associated substitutions: 48-week results from VIKING-4, a randomized study. *Antivir Ther.* 2015;20:343–348.

Allavena C, Rodallec A, Leplat A, et al. Interest of proviral HIV-1 DNA genotypic resistance testing in virologically suppressed patients candidate for maintenance therapy. *J Virol Methods.* 2018;251:106–110.

Antiretroviral Therapy Cohort Collaboration. Survival of HIV-positive patients starting antiretroviral therapy between 1996 and 2013: a collaborative analysis of cohort studies. *Lancet HIV.* 2017;4:e349–e356.

Armenia D, Bouba Y, Gagliardini R, et al. Virological response and resistance profile in highly treatment-experienced HIV-1-infected patients switching to dolutegravir plus boosted darunavir in clinical practice. *HIV Med.* 2021;22(6):519–525.

Armenia D, Forbici F, Bertoli A, et al. Bictegravir/emtricitabine/tenofovir alafenamide ensures high rates of virological suppression maintenance despite previous resistance in PLWH who optimize treatment in clinical practice. *J Glob Antimicrob Resist.* 2022;30:326–334.

Armenia D, Zaccarelli M, Borghi V, et al. Resistance detected in PBMCs predicts virological rebound in HIV-1 suppressed patients switching treatment. *J Clin Virol.* July 2018;104:61–64.

Avila-Rios S, Garcia-Moralis C, Matias-Florentino M, et al; HIVDR MexNet Group. Pretreatment HIV-drug resistance in Mexico and its impact on the effectiveness of first-line antiretroviral therapy: a nationally representative 2015 WHO survey. *Lancet HIV.* 2016b;3:e579–e591.

Avila-Rios S, Parkin N, Swanstrom R, et al. Next-generation sequencing for HIV drug resistance testing: laboratory, clinical, and implementation considerations. *Viruses.* 2020;12(6):617.

Avila-Rios S, Sued O, Rhee SY, et al. Surveillance of HIV transmitted drug resistance in Latin America and the Caribbean: a systematic review and meta-Analysis. *PLoS One.* 2016a;11:e0158560.

Ba S, Raugi DN, Smith RA, et al; University of Washington-Dakar HIV-2 Study Group. A trial of a single-tablet regimen of elvitegravir, cobicistat, emtricitabine, and tenofovir disoproxil fumarate for the initial treatment of Human Immunodeficiency Virus Type 2 infection in a resource-limited setting: 48-week results from Senegal, West Africa. *Clin Infect Dis.* 2018;67(10):1588–1594.

Babiker A, Castro nee Green H, Compagnucci A, et al. First-line antiretroviral therapy with a protease inhibitor versus non-nucleoside reverse transcriptase inhibitor and switch at higher versus low viral load in HIV-infected children: an open-label, randomized phase 2/3 trial. *Lancet Infect Dis.* 2011;11(4):273–283.

Bachmann N, von Braun A, Labhardt ND, et al. Importance of routine viral load monitoring: higher levels of resistance at ART failure in Uganda and Lesotho compared with Switzerland. *J Antimicrob Chemother.* 2019;74(2):468–472.

Baeten JM, Palanee-Phillips T, Mgodi NM, et al. Safety, uptake, and use of a dapivirine vaginal ring for HIV-1 prevention in African women (HOPE): an open label, extension study. *Lancet HIV.* 2021;8(2):e87–e95.

Bailey AJ, Rhee SY, Shafer RW. Integrase strand transfer inhibitor resistance in integrase strand transfer inhibitor-naïve persons. *AIDS Res Hum Retroviruses.* 2021;37(10):736–743.

Bajema KL, Nance RM, Delaney JAC, et al. Substantial decline in heavily treated therapy-experienced persons with HIV with limited antiretroviral treatment options. *AIDS.* 2020;34(14):2051–2059.

Balakrishna S, Loosli T, Zaheri M, et al. Frequency matters: comparison of drug resistance mutation detection by Sanger and next-generation sequencing in HIV-1. *J Antimicrob Chemother.* 2023;78(3):656–664.

Bamford A, Foster C, Lyall H. Infant feeding: emerging concepts to prevent HIV transmission. *Curr Opin Infect Dis.* 2024;37(1):8–16.

Bavaro DF, De Vito A, Pasculli G, et al. Early versus delayed antiretroviral therapy based on genotypic resistance test: results from a large retrospective cohort study. *J Med Virol.* 2022;94(8):3890–3899.

Baxter JD, Dunn D, Tostevin A, et al. Transmitted HIV-1 drug resistance in a large international cohort using next-generation sequencing: results from the Strategic Timing of Antiretroviral Treatment (START) study. *HIV Med.* 2021;22(5):360–371.

Bennett DE, Camacho RJ, Otelea D, et al. Drug resistance mutations for surveillance of transmitted HIV-1 drug resistance: 2009 update. *PLoS One.* 2009;4(3):e4724.

Benson C, Wang X, Dunn K, et al. Antiretroviral adherence, drug resistance, and the impact of social determinants of health in HIV-1 patients in the US. *AIDS Behav.* 2020;24(12):3562–3573.

Bertagnolio S, Jordan MR, Giron A, Inzaule S. Epidemiology of HIV drug resistance in low- and middle-income countries and WHO global strategy to monitor its emergence. *Curr Opin HIV AIDS.* 2022;17(4):229–239.

Bishop MD, Korutaro V, Boyce CL, et al. Characterizing HIV drug resistance in cases of vertical transmission in the VESTED randomized antiretroviral treatment trial. *J Acquir Immune Defic Syndr.* 2024;96(4):385–392.

Blair H. Ibalizumab: a review in multidrug-resistant HIV-1 infection. *Drugs.* 2020;80(2):189–196.

Boltz VF, Zheng Y, Lockman S, et al. Role of low-frequency HIV-1 variants in failure of nevirapine-containing antiviral therapy in women previously exposed to single-dose nevirapine. *Proc Natl Acad Sci USA.* 2011;108:9202–9207.

Borghetti A, Cicculo A, Lombardi F, et al. Transmitted drug resistance to NRTIs and risk of virological failure in naïve patients treated with integrase inhibitors. *HIV Med.* 2021;22(1):22–27.

Boukli N, Boyd A, Collot M, Meynard JL, Girard PM, Morand-Joubert L. Utility of HIV-1 DNA genotype in determining antiretroviral resistance in patients with low or undetectable HIV RNA viral loads. *J Antimicrob Chemother.* 2018;73(11):3129–3136.

Boyce CL, Sils T, Ko D, et al. Maternal human immunodeficiency virus (HIV) drug resistance is associated with vertical transmission and is prevalent in infected infants. *Clin Infect Dis.* 2022;74(11):2001–2009.

Boyd MA, Boffito M, Castagna A, Estrada V. Rapid initiation of antiretroviral therapy at HIV diagnosis: definition, process, knowledge gaps. *HIV Medicine.* 2019;20(Suppl):3–11.

Boyer PL, Clark PJ, Hughes SH. HIV-1 and HIV-2 reverse transcriptases: different mechanisms of resistance to nucleoside reverse transcriptase inhibitors. *J Virol.* 2012;86(10):5885–94.

Briand C, Dollfus C, Faye A, et al. Efficacy and tolerance of dolutegravir-based combined ART in perinatally HIV-1-infected adolescents: a French multicentre retrospective study. *J Antimicrob Chemother.* 2017;72(3):837–843.

Capetti AF, De Socio GV, Cossu MV, et al. Durability of dolutegravir plus boosted darunavir as salvage or simplification of salvage regimens in HIV-1 infected, highly treatment-experienced subjects. *HIV Clin Trials.* 2018;19(6):242–248.

Carr A, Richardson R, Liu Z. Success and failure of initial antiretroviral therapy in adult: an updated systematic review. *AIDS.* 2019;33(3):443–453.

Castagna A, Maggiolo F, Penco G, et al. Dolutegravir in antiretroviral-experienced patients with raltegravir-and/or elvitegravir-resistant HIV-1: 24-week results of the phase III VIKING-3 Study. *J Infect Dis.* 2014;210: 354–362.

Castro H, Pillay D, Cane P, et al; UK Collaborative Group on HIV Drug Resistance. Persistence of HIV-1 transmitted drug resistance mutations. *J Infect Dis.* 2013;208:1459–1463.

Centers for Disease Control and Prevention. Monitoring HIV drug resistance with CADRE. https://www.cdc.gov/globalhivtb/images/2024CADRE_Factsheet_MonitoringHIV.pdf. Published May, 2024. Accessed June 4, 2024.

Cervo A, Russo A, Di Carlo D et al. Long-acting combination of cabotegravir plus rilpivirine: a picture of potential eligible and ineligible HIV-positive individuals from the Italian ARCA cohort. *J Glob Antimicrob Resist.* 2023;34:141–144.

Charpentier C, Storto A, Soulié C, et al. Prevalence of genotypic baseline risk factors for cabotegravir + rilpivirine failure among ARV-naïve patients. *J Antimicrob Chemother.* 2021;76(11):2983–2987.

Chu C, Armenia D, Walworth C, Santoro MM, Shafer RW. Genotypic resistance testing of HIV-1 DNA in peripheral blood mononuclear cells. *Clin Micro Rev.* 2022;35(4):e0005222.

Clutter DS, Zhou S, Varghese V, et al. Prevalence of drug resistant minority variants in untreated HIV-1-infected individuals with and those without transmitted drug resistance detected by Sanger sequencing. *J Infect Dis.* 2017;216(3):387–391.

Coffey S, Bacchetti P, Sachdev D, et al. RAPID antiretroviral therapy: high virologic suppression rates with immediate antiretroviral therapy initiation in a vulnerable urban clinic population. *AIDS.* 2019;33(5):825–832.

Coffin JM. HIV population dynamics in vivo: implications for genetic variation, pathogenesis, and therapy. *Science.* 1995;267(5197): 483–489.

Colasanti J, Sumitani J, Mehta CC, et al. Implementation of a rapid entry program decreases time to viral suppression among vulnerable persons living with HIV in the Southern United States. *Open Forum Infect Dis.* 2018;5(6):ofy104.

Cozzi-Lepri A, Noguera-Julian M, Di Giallonardo F; CHAIN Minority HIV-1 Variants Working Group. Low-frequency drug-resistant HIV-1 and risk of virological failure to first-line NNRTI-based ART: a multicohort European case-control study using centralized ultrasensitive 454 pyrosequencing. *J Antimicrob Chemother.* 2015;70:930–940.

Curanovic D, Martens S, Rodriguez M, et al. HIV-1 DNA testing in viremic patients identifies more drug resistance than HIV-1 RNA testing. *Open Forum Infect Dis.* 2023;10(4):ofad146.

Cutrell AG, Schapiro JM, Perno CF, et al. Exploring predictors of HIV-1 virologic failure to long-acting cabotegravir and rilpivirine: a multivariable analysis. *AIDS.* 2021;35(9):1333–1342.

D'Antoni ML, Andreatta K, Acosta R, et al. Brief report: bictegravir/emtricitabine/tenofovir alafenamide efficacy in participants with preexisting primary integrase inhibitor resistance through 48 weeks of phase 3 clinical trials. *J Acquir Immune Defic Syndr.* 2022;89(4):433–440.

da Silveira Gouvêa MIF, de Lourdes Benamor Teixeira M, Fuller T, et al. Resistance rates among antiretroviral regimens in pregnant people living with HIV. *HIV Med.* 2023;24(9):1020–1025.

Dauwe K, Staelens D, Vancoillie L, et al. Deep sequencing of HIV-1 RNA and DNA in newly diagnosed patients with baseline drug resistance showed no indications for hidden resistance and is biased by strong interference of hypermutation. *J Clin Micro.* 2016;54:1605–1615.

Davy-Mendez T, Eron JJ, Brunet L, et al. New antiretroviral agent use affects prevalence of HIV drug resistance in clinical care populations. *AIDS.* 2018;32(17):2593–2603.

D^{2}EFT Study Group. Dolutegravir plus boosted darunavir versus recommended standard-of-care antiretroviral regimens in people with HIV-1 for whom recommended first-line non-nucleoside reverse transcriptase inhibitor therapy has failed (D^{2}EFT): an open-label, randomized, phase 3b/4 trial. *Lancet HIV.* 2024;May 21:S2352-3018(24)00089-4.

Deeks SF, Wrin T, Liegler T, et al. Virologic and immunologic consequences of discontinuing combination antiretroviral-drug therapy in HIV-infected patients with detectable viremia. *N Engl J Med.* 2001;344:472–480.

Delaugerre C, Bruan J, Charreau I, et al; ANRS 138-EASIER study group. Comparison of resistance mutation patterns in historical plasma HIV RNA genotypes with those in current proviral HIV DNA genotypes among extensively treated patients with suppressed replication. *HIV Medicine.* 2012a:13:517–525.

Delaugerre C, Chaix ML, Blanche S, et al; ANRS French Perinatal Cohort. Perinatal acquisition of drug-resistant HIV-1 infection mechanisms and long-term outcome. *Retrovirology.* 2009; 6:85.

Delaugerre C, Gallien S, Flandre P, et al. Impact of low-level viremia on HIV-1 drug resistance evolution among antiretroviral treated patients. *PLoS One.* 2012b;7(5):e36673.

De Meyer S, Vangeneugden T, Van Baelen B, et al. Resistance profile of darunavir: combined 24-week results from the POWER trials. *AIDS Res Human Retroviruses.* 2008;24(3):379–388.

Department of Health and Human Services (DHHS) Panel on Antiretroviral Guidelines for Adults and Adolescents. Guidelines for the use of antiretroviral agents in adults and adolescents with HIV. http://www.aidsinfo.nih.gov/ContentFiles/AdultandAdolescentGL.pdf. Published 2024. Accessed June 2, 2024.

Derache A, Shin HS, Balamane M, et al. HIV drug resistance mutations in proviral DNA from a community treatment program. *PLoS One.* 2015;10(1):30117430.

de Salazar A, Viñuela L, Fuentes A, et al. Transmitted drug resistance to integrase-based first-line human immunodeficiency virus antiretroviral regimens in Mediterranean Europe. *Clin Infect Dis.* 2023;76(9):1628–1635.

Devereux HL, Loveday C, Youle M, et al. Substantial correlation between HIV type 1 drug-associated resistance mutations in plasma and peripheral blood mononuclear cells in treatment-experienced patients. *AIDS Res Human Retrovirus*. 2000;16(11):1025–1030.

Devereux HL, Youle M, Johnson MA, Loveday C. Rapid decline in detectability of HIV-1 drug resistance mutations after stopping therapy. *AIDS*. 1999;13:F123–127.

Dolling DI, Dunn DT, Sutherland KA, et al; UHDRD (UKHDRD) and the UCHCS (UK). Low frequency of genotypic resistance in HIV-1-infected patients failing an atazanavir-containing regimen: a clinical cohort study. *J Antimicrob Chemother*. 2013;68:2339–2343.

Drescher SM, von Wyl V, Yang WL, et al. Treatment-naïve individuals are the major source of transmitted HIV-1 drug resistance in men who have sex with men in the Swiss HIV Cohort Study. *Clin Infect Dis*. 2014;58(2):285–294.

Eberle J, Gurtler L. HIV types, groups, subtypes and recombinant forms: errors in replication, selection pressure and quasispecies. *Intervirology*. 2012b;55:79–83.

Eberle J, Gurtler L. The evolution of drug resistance interpretation algorithms: ANRS, REGA and extension of resistance analysis to HIV-1 group O and HIV-2. *Intervirology*. 2012a;55(2):128–133.

El Bouzidi K, White E, Mbisa JL, et al. Protease mutations emerging on darunavir in protease inhibitor-naïve and experienced patients in the UK. *J Int AIDS Soc*. 2014;17(4 Suppl 3):19739.

Ellis KE, Nawas GT, Chan C, et al. Clinical outcomes following the use of archived proviral HIV-1 DNA genotype to guide antiretroviral therapy adjustment. *Open Forum Inf Dis*. 2019;7(1):ofz533.

Elvstam O, Medstrand P, Yilmaz A, et al. Virological failure and all-cause mortality in HIV-positive adults with low-level viremia during antiretroviral treatment. *PLoS One*. 2017;12(7):e0180761.

Emu B, Fessel K, Schrader S, et al. Phase 3 study of ibalizumab for multidrug-resistant HIV-1. *N Engl J Med*. 2018;379:645–654.

Eron JJ, Clotet B, Durant J, et al; VIKING Study Group. Safety and efficacy of dolutegravir in treatment-experienced subjects with raltegravir-resistant HIV type 1 infection: 24-week results of the VIKING study. *J Infect Dis*. 2013;207:740–748.

Eron JJ, Young B, Cooper DA, et al. Switch to a raltegravir-based regimen versus continuation of a lopinavir-ritonavir-based regimen in stable HIV-infected patients with suppressed viraemic (SWITCHMRK 1 and 2): two multicenter-double-blind, randomized controlled trials. *Lancet*. 2010;375(9712):396–407.

Esber A, Polyak C, Kiweewa F, et al. Persistent low-level viremia predicts subsequent virologic failure: is it time to change the third 90? *Clin Infect Dis*. 2019;69(5):805–812.

Eshleman SH, Fogel JM, Piwowar-Manning E, et al. Characterization of human immunodeficiency virus (HIV) infections in women who received injectable cabotegravir or tenofovir disoproxil fumarate/emtricitabine for HIV prevention: HPTN084. *J Infect Dis*. 2022;225(10):1741–1749.

European AIDS Clinical Society (EACS) Guidelines version 12.0, October 2023. https://www.eacsociety.org/guidelines/eacs-guidelines/. Accessed June 2, 2024.

Fleming J, Mathews WC, Rutstein RM, et al; HIV Research Network. Low-level viremia and virologic failure in persons with HIV infection treated with antiretroviral therapy. *AIDS*. 2019;33:2005–2012.

Fogel JM, Mwatha A, Richardson P, et al. Impact of maternal and infant antiretroviral drug regimens on drug resistance in HIV-infected breastfeeding infants. *Pediatr Infect Dis*. 2013;32(4):e164–e169.

Fogel JM, Wilson EA, Piwowar-Manning E, et al. HPTN 071 (PopART) Study Team. HIV drug resistance in a community-randomized trial of universal testing and treatment: HPTN 071 (PopART). *J Int AIDS Soc*. 2022;25(7):e25941.

Ford N, Migone C, Calmy A, et al. Benefits and risks of rapid initiation of antiretroviral therapy. *AIDS*. 2018;32(1):17–23.

Gaitan N, D'Antoni M, Acosta R, et al. HIV drug resistance mutations in proviral DNA using next-generation sequencing and routine HIV RNA genotyping. *J Acquir Immune Defic Syndr*. 2023;93(3):213–218.

Gandhi RT, Bedimo R, Hoy JF, et al. Antiretroviral drugs for treatment and prevention of HIV infection in adults: 2022 recommendations of the International Antiviral Society-USA Panel. *JAMA*. 2023;329(1):63–84.

Gartland M, Cahn P, DeJesus E, et al. Week 96 genotypic and phenotypic results of the fostemsavir phase 3 BRIGHTE study in heavily treatment-experienced adults living with multidrug-resistance HIV-1. *Antimicrob Agents Chemother*. 2022;66:e0175121.

Geretti AM, White E, Orkin C, et al. Virological outcomes of boosted protease inhibitor-based first-line ART in subjects harbouring thymidine analogue-association mutations as the sole form of transmitted drug resistance. *J Antimicrob Chemother*. 2019;74:746–753.

Gibas KM, van den Berg P, Powell VE, Krakower DS. Drug resistance during HIV pre-exposure prophylaxis. *Drugs*. 2019;79(6):609–619.

Girometti N, McCormack S, Tittle V, McOwan A, Whitlock G; 56 Dean Street Collaborative Group. Rising rates of recent preexposure prophylaxis exposure among men having sex with men newly diagnosed with HIV: antiviral resistance patterns and treatment outcomes. *AIDS*. 2022;36(4):561–566.

Gonzalez-Serna A, Min JE, Woods C, et al. Performance of HIV-1 drug resistance testing at low-level viremia and its ability to predict future virologic outcomes and viral evolution in treatment-naïve individuals. *Clin Infect Dis*. 2014;58:1165–1173.

Gottlieb GS, Dia Badiane NM, Hawed SE, et al; University of Washington-Dakar HIV-2 Study Group. Emergence of multiclass drug resistance in HIV-2 in antiretroviral-treated individuals in Senegal: implications for HIV-2 treatment in resource-limited West Africa. *Clin Infect Dis*. 2009;48(4):476–483.

Gregson J, Tang M, Ndembi N, et al; TenoRes Study Group. Global epidemiology of drug resistance after failure of WHO recommended first-line regimens for adult HIV-1 infection: a multicentre retrospective cohort study. *Lancet Infect Dis*. 2016;16(5):565–575.

Günthard HF, Calvez V, Paredes R, et al. Human immunodeficiency virus drug resistance: 2018 recommendations of the International Antiviral Society–USA Panel. *Clin Infect Dis*. 2019 Jan 15;68(2):177–187.

Gupta RK, Gregson J, Parkin N, et al. HIV-1 drug resistance before initiation or re-initiation of first-line antiretroviral therapy in low-income and middle-income countries: a systematic review and meta-regression analysis. *Lancet Inf Dis*. 2018;18:346–355.

Hermans LE, Moorhouse M, Carmona S, et al. Effect of HIV-1 low-level viraemia during antiretroviral therapy on treatment outcomes in WHO-guided South African treatment programmes: a muticentre cohort study. *Lancet Infect Dis*. 2018;18(2):130–131.

Hikichi Y, Grover JR, Schäfer A, et al. Epistatic pathways can drive HIV-1 escape from integrase strand transfer inhibitors. *Sci Adv*. 2024;10(9):eadn0042.

Hoffman C, Wolf E, Braun P, et al. Temporal variability of multi-class resistant HIV-1 in proviral DNA. Abstract 513. Presented at the Conference on Retroviruses and Opportunistic Infections. Virtual; 2022. https://www.croiconference.org/search-abstracts/

Huber M, Metzner KJ, Geissberger FD, et al. A rapid and versatile tool for HIV-1 drug resistance genotyping by deep sequencing. *J Virol Methods*. 2017;240:7–13.

Inzaule SC, Hamers RL, Noguera-Julian M, et al. Clinically relevant thresholds for ultrasensitive HIV drug resistance testing: a multi-country nested case-control study. *Lancet HIV*. 2018;5:e638–e646.

Jablonowska E, Siwak E, Bociaga-Jasik M, et al. Real-life study of dual therapy based on dolutegravir and ritonavir-boosted darunavir in HIV-1-infected treatment-experienced patients. *PLoS One*. 2019;14(1):e0210476.

Jain V, Sucupira MC, Bacchetti P, et al. Differential persistence of transmitted HIV-1-drug resistance mutation classes. *J Infect Dis*. 2011;203:1174–1181.

Johnson KA, Chen MJ, Kohn R, et al. Acute HIV at the time of initiation of pre-exposure or post-exposure prophylaxis: impact on drug resistance and clinical outcomes. *J Acquir Immune Defic Syndr*. 2021;87(2):818–825.

Joya C, Won SH, Schofield C, et al. Persistent low-level viremia while on antiretroviral therapy is an independent risk factor for virologic failure. *Clin Infect Dis*. 2019;69(12):2145–2152.

Kagan RM, Dunn KJ, Snell GP, et al. Trends in HIV-1 drug resistance mutations from a US reference laboratory from 2006 to 2017. *AIDS Res Hum Retroviruses*. 2019;35(8):698–709.

Kessler HH, Stelzl E, Blazic A, Mehta SR, et al. Antiretroviral treatment simplification with 2–drug regimens: impact of transmitted drug resistance mutations. *Open Forum Infect Dis*. 2020 Jan;7(1):ofz535.

Keys JR, Zhou S, Anderson JA, et al. Primer ID informs next-generation sequencing platforms and reveals preexisting drug resistance mutations in the HIV-1 reverse transcriptase coding domain. *AIDS Res Hum Retroviruses*. 2015;31(6):658–668.

Kirichenko A, Kireev D, Lopatukhin A, et al. Prevalence of HIV-1 drug resistance in Eastern European and Central Asian countries. *PLoS One*. 2022;17(1):e0257731.

Knyphausen F, Scheufele R, Kücherer C, et al. First line treatment response in patients with transmitted HIV drug resistance and well-defined time point of HIV infection: updated results from the german HIV-1 Seroconverter Study. *PLoS One*. 2014;9:e95956.

Kozal M, Aberg J, Pialoux G, et al. Fostemsavir in adults with multidrug-resistant HIV-1 infection. *New Eng J Med*. 2020;382:1232–1243.

Landovitz RJ, Tao L, Yang J, et al; Global F/TDF PrEP Study Team. HIV-1 incidence, adherence, and drug resistance in individuals taking daily emtricitabine/tenofovir disoproxil fumarate for HIV-1 pre-exposure prophylaxis: pooled analysis from 72 global studies. *Clin Infect Dis*. 2024;79(5):1197–1207. doi:10.1093/cid/ciae143

Lapointe HR, Dong W, Lee GQ, et al. High drug resistance testing by high-multiplex "wide" sequencing on the MiSeq instrument. *Antimicrobial Agents Chemo*. 2015;59:6824–6833.

Laprise C, de Pokomandy A, Baril JG, Dufresne S, Trottier H. Virologic failure following persistent low-level viremia in a cohort of HIV-positive patients: results from 12 years of observation. *Clin Infect Dis*. 2013;57(10):1489–1496.

Lathouwers E, Seyedkazemi S, Lou D, et al. Pooled resistance analyses of darunavir once-daily regimens and formulations across 10 clinical studies of treatment-naïve and treatment-experienced patients with human immunodeficiency virus-1 infection. *HIV Res Clin Prac*. 2020;21:83–89.

Laurent C, Yaya I, Cuer B, et al.; CohMSM-PrEP Study Group. Human immunodeficiency virus seroconversion among men who have sex with men who use event-driven or daily oral pre-exposure prophylaxis (CohMSM-PrEP): a multi-country demonstration study from West Africa. *Clin Infect Dis*. 2023;77(4):606–614.

Le Hingrat Q, Collin G, Bachelard A, et al. Ibalizumab shows in-vitro activity against group A and group B HIV-2 clinical isolates. *AIDS*. 2022;36(8):1055–1060.

Levy DN, Aldrovandi GM, Kutsch O, Shaw GM. Dynamics of HIV-1 recombination in its natural target cells. *PNAS*. 2004;101: 4204–4209.

Levy L, Peterson JM, Kudrick LD, et al.; Global Evaluation of Microbicide Sensitivity (GEMS) project. Casting a wide net: HIV drug resistance monitoring in pre-exposure prophylaxis seroconverters in the global evaluation of microbicide sensitivity project. *Glob Health Sci Pract*. 2022;10(2):e2100122.

Li JZ, Gallien S, Do TD, et al. Prevalence and significance of HIV-1 drug resistance mutations among patients on antiretroviral therapy with detectable low-level viremia. *Antimicrobial Agents Chemo*. 2012;56(11):5998–6000.

Li JZ, Paredes R, Ribaudo H, et al. Minority HIV-1 drug resistance mutations and the risk of NNRTI-based antiretroviral treatment failure: a systematic review and pooled analysis. *JAMA*. 2011;305(13):1327–1335.

Li X, Brown TT, Ho KS, et al. Recent trends and effectiveness of antiretroviral regimens among men who have sex with men living with HIV in the United States: the Multicenter AIDS Cohort Study (MACS) 2008–2017. *Open Forum Infect Dis*. 2019;6:ofz333.

Llibre JM, Arribas JR, Domingo P, et al. Clinical implications of fixed-dose coformulations of antiretrovirals on the outcome of HIV-1 therapy. *AIDS*. 2011;25(14):1683–1690.

Lodi S, Gunthard HF, Dunn D, et al. Effect of immediate initiation of antiretroviral treatment on the risk of acquired HIV drug resistance. *AIDS*. 2018;32(3):327–335.

Lombardi F, Giacomelli A, Armenia D, et al. Prevalence and factors associated with HIV-1 multi-drug resistance over the past two decades in the Italian ARCA database. *Int J Antimicrob Agents*. 2021;57(2):106252.

Lubke N, Di Cristanziano V, Sierra S, et al.; Resina Study Group. Proviral DNA as a target for HIV-1 resistance analysis. *Intervirology*. 2015;58:184–189.

Lv S, Sun L, Li T, et al. Role of proviral HIV-1 DNA genotyping for people living with HIV (PLWH) who had low-level viremia while receiving antiretroviral therapy. *Infect Drug Resist*. 2023;16:4697–4706.

Macdonald V, Mbuagbaw L, Jordan MR, et al. Prevalence of pretreatment HIV drug resistance in key populations: a systematic review and meta-analysis. *J Int AIDS Soc*. 2020;23(12):e25656.

Machnowska P, Meixenberger K, Schmidt D, et al.; German HIV-1 Seroconverted Study Group. Prevalence and persistence of transmitted drug resistance mutations in the German hIV-1 Seroconverter Study Cohort. *PLoS One*. 2019;14(1):e0209605.

Mackie NE, Phillips AN, Kaye S, et. al; UK Resistance Database and the UK Collaborative HIV Cohort Study. Antiretroviral drug resistance in HIV-1-infected patients with low-level viremia. *J Infect Dis*. 2010;210(9):1303–1307.

Malet I, Delelis O, Nguyen T, et. al. Variability of the HIV-1 3′ polypurine tract (3′PPT) region and implication in integrase inhibitor. *J Antimicrob Chemother*. 2019;74(12):3440–3444.

Manyana S, Gounder L, Pillay M, et al. HIV-1 drug resistance genotyping in resource limited settings: current and future perspectives in sequencing technologies. *Viruses*. 2021;13(6):1125.

Marcelin AG, Charpentier C, Bellecave P, et al. Factors associated with the emergency of integrase resistance mutations in patients failing dual or triple integrase inhibitor-based regimens in a French national survey. *J Antimicrob Chemother*. 2021;76(9):2400–2406.

Margot N, Naik V, VanderVeen L, et al. Resistance analyses in highly treatment-experienced people with human immunodeficiency virus (HIV) treated with the novel capsid HIV inhibitor lenacapavir. *J Infect Dis*. 2022;226:1985–1991.

Margot N, Pennetzdorfer N, Naik V, et al. Cross-resistance to entry inhibitors and lenacapavir resistance through week 52 in study CAPELLA. *Antivir Ther*. 2023;28(6):13596535231220754. doi:10.1177/13596535231220754

Margot N, Ram R, McNicholl I, et al. Differential detection of M184V/I between plasma historical HIV genotypes and HIV proviral DNA from PBMCs. *J Antimicrob Chemother*. 2020;75:2249–2252.

Margot NA, Wong P, Kulkarni R, et al. Commonly transmitted HIV-1 drug resistance mutations in reverse-transcriptase and protease in antiretroviral treatment-naïve patients and response to regimens containing tenofovir disoproxil fumarate or tenofovir alafenamide. *J Infect Dis*. 2017;215(6):920–927.

Martin TCS, Abrams M, Anderson C, Little SJ. Rapid antiretroviral therapy among individuals with acute and early HIV. *Clin Inf Dis*. 2021; 73(1):130–133.

Marzinke MA, Fogel JM, Wang Z, et al. Extended analysis of HIV infection in cisgender men and transgender women who have sex with men receiving injectable cabotegravir for HIV prevention: HPTN 083. *Antimicrob Agents Chemother*. 2023;67:e0005323.

Marzinke MA, Grinsztejn B, Fogel JM, et al. Characterization of human immunodeficiency virus (HIV) infection in cisgender men and transgender women who have sex with men receiving injectable cabotegravir for HIV prevention: HPTN083. *J Infect Dis*. 2021;224(9):1581–1592.

Mateo-Urdiales A, Johnson S, Smith R, Nachega JB, Eshun-Wilson I. Rapid initiation of antiretroviral therapy for people living with HIV. *Cochrane Database Syst Rev*. 2019;6(6):CD012962.

Matheron S, Descamps D, Gallien S, et al. First-line raltegravir/emtricitabine/tenofovir combination in human immunodeficiency virus type 2 (HIV-2) infection: a phase 2, noncomparative trial (ANRS 159 HIV-2). *Clin Infect Dis*. 2018;67 (8):1161–1167.

Mbunkah HA, Bertagnolio S, Hamers RL; WHO HIVResNet Working Group. Low-abundance drug-resistant HIV-1 variants in antiretroviral drug-native individuals: a systematic review of detection methods, prevalence, and clinical impact. *J Infect Dis*. 2020;221:1584–1597.

McClung RP, Ocfemia CB, Saduvala N, et al. US HIV drug resistance: implications for current and future PrEP regimens. Abstract. Presented at the Conference on Retroviruses and Opportunistic Infections. Boston, MA; 2020. https:// www.croiconference.org/search-abstracts/

McClung RP, Oster AM, Ocfemia MCB, et al. Transmitted drug resistance among human immunodeficiency virus (HIV)-1 diagnoses in the United States, 2014–2018. *Clin Infect Dis.* 2022;74(6):1055–1062.

McCluskey SM, Siedner MJ, Marconi VC. Management of virologic failure and HIV drug resistance. *Infect Dis Clin North Am.* 2019;33(3):707–742.

Metzner KJ, Rauch P, von Wyl V, et al. Efficient suppression of minority drug-resistant HIV type 1 (HIV-1) variants present at primary HIV-1 infection by ritonavir-boosted protease inhibitor-containing antiretroviral therapy. *J Infect Dis.* 2010;201:1063–1071.

Miller MD, Margot N, Lu B, et al. Genotypic and phenotypic predictors of the magnitude of response to tenofovir disoproxil fumarate treatment in antiretroviral-experienced patients. *J Infect Dis.* 2004;189:837–846.

Miranda MNS, Pingarilho M, Pimentel V, et al. Trends of transmitted and acquired drug resistance in Europe from 1981 to 2019: a comparison between the populations of late presenters and non-late presenters. *Front Microbiol.* 2022;13:846943.

Misra K, Huang J, Udeagu CC, et al. Pre-exposure prophylaxis use history in people with antiretroviral resistance at HIV diagnosis: findings from New York City HIV Surveillance and Partner Services, 2015–2022. *Clin Infect Dis.* 2024;78(5):1240–1245.

Moranguinho I, Taveira N, Bártolo I. Antiretroviral treatment of HIV-2 infection: available drugs, resistance pathways, and promising new compounds. *Int J Mol Sci.* 2023;24(6):5905.

Nance RM, Delaney JAC, Simoni JM, et al. HIV viral suppression trends over time among HIV-infected patients receiving care in the United States, 1997 to 2015. *Ann Int Med.* 2018;169:376–384.

Nel A, van Neikerk N, Van Baelen B, et al. Safety, adherence, and HIV-1 seroconversion among women using the dapivirine vaginal ring (DREAM): an open-label, extension study. *Lancet HIV.* 2021;8(2):e77–-e86.

New York State Department of Health AIDS Institute. Diagnosis and management of HIV-2 in adults. https://www.hivguidelines.org/guideline/hiv-2/?mycollection=hiv-testing-acute-infection. Published 2012. Accessed June 4, 2024.

Noguera-Julian M, Edgil D, Harrigan PR, et al. Next-generation human immunodeficiency virus sequencing for patient management and drug resistance surveillance. *J Infect Dis.* 2017 Dec 1;216(Suppl 9):S829–S833.

Nowicka-Sans B, Gong YF, McAuliffe B, et al. In vitro antiviral characteristics of HIV-1 attachment inhibitor BMS-626529, the active component of the prodrug BMS-663068. *Antimicrob Agents Chemother.* 2012;56(7):3498–3507.

Pacheco P, Marques N, Rodrigues P, et al. Safety and efficacy of triple therapy with dolutegravir plus 2 nucleoside reverse transcriptase inhibitors in treatment naïve Human Immunodeficiency Virus type 2 patients: results from a 48-week phase 2 study. *Clin Infect Dis.* 2023;77(5):740–748.

Paquet A, Solberg OD, Napolitano LA, et al. A decade of HIV-1 drug resistance in the United States: trends and characteristics in a large protease/reverse transcriptase and co-receptor tropism database from 2003 to 2012. *Antivir Ther.* 2014;19(4):435–441.

Paredes R, Tzou PL, van Zyl G, et al. Collaborative update of a rule-based expert system for HIV-1genotypic resistance test interpretation. *PLoS One.* 2017;12(7):e0181357.

Parikh UM, Mellors JW. How could HIV-1 drug resistance impact preexposure prophylaxis for HIV prevention? *Curr Opin HIV AIDS.* 2022;17(4):213–221.

Parikh UM, Mellors JW. Should we fear resistance from tenofovir/emtricitabine preexposure prophylaxis? *Curr Opin HIV AIDS.* 2016;11:49–55.

Parikh UM, Penrose KJ, Heaps AL et al.; MTN-020 Study Team. HIV-1 drug resistance among individuals who seroconverted in the ASPIRE dapivirine ring trial. *J Int AIDS Soc.* 2021; 24(11):e25833.

Parkin NT, Hellmann NS, Whitcomb JM, et al. Natural variation of drug susceptibility in wild-type human immunodeficiency virus type 1. *Antimicrobial Agents Chemother.* 2004;48:437–443.

Paton NI, Musaazi J, Kityo C, et al. Efficacy and safety of dolutegravir or darunavir in combination with lamivudine plus either zidovudine or tenofovir for second-line treatment of HIV infection (NADIA): week 96 results from a prospective, multicentre, open-label, factorial, randomized, non-inferiority trial. *Lancet HIV.* 2022;9(6):e381–e393.

Petropoulos CJ, Parkin NT, Limoli KL, et al. A novel phenotypic drug susceptibility assay for human immunodeficiency virus type 1. *Antimicrob Agents Chemo.* 2000;44(4):920–928.

Peuchant O, Thiebaut R, Capdepont S, et al. Transmission of HIV-1 minority-resistance variants and response to first-line antiretroviral therapy: transmission of minority resistant HIV-1. *AIDS.* 2008;22(12):1417–1423.

Pilcher CD, Ospina-Norvell C, Dasgupta A, et al. The effect of same-day observed initiation of antiretroviral therapy on HIV viral load and treatment outcomes in a US public health setting. *J Acquir Immune Defic Syndr.* 2017;74(1):44–51.

Pingen M, Wensing A, Fransen K, et al. Persistence of frequently transmitted drug-resistant HIV-1 variants can be explained by high viral replication capacity. *Retrovirology.* 2014;11:105.

Porter DP, Toma J, Tan Y, et al. Clinical outcomes of virologically-suppressed patients with pre-existing HIV-1 drug resistance mutations switching to rilpivirine/emtricitabine/tenofovir disoproxil fumarate in the SPIRIT study. *HIV Clin Trials.* 2016;17(1):29–37.

Poschman K, Spencer EC. Prevalence of HIV-1 antiretroviral drug resistance in Florida, 2015–2016. Abstract 526. Presented at the Conference on Retroviruses and Opportunistic Infections. Boston, MA; 2020. https://www.croiconference.org/search-abstracts/

Pou C, Noguera-Julian M, Perez-Alvarez S, et al. Improved prediction of salvage antiretroviral therapy outcomes using ultrasensitive HIV-1 drug resistance testing. *Clin Infect Dis.* 2014;59(4):578–588.

Puertas MC, Ploumidis G, Ploumidis M, et al. Pan-resistant HIV-emergence in the era of integrase strand-transfer inhibitors: a case report. *Lancet Microbe.* 2020;1(3):e130–e135.

Raccagni AR, Bruzzesi E, Gianotti N, et al. Failure of on-demand preexposure prophylaxis: the risk of HIV drug resistance. *Sex Transm Infect.* 2022 May;98(3):234.

Rambaut A, Posada D, Crandall KA, Holmes EC. The causes and consequences of HIV evolution. *Nature Rev Gen.* 2004;5:52–61.

Rauschning D, Ehren I, Heger E, et al. Optimizing antiretroviral therapy in heavily ART-experienced patients with multi-class resistant HIV-1 using proviral DNA genotypic resistance testing. *Viruses.* 2023;15(7):1444.

Raymond S, Piffaut M, Bigot J, et al. Sexual transmission of an extensively drug-resistance HIV-1 strain. *Lancet HIV.* 2020;7(8):e529–e530.

Requena S, Trevino A, Cabeza T; Spanish HIV-2 Study Group. Drug resistance mutations in HIV-2 patients failing raltegravir and influence on dolutegravir response. *J Antimicrob Chemother.* 2017;72(7):2083–2088.

Rhee SY, Blanco JL, Jordan MR, et al. Geographic and temporal trends in the molecular epidemiology and genetic mechanisms of transmitted HIV-1 drug resistance: an individual-patient-and sequence-level meta-analysis. *PLoS Med.* 2015;12(4):e1001810. http://doi:10.1371/journal.pmed.1001810

Rhee SY, Clutter D, Feddel WJ, et al. Trends in the molecular epidemiology and genetic mechanisms of transmitted human immunodeficiency virus type 1 drug resistance in a large US clinic population. *Clin Infect Dis.* 2019a;68(2):213–221.

Rhee SY, Clutter D, Hare CB, et al. Virological failure and acquired genotypic resistance associated with contemporary antiretroviral treatment regimens. *Open Forum Infect Dis.* 2020a Aug 6;7(9):ofaa316.

Rhee SY, Fessel WJ, Liu TF, et al. Predictive value of HIV-1 genotypic resistance test interpretation algorithms. *J Infect Dis.* 2009;200(3):453–463.

Rhee SY, Grant PM, Tzou PL, et al. A systematic review of the genetic mechanisms of dolutegravir resistance. *J Antimicrob Chemother.* 2019b;74:3135–3149.

Rhee SY, Kassaye SH, Barrow G et al. HIV-1 transmitted drug resistance surveillance: shifting trends in study design and prevalence estimates. *J Int AIDS Soc.* 2020b;23(9):e25611.

Rhee SY, Parkin N, Harrigan PR, et al. Genotypic correlates of resistance to the HIV-1 strand transfer integrase inhibitor cabotegravir. *Antiviral Res.* 2022;208:105427.

Rhee SY, Tzou PL, Shafer RW. Temporal trends in HIV-1 mutations used for the surveillance of transmitted drug resistance. *Viruses.* 2021;13(5):879.

Rich SN, Poschman K, Hu H, et al. Sociodemographic, ecological, and spatiotemporal factors associated with HIV drug resistance in Florida: a retrospective analysis. *J Infect Dis.* 2020;223(5):866–875.

Rodriguez AE, Wawrzyniak AJ, Tookes HE, et al. Implementation of an immediate HIV treatment initiation program in a public/academic medical center in the US South: the Miami Test and Treat Rapid Response Program. *AIDS Behav.* 2019;23(Suppl 3):287–295.

Rodriguez MA, Mills A, Stoker A, et al. HIV-1 DNA resistance testing informs the successful switch to a single tablet regimen. *J AIDS Clin Res.* 2021;12(1). https://www.hilarispublisher.com/open-access/hiv1-dna-resistance-testing-informs-the-successful-switchto-a-single-tablet-regimen.pdf. Accessed June 6, 2024.

Rolle CP, Berhe M, Singh T, et al. Sustained virologic suppression with dolutegravir/lamivudine in a test-and-treat setting through 48 weeks. *Open Forum Infect Dis.* 2023;10(3):ofad101.

Rolle CP, Nguyen V, Patel K, et al. Real-world efficacy and safety of switching to bictegravir/emtricitabine/tenofovir alafenamide in older people living with HIV. *Medicine (Baltimore).* 2021;100(38):e27330.

Rose R, Gartland M, Li Z, et al. Clinical evidence for a lack of cross-resistance between temsavir and ibalizumab or maraviroc. *AIDS.* 2022;36(1):11–18.

Saladini F, Giammarino F, Maggiolo F, et al. Residual phenotypic susceptibility to doravirine in multidrug-resistant HIV-1 from subjects enrolled in the PRESTIGIO Registry. *Int J Antimicrob Agents.* 2023;61(3):106737.

Sax PE, Andreatta K, Molina JM, et al. High efficacy of switching to bictegravir/emtricitabine/tenofovir alafenamide in people with suppressed HIV and pre-existing M184V/I. *AIDS.* 2022;36(11):1511–1520.

Scarsi KK, Havens JP, Podany AT, et al. HIV-1 integrase inhibitors: a comparative review of efficacy and safety. *Drugs.* 2020;80:1649–1676.

Scherrer AU, von Wyl V, Yang WL, et al. Emergence of acquired HIV-1 drug resistance almost stopped in Switzerland: a 15-year prospective cohort analysis. *Clin Infect Dis.* 2016;62:1310–1317.

Shafran SD, Hughes CA. Bictegravir/emtricitabine/tenofovir alafenamide in patients with genotypic NRTI resistance. *HIV Med.* 2023;24(3):361–365.

Siefried KJ, Mao L, Kerr S, et al.; PAART study investigators. Socioeconomic factors explain suboptimal adherence to antiretroviral therapy among HIV-infected Australian adults with viral suppression. *PLoS One.* 2017;12:e0174613.

Siliciano JD, Siliciano RF. Recent trends in HIV-1 drug resistance. *Curr Opin Virology.* 2013;3:487–494.

Smith J, Bansi-Matharu L, Cambiano V, et al. Predicted effects of the introduction of long-acting injectable cabotegravir pre-exposure prophylaxis in sub-Saharan Africa: a modelling study. *Lancet HIV.* 2023;10:e254–265.

Smith RA, Raugi DN, Nixon RS, et al. Antiviral activity of lenacapavir against HIV-2 isolates and drug-resistance HIV-2 mutants. *J Infect Dis.* 2024;229(5):1290–1294.

Smith RA Wu VH, Song J, et al. Spectrum of activity of raltegravir and dolutegravir against novel treatment-associated mutations in HIV-2 integrase: a phenotypic analysis using an expanded panel of site-directed mutants. *J Infect Dis.* 2022;226(3):497–509.

Stella G, Volpicelli L, Di Carlo D, et al. Impact of pre-existent drug resistance on virological efficacy of single-tablet regimens in people living with HIV. *Int J Antimicrob Agents.* 2022;60(3):106636.

Swenson LC, Min JE, Woods CK, et al. HIV drug resistance detected during low-level viremia is associated with subsequent virologic failure. *AIDS.* 2014 May 15;28(8):1125–1134.

Teo C, Norhisham N, Lee O, et al. Towards next-generation sequencing for HIV-1 drug resistance testing in a clinical setting. *Viruses.* 2022;14(10):2208.

Toni TA, Asahchop EL, Moisi D, et al. Detection of human immunodeficiency virus (HIV) type 1 M184V and K103N minority variants in patients with primary HIV infection. *Antimicrob Agents Chemother.* 2009;53:1670–1672.

Tzou PH, Rhee SY, Descamps, et al; WHO HIVResNet Working Groups. Integrase strand transfer inhibitor (INSTI)-resistance mutations for the surveillance of transmitted HIV-1 drug resistance. *J Antimicrob Chemother.* 2020;75:170–182.

United Nations Programme on HIV/AIDS (UNAIDS). *The Path That Ends AIDS: UNAIDS Global AIDS Update 2023.* Geneva: Joint United Nations Programme on HIV/AIDS; 2023. License: CC BY-NC-SA 3.0 IGO. https://www.unaids.org/sites/default/files/media_asset/2023-unaids-global-aids-update_en.pdf. Accessed May 29, 2024.

U.S. Department of Health and Human Services (DHHS). Panel on Antiretroviral Guidelines for Adults and Adolescents. Guidelines for the use or antiretroviral agents in adults and adolescents with HIV. Department of Health and Human Services. https://clinicalinfo.hiv.gov/en/guidelines/adult-and-adolescent-arv. Last updated February 24, 2024a. Accessed June 10, 2024.

USDHHS. Panel on Antiretroviral Therapy and Medical Management of Children Living with HIV. Guidelines for the use of antiretroviral HIV infection. Department of Health and Human Services. https://clinicalinfo.hiv.gov/en/guidelines/pediatric-arv. Last updated January 31, 2024b. Accessed June 10, 2024.

USDHHS. Panel on Treatment of HIV During Pregnancy and Prevention of Perinatal Transmission. Recommendations for the use of antiretroviral drugs during pregnancy and interventions to reduce perinatal HIV United States. Department of Health and Human Services. https://clinicalinfo.hiv.gov/en/guidelines/perinatal. Last updated January 31, 2024c. Accessed June 10, 2024.

Vandenhende MA, Perrier A, Bonnet F, et al. Risk of virological failure in HIV-1-infected patients experiencing low-level viraemia under active antiretroviral therapy (ANRS CO3 cohort study). *Antivir Ther.* 2015;20(6):655–660.

Van Wyk J, Orkin C, Rubio R, et al. Durable suppression and low rate of virologic failure 3 years after switch to dolutegravir + rilpivirine 2-drug regimen: 148-week results from the SWORD-1 and SWORD-2 randomized clinical trials. *J Acquir Immune Defic Syndr.* 2020;85(3):325–330.

Van Zyl G, Bale MJ, Kearney MF. HIV evolution and diversity in ART-treated patients. *Retrovirology.* 2018;15(1):14.

Varghese V, Shahriar R, Rhee SY, et al. Minority variants associated with transmitted and acquired HIV-1 non-nucleoside RT (NNRTI) resistance: implications for the use of second generation NNRTIs. *J Acquir Immune Defic Syndr.* 2009;52(3):309–315.

Verhofstede C, Noe A, Demecheleer E, et al. Drug-resistance variants that evolve during nonsuppressive therapy persist in HIV-1-infected peripheral blood mononuclear cells after long-term highly active antiretroviral therapy. *J Acquir Immune Defic Synd.* 2004;35:473–483.

Viani RM, Ruel T, Alvero C, et al. Long-term safety and efficacy of dolutegravir in treatment-experienced adolescents with human immunodeficiency virus infection: results of the IMPAACT P1093 study. *J Pediatric Infect Dis Soc.* 2020;9(2):159–165.

Villalobos C, Ceballos ME, Ferres M, Palma C. Drug resistance mutations in proviral DNA of HIV-infected patients with low level of viremia. *J Clin Virol.* 2020;132:104657.

Vingerhoets J, Tambuyzer L, Azijn H, et al. Resistance profile of etravirine: combined analysis of baseline genotypic and phenotypic data from the randomized, controlled phase III clinical studies. *AIDS.* 2010 Feb 20;24(4):503–514.

Visseaux B, Charpentier C, Hurtado-Nedelec M, et al. In vitro phenotypic susceptibility of HIV-2 clinical isolates to CCR5 inhibitors. *Antimicrob Agents Chemother.* 2012;56(1):137–139.

Volpe LJ, Powis KM, Legbedze J, et al. A counseling and monitoring approach for supporting breastfeeding women living with HIV in Botswana. *J Acquir Immune Defic Syndr.* 2022;89(2):e16.

Waitt C, Olagunju A, Nakalema S, et al. Plasma and breast milk pharmacokinetics of emtricitabine, tenofovir and lamivudine using dried blood and breast milk spots in nursing African mother-infant pairs. *J Antimicrob Chemother.* 2018;73(4):1013–1019.

Waters L, Winston A, Reeves I, et al. BHIVA guidelines on antiretroviral treatment for adults living with HIV-1. *HIV Med.* 2022;23 Suppl 5:3–115. https://www.bhiva.org/HIV-1-treatment-guidelines. Accessed June 2, 2024.

Wensing AM, Calvez V, Ceccherini-Silberstein F, et al. 2022 update of the drug resistance mutations in HIV-1. *Top Antivir Med.* 2022;30(4):559–574.

Westby J, Lewis M, Whitcomb J, et al. Emergence of CXCR4-using human immunodeficiency virus type 1 (HIV-1) variants in a minority of HIV-1-infected patients following treatment with the CCR5 antagonist maraviroc is from a pretreatment CXCR4-using virus reservoir. *J Virol.* 2006 May;80(10):4909–4920.

Weyland C, Mirani G, Gillespie SL, Paul ME. A case of in utero transmission of drug-resistant HIV in the United States. *Pediatr Infect Dis J.* 2022;41(1):57–59.

Wheeler WH, Ziebell RA, Zabina H, et al. Prevalence of transmitted drug resistance associated mutations and HIV-1 subtypes in new HIV-1 diagnoses, US—2006. *AIDS.* 2010;24:1203–1212.

Winters B, van Craenenbroeck E, van der Borght K, et al. Clinical cutoffs for HIV-1 phenotypic resistance estimates: update based on recent pivotal clinical trial data and a revised approach to viral mixtures. *J Virologic Methods.* 2009;162:101–108.

Wirden M, Soulie C, Valantin MA, et al. Historical HIV-RNA resistance test results are more informative than proviral DNA genotyping in cases of suppressed or residual viraemia. *Antimicrob Chemother.* 2011;66:709–712.

World Health Organization (WHO). Consolidated guidelines on HIV prevention, testing, treatment, service delivery and monitoring: recommendations for a public health approach. https://www.who.int/publications/i/item/9789240031593. Published 2021. Accessed June 12, 2024.

WHO. *HIV Drug Resistance: Brief Report 2024.* Geneva: World Health Organization; 2024. License: CC BY-NC-SA 3.0 IGO. https://www.who.int/publications/i/item/9789240086319. Accessed June 12, 2024.

WHO. What ARV regimen to start with in adults, adolescents, and pregnant women living with HIV-2? http://apps.who.int/iris/bitstream/10665/90772/1/WHO_HIV_2013.36_eng.pdf?ua=1. Published 2013. Accessed June 12, 2024.

Yanik EL, Napravnik S, Hurt CB, et al. Prevalence of transmitted antiretroviral drug resistance differs between acutely and chronically HIV-infected patients. *J Acquir Immun Defic Syndr.* 2012;61:258–262.

Zaccarelli M, Santoro MM, Armenia D, et al. Genotypic resistance test in proviral DNA can identify resistance mutations never detected in historical genotypic test in patients with low level or undetectable HIV-RNA. *J Clin Virol.* 2016 Sep;82:94–100.

Zhou N, Nowicka-Sans B, McAuliffe B, et al. Genotypic correlates of susceptibility to HIV-1 attachment inhibitor BMS-626529, the active agent of the prodrug BMS-663068. *J Antimicrob Chemother.* 2014;69(3):573–581.

18.

THE HIV RESERVOIR AND CURE AND REMISSION STRATEGIES

Boris Juelg, Rajesh Gandhi, and Nikolaus Jilg

LEARNING OBJECTIVES

Upon completion of this chapter, the reader should be able to:

- Identify key hurdles for HIV eradication strategies and explain approaches that might overcome these challenges.
- Discuss new antiretroviral drugs in development.
- Discuss current research on preventive and therapeutic vaccines, immunomodulatory agents, and gene therapy approaches.

THE HIV RESERVOIR AND CURE AND REMISSION STRATEGIES

WHAT'S NEW?

Novel strategies to promote HIV latency reversal and approaches to boost HIV-specific immunity are being evaluated in clinical trials aimed at eradicating HIV. A new generation of broadly neutralizing antibodies has demonstrated potency at suppressing HIV-1 viremia in clinical trials and may play a role in immunotherapy and prevention. Latency-reversing agents (e.g., histone deacetylase inhibitors) and gene therapy strategies using modified hematopoietic stem cells and CRISPR are being evaluated in trials.

KEY POINTS

- HIV-1 persists quiescently in cellular reservoirs not detected by the immune system because of the lack of active viral replication; these reservoirs represent the biggest obstacle to cure approaches.
- Reversal of HIV-1 latency and induction of virus expression by a variety of interventions may render infected cells susceptible to immune recognition and active clearance.
- Strategies to boost immune responses via active or passive immunization, immunomodulation, or gene therapy are being evaluated with the aim of achieving HIV-1 control or remission without antiretroviral therapy (ART) and viral eradication.

INTRODUCTION

Currently available antiretroviral medications consistently achieve durable suppression of HIV but do not eliminate the latent reservoir of infection; as a result, people with HIV must take antiretroviral medications for a lifetime to prevent HIV rebound, clinical progression, and transmission. HIV reservoir reduction and cure/remission approaches therefore remain of high interest to the scientific and public health communities, in addition to the development of new antiretroviral drugs, and various strategies targeting immune dysregulation and T-cell homeostasis. Ongoing clinical research is being conducted to evaluate immunomodulators and therapeutic vaccines.

WHY SHOULD WE TRY TO CURE HIV?

Although current ART is highly effective at controlling HIV-1 replication, it does not eradicate or cure the infection. There are several compelling reasons for trying to cure HIV-1. First, despite efforts to expand access to treatment, many people with HIV (PWH) worldwide are not receiving ART, leading to ongoing transmission of the virus. Second, because current ART does not eradicate HIV-1, PWH must take ART for many decades, which may pose difficulties with sustained adherence, substantial cost, and the potential for long-term side effects. Third, PWH have increased rates of cardiovascular disease, liver disease, neurocognitive disorders, and other chronic noninfectious complications that may be driven by elevated levels of inflammation that persist despite suppressive ART. Fourth, many PWH treated with ART alone do not achieve immune restoration despite viral suppression; in a large trial of adults with HIV achieving virologic suppression for 3 years with $CD4^+$ T-cell counts of 200 cells/µL or less, these individuals had significantly greater mortality compared to PWH with $CD4^+$ T-cell counts of more than 200 cells/µL (adjusted hazard ratio 2.6) (Engsig et al., 2014). Given significant evidence that $CD4^+$ T-cell counts have been correlated with normal life expectancy (ART Collaboration Cohort, 2008; Lewden et al., 2007), attention has thus turned to strategies that reduce chronic immune activation and reverse loss of normal T-cell homeostasis seen in HIV. Finally, HIV-1 infection continues to be associated with stigma and social isolation, which adversely affects quality of life. Given these limitations of current ART, there is a concerted effort to find a cure for HIV-1.

While complete viral eradication, or a "sterilizing cure," is the ultimate goal, an intermediate aim is achieving a "functional cure" or "ART-free remission," in which the host controls the virus without the need for ART. Several clinical observations indicate that "sterilizing" and "functional" cures are possible. The most compelling and visible example is that of the "Berlin patient." This man with HIV-1 and virologic suppression on ART received, as treatment for acute myelogenous leukemia, allogeneic hematopoietic stem cell transplants from a donor who carried a homozygous deletion in CCR5 (CCR5Δ32/Δ32), the coreceptor for HIV-1, thereby making his new $CD4^+$ T-cells resistant to infection (Hutter et al., 2009). Following discontinuation of ART, no HIV-1 RNA was subsequently detected in the Berlin patient's peripheral blood; moreover, multiple attempts to detect HIV-1 RNA or proviral DNA in cellular reservoirs and other tissue compartments were negative (Yuki et al., 2013).

More recently, these findings were replicated in the "London patient," who underwent a similar allogeneic stem cell transplantation with cells that did not express CCR5; following the transplant, no replication-competent virus in blood, cerebrospinal fluid (CSF), intestinal tissue, or lymphoid tissue was detected at 30 months following ART discontinuation (Gupta et al., 2020). Since then, cases involving other PWH (a total of 7 at the time of this writing) have been reported with similar outcomes. Because of the risk of stem cell transplantation, however, this intensive approach is not appropriate in PWH who do not have a hematologic malignancy.

Another notable "proof of concept" came from studies of early ART initiation during acute HIV-1 infection. The VISCONTI study identified 14 PWH whose viremia remained controlled for years after the interruption of ART that had been initiated during primary infection (Saez-Cirion et al., 2013). Further, the CHAMP (Control of HIV After Antiretroviral Medication Pause) study, which combined more than 700 PWH who discontinued ART, reported posttreatment controller (PTC) rates of up to 13% in early ART-treated individuals (Namazi et al., 2018); of note, <5% of PTCs were identified in those who initiated ART during chronic stages of infection. Finally, exceptional elite controllers—individuals who appear to have achieved "natural cures"—have been reported (Jiang et al., 2020; Turk et al., 2022).

Along these lines, the "Mississippi baby," a child born to a woman with HIV, was started on ART 30 hours after delivery and quickly achieved virologic suppression (Persaud et al., 2013). The child was lost to follow-up, however, and ART was discontinued. Despite stopping ART, the virus remained undetectable for 27 months, but the child ultimately experienced virologic rebound (Luzuriaga et al., 2015). There have been other reports of children who have controlled HIV after stopping antiretroviral therapy, but these cases are rare (Persaud et al., 2024).

These examples demonstrate that it is possible, under extraordinary circumstances, to eradicate HIV-1 (in the cases of people who receive stem cell transplantation for malignancy) or to control HIV-1 without ART (in PWH in the VISCONTI and CHAMP cohorts and, temporarily, the "Mississippi baby" and other early-treated PWH). The challenge now is to extend insights from these remarkable cases and cohorts to the development of practical interventions that will lead to ART-free remission in the global population of people living with HIV.

EARLY ESTABLISHMENT AND PERSISTENCE OF THE LATENT HIV-1 RESERVOIR

In 1995, investigators identified integrated provirus as a persistent reservoir of infection in the resting $CD4^+$ T cells of PWH (Chun et al., 1995). While most activated memory $CD4^+$ T cells are destroyed during viral replication, a small fraction of infected cells survives to return to a resting and memory state. In the resting memory state, HIV-1 gene expression is shut down, resulting in latent infection of $CD4^+$ T cells (Nabel and Baltimore, 1987). As these cells do not express viral proteins, they remain hidden from the host immune response; moreover, currently approved antiviral drugs only act against the virus during active replication. Although HIV infected $CD4^+$ T cells continuously leave the quiescent memory state, the pool of infected cells persists, perhaps in part because of homeostatic proliferation. It has also been suggested that specific $CD4^+$ T-cell memory subsets, including central memory (TCM), transitional memory (TTM), and memory stem cells (TSCM), harbor the majority of integrated HIV-1 DNA and that eradication therapies may require targeting of specific $CD4^+$ T-cell populations (Buzon et al., 2014).

Reactivation of latently infected cells leads to viral gene expression and active viral replication. In PWH on long-term ART, the percentage of latently infected cells is extremely low: less than 1 per million resting memory $CD4^+$ T cells harbor replication-competent HIV-1 (Finzi et al., 1997; Wong et al., 1997). Nevertheless, after a more rapid decline in the first year after infection, this latent pool decays very slowly: the mean half-life of this reservoir is approximately 44 months, and, as a result, suppressive ART would need to be maintained for more than 60 years to achieve viral eradication even if an infected person had only 100,000 latently infected cells (Besson et al., 2014; Finzi et al., 1999). Longitudinal studies of the reservoir are time-consuming, technically demanding, and challenged by in-person, between-person, and testing heterogeneity (e.g., expansion and contraction of infected T-cell clones were shown to occur even after years on ART), as well as difficulties in comparing different testing methods (Banga and Perreau, 2024; Einkauf et al., 2022; Guo et al., 2022; Hossain et al., 2024; Inderbitzin et al., 2022;). In addition, it is conceivable that latent infection may persist in cells other than $CD4^+$ T cells—but it remains unclear to what extent these cells may play a role in persistence of the HIV reservoir (Veenhuis et al., 2023).

It was initially believed that early suppression of viral replication during primary infection might prevent reservoir formation. However, Chun et al. demonstrated that ART initiated within 10 days of primary infection did not prevent the generation of latently infected CD4$^+$ T cells (Chun et al., 1998), pointing toward an early seeding of the reservoir. Additional data from the rhesus macaque model demonstrate that the latent reservoir is established within days of virus exposure, even before virus can be detected in peripheral blood (Whitney et al., 2014); the implication of this finding is that it may be practically impossible to treat or even diagnose HIV-1 infection early enough to avoid reservoir seeding. Several studies, however, have demonstrated that initiating ART during the acute/early phase of the infection results in a smaller HIV-1 reservoir (Ananworanich et al., 2012; Gantner et al., 2023; Garcia-Broncano et al., 2019; Hocqueloux et al., 2013; Saez-Cirion et al., 2013), and may preserve functionality of CD8$^+$ T cells (Takata et al., 2022), suggesting that early treatment could be beneficial by reducing the barrier to cure (Henrich and Gandhi, 2013; Strain et al., 2005).

Persistence of the HIV-1 latent reservoir represents the biggest obstacle for cure approaches. For this reason, a deeper understanding of how latency is maintained and how this state can be reversed is critical to inform HIV eradication strategies (Deeks et al., 2021).

"KICK AND KILL" AND "BLOCK AND LOCK"

In order to achieve viral eradication, or at least a state of HIV-1 suppression that does not require continuous ART, different strategies have been proposed, including modification of the host immune response to achieve enhanced control of viral replication, interventions to prevent reactivation of virus latency (Mousseau et al., 2015), and gene therapy to increase the resistance of target cells to HIV-1 infection (Tebas et al., 2014). Currently, the strategy receiving the most attention is the "shock and kill" or "kick and kill" approach (Landovitz et al., 2023). In this strategy, the first step is to flush out HIV-1 from the latent reservoir by activating proviral DNA expression in resting cells, leading to de novo viral protein production (the "shock" or "kick"). If this "kick" is successful, the next step is to enhance immune recognition and elimination of infected cells (the "kill"). This two-step approach, however, requires a latency-reversing strategy and an antiviral immune response in order to clear infected cells; both tasks are encumbered by substantial challenges. A strategy that aims to achieve the opposite is named "block and lock." Here, HIV is locked into its latent form, eliminating or at least reducing the chance of viral reactivation and replication. The "block and lock" approach is supported by the recognition that some exceptional elite controllers no longer have replication-competent HIV and therefore have been cured of HIV without antiretroviral therapy, perhaps because their immune system has eliminated HIV proviruses from parts of the genome where the virus was expressed (Jiang et al., 2020; Turk et al., 2022).

LATENCY REVERSAL APPROACHES

Latently infected CD4$^+$ T cells evade immune surveillance, as they do not express HIV-1 proteins (Hermankova et al., 2003). Reversal of HIV-1 latency and induction of virus expression may render infected cells susceptible to attack by cytolytic T lymphocytes or to destruction by viral cytopathic effects (Chun et al., 1997; Deeks, 2012). Several latency-reversing agents (LRAs) have been identified, perhaps the most promising being histone deacetylase inhibitors (HDACi) and toll-like receptor (TLR) agonists (Kim et al., 2018). HDACi are currently approved as anticancer drugs, and several have been evaluated in ART-suppressed PWH for their latency-reversing potential (Archin et al., 2014; Elliott et al., 2014; Rasmussen et al., 2014). Vorinostat, the first HDACi to be studied in PWH on ART, was found to induce viral expression by an average of 4.8-fold in resting CD4$^+$ T cells after a single dose (Archin et al., 2014). Two other HDACi agents—panobinostat and romidepsin—have also been found to induce virus expression in PWH on suppressive ART (Rasmussen et al., 2014; Sogaard et al., 2015). Following administration of romidepsin, plasma HIV-1 RNA levels became detectable in some individuals, suggesting that the LRA was inducing virus production (Sogaard et al., 2015). However, the size of the HIV-1 reservoir, based on measurements of HIV-1 DNA and virus outgrowth assay, remained unchanged following 3 weekly infusions of romidepsin. In addition, romidepsin alone failed to increase HIV-1 expression in persons on ART (McMahon et al., 2019); therefore clinical studies of romidepsin in combination with other agents or strategies are being explored (Mothe et al., 2020) and are discussed later in this chapter. In an exploratory randomized controlled trial, panobinostat in combination with pegylated interferon-α2a led to structural transformation of the HIV reservoir with reduced frequency of intact proviruses in general and particularly in genetic regions that are activated by panobinostat (Armani-Tourret et al., 2024).

TLR agonists are another group of drugs under investigation. The TLR7 agonist vesatolimod was shown to induce transient increases in plasma viral load and decreases in cellular viral DNA levels in simian immunodeficiency virus (SIV)-infected rhesus macaques (Whitney et al., 2015). In a separate study in monkeys treated with ART during acute simian-human immunodeficiency virus (SHIV) infection, a combination of a TLR-7 agonist with a broadly neutralizing antibody (PGT121) led to virologic control in 5 of 11 animals even after the interventions and ART were stopped (Borducchi et al., 2018). Trials using vesatolimod in ART-treated PWH are being conducted (Riddler et al., 2021; SenGupta et al. 2021); one study in ART-suppressed PWH with low pre-ART viral loads demonstrated a modest increase in time to viral rebound after analytical treatment interruption (ATI) in the vesatolimod group (SenGupta et al., 2021). Further, the TLR9 agonist lefitolimod increased HIV-1 transcription and enhanced cytotoxic natural killer (NK) cell activation in a small group of ART-suppressed individuals, but subsequently failed to increase the time to viral rebound when ART was held during an ATI (Vibholm et al., 2017;

Vibholm et al., 2019). Another small, randomized placebo-controlled trial studying ART-free virological control after lefitolimod alone versus lefitolimod in combination with two broadly neutralizing anti-HIV-1 antibodies (bNAbs) found no benefit of either using lefitolimod alone or in combination with bNAb treatment (Gunst et al., 2023). Overall, it remains uncertain whether a single agent will be sufficient to effectively and completely purge the pool of replication-competent, integrated, latent HIV-1; rather, a combination of LRAs targeting distinct pathways, and potentially different cell types, might be required (Laird et al., 2015, Armani-Tourret et al. 2024).

LATENCY SILENCING

In contrast to activating latency, it has been proposed that reinforcing a deep state of latency by permanently silencing HIV transcription could be an alternative approach for a functional cure (Mori and Valente, 2020). This concept, also known as the "block and lock" or "soothe and snooze" strategy, would apply latency-promoting agents to block the reactivation of latently infected HIV-1 proviruses, as described above. A potential agent that has been studied is the Tat inhibitor didehydro-cortistatin A, which, when added to ART, reduced viral mRNA in tissues of HIV-1–infected humanized mice and significantly delayed viral rebound following ART interruption (Kessing et al., 2017). More in vivo studies are needed to further determine the role of these interventions in HIV cure.

IMMUNE-ENHANCING AND/OR MODULATING STRATEGIES

While latency reversal will be crucial for eradication strategies, inducing viral replication alone will most likely not be sufficient to eliminate HIV infection. Indeed, in an in vitro model, reversal of latency alone did not result in clearance of infected cells (Shan et al., 2012). For this reason, it is anticipated that, following reactivation, cells harboring the reservoir will need to be actively cleared, perhaps through a second line of attack by the host immune system. Strategies to enhance immune responses via active or passive immunization or via immunomodulation have been proposed. For example, it has been hypothesized that boosting T-cell responses will lead to enhanced viral control—similar to what is seen in so-called HIV-1 elite controllers, individuals who maintain undetectable viral loads in the absence of ART, where antiviral T-cells have been associated with viral suppression (Deeks and Walker, 2007; McMichael et al., 2010). Vaccination strategies will be discussed later in this chapter; what follows next are other immunomodulatory approaches.

IMMUNE MODULATION: CHECKPOINT INHIBITORS

Given the challenge that the cellular dysfunction in PWH, known as T-cell exhaustion, poses for therapeutic vaccination strategies, novel immune-modulating concepts have been developed to reverse this state of exhaustion by inhibiting immune checkpoints (Gubser et al., 2022; Lee and Whitney, 2024). During progressive HIV-1 infection with persistent antigen exposure, increased expression of inhibitory receptors like PD-1 on HIV-1–specific T cells is associated with greater immune dysfunction (Day et al., 2006; Khaitan and Unutmaz, 2011), and it is thought that anti-PD-1 antibodies may be able to restore the function of exhausted $CD4^+$ and $CD8^+$ T cells by restoring host cell pathways needed for T-cell activation (Porichis and Kaufmann, 2012). Inhibiting the PD-1 pathway has shown efficacy in reversing T-cell exhaustion in the cancer field (Topalian et al., 2012), and data suggest that PD-1 blockade restores the ability of antiviral T cells to inhibit HIV-1 replication in animal models, including non-human primates (Palmer et al., 2013; Velu et al., 2009; Velu et al., 2022). Moreover, PD-1 is believed to play an important role in the establishment and maintenance of latently infected cells (Evans et al., 2018) and PD1-blockade might therefore lead to increased HIV transcription, a key step in latency reversal, and this may be true for other immune checkpoint pathways as well (Gubser et al., 2022). Ex vivo, a PD-L1 antibody (BMS-936559) was not sufficient to increase latency reversal measured by HIV virion production from $CD4^+$ T cells (Bui et al., 2019). Dose-escalation of this antibody delayed viral load rebound after ARV cessation in rhesus macaques and significantly lowered the viral load set point (Mason et al., 2014). In a phase 1 randomized clinical trial in 8 PWH on ART with $CD4^+$ T-cell counts of greater than 350 cells/mm^3 and detectable viral load who received a single infusion of BMS-936559, two participants demonstrated an increase in HIV-specific T-cell responses. However, the trial was stopped prior to full enrollment as there was concern about antibody-associated retinal toxicity in animal studies (Gay et al., 2017). Another checkpoint inhibitor trial (ACTG 5370) was stopped early because of concern for two possible immune-related adverse event complications (Hardy, 2020). However, these studies did demonstrate, as a proof of concept, the potential utility of immune checkpoint inhibitors in targeting the HIV reservoir. Intriguingly, repeated doses of the anti-PD-1 antibody pembrolizumab in a single individual with HIV and lung cancer were associated with an increase in functional HIV-specific $CD8^+$ T cells and a decline in cell-associated HIV-DNA (Guihot et al., 2018), and a recent trial in people with cancer on ART showed measurable latency reversal in the absence of clonal expansion after a single infusion of pembrolizumab (Uldrick et al., 2022).

Other immune checkpoint inhibitors have been approved as cancer therapies, including nivolumab, an anti-PD-1 antibody, which, as described in a case report, appeared to decrease the HIV reservoir (as suggested by a decrease in cell-associated HIV-DNA, increase in HIV-RT and Nef-specific $CD8^+$ cells, and increase in T-cell activation) in a man with non–small-cell carcinoma and well-controlled HIV infection (Guihot et al., 2018). An observational study of 32 PWH who were treated for cancer with monoclonal antibodies against PD-1 failed to demonstrate increased immune responses to HIV, but found substantial induction of other immune checkpoint pathways, potentially indicating compensatory mechanism with inhibition of a single immune checkpoint pathway (Baron et al. 2022). In another study with either anti-PD-1 monotherapy or the combination of both anti-PD-1 and anti-CTLA-4, a modest increase in cell-associated HIV RNA was detected in the few participants receiving combination therapy (Rasmussen et al., 2021).

Remaining concerns with immune checkpoint inhibitors, mainly informed by experiences in treatment for malignant diseases, are variable response rates, development of resistance to therapy, and, particularly, induction of autoimmune disease (Wykes and Lewin, 2018).

T-CELL TRAFFICKING

Early HIV infection of lymphocytes within gut-associated lymphoid tissue (GALT) and subsequent depletion of gut $CD4^+$ T cells appears to significantly contribute to the immune dysfunction observed in chronic HIV infection. Durable suppression of HIV replication with ART does not significantly reverse the damage caused to GALT during early infection. Accordingly, therapies aimed at attenuating HIV-mediated destruction of GALT may serve as an effective strategy to treat and/or prevent HIV-related immune dysfunction and has been suggested as a potential cure strategy. One such approach involves disruption of the interaction between $\alpha_4\beta_7$ gut-homing receptors on $CD4^+$ T cells and the gut endothelial cell adhesion molecules to which these receptors bind via interaction with mucosal addressing cell adhesion molecules (MAdCAM). HIV interacts with $\alpha_4\beta_7$ via the V2 domain of the gp120 subunit, and $CD4^+$ T cells with high expression of $\alpha_4\beta_7$ appear to be preferentially infected during acute HIV or SIV infection. Treatment of SIV-infected ART-suppressed macaques with an anti-$\alpha_4\beta_7$ integrin monoclonal antibody resulted in persistent viral control following ART cessation (Byrareddy et al., 2016). However, other studies in macaques were unable to show this effect (Abbink et al., 2019; Iwamoto et al., 2019).

A commercially available humanized anti-$\alpha_4\beta_7$ mAb, vedolizumab (Act-1), is currently Food and Drug Administration (FDA) approved for use in inflammatory bowel disease. This antibody blocks binding to MAdCAM at the b7 chain of $\alpha_4\beta_7$, thereby inhibiting the migration of lymphocytes into the gastrointestinal tract and reducing local inflammatory responses. In a phase 1 study evaluating vedolizumab in 20 participants with HIV undergoing analytical treatment interruption, the median duration of plasma viremia <400 copies/mL was only 5.4 weeks, failing to show sustained viral suppression (Sneller et al., 2019). Similarily, vedolizumab dosed during ART initiation demonstrated that although the therapy was safe and well tolerated, it had no substantial impact on viral remission after participants underwent an ATI (Jimenez-Leon et al., 2024); other studies are ongoing (ClinicalTrials.gov identifiers: NCT03147859 and NCT04120415).

In contrast to preventing trafficking of HIV target cells into anatomic sites of high viral replication, an alternative approach is promoting cytotoxic $CD8^+$ T-cell migration into lymph node follicles to clear infected cells. In the non-human primate model, administration of an interleukin-15 super-agonist resulted in an increase of CXCR5 expression on $CD8^+$ T cells and an increased frequency of such cells in the lymphoid tissues (Webb et al., 2018). A phase 1 trial that evaluated different doses of the IL-15 superagonist N-803 in ART-suppressed PWH demonstrated that while transcription in memory $CD4^+$ T cells and intact proviral DNA initially increased after N-803 treatment, the frequency of PBMCs with an inducible HIV provirus shows a small but significant decrease that persisted for up to 6 months after therapy (Miller et al., 2022). This concept is now being further examined in humans, also combining IL15-agonists with monoclonal anti-HIV antibodies (ClinicalTrials.gov identifiers: NCT04505501, NCT04340596, and NCT05245292).

CYTOKINES

IL-2, an autocrine T-cell growth factor, is produced by $CD4^+$ T cells, and expression was found to be lower in PWH. Based on promising phase 2 trials showing increased $CD4^+$ T-cell counts in participants receiving recombinant IL-2 (rIL-2) (Pett et al., 2010), two phase 3 trials were performed. In the ESPRIT study, 4,111 PWH with $CD4^+$ T-cell counts of 300 cells/µL or more were randomly assigned to receive either SQ IL-2 (three 5-day cycles 8 weeks apart) with ART or ART alone (Abrams et al., 2009). Although the rIL-2 group had significantly higher $CD4^+$ T-cell counts, this difference declined with time, and clinical outcomes (including opportunistic infection/death and all-cause mortality) did not significantly differ between the two groups. In addition, there were more grade 4 adverse events in the group receiving IL-2, most notably deep venous thrombosis. Subsequent analysis also raised concern for an increased incidence of pneumonia in patients who received rIL-2 less than 180 days previously (Pett et al., 2011). The second IL-2 phase 3 trial, SILCAAT, randomly assigned 1,695 patients with $CD4^+$ T-cell counts of 50–299 cells/mm^3 to similar treatment arms, except the IL-2 group received six cycles at a lower dose (Abrams et al., 2009). $CD4^+$ T-cell counts were again higher in the IL-2 group, but statistically significant differences in opportunistic infection/death, all-cause mortality, and grade 4 clinical events were not seen.

Additionally, IL-2 has been studied as a means to reduce the viral reservoir. One randomized trial did not show an impact of rIL-2 with ART on proviral DNA in blood, lymph nodes, and CSF compared to ART alone (Stellbrink et al., 2002). Other potential uses of rIL-2, such as a means to delay ART initiation, facilitate ART treatment interruption, or as a vaccine adjunct, have also been studied. However, in the STALWART study, a phase 2 trial involving participants not on ART with $CD4^+$ T-cell counts greater than 300 cells/µl, rIL-2 use was associated with more opportunistic disease and death and a statistically significant increase in grade 3 or grade 4 events (Tavel et al., 2010). In summary, IL-2 currently does not appear to confer clinical benefit to PWH, regardless of whether they are on ART, although this continues to be an area of investigation.

Other cytokines being studied for use in HIV include IL-7, IL-15, and IL-21 (Gunst et al., 2023). IL-7 plays a key role in T-cell homeostasis, leading to expansion and survival of naive and memory T-cells and preventing apoptosis of CD4+ and CD8+ T cells in PWH in vitro. In early clinical trials, human recombinant IL-7 therapy was well tolerated and induced a significant and dose-dependent increase in functional naive and memory CD4+ and CD8+ T cells in lymphopenic PWH on ART (Levy et al., 2009; Sereti et al., 2009). In a randomized, placebo-controlled trial of recombinant IL-7 in ART-treated PWH, there were brisk T-cell increases of naive and central memory T cells (averaging 323 cells/μL at 12 weeks), with a durable response seen up to 1 year (Levy et al., 2012). IL-7, however, appears to have a minimal impact on the latent HIV reservoir. A follow-up study of peripheral blood monocytes collected from 10 participants who participated in an IL-7 treatment trial failed to demonstrate activation of latently infected resting memory CD4+ T cells (Vandergeeten et al., 2013).

In macaque models, IL-21 has demonstrated beneficial immune responses, such as improved NK and T-cell cytotoxicity and reduced levels of intestinal T-cell proliferation and microbial translocation. With this novel mechanism of action, it appears to be a promising treatment for augmenting immune response while ameliorating intestinal immune activation (Pallikkuth et al., 2011, 2013).

IL-15, like IL-2, has lymphocyte stimulatory activity and is significantly increased in PWH with a virologic and immunologic response to ART compared to ART-naive patients (Forcina et al., 2004). This has prompted interest in its role in immune therapy (Harwood and O'Connor, 2021). A recent phase 1 study demonstrated safety of N-803, a long-acting IL-15 superagonist, and a possible effect on the reservoir in PWH (Miller et al., 2022).

CHIMERIC ANTIGEN RECEPTOR T-CELLS

An alternative approach, which circumvents the problem of eliciting immune responses in PWH, is the adoptive transfer of T cells with molecularly cloned high-affinity T-cell receptors and superior antiviral activity, targeting conserved and vulnerable regions of the virus (Varela-Rohena et al., 2008). Chimeric antigen receptor transduced T (CAR T) cells, which combine the specificity of an antibody with the signaling of a T-cell receptor, have shown promise in cancer (Hombach et al., 2013) and are being studied in HIV (Choudhary et al., 2022; Lam and Bollard, 2013; Leibman et al., 2017). Clinical trials testing chimeric antigen receptor (CAR) T-cell therapy in ART-suppressed individuals include bNAb-based CAR (Liu et al., 2021; Mao et al., 2024) and a CD4-CAR T-cell modified by zinc-finger nuclease CCR5 disruption to induce HIV resistance (ClinicalTrials.gov identifier: NCT03617198).

MONOCLONAL ANTIBODY THERAPY

During the past decade, multiple monoclonal antibodies (mAbs) have been developed against various viral targets, including viral membrane targets (e.g., gp120 and gp41), the CD4+ receptor, and the CCR5 coreceptor (Chen and Dmitrov, 2012). Very few of these mAbs showed clinical benefit, despite efficacy in nonhuman primate models, largely owing to the virus's ability to rapidly develop resistant variants. Nonetheless, several promising compounds and treatment approaches have recently evolved.

Leronlimab (PRO 140), a humanized CCR5 mAb, had potent activity in early clinical trials. Currently in phase 2b/3 study, participants who are suppressed on a stable ART regimen are switched to weekly subcutaneous injections of leronlimab as a single-agent maintenance therapy in patients with exclusively CCR5-tropic HIV-1. Preliminary results showed a failure rate of 65% in the 350 mg dose arm. (Dhody et al., 2018; Dhody and Kazempour, 2019). However, in phase 2b/3, PRO 140 subcutaneous injections were added to a failing ART regimen. Of 52 participants, 64% versus 23% (p = 0.0032) had at least 0.5 log viral load drop after 1 week (Dhody et al., 2018) with no treatment-related resistance. In February 2024, a partial clinical hold on leronlimab's clinical development program for HIV, originally placed on the program in March 2022, was lifted by the FDA.

UB-421 is a humanized IgG1 monoclonal antibody that inhibits attachment of HIV-1 virus and entry into the cells by competitively binding to the CD4+ receptor. In a phase 2 nonrandomized trial, 29 participants who had undetectable viral loads were enrolled and received either 10 mg/kg dosing every week or 25 mg/kg biweekly after stopping their ART for 8 weeks, with 94% of participants maintaining virologic suppression (Wang et al., 2019). A phase 2 study that evaluated the efficacy of UB-421 in combination with standard ART in reducing the HIV reservoir in PWH was recently completed and results are pending (ClinicalTrials.gov identifier: NCT03743376). Another study assessing the efficacy of UB-421 administered as an add-on to the standard ART in ART-treated PWH with stably suppressed HIV-1 plasma viral loads is ongoing (ClinicalTrials.gov identifier: NCT04404049).

BROADLY NEUTRALIZING ANTIBODIES

HIV-1 immunotherapy with first-generation mAbs in the preclinical and clinical settings was largely ineffective. However, the recent identification of novel broadly neutralizing anti-HIV-1 antibodies (bNAbs), which are able to neutralize the majority of viral strains at very low concentrations, may provide another approach to target the HIV-1 reservoir. In preclinical studies, administration of bNAbs was shown to reduce plasma viremia in chimeric SHIV-infected macaques (Barouch et al., 2013b; Shingai et al., 2013; Julg et al., 2017). In fact, one particular bNAb, PGT121, also resulted in substantial reductions of proviral DNA in peripheral blood, lymph nodes, and gastrointestinal mucosa (Barouch et al., 2013b). Multiple different bNAbs have been tested in PWH and have shown promising reductions in plasma viremia (Caskey et al., 2015; Caskey et al., 2017; Julg et al., 2022; Lynch et al., 2015; Stephenson et al., 2021). As a potential mechanism, it has been suggested that clearance of infected cells expressing viral antigen on their surfaces (Lu et al., 2016) is mediated through interactions between the Fc component of the antibody and its receptor on innate immune effectors cells like NK cells and macrophages (Bruel et al., 2016).

VRC01 is a bNAb that targets the CD4-binding site of the HIV envelope glycoprotein. In a phase 1 randomized placebo-controlled trial, VRC01 was safe and well tolerated, but did not have any significant effects on low-level plasma or cellular HIV-1 viremia in individuals on effective ART (Riddler et al., 2018); nevertheless, VCR01 is undergoing phase 2b studies. A phase 1 study evaluating a long-acting form of VRC01 (VRC01LS) demonstrated that VRC01LS was safe, well tolerated, had a 4-fold greater half-life, and elicited HIV-1 neutralizing activity (Gaudinski et al., 2018). Similarly, other bNAbs with half-life extending modifications, such as 3BNC117-LS, VRC07-523LS, 10-1074-LS, PGT121.414.LS, and PGDM1400LS, are currently being evaluated (ClinicalTrials.gov identifier: NCT05184452). A recent analysis on the impact of the half-life extending LS mutation on antibody pharmacokinetics that included data from 16 clinical trials suggested a favorable pharmacokinetic profile of LS variants regardless of HIV epitope specificity, supporting lower dosages and/or less frequent dosing of LS variants to achieve similar levels of antibody exposure in future clinical applications (Mayer et al., 2024).

Administration of the antibodies 3BNC117 and VRC01 resulted in delayed viral rebound after ART cessation compared with historical controls, but effects were modest and generally transient (Bar et al., 2016; Scheid et al., 2016). Not surprisingly, the rapid selection of archived resistant viral strains reduced the therapeutic efficacy of single bNAbs; for this reason, bNAb combinations were proposed, and several clinical trials that combined the bNAbs 3BNC117 and 10–1074 demonstrated effective suppression of viral rebound for extended periods (Gaebler et al., 2022; Mendoza et al., 2018, Sneller et al., 2022). The ongoing RIO study is a placebo-controlled randomized two-arm phase 2 trial that tests if the use of long-acting 3BNC117LS and 10–1074LS in PWH who initiated ART during early HIV infection will prevent HIV rebound during ATI (ClinicalTrials.gov identifier: NCT04319367).

In addition, next-generation antibodies that incorporate the antigen specificity of different bNAbs by binding to multiple nonoverlapping sites on the virus or attaching to both virus and $CD4^+$ receptors have been engineered (Huang et al., 2016; Xu et al., 2017). The administration of three bNAbs targeting the CD4 binding site (VRC07-523LS), the V3-glycan (PGT121), and the V2 apex (PGDM1400) resulted in a robust reduction of plasma HIV RNA levels in viremic individuals not on ART. Viral rebound, however, occurred quickly and demonstrated partial to complete resistance to PGDM1400 and PGT121, suggesting rapid selection of viral escape variants (Julg et al., 2022). Triple combinations of bNAbs or a tri-specific antibody (Xu et al., 2017) are currently being evaluated in additional early phase clinical trials (ClinicalTrials.gov identifiers: NCT03721510 and NCT03705169).

These results will need to be studied further, especially with regard to their impact on the latent reservoir and immune dysregulation, as chronic antigen stimulation should be reduced by these antibodies. Further, the lack of accessibility of antibodies to certain anatomic reservoir sites, such as the central nervous system, will need to be overcome.

DUAL-AFFINITY RETARGETING

A novel method to combine antibody and T-cell activity against HIV-1-infected cells is through bispecific protein constructs (dual-affinity retargeting [DARTs]), which are designed to latch onto HIV-1 envelope proteins on the surface of infected cells while also binding to CD3 on T cells. This approach directs cytotoxic T cells to eliminate infected cells while obviating the need for the T cells to specifically bind to HIV-1 surface antigens (Pegu et al., 2015; Sung et al., 2015). Early in vitro studies of this approach are promising, and a first-in-human phase 1 safety study of the DART *MGD014* (A32 x anti-CD3) in PWH showed a favorable safety profile (Nordstrom et al., 2022). A combination study with a second DART (*MGD020*) in PWH on ART is planned.

COMBINATION STRATEGIES

The first randomized human trial using the "shock and kill" cure strategy was the RIVER study that combined a therapeutic vaccine ChAdV63.HIVconsv prime with MVA. HIVconsv boost, followed by administration of the LRA vorinostat. Disappointingly, no significant change in the viral reservoir was observed (Fidler et al., 2020). Another trial tested the combination of the HDACi romidepsin and the MVA.HIVconsv vaccine in early treated PWH and a sustained suppression of viremia up to 32 weeks was reported (Mothe et al., 2020). In a randomized phase 1b/2a trial, the impact of latency reservoir romidepsin followed by 3BNC117 on reservoir size and time to viral rebound was compared to romidepsin alone. Twenty patients were enrolled; the combination did not reduce the reservoir size or delay viral rebound (Gruell et al., 2022). Another phase 2a trial that evaluated the efficacy of the TLR9-agonist lefitolimid with the bNAbs 3BNC117 and 10-1074 showed that the groups receiving dual bNAb treatment had a significant delay in the time to viral rebound during ATI, as compared to placebo or lefitolimod only, but that the addition of lefitolimod to dual bNAb treatment did not confer any additional effect on viral control (Gunst et al., 2023). Another study combining these bNAbs with peg-IFN-α2b resulted in 20% of participants maintaining viral suppression off ART after all study treatment had been discontinued. The latter, however, did not result in changes in the reservoir size (Tebas et al., 2023). In another study, 10-1074 in combination with the bNAb VRC07-523LS and the IL-15 superagonist N-803 is being evaluated during an ATI (ClinicalTrials.gov identifier: NCT04340596). A recent trial exploring the combination of (i) latency reversal agents, (ii) therapeutic vaccines, and (iii) bNAbs in PWH who had initiated ART within 6 months of HIV infection found that 5 of 10 participants had viral load set points <1,000 copies/mL after ART interruption, suggesting enhanced immune control (Peluso et al., 2023) (ClinicalTrials.gov identifier: NCT04357821). Additional studies combining bNAbs, therapeutic vaccines, and/or LRAs are planned or currently enrolling (ClinicalTrials.gov identifiers: NCT06484335, NCT06071767, NCT04983030, NCT05281510).

OTHER IMMUNOMODULATORY TREATMENTS

Because T-cell activation is controlled by several signaling pathways, inhibitors of these pathways may also play a role in reducing the size of the latent viral reservoir. Early preclinical research has shown that mTOR inhibitors (e.g., sirolimus, temsirolimus, and everolimus) may play a role in reducing T-cell activation and inflammation (Heredia et al., 2015; Martin and Siciliano, 2015; Palmer et al., 2015), although clinical trial data are lacking. A phase 4 study evaluated the impact of everolimus on HIV persistence post kidney or liver transplant in patients who were stable on ART. The study failed to demonstrate significant change in low-level viremia or CD4$^+$ T-cell associated HIV-DNA or RNA levels 6 months after initiation of everolimus. However, the authors noted that participants who achieved a higher everolimus trough level of 5 ng/mL during the first 2 months had significant sustained reduction in cellular RNA levels at 12 months. This study supported the hypothesis that there is a mechanistic interaction between mTOR inhibitor use and HIV persistence (Henrich et al., 2021). Other immunomodulators such as the janus-kinase (JAK 1/2) inhibitor ruxolitinib resulted in reduced immune activation in PWH on ART (Marconi et al., 2022) and the JAK 1/2 inhibitor baricitinib is currently being evaluated for reduction of HIV in the central nervous system (ClinicalTrials.gov identifier: NCT05452564) based on promising preclinical data.

GENE MODIFICATION

Gene therapy, also referred to as "intracellular immunization," involves the insertion of protective genes either mechanically or by viral vectors. Gene therapy research has focused on two areas: the disruption of cellular genes involved in HIV entry, such as the CCR5 coreceptor, and the introduction of genes to disrupt HIV replication. The goal of gene therapy in HIV is to have the target cells produce gene products that protect them and their progeny from HIV infection. The use of various technologies, including CRISPR, ribozymes, aptamers, RNA-based interference strategies, and zinc-finger nucleases, is currently being investigated.

RENDERING THE HOST'S CD4$^+$ T CELLS RESISTANT TO INFECTION

The Berlin patient, the London patient, and others appear to be cured from HIV-1 after receiving stem cell transplants from CCR5Δ32 homozygous donors, which inspired attempts to generate HIV-1 resistant cells through gene therapy. Zinc-finger nucleases (ZFNs) are bioengineered restriction enzymes with two functional domains—one that recognizes DNA and another that cleaves it. ZFNs can bind specific DNA sequences, produce a double-stranded break, and then lead to permanent gene disruption when cellular repair pathways lead to the addition or deletion of nucleotides at the break site. ZFNs have been shown to disrupt CCR5 expression in human stem cells administered in a mouse model of HIV and to be associated with lower HIV viral loads after HIV challenge (Holt et al., 2010; Perez et al., 2008), and have entered evaluation in clinical trials.

SB-728T, an infusion of ZFN-modified autologous CD4$^+$ T cells with the ability to knock out CCR5 expression, increased CD4$^+$ T-cell counts, decreased proviral DNA, and restored the CD4$^+$-depleted population of the gut mucosa in PWH with CD4$^+$ T-cell counts >200 cells/μL (June et al., 2012; Lalezar et al., 2012). One participant with the highest level of CCR5 modification had an undetectable viral load when ART treatment interruption occurred. Using the ZFN strategy, researchers modified the CCR5 gene ex vivo in autologous CD4$^+$ T cells in 12 PWH and infused the cells back into the autologous donors (Tebas et al., 2014). The study found that genetically modified CD4$^+$ T cells were significantly increased and persisted in vivo with a half-life of nearly a year. While no dramatic difference was seen in viral load set points following interruption of ART in 6 study participants, the modified cells appeared to be protected from HIV-1 infection as unmodified cells showed a faster depletion. Six of these patients underwent 12-week ART interruption, but in only 1 patient (heterozygous for the CCR5Δ32 mutation) did the viral load decline to an undetectable level prior to ART re-initiation.

Additional studies of SB-728T are underway, with one examining CCR5Δ32 heterozygotes and another examining the use of cyclophosphamide prior to CD4$^+$ T-cell infusion to decrease the number of existing CD4$^+$ T cells. Early data from the latter trial demonstrated that cyclophosphamide treatment is well tolerated with a dose-related increase in total CD4$^+$ T-cell count and engraftment of CCR5-modified cells (Blick et al., 2014). While this approach did not lead to durable suppression of HIV after cessation of ART, it did appear to delay viral load rebound in study participants (Tebas et al., 2021). Additional research investigating HIV-1 coreceptor modulation is ongoing.

Data in SHIV-infected and ART-suppressed pigtail macaques demonstrated that CCR5 gene-edited hematopoietic stem/progenitor cells (HSPCs) persisted following transplantation and expansion through virus-dependent positive selection, resulting in a significant reduction of tissue-associated SHIV DNA and RNA levels in the transplanted animals compared to controls (Peterson et al., 2018). Gene editing techniques carry a risk for off-target effects causing mutations at unintended sites in the genome, a currently relevant hurdle to their use in clinical trials (Cradick et al., 2013). The safety and feasibility of administration of clustered regularly interspaced short palindromic repeat (CRISPR)/Cas9 CCR5 gene-modified CD34$^+$ HSPC and ZFN CCR5 modified autologous CD4$^+$ T cells in ART-suppressed PWH is currently being evaluated. Of note, a 2019 report describes the case of an individual with HIV and acute lymphoblastic leukemia who was treated with an allogeneic bone marrow transplant in which the CCR5Δ32 mutation was introduced using CRISPR/Cas9. Cells with the deletion were only found in a small percentage of bone-marrow-engrafted cells. While the leukemia was subsequently in remission, the patient experienced viral rebound shortly after interrupting

ART (Xu et al., 2019), perhaps because too few cells carried the protective mutation.

EXCISING THE HIV-1 PROVIRUS FROM THE HOST CELL GENOME

The CRISPR/Cas9 system permits targeted and precise genome editing in diverse cell types and organisms, including human cells (Cong et al., 2013; Maslennikova and Mazurov, 2022). Several research groups have successfully applied gene editing technology to excise HIV-1 provirus from the host cell genome in vitro (Ebina et al., 2013; Hu et al., 2014; Liao et al., 2015). Importantly, the disruption of provirus expression not only restricted transcriptionally active provirus but also blocked the expression of latently integrated provirus (Ebina et al., 2013). Moreover, inserting the stably expressed CRISPR/Cas9 system into a T-cell line conferred long-term protection against HIV-1 infection (Liao et al., 2015). These results from in vitro cell culture models are promising, and this technology may open new avenues to developing antiviral therapies in the future.

RIBOZYMES, RNA-BASED INTERFERENCE, AND APTAMERS

Ribozymes are small, catalytically active RNA molecules that can be engineered to target specific RNA sequences. They target viral RNA during uncoating and after transcription of HIV, leading to RNA degradation. Although in vitro studies of ribozyme gene therapy have been promising, retroviral vectors delivering ribozymes targeting viral targets (e.g., Tat and Rev) have been plagued by problems with low transduction efficiency (Mitsuyasu et al., 2009).

RNA interference utilizes short RNAs that mediate the degradation of mRNAs in a sequence-specific manner: antisense oligonucleotides bind mRNA and trigger degradation through an RNase H-dependent pathway or block ribosome binding, thus preventing gene expression. Clinical research in this field has been limited by the ability to deliver the RNAs to the correct target cells, poor cellular uptake and stability, and viral escape (Zhou and Rossi, 2011). VRX496 (Lexgenleucel-T), antisense Env in a lentiviral vector, has been delivered via autologous $CD4^+$ T-cell infusion to both PWH on failing regimens and PWH on a fully suppressive ART regimen. In one trial, 17 participants received Lexgenleucel-T over 16 weeks, with ART interruption 1 month later in 13 of these individuals (Tebas et al., 2013). Six of eight participants analyzed were noted to have a decrease in viral load set point. The use of a short-interfering RNA targeting a unique triple repeat of NF-κB was also shown to achieve long-term suppression of HIV-1 (Singh et al., 2014).

Aptamers are single-stranded RNA or DNA molecules that bind viral proteins, preventing them from carrying out their function in the viral life cycle (Figure 18.1). In clinical trials, when used alone, they have not been shown to be effective. However, strategies combining aptamers, ribozymes, and RNA interference, based on in vitro efficacy, have shown potent inhibition of HIV-1 in vitro (Brake et al., 2008; Centlivre et al., 2013).

OTHER GENE STRATEGIES

A strategy to render T-cells resistant to HIV replication is the use of MazF-T (i.e., autologous $CD4^+$ T cells modified with the MazF endoribonuclease gene) (Saito et al., 2014). Modified stem cells are being evaluated for PWH with hematologic malignancies. Although promising, it will be difficult to develop these and other gene strategies for widespread use because of high technical demands and costs. Gene therapy could also hypothetically be used to inhibit viral fusion. C46, a peptide with structural similarity to enfuvirtide, has been engineered for expression on autologous T-cells and was well tolerated in clinical trials, although clinical efficacy has not yet been demonstrated (van Lundzen et al., 2007). A dual-cassette, lentiviral vector expressing CCR5 shRNA (knockdown) and C46 (CAL-1) has been shown in preclinical studies to be nontoxic and to protect gene-modified cells from both CXCR4- and CCR5-tropic HIV-1 strains (Wolstein et al., 2014). The results of a phase 1/2a clinical trial using autologous, CAL-1–modified $CD4^+$ T cells and hematopoietic progenitor/stem cells with and without bone marrow precondition (busulfan) in PWH demonstrated safety, but only transient evidence of bone marrow engraftment (Mitsuyasu et al., 2020).

NOVEL NONCURATIVE ANTIRETROVIRAL DRUGS

Antiretroviral therapy remains the mainstay of treatment for PWH. Novel drugs, both within existing and new classes, are in various stages of development and testing (Figure 18.2). Fostemsavir, an oral attachment inhibitor binding to HIV-1 gp120 and, thereby, blocking viral attachment to host $CD4^+$ T cells, was approved by the FDA in 2020 (Kozal et al., 2020). Lenacapavir (LEN), an HIV capsid inhibitor, has been approved for treatment of multidrug-resistant HIV and was recently demonstrated to have excellent potency for HIV pre-exposure prophylaxis (see PrEP section in Chapter 14). Oral LEN is also being studied in combination with oral bictegravir and as part of a weekly combination with islatravir (ISL).

Islatravir is a nucleoside reverse transcriptase translocation inhibitor in clinical development. MK-8591 triphosphate (MK-8591 TP) is the active phosphorylated form, which has a half-life of 78–128 hours in human peripheral blood mononuclear cells. In an open-label study, a single dose of MK-8591 in HIV-1 treatment-naive participants showed a greater than 1 $\log_{10}$ viral load decline after 7–10 days (Schurmann et al., 2020). A phase 2 randomized trial to evaluate the safety, tolerability, and ARV activity of MK-8591 in combination with doravirine and lamivudine is underway. Primate studies demonstrated clinically relevant drug levels for more than 6 months after single a single dose of parenterally administered MK-8591, supporting evaluation of extended dosing formulations, which may have utility as PrEP or maintenance treatment (Barrett et al., 2018). Islatravir showed further promise in later-stage clinical trials. In 2022, however, following multiple occurrences of lymphopenia, with decreased $CD4^+$ T

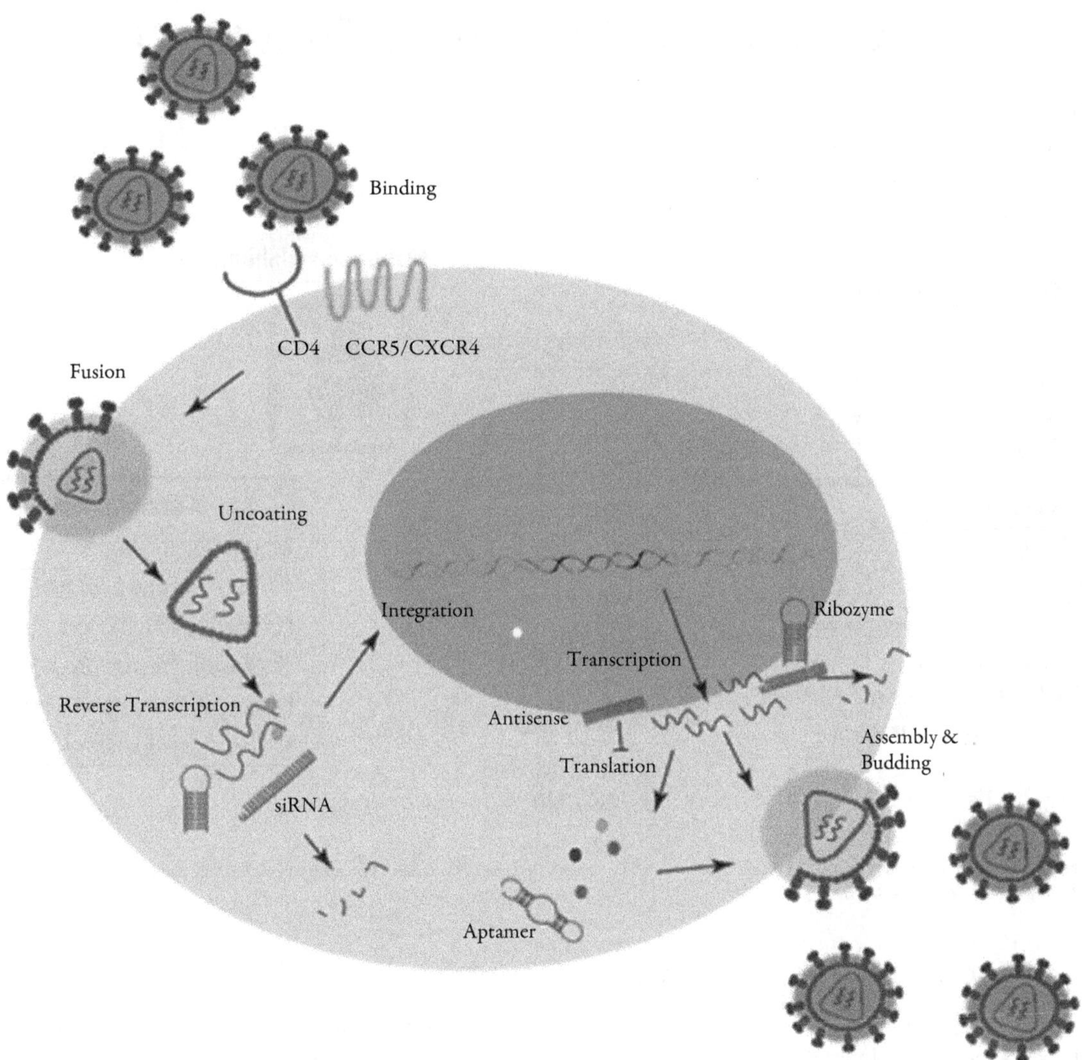

Figure 18.1 Schematic diagram of the HIV viral life cycle in host cell and gene therapy targets. SOURCE: Zeller S, et al. *Yale J Biol Med.* 2011;84(3):301–309.

cells, ISL studies were placed on clinical hold. The trials have been subsequently reopened and are using a lower dose of ISL; these studies are evaluating the drug for HIV treatment rather than prophylaxis.

Other drugs target different stages of the viral life cycle. Figure 18.2 depicts examples of some of the agents that are being evaluated, including broadly neutralizing antibodies.

CONCLUSION

Although antiretroviral medications effectively treat HIV-1 infection, there are many compelling reasons to attempt to cure HIV-1, not least of which is the stigma and isolation experienced by many people with HIV. The major barrier to HIV-1 cure is the persistence of a long-lived population of latently infected cells in PWH on suppressive treatment. Current efforts to cure HIV-1 infection are centered on flushing HIV-1 out of the latent reservoir, along with enhancing immune mechanisms to clear infected cells. The scientific community is still in the early days of this difficult undertaking, and it is too soon to tell whether the approaches being pursued will be effective. Nevertheless, just as the development of combination ART was based on a series of advances that culminated in the eventual ability to successfully treat HIV-1, the stepwise progress currently being made will hopefully lead to an even greater breakthrough: the capability to eradicate or control HIV-1 without the need for lifelong therapy.

RECOMMENDED READING

Ahlenstiel CL, Suzuki K, Marks K, et al. Controlling HIV-1: non-coding RNA gene therapy approaches a functional cure. *Front Immunol.* 2015;6:474.

Arthos JA, Cicala C, Nawaz F, et al. The role of integrin $\alpha_4\beta_7$ in HIV pathogenesis and treatment. *Curr Opin HIV AIDS.* 2018;15:127–135.

Barouch DH, Deeks SG. Immunologic strategies for HIV-1 remission and eradication. *Science.* 2014; 45(6193):169–174.

Chomont N, El-Far M, Ancuta P, et al. HIV reservoir size and persistence are driven by T cell survival and homeostatic proliferation. *Nat Med.* 2009;15(8):893–900.

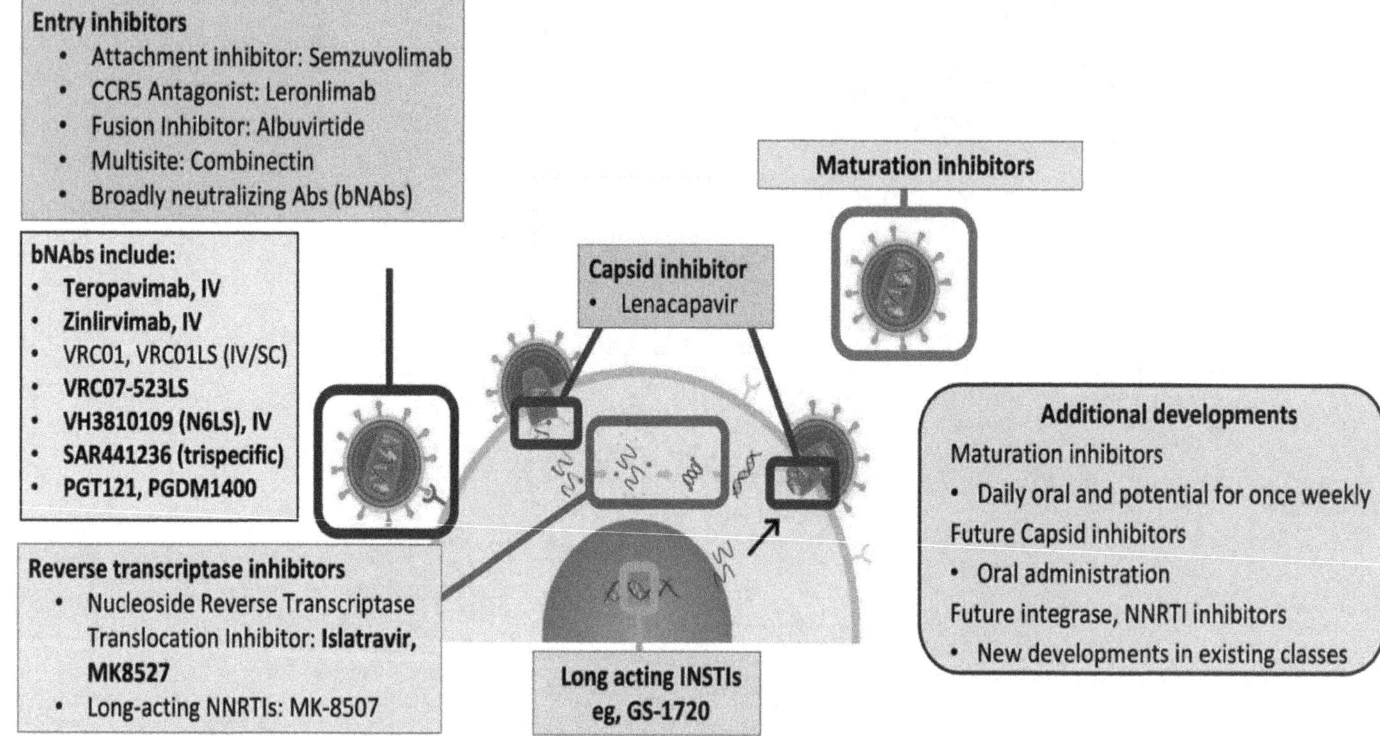

Figure 18.2 New drugs continue to be developed. SOURCE: Courtesy of Ben J Barnett, MD, and Rajesh Gandhi, MD. Adapted from PRIME Education. https://primeinc.org/virtual/treating-hiv-today-tomorrow-look-down-pipeline. October 18, 2023.

Choudhary MC, Cyktor JC, Riddler SA. Advances in HIV-1-specific chimeric antigen receptor cells to target the HIV-1 reservoir. *J Virus Erad.* 2022 Jun 18;8(2):100073.

Deeks SG, Archin N, Cannon P, et al. International AIDS Society (IAS) Global Scientific Strategy working group. Research priorities for an HIV cure: International AIDS Society Global Scientific Strategy 2021. *Nat Med.* December 2021;27(12):2085–2098.

Frater J. New approaches in HIV eradication research. *Curr Opin Infect Dis.* 2011;24(6):593–598.

Gubser C, Chiu C, Lewin SR, Rasmussen TA. Immune checkpoint blockade in HIV. *EBioMedicine.* 2022 Feb;76:103840.

Kitchen SG, Shimizu S, A DS. Stem cell-based anti-HIV gene therapy. *Virology.* 2011;411:260–272.

Levy J. Not an HIV cure but encouraging new directions. *N Engl J Med.* 2009;360:724–725.

Lewin S, Rouzioux C. HIV cure and eradication: how will we get from the laboratory to effective clinical trials? *AIDS.* 2011;25:885–897.

Olender SA, Taylor BS, Wong M, et al. CROI 2015: advances in antiretroviral therapy. *Top Antivir Med.* 2015;23(1):28–45.

Pace P, Markowitz M. Monoclonal antibodies to host cellular receptors for the treatment and prevention of HIV-1 infection. *Curr Opin HIV AIDS.* 2015;10(3):144–150.

Wykes MN, Lewin SR. Immune checkpoint blockade in infectious diseases. *Nat Rev Immunol.* February 2018;18(2):91–104.

THERAPEUTIC AND PREVENTIVE VACCINES

LEARNING OBJECTIVE

Discuss the progression and status of research in HIV vaccines.

WHAT'S NEW?

HIV vaccine research has seen a resurgence in recent years, with different classes of vaccines showing promise in clinical trials.

KEY POINTS

- Therapeutic immunization is a strategy for boosting anti-HIV-1 immunity in chronically infected PWH.
- Recent therapeutic vaccines under study have provided more durable and diverse immune responses and lowering of viral load set points.
- Many different types of vaccines have progressed to phase 2 trials, including DNA, subunit, and dendritic cell vaccines; additionally, novel vaccine concepts using mRNA are being explored.

OVERVIEW OF EARLY THERAPEUTIC VACCINE TRIALS, 1990–2015

Therapeutic immunization aims to induce a cellular immune response through vaccination with components of HIV-1 that will help contain viral replication through reconstitution of anti-HIV-1 immune responses. Data support the observation that the cellular immune response is critical in controlling

HIV-1 replication, as reported in persons with primary HIV-1 infection and in HIV long-term nonprogressors (Borrow et al., 1994; Cao et al., 1995; Kroup et al., 1994; Rosenberg et al., 1997). Therapeutic vaccines can potentially be of benefit to ART-naive PWH by delaying progression to AIDS and time to initiation of ART. Among PWH on ART, development of a durable vaccine may intensify the effects of ART (accelerate response time to therapy, decrease risk of transmission, potentiate the immune effects of ART, and reduce proviral DNA), simplify ART regimens, and support regimens with treatment interruption (Ensoli et al., 2014).

Clinical therapeutic vaccine research for HIV started prior to the introduction of ART, first with a gp120-depleted inactivated HIV-1 preparation and then with vectors expressing viral proteins (e.g., Gag p17 and p24). Clinical trials of these agents largely failed to show efficacy and a sustained HIV-1-specific response (Hardy et al., 2007). Subsequent vaccines with recombinant HIV-1 glycoproteins (e.g., gp120 and gp160) also fared poorly, not altering the decline in CD4$^+$ T-cell count or halting disease progression in HIV-1-infected individuals in phase 2 trials (Eron et al., 1996; Pontesilli et al., 1998; Sandstrom et al., 1999; Tsoukas et al., 1998). In one of the largest of these trials, 608 PWH with CD4$^+$ T-cell counts of greater than 400 cells/mm^3 were repeatedly immunized with a recombinant gp160 vaccine (VaxSyn HIV-1) or placebo and followed for 3–5 years. Although the vaccine had excellent immunogenicity (~70%), it failed to show a difference in reaching the primary clinical endpoints of preventing a 50% decline in CD4$^+$ T-cell count or disease progression to Walter Reed stages 4, 5, and 6 (Birx et al., 2000).

ANRS 093, a study enrolling 70 PWH, compared ART to immunization with recombinant canarypox vector expressing several HIV genes (Env, Gag, Pol, and Nef) and lipo-6T (HIV-1 lipopepides) followed by SQ IL-2. The vaccine elicited a statistically significant INF-γ-producing CD8 $^+$ T-cell response that correlated with virologic control (Levy et al., 2005). The vaccine group had a lower viral set point and therefore a significantly greater number of days off ART (Levy et al., 2006), but the results of this study continue to await validation in larger trials.

In ACTG 5197, administration of a replication-defective adenovirus type 5 HIV-1 Gag vaccine to PWH with CD4$^+$ T-cell counts >500 cells/mm^3 failed to be sufficiently immunogenic and lacked statistically significant efficacy (Schooley et al., 2010). The finding that the plasma viral load was 0.5 $\log_{10}$ lower in the vaccine arm at 16 weeks post-ART interruption prompted further analysis of the HLA class I alleles in all 110 participants, because HLA classes have previously been shown to influence viral evolution and disease progression. Vaccinated PWH with neutral HLA alleles in this cohort had a lower plasma viral load than those of both PWH vaccinated with protective alleles and placebo participants with neutral alleles (Li et al., 2011).

A novel therapeutic vaccine strategy with promising results targeted Tat, a transactivator of HIV gene expression essential for viral replication which is relatively conserved among HIV-1 subtypes. This vaccine is aimed at PWH on ART with the hope of decreasing viral reservoirs and restoring immune homeostasis. In phase 2 trials, 168 PWH who were controlled on ART and anti-Tat antibody negative at baseline were administered the vaccine 3 or 5 times monthly and showed specific and durable immune responses when followed for up to 144 weeks (Ensoli et al., 2015). Most (79%) developed anti-Tat antibodies, which was associated with significant reduction of proviral DNA after week 72. The vaccine was also associated with a restoration of T, B, and NK cells and CD4$^+$ and CD8$^+$ T-cell central memory subsets.

A multinational phase 2 trial examined the safety and immunogenicity of Vacc-4x, a peptide-based HIV-1 therapeutic vaccine targeting the conserved domains of p24Gag (Pollard et al., 2014). In chronically infected PWH who were virologically suppressed on ART, the Vacc-4x vaccine did not alter time to ART resumption or lead to significant changes in CD4$^+$ T-cell count at week 28 during treatment interruption. However, there was a statistically significant difference in HIV viral load at both week 48 (23,000 vs. 71,800 copies/mL) and week 52 (19,500 vs. 51,000 copies/mL). Despite this series of often discouraging HIV vaccine trial outcomes, promise remains and new therapeutic vaccine approaches are being developed, examples of which are discussed below.

T-CELL VACCINES

The ability to enhance the host's immune responses by therapeutic vaccination faces several key challenges. The majority of PWH have dysfunctional virus-specific effector cells (Sauce et al., 2013) as a result of continuous antigenic stimulation prior to treatment, and ART only incompletely restores T-cell functionality on an epigenetic level (Youngblood et al., 2013). Further, in PWH who initiate ART during chronic infection, almost all of the proviral sequences in the latent reservoir contain escape mutations that prevent killing of infected cells by cytotoxic T lymphocytes (Deng et al., 2015; Papuchon et al., 2013). The implication is that an effective vaccination strategy, instead of just expanding preexisting responses that already had failed to control the infection, would need to improve the quality and functionality of HIV-1-specific immune response and elicit CD8 $^+$ T-cell responses against previously untargeted epitopes or unmutated regions of the virus to avoid escape (Chen and Julg, 2020). To achieve this goal, multiple approaches are currently being tested in preclinical and clinical studies, including the following:

- Viral-vector–based vaccines, such as adenovirus (human and chimpanzee serotypes), poxvirus modified vaccinia Ankara (MVA), vesicular stomatitis virus, arenaviruses, and modified cytomegalovirus (CMV): Some of these approaches to deliver HIV-1 antigens have demonstrated robust immunogenicity, inducing broad and durable cellular immune responses, which were able to protect monkeys against SIV infection in preclinical challenge studies (Barouch et al., 2012; Barouch et al., 2013a; Hansen et al., 2011; Hansen et al., 2013), but, more importantly, significantly reduced the viral load set points in SIV-infected macaques following ART cessation when combined with a TLR7 agonist (Borducchi et al.,

2016). A phase 1/2a clinical trial of an Ad26 prime/MVA boost combination with mosaic HIV inserts in a cohort that initiated ART during acute infection, however, did not lead to viremic control after treatment interruption (Colby et al., 2020). It did, however, result in robust HIV-specific T-cell expansion in PWH who had initiated ART during the chronic phase of infection (Marconi et al., 2022). Other ChAdOx1 and/or MVA-vectored vaccines expressing tHIVconsv immunogens are being evaluated for safety and efficacy in adults with HIV (ClinicalTrials.gov identifiers: NCT03844386 and NCT05604209). A prototype human CMV-based HIV vaccine (ClinicalTrials.gov identifier: NCT04725877, NCT05854381) and arenavirus-based HIV vaccine (ClinicalTrials.gov identifiers: NCT06430905) are currently being tested.

- Plasmid DNA expressing HIV-1 genes (Hallengard et al., 2011; Rodriguez et al., 2013; Sneller et al., 2017): A phase 2 trial evaluating the PENNVAX-GP vaccine, a synthetic plasmid expressing HIV Gag, Pol, and Env, demonstrated modest effects on markers of the viral reservoir in vaccinees with greatest Gag-specific T-cell responses by IFNg ELISPOT. Another vaccine with HIV-derived conserved element (CE) p24 Gag DNA showed promising immunogenicity in macaques (Hu et al., 2016), and elicited new conserved element-directed cellular immune response in approximately half the treated PWH on ART in a phase 1/2a trial (Jacobson et al., 2024). The DNA plasmid vaccine GTU-multi-HIV-B, aimed at inducing immune responses to HIV-1 regulatory genes, has shown efficacy in HIV-1 subtype C PWH not on ART. In a population of 63 participants, the vaccine was deemed safe and was associated with a statistically significant decline in log pHIV-RNA with an increase in $CD4^+$ T-cell counts nearing significance compared to placebo, especially after intramuscular injections (Vardas et al., 2012). The GTU-multi-HIV-B DNA vaccine and LIPO-5 vaccine in a prime-boost strategy in PWH virologically suppressed on ART elicited strong and polyfunctional HIV-specific $CD4^+$ and $CD8^+$ T-cell responses, but these responses were not able to control viremia following antiretroviral treatment interruption (Levy et al., 2021). The AELIX-002 trial evaluated in 45 early ART-treated individuals a combination of DNA, MVA and ChAdOx1 vaccines expressing immunogens designed to induce T-cell responses associated with better viral control. The vaccines did not prevent viral rebound during analytical treatment interruption but plasma viral loads and time off ART positively correlated with vaccine-induced T-cell responses (Bailón et al., 2022).
- mRNA vaccines: The unprecedented success of mRNA-based vaccines against SARS-CoV-2 has channeled subsequent efforts to develop mRNA-based vaccines against other pathogens including HIV-1. Several studies are currently evaluating the ability of mRNA vaccines to induce potent neutralizing antibodies against HIV (ClinicalTrials.gov identifiers: NCT05903339, NCT05217641, NCT05001373, NCT05414786).
- Dendritic cell–based vaccines to deliver HIV-1 antigens: Significant attention has also focused on dendritic cells as cellular adjuvants for therapeutic HIV-1 vaccines because they have been shown to elicit strong $CD4^+$ and $CD8^+$ T-cell responses in vivo. One uncontrolled study of immunization of 18 treatment-naive PWH with dendritic cells pulsed with inactivated autologous virus reported a 90% decrease in viral load during the course of a year (Lu et al., 2004). A subsequent randomized controlled trial of 24 treatment-naive participants with a similar vaccine, however, showed a weak HIV-1-specific response and a modest decrease in viral load compared to placebo (Garcia et al., 2011). In a trial of chronically infected PWH on ART with $CD4^+$ T-cell counts >450 cells/mm^3, the use of a monocyte-derived dendritic cell pulse with heat-inactivated whole HIV helped lower plasma viral load set point after treatment interruption, with an associated increased in HIV-1-specific T-cell responses compared to placebo (Garcia et al., 2013). Other trials also demonstrated better vaccine responses and control of viral replication (Levy et al., 2014). Dendritic cells expressing the HIV proteins Gag, Tat, Rev, and Nef administered as a vaccine have been shown to elicit potent antiviral T-cell responses in PWH on ART, including a Gag-specific IFN-γ response that correlated with HIV-1 inhibitory activity (van Gulck et al., 2012). An ongoing trial aims to test if autologous dendritic cells loaded with a conserved HIV Gag and Pol peptide pool or inactivated autologous HIV will yield broader T-cell responses (ClinicalTrials.gov identifier: NCT03758625).

Although no therapeutic vaccine is currently FDA approved, the future of therapeutic vaccine research for both naive and ART-treated PWH remains promising. Recent data have been encouraging, but the results of therapeutic vaccine trials have yet to yield a therapeutic vaccine strategy that can be implemented. In addition to further clinical trials of the vaccines discussed previously, additional studies investigating the heterogeneity of response to vaccines (e.g., genetic determinants) and the immunologic correlates of vaccine efficacy are needed for the field to advance. Some of the key vaccines in development are highlighted in Table 18.1.

PREVENTIVE VACCINES

Although a preventive HIV-1 vaccine would help control the worldwide HIV/AIDS pandemic, there have been many obstacles to its development. HIV-1 has significant genetic and antigenic diversity, making it difficult to target with a vaccine. The failure to induce broadly neutralizing antibodies against the virus and the lack of clear immune correlates of protection have also been challenges. Additionally, the SIV/SHIV nonhuman primate models on which preclinical testing of the

Table 18.1 SELECT THERAPEUTIC VACCINE TRIALS

VACCINE*	DESCRIPTION	STAGE OF DEVELOPMENT	REGISTRATION NUMBER
Ad26.Mos4.HIV, MVA-BN-HIV, PGT121, PGDM1400, VRC07-523LS	Viral vector vaccine +/- broadly neutralizing antibodies	Phase 1/2	NCT04983030
HVRRICANE	DNA vaccine (HIVIS DNA) + viral vector vaccine (MVA-CMDR) +/– TLR4 agonist	Phase 1	NCT04301154
DC-HIV04	Dendritic cell vaccine (a1DC or pgDC) + inactivated whole autologous HIV or conserved HIV peptides	Phase 1	NCT03758625
NETI	Recombinant HIV envelope protein VRC-HIVRGP096-00-VP (Trimer 4571) therapeutic vaccination	Phase 1	NCT04985760
ChAdOx1.HIVconsv62–MVA.tHIVconsv4 (C62-M4), ChAdOx1.tHIVconsv1+C62-MVA. tHIVconsv3+M4 (C1C62-M3m4)	Viral vector vaccines with conserved T-cell epitopes	Phase 1	NCT05604209
ICVAX	PD-1-enhanced HIV DNA vaccine	Phase 1	NCT06253533
BELIEVE	BCG vaccination effect on latent reservoir size in treated HIV-1 infection	Phase 2a	NCT05004038

* https://www.treatmentactiongroup.org/cure/trials/.

vaccines is typically done have often showed promising results not reproduced in human clinical trials.

Multiple phase 1 and 2 vaccine trials were conducted dating back to 1987, but very few reached phase 2b/3. Initial trials used recombinant proteins to induce neutralizing antibodies. In two large randomized controlled trials, VAX003 and VAX004, involving vaccination with recombinant gp120 subunits, there were no statistically significant reductions in HIV infection in the vaccinated groups (Flynn et al., 2005; Pitisuttithum et al., 2006). In subsequent analysis, these vaccines seemed to fail because of a lack of a broad neutralizing antibody response.

Vaccine development subsequently shifted toward the use of live viral or bacterial vectors engineered to carry genes encoding the HIV antigens. These antigens are expressed in the cytoplasm of the target cell, broken down, and then presented on the surface of the cell, priming a $CD8^+$ response. In the STEP trial, HIV-negative participants received immunization with three injections of a replication-incompetent recombinant adenovirus vector expressing HIV-1 Gag, Pol, and Nef (Buchbinder et al., 2008). The vaccine did not show any benefit in preventing transmission or reducing early viral load after infection.

Surprisingly, however, vaccinated persons who were seropositive for AD-5 or who were uncircumcised had higher rates of HIV-1 infection than placebo, a finding prompting discontinuation of a contemporaneous clinical trial with the same vaccine. Subsequent genetic sequencing of the HIV-1 strains from the vaccine and placebo groups revealed that the virus infecting the vaccine group had different epitopes from those in the placebo group (Rolland et al., 2011). The divergence was confined to the vaccine components of the virus, supporting the notion of selective pressure from vaccine-induced T-cell responses.

More recent vaccine strategies have used a heterologous prime-boost strategy to activate both cellular and humoral immune arms by priming with a certain vaccine (e.g., DNA vaccine) and then boosting the immune response with another type of vaccine (e.g., live vector vaccine) (Girard et al., 2011). The RV144 trial, a phase 3 randomized controlled trial, primed participants with two successive doses of a canarypox vector (ALVAC) encoding Gag/Pro and Env antigens followed by two additional immunizations with this vector and AIDSVAX B/E, a bivalent HIV gp120 envelope glycoprotein derived from a subtype B and subtype E envelope (Rerks-Ngarm et al., 2009). In the placebo group, 74 of 7,325, and in the vaccine group, 51 of 7,347, developed HIV-1 infection at 96 weeks, offering a mildly statistically significant 31% efficacy. These results were encouraging, but there was not a significant broadly neutralizing antibody response, and the vaccine efficacy peaked in the first 6–12 months (50%–60%) only to decrease thereafter. Analysis of the RV144 trial, however, showed two immune correlates of infection risk after vaccination (Haynes et al., 2012). Binding of IgG antibodies to the variable regions of Env inversely correlated with infection rates, while plasma IgA binding to Env was directly correlated.

Building on the RV144 data, the HIV Vaccine Trials Network implemented HVTN 100, a phase 1/2, randomized controlled, double-blind trial in South Africa that compared a canarypox vector, ALVAC-HIV[vCP2438], in combination with an envelope glycoprotein (gp120), both adapted to circulating strains in South Africa and paired with a more potent adjuvant to placebo. This combination induced strong humoral and cellular responses (Bekker et al., 2018). These encouraging results led to the development of HVTN 702, a phase 2b/3 efficacy trial which randomly assigned 5,404 adults without HIV-1 infection to receive ALVAC-HIV/bivalent subtype C gp120–MF59 adjuvant (2,704 participants) or placebo (2,700 participants). During an interim analysis, non-efficacy criteria were met and further vaccinations were subseqüently halted (Gray et al., 2021).

Another strategy was evaluated in the APPROACH trial, a multicenter, randomized, double-blind, placebo-controlled phase 1/2a trial in Africa, South Africa, Thailand, and the United States (Barouch et al., 2018). The participants received Ad26.Mos.HIV expressing mosaic HIV-1 envelope (Env)/Gag/Pol antigens and aluminum-adjuvanted clade C Env gp140 protein or placebo. Researchers evaluated the vaccine safety, tolerability, and antibody responses at weeks 28 and 52. A parallel study was also conducted in rhesus monkeys. It elicited Env-specific binding antibody responses (100%) and antibody-dependent cellular phagocytosis responses (80%) at week 52 and T-cell responses at week 50 (83%) in humans. The most common adverse event was injection site reaction (69%–88%).

After these results, two large global trials were initiated to evaluate Ad 26 viral vaccines that express mosaic Env/Gag and Pol antigens. In sub-Saharan Africa, the HVTN 705 (Imbokodo trial) investigated a trivalent Ad26 construct boosted with a clade C gp140 glycoprotein. Imbokodo recruited 2,637 young women in five southern African countries. There were 14% fewer infections in women who received the vaccine compared to placebo, but this did not reached statistical significance (Gray et al., 2024). Correlates of protection analyses are ongoing at this point. In the Americas and Europe, HVTN 706 (Mosaico trial) was evaluating a tetravalent Ad26 vector boosted with a bivalent mosaic clade C gp140 glycoprotein with alum adjuvant (Mosaico study) in 3,887 volunteers. Based on interim analyses, the study was discontinued in January 2023 due to lack of efficacy (https://www.jnj.com/media-center/press-releases/janssen-and-global-partners-to-discontinue-phase-3-mosaico-hiv-vaccine-clinical-trial).

More recently, BG505 SOSIP.644 and related native-like soluble trimers with different adjuvants are being evaluated in several clinical trials (ClinicalTrials.gov identifiers: NCT04177355 and NCT04915768). In addition, "germline-targeting" recombinant Env immunogen, with the goal to specifically stimulate proliferation of B-cells expressing certain bNAb-like B-cell receptors, is being explored, and a recent proof of concept phase 1 clinical trial testing the vaccine candidate eOD-GT8 60mer adjuvanted with AS01B showed a favorable safety profile with induction of VRC01-class bNAb precursors in 97% of vaccine recipients (Leggat et al., 2022). Additional studies are currently exploring these concepts (ClinicalTrials.gov identifier: NCT05471076).

Further, the HIV Vaccine Trial Network study HVTN302 is now evaluating three different HIV vaccines that are using the mRNA vaccine technology (Clinical Trials.gov identifier: NCT05217641) as well as the IAVI G002 study (ClinicalTrials.gov identifier: NCT05001373) that is evaluating germline-targeting prime and directional boost regimens with eOD-GT8 60mer mRNA and Core-g28v2 60mer to guide generation of bNAbs.

An alternative approach to actively inducing immune responses against HIV-1 is to utilize passive immunization with bNAbs. The Antibody Mediated Prevention (AMP) trials evaluated regular infusions of the bNAb VRC01 compared to placebo among 1,924 women in sub-Saharan Africa in HVTN 703/HIV Prevention Trials Network [HPTN] 084 and 2,699 men and transgender people in the Americas and Europe in HVTN 704/HPTN 085. While overall no infection prevention was observed, the pooled prevention efficacy against viral isolates highly susceptible to VRC01 was 75.4% (Corey et al., 2021).

In summary, recent progress has been made toward the development of a preventive HIV vaccine. Key issues remain the identification of the correlates of immunity, induction of broadly neutralizing antibody responses, and the durability of these responses. It is hoped that ongoing studies will provide insight into the correlates of immunity and eventually lead to an effective preventive vaccine strategy.

RECOMMENDED READING

Ensoli B, Cafaro A, Monini P, et al. Challenges in HIV vaccine research for treatment and prevention. *Front Immunol.* 2014;5:417.

Gilliam BL, Redfield RR. Therapeutic HIV vaccines. *Curr Top Med Chem.* 2003;3(13):2536–1553.

Gotch FM, Imami N, Hardy G. Candidate vaccines for immunotherapy in HIV. *HIV Med.* 2001;2:260–265.

Haynes BF, Wiehe K, Borrow P, et al. Strategies for HIV-1 vaccines that induce broadly neutralizing antibodies. *Nat Rev Immunol.* August 12, 2022:1–17.

Levy Y. Therapeutic HIV vaccines: an update. *Curr HIV/AIDS Rep.* 2005;2(1):5–9.

Van Gulck E, Van Tendeloo VF, Berneman ZN, et al. Role of dendritic cells in HIV immunotherapy. *Curr HIV Res.* 2010;8(4):310–322.

ACKNOWLEDGMENTS

This chapter is based on previous versions with contributions from Drs. David Margolis, Adrian Majid, Bruce Gilliam, Niyati Jakharia, and Rohit Talwani.

REFERENCES

Abbink P, Mercado NB, Nkolola JP, et al. Lack of therapeutic efficacy of an antibody to $\alpha4\beta7$ in SIVmac251-infected rhesus macaques. *Science.* 2019;365(6457):1029–1033. doi:10.1126/science.aaw8562

Abrams D, Levy Y, Losso MH, et al.; INSIGHT-ESPRIT Study Group; SILCAAT Scientific Committee. Interleukin 2 therapy in patients with HIV infection. *N Engl J Med.* 2009;361(16):1548–1559.

Ananworanich J, Schuetz A, Vandergeeten C, et al. Impact of multi-targeted antiretroviral treatment on gut T cell depletion and HIV reservoir seeding during acute HIV infection. *PLoS One.* 2012;7(3):e33948.

Archin NM, Bateson R, Tripathy MK, et al. HIV-1 expression within resting CD4$^{\backslash+\backslash+}$ T cells after multiple doses of vorinostat. *J Infect Dis.* 2014;210(5):728–735.

Armani-Tourret M, Gao C, Hartana CA, et al. Selection of epigenetically privileged HIV-1 proviruses during treatment with panobinostat and interferon-α2a. *Cell*. 2024;187(5):1238–1254.e14.

ART Collaboration Cohort. Life expectancy of individuals on combination antiretroviral therapy in high-income countries: a collaborative analysis of 14 cohort studies. *Lancet*. 2008;372:293–299.

Bailón L, Llano A, Cedeño S; AELIX002 Study Group. Safety, immunogenicity and effect on viral rebound of HTI vaccines in early treated HIV-1 infection: a randomized, placebo-controlled phase 1 trial. *Nat Med*. 2022;28(12):2611–2621.

Banga R, Perreau, M. The multifaceted nature of HIV tissue reservoirs. *Curr Opin HIV AIDS*. 2024;19(3):116–123.

Bar KJ, Sneller MC, Harrison LJ, et al. Effect of HIV antibody VRC01 on viral rebound after treatment interruption. *N Engl J Med*. 2016;375:2037–2050.

Baron M, Soulie C, Lavole A, et al. Impact of anti-PD-1immunotherapy on HIV reservoir and anti-viral immune responses in people living with HIV and cancer. *Cells*. 2022;11(6):1015.

Barouch DH, Liu J, Li H, et al. Vaccine protection against acquisition of neutralization-resistant SIV challenges in rhesus monkeys. *Nature*. 2012;482(7383):89–93.

Barouch DH, Stephenson KE, Borducchi EN, et al. Protective efficacy of a global HIV-1 mosaic vaccine against heterologous SHIV challenges in rhesus monkeys. *Cell*. 2013a;155(3):531–539.

Barouch DH, Tomaka FL, Wegmann F, et al. Evaluation of a mosaic HIV-1 vaccine in a multicentre, randomised, double-blind, placebo-controlled, phase 1/2a clinical trial (APPROACH) and in rhesus monkeys (NHP 13–19). *Lancet*. 2018;392 (10143):232–243.

Barouch DH, Whitney JB, Moldt B, et al. Therapeutic efficacy of potent neutralizing HIV-1-specific monoclonal antibodies in SHIV-infected rhesus monkeys. *Nature*. 2013b;503(7475):224–228.

Barrett SE, Teller RS, Forster SP, et al. Extended-duration MK-8591-eluting implant as a candidate for HIV treatment and prevention. *Antimicrob Agents Chemother*. September 24, 2018; 62(10):e01058-18. doi:10.1128/AAC.01058-18

Bekker L-G, Moodie Z, Grunenberg N, et al. Subtype C ALVAC-HIV and bivalent subtype C gp120/MF59 HIV-1 vaccine in low-risk, HIV-uninfected, South African adults: a phase 1/2 trial. *Lancet HIV*. 2018;5(7):PE366–E378.

Besson GJ, Lalama CM, Bosch RJ, et al. HIV-1 DNA decay dynamics in blood during more than a decade of suppressive antiretroviral therapy. *Clin Infect Dis*. 2014;59(9):1312–1321.

Birx D, Loomis-Price LD, Aronson N, et al. Efficacy of recombinant human immunodeficiency virus (HIV) gp160 as a therapeutic vaccine in early-stage HIV-1-infected volunteers. *J Infect Dis*. 2000;181:881–889.

Blick G, Lalezari J, Hsu R, et al. Cyclophosphamide enhances SB-728T engraftment to levels associated with HIV-RNA control. Abstract 141. Paper presented at the 21st Conference on Retroviruses and Opportunistic Infections. Boston, MA; March 2014.

Borducchi E, Abbink P, Nkolola J, et al. PGT121 combined with GS-9620 delays viral rebound in SHIV-infected rhesus monkeys. Abstract 73LB. The Conference on Retroviruses and Opportunistic Infections. Boston, MA; March 4–7, 2018.

Borducchi EN, Cabral C, Stephenson KE, et al. Ad26/MVA therapeutic vaccination with TLR7 stimulation in SIV-infected rhesus monkeys. *Nature*. December 8, 2016;540(7632):284–287.

Borrow P, Lewicki H, Hahn BH, et al. Virus specific CD8 cytotoxic T-lymphocyte activity associated with control of viremia in primary human immunodeficiency virus type 1 infection. *J Virol*. 1994;68:6103–6110.

Brake OT, Hooft K, Liu YP, et al. Lentiviral vector design for multiple shRNA expression and durable HIV-1 inhibition. *Mol Ther*. 2008;16:557–564.

Bruel T, Guivel-Benhassine F, Amraoui S, et al. Elimination of HIV-1 infected cells by broadly neutralizing antibodies. *Nat Commun*. 2016;7:10844.

Buchbinder SP, Mehrotra DV, Duerr et al. Efficacy assessment of a cell-mediated immunity HIV-1 vaccine (the Step Study): a double-blind, randomised, placebo-controlled, test-of-concept trial. *Lancet*. 2008 Nov 29;372(9653):1881–1893.

Bui JK, Cyktor JC, Fyne E, et al. Blockade of the PD-1 axis alone is not sufficient to activate HIV-1 virion production from CD4+ T cells of individuals on suppressive ART. *PLoS One*. 2019;14(1):e0211112.

Buzon MJ, Sun H, Li C, et al. HIV-1 persistence in CD4$^{\backslash+\backslash+}$ T cells with stem cell-like properties. *Nat Med*. 2014;20(2):139–142.

Byrareddy SN, Arthros J, Cicala C, et al. Sustained virologic control in SIV$^{\backslash+}$ macaques after antiretroviral and α4β7 antibody therapy. *Science*. 2016;354:197–202.

Cao Y, Qin L, Zhang L, et al. Virologic and immunologic characterization of long-term survivors of human immunodeficiency virus type 1 infection. *N Engl J Med*. 1995;332:201–208.

Caskey M, Klein F, Lorenzi JC, et al. Viraemia suppressed in HIV-1–infected humans by broadly neutralizing antibody 3BNC117. *Nature*. 2015;522(7557):487–491.

Caskey M, Schoofs T, Gruell H, et al. Antibody 10-1074 suppresses viremia in HIV-1-infected individuals. *Nat Med*. 2017;23(2):185–191.

Centlivre M, Legrand N, Klamer S, et al. Preclinical in vivo evaluation of the safety of a multi-shRNA-based gene therapy against HIV-1. *Mol Ther Nucleic Acids*. 2013; 2:e120.

Chen W, Dmitrov D. Monoclonal antibody-based candidate therapeutics against HIV type 1. *AIDS Res Hum Retroviruses*. May 2012;28(5):425–434.

Chen Z, Julg B. Therapeutic vaccines for the treatment of HIV. *Transl Res*. 2020;223:61–75.

Choudhary MC, Cyktor JC, Riddler SA. Advances in HIV-1-specific chimeric antigen receptor cells to target the HIV-1-reservoir. *J Virus Erad*. 2022;8(2):100073.

Chun TW, Engel D, Berrey MM, et al. Early establishment of a pool of latently infected, resting CD4$^{\backslash+}$($^{\backslash+}$) T cells during primary HIV-1 infection. *Proc Natl Acad Sci USA*. 1998;95(15):8869–8873.

Chun TW, Finzi D, Margolick J, et al. In vivo fate of HIV-1–infected T cells: quantitative analysis of the transition to stable latency. *Nat Med*. 1995;1(12):1284–1290.

Chun TW, Stuyver L, Mizell SB, et al. Presence of an inducible HIV-1 latent reservoir during highly active antiretroviral therapy. *Proc Natl Acad Sci USA*. 1997;94(24):13193–13197.

ClinicalTrials.gov. NCT03147859.

ClinicalTrials.gov. NCT03307915.

ClinicalTrials.gov. NCT03367754.

ClinicalTrials.gov. NCT03560258.

ClinicalTrials.gov. NCT03617198.

ClinicalTrials.gov. NCT03705169.

ClinicalTrials.gov. NCT03721510.

ClinicalTrials.gov. NCT03743376.

ClinicalTrials.gov. NCT03758625.

ClinicalTrials.gov. NCT03837756.

ClinicalTrials.gov. NCT03844386.

ClinicalTrials.gov. NCT03964415.

ClinicalTrials.gov. NCT04120415.

ClinicalTrials.gov. NCT04301154.

ClinicalTrials.gov. NCT04319367.

ClinicalTrials.gov. NCT04340596.

ClinicalTrials.gov. NCT04357821.

ClinicalTrials.gov. NCT04404049.

ClinicalTrials.gov. NCT04505501.

ClinicalTrials.gov. NCT04725877.

ClinicalTrials.gov. NCT04983030.

ClinicalTrials.gov. NCT04985760.

ClinicalTrials.gov. NCT05004308.

ClinicalTrials.gov. NCT05184452.

ClinicalTrials.gov. NCT05217641.

ClinicalTrials.gov. NCT05245292.

ClinicalTrials.gov. NCT05281510.

ClinicalTrials.gov. NCT05471076.

ClinicalTrials.gov. NCT05604209.

ClinicalTrials.gov. NCT06071767.

ClinicalTrials.gov. NCT06253533.

ClinicalTrials.gov. NCT06484335.

Colby DJ, Sarnecki M, Barouch DH, et al. Safety and immunogenicity of Ad26 and MVA vaccines in acutely treated HIV and effect on viral rebound after antiretroviral therapy interruption. *Nat Med.* 2020;26(4):498–501.

Cong L, Ran FA, Cox D, et al. Multiplex genome engineering using CRISPR/Cas systems. *Science.* 2013;339(6121):819–823.

Corey L, Gilbert PB, Juraska M; HVTN 704/HPTN 085 and HVTN 703/HPTN 081 Study Teams. Two randomized trials of neutralizing antibodies to prevent HIV-1 acquisition. *N Engl J Med.* 2021;384(11):1003–1014.

Cradick TJ, Fine EJ, Antico CJ, et al. CRISPR/Cas9 systems targeting β-globin and CCR5 genes have substantial off-target activity. *Nucleic Acids Res.* 2013;41(20):9584–9592.

Day CL, Kaufmann DE, Kiepiela P, et al. PD-1 expression on HIV-specific T cells is associated with T cell exhaustion and disease progression. *Nature.* 2006;443(7109):350–354.

Deeks SG. HIV: shock and kill. *Nature.* 2012;487(7408):439–440.

Deeks SG, Walker BD. Human immunodeficiency virus controllers: mechanisms of durable virus control in the absence of antiretroviral therapy. *Immunity.* 2007;27(3):406–416.

Deng K, Pertea M, Rongvaux A, et al. Broad CTL response is required to clear latent HIV-1 due to dominance of escape mutations. *Nature.* 2015;517(7534):381–385.

Dhody K, Kazempour K. PRO 140 SC: long-acting, single-agent, maintenance therapy for HIV-1 infection. Abstract 486. Paper presented at Conferences on Retroviruses and Opportunistic Infections (CROI). Seattle, WA; March 2019.

Dhody K, Kazempour K, Pourhassan N, Maddon PJ. Primary efficacy results of PRO 140 SC in a pivotal phase 2b/3 study. ASM Microbe 2018, June 7–11, 2018, Atlanta, GA. Abstract AAR LB15.

Dhody K, Pourhassan N, Kazempour K, et al. PRO 140, a monoclonal antibody targeting CCR5, as a long-acting, single-agent maintenance therapy for HIV-1 infection. *HIV Clin Trials.* 2018;19(3):85–93.

Ebina H, Misawa N, Kanemura Y, et al. Harnessing the CRISPR/Cas9 system to disrupt latent HIV-1 provirus. *Sci Rep.* 2013;3:2510.

Einkauf KB, Osborn MR, Gao C, et al. Parallel analysis of transcription, integration, and sequence of single HIV-1 proviruses. *Cell.* 2022;185(2):266–282.e15.

Elliott JH, Wightman F, Solomon A, et al. Activation of HIV transcription with short-course vorinostat in HIV-positive patients on suppressive antiretroviral therapy. *PLoS Pathog.* 2014;10(10):e1004473.

Engsig FN, Zangerle R, Katsarou O, et al. Long-term mortality in HIV-positive individuals virally suppressed for >3 years with incomplete CD4 recovery. *Clin Infect Dis.* 2014;58(9):1312–1321.

Ensoli B, Cafaro A, Monini P, et al. Challenges in HIV vaccine research for treatment and prevention. *Front Immunol.* 2014;5:417.

Ensoli F, Cafaro A, Casabianco A, et al. HIV-1 Tat immunization restores immune homeostasis and attacks the HAART-resistant blood HIV DNA: results of a randomized phase II clinical exploratory clinical trial. *Retrovirology.* 2015;12:33.

Eron JJ Jr, Ashby MA, Giordano MF, et al. Randomized trial of MNrgp120 HIV-1 vaccine in symptomless HIV-1 infection. *Lancet.* 1996;348:1547–1551.

Evans VA, van der Sluis RM, Solomon A, et al. Programmed cell death-1 contributes to the establishment and maintenance of HIV-1 latency. *AIDS.* 2018;32(11):1491–1497.

Fidler S, Stöhr W, Pace M, et al; RIVER trial study group. Antiretroviral therapy alone versus antiretroviral therapy with a kick and kill approach, on measures of the HIV reservoir in participants with recent HIV infection (the RIVER trial): a phase 2, randomised trial. *Lancet.* 2020 Mar 14;395(10227):888–898.

Finzi D, Blankson J, Siliciano JD, et al. Latent infection of CD4\+\+ T cells provides a mechanism for lifelong persistence of HIV-1, even in patients on effective combination therapy. *Nat Med.* 1999;5(5):512–517.

Finzi D, Hermankova M, Pierson T, et al. Identification of a reservoir for HIV-1 in patients on highly active antiretroviral therapy. *Science.* 1997;278(5341):1295–1300.

Flynn NM, Forthal DN, Harro CD, et al. Placebo-controlled phase 3 trial of a recombinant glycoprotein 120 vaccine to prevent HIV-1 infection. *J Infect Dis.* 2005;191:654–665.

Forcina G, d'Ettorre G, Mastroianni C, et al. Interleukin-15 modulated interferon-γ and β-chemokine production in patients with HIV infection: implications for immune-based therapy. *Cytokine.* 2004;25:283–290.

Gaebler C, Nogueira L, Stoffel E, et al. Prolonged viral suppression with anti-HIV-1 antibody therapy. *Nature.* 2022;606(7913):368–374.

Gantner P, Buranapraditkun S, Pagliuzza A, et al. HIV rapidly targets a diverse pool of $CD4^+$ T cells to establish productive and latent infections. *Immunity.* 2023;56(3):653–668.e5.

Garcia F, Climent N, Assoumou L, et al. A therapeutic dendritic cell-based vaccine for HIV-1 infection. *J Infect Dis.* 2011;203:473–478.

Garcia F, Climent N, Guardo AC, et al. A dendritic cell-based vaccine elicits T cell responses associated with control of HIV-1 replication. *Sci Transl Med.* 2013;5:166ra62.

Garcia-Broncano P, Maddali S, Einkauf KB, et al. Early antiretroviral therapy in neonates with HIV-1 infection restricts viral reservoir size and induces a distinct innate immune profile. *Sci Transl Med.* 2019;11(520):eaax7350.

Gaudinski MR, Coates EE, Houser K, et al. Safety and pharmacokinetics of the Fc-modified HIV-1 human monoclonal antibody VRC01LS: a phase 1 open-label clinical trial in healthy adults. *PLoS Med.* 2018 Jan 24;15(1):e1002493. doi:10.1371/journal.pmed.1002493. eCollection January 2018.

Gay CL, Bosch RJ, Ritz J, et al. Clinical trial of the anti-PDL-L1 antibody BMS-936559 in HIV-1 infected participants on suppressive antiretroviral therapy. *J Infect Dis.* June 1, 2017;215(11):1725–1733.

Girard MP, Osmanov S, Assossou OM, Kieny MP. Human immunodeficiency virus (HIV) immunopathogenesis and vaccine development: a review. *Vaccine.* 2011;29:6191–6218

Gray GE, Bekker LG, Laher F, et al. Vaccine efficacy of ALVAC-HIV and bivalent subtype C gp120-MF59 in adults. *N Engl J Med.* 2021;384(12):1089–1100.

Gray GE, Mngadi K, Lavreys L; Imbokodo/HVTN 705/HPX2008 Study Group. Mosaic HIV-1 vaccine regimen in southern African women (Imbokodo/HVTN 705/HPX2008): a randomised, double-blind, placebo-controlled, phase 2b trial. *Lancet Infect Dis.* 2024;19:S1473-3099(24)00358-X.

Gruell H, Gunst JD, Cohen YZ, et al. Effect of 3BNC117 and romidepsin on the HIV-1 reservoir in people taking suppressive antiretroviral therapy (ROADMAP): a randomised, open-label, phase 2A trial. *Lancet Microbe.* 2022;2(3):e203–e214.

Gubser C, Chiu C, Lewin SR, et al. Immune checkpoint blockade in HIV. *EBioMedicine.* 2022;76:103840.

Guihot A, Marcelin AG, Massiani MA, et al. Drastic decrease of the HIV reservoir in a patient treated with nivolumab for lung cancer. *Ann Oncol.* 2018;29:517–518.

Gunst JD, Højen JF, Pahus MH, et al. Impact of a TLR9 agonist and broadly neutralizing antibodies on HIV-1 persistence: the randomized phase 2a TITAN trial. *Nat Med.* 2023;29(10):2547–2558.

Guo S, Luke BT, Henry AR, et al. HIV infected CD4+ T-cell clones are more stable than uninfected clones during long-term antiretroviral therapy. *PLoS Pathog.* 2022;18(8):e1010726.

Gupta RK, Peppa D, Hill AL, et al. Evidence for HIV-1 cure after CCR5Δ32/Δ32 allogeneic haemopoietic stem-cell transplantation 30 months post analytical treatment interruption: a case report. *Lancet HIV.* 2020;7(5):e340–e347.

Hallengard D, Haller BK, Maltais AK, et al. Comparison of plasmid vaccine immunization schedules using intradermal in vivo electroporation. *Clin Vaccine Immunol.* 2011;18(9):1577–1581.

Hansen SG, Ford JC, Lewis MS, et al. Profound early control of highly pathogenic SIV by an effector memory T cell vaccine. *Nature.* 2011;473(7348):523–527.

Hansen SG, Piatak M Jr, Ventura AB, et al. Immune clearance of highly pathogenic SIV infection. *Nature.* 2013;502(7469):100–104.

Hardy GA, Imami N, Nelson MR. A phase I, randomized study of combined IL-2 and therapeutic immunization with antiretroviral therapy. *J Immune Based Therapies Vaccines*. 2007;5:6.
Hardy WD. A5370 Safety and immunotherapeutic activity of an anti-PD-1 antibody (cemiplimab) in HIV-1 diagnosed participants on suppressive cART: a phase I/II, double-blind, placebo-controlled, ascending multiple dose study. Presented at Pre-CROI Community HIV Cure Research Workshop. Boston, MA; March 7, 2020. https://www.treatmentactiongroup.org/wp-content/uploads/2020/03/final_A5370_CROI_Presentations_030720.pdf. Accessed August 27, 2024.
Harwood O, O'Connor S. Therapeutic potential of IL-15 and N-803 in HIV/SIV infection. *Viruses*. 2021;13(9):1750.
Haynes BF, Gilbert PB, McElrath MJ, et al. Immune-correlates analysis of and HIV-1 vaccine efficacy trial. *N Engl J Med*. 2012;366:1275–1286.
Henrich TJ, Gandhi RT. Early treatment and HIV-1 reservoirs: a stitch in time? *J Infect Dis*. 2013;208(8):1189–1193.
Henrich TJ, Schreiner C, Cameron C, et al. Everolimus, an mTORC1/2 inhibitor, in ART-suppressed individuals who received solid organ transplantation: a prospective study. *Am J Transplant*. 2021;21(5):1765–1779.
Heredia A, Le N, Gartenhaus RB, et al. Targeting of mTOR catalytic site inhibits multiple steps of the HIV-1 lifecycle and suppresses HIV-1 viremia in humanized mice. *Proc Natl Acad Sci USA*. 2015;112(30):9412–9417.
Hermankova M, Siliciano JD, Zhou Y, et al. Analysis of human immunodeficiency virus type 1 gene expression in latently infected resting CD4\+ T lymphocytes in vivo. *J Virol*. 2003;77(13):7383–7392.
Hocqueloux L, Avettand-Fenoel V, Jacquot S, et al. Long-term antiretroviral therapy initiated during primary HIV-1 infection is key to achieving both low HIV reservoirs and normal T cell counts. *J Antimicrobial Chemother*. 2013;68(5):1169–1178.
Holt N, Wang J, Kim K, et al. Human hematopoietic stem/progenitor cells modified by zinc-finger nucleases targeted to CCR5 control HIV-1 in vivo. *Nat Biotechnol*. 2010;28(8):839–847.
Hombach AA, Holzinger A, Abken H. The weal and woe of costimulation in the adoptive therapy of cancer with chimeric antigen receptor (CAR)-redirected T cells. *Curr Mol Med*. 2013;13(7):1079–1088.
Hossain T, Lungu C, de Schrijver S, et al. Specific quantification of inducible HIV-1 reservoir by RT-LAMP. *Commun Med*. 2024;4(1):123.
Hu W, Kaminski R, Yang F, et al. RNA-directed gene editing specifically eradicates latent and prevents new HIV-1 infection. *Proc Natl Acad Sci*. 2014;111(31):11461–11466.
Hu X, Valentin A, Dayton F, et al. DNA prime-boost vaccine regimen to increase breadth, magnitude, and cytotoxicity of the cellular immune responses to subdominant Gag epitopes of simian immunodeficiency virus and HIV. *J Immunol*. 2016;197(10):3999–4013.
Huang Y, Yu J, Lanzi A, et al. Engineered bispecific antibodies with exquisite HIV-1-neutralizing activity. *Cell*. 2016;165:1621–1631.
Hutter G, Nowak D, Mossner M, et al. Long-term control of HIV by CCR5 Delta32/Delta32 stem-cell transplantation. *N Engl J Med*. 2009;360(7):692–698.
Inderbitzin A, Loosli T, Optiz L, et al. Transcriptome profiles of latently- and reactivated HIV-1 infected primary CD4+ T cells: a pooled data-analysis. *Front Immunol*. 2022;13:915805.
Iwamoto N, Mason RD, Song K, et al. Blocking α4β7 integrin binding to SIV does not improve virologic control. *Science*. 2019;365(6457):1033–1036.
Jacobson JM, Felber BK, Chen H, Pavlakis; ACTG 5369 Study Team. The immunogenicity of an HIV-1 Gag conserved element DNA vaccine in people with HIV and receiving antiretroviral therapy. *AIDS*. 2024;38(7):963–973.
Jiang, C, Lian X, Gao C, et al. Distinct viral reservoirs in individuals with spontaneous control of HIV-1. *Nature*. 2020;585(7824):261–267.
Jimenez-Leon MR, Gasca-Capote C, Roca-Oporto C, et al. Vedolizumab and ART in recent HIV-1 infection unveil the role of α4β7 in reservoir size. *JCI Insight*. 2024;9(16):e182312.
Julg B, Pequ A, Abbink P, et al. Virologic control by the CD4-binding site antibody N6 in simian-human immunodeficiency virus-infected rhesus monkeys. *J Virol*. July 27, 2017;91(16):e00498–17.
Julg B, Stephenson KE, Wagh K, et al. Safety and antiviral activity of triple combination broadly neutralizing monocloncal antibody therapy against HIV-1: a phase 1 clinical trial. *Nat Med*. 2022;28(6):1288–1296.
June C, Tebas P, Stein D, et al. Induction of acquired CCR5 deficiency with zinc finger nuclease-modified autologous CD4 T cells (SB-728-T) correlates with increases in CD4 count and effects on viral load in HIV-infected subjects. Abstract 155. Paper presented at the 19th Conference on Retroviruses and Opportunistic Infection. Seattle, WA; February 2012.
Kessing CF, Nixon CC, Li C, et al. In vivo suppression of HIV rebound by didehydro-cortistatin A, a "block-and-lock" strategy for HIV-1 treatment. *Cell Rep*. 2017 Oct 17;21(3):600–611.
Khaitan A, Unutmaz D. Revisiting immune exhaustion during HIV infection. *Current HIV/AIDS Reports*. 2011;8(1):4–11.
Kim Y, Anderson JL, Lewin SR. Getting the "kill" into "shock and kill": strategies to eliminate latent HIV. *Cell Host Microbe*. 2018;23(1):14–26.
Kozal M, Aberg J, Pialoux G, et al. Fostemsavir in adults with multidrug-resistant HIV-1 infection. *N Engl J Med*. 2020;382(13):1232–1243.
Kroup RA, Safrit JT, Cao Y, et al. Temporal association of cellular immune responses with the initial control of viremia in primary human immunodeficiency virus type 1 syndrome. *J Virol*. 1994;68:4650–4655.
Laird GM, Bullen CK, Rosenbloom DI, et al. Ex vivo analysis identifies effective HIV-1 latency-reversing drug combinations. *J Clin Invest*. 2015;125(5):1901–1912.
Lalezari J, Mitsuyasu R, Wang S, et al. A single infusion of zinc finger nuclease CCR5 modified autologous CD4 T cells (SB-728T) increased CD4 counts and leads to decrease in HIV proviral load in an aviremic HIV-infected subject. Abstract 433. Paper presented at the 19th Conference on Retroviruses and Opportunistic Infection. Seattle, WA; February 2012.
Lam S, Bollard C. T cell therapies for HIV. *Immunotherapy*. 2013;5(4):407–414.
Landovitz RJ, Scott H, Deeks SG. Prevention, treatment and cure of HIV infection. *Nat Rev Microbiol*. 2023;21(10):657–670.
Lee J, Whitney JB. Immune checkpoint inhibition as a therapeutic strategy for HIV eradication: current insights and future directions. *Curr Opin HIV AIDS*. 2024;19(4):179–186.
Leggat DJ, Cohen KW, Willis JR, et al. Vaccination induces HIV broadly neutralizing antibody precursors in humans. *Science*. 2022;378(6623):eadd6502.
Leibman RS, Richardson MW, Ellebrecht CT, et al. Supraphysiologic control over HIV-1 replication mediated by CD8 T cells expressing a re-engineered CD4-based chimeric antigen receptor. *PLoS Pathog*. 2017 Oct 12;13(10):e1006613.
Levy Y, Durier C, Lascauz AS, et al. Sustained control of viremia following therapeutic immunization in chronically HIV-1 infected individuals. *AIDS*. 2006;20:405–413.
Levy Y, Gahery-Segard H, Durier C, et al. Immunologic and virologic efficacy of therapeutic immunization combined with interleukin-2 in chronically HIV-1 infected patients. *AIDS*. 2005;19:279–286.
Levy Y, Lacabaratz C, Lhomme E, et al. A randomized placebo0controlled efficacy study of a prime boost therapeutic vaccination strategy in HIV-1-infected individuals: VRI01 ANRS 149 LIGHT phase II trial. *J Virol*. 2021;95(9):e02165–20.
Levy Y, Lacabaratz C, Weiss L, et al. Enhanced T cell recovery in HIV-1 infected adults through IL-7 treatment. *J Clin Invest*. 2009;119(4):997–1007.
Levy Y, Sereti I, Tambussi G, et al. Effects of recombinant human interleukin 7 on T-cell recovery and thymic output in HIV-infected patients receiving antiretroviral therapy: results of a phase I/ IIa randomized, placebo-controlled multicenter study. *Clin Infect Dis*. 2012;55(2):291–300.

Levy Y, Thiebaut R, Montes M, et al. Dendritic cell-based therapeutic vaccine elicits polyfunctional HIV-specific T-cell immunity associated with control of viral load. *Eur J Immunol.* 2014;44:2802–2810.

Lewden C, Chene G, Morlat P, et al. HIV-infected adults with a CD4 cell count greater than 500 cells/µl on long-term combination antiretroviral therapy reach same mortality rates as the general population. *J AIDS.* 2007;46(1):72–77.

Li J, Brumme Z, Brumme C, et al. Factors associated with viral rebound in HIV-1 infected individuals enrolled in a therapeutic HIV-1 Gag vaccine trial. *J Infect Dis.* 2011;203:976–983.

Liao HK, Gu Y, Diaz A, et al. Use of the CRISPR/Cas9 system as an intracellular defense against HIV-1 infection in human cells. *Nat Commun.* 2015;6:6413.

Liu B, Zhang W, Xia B, et al. Broadly neutralizing antibody-derived CAR T cells reduce viral reservoir in individuals infected with HIV-1. *J Clin Invest.* 2021;131(19):e150211.

Lu CL, Murakowski DK, Bournazos S, et al. Enhanced clearance of HIV-1–infected cells by broadly neutralizing antibodies against HIV-1 in vivo. *Science.* 2016;352:1001–1004.

Lu W, Arraes C, Ferreira WT, et al. Therapeutic dendritic cell vaccination for chronic HIV-1 infection. *Nat Med.* 2004;10:1359–1365.

Luzuriaga K, Gay H, Ziemniak C, et al. Viremic relapse after HIV-1 remission in a perinatally infected child. *N Engl J Med.* 2015;372(8):786–788.

Lynch RM, Boritz E, Coates EE, et al. Virologic effects of broadly neutralizing antibody VRC01 administration during chronic HIV-1 infection. *Sci Ttransl Med.* 2015;7(319):319ra206.

Mao Y, Liao Q, Zhu Y, et al. Efficacy and safety of novel multifunctional M10 CAR-T cells in HIV-1-infected patients: a phase I, multicenter, single-arm, open-label study. *Cell Discov.* 2024;10(1):49.

Marconi VC, Moser C, Gavegnano C, et al. Randomized Trial of Ruxolitinib in Antiretroviral-Treated Adults With Human Immunodeficiency Virus. *Clin Infect Dis.* 2022;74(1):95-104.

Martin AR, Siciliano RF. Immune modulation with rapamycin as a potential strategy for HIV-1 eradication. Abstract 415. Paper presented at the 22nd Conference on Retroviruses and Opportunistic Infections. Seattle, WA; February 2015.

Mascolini M. Primary efficacy results of PRO 140 SC in a pivotal phase 2b/3 study in heavily treatment-experienced HIV-1 patients. Paper presented at ASM Microbe. Atlanta, GA; June 2018.

Maslennikova A, Mazurov D. Application of CRISPR/Cas genomic editing tools for HIV therapy: toward precise modifications and multilevel protection. *Front Cell Infect Microbiol.* 2022;12:880030.

Mason SW, Sanisetty S, Osuna Gutierrez C, et al. Viral suppression was induced by anti-PD-L1 following ARV-interruption in SIV-infected monkeys. Abstract 318LB. Paper presented at the 21st Conference on Retroviruses and Opportunistic Infections. Boston, MA; March 2014.

Mayer BT, Zhang L, deCamp AC, et al. Impact of LS mutation on pharmacokinetics of preventive HIV broadly neutralizing monoclonal antibodies: a cross-protocol analysis of 16 clinical trials in people without HIV. *Pharmaceutics.* 2024;16(5):594.

McMahon DK, Zheng L, Cyktor JC, et al. Multidose IV romidepsin: no increased HIV-1 expression in persons on ART, ACTG A5315. CROI Abstract 26. In Special issue: abstracts from the 2019 Conference on Retroviruses and Opportunistic Infections. *Top Antivir Med.* 2019;27(Suppl 1):11s–12s.

McMichael AJ, Borrow P, Tomaras GD, The immune response during acute HIV-1 infection: clues for vaccine development. *Nat Rev Immunol.* 2010;10(1):11–23.

Mendoza P, Gruell H, Nogueira L, et al. Combination therapy with anti-HIV-1 antibodies maintains viral suppression. *Nature.* 2018;561(7724):479–484.

Miller JS, Davis BZ, Helgeson E, et al. Safety and virologic impact of the IL-15 superagonist N-803 in people with HIV-a phase 1 trial. *Nat Med.* 2022;28(2):3920400.

Mitsuyasu RT, Lalezari J, Burke B, et al. Phase I study of gene-modified CD4+ T cells and CD34+ cells with or without busulfan in HIV+ adults. CROI Abstract 338. In Special issue: abstracts from the 2020 Conference on Retroviruses and Opportunistic Infections. *Top Antivir Med.* 2020;28(1):116.

Mitsuyasu RT, Merigan TC, Carr A, et al. Phase 2 gene therapy trial of anti-HIV ribozyme in autologous CD34\+ cells. *Nat Med.* 2009;15(3):285–292.

Mori L, Valente ST. Key players in HIV-1 transcriptional regulation: targets for a functional cure. *Viruses.* 2020;12(5):529.

Mothe B, Rosás-Umbert M, Coll P, et al. HIVconsv vaccines and romidepsin in early-treated HIV-1-infected individuals: safety, immunogenicity and effect on the viral reservoir (study BCN02). *Front Immunol.* 2020;11:823.

Mousseau G, Kessing CF, Fromentin R, et al. The Tat inhibitor didehydro-cortistatin A prevents HIV-1 reactivation from latency. *MBio.* 2015;6(4):e00465. doi:10.1128/mBio.00465-15

Nabel G, Baltimore D. An inducible transcription factor activates expression of human immunodeficiency virus in T cells. *Nature.* 1987;326(6114):711–713.

Namazi G, Fajnzylber JM, Aga E, et al. The Control of HIV After Antiretroviral Medication Pause (CHAMP) study: posttreatment controllers identified from 14 clinical studies. *J Infect Dis.* 2018;218(12):1954–1963.

Nordstrom JL, Ferrari G, Margolis DM. Bispecific antibody-derived molecules to target persistent HIV infection. *J Virus Erad.* 2022;8(3):100083.

Pallikkuth S, Micci L, Ende ZS, et al. Maintenance of intestinal Th17 cells and reduced microbial translocation in SIV-infected rhesus macaques treated with interleukin (IL)-21. *PLoS Pathog.* 2013;9:e1003471.

Pallikkuth, S, Rogers K, Villinger F, et al. Interleukin-21 administration to rhesus macaques chronically infected with simian immunodeficiency viruses increases cytotoxic effector molecules in T cells and NK cells and enhances B cell function without increasing immune activation or viral replication. *Vaccine.* 2011;29:9929–9938.

Palmer BE, Neff CP, Lecureux J, et al. In vivo blockade of the PD-1 receptor suppresses HIV-1 viral loads and improves CD4\+ T cell levels in humanized mice. *J Immunol.* 2013;190(1):211–219.

Palmer CS, Ostrowski M, Zhou J, et al. The mTORC1 inhibitors, temsirolimus and everolimus, suppress HIV-patient-derived CD4\+ T-cell death and activation in vitro. Abstract 320. Paper presented at the 22nd Conference on Retroviruses and Opportunistic Infections. Seattle, WA; February 2015.

Papuchon J, Pinson P, Lazaro E, et al. Resistance mutations and CTL epitopes in archived HIV-1 DNA of patients on antiviral treatment: toward a new concept of vaccine. *PLoS One.* 2013;8(7):e69029.

Pegu A, Asokan M, Wu L, et al. Activation and lysis of human CD4 cells latently infected with HIV-1. *Nature Commun.* 2015;6:8447.

Peluso M, Deitchman A, Magombedze G, et al. Rebound dynamics following immunotherapy with an HIV vaccine, TLR-9 agonist, and broadly neutralizing antibodies. Abstract 435. Paper presented at the Conference on Retroviruses and Opportunistic Infections. Seattle, WA; February 19–22, 2023.

Perez EE, Wang J, Miller JC, et al. Establishment of HIV-1 resistance in CD4\+ T cells by genome editing using zinc-finger nucleases. *Nat Biotechnol.* 2008;26(7):808–816.

Persaud D, Colletti A, Nelson BS, et al. ART-free HIV-1 remission in very early treated children: results from IMPAACT P1115. Abstract 184. Conference on Retroviruses and Opportunistic Infections in Denver, CO; March 6, 2024. https://www.croiconference.org/abstract/art-free-hiv-1-remission-in-very-early-treated-child. Accessed August 27, 2024.

Persaud D, Gay H, Ziemniak C, et al. Absence of detectable HIV-1 viremia after treatment cessation in an infant. *N Engl J Med.* 2013;369(19):1828–1835.

Peterson CW, Wang J, Deleage C, et al. Differential impact of transplantation on peripheral and tissue-associated viral reservoirs: implications for HIV gene therapy. *PLoS Pathog.* April 19, 2018;14(4):e1006956.

Pett SL, Carey C, Lin E, et al. Predictors of bacterial pneumonia in Evaluation of Subcutaneous Interleukin-2 in Randomized International TRIAL (ESPRIT). *HIV Med.* 2011;12(4):219–227.

Pett SL, Kelleher AD, Emery S. Role of interleukin-2 in patients with HIV infection. *Drugs*. 2010;70(9):1115–1130.

Pitisuttithum P, Gilbert P, Gurwith M, et al. Randomized, double-blind, placebo-controlled efficacy trial of a bivalent recombinant glycoprotein 120 HIV-1 vaccine among injection drug users in Bangkok, Thailand. *J Infect Dis*. 2006;194:1661–1671.

Pollard RB, Rockstroh JK, Pantaleo G, et al. Safety and efficacy of the peptide-based therapeutic vaccine for HIV-1, Vacc-4x: a phase 2 randomised double-blind, placebo-controlled trial. *Lancet Infect Dis*. 2014;14(4):291–300.

Pontesilli I, Guerra ES, Ammassari A, et al. Phase II controlled trial of post-exposure immunization with recombinant gp160 versus antiretroviral therapy in asymptomatic HIV-1 infected adults. *AIDS*. 1998;12:473–480.

Porichis F, Kaufmann DE. Role of PD-1 in HIV pathogenesis and as a target for therapy. *Curr HIV/AID Rep*. 2012;9(1):81–90.

Rasmussen TA, Brinkmann CR, Olesen R, et al. Panobinostat, a histone deacetylase inhibitor, for latent-virus reactivation in HIV-infected patients on suppressive antiretroviral therapy: a phase 1/2, single group, clinical trial. *Lancet HIV*. 2014;1(1):e14–e21.

Rasmussen TA, Rajdev L, Rhodes A, et al. Impact of anti-PD-1 and anti-CTLA-4 on the human immunodeficiency virus (HIV) reservoir in people living with HIV with cancer on antiretroviral therapy: the AIDS Malignancy Consortium 095 study. *Clin Infect Dis*. 2021;73(7):e1973–e1981.

Rerks-Ngarm S, Pitisuttithum P, Nitayaphan S, et al. Vaccination with ALVAC and AIDSVAX to prevent HIV-1 infection in Thailand. *N Engl J Med*. 2009;361(23):2209–2220.

Riddler SA, Para M, Benson CA, et al. Vesatolimod, a Toll-like receptor 7 agonist, induces immune activation in virally suppressed adults living with human immunodeficiency virus-1. *Clin Infect Dis*. 2021;72(11):e815–e824.

Riddler SA, Zheng L, Durand CM, et al. Randomized clinical trial to assess the impact of the broadly neutralizing HIV-1 monoclonal antibody VRC01 on HIV-1 persistence in individuals on effective ART. *Open Forum Infect Dis*. 2018;5(10):ofy242.

Rodriguez B, Asmuth DM, Matining RM, et al. Safety, tolerability, and immunogenicity of repeated doses of dermavir, a candidate therapeutic HIV vaccine, in HIV-infected patients receiving combination antiretroviral therapy: results of the ACTG 5176 trial. *J Acquir Immune Defic Syndr*. 2013;64(4):351–359.

Rolland M, Tovanbutra S, Decamp AC, et al. Genetic impact of vaccination on breakthrough HIV-1 sequences from the STEP trial. *Nat Med*. 2011;17(3):366–371.

Rosenberg ES, Billingsley JM, Caliendo AM, et al. Vigorous HIV-1-specific CD4R T cell responses associated with control of viremia. *Science*. 1997;278:1447–1450.

Saez-Cirion A, Bacchus C, Hocqueloux L, et al. Post-treatment HIV-1 controllers with a long-term virological remission after the interruption of early initiated antiretroviral therapy ANRS VISCONTI study. *PLoS Pathog*. 2013;9(3):e1003211.

Saito N, Chono H, Shibata H, et al. CD4$^{\+}$ T cells modified by endoribonuclease MazF are safe and can persist in SHIV-infected rhesus macaques. *Mol Ther Nucleic Acids*. 2014;3(6):e168.

Sandstrom E, Wahren B; Nordic Vac-04 Study Group. Therapeutic immunization with recombinant gp160 in HIV-1 infection: a randomized double-blind placebo-controlled trial. *Lancet*. 1999;353:1735–1742.

Sauce D, Elbim C, Appay V. Monitoring cellular immune markers in HIV infection: from activation to exhaustion. *Curr Opin HIV AIDS*. 2013;8(2):125–131.

Scheid JF, Horwitz JA, Bar-On Y, et al. HIV-1 antibody 3BNC117 suppresses viral rebound in humans during treatment interruption. *Nature*. 2016;535(7613):556–560.

Schooley RT, Spritzler J, Wang H, et al.; AIDS Clinical Trials Group 5197. A placebo-controlled trial of immunization of HIV-1-infected persons with a replication-deficient adenovirus type 5 vaccine expressing the HIV-1 core protein. *J Infect Dis*. 2010;202(5):705–716.

Schürmann D, Rudd DJ, Zhang S, et al. Safety, pharmacokinetics, and antiretroviral activity of islatravir (ISL, MK-8591), a novel nucleoside reverse transcriptase translocation inhibitor, following single-dose administration to treatment-naive adults infected with HIV-1: an open-label, phase 1b, consecutive-panel trial. *Lancet HIV*. 2020;7(3):e164–e172.

SenGupta D, Brinson C, DeJesus E, et al. The TLR7 agonist vesatolimod induced a modest delay in viral rebound in HIV controllers after cessation of antiretroviral therapy. *Sci Transl Med*. 2021;13(599):eabg3071.

Sereti I, Dunham RM, Spritzler J, et al. IL-7 administration drives T cell entry and expansion in HIV-1 infection. *Blood*. 2009;113(25):6304–6314.

Shan L, Deng K, Shroff NS, et al. Stimulation of HIV-1-specific cytolytic T lymphocytes facilitates elimination of latent viral reservoir after virus reactivation. *Immunity*. 2012;36(3):491–501.

Shingai M, Nishimura Y, Klein F, et al. Antibody-mediated immunotherapy of macaques chronically infected with SHIV suppresses viraemia. *Nature*. 2013;503(7475):277–280.

Singh A, Palanichamy JK, Ramalingam P, et al. Long-term suppression of HIV-1 C virus production in human peripheral blood mononuclear cells by LTR heterochromatization with a short double-stranded RNA. *J Antimicrob Chemother*. 2014;69:405–415.

Sneller MC, Blazkova J, Justement JS, et al. Combination anti-HIV antibodies provide sustained virological suppression. *Nature*. 2022;606(7913):375–381.

Sneller MC, Clarridge KE, Seamon C, et al. An open-label phase 1 clinical trial of the anti-α4β7 monoclonal antibody vedolizumab in HIV-infected individuals. *Sci Transl Med*. 2019;11(509):eaax3447.

Sneller MC, Justement JS, Gittens KR, et al. A randomized controlled safety/efficacy trial of therapeutic vaccination in HIV-infected individuals who initiated antiretroviral therapy early in infection. *Sci Transl Med*. 2017;9(419):eaan8848.

Sogaard OS, Graversen ME, Leth S, et al. The depsipeptide romidepsin reverses HIV-1 latency in vivo. *PLoS Pathog*. 2015;11(9):e1005142.

Stellbrink HJ, van Lundzen J, Westby M, et al. Effects of interleukin-2 plus highly active antiretroviral therapy on HIV-1 replication and proviral DNA (COSMIC trial). *AIDS*. 2002;16:1479–1487.

Stephenson KE, Julg B, Tan CS, et al. Safety, pharmacokinetics and antiviral activity of PGT121, a broadly neutralizing monoclonal antibody against HIV-1: a randomized, placebo-controlled, phase 1 clinical trial. *Nat Med*. 2021;27(10):1718–1724.

Strain MC, Little SJ, Daar ES, et al. Effect of treatment, during primary infection, on establishment and clearance of cellular reservoirs of HIV-1. *J Infect Dis*. 2005;191(9):1410–1418.

Sung JA, Pickeral J, Liu L, et al. Dual-affinity re-targeting proteins direct T cell-mediated cytolysis of latently HIV-infected cells. *J Clin Invest*. 2015;125(11):4077–4090.

Takata H, Kakzau JC, Mitchell JL, et al. Long-term antiretroviral therapy initiated in acute HIV infection prevents residual dysfunction of HIV-specific CD8+ T cells. *EBioMedicine*. 2022;84:104253.

Tavel JA; INSIGHT STALWART Study Group. Effect of intermittent IL-2 alone or with peri-cycle antiretroviral therapy in early HIV-1 infection: the STALWART study. *PLoS One*. 2010;5(2):e9334.

Tebas P, Azzoni L, Papasavvas E, et al. Beat2 Primary Trial Outcomes: Peg-Ifn-A2b +3bnc117 & 10-1074 In Chronic HIV Infection. Abstract 431. Conference on Retroviruses and Opportunistic Infections. February 19–22, 2023. Seattle, WA.

Tebas P, Jadlowski J, Shaw P, et al. CCR5-edited CDr+ T cells augment HV-specific immunity to enable post-rebound control of HIV replication. *J Clin Invest*. 2021;131(7):e144486.

Tebas P, Stein D, Binder-Scholl G, et al. Antiviral effects of autologous CD4 T cells genetically modified with a conditionally replicating lentiviral vector expressing long antisense to HIV. *Blood*. 2013;121(9):1524–1533.

Tebas P, Stein D, Tang WW, et al. Gene editing of CCR5 in autologous CD4 T cells of persons infected with HIV. *N Engl J Med*. 2014;370(10):901–910.

Topalian SL, Hodi FS, Brahmer JR, et al. Safety, activity, and immune correlates of anti-PD-1 antibody in cancer. *N Engl J Med*. 2012;366(26):2443–2454.

Tsoukas CM, Raboud J, Bernard NF, et al. Active immunization of patients with HIV infection: a study of VaxSyn, a recombinant HIV envelope subunit vaccine, on progression of immunodeficiency. *AIDS Res Hum Retroviruses.* 1998;14:483–490.

Turk G, Seiger K, Lian X, et al. A possible sterilizing cure of HIV-1 infection without stem cell transplantation. *Ann Intern Med.* 2022;175(1):95–100.

Uldrick TS, Adams SV, Fromentin R, et al. Pembrolizumab induces HIV latency reversal in people living with HIV and cancer on antiretroviral therapy. *Sci Transl Med.* 2022;14(629):eabl3836.

Van Gulck E, Vlieghe E, Vekemans M, et al. mRNA-based dendritic cell vaccination induced potent antiviral responses in HIV-1 infected patients. *AIDS.* 2012;26:F1–F12.

Van Lundzen J, Glausinger T, Stahmer I, et al. Transfer of autologous gene-modified T cells in HIV-infected patients with advanced immunodeficiency and drug-resistant virus. *Mol Ther.* 2007;15:1024–1033.

Vandergeeten C, Fromentin R, DaFronseca S, et al. Interleukin-7 promotes HIV persistence during antiretroviral therapy. *Blood.* 2013;121(21):4321–4329.

Vardas E, Stanescu I, Leinonen M, et al. Indicators of a therapeutic effect in FIT-06, a phase II trial of a DNA vaccine, GTU-Multi-HIVB, in untreated HIV-1 infected subjects. *Vaccine.* 2012;30(27):4046–4054.

Varela-Rohena A, Molloy PE, Dunn SM, et al. Control of HIV-1 immune escape by CD8 T cells expressing enhanced T cell receptor. *Nat Med.* 2008;14(12):1390–1395.

Veenhuis RT, Abreu CM, Costa PAG, et al. Monocyte-derived macrophages contain persistent latent HIV reservoirs. *Nat Microbiol.* 2023;8(5):833–844.

Velu V, Titanji K, Ahmed H, et al. PD-1 blockade following ART interruption enhances control of pathogenic SIV in rhesus macaques. *Proc Natl Acad Sci USA.* 2022;119(33):e2202148119.

Velu V, Titanji K, Zhu B, et al. Enhancing SIV-specific immunity in vivo by PD-1 blockade. *Nature.* 2009;458(7235):206–210.

Vibholm L, Konrad CV, Schleimann MH, et al. Effects of 24-week Toll-like receptor 9 agonist treatment in HIV type 1+ individuals. *AIDS.* 2019;33(8):1315–1325.

Vibholm L, Schleimann MH, Hojen JF, et al. Short-course toll-like receptor 9 agonist treatment impacts innate immunity and plasma viremia in individuals with human immunodeficiency virus infection. *Clin Infect Dis.* June 15, 2017;64(12):1686–1695.

Wang CY, Wong WW, Tsai HC, et al. Effect of anti-CD4 antibody UB-421 on HIV-1 rebound after treatment interruption. *N Engl J Med.* 2019;380(16):1535–1545.

Webb GM, Li S, Mwakalundwa G, et al. The human IL-15 superagonist ALT-803 directs SIV-specific CD8^{+} T cells into B-cell follicles. *Blood Adv.* 2018;2:76–84.

Whitney JB, Hill AL, Sanisetty S, et al. Rapid seeding of the viral reservoir prior to SIV viraemia in rhesus monkeys. *Nature.* 2014;512(7512):74–77.

Whitney JB, Osuna CE, Sanisetty S, et al. Treatment with a TLR7 agonist induces transient viremia in SIV-infected ART-suppressed monkeys. Conference on Retroviruses and Opportunistic Infections. Seattle, WA; 2015.

Wolstein O, Boyd M, Millington M, et al. Preclinical safety and efficacy of an anti-HIV-1 lentiviral vector containing a short hairpin RNA to CCR5 and the C46 fusion inhibitor. *Mol Ther Methods Clin Dev.* 2014;1:11.

Wong JK, Hezareh M, Gunthard HF, et al. Recovery of replication-competent HIV despite prolonged suppression of plasma viremia. *Science.* 1997;278(5341):1291–1295.

Wykes MN, Lewin SR. Immune checkpoint blockade in infectious diseases. *Nat Rev Immunol.* 2018;18(2):91–104.

Xu L, Pequ A, Rao E, et al. Trispecific broadly neutralizing HIV antibodies mediate potent SHIV protection in macaques. *Science.* 2017;358:85–90.

Xu L, Wang J, Liu Y, et al. CRISPR-edited stem cells in a patient with HIV and acute lymphocytic leukemia. *N Engl J Med.* 2019;381(13):1240–1247.

Youngblood B, Noto A, Porichis F, et al. Cutting edge: prolonged exposure to HIV reinforces a poised epigenetic program for PD-1 expression in virus-specific CD8 T cells. *J Immunol.* 2013;191(2):540–544.

Yukl SA, Boritz E, Busch MB, et al. Challenges in detecting HIV persistence during potentially curative interventions: a study of the Berlin patient. *PLoS Pathog.* 2013;9(5):e1003347.

Zhou J, Rossi JJ. Current progress in the development of RNAi based therapeutics for HIV-1. *Gene Ther.* 2011;18:1134–1138.

19.

OPPORTUNISTIC INFECTIONS

Lisa Y. Armitige, Karen Vigil, and Rita Wilson Dib

LEARNING OBJECTIVE

Upon completion of this chapter, the reader should be able to:

- Recognize and manage the most common opportunistic infections found in people with HIV (PWH).
- Describe optimal timing of ART initiation in PWH who are diagnosed with opportunistic infections involving the central nervous system.

Opportunistic infections (OIs) are infections that occur more frequently or present with more severe manifestations in the context of immunosuppression. A wide variety of pathogens and clinical syndromes have been described among people with advanced HIV/AIDS. On average, these OIs and other opportunistic conditions (e.g., certain cancers such as Kaposi sarcoma, CNS lymphoma, and invasive cervical cancer) develop several years after HIV acquisition if HIV infection is left undiagnosed/untreated. Thus, some PWH present with an OI as the "sentinel event" leading to a diagnosis of HIV, or may present with an OI as a complication of unsuccessful HIV treatment and ongoing viremia with the progression of immunosuppression. This chapter covers key OIs that HIV providers should be familiar with. It does not capture the entirety of conditions that PWH may develop; resources such as the US DHHS Guidelines for the Prevention and Treatment of Opportunistic Infections in Adults and Adolescents with HIV offer comprehensive details on the prevention and management of multiple OIs (DHHS, 2024b). Due to the importance of drug interactions between OI treatment and ART, this chapter focuses on several mycobacterial OIs; additionally, due to high morbidity and mortality associated with several virus-associated OIs causing end-organ disease, the diagnosis and management of several viral OIs is also described.

PNEUMOCYSTIS PNEUMONIA

EPIDEMIOLOGY

Pneumocystis jirovecii is a ubiquitous fungal organism that primarily causes pulmonary disease (i.e., Pneumocystis pneumonia, or PCP) in immunocompromised people. Among PWH, the incidence of PCP has decreased significantly with widespread use of effective ART, such that most cases now occur in people with undiagnosed HIV or people not consistently adherent to treatment: overall annual incidence in PWH ranges from 0.9 to 5.4 cases per 1,000 person-years (Cilloniz et al., 2019; DHHS, 2024b). Risk increases when $CD4^+$ cell count falls below 200 cells/mm^3.

CLINICAL PRESENTATION

PCP generally presents as subacute progressive dyspnea, fever, and nonproductive cough (with or without fatigue) over days to weeks. Clinical assessment may reveal minimal abnormalities on pulmonary exam in cases of mild disease; however, upon exertion individuals may exhibit tachypnea, tachycardia, and diffuse dry rales (and possibly oxygen desaturation). Hypoxemia ranges from mild to severe. Chest radiograph findings range from normal (in cases of early disease) to diffuse symmetrical "ground-glass" interstitial infiltrates bilaterally (see Figure 19.1); alveolar infiltrates in a perihilar distribution may also be seen. Computed tomography should be considered when chest radiograph is unrevealing.

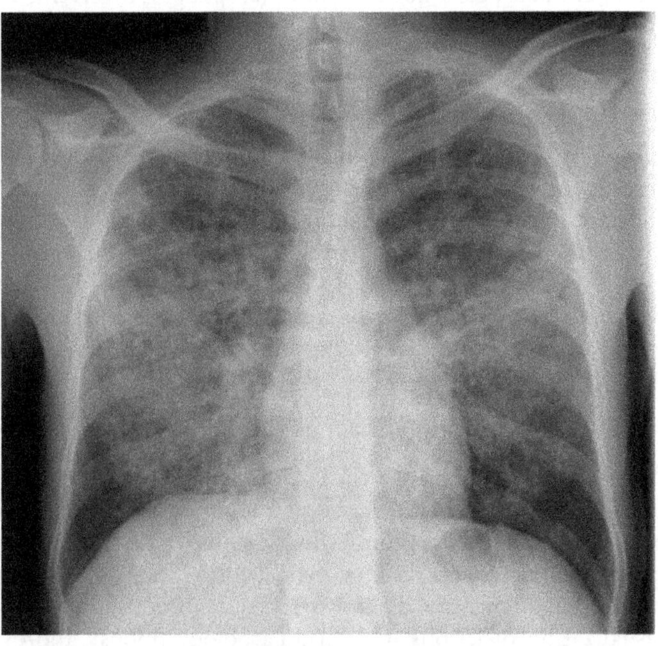

Figure 19.1 Chest radiograph of person with HIV and *Pneumocystis* pneumonia. SOURCE: Reproduced with permission from National HIV Curriculum (https://www.hiv.uw.edu).

DIAGNOSIS

Definitive diagnosis is made with histopathologic or cytopathologic demonstration of the organism in tissue, bronchoalveolar lavage fluid, or induced sputum samples. Molecular techniques (i.e., PCR) have been increasingly utilized; however, their use is not standardized at this time; because a positive PCR does not distinguish between colonization and true infection, interpretation must be guided by overall clinical context. Additionally, there has been interest in the 1,3 ß-D-glucan assay. However, its use as a sole indicator for diagnostic purposes is limited by lack of specificity.

TREATMENT

Trimethoprim-sulfamethoxazole (TMP-SMX) for 21 days remains first-line therapy for PCP; dosing by disease severity is provided in the 2024 DHHS guidelines. Empiric treatment may be initiated in acutely ill PWH in whom there is a high index of clinical suspicion. Adjunctive steroids are recommended in moderate-to-severe disease, and should be started as soon as possible. Indications and recommendations for primary and secondary prevention are detailed in the DHHS OI guidelines (DHHS, 2024b).

FUNGAL INFECTIONS

CANDIDIASIS

Epidemiology

Oropharyngeal and esophageal candidiasis are common in PWH and are typically caused by *Candida albicans*, although other species have been reported. Risk increases when $CD4^+$ cell count falls below 200 cells/mm^3 (esophageal involvement generally occurs at lower $CD4^+$ counts).

Clinical Presentation

Oropharyngeal candidiasis most commonly presents with thick, white lesions which may appear on buccal surfaces, the hard or soft palate, tongue, or oropharyngeal mucosa (see Figure 19.2). It can also manifest as angular cheilosis. Lesions can be readily scraped off with a tongue depressor. For PWH with esophageal involvement, retrosternal pain or burning with painful and difficult swallowing are often described.

Diagnosis

Candidiasis is primarily a clinical diagnosis, and laboratory testing is rarely needed. If necessary, lesion scrapings may be examined using a potassium hydroxide preparation to visualize the characteristic yeast or hyphal forms. For esophageal candidiasis, definitive diagnosis rests on direct endoscopic visualization of lesions with histopathology (biopsy and/or brushings) confirming *Candida* in affected tissue, along with confirmation by fungal culture and speciation. Importantly, esophageal candidiasis should be differentiated from other forms of infectious esophagitis that may be caused by other opportunistic pathogens and noninfectious conditions (Mohamed et al., 2019).

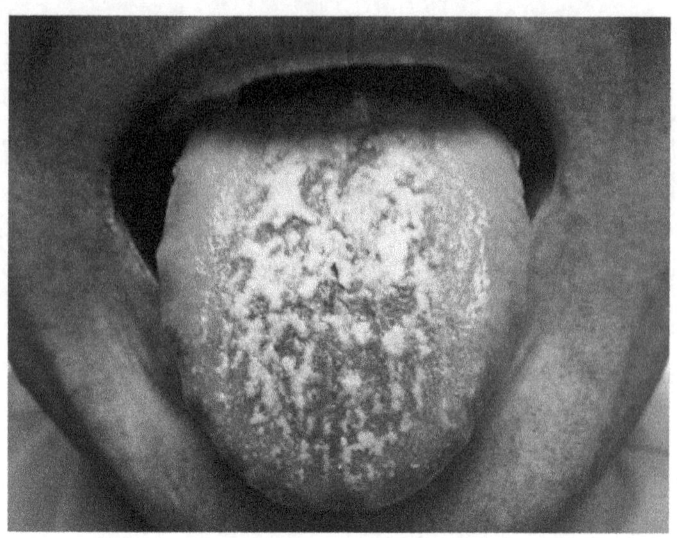

Figure 19.2 Pseudomembranous candidiasis involving the tongue. SOURCE: Reproduced with permission from National HIV Curriculum (https://www.hiv.uw.edu).

Treatment

Oral fluconazole is the treatment of choice for candidiasis: 1–2 weeks of therapy are recommended for oropharyngeal disease, and 2–3 weeks of therapy are recommended for esophageal disease. Routine primary prophylaxis is not recommended, and secondary prophylaxis is similarly not recommended by many HIV specialists unless in cases of frequent or severe recurrences (DHHS, 2024b).

CRYPTOCOCCOSIS

Epidemiology

Cryptococcal disease is one of the most important opportunistic infections affecting people with advanced HIV and remains a major contributor to morbidity and mortality; globally, it accounts for 1 in 5 AIDS-related deaths (Sati et al., 2023). The most common causative agent is *Cryptococcus neoformans*, although *C. gattii* is occasionally identified. In the 2022 World Health Organization Fungal Priority Pathogens List (FPPL), *C. neoformans* was ranked the number 1 key priority pathogen (WHO, 2022). The vast majority of cases in PWH are observed in people with $CD4^+$ cell counts <100 cells/mm^3, and U.S. guidelines recommend routine screening with serum cryptococcal antigen for newly diagnosed, asymptomatic PWH with $CD4^+$ cell count ≤100 cells/mm^3 (DHHS, 2024b).

Clinical Presentation

Cryptococcosis typically presents as subacute meningitis or meningoencephalitis with fever, malaise, and worsening headache over several weeks. Photophobia and neck stiffness occur in less than one-third of individuals. For people with encephalitis and increased intracranial pressure, altered mental status and lethargy may be observed. Although central nervous system (CNS) involvement is the most widely recognized manifestation of disseminated cryptococcosis, any organ may be involved, including the skin and pulmonary system.

Diagnosis

Initial evaluation should include neurologic exam and serum cryptococcal antigen, as well as lumbar puncture to assess for elevated intracranial pressure and cerebrospinal fluid analysis (including cryptococcal antigen as well as culture and/or Gram stain/India ink preparation). Imaging is often performed to help assess for increased pressure and/or central nervous system mass lesions. Cerebrospinal fluid (CSF) evaluation generally reveals an abnormal white blood cell count and differential, elevated protein and low-normal glucose.

Treatment

Treatment consists of three phases: induction, consolidation, and maintenance. For the induction phase, U.S. guidelines recommend intravenous liposomal amphotericin B plus oral flucytosine for 2 weeks. For stable patients, repeat lumbar puncture and CSF culture should be obtained, with a transition to the consolidation phase involving daily fluconazole for 8 or more weeks as indicated by repeat testing results (total duration and dosing should be guided by clinical status and CSF results) (DHHS, 2024b). Lower doses of fluconazole are then used for the maintenance phase and should be continued until at least one year from initiation of antifungal therapy. For more information, refer to Chapter 28, "Neurological Complications of HIV Infection."

COCCIDIODOMYCOSIS AND HISTOPLASMOSIS

Epidemiology

Of endemic mycosis, coccidioidomycosis and histoplasmosis are commonly encountered in the United States: national surveillance data indicate that 20,000 cases of coccidioidomycosis and 1,100 cases of histoplasmosis were reported in 2019 (Smith et al., 2022). Coccidioidomycosis (also known as Valley fever) is most often acquired in the southwestern and western United States, and histoplasmosis is primarily acquired in the southcentral, central, and eastern United States. People with HIV can develop disseminated infection: the risk of symptomatic disease increases at CD4 counts <250 cells/mm^3 and <150 cells/mm^3 for coccidioidomycosis and histoplasmosis, respectively.

Clinical Presentation

Four main syndromes of coccidioidomycosis have been described: focal pneumonia, diffuse pneumonia, extrathoracic involvement (e.g., meningitis, osteoarticular infection), and positive serologic tests without evidence of localized infection. In contrast, clinical manifestations of progressive disseminated histoplasmosis are generally systemic in nature and include fever, fatigue, and weight loss. Hepatosplenomegaly may be observed on physical exam and/or imaging. Pulmonary symptoms may occur in half of patients with histoplasmosis; CNS, gastrointestinal, and dermatologic involvement are less common.

Diagnosis

The diagnosis of coccidioidomycosis is based on serology, histology, culture, and clinical presentation including exposure history. Given the heightened biosafety risk, laboratory personnel should handle culture specimens securely and carefully. For histoplasmosis, antigen detection in blood or urine may facilitate timely diagnosis; cases of suspected pulmonary or CNS involvement may require fluid specimens acquired via bronchoalveolar lavage or lumbar puncture (a positive CSF antibody test is also considered diagnostic for *Histoplasma* meningitis). In PWH with severe disseminated histoplasmosis, peripheral blood smears and histopathological examination of biopsy material from affected tissue may show the characteristic yeast forms. Cultures may be obtained but typically require several weeks to demonstrate organism growth.

Treatment

Recommendations for prevention and treatment are covered extensively according to disease severity and organ involvement in the DHHS guidelines (DHHS, 2024b).

PROTOZOAN/PARASITIC INFECTIONS

TOXOPLASMOSIS

Epidemiology

Toxoplasmosis is a common opportunistic CNS infection among people with advanced HIV/AIDS who are not on appropriate prophylaxis. In PWH with immunosuppression (particularly CD4 cell counts <100 cell/mm^3) and previous exposure to *Toxoplasma gondii* oocysts, latent tissue cysts of the parasite reactivate and cause clinically apparent disease. The most common site of reactivation is the CNS.

Clinical Presentation

People with toxoplasmic encephalitis (TE) often present with headaches and/or other focal neurologic symptoms (including motor weakness) or seizures. Fever may or may not be present. Mental status changes range from changes in affect to confusion to coma.

Diagnosis

Diagnosis requires a clinically compatible syndrome, identification of one or more ring-enhancing mass lesions on brain imaging (MRI is more sensitive than CT; see Figure 19.3), and detection of the organism in a clinical sample. Most PWH with TE are seropositive for anti-toxoplasma immunoglobulin (IgG) antibodies. Given high mortality if left untreated, therapy is typically initiated presumptively and brain biopsy is rarely undertaken; however, if no clinical and radiologic improvement is seen within 10–14 days, alternative diagnoses should be considered (DHHS, 2024b; Vidal, 2019). If lumbar puncture can be performed safely, testing can be done for *T. gondii* PCR, although the diagnostic sensitivity of this assay wanes once anti-toxoplasma therapy has been started.

Treatment

First-line therapy for initial treatment of TE consists of pyrimethamine plus sulfadiazine plus leucovorin, typically given for 6 weeks (pyrimethamine plus clindamycin plus leucovorin is an alternative). Given tolerability and access challenges, trimethoprim-sulfamethoxazole has also been utilized. After initial therapy is completed, patients should be continued on chronic maintenance therapy until ART-mediated immune reconstitution is achieved. Primary prophylaxis is indicated for Toxoplasma-seropositive PWH who have CD4 counts <100 cells/mm^3. Additional details are outlined in DHHS guidelines (DHHS, 2024b). For more information, see Chapter 28, "Neurological Complications of HIV Infection."

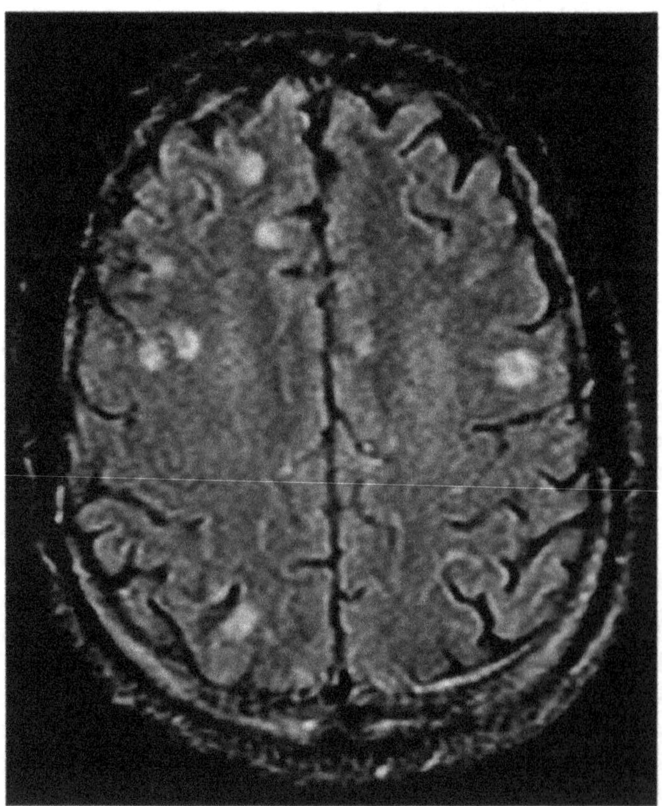

Figure 19.3 Brain magnetic resonance imaging (MRI) of person with HIV and *Toxoplasma* encephalitis. SOURCE: Reproduced with permission from National HIV Curriculum (https://www.hiv.uw.edu).

CRYPTOSPORIDIOSIS AND CYSTOISOSPORIASIS (FORMERLY ISOSPORIASIS)

Epidemiology

Cryptosporidiosis is caused by the protozoan parasite *Cryptosporidium* and remains a common cause of chronic diarrhea in people with advanced HIV/AIDS, especially in resource-limited areas. The risk of severe or prolonged disease is associated with a CD4$^+$ cell count below 100 cells/mm^3. *Cystoisospora belli* primarily affects PWH with CD4$^+$ cell counts below 250 cells/mm^3.

Clinical Presentation

Because infection typically targets the small bowel mucosa, individuals generally present with acute or subacute watery diarrhea (in severe cases, diarrhea may be continuous and voluminous) with or without malaise, nausea/vomiting, and abdominal cramping. The biliary tract and pancreatic duct may also be affected in some cases of prolonged disease.

Diagnosis

Diagnosis of cryptosporidiosis may be made by microscopy, fecal immunoassays, or PCR testing—PCR and other molecular diagnostic methods are increasingly utilized given their favorable sensitivity and operational benefits. Laboratories should be alerted to the potential diagnosis of *Cryptosporidium* and specific testing should be requested, since routine ova and parasite testing may not detect cryptosporidia oocysts. For cystoisosporiasis, infection is generally diagnosed by detecting *Isospora* oocysts in fecal specimens (testing may be enhanced by use of more sensitive methods such as modified acid-fast techniques and UV fluorescent microscopy).

Treatment

Management involves supportive care as well as pharmacotherapy: rehydration and correction of electrolyte abnormalities are important for people with severe disease, and antimotility interventions may also be offered if indicated. With cryptosporidiosis, ART is the mainstay of pharmacotherapy and should be initiated promptly for PWH not already receiving HIV treatment. Antimicrobial therapy may be initiated for people with severe symptoms or persistent symptoms despite ART initiation; for cryptosporidiosis, U.S. guidelines recommend nitazoxanide or paromomycin given for at least 2 weeks (DHHS, 2024b). For cystoisosporiasis, U.S. guidelines recommend trimethoprim-sulfamethoxazole for seven to ten days (DHHS, 2024b).

MICROSPORIDIOSIS

Epidemiology

Microsporidia are a group of small, intracellular parasites closely related to fungi. Overall prevalence has declined with widespread ART, and clinical disease related to microsporidiosis is typically seen in PWH with $CD4^+$ cell counts below 100 cells/mm^3.

Clinical Presentation

Microsporidiosis most commonly manifests as a gastrointestinal tract infection with diarrhea, although cases of encephalitis, keratoconjunctivitis, sinusitis, and disseminated infection have been observed. Presentation varies by species.

Diagnosis

Diagnosis can be established from clinical or tissue samples using light microscopy and special staining. Species can be identified by morphology, staining with species-specific antibodies, or PCR using species- or genus-specific primers.

Treatment

As with cryptosporidiosis, ART is the mainstay of treatment for microsporidiosis and should be initiated promptly for PWH not already receiving HIV treatment. Management also includes supportive care with fluids and nutritional support to address dehydration and malnutrition, and antimotility agents as indicated. Additional species-specific pharmacotherapy interventions are described in U.S. guidelines (DHHS, 2024b).

MYCOBACTERIAL INFECTIONS

LEARNING OBJECTIVE

Discuss the available tests and treatment modalities to appropriately manage PWH coinfected with *Mycobacterium tuberculosis*, *M. avium* complex, and *M. kansasii*, the most common mycobacterial diseases associated with HIV infection.

WHAT'S NEW

- Shorter regimens for multidrug-resistant tuberculosis (MDR-TB) have shown efficacy in PWH.
- If tenofovir alafenamide (TAF) is used with any of the rifamycins (rifampin, rifabutin, rifapentine), the patient should be monitored for evidence of HIV treatment failure.
- Primary prophylaxis to prevent disseminated *Mycobacterium avium complex* (MAC) disease is no longer recommended for PWH who immediately initiate antiretroviral therapy (ART).

KEY POINTS

- HIV infection markedly increases the likelihood of a person progressing from LTBI to active TB disease.
- Rifamycins are a critical component of effective TB therapy in PWH but have many drug-drug interactions.
- MAC should be treated with multidrug therapy, including clarithromycin and ethambutol optimally.
- Optimal treatment of MAC disease should include medications for both MAC and HIV (to reconstitute the immune system).
- *Mycobacterium kansasii* infection closely resembles TB, with more frequent pulmonary presentation than MAC.
- Diagnosis and treatment of *M. kansasii* as outlined in the American Thoracic Society (2020) guidelines are the same for PWH and people without HIV.

MYCOBACTERIUM TUBERCULOSIS

Epidemiology

There were 10.6 million new cases of TB worldwide in 2022, with 0.63 million TB cases among PWH. TB case numbers declined during COVID-19 but have rebounded and increased annually since 2020 (WHO, 2024). In 2022, TB was second only to COVID-19 as a cause of death from a single infectious organism, causing almost twice as many deaths as HIV (WHO, 2024). PWH are 16 times more likely to develop active TB than the general population (WHO, 2023). Recognition of the vulnerability of PWH to TB and increased awareness of the need to rapidly diagnose and treat people with TB/HIV coinfection have led to a steady decrease in HIV-associated TB deaths since numbers peaked globally in 2004. Deaths from TB in PWH declined from 540,000 in 2004 to 209,000 in 2019, which, despite these gains, remains substantial at 2.7 (2.4–3.1) per 100,000 PWH population. Deaths from TB-associated HIV increased for the first time since 2004 (rising to 214,000 in 2020), reflecting the global impact of the COVID-19 pandemic on healthcare access worldwide, but have since declined to 167,000 in 2022 (WHO, 2024).

The total number of TB cases in the United States peaked in 1992 and has been steadily declining, with a slower progression noted in 2020 in the setting of the COVID-19 pandemic and a suspected state of underdiagnosis (CDC, 2020). The Centers for Disease Control and Prevention (CDC, 2012) recommends testing for HIV in all persons with active TB. HIV testing was completed for 89.5% of reported TB cases in the United States, with 4.3% of total cases reported to have HIV coinfection in 2022 (CDC, 2022). This has decreased significantly compared to a peak in 1992, when nearly two-thirds of persons with TB aged 25–44 years had HIV. Attention to screening and treatment of tuberculosis, as well as increasing focus on HIV treatment in the United States, has resulted in a decrease in HIV-associated TB cases and a faster decline than in the general population (CDC, 2022).

Unlike other HIV-related opportunistic infections, $CD4^+$ T-cell count does not predict risk of TB infection. Rates of TB in PWH are higher than those in people without HIV at all $CD4^+$ T-cell counts.

Clinical Presentation

Infection with *M. tuberculosis* generally occurs after inhalation of infectious particles coughed into the air by a person with active pulmonary TB disease. A less common route of infection involves ingestion of unpasteurized dairy products produced from the milk of cows with *Mycobacterium bovis* (bovine TB). Once infected, individuals will either progress to active disease (progressive primary disease) or their immune system will contain growth of the organism but not kill it (LTBI). Host immune factors play a major role in which route initial infection will take. Host factors also play a role in whether individuals with LTBI will progress to active TB disease (post-primary or reactivation disease).

TB in PWH typically presents as pulmonary disease. Often, the upper lobes of the lungs are involved, and cavitary lesions are characteristic. Pulmonary disease is frequently accompanied by constitutional symptoms such as fever, night sweats, and weight loss. These findings are more typical of reactivation disease rather than progressive primary infection found when there is poor containment of the infecting organism by the immune system.

$CD4^+$ T-cell count plays a pivotal role in the containment of *M. tuberculosis*. As HIV infection progresses and there is a decline in the number of these cells, there is less containment of infecting organisms. The clinical presentation of TB in PWH differs based on the $CD4^+$ T-cell count, such that PWH with $CD4^+$ T-cell counts >350 cells/mm^3 often present with the classically described pulmonary presentation. As the $CD4^+$ T-cell count decreases, however, the clinical presentation can look more like a progressive primary disease. In PWH with $CD4^+$ T-cell counts <200 cells/mm^3, pulmonary lesions may involve any lobe of the lungs and range from infiltrates to pneumonia. Cavitary lesions become less common with advanced HIV disease, and a number of persons with HIV and TB will have no abnormalities on chest radiograph at all.

Another feature of HIV-associated TB is extrapulmonary disease. Extrapulmonary disease is found in up to 50% of individuals in some series. Lymph node disease is the most common extrapulmonary site. Disseminated (miliary) disease and mycobacteremia are far more common in PWH with low $CD4^+$ T-cell counts.

Diagnosis

Diagnosis of TB infection in PWH requires a high index of suspicion. Recent advances in diagnostic testing modalities for TB, such as interferon-gamma release assays (IGRAs), have not translated into a major improvement in the diagnosis of TB infection in PWH. Diagnosis of TB disease requires HIV providers to remain vigilant.

Traditionally, screening for TB infection has been performed with the tuberculin skin test (TST). The test involves injection of 0.1 ml (comprising 5 tuberculin units) of purified protein derivative subcutaneously into the volar surface of the forearm. Individuals who have been previously infected with *M. tuberculosis* develop a delayed-type hypersensitivity reaction to the injected proteins. Induration caused by this reaction is measured after 48–72 hours. A TST measurement of 5 mm of induration or greater is considered positive in PWH. Sensitivity of this test has always been poor in PWH, and it can be as low as 30% in patients with TB and $CD4^+$ T-cell counts <200 cells/mm^3. It is also important to note that the TST will not distinguish between persons with LTBI and those with active TB, and it may be falsely positive in persons vaccinated with Bacillus Calmette–Guérin (BCG) because of the cross-reaction with antigens found in the BCG vaccine.

IGRAs are diagnostic in vitro blood tests based on immune responses to antigens unique to *M. tuberculosis*. IGRAs have the benefits of negating the false positive results seen with BCG vaccination and involving only a single visit for blood draw. There are two commercially available U.S. Food and Drug Administration–approved IGRAs: the QuantiFERON-TB Plus (QFT-Plus) and the T.SPOT.TB (T-spot). The QFT-Plus assay replaced the QFT Gold In Tube (QFT-GIT) and tests the $CD4^+$ and $CD8^+$ cellular immune responses to *M. tuberculosis*–specific antigens. Evidence consistently indicates that the QFT-Plus and QFT-GIT assays perform similarly. Meta-analyses (Cattamanchi et al., 2011; Santin et al., 2012) showed the sensitivity to be approximately 60% for the QFT-GIT and 70% for the T-SPOT.TB assay in detecting *M. tuberculosis* infection. A separate meta-analysis which included 20 studies addressing IGRA use in active TB showed a pooled sensitivity for both IGRAs to be 75%, with a pooled specificity of 82% (Ma et al., 2021). Although this appears to be an improvement over the TST, there was not a significant difference in head-to-head sensitivity with either test compared to the TST. Studies highlight the fact that there are still many cases of LTBI or active TB disease that may be missed by these tests and a high index of suspicion is still warranted. As highlighted in the recommendations on IGRAs outlined by the ATS/CDC/IDSA guidelines (Nahid et al., 2016), these tests are most useful in BCG-vaccinated populations (adding greater specificity) and in populations with poor rates of follow-up (negating the need for a return visit for reading). These same guidelines state clearly that routine testing with both a TST and an IGRA is not generally recommended.

PWH should be screened for TB infection by a TST or IGRA at the time of initial HIV diagnosis and, if at high risk for exposure, regularly thereafter. Individuals who travel to countries with a high TB burden or who reside in areas with high rates of TB should be tested annually. All others should be tested when there is suspicion of exposure to an active case after their initial screening. Individuals with $CD4^+$ T-cell counts <200 cells/mm^3 at HIV diagnosis should be tested at baseline and, if they test negative, should undergo repeat screening after $CD4^+$ T-cell count recovery to >200 cells/mm^3 to confirm they are truly negative.

An individual with a positive TB test (TST or IGRA) without clinical or radiographic evidence of active TB disease should be given a diagnosis of LTBI. PWH with LTBI are at very high risk for advancing to active TB. Individuals with LTBI without HIV have a 5%–10% lifetime risk of developing active TB, whereas PWH and LTBI are 18 (range: 15–21) times more likely to progress to active disease than persons without HIV (WHO, 2024). LTBI treatment in this population is paramount and has formed the cornerstone of progress in reducing global HIV-associated TB cases and deaths.

Diagnosis of active TB disease requires the utilization of many pieces of data. A thorough clinical history is useful in most cases. Important information to note includes exposure to an individual with active TB disease, residence in high-risk settings such as jails or homeless shelters, and a prior diagnosis of untreated LTBI. Signs and symptoms of active disease may include a cough lasting over 3 weeks, unexplained weight loss, fevers, and/or night sweats. There are no physical exam findings specific for TB, but a thorough physical exam may reveal suspicious lymphadenopathy, draining fistulas, abnormal respiratory sounds, or signs of meningitis.

Tests such as the TST and IGRA can add to available data but cannot be relied on entirely. One may also consider performing more than one of these tests to increase sensitivity, especially when the individual has a low $CD4^+$ T-cell count. While performing both an IGRA and a TST is not generally recommended for routine screening purposes, when increased sensitivity is desired, performing both tests can be helpful in making a diagnosis. In general, a positive TST or IGRA result should be taken as evidence of infection.

All PWH suspected of having active TB should receive a chest radiograph because the lungs are the most common entry point and a frequent site of infection. Though chest radiographs can be normal in patients with culture-positive pulmonary TB, a high-resolution computed tomography (CT) scan may show early miliary-type lesions. Any person with respiratory symptoms, regardless of chest radiograph findings, should have sputum collected (at least 3 specimens) 8–24 hours apart, with at least one sputum being an early morning specimen and, preferably, at least one observed.

Individuals with low $CD4^+$ T-cell counts are more likely to have extrapulmonary TB with infected tissues that are more difficult to access and that have fewer organisms. It may be necessary to obtain biopsy specimens from lymph nodes, bone marrow, or pulmonary parenchyma to make the diagnosis. CSF, ascitic fluid, or abscess fluid may provide important diagnostic information. In patients with suspected TB lymphadenitis, excisional biopsy is preferred over fine-needle aspiration of peripheral lymph nodes, as needle aspiration can lead to lymphocutaneous fistulas. All tissue specimens from suspected sites of infection should be submitted for smear and culture analysis for acid-fast bacilli and, if indicated, histopathologic analysis searching for characteristic granulomas on pathology. When available, nucleic acid amplification tests significantly improve sensitivity in detecting *M. tuberculosis* organisms in clinical specimens.

Treatment

Treatment of LTBI in PWH is essentially the same as that in people without HIV. The mainstay for treatment of LTBI in PWH has been 9 months of isoniazid (INH) dosed daily, self-administered, or intermittently (twice weekly) by directly observed therapy (DOT). Treatment with INH for 6–9 months has been shown to be effective in multiple studies. When used, INH doses should be supplemented with pyridoxine 25–50 mg to minimize the likelihood of peripheral neuropathy. While treatment with INH has the benefit of compatibility with nearly all ART regimens, completion rates tend to be lower due to longer courses of treatment for LTBI. Newer, shorter treatment regimens using rifamycins have been shown to be equally effective with increased rates of completion.

The most recently approved treatment regimens for LTBI include INH-rifapentine (3HP) dosed weekly and INH-rifampin (3HR) dosed daily. The 3HP regimen can be given by DOT or self-administered and is highly desirable as it can provide cure for LTBI with only 12 weekly doses. Initially, 3HP was contraindicated in any patients taking antiretroviral medication, but newer pharmacokinetic data showed rifapentine use to be compatible with raltegravir-, dolutegravir-, and efavirenz-based regimens in virally suppressed individuals (Borisov et al., 2018). The 3HR regimen can also cure LTBI in 12 weeks but requires daily dosing of both INH and rifampin. Both 3HP and 3HR showed similar effectiveness when compared with 9-month courses of INH. The 3HR regimen has more treatment limitations owing to the potential for drug-drug interactions between rifampin and most ARVs. Rifampin taken for 4 months is an acceptable and effective LTBI regimen, especially in patients who are intolerant of INH or who are exposed to an INH-resistant case. Rifampin interacts with many commonly used antiretroviral agents. This interaction excludes all of the nucleoside analogues *except* tenofovir alafenamide (TAF), and all rifamycins decrease serum TAF levels. Therefore, if TAF is used with any of the rifamycins (rifampin, rifabutin, rifapentine), the patient should be monitored for evidence of HIV treatment failure.

In many cases, rifabutin can be substituted for rifampin; however, there have been no studies utilizing rifabutin for the treatment of LTBI in PWH. CDC guidelines for LTBI treatment endorse use of rifabutin in place of rifampin when unacceptable drug-drug interactions exist, though DHHS guidelines caution against substituting rifabutin for rifampin due to a lack of studies. The BRIEF-TB study evaluated 1 month of daily INH/rifapentine (1HR) for the treatment of LTBI in PWH. Endpoints of the study included progression to active TB disease, death from TB, or death from other causes. Though the outcomes of treatment with 1 month of daily INH/rifapentine were similar to treatment with 9 months of INH, only 21% of enrollees had a positive screening TST at baseline, indicating a low risk of progression in the study group as a whole (Swindells et al., 2019). While the CDC does not endorse the use of 1HR, DHHS guidelines suggest its use as an alternate LTBI treatment regimen. When a rifamycin is used to treat a PWH on ART, drug-drug interactions must be carefully considered. Specific guidance is available in a regularly updated document at https://hivinfo.nih.gov/.

Treatment of active TB disease in PWH is also essentially the same as that for people without HIV. All individuals diagnosed in the United States with active TB should be started on a four-drug regimen consisting of isoniazid, rifampin, ethambutol, and pyrazinamide, unless there is known resistance or baseline severe impairment of hepatic or renal function. After 2 months of this four-drug therapy (initial phase) and if the patient's organism is not resistant, the regimen can be reduced to INH and rifampin for the duration of treatment (continuation phase). Length of treatment will depend on the site and extent of disease. Most cases can be treated with 6–9 months of total therapy, whereas infections involving the bones or meninges should be treated for a total of 9–12 months. Infections of the CNS should be treated with steroids in addition to anti-TB medications. Prior recommendations were to treat infectious of the pericardium with steroids; however, subsequent data suggested that the addition of steroids in these cases does not impact outcomes (Nahid et al., 2016).

The most significant differences between treatment of patients with and without HIV involve use of the rifamycins and frequency of dosing. As previously noted, there is significant interaction between rifampin and most antiretrovirals, so care must be taken in introducing this class of medications into the regimen. Treatment regimens for active TB that do not contain a rifamycin have very high rates of relapse. Hence, every effort should be made to include a rifamycin in the treatment of PWH and TB. Regularly updated guidance on how to manage drug interactions can be found at https://hivinfo.nih.gov/. Use of rifabutin in place of rifampin for treating active TB allows the most flexibility in choosing concomitant treatment for HIV infection.

DOT is highly recommended for all cases of active TB treated in the United States to support the individual's efforts at cure. Newer technologies involving directly observed therapy by synchronous or nonsynchronous video (VDOT) allow more flexibility while maintaining the support afforded by DOT. Daily rather than intermittent dosing of TB medications is recommended for the treatment of active TB, especially in PWH. Highly intermittent dosing of TB therapy (once- or twice-weekly dosing) is associated with an increased risk of relapse with rifampin-resistant disease and should be avoided in PWH (Nahid et al., 2016). This is especially noted in patients with $CD4^+$ T-cell counts <100 cells/mm^3 (Nahid et al., 2016).

The question of when to initiate ART in a PWH and TB is not a trivial one. Treatment for both diseases simultaneously can result in a large pill burden, potential for multiple drug interactions, and potential for multiple drug toxicities. Although it is clear that PWH who are diagnosed with TB should be started immediately on anti-TB medications, until recently the timing of adding ART was less clear. Several studies (Blanc et al., 2011; Havlir et al., 2011; Karim et al., 2011; Martinson et al., 2011) conducted at multiple sites have shown a survival benefit (reduced mortality) when starting ART within 2 weeks of starting TB medications in patients with $CD4^+$ T-cell counts <50 cells/mm^3. Of note, a single study (Mfinanga et al., 2014) showed that ART could be delayed until completion of 6 months of TB therapy in patients with $CD4^+$ T-cell counts >220 cells/mm^3. At $CD4^+$ T-cell counts >50 cells/mm^3, the incidence of IRIS events increased. Although these same studies did not show a survival benefit to starting ART earlier in patients with $CD4^+$ T-cell counts ≥50 cells/mm^3, there was no demonstration of harm, and there were many other documented benefits to starting ART. Expert opinion is that ART should be started by 8 weeks of starting treatment for TB in patients with $CD4^+$ T-cell counts ≥50 cells/mm^3.

With HIV and TB coinfection, IRIS can be unmasking or paradoxical. Unmasking IRIS involves "unmasking" of previously undetected TB following ART initiation. Paradoxical IRIS presents as worsening signs and symptoms in individuals with adequately treated TB after they have been started on ART. Optimal timing of ART has yet to be established. If IRIS does occur in the course of treatment, it is important that both antiretroviral and TB treatment be continued. Mild cases of IRIS can be observed or treated with nonsteroidal anti-inflammatory agents or, if more severe, a short course of steroids may be necessary. A randomized trial showed lower incidence of TB-associated IRIS in PWH, TB, and median $CD4^+$ T-cell counts 50 cells/mm^3 started empirically on steroids (Meintjes et al., 2018). In patients where TB-associated IRIS is likely, empiric steroids may be considered.

Special consideration should be given to PWH and TB meningitis. IRIS involving central nervous system disease leads to worse outcomes. PWH and TB meningitis must be monitored carefully and treated with steroid therapy and a slow wean to reduce the inflammatory effects associated with disease. Treatment with antiretroviral drugs should be added with careful monitoring of the patient with TB meningitis for any evidence of IRIS. Additional information on IRIS can be found in Chapter 20.

Drug-resistant TB disease in PWH requires individualized therapy and should be approached with an expert in drug-resistant TB. Patients with multidrug-resistant or extensively drug-resistant TB should have ART initiated within 2–4 weeks after initiation of MDR TB drug therapy. Standard MDR treatment duration can range from 18 to 24 months. It can be shortened to 6–12 months when bedaquiline is part of the regimen (Gill et al., 2022); however, bedaquiline has significant interactions with several antiretroviral agents. The Nix-TB trial utilized the BPaL regimen (bedaquiline, pretomanid, linezolid) as a salvage regimen in patients with extensively drug-resistant TB or failure to respond to other TB therapy. Over half of the 109 participants were PWH. The study showed 92% positive outcomes (compared to 55% in the standard of care arm) (Conradie et al., 2022). The TB-PRACTECAL study sought to optimize the BPaL regimen by adding either moxifloxacin (BPaLM) or clofazimine (BPaLC). This study had 23% PWH in each arm and showed excellent outcomes with less associated toxicity (Nyang'wa et al., 2022). BPaLM offers a shorter, all-oral regimen with excellent outcomes for PWH and MDR TB and has become the regimen of choice in individuals with coinfection.

Prevention

As discussed, PWH should be screened for TB by a TST or IGRA at the time of diagnosis and as needed thereafter. PWH who are found to have a positive TST or IGRA without evidence of active disease should be treated for LTBI to prevent progression to active disease.

PWH who are contacts to a case with infectious pulmonary TB and have no evidence of active disease should be treated with a full course of therapy for LTBI, even with a negative TST or IGRA diagnostic test. As outlined previously, available diagnostic tests are not sensitive enough to rule out TB infection, and patients exposed to an infectious case are highly susceptible. Active disease should be ruled out in all patients prior to initiation of treatment for LTBI.

People who have a history of untreated or inadequately treated TB who do not have evidence of currently active disease should receive treatment for LTBI. This may manifest as old fibrotic lesions on chest x-ray noted during routine screening.

MYCOBACTERIUM AVIUM COMPLEX

Epidemiology

MAC, also known as MAI, consists of *M. avium* and *M. intracellulare*, two organisms so similar that they can only be differentiated using DNA probes. MAC infections are the most common nontuberculous mycobacteria (NTM) infections in both PWH and people without HIV infection (Griffith et al., 2007). These organisms are ubiquitous and are found environmentally in water, soil, and animal sources. Despite the many places from which the organisms can be isolated, the actual route of infection in PWH is unclear. There is no evidence for human-to-human or animal-to-human transmission.

Disseminated disease is the most common presentation of MAC infection associated with HIV, and occurs almost exclusively in people with profound immunosuppression who are not yet receiving ART. Disseminated disease is most commonly found in PWH with $CD4^+$ T-cell counts < 50 cells/mm^3. Having high HIV RNA levels (>100,000 copies/mm^3) has also been identified as a risk factor. The incidence of disseminated MAC has declined steadily since the introduction of combination ART, with most cases occurring in individuals who have not accessed care or who have poor adherence to ART.

Clinical Presentation

As stated previously, the most common presentation of MAC infection in PWH is disseminated disease. Symptoms tend to be nonspecific and typically include fever, night sweats, anorexia, weight loss, and gastrointestinal symptoms such as nausea, vomiting, diarrhea, and abdominal pain. It is important to remember that these same symptoms can be associated with other OIs, such as TB and fungal disease.

Disseminated MAC infection tends to involve the reticuloendothelial system, and, subsequently, physical exam findings may include hepatomegaly, splenomegaly, and lymphadenopathy. Pulmonary disease is rare, even with disseminated disease, but occasionally can manifest as nodules, infiltrates, cavities, or mediastinal/hilar adenopathy. Pulmonary findings are more likely to be associated with infection due to *M. tuberculosis* or *M. kansasii*.

Immune reconstitution in patients newly started on ART may "unmask" preexisting, previously undetected disease. The presentation in these cases may manifest as disseminated disease or perhaps localized disease.

Diagnosis

Isolation of MAC from a normally sterile site, such as the blood or tissue, should be considered diagnostic for disseminated disease. In the absence of a positive blood culture, other more invasive approaches (e.g., lymph node, liver, or bone marrow biopsy) may be necessary to obtain an adequate specimen for diagnosis.

Isolation of MAC from nonsterile sites such as the respiratory or gastrointestinal tracts may represent true pathology but can also represent colonization. In these cases, it is important to make an effort to determine if other pathogens may be at play.

Treatment

Optimally, the approach to treatment of disseminated MAC disease should include treatment of both MAC and HIV. Similar to treatment of TB and other NTM infections, treatment of MAC infection should include multidrug therapy, and ART should be started and optimized as soon as possible. Drug susceptibility testing should be performed, as macrolide susceptibility is associated with greater treatment success when using this class of drug. It should be noted that only macrolide and amikacin susceptibilities are associated with treatment outcomes.

Clarithromycin should be the first drug added to a MAC treatment regimen. Studies have shown treatment with clarithromycin to be associated with faster clearance of bacteremia than treatment with azithromycin. In the event of clarithromycin intolerance or a prohibiting drug interaction with other medications, azithromycin may constitute an alternative.

The second drug added should be ethambutol. Addition of ethambutol to a macrolide is associated with decreased relapse in the treatment of MAC. Rifabutin can also be added to the MAC regimen, especially in situations where the risk of mortality is high and/or emergence of resistance is likely. The addition of rifabutin also adds the potential for significant interaction with many antiretrovirals and can lower the serum drug levels of clarithromycin when used in combination. Therefore, prior to adding rifabutin as treatment of a mycobacterial infection, TB must be ruled out to prevent the emergence of rifampin-resistant TB disease.

Based on data from people without HIV, fluoroquinolones such as moxifloxacin or levofloxacin and injectable antibiotics such as amikacin and streptomycin can be utilized if there is a need for additional medication options owing to resistance, intolerance, or toxicity. While there are in vitro data showing susceptibility to these drugs, there are no randomized controlled trials evaluating their efficacy in the setting of macrolide susceptibility or effective ART. Additional agents that can be considered in the setting of refractory disease include bedaquiline, tedizolid, linezolid, and omadacycline.

The occurrence of IRIS has been documented with treatment of MAC disease, as it has with TB. It generally presents as a recurrence of fever and worsening lymphadenitis with negative blood cultures. Mild cases can be simply monitored or treated with a nonsteroidal anti-inflammatory agent or, in severe cases, a short course of steroids. Treatment for both MAC and HIV should be continued during management of IRIS.

Treatment of disseminated disease should continue for 12 months. Repeat blood cultures should be reserved for those without a clinical response after 4–8 weeks of treatment. PWH who complete a 12-month course of therapy, remain free of signs or symptoms of disease, and who show a sustained increase in $CD4^+$ T-cell count to >100 cells/mm^3 for at least 6 months have a low risk of relapse. If a previously treated person experiences a decrease in $CD4^+$ T-cell count <100 cells/mm^3 or is not on fully suppressive ART, preventive (secondary) prophylactic treatment should be reinitiated.

Prevention/Prophylaxis

No direct route for infection with MAC has been identified and, thus, there is no specific action known to prevent exposure to MAC. Primary prophylaxis to prevent disseminated MAC disease *is no longer recommended* for PWH who immediately initiate ART. If primary prophylaxis is initiated, it should be discontinued once the patient is on a fully suppressive ART regimen. Primary prophylaxis for disseminated MAC is reserved for people with a $CD4^+$ T-cell count <50 cells/mm^3 who are not receiving ART, remain viremic, or for whom a fully suppressive ART regimen is not an option. Before starting primary prophylaxis, disseminated MAC should be ruled out.

Azithromycin dosed at 1,200 mg weekly is the preferred regimen for both primary and secondary prophylaxis. Clarithromycin dosed at 500 mg twice daily is effective but, because of the increased pill burden and higher number of drug interactions, is considered an alternative. Azithromycin 600 mg twice weekly is another alternative. Rifabutin is an alternative when there is evidence of macrolide-resistant disease and secondary prophylaxis is needed or when there is macrolide intolerance, but it is less effective in this capacity and adds increased risk of drug interactions with many ARVs. Rifabutin should not be added to clarithromycin, as the combination is no more effective than clarithromycin alone. Addition of rifabutin to azithromycin is more effective than azithromycin alone, but the combination adds increased cost, increased toxicity, increased drug interactions, and no proven survival benefit. Rifampin in combination with azithromycin is not recommended. In any case, before the use of rifabutin, every effort should be made to rule out active TB.

MYCOBACTERIUM KANSASII

Epidemiology

Mycobacterium kansasii infection is the second most common NTM infection in PWH (after MAC infection). Tap water appears to be the most likely environmental reservoir for strains causing human disease (Griffith, 2002). Lung disease caused by *M. kansasii* closely resembles disease caused by *M. tuberculosis* in both people with and without HIV. Despite its similarities to TB, there is no evidence of human-to-human transmission of *M. kansasii*. Similar to MAC, infection with *M. kansasii* is most common in individuals with $CD4^+$ T-cell counts <50 cells/mm^3.

Clinical Presentation

Unlike MAC disease, which is most commonly disseminated and rarely pulmonary, *M. kansasii* can be disseminated but is more commonly pulmonary. Radiographically, *M. kansasii* infection closely resembles *M. tuberculosis* infection, with symptoms that include cough, fever, night sweats, weight loss, and hemoptysis.

Diagnosis

Diagnosis requires isolation of the organism from a sterile site or meeting the criteria outlined in the guidelines set forth by the American Thoracic Society (ATS) (Griffith et al., 2007). Briefly, the ATS criteria for both people with and without HIV require that the individual have pulmonary symptoms with suggestive radiography, exclusion of other diagnoses, positive culture results from two separate expectorated sputa, or at least one bronchoalveolar lavage specimen or bronchial biopsy with suggestive histopathology.

Mycobacterium kansasii, like other mycobacteria, will stain positive by acid-fast staining, which, when isolated from the sputum of a person with pulmonary lesions, can trigger an unnecessary public health investigation for TB. Testing with a nucleic acid amplification test can rule out TB in these cases.

Treatment

Most studies guiding treatment of *Mycobacterium kansasii* infection are conducted in individuals without HIV. *Mycobacterium kansasii* responds well to anti-TB medications with the exception of pyrazinamide (the organism is widely resistant). Treatment with a rifamycin, ethambutol, and either isoniazid or a macrolide is recommended for at least 12 months. Prior studies suggested treatment for 12 months after culture conversion, but there is no evidence that treatment for longer than 12 total months prevents relapse (Daley et al., 2020). Two studies demonstrated good outcomes with clarithromycin substituted for isoniazid (Griffith et al., 2003; Moon et al., 2019). Rifamycins in the treatment regimen of patients with *M. kansasii* (unlike patients with MAC disease) provide clear benefit and prevent relapse. The choice and dose of rifamycin should be guided by a person's ART, with special attention to potential drug interactions.

As with infections caused by other mycobacteria, IRIS has been documented with treatment of *M. kansasii*. Mild cases can be monitored or treated with a nonsteroidal anti-inflammatory agent or, in severe cases, a short course of steroids. Treatment for both *M. kansasii* and HIV should be continued during management of IRIS.

RECOMMENDED READING

Griffith DE, Aksamit T, Brown-Elliott BA, et al. An official ATS/IDSA statement: Diagnosis, treatment, and prevention of nontuberculous mycobacterial diseases. *Am J Respir Crit Care Med*. 2007; 175:367–416.

U.S. Department of Health and Human Services. Guidelines for prevention and treatment of opportunistic infections in HIV-infected adults and adolescents. https://clinicalinfo.hiv.gov/sites/default/files/guidelines/documents/adult-adolescent-oi/guidelines-adult-adolescent-oi.pdf. Published August 15, 2024. Accessed August 15, 2024.

U.S. Department of Health and Human Services, Panel on Antiretroviral Guidelines for Adults and Adolescents. Guidelines for the use of antiretroviral agents in HIV-1-infected adults and adolescents. https://clinicalinfo.hiv.gov/sites/default/files/guidelines/documents/adult-adolescent-arv/guidelines-adult-adolescent-arv.pdf. Published 2024. Accessed August 15, 2024.

VIRAL INFECTIONS

LEARNING OBJECTIVE

Discuss the established and evolving science regarding diagnosis, treatment, and prophylaxis of opportunistic viral infections associated with HIV to improve quality of life and length of survival.

WHAT'S NEW?

A new recombinant zoster vaccine (RZV) was approved in October 2017. In October 2021, the Advisory Committee on Immunization Practices (ACIP) recommended 2 RZV doses for prevention of herpes zoster and related complications in immunodeficient or immunosuppressed adults aged ≥18 years.

KEY POINTS

HERPES SIMPLEX VIRUS

- Herpes simplex virus (HSV) is a prevalent disease in PWH, typically presenting with orolabial, genital, and/or anorectal ulcers that may be very severe in the setting of advanced immunosuppression. HSV can also manifest as proctitis (particularly in men who have sex with men), esophagitis, keratitis, meningitis, encephalitis, radiculitis, and retinitis (presenting as acute retinal necrosis).
- Treatment is generally with acyclovir or one of its derivatives. Acyclovir resistance is more common among PWH. HSV suppression should be considered for individuals with frequent or severe recurrent episodes.

VARICELLA ZOSTER VIRUS

- Varicella zoster reactivation disease in PWH is often more severe, multi-dermatomal, or disseminated. Severe complications such as progressive outer retinal necrosis must be treated quickly to prevent permanent sequelae. For mild disease, oral therapy with acyclovir or a derivative is appropriate; in severe cases, intravenous therapy is required.

CYTOMEGALOVIRUS

- Cytomegalovirus may cause a variety of clinical manifestations in PWH with $CD4^+$ T-cell counts of less than 50 cells/mm^3. Retinitis and colitis are the most common. Ganciclovir (or the oral prodrug valganciclovir), cidofovir, or foscarnet are commonly used therapies, but they carry significant risk of toxicity. Primary prophylaxis is not recommended.

JC VIRUS

- Reactivation of the polyomavirus JC (JCV) causes progressive multifocal leukoencephalopathy (PML), a progressive, demyelinating disease of the central nervous system that leads to relatively rapid progression of neurologic deficits with dementia, coma, and death. Diagnosis is generally made clinically with the support of suggestive magnetic resonance imaging (MRI) findings and JCV polymerase chain reaction (PCR) in the CSF. Definitive diagnosis is made by brain biopsy. No specific antiviral therapy exists for JCV. ART often results in stabilization or regression of disease.

HERPESVIRUS

Herpes Simplex Virus

HSV-1 and HSV-2 are highly prevalent in PWH, with seroprevalence rates differing by country, gender, and age ranges (Bradley et al., 2018; Xu et al., 2006). HSV-2 rates are significantly higher (59.7%–80.5%) when compared with the general population (19.2%–40.8%) (Lama et al., 2006; Patel et al., 2012). Classically, HSV-1 infection manifests with orolabial ulcers, whereas HSV-2 causes genital ulcers; currently, however, both are increasingly recognized as causing genital infection, especially in young women and men who have sex with men (MSM). Primary HSV-1 genital infections present with lesions identical to HSV-2 (Ryder et al., 2009).

The primary mode of transmission is through direct contact with oral or genital secretions. Although clinical HSV disease is common in the absence of HIV infection, manifestations are more common, more severe, or atypical in the setting of HIV infection.

Clinical Presentation

The classical presentation of herpes infection is large, painful, grouped vesicles with an erythematous base, typically in the orolabial, genital, and anorectal regions; they may, however, involve any area of the body. Inguinal lymphadenopathy is commonly seen in primary infection (Corey and Holmes, 1983). In patients with advanced HIV-associated immunosuppression, anogenital lesions may be severe, and they may be refractory to treatment or secondary to acyclovir-resistant virus (Safrin et al., 1994). Dissemination is possible, but rare. Hypertrophic genital herpes, which is an atypical presentation, often resembles neoplasia and requires biopsy to confirm the diagnosis (Yudin and Kaul, 2008). Proctitis (particularly in MSM), keratitis, meningitis, encephalitis, radiculitis, and retinitis (presenting as acute retinal necrosis) are possible complications. HSV esophagitis may occur in people with CD4+ T-cell counts of less than 50 cells/mm^3 and typically presents with retrosternal chest pain and odynophagia.

Reactivation of HSV is more common in PWH. Recurrent lesions are often more frequent, more extensive, and of longer duration. In addition, there is prolonged shedding of the virus even in the absence of lesions, especially in PWH with lower CD4+ T-cell counts and higher plasma HIV-1 RNA levels.

Diagnosis

HSV DNA PCR and viral culture are the recommended modalities for diagnosis for all suspected HSV mucosal infections, with PCR having the highest sensitivity (Workowski et al., 2021). Type-specific serological assays are available and may be considered, but false positive HSV-2 serologic tests have been reported with enzyme immunoassay antibody tests with low index values (1.1 to 3.5), and repeat testing is recommended in such cases for confirmation (Workowski et al., 2021). Culture specimens can also be tested for antiviral drug susceptibility.

Prevention

Latex condoms, when consistently used, decrease the acquisition of HSV-2 by 30% (Martin et al., 2009). Suppressive therapy with oral acyclovir, valacyclovir, or famciclovir is recommended for severe or frequent recurrences in PWH. Annual assessment is recommended to determine whether supportive therapy should be continued. There is no vaccine available for prevention of HSV infection.

Treatment

Table 19.1 shows the current treatment recommendations from the Guidelines for the Prevention and Treatment of Opportunistic Infections in Adults and Adolescents with HIV (DHHS, 2024b). Oral acyclovir, valacyclovir, and famciclovir are comparable alternatives. In people with extensive mucocutaneous lesions, intravenous acyclovir is recommended. Failure of resolution of herpes lesions in 7–10 days after starting anti-HSV therapy raises suspicion for acyclovir resistance, and viral culture of the lesion with phenotypic testing and susceptibility testing should be performed (DHHS, 2024b).

Resistance to acyclovir has been reported in up to 5% of PWH with HSV-2 infection and is more frequent in patients with prolonged acyclovir use. Acyclovir inhibits HSV-specific DNA polymerase after incorporation into the growing DNA, resulting in chain termination owing to the absence of the 3′ hydroxyl group. It requires phosphorylation by a virally encoded thymidine kinase in order to be active. Altered, reduced, or absent thymidine kinase or altered viral DNA polymerase confers resistance to acyclovir and all others in the class, including ganciclovir. In these cases, foscarnet is the drug of choice. Cidofovir is a reasonable alternative for thymidine kinase negative HSV (LoPresti et al., 1998). Pritelivir, a helicase-primase inhibitor, is a novel agent being studied in clinical trials for treatment of acyclovir-resistant herpes in immunocompromised populations. Prolonged application (21–28 days or longer) of topical agents like trifluridine, foscarnet, cidofovir, and imiquimod can effectively treat external lesions, based on expert opinion.

Table 19.1 HSV TREATMENT RECOMMENDATIONS

CONDITION	FIRST CHOICE TREATMENT	ALTERNATIVE TREATMENT
Orolabial lesions	**Valacyclovir 1 g by mouth twice daily. *or* Famciclovir 500 mg by mouth twice daily *or* Acyclovir 400 mg by mouth 3 times per day for 5–10 days**	
Initial or recurrent genital lesions	**Valacyclovir 1 g by mouth twice daily *or* Famciclovir 500 mg by mouth twice daily *or* Acyclovir 400 mg by mouth 3 times per day for 5–10 days**	
Severe mucocutaneous lesions	**Acyclovir 5 mg/kg IV every 8 hours until lesions regress, then switch to acyclovir 400 mg by mouth 3 times per day until lesions are healed**	
Esophagitis	**Valacyclovir 1 g by mouth 3 times per day *or* Famciclovir 500 mg by mouth 3 times per day *or* Acyclovir 400 mg by mouth 5 times daily for 14–21 days**	
Encephalitis and hepatitis	**Acyclovir 10–15 mg/kg IV every 8 hours for 21 days**	
Acyclovir-resistant herpes	**Foscarnet 90–120 mg/kg/day IV 2–3 times daily until clinical response Cidofovir 5 mg/kg/week IV for 3 weeks, then 5 mg/kg every other week with saline hydration and probenecid 2 g by mouth 3 hours before the dose, followed by 1 g 2 hours and 8 hours after the dose (total of 4 g) until clinical response (off label)**	**Topical trifluridine *or* Cidofovir 1% gel *or* Topical imiquimod 5% 3 times weekly for 21–28 days or longer based on clinical response**

Prophylaxis

Condoms are recommended to prevent transmission of HSV-2. The use of 1% tenofovir vaginal gel has been shown to be associated with a 50% risk reduction of HSV-2 acquisition in women at high risk of HIV infection (Bender Ignacio et al., 2015). However, this has not been confirmed in other studies. Additionally, in patients taking oral tenofovir, the rates of vaginal shedding of HSV-1 and HSV-2 are similar. Suppressive therapy with oral acyclovir, valacyclovir, or famciclovir is effective in preventing genital herpes recurrences, and should be discussed with all patients with HSV-2 (Table 19.2). Immune reconstitution improves the frequency and severity of clinical episodes of genital herpes, but does not decrease shedding.

In individuals with $CD4^+$ T-cell count less than 250 cells/mm^3 who will start ART, there is an increased risk of HSV-2 shedding and genital ulcer diseases in the first 6 months. It is recommended to give suppressive antiviral therapy because it decreases the risk of genital ulcer diseases by 60%.

VARICELLA ZOSTER VIRUS

Varicella zoster virus (VZV) typically causes initial infection in childhood (chickenpox) and later reactivates, causing herpes zoster. The prevalence of herpes zoster is 3%–5% in the general population, but 15–25 times higher in PWH (Buchbinder et al., 1992). In the era of combination ART, the risk of reactivation and disease declined among PWH but remained 3-fold higher than the general population (Grabar et al., 2015).

Clinical Presentation

Initial clinical presentation is similar to that of immunocompetent patients, manifesting as a prodrome of cutaneous burning or pain, followed by eruption of grouped vesicles on an erythematous base along a dermatome. PWH are at increased risk for multi-dermatomal or disseminated zoster, including neurologic and ophthalmologic complications. Approximately 20%–30% of PWH will experience subsequent episodes of herpes zoster, either in the same or in different dermatomes. The probability of a recurrence of herpes zoster within 1 year of the index episode is 10% (Gebo et al., 2005). Postherpetic neuralgia is reported in 10%–15% of PWH (Gebo et al., 2005; Harrison et al., 1999).

Atypical VZV presentations such as chronic hyperkeratotic lesions or chronic disseminated ecthyma have also been reported. Meningitis, multifocal leukoencephalitis, ventriculitis, myelitis, cranial nerve palsies, and focal brainstem lesions are possible neurological complications. Involvement of the ophthalmic division of the trigeminal nerve causes anterior uveitis, corneal scarring, and vision loss. Ocular involvement with acute retinal necrosis and progressive outer retinal necrosis are syndromes similar to CMV retinitis, but involving faster progression that typically occurs at $CD4^+$ T-cell counts of less than 100 cells/mm^3 and may result in retinal blindness (Engstrom et al., 1994).

Table 19.2 **HSV SUPPRESSIVE THERAPY RECOMMENDATIONS**

CONDITION	FIRST CHOICE TREATMENT
Genital lesions	Valacyclovir 500 mg by mouth twice daily *or* Famciclovir 500 mg by mouth twice daily *or* Acyclovir 400–800 mg by mouth twice daily or 3 times per day

Diagnosis

The diagnosis of VZV is made clinically. Laboratory confirmation is possible using viral culture, direct immunofluorescence testing, and PCR testing, which is the most sensitive assay.

Treatment

VZV treatment is summarized in Table 19.3.

Table 19.3 **VZV TREATMENT RECOMMENDATIONS**

CONDITION	FIRST CHOICE TREATMENT
VZV infection, immunocompromised patients	SEVERE: Acyclovir 10–15 mg/kg IV every 8 hours for 7–10 days. May switch to oral if no evidence of visceral involvement. UNCOMPLICATED: Valacyclovir (1 g by mouth 3 times per day), *or* famciclovir (500 mg by mouth 3 times per day) for 5 to 7 days
Herpes zoster, acute localized dermatomal	Valacyclovir 1 g 3 times per day *or* Famciclovir 500 mg 3 times per day *or* Acyclovir 800 mg by mouth 5 times daily, each administered for 7–10 days Consider longer duration if lesions slow to resolve.
Herpes zoster, extensive cutaneous lesion or visceral involvement	Acyclovir 10–15 mg/kg IV every 8 hours After clinical improvement is evident, switch to oral therapy: Valacyclovir 1 g 3 times per day *or* Famciclovir 500 mg 3 times per day *or* Acyclovir 800 mg 5 times daily each administered for 10–14 days
Acute retinal necrosis	Acyclovir 10 mg/kg IV every 8 hours for 10–14 days; followed by oral valacyclovir 1 g 3 times per day for 6 weeks *plus* Ganciclovir 2 mg/0.05 mL intravitreal twice weekly × 1 or 2 doses.
Progressive outer retinal necrosis	Ganciclovir 5 mg/kg IV *and/or* Foscarnet 90 mg/kg IV every 12 hours *plus* Ganciclovir 2 mg/0.05 ml intravitreal twice weekly × 1 or 2 doses.
Acyclovir-resistant VZV infection	Foscarnet 90 mg/kg IV every 12 hours.

Prevention

Long-term prophylaxis or suppressive treatment is not recommended. Postexposure prophylaxis is recommended for PWH susceptible to VZV and in close contact with a person who has active varicella or herpes zoster. The preferred regimen is a single intramuscular dose of varicella zoster immune globulin dosed on body weight (maximum of 625 IU) administered as soon as possible, within 10 days after exposure. Alternatively, a 5- to 7-day course of acyclovir or valacyclovir could be given starting 7–10 days after exposure.

RZV, a recombinant herpes zoster vaccine, is the only FDA-approved vaccine available for the prevention of zoster in the United States. A small phase 1/2a, randomized, observer-masked, placebo-controlled study evaluated the safety and immunogenicity of RZV in 123 PWH. The vaccine was found to have a clinically acceptable safety profile and elicited strong gE-specific cell-mediated and anti-gE humoral immune responses that persisted at least one year after the last vaccination (Berkowitz et al., 2015). In October 2021, the ACIP recommended 2 RZV doses administered 2 to 6 months apart for prevention of herpes zoster and related complications in immunodeficient or immunosuppressed adults aged ≥18 years. ZVL, a one-dose attenuated life virus vaccine, is no longer available in the United States. It should be noted that ZVL was contraindicated in PWH with $CD4^+$ T-cell counts <200 cells/mm^3 as it could lead to disseminated ZVL vaccine strain infection. PWH vaccinated with ZVL should be revaccinated with RZV.

CYTOMEGALOVIRUS

Cytomegalovirus (CMV) is a DNA herpesvirus and the largest among them with the longest genome. It is typically acquired from close contact during youth or adolescence. In the general population, the percentage of people with evidence of previous CMV infection ranges from 40% to 100% and varies with ethnicity and country. Active disease associated with HIV typically results from reactivation of latent infection in the setting of advanced immunosuppression (i.e., $CD4^+$ T-cell counts less than 50 cells/mm^3) (Dieterich et al., 1991). Other risk factors for CMV disease include plasma HIV RNA levels above 100,000 copies/mL and the presence of other OIs.

Before the use of ART, CMV retinitis was the most common intraocular infection in people with AIDS, occurring in 21%–40% of patients (Whitcup, 2000). Since combination ART was introduced, rates of CMV retinitis have declined by up to 83%, and the overall rates of CMV end-organ disease have declined by 95% (Jabs et al., 2009; Schwarcz et al., 2013; Ude et al., 2022).

Clinical Presentation and Diagnosis

CMV can infect different organs of the body. Retinitis accounts for 85% of CMV manifestations and is the leading cause of vision loss among people with AIDS. Other clinical syndromes include esophagitis, colitis, polyradiculopathy, ventriculoencephalitis, pneumonitis, adrenalitis, and pancreatitis.

Chorioretinitis

CMV chorioretinitis presents with painless progressive loss of vision, floaters, and/or visual field cut defects. Symptoms are initially unilateral, but without treatment, can progress to the contralateral side. The diagnosis is exclusively made by recognition of typical retinal changes during a funduscopic examination: creamy or yellow-white granular areas with perivascular exudates and hemorrhage. These lesions initially are found in the periphery of the fundus and later involve the macula and optic disc, resulting in blindness.

Colitis

CMV colitis is the second most common manifestation of CMV infection in people with AIDS. Patients present with severe diarrhea, abdominal pain and cramping, anorexia, weight loss, and fever. The diagnosis is made by detection of mucosal ulcerations on colonoscopy, coupled with histologic evidence of intracytoplasmic or intranuclear inclusions. A positive culture or positive PCR in tissue or stool does not confirm the diagnosis. Mucosal hemorrhage and perforation rarely occur but are life-threatening.

Esophagitis

CMV esophagitis causes odynophagia, nausea, fever, and retrosternal pain. Diagnosis is made by endoscopic examination revealing diffuse inflammation of the esophagus and/or esophageal ulcers. Biopsy specimens also reveal intranuclear inclusions. A positive culture or tissue PCR itself does not establish a diagnosis.

CMV Polyradiculopathy

CMV polyradiculopathy presents with sacrolumbar radicular pain and lower limb paresthesia that may develop into progressive flaccid paralysis of the legs with decreasing and ultimately absent tendon reflexes. Urinary retention and stool incontinence may occur. If untreated, the condition rapidly advances up the spine, causing ascending sensory loss and growing flaccidity in the upper limbs, similar to Guillain–Barré paralysis. The CSF may reveal pleocytosis with a predominance of polymorphonuclear cells, elevated protein, and moderately low glucose. Lumbar MRI may show gadolinium enhancement of the cauda equina in 33% of patients. Diagnosis is made by viral culture, CMV antigen assays, and detection of CMV DNA by CSF PCR.

Ventriculoencephalitis

CMV ventriculoencephalitis is a late manifestation of CMV disease. The course is acute, consisting of cranial nerve palsies, nystagmus, and other focal neurologic deficits that rapidly lead to death. CT and MRI scans show white matter enhancement. MRI with gadolinium may reveal a characteristic periventricular ring-like enhancement. Viral culture of the CSF is not always positive; however, high levels of CMV DNA can often be detected in CSF using PCR.

Dementia

CMV dementia can present similarly to HIV-associated dementia but is caused by CMV encephalitis. Patients exhibit lethargy and confusion with or without fever. CSF analysis is significant for pleocytosis that may be polymorphonuclear with low to normal glucose, and normal to high protein. CT and MRI scans may show cerebral atrophy.

Pneumonia

CMV pneumonitis is uncommon in patients with AIDS. Symptoms include shortness of breath, dyspnea, dry nonproductive cough, and hypoxia. Imaging studies show diffuse interstitial infiltrates. A definitive diagnosis is made when multiple CMV inclusion bodies are seen in lung tissue. CMV may be isolated from bronchial washing or bronchoalveolar lavage fluid from approximately 50% of PWH undergoing bronchoscopy; however, the clinical significance of CMV isolation from these fluids and respiratory secretions remains controversial due to viral shedding.

CMV viremia is common in asymptomatic persons with low CD4+ T-cell counts (<100 cells/mm^3). Viremia is typically present in active disease but may also be present without end-organ disease, so this type of testing is of limited value. The absence of CMV antibody may be helpful in excluding CMV disease; however, rarely, active disease can present during primary CMV infection with negative antibodies, and immunoglobin G antibody tests may revert to negative in individuals with advanced immunosuppression.

Treatment

Table 19.4 shows the current CMV treatment recommendations from the Guidelines for the Prevention and Treatment of Opportunistic Infections (DHHS 2024b).

For CMV chorioretinitis, treatment consists of an induction phase of high-dose drug given for at least 2 weeks. Once retinitis is stable, patients are placed on chronic maintenance therapy until there is evidence of immune recovery (sustained CD4+ T-cell counts >100 cells/mm^3 for ≥6 months). In the absence of ART-mediated immune reconstitution, most patients will have a reactivation of CMV infection despite suppressive therapy and will require reinduction therapy. Intraocular treatment may be useful in salvage therapy for

Table 19.4 CMV TREATMENT RECOMMENDATIONS

CONDITION	FIRST CHOICE TREATMENT	ALTERNATIVE TREATMENT
CMV retinitis	*For sight-threatening lesions*: Intravitreal injections Ganciclovir or foscarnet *plus* Valganciclovir 900 mg by mouth twice daily for 14–21 days, then once daily *For small peripheral lesions*: Valganciclovir 900 mg by mouth twice daily for 14–21 days, then 900 mg once daily *or* any of the alternative treatments	Intravitreal injections Ganciclovir or foscarnet *plus* Ganciclovir 5 mg/kg IV every 12 hours for 14–21 days, then 5 mg/kg IV daily *or* Ganciclovir 5 mg/kg IV every 12 hours for 14–21 days, then valganciclovir 900 mg by mouth daily Foscarnet 60 mg/kg IV every 8 hours or Foscarnet 90 mg/kg IV every 12 hours for 14–21 days, then 90–120 mg/kg IV every 24 hours *or* Cidofovir 5 mg/kg/week IV for 2 weeks, then 5 mg/kg every other week with saline hydration and probenecid 2 g by mouth 3 hours before the dose, followed by 1 g 2 hours and 8 hours after the dose (total of 4 g)
Secondary prophylaxis (previously called maintenance therapy) for CMV retinitis	Valganciclovir 900 mg by mouth daily *or* Ganciclovir implant (replaced every 6–8 months if CD4+ count remains <100 cells/mm^3) *plus* Valganciclovir 900 mg by mouth daily until immune recovery	Ganciclovir 5 mg/kg IV 5–7 times weekly *or* Foscarnet 90–120 mg/kg body weight IV once daily *or* Cidofovir 5 mg/kg body weight IV every other week as above
CMV colitis or esophagitis	Ganciclovir IV *or* Foscarnet IV for 21–28 days	–
CMV neurological disease	Ganciclovir IV *plus* Foscarnet IV until symptomatic improvement	–

CMV = cytomegalovirus; IV = intravenous.

patients who cannot tolerate systemic antivirals. Otherwise, any local treatment should be accompanied by systemic anti-CMV therapy. Systemic therapy has been shown to decrease CMV involvement of the contralateral eye, reduce the risk of CMV disease in other organs, and increase survival rates. Intraocular therapy alone has been associated with progression of CMV to the contralateral eye as well as with systemic disease (Martin et al., 1994).

Maribavir has emerged as a salvage therapy for refractory or resistant CMV infections. PWH with asymptomatic CMV viremia were included in the phase 1 trial that demonstrated safety, tolerability, and efficacy.

Ganciclovir and valganciclovir, foscarnet, and cidofovir carry a significant toxicity risk. Ganciclovir and valganciclovir can cause neutropenia, thrombocytopenia, nausea, diarrhea, renal dysfunction, and central venous catheter infection. Foscarnet more commonly causes nephrotoxicity, electrolyte abnormalities, seizures, genital ulcers, and central venous catheter infection. Cidofovir, when used, is associated with nephrotoxicity and intraocular hypotony. Maribavir has been associated with dose-related taste disturbance and diarrhea.

Prevention/Prophylaxis

In PWH with $CD4^+$ T-cell counts of less than 100 cells/mm^3, early recognition of the manifestations of end-organ CMV disease is the best modality for early diagnosis and prevention of further disease progression. Primary prophylaxis against CMV is not recommended. Patients with $CD4^+$ T-cell counts of less than 100 cells/mm^3 should have an annual ophthalmology exam. Secondary prophylaxis using valganciclovir should be given until $CD4^+$ T-cell count has been greater than 100 cells/mm^3 for 3–6 months and lesions are not life-threatening. If $CD4^+$ T-cell count decreases to less than 100 cells/mm^3, secondary prophylaxis should be reinstituted.

HUMAN HERPESVIRUS-8

The prevalence of human herpesvirus-8 (HHV-8) ranges between 1% and 5% in the general population, but it is between 20% and 77% in MSM (Pauk et al., 2000). HHV-8 is associated with all forms of Kaposi's sarcoma, primary effusion lymphoma, and lymphoproliferative disorders such as multicentric Castleman's disease (see Chapter 25, "Malignancies in HIV."

JOHN CUNNINGHAM VIRUS (JCV)

Reactivation of the polyomavirus JC virus (JCV) causes progressive multifocal leukoencephalopathy (PML), a disease characterized by focal demyelination. Approximately 85% of adults are seropositive for JCV worldwide. Most individuals usually are exposed to JCV in childhood, which causes asymptomatic infection and a chronic asymptomatic carrier state (Antonsson et al., 2010; Knowles, 2006). The incidence of PML has decreased significantly since the widespread use of ART. However, PML has also been reported in PWH with $CD4^+$ T-cell counts of greater than 300 cells/mm^3 and as a complication of IRIS (Berger et al., 1998; Cinque et al., 2003).

Clinical Presentation

The clinical presentation of PML depends on the location of brain lesions, and specific deficits vary across individuals. Commonly involved areas include the occipital lobe (causing hemianopsia); the frontal and parietal lobes (leading to aphasia, hemiparesis, and hemisensory deficits); and the cerebellar peduncles and deep white matter (causing dysmetria and ataxia) (Richardson and Webster, 1983). The spinal cord is rarely involved, and optic nerves are usually spared (Bernal-Cano et al., 2007). Patients can present with symptoms ranging from diffuse encephalopathy to focal deficits such as ataxia, hemiparesis, or speech difficulties. Symptoms tend to progress over several weeks to months. Seizures are seen in 20% of cases. Headache and fever are unusual in PML and if present, raise the possibility of another OI.

Diagnosis

MRI of the brain demonstrates distinct white matter lesions in areas of the brain corresponding to the clinical deficits. The lesions are usually white on T2 images, and they are also characteristically dark on T1 images. JCV DNA PCR in CSF is recommended to confirm diagnosis and has a sensitivity of 70%–80% and specificity of 100% (Cinque, 1997). Brain biopsy, used to make a definitive diagnosis, will reveal typical findings of focal myelin loss with characteristic astrocytes and lipid-laden macrophages. Because of high JCV seroprevalence, serological testing is not recommended.

Prevention

Early initiation of ART to prevent HIV-related immunosuppression is the only effective modality for prevention of PML.

Treatment

Initiation of effective ART is the treatment of choice. It prolongs survival and improves neurologic deficits when immune reconstitution is achieved. The early use of an optimized ART regimen after PML diagnosis appeared to improve survival (Gasnault et al., 2011). Other treatments have been attempted with no improvement in survival. Recrudescence after remission of PML with ART is extremely rare, but a few cases have been reported (Cinque et al, 2001; Crossley et al., 2016).

PML-IMMUNE RECONSTITUTION INFLAMMATORY SYNDROME

PML-IRIS may occur after initiating ART in people with advanced HIV infection and low $CD4^+$ T-cell counts. These cases may present with clinical and radiological findings different from classical PML. Radiologic findings of lesions with contrast enhancement, edema, and mass effect have been reported (Post et al., 2013). Both new onset and paradoxical worsening of PML can occur in ART-induced IRIS, and in many studies, empiric use of corticosteroids has been somewhat beneficial. The dose and duration of adjuvant corticosteroid treatment is yet to be established (Cinque et al., 2009; Fournier et al., 2017; Tan et al., 2009).

TIMING OF ANTIRETROVIRAL THERAPY INITIATION AND IMPACT ON OPPORTUNISTIC INFECTIONS

LEARNING OBJECTIVES

- Describe issues concerning ART initiation in the context of OIs.
- Summarize recommendations for starting ART in the setting of an OI.

KEY POINTS

- Early initiation of ART was associated with a decrease in AIDS progression and death in ACTG A5164.
- Early initiation of ART near the time of starting treatment for an OI should be considered for most patients, with the exception of PWH with cryptococcal or tuberculous meningitis.

The appropriate timing of ART initiation in the setting of an acute or ongoing OI has been debated. While immediate initiation of ART in the presence of an OI may lead to better clinical outcomes as the immune system recovers, it is important to consider potential complications. Rapidly decreasing HIV RNA levels have been associated with the development of immune reconstitution inflammatory syndrome (IRIS), potentially exacerbating the existing OI. Additionally, considerations extend to increased pill burden, potential drug-drug interactions, additive toxicity, and adverse events. Another practical concern is ensuring continuity of care if ART is started in a hospital setting for a newly diagnosed patient with HIV who does not yet have established outpatient care. This is particularly troublesome for people who do not have health insurance in place or otherwise do not have affordable access to ART after hospital discharge.

In the absence of pathogen-specific therapies, some opportunistic conditions such as cryptosporidiosis, microsporidiosis, and PML can only be managed with ART. This mandates early ART initiation in the presence of a concomitant OI. Further, patients with mild to moderate Kaposi's sarcoma (KS) may achieve remission through the receipt of ART without requiring chemotherapy. However, OIs with available targeted therapies may resolve with their corresponding therapies in the absence of ART. These include *Pneumocystis* pneumonia, *Cryptococcus neoformans* meningitis, and *Mycobacterium tuberculosis* meningitis. The optimal time to start ART has been a point of controversy for patients in this situation.

CLINICAL TRIAL RESULTS

The AIDS Clinical Trials Group (ACTG) A5164 study was designed to address the question of optimal timing of ART initiation for individuals presenting with AIDS-defining OIs or serious bacterial infections (SBIs), other than tuberculosis, for which effective antimicrobial therapies were available. This was a randomized, open-label strategy trial to evaluate early (defined as within 14 days of starting acute OI treatment) versus deferred (given after OI treatment is completed) initiation of ART in patients starting treatment of acute OIs or SBIs, using clinical and virologic endpoints at 48 weeks (Zolopa et al., 2009); 282 patients (141 in each arm) had evaluable results. Most participants were from racial/ethnic minority groups (73%), male (85%), with a median age of 38 years, median $CD4^+$ T-cell count of 29 cells/mm^3, and median HIV RNA level of 5.07 $\log_{10}$ copies/mL. The most common recorded infections were *Pneumocystis* pneumonia (63%), cryptococcal meningitis (12%), and SBIs (12%). ART was initiated at a mean of 12 days after starting OI treatment in the "early" arm versus 45 days after OI treatment in the "deferred" arm.

The study found a statistically significant decrease in the proportion of participants experiencing a second AIDS-defining disease and/or death (composite endpoint) in the early treatment arm (14.2%) compared to the deferred arm (24.1%) (odds ratio [OR] 0.51; 95% CI: 0.27–0.94). Time to AIDS progression and death was also longer in the early treatment arm compared to the deferred group (hazard ratio 0.53; 95% CI: 0.30–0.92). The impact of these differences was seen most prominently in the first 6 months after the diagnosis of the OI. The rate of adverse events was not different, and IRIS was reported in 8 participants in the early arm versus 12 in the deferred arm. These findings substantiated the fact that early initiation of ART during treatment for an acute OI or SBI is life-saving or, at least, serious morbidity–reducing if there are no major contraindications to starting ART. A cost-effectiveness analysis was supportive of this early treatment strategy (Sax et al., 2010).

The overall rates of IRIS in the A5164 cohort were lower than those observed in previously published retrospective trials, possibly because of the types of OIs included (mostly *Pneumocystis* pneumonia)—PWH with *M. tuberculosis* infection were excluded. The presence of fungal infections (*Cryptococcus* or *Histoplasma*), lower baseline $CD4^+$ T-cell counts, and higher baseline HIV RNA levels were found to be associated with IRIS in A5164. The occurrence of IRIS was also associated with higher $CD4^+$ T-cell counts and lower HIV RNA levels while on ART. Early initiation of ART did not increase the incidence of IRIS.

Recommendations regarding timing of ART initiation specifically in the setting of meningitis due to *C. neoformans* or *M. tuberculosis* are more complex and warrant ART deferral. In a study evaluating *C. neoformans* meningitis–related IRIS (Sungkanuparph et al., 2009), analysis of 101 participants employed a different methodology than ACTG 5164 and found no association between the timing of ART initiation and diagnosis of IRIS. Rather, it found that an increased baseline serum cryptococcal antigen titer was a risk factor for IRIS. In contrast, a study of 54 participants in Zimbabwe showed that early ART initiation (within 72 hours of diagnosis) versus delayed initiation (after 10 weeks of treatment with fluconazole alone) in persons with cryptococcal meningitis was associated with increased mortality. In this population, optimal management of increased intracranial pressure (i.e., decreasing CSF volume by lumbar puncture or other sterile procedure) was not always provided (Makadzange et al., 2010). Further, the 2014 Cryptococcal Optimal ART Timing Trial of 177 participants with HIV from Uganda and South Africa reported increased mortality (hazard ratio, 1.73) at 26 weeks for participants who started ART within 1 or 2 weeks compared to those who deferred ART for 5 weeks (Boulware et al., 2014). Participants in the early group started ART at a median of 8 days after being on antifungal therapy, while participants in the deferred group started ART at a median of 36 days. Most of the increase in mortality was observed within the first 8–30 days. Differences in mortality were especially pronounced in people who had white blood cell (WBC) counts of less than five cells/μL in their CSF, although it was unclear if the increase in mortality in this study was due to progression of cryptococcal disease or IRIS. Current U.S. Department of Health and Human Services (DHHS, 2024a) guidelines recommend a short delay in initiating ART in the presence of cryptococcal meningitis.

For patients with concomitant TB meningitis, immediate initiation of ART was associated with high rate of severe adverse events compared with initiating ART 2 months after the start of treatment in a cohort from Vietnam (Török et al., 2011). Different public and governmental guidelines recommend delaying ART between 2–8 weeks, with decision-making contingent on patient clinical status, initial CD4 levels, and access to care.

Implementation of the findings of A5164 and similar studies may prove difficult in practice, particularly in settings in which PWH may not have established linkage to primary care and have limited access to ongoing treatment with ART after the resolution of the acute OI. However, effective implementation of early ART was accomplished and published by an academic medical center, and this may be a model for bringing early ART to various "real-world" populations (Geng et al., 2011).

RECOMMENDATIONS OF GUIDELINES

The U.S. guidelines for prevention and treatment of OIs in adults and adolescents with HIV are regularly updated and available at: (https://clinicalinfo.hiv.gov/en/guidelines/hiv-clinical-guidelines-adult-and-adolescent-opportunistic-infections/whats-new). These provide recommendations regarding the timing of ART initiation in the setting of specific opportunistic conditions, and should be referenced for guidance in the treatment of PWH with those conditions. Guidelines generally reiterate the findings of A5164, suggesting that (unless contraindications are present) early initiation of ART near the time of treatment of an OI should be considered for most people with an acute OI. Other elements that should be considered include degree of immunosuppression, availability of treatment for the OI, drug-drug interactions and overlapping toxicities, and the risk and potential consequences of IRIS.

For PWHs with coinfections such as PML, cryptosporidiosis, microsporidiosis, and fungal infections other than meningitis caused by *C. neoformans*, it is recommended that ART be started as soon as possible. For *Pneumocystis* pneumonia and invasive SBIs, guidelines recommend starting ART within 2 weeks of diagnosis, although the panel notes that no patients with respiratory failure requiring mechanical ventilation were enrolled in the A5164 study. For *Toxoplasma gondii* encephalitis, the panel cites expert opinion to start ART within 2 or 3 weeks after diagnosis and initiation of specific treatment for toxoplasmosis based on data from A5164, which studied only 5% of participants diagnosed with toxoplasmosis. For Bartonella central nervous system or ophthalmic infection, the data are not evident, but experts recommend delaying ART for 2–4 weeks from starting targeted bartonella therapy due to risk of IRIS. For disseminated *Mycobacterium avium* complex, the panel cites starting ART after the first 2 weeks of antimycobacterial therapy in order to decrease the overall initial pill burden and to decrease the possibility for IRIS. For cytomegalovirus (CMV) retinitis, the panel notes that many experts would not delay ART for more than 2 weeks after starting CMV-specific treatment. The presence of disease caused by herpes simplex virus (HSV) or varicella zoster virus (VZV) does not preclude ART initiation.

For cryptococcal meningitis, the panel notes that it would be prudent to defer ART at least until the initial 2-week induction phase is complete and CSF cultures have sterilized. Most experts consider initiation after 4–6 weeks of antifungal therapy and possibly delay until the completion of the consolidation phase at 10 weeks, especially if the patient has increased intracranial pressure or a low CSF WBC count. The panel also notes that if ART is started prior to 10 weeks of antifungal treatment, the clinician should be prepared to promptly investigate and treat manifestations of IRIS, including increased intracranial pressure. Lastly, there is very limited randomized clinical trial evidence to guide the optimal time for ART initiation in the setting of concomitant tuberculous meningitis. Expert opinion remains relevant in managing these patients.

SUMMARY

Although substantial barriers to early initiation of ART in the setting of an acute OI exist, the weight of the available evidence falls on the side of starting ART as soon as possible for most patients with acute OIs and invasive SBIs, with the notable exception of meningitis due to *C. neoformans* or *M. tuberculosis*.

RECOMMENDED READING

Abdool Karim SS, Naidoo K, Grobler A, et al. Timing of initiation of antiretroviral drugs during tuberculosis therapy. *N Engl J Med.* 2010 Feb 25;362(8):697–706. http://www.ncbi.nlm.nih.gov/pubmed/20181971

Blanc FX, Sok T, Laureillard D, et al. Earlier versus later start of antiretroviral therapy in HIV-positive adults with tuberculosis. *N Engl J Med.* 2011 Oct 20;365(16):1471–1481. http://www.ncbi.nlm.nih.gov/pubmed/22010913

Boulware DR, Meya DB, Muzoora C, et al. Timing of antiretroviral therapy after diagnosis of cryptococcal meningitis. *N Engl J Med.* 2014 Jun 26;370(26):2487–2498.

Mfinanga SG, Kirenga BJ, Chanda DM, et al. Early versus delayed initiation of highly active antiretroviral therapy for HIV-positive adults with newly diagnosed pulmonary tuberculosis (TB-HAART): a prospective, international, randomised, placebo-controlled trial. *Lancet Infect Dis.* July 2014;14(7):563–571. http://www.ncbi.nlm.nih.gov/pubmed/24810491

Temprano ANRS Study Group; Danel C, Moh R, Gabillard D, et al. A trial of early antiretrovirals and isoniazid preventive therapy in Africa. *N Engl J Med.* 2015 Aug 27;373(9):808–822. http://www.ncbi.nlm.nih.gov/pubmed/26193126

Zolopa A, Andersen J, Powderly W, et al. Early antiretroviral therapy reduces AIDS progression/death in individuals with acute opportunistic infections: a multicenter randomized strategy trial. *PLoS One.* 2009;4(5):e5575.

REFERENCES

American Thoracic Society. Targeted tuberculin testing and treatment of latent tuberculosis infection. http://www.cdc.gov/mmwr/preview/mmwrhtml/rr4906a1.htm. Published June 2020. Accessed September 13, 2024.

Antonsson A, Green AC, Mallitt KA, et al. Prevalence and stability of antibodies to the BK and JC polyomaviruses: a long-term longitudinal study of Australians. *J Gen Virol.* 2010;91(Pt 7):1849–1853.

Bender Ignacio RA, Perti T, Magaret AS, et al., Oral and vaginal tenofovir for genital herpes simplex virus type 2 shedding in immunocompetent women: a double-blind, randomized, cross-over trial. *J Infect Dis.* 2015 212(12): 1949–1956.

Berger JR, Levy RM, Flomenhoft D. Predictive factors for prolonged survival in acquired immunodeficiency syndrome-associated progressive multifocal leukoencephalopathy. *Ann Neurol.* 1998;44:341–349.

Berkowitz EM, Moyle G, Stellbrink HJ, et al. Safety and immunogenicity of an adjuvanted herpes zoster subunit candidate vaccine in HIV-positive adults: a phase 1/2a randomized, placebo-controlled study. *J Infect Dis.* 2015;211(8):1279–1287.

Bernal-Cano F, Joseph JT, Koralnik IJ. Spinal cord lesions of progressive multifocal leukoencephalopathy in an acquired immunodeficiency syndrome patient. *J Neurovirol.* 2007;13(5):474–476. https://www.ncbi.nlm.nih.gov/pubmed/17994433

Blanc FX, Sok T, Laureillard, D, et al. Earlier versus later start of antiretroviral therapy in HIV-positive adults with tuberculosis. *N Engl J Med.* 2011;365(16):1471–1481.

Borisov AS, Bamrah Morris S, et al. Update of recommendations for use of once-weekly isoniazid-rifapentine regimen to treat latent mycobacterium tuberculosis infection. *MMWR.* 2018 Jun 29;67(25):723–726.

Boulware DR, Meya DB, Muzoora C, et al. Timing of antiretroviral therapy after diagnosis of cryptococcal meningitis. *N Engl J Med.* 2014;370(26):2487–2498.

Bradley J, Floyd S, Piwowar-Manning E, Laeyendecker O, et al. Sexually transmitted bedfellows: exquisite association between HIV and herpes simplex virus type 2 in 21 communities in Southern Africa in the HIV Prevention Trials Network 071 (PopART) Study. *J Infect Dis.* 2018;2;218(3):443–452. doi:10.1093/infdis/jiy178. PMID: 29659909; PMCID: PMC6049005.

Buchbinder SP, Katz MH, Hessol NA, et al. Herpes zoster and human immunodeficiency virus infection. *J Infect Dis.* 1992;166(5):1153–1156. doi:10.1093/infdis/166.5.1153

Cattamanchi A, Smith R, Steingart KR, et al. Interferon-gamma release assays for the diagnosis of latent tuberculosis infection in HIV-infected individuals: a systematic review and meta-analysis. *J Acquir Immune Defic Syndr.* 2011;56(3):230–238.

Centers for Disease Control and Prevention (CDC). *Recommendations for Human Immunodeficiency Virus (HIV) Screening in Tuberculosis (TB) Clinics, Factsheet.* Atlanta, GA: U.S. Department of Health and Human Services, CDC; 2012. https://www.cdc.gov/tb/publications/factsheets/testing/HIVscreening.pdf

Centers for Disease Control and Prevention (CDC). *Reported Tuberculosis in the United States, 2020.* Atlanta, GA: U.S. Department of Health and Human Services, CDC; 2022.

Cilloniz C, Dominedo C, Alvarez-Martinez MJ, et al. Pneumocystis pneumonia in the twenty-first century: HIV-infected versus HIV-uninfected patients. *Expert Rev Anti Infect Ther.* 2019;17(1):787–801.

Cinque P. Cytomegalovirus infections of the nervous system. *Intervirology.* 1997;40(2–3):85–97.

Cinque P, Bossolasco S, Brambilla AM, et al. The effect of highly active antiretroviral therapy-induced immune reconstitution on development and outcome of progressive multifocal leukoencephalopathy: study of 43 cases with review of the literature. *J Neurovirol.* 2003;9(Suppl 1):73–80.

Cinque P, Koralnik IJ, Gerevini S, et al. Progressive multifocal leukoencephalopathy in HIV-1 infection. *Lancet Infect Dis.* 2009;9(1):625–636.

Cinque P, Pierotti C, Vigano MG, et al. The good and evil of HAART in HIV-related progressive multifocal leukoencephalopathy. *J Neurovirol.* 2001;7(4):358–363.

Conradie F, Diacon AH, Ngubane N, et al. 2022. Treatment of highly drug-resistant pulmonary tuberculosis. *N Engl J Med.* 2020;382:893–902.

Corey L, Holmes KK. Genital herpes simplex virus infections: current concepts in diagnosis, therapy and prevention. *Ann Intern Med.* 1983;98(6):973–983.

Crossley KM, Agnihotri S, Chaganti J, et al. Recurrence of progressive multifocal leukoencephalopathy despite immune recovery in two HIV seropositive individuals. *J Neurovirol.* 2016;22(4):541–545.

Daley CL, Iaccarino JM, Lang C, et al. Treatment of nontuberculous mycobacterial pulmonary disease: an official ATS/ERS/ESCMID/IDSA clinical practice guideline. *Clin Infect Dis.* 2020;71(4):e1–e36.

DHHS, Panel on Antiretroviral Guidelines for Adults and Adolescents. Guidelines for the use of antiretroviral agents in adults and adolescents with HIV. Department of Health and Human Services. https://clinicalinfo.hiv.gov/en/guidelines/adult-and-adolescent-arv. Published September 12, 2024a. Accessed September 13, 2024.

DHHS, Panel on Guidelines for the Prevention and Treatment of Opportunistic Infections in Adults and Adolescents with HIV. Guidelines for the prevention and treatment of opportunistic infections in adults and adolescents with HIV. National Institutes of Health, Centers for Disease Control and Prevention, HIV Medicine Association, and Infectious Diseases Society of America. https://clinicalinfo.hiv.gov/en/guidelines/adult-and-adolescent-opportunistic-infection. Published August 15, 2024b. Accessed September 11, 2024.

Dieterich DT, Kim MH, McMeeding A, et al. Cytomegalovirus appendicitis in a patient with acquired immune deficiency syndrome. *Am J Gastroenterol.* 1991;86(7):904–906.

Engstrom RE, Holland GN, Margolis TP, et al. The progressive outer retinal necrosis syndrome. A variant of necrotizing herpetic retinopathy in patients with AIDS. *Ophthalmology.* 1994;101(9):1488–1502.

Fournier A, Martin-Blondel G, Lechapt-Zalcman E, et al. Immune reconstitution inflammatory syndrome unmasking or worsening AIDS-related progressive multifocal leukoencephalopathy: a literature review. *Front Immunol.* 2017;8:577.

Gasnault J, Costagliola D, Hendel-Chavez H, et al. Improved survival of HIV-1-infected patients with progressive multifocal

leukoencephalopathy receiving early 5-drug combination antiretroviral therapy. *PLoS One*. 2011;6(6):e20967.
Gebo KA, Kalyani R, Moore RD, et al. The incidence of, risk factors for, and sequelae of herpes zoster among HIV patients in the highly active antiretroviral therapy era. *J Acquir Immune Defic Syndr*. 2005;40(2):169–174.
Geng EH, Kahn JS, Chang OC, et al. The Effect of AIDS Clinical Trials Group Protocol 5164 on the time from *Pneumocystis jirovecii* pneumonia diagnosis to antiretroviral initiation in routine clinical practice: a case study of diffusion, dissemination, and implementation. *Clin Infect Dis*. 2011;53(10):1008–1014.
Gill CM, Dolan L, Piggot LM, et al. New developments in tuberculosis diagnosis and treatment. *Breathe*. 2022;8(1):210149.
Grabar S, Tattevin P, Selinger-Leneman H, de La Blanchardiere A, et al. Incidence of herpes zoster in HIV-infected adults in the combined antiretroviral therapy era: results from the FHDH-ANRS CO4 cohort. *Clin Infect Dis*. 2015 Apr 15;60(8):1269–1277. doi:10.1093/cid/ciu1161
Griffith DE. Management of disease due to *Mycobacterium kansasii*. *Clin Chest Med*. 2002;23:613–621.
Griffith DE, Brown-Elliott BA, Wallace RJ Jr. 2003. Thrice-weekly clarithromycin-containing regimen for treatment of *Mycobacterium kansasii* lung disease: results of a preliminary study. *Clin Inf Dis*. 2003;37(9): 1178–1182.
Harrison RA, Soong S, Weiss HL, et al. A mixed model for factors predictive of pain in AIDS patients with herpes zoster. *J Pain Symptom Manage*. 1999;17(6):410–417.
Havlir DV, Kendall MA, Ive P, et al. Timing of antiretroviral therapy for HIV-1 infection and tuberculosis. *N Engl J Med*. 2011 Oct 20;365(16):1482–1491. http://www.ncbi.nlm.nih.gov/pubmed/22010914
Jabs DA, Martin BK, Forman MS; Cytomegalovirus Retinitis and Viral Resistance Research Group. Mortality associated with resistant cytomegalovirus among patients with cytomegalovirus retinitis and AIDS. *Ophthalmology*. 2010;117(1):128-132.e2. doi:10.1016/j.ophtha.2009.06.016.
Karim SSA, Naidoo K, Grobler A, et al. Integration of antiretroviral therapy with tuberculosis treatment. *N Engl J Med*. 2011; 365(16):1492–1501.
Knowles WA. Discovery and epidemiology of the human polyomaviruses BK virus (BKV) and JC virus (JCV). *Adv Exp Med Biol*. 2006;577:19–45.
Lama JR, Lucchetti A, Suarez L, Laguna-Torres VA, et al. Peruvian HIV Sentinel Surveillance Working Group. Association of herpes simplex virus type 2 infection and syphilis with human immunodeficiency virus infection among men who have sex with men in Peru. *J Infect Dis*. 2006;194(10):1459–1466.
LoPresti AE, Levine JF, Munk GB, Tai CY, Mendel DB. Successful treatment of an acyclovir- and foscarnet- resistant herpes simplex virus type 1 lesion with intravenous cidofovir. *Clin Infect Dis*. 1998;26(2):512.
Ma Y, Xu Y, Cao X, Chen X, Zhong Y. Diagnostic value of interferon-γ release assay in HIV-infected individuals complicated with active tuberculosis: a systematic review and meta-analysis. *Epidemiol Infect*. 2021;149:e204, 1–9.
Makadzange AT, Ndhlovu CE, Takarina K, et al. Early versus delayed initiation of antiretroviral therapy for concurrent HIV infection and cryptococcal meningitis in Sub-Saharan Africa. *Clin Infect Dis*. 2010;50(11):1532–1538.
Martin DF, Parks DJ, Mellow SD, et al. Treatment of cytomegalovirus retinitis with an intraocular sustained-release ganciclovir implant: a randomized controlled clinical trial. *Arch Ophthalmol*. 1994;112(12):1531–1539.
Martin ET, Krantz E, Gottlieb SL, et al. A pooled analysis of the effect of condoms in preventing HSV-2 acquisition. *Arch Intern Med*. 2009;169(13):1233–1240.
Martinson NA, Hoffmann CJ, Chaisson RE. Epidemiology of tuberculosis and HIV. *Proc Am Thorac Soc*. 2011;8:288–293.
Meintjes G, Stek C, Blumenthal L, et al. Prednisone for the prevention of paradoxical tuberculosis-associated IRIS. *N Engl J Med*. 2018;379:1915–1925.
Mfinanga SG, Kirenga BJ, Chanda DM, et al. Early versus delayed initiation of highly active antiretroviral therapy for HIV-positive adults with newly diagnosed pulmonary tuberculosis (TB-HAART): a prospective, international, randomised, placebo-controlled trial. *Lancet Infect Dis*. 2014;14:563–571.
Mohamed AA, Lu XL, Mounmin FA. Diagnosis and treatment of esophageal candidiasis: current updates. *Can J Gastroenterol Hepatol*. 2019;3585136. doi:10.1155/2019/3585136Moon SM, Choe J, Jhun BW, et al. 2019. Treatment with a macrolide-containing regimen for Mycobacterium kansasii pulmonary disease. *Respir Med*. 2019;148:37–42.
Nahid P, Dorman SE, Alipanah N, et al. Official American Thoracic Society/Centers for Disease Control and Prevention/Infectious Diseases Society of America clinical practice guidelines: treatment of drug-susceptible tuberculosis. *Clin Infect Dis*. 2016;63(7):e147–e195. http://doi:10.1093/cid/ciw376.
Nyang'wa B-T, Berry C, Kazounis E, et al. 2022. A 24-week, all-oral regimen for rifampin-resistant tuberculosis. *N Engl J Med*. 2022;387:2331–2343.
Patel P, Bush T, Mayer KH, Desai S, et al. Prevalence and risk factors associated with herpes simplex virus-2 infection in a contemporary cohort of HIV-infected persons in the United States. *Sex Transm Dis*. 2012 Feb;39(2):154–160. doi:10.1097/OLQ.0b013e318239d7fd
Pauk J, Huang ML, Brodie SJ, et al. Mucosal shedding of human herpesvirus 8 in men. *N Engl J Med*. 2000;343(19):1369–1377.
Post MJD, Thurnher MM, Clifford DB, et al. CNS-immune reconstitution inflammatory syndrome in the setting of HIV infection, part 2: discussion of neuro-immune reconstitution inflammatory syndrome with and without other pathogens. *AJNR Am J Neuroradiol*. 2013;34(7):1308–1318.
Richardson EP Jr, Webster HD. Progressive multifocal leukoencephalopathy: its pathological features. *Prog Clin Biol Res*. 1983:105:191–203.
Ryder N, Jin F, McNulty AM et al. Increasing role of herpes simplex virus type 1 in first-episode anogenital herpes in heterosexual women and younger men who have sex with men, 1992–2006. *Sex Transm Infect*. 2009;85(6):416–419.
Safrin S, McKinley G, McKeough M, et al. Treatment of acyclovir-unresponsive cutaneous herpes simplex virus infection with topically applied SP-303. *Antiviral Res*. 1994;25(3–4):185–192.
Santin M, Munoz L, Rigau D. Interferon-γ release assays for the diagnosis of tuberculosis and tuberculosis infection in HIV-infected adults: a systematic review and meta-analysis. *PLoS One*. 2012;7(3):332482.
Sati H, Alastruey-Izquierdo A, Perfect J, et al. HIV and fungal priority pathogens. *Lancet HIV*. 2023;10(11):e750–d754.
Sax PE, Sloan CE, Schackman BR, et al. Early antiretroviral therapy for patients with acute aids-related opportunistic infections: a cost-effectiveness analysis of ACTG A5164. *HIV Clin Trials*. 2010;11(5):248–259.
Schwarcz L, Chen MJ, Vittinghoff E, Hsu L, Schwarcz S. Declining incidence of AIDS-defining opportunistic illnesses: results from 16 years of population-based AIDS surveillance. *AIDS*. 2013 Feb 20;27(4):597–605. doi:10.1097/QAD.0b013e32835b0fa2
Smith DJ, Williams SL, Endemic Mycoses State Partners Group, Benedict KM, Jackson BR, Toda M. Surveillance for coccidioidomycosis, histoplasmosis, and blastomycosis—United States, 2019. *MMWR Surveill Summ*. 2022;71(SS-7):1–14.
Sungkanuparph S, Filler SG, Chetchotisakd P, et al. Cryptococcal immune reconstitution inflammatory syndrome after antiretroviral therapy in AIDS patients with cryptococcal meningitis: a prospective multicenter study. *Clin Infect Dis*. 2009;49(6):931–934.
Swindells S, Ramchandani R, Gupta A, et al. One month of rifapentine plus isoniazid to prevent HIV-related tuberculosis. *N Engl J Med*. 2019;380:1001–1011. http://doi10.1056/NEJMoa1806808
Tan K, Roda R, Ostrow L, et al. PML-IRIS in patients with HIV infection: clinical manifestations and treatment with steroids. *Neurology*. 2009;72(17):1458–1464.

Török ME, Yen NT, Chau TT, Mai NT, et al. Timing of initiation of antiretroviral therapy in human immunodeficiency virus (HIV)–associated tuberculous meningitis. *Clin Infect Dis.* 2011 Jun;52(11):1374–1383. doi:10.1093/cid/cir230
Ude IN, Yeh S, Shantha JG. Cytomegalovirus retinitis in the highly active anti-retroviral therapy era. *Ann Eye Sci.* 2022;7:5. doi:10.21037/aes-21-18
Vidal JE. HIV-related cerebral toxoplasmosis revisited: current concepts and controversies of an old disease. *J Int Assoc Provid AIDS Care.* 2019;18:2325958219867315. doi:10.1177/2325958219867315
Whitcup SM. Cytomegalovirus retinitis in the era of highly active antiretroviral therapy. *JAMA.* 2000;283(5):653–657.
Workowski KA, Bachmann LH, Chan PA, et al. Sexually transmitted infections treatment guidelines, 2021. *MMWR Recomm Rep.* 2021;20(4):1–187.
World Health Organization (WHO). *Fungal Priority Pathogens List to Guide Research, Development and Public Health Action.* Geneva: World Health Organization; 2022. License: CC BY-NC-SA 3.0 IGO. https://www.who.int/publications/i/item/9789240060241. Accessed September 1, 2024.
World Health Organization (WHO). Global tuberculosis report 2023. https://www.who.int/teams/global-tuberculosis-programme/data. Published 2024. Accessed June 22, 2024.
WHO. Tuberculosis factsheet 2023. https://www.who.int/news-room/fact-sheets/detail/tuberculosis. Published 2023. Accessed June 22, 2024.
Xu F, Sternberg MR, Kottiri BJ, McQuillan GM, et al. Trends in herpes simplex virus type 1 and type 2 seroprevalence in the United States. *JAMA.* 2006;296(8):964–73.16926356.
Yudin MH, Kaul R. Progressive hypertrophic genital herpes in an HIV-infected woman despite immune recovery on antiretroviral therapy. *Infect Dis Obstet Gynecol.* 2008;2008:592532. doi:10.1155/2008/592532
Zolopa A, Andersen J, Powderly W, et al. Early antiretroviral therapy reduces AIDS progress/death in individuals with acute opportunistic infections: a multicenter randomized strategy trial. *PLoS One.* 2009;4(5):e5575.

20.

IMMUNE RECONSTITUTION INFLAMMATORY SYNDROME (IRIS)

Dagan Coppock

LEARNING OBJECTIVES

Upon completion of this chapter, the reader should be able to:

- Explain the epidemiology of immune reconstitution inflammatory syndrome (IRIS) and its associated opportunistic infections.
- Recognize timing considerations regarding opportunistic infection (OI) treatment and antiretroviral therapy (ART) initiation as they relate to the risk for IRIS.
- Discuss the management approaches to IRIS, based upon its presentation and the underlying opportunistic infection.
- Review the current status of research and clinical recommendations regarding IRIS.

WHAT'S NEW?

- For individuals starting antiretroviral therapy (ART) after a diagnosis of mpox, early data suggest that IRIS may be a possibility. Despite this possibility, current guidelines recommend early initiation of ART. If treatment for mpox is warranted, treatment should be started concurrently with ART.

KEY POINTS

- IRIS is associated with either worsening of a recognized infection (paradoxical IRIS) or an unrecognized infection (unmasking IRIS), which occurs in the setting of improved immunologic function.
- Most people presenting with IRIS should be maintained on ART, along with treatment for the associated infection.

INTRODUCTION

The hallmark of HIV pathogenesis is the gradual destruction of the cell-mediated immune system over a period of many years, as evidenced by a progressive and profound decline in $CD4^+$ T lymphocytes. This decline leads to increased susceptibility to opportunistic infections (OIs), malignancies, and the development of acquired immunodeficiency syndrome (AIDS). ART can suppress HIV replication, and allows for regeneration of the immune system. Even people with advanced AIDS have a marked improvement in both quantity and quality of their immune system after starting ART. In a subset of people with HIV (PWH) initiating ART, the harmonious, gradual reconstitution of the immune system does not occur; rather, there is a rapid immunologic recovery with an abrupt transition to a pathologic inflammatory state, often causing clinical deterioration. Opportunistic and other infections, previously unrecognized or tolerated by the failing immune system, suddenly become the targets of this overzealous immunologic recovery. In this inflammatory state, people can clinically worsen despite an otherwise excellent response to ART, as evidenced by a decreased viral load and increased $CD4^+$ T-cell counts. This inflammatory response has been termed *immune reconstitution inflammatory syndrome* (IRIS) (French et al., 2004), which is used as an umbrella term encompassing two clinical entities: (1) paradoxical IRIS, an exacerbation of a known OI; and (2) unmasking IRIS, a flare of an undiagnosed (subclinical) OI.

INCIDENCE AND ASSOCIATED OPPORTUNISTIC INFECTIONS

The incidence of IRIS is dependent on the population being studied. It occurs more frequently in persons with specific OIs, a higher HIV viral load, and more significant immunosuppression (Müller et al., 2010). The HIV Outpatient Study—an eight-city, U.S.-wide, prospective cohort study—evaluated 2,610 persons with 370 cases of IRIS (occurring in 276 people) who initiated or resumed ART and, during the next 6 months, demonstrated a decline in plasma HIV ribonucleic acid (RNA) viral load of at least 0.5 $\log_{10}$ copies/mL or an increase of at least 50% in $CD4^+$ T-cell count per microliter. In this cohort, incidence of IRIS was 10.6%, with the most common IRIS-defining diagnoses including candidiasis (23%), cytomegalovirus (CMV) infection (3.5%), disseminated *Mycobacterium avium* intracellular (3.2%), *Pneumocystis* pneumonia (2.7%), *Varicella zoster* (2.4%), Kaposi's sarcoma (KS) (2.4%), non-Hodgkin's lymphoma (2.2%), and *Mycobacterium tuberculosis* (0.3%). IRIS was independently associated with $CD4^+$ T-cell counts of less than 50 cells/mL (versus at least 200 cells/mL, with odds ratio [OR] of 5.0) and a viral load of at least 5.0 $\log_{10}$ copies/

mL (versus less than 4.0 $\log_{10}$ copies/mL, with OR of 2.3) (Novak et al., 2012). In contrast, a study from the University of Washington HIV Cohort demonstrated a higher rate of IRIS in people with KS (29%), with no evident cases in people with CMV disease or *Candida* esophagitis. In this study, the highest IRIS-associated morbidity was in cases of visceral KS. The differences in clinical characteristics between these two studies may reflect population and geographic variability.

IRIS AND ANTIRETROVIRAL THERAPY

In addition to potential demographic factors that might affect the presentation of IRIS, choice of ART regimen may also play a role. The AIDS Clinical Trial Group (ACTG) reported the incidence and associations with IRIS in ACTG 5202, which was a phase 3b, randomized clinical trial conducted in the United States that compared the safety, tolerability, and efficacy of four commonly used, once-daily, initial ART regimens. Two dual nucleoside/nucleotide reverse transcriptase inhibitor fixed-dose combinations (tenofovir disoproxil fumarate/emtricitabine or abacavir/lamivudine) were compared when used in combination with either the non-nucleoside reverse transcriptase inhibitor (NNRTI) efavirenz or a ritonavir-boosted protease inhibitor, atazanavir/ritonavir. Among 1,848 eligible participants who enrolled in this study, IRIS events occurred in 52 participants by week 48, with 4 participants having two events. Incidence rates were 6.05 (95% confidence interval [CI]: 4.57–8.00) and 3.30 (95% CI: 2.51–4.33) cases/100 person-years (py) through 24 and 48 weeks, respectively. IRIS occurred 1–298 days after ART initiation, with 75% of cases occurring within 67 days, and 3 cases after 24 weeks. IRIS events included the following associated OIs or other clinical diagnoses: *Mycobacterium avium* complex (MAC) (n = 11); *Varicella zoster* virus (n = 11); herpes simplex virus (n = 8); KS (n = 5); hepatitis C virus (HCV), tuberculosis (TB), and *Pneumocystis jirovecii* pneumonia (PCP) (n = 4 each); toxoplasmosis and cryptococcosis (n = 2 each); and CMV-associated colitis, progressive multifocal leukoencephalopathy (PML), *Mycobacterium kansasii*, eosinophilic folliculitis, and swollen lymph node (n = 1 each). The most commonly reported symptoms were fever and pain. There were no deaths from IRIS in this cohort. Among participants with IRIS, the median baseline HIV RNA was 4.9 $\log_{10}$ copies/mL, and the median CD4$^+$ T-cell count was 49 cells/mm^3. Fifty percent had prior AIDS-related illnesses. In univariate Cox proportional hazards models, an increased risk of IRIS was associated with baseline prior AIDS-related illness, higher HIV RNA level, lower CD4$^+$ T-cell count and percentage, lower CD8$^+$ T-cell count and higher percentage, and lower CD4$^+$:CD8$^+$ T-cell ratio (all $p \leq 0.01$). No significant association was observed with sex, age, or race/ethnicity ($p > 0.19$). Of note, IRIS events were more common with abacavir/lamivudine relative to tenofovir/emtricitabine for participants with low CD4$^+$ T-cell counts. This finding may reflect the more rapid CD4$^+$ T-cell increases observed with abacavir/lamivudine regimens (Fischl et al., 2010).

Early observational data raised concerns regarding INSTI-based regimens and their associations with IRIS; however, subsequent clinical trial data do not bear out these findings. In a retrospective cohort trial, 2,287 persons with CD4$^+$ T-cell counts below 200/mm^3 were evaluated by ART regimen. Cohorts consisted of participants receiving either INSTI-based or non-INSTI-based ART regimens. The odds ratio for developing IRIS was 1.99 (1.09–3.47) (p = 0.04) for the INSTI-based group (Dutertre et al., 2017). However, a clinical trial that evaluated standard two-nucleoside reverse transcriptase inhibitor/one-non-nucleoside reverse transcriptase inhibitor therapy compared with standard therapy intensified with raltegravir demonstrated no difference in the occurrence of IRIS between groups (86 [9.5%] with standard ART versus 89 [9.9%] among participants with raltegravir-intensified ART, p = 0.79) (Kityo et al., 2019). In a trial that compared efavirenz-based versus dolutegravir-based therapy, there were two reported cases of IRIS (one associated with KS, one associated with pulmonary tuberculosis) in the efavirenz group, while there were no reported cases in the dolutegravir group (NAMSAL, 2019). In summary, although INSTIs do lead to a more rapid reduction in viral load, available trials do not support the concern that they induce IRIS more than non-INSTI-based regimens.

ETIOLOGY AND PATHOGENESIS

Recovery of pathogen-specific T-cell responses and increased production of proinflammatory chemokines and cytokines produced by the innate immune response after commencing ART may contribute to the immunopathogenesis of IRIS. Higher T-cell responses to nonstructural antigens of HCV in enzyme-linked immunosorbent spot assays and higher serum levels of antibodies to a mixture of virus proteins were demonstrated in PWH and HCV coinfection who experienced an increase in serum liver enzyme levels after commencing ART (Cameron et al., 2011). People who develop TB IRIS have lower plasma levels of the chemokine CCL2 before commencing ART (Oliver et al., 2010).

The identification of biomarkers could be used to help diagnose IRIS in the future and predict which persons might be at high risk. A cohort of 45 treatment-naive PWH with baseline CD4$^+$ T-cell counts of 100 cells/μL or less who were started on ART, suppressed HIV RNA to less than 50 copies/mL, and were seen every 1–3 months for 1 year were retrospectively evaluated for suspected or confirmed IRIS. Pre-ART levels of both D-dimer and the inflammatory biomarker C-reactive protein (CRP) were higher in IRIS cases versus controls (Porter et al., 2010). In another study, individuals with elevated baseline levels of CRP and the fibrosis biomarker hyaluronic acid were more likely to progress to AIDS, develop IRIS, or die within the first month after starting ART (Boulware et al., 2011). Large prospective studies to elucidate the predictive and diagnostic values of IRIS biomarkers are needed.

GUIDELINES FOR ART INITIATION

Current U.S. guidelines recommend early initiation of ART with the exception of select clinical scenarios including some OI-related circumstances (DHHS, 2024). For cryptococcal meningitis, the initiation of ART is typically delayed until an individual receives 4–6 weeks of antifungal therapy (DHHS, 2024). For tuberculous meningitis, the DHHS guidelines recommend initiation within 2–8 weeks of initiating tuberculosis treatment, while the Infectious Diseases Society of America guidelines recommend a delay of 8 weeks for all individuals (Nahid, 2016). For pulmonary TB, both guidelines stratify initiation based on CD4 count (Nahid et al., 2016; DHHS, 2024). ART can be initiated within 2 weeks of starting TB treatment for persons with a $CD4^+$ T-cell count less than 50 cells/mm^3, and between 2 and 8 weeks for persons with a $CD4^+$ T-cell count greater than 50 cells/mm^3. The evidence supporting these guidelines, as well as for other OIs, is discussed below.

ART INITIATION AND THE RISK OF NON-TUBERCULOSIS-ASSOCIATED IRIS

The timing of ART initiation and its association with OI-specific IRIS remains a concern for clinicians. In the ACTG 5164 study, 282 participants with an acute OI and a baseline median $CD4^+$ T-cell count of 29 cells/mm^3 were prospectively randomly assigned to immediate (<14 days) versus delayed (>28 days) initiation of ART. In this study, which included participants diagnosed with PCP (63%), cryptococcal meningitis (12%), and bacterial infections (12%), earlier initiation of ART resulted in less progression to AIDS and/or death and no increase in adverse events or loss of virologic response compared to deferred ART. Participants with or on treatment for TB were excluded. Rates of IRIS in this study were low (7%) and did not differ by timing of ART (Zolopa et al., 2009). IRIS was reported in 23 cases and confirmed in 20: 8 participants in the immediate arm and 12 in the deferred arm. There was no evidence of an association of IRIS with the entry OI/bacterial infection: 13 (65%) IRIS cases were in participants with PCP, who comprised 63% of the study population. IRIS developed a median of 33 days (interquartile range 26–72 days) after initiation of ART. There was no significant difference in the frequency of IRIS between participants who received corticosteroids during the treatment of their OI and those who did not receive corticosteroids: 9/150 (6%) versus 11/112 (9.8%), respectively ($p = 0.35$).

In contrast to the above study, early initiation of ART has been demonstrated in clinical trials focusing on cryptococcal meningitis. In a trial of patients treated for cryptococcal meningitis with fluconazole, ART initiation within 72 hours was associated with a higher rate of mortality compared to waiting for at least 10 weeks (Makadzange et al., 2010). A clinical trial conducted in Botswana compared the early (within 7 days) and late (after 28 days) ART initiation in patients being treated for cryptococcal meningitis (Bisson et al., 2013). There was no difference in mortality between the two arms. However, the incidence of IRIS was higher in patients in the early initiation arm. Benefits to delayed initiation were also seen in a study conducted in Uganda and South Africa (Boulware et al., 2014). In this study, patients were randomly assigned to receive ART within 48 hours of assignment or 4 weeks after assignment, and 177 patients underwent assignment after a median of 8 days of amphotericin. The 26-week mortality with early ART initiation was significantly higher than with delayed ART initiation (45% versus 30%; hazard ratio for death 1.73; P = 0.03). Based on the above findings, the DHHS currently recommends delaying ART initiation by 4–6 weeks after starting antifungal treatment.

IRIS related to JC polyomavirus infection remains a clinical challenge, as ART initiation and immune reconstitution are the only available treatment. Prior to ART, JC virus infection led to PML in people with advanced HIV infection. However, approximately 15% of individuals experienced an exacerbation of PML after ART was started (Martin-Blondel et al., 2011). A review of 54 cases of PML IRIS evaluated the mortality of persons as stratified by steroid use. Of the 12 persons receiving steroids and 42 persons not receiving steroids, 5 and 14 died, respectively, suggesting a high mortality of PML IRIS, regardless of steroid use (Tan et al., 2009).

In people coinfected with HIV and viral hepatitis, IRIS is a frequent concern. Up to 25% of PWH and HBV or HCV coinfection experience a flare of hepatitis and/or elevation of serum liver enzyme levels after commencing ART (Cameron et al., 2011; Crane et al., 2009). Hepatitis flares in PWH and HBV coinfection are associated with a higher plasma HBV DNA level before ART (Crane et al., 2009), suggesting that pathogen load is an important determinant of disease. Even when ART with activity against HBV is selected for treatment, HBV IRIS can still occur, complicating the differential of a hepatitis flare (Crane et al., 2008). For individuals who are HBV/HCV-coinfected, the use of direct-acting antivirals (DAAs) for HCV treatment has been associated with HBV reactivation (Bersoff-Matcha et al., 2017). For people who are HIV/HBV/HCV-coinfected, DHHS (2024) guidelines recommend first initiating ART with activity against HBV prior to the initiation of DAAs.

During the 2022 mpox outbreak, 36%–42% of infected individuals were people with HIV (Mitjà et al., 2023c). A case series from that outbreak included data on a population of 382 individuals, known to be living with HIV, with confirmed cases of mpox (Mitjà et al., 2023a, 2023b). IRIS was suspected in 21 of the 85 individuals who were initiated on ART. Of those 21 cases with IRIS, 57% died. DHHS guidelines note that "[d]ata are insufficient to inform recommendations on identification and management of dysregulated immune responses in the setting of mpox infection in people with advanced HIV" (DHHS, 2024, n.p.). For individuals infected with mpox who are not on ART, they recommend initiating ART as soon as possible. For individuals infected with advanced HIV who warrant mpox treatment, they recommend concurrent initiation of mpox treatment and ART.

TUBERCULOSIS-IRIS

For individuals with HIV and TB coinfection, unmasking and paradoxical IRIS can lead to two distinct clinical scenarios. In the context of TB, unmasking IRIS is the development of overt TB in people who initially screened negative for this infection, typically seen within the first 60 days following ART initiation (Dheda et al., 2004; Shelburne et al., 2006). It is thought to be due to an increase in circulating memory T-cells that were sequestered in lymphatic tissue prior to therapy. Alternatively, paradoxical IRIS involves worsening of signs and symptoms of TB in individuals with a known history of TB after they have been started on ART.

The HIV-CAUSAL Collaboration demonstrated that the incidence of TB decreased after ART initiation but not among persons aged older than 50 years or those with a CD4$^+$ T-cell count of less than 50 cells/mm^3. Despite an overall decrease in TB incidence, the increased rate during 3 months of ART suggested unmasking IRIS. This was a multinational cohort study among PWH from high-income countries. Among 65,121 individuals, 712 developed TB during 28 months of median follow-up (incidence, 3.0 cases per 1,000 py). The hazard ratio (HR) for TB for ART versus no ART was 0.56 (95% CI: 0.44–0.72) overall, 1.04 (95% CI: 0.64–1.68) for individuals aged older than 50 years, and 1.46 (95% CI: 0.70–3.04) for people with a CD4$^+$ T-cell count of less than 50 cells/mm^3. Compared with people who had not started ART, HRs differed by time since ART initiation: 1.36 (95% CI: 0.98–1.89) for initiation less than 3 months previously and 0.44 (95% CI: 0.34–0.58) for initiation 3 months or more previously. Compared with people who had not initiated ART, HRs less than 3 months after ART initiation were 0.67 (95% CI: 0.38–1.18), 1.51 (95% CI: 0.98–2.31), and 3.20 (95% CI: 1.34–7.60) for people aged younger than 35 years, 35–50 years, and older than 50 years, respectively, and 2.30 (95% CI: 1.03–5.14) for people with a CD4$^+$ T-cell count of less than 50 cells/mm^3 (HIV-CAUSAL Collaboration, 2012).

In a South African cohort of 498 persons with advanced HIV, symptomatic individuals were screened for TB by chest X-ray and/or sputum examination. People who screened positive were initiated on anti-TB therapy prior to starting ART. Individuals who screened negative and went on to develop unmasking IRIS were found to have significantly elevated levels of interferon-γ (IFN-γ) and CRP at baseline prior to ART compared to non-IRIS, non-TB controls. These results suggest the presence of subclinical TB infection despite negative screening done prior to the initiation of ART (Haddow et al., 2009). Persons who exhibit paradoxical IRIS have been reported to have elevated tuberculin-specific effector memory CD4$^+$ T-cells prior to initiation of ART. Following ART, increased levels of Th1-associated cytokines, IFN-γ, and tumor necrosis factor-α most likely contribute to the overwhelming inflammatory reaction to the TB antigen present (Bourgarit et al., 2009). PWH with latent TB (defined as >5 mm skin test induration or positive IFN-γ release assay and no active disease) are at increased risk for progression to active TB compared to the HIV-negative population. This underscores the need to identify and treat people with latent disease. Active TB in PWH requires immediate treatment. However, defining the optimal timing of ART has been a challenge.

TIMING OF ART WITH TB IRIS

With regard to ART initiation, the incidence of TB IRIS has been evaluated both from the standpoint of interval to initiation as well as baseline CD4$^+$. In general, current DHHS guidelines recommend an early approach to ART initiation. There have been several trials evaluating various approaches to treatment initiation. A few foundational trials are reviewed below.

In the SAPiT trial, there were no differences in rates of AIDS or death between people who started ART within 4 weeks after initiating TB treatment and those who started ART at 8–12 weeks (i.e., within 4 weeks after completing the intensive phase of TB treatment) (Abdool Karim, 2010). However, in people with baseline CD4$^+$ T-cell counts of less than 50 cells/mm^3, the rate of AIDS or death was lower in the earlier therapy group than in the later therapy group (8.5 vs. 26.3 cases per 100 py, a strong trend favoring the earlier treatment arm [p = 0.06]). For all people, regardless of CD4$^+$ T-cell count, earlier therapy was associated with a higher incidence of IRIS and of adverse events that required a switch in antiretroviral drugs compared to those who started therapy later. In this study, 2 deaths were attributed to IRIS.

In the CAMELIA study, people who had CD4$^+$ T-cell counts of less than 200 cells/mm^3 were randomly assigned to initiate ART at 2 or 8 weeks after initiation of TB treatment (Blanc et al., 2011). Study participants had a median CD4$^+$ T-cell count of 25 cells/mm^3 and high rates of disseminated TB disease. ART initiated at 2 weeks resulted in a 38% reduction in mortality (p = 0.006) compared with that of therapy initiated at 8 weeks. A significant reduction in mortality was seen in people with CD4$^+$ T-cell counts of 50 cells/mm^3 or less and in people with CD4$^+$ T-cell counts of 51–200 cells/mm^3. Overall, 6 deaths were associated with TB IRIS.

The ACTG 5221 (STRIDE) trial, a multinational study, randomly assigned ART-naive individuals with confirmed or probable TB and CD4$^+$ T-cell counts of less than 250 cells/mm^3 to earlier (<2 weeks) or later (8–12 weeks) ART (Havlir et al., 2011). At study entry, participants' median CD4$^+$ T-cell count was 77 cells/mm^3. The rates of mortality and AIDS diagnoses were not different between the earlier and later arms, although higher rates of IRIS were seen in the earlier arm. However, a significant reduction in AIDS or death was seen in the subset of people with CD4$^+$ T-cell counts of less than 50 cells/mm^3 who were randomly assigned to the earlier ART arm (p = 0.02).

Though the above studies focus on pulmonary TB, central nervous system TB is seen as a unique entity. A clinical trial conducted in Vietnam explored outcomes in HIV-associated TB meningitis (Török et al., 2018). For the study population, individuals were randomly assigned to ART immediately or 2 months after the initiation of tuberculosis treatment. The investigators found that immediate ART did not improve outcomes. Further, there were significantly more grade 4 adverse events in the immediate initiation ART. Based on this data, the American Thoracic Society/Centers for Disease Control/Infectious Diseases Society of America guidelines support an 8-week delay in ART initiation with TB meningitis (Nahid et al., 2016). However, the DHHS guidelines state that it is unclear if the findings are generalizable to higher-resourced countries and make different recommendations, as below (DHHS, 2024).

Given the above data, DHHS guidelines recommend that, when TB meningitis is not suspected, ART should be initiated within 2 weeks of starting tuberculosis treatment when an individual's $CD4^+$ T-cell count is less than 50 cells/mm^3 and within 2–8 weeks for higher $CD4^+$ counts (DHHS, 2024). However, for individuals with TB meningitis, ART should be delayed until the meningitis is under control and the individual has received at least 2 weeks of TB treatment.

PREVENTION AND TREATMENT OF IRIS

When IRIS occurs, regardless of the OI, ART should be continued (DHHS, 2024). Otherwise, the underlying OI should be treated as soon as possible. Management of IRIS is dependent on the OI in question. For paradoxical TB, both preventive and management strategies have been evaluated. Regarding prevention, a trial was conducted in which PWH (baseline CD4 counts <100 cells/microliter) who were initiating ART and had initiated TB treatment within 30 days were started on either prednisone or placebo (Meintjes et al., 2010; Stek et al., 2018). Those who received prednisone had a lower incidence of TB-associated IRIS. Based on these findings, DHHS guidelines recommend prednisone be offered to individuals with a CD4 count <100 cells/microliter who are within 30 days of initiated TB therapy. For paradoxical TB management, milder disease can be managed symptomatically, while more severe disease should be managed with steroids. In a randomized, double-blind, placebo-controlled trial of prednisone, the combined endpoint of days of hospitalization and outpatient therapeutic procedures was significantly reduced in the intervention arm (Meintjes et al., 2010). However, patients with life-threatening TB-IRIS were excluded.

In other forms of IRIS, corticosteroids are often used, although data are less robust. In MAC-associated IRIS, adjunctive low-dose steroids may be of benefit in people experiencing persistent symptoms (Wormser et al., 1994). While data to support corticosteroid use in cryptococcal meningitis IRIS are sparse, European Confederation of Medical Mycology/International Society for Human and Animal Mycology guidelines suggest considering their use in the setting of increased intracranial pressure when therapeutic lumbar punctures are ineffective (Chang et al., 2024). Corticosteroid or other anti-inflammatory therapies may also be effective for treating some forms of IRIS, such as PML-associated IRIS (Martin-Blondel et al., 2011).

In summary, in unmasking IRIS, management should focus on the diagnosis and treatment of the underlying OI. In paradoxical IRIS, treatment for the OI should be continued and alternate diagnoses should be excluded to ensure the individual is receiving appropriate therapy. IRIS is typically managed supportively. If at all possible, ART should be continued without interruption. In certain conditions, corticosteroids may be used adjunctively to manage IRIS-related symptoms.

REFERENCES

Abdool Karim SS. Timing of initiation of antiretroviral drugs during tuberculosis therapy. *N Engl J Med.* 2010 Feb 5;362(8):697–706.

Bersoff-Matcha SJ, Cao K, et al. Hepatitis B virus reactivation associated with direct-acting antiviral therapy for chronic hepatitis C virus: a review of cases reported to the US Food and Drug Administration adverse event reporting system. *Ann Intern Med.* 2017;166(11):792–798.

Bisson GP, Molefi M, Bellamy S, et al. Early versus delayed antiretroviral therapy and cerebrospinal fluid fungal clearance in adults with HIV and cryptococcal meningitis. *Clin Infect Dis.* 2013;56(8):1165–1173.

Blanc FX, Sok T, Laureillard D, et al. Earlier versus later start of antiretroviral therapy in HIV-infected adults with tuberculosis. *N Engl J Med.* 2011 Oct 20;365(16):1471–1481.

Boulware DR, Hullsiek KH, Puronen CE, et al.; INSIGHT Study Group. Higher levels of CRP, D-dimer, IL-6, and hyaluronic acid before initiation of antiretroviral therapy (ART) are associated with increased risk of AIDS or death. *J Infect Dis.* 2011 Jun 1;203(11):1637–1646.

Boulware DR, Meya DB, Muzoora C, et al. Timing of antiretroviral therapy after diagnosis of cryptococcal meningitis. *N Engl J Med.* 2014;370(26):2487–2498.

Bourgarit A, Carcelain G, Samri A, et al. TB-associated immune restoration syndrome in HIV-1-infected patients involves tuberculin-specific CD4 Th1 cells and can be predicted by KIR-negative gamma delta T cells. Abstract 772. Paper presented at the 16th Conference on Retroviruses and Opportunistic Infections. Montréal, Canada; February 8–11, 2009.

Cameron BA, Emerson CR, Workman C, et al. Alterations in immune function are associated with liver enzyme elevation in HIV and HCV co-infection after commencement of combination antiretroviral therapy. *J Clin Immunol.* 2011;31:1079–1083.

Chang CC, Harrison TS, Bicanic TA et al. Global guideline for the diagnosis and management of cryptococcosis: an initiative of the ECMM and ISHAM in cooperation with the ASM. *Lancet Infect Dis.* 2024;24(8):e495–e512.

Crane M, Matthews G, Lewin SR. Hepatitis virus immune restoration disease of the liver. *Curr Opin HIV AIDS.* 2008;3(4):446–452.

Crane M, Oliver B, Matthews G, et al. Immunopathogenesis of hepatic flare in HIV/hepatitis B virus (HBV)-coinfected individuals after the initiation of HBV-active antiretroviral therapy. *J Infect Dis.* 2009;199:974–981.

Dheda K, Lampe FC, Johnson MA, et al. Outcome of HIV-associated tuberculosis in the era of highly active antiretroviral therapy. *J Infect Dis.* 2004;190(9):1670.

Dutertre M, Cuzin L, Demonchy E, et al. Initiation of antiretroviral therapy containing integrase inhibitors increases the risk of IRIS requiring hospitalization. *JAIDS.* 2017;76(1):e23–e26.

Fischl M, Mollan K, Pahwa S, et al. IRIS among US subjects starting ART in AIDS Clinical Trials Group Study A5202. Abstract 791. Paper presented at the 15th Conference on Retroviruses and Opportunistic Infections. San Francisco, CA; February 16–19, 2010.

French MA, Price P, Stone SF. Immune restoration disease after antiretroviral therapy. *AIDS.* 2004;18:1615–1627.

Haddow L, Borrow P, Dibben O, et al. Cytokine profiles predict unmasking TB immune reconstitution inflammatory syndrome and are associated with unmasking and paradoxical presentations of TB immune reconstitution inflammatory syndrome. Abstract 773. Paper

presented at the 16th Conference on Retroviruses and Opportunistic Infections. Montréal, Canada; February 8–11, 2009.
Havlir DV, Kendall MA, Ive P, et al. Timing of antiretroviral therapy for HIV-1 infection and tuberculosis. *N Engl J Med*. October 20, 2011;365(16):1482–1491.
HIV-CAUSAL Collaboration. Impact of antiretroviral therapy on tuberculosis incidence among HIV-positive patients in high-income countries. *Clin Infect Dis*. May 2012;54(9):1364–1372.
Kityo C, Szubert AJ, Siika A, et al. Raltegravir-intensified initial antiretroviral therapy in advanced HIV disease in Africa: a randomized controlled trial. *PLoS Med*. 2019;15(12):e1002706.
Makadzange AT, Ndhlovu CE, Takarinda K, et al. Early versus delayed initiation of antiretroviral therapy for concurrent HIV infection and cryptococcal meningitis in sub-Saharan Africa. *Clin Infect Dis*. 2010;50:1532–1538.
Martin-Blondel G, Delobel P, Blancher A, et al. Pathogenesis of the immune reconstitution inflammatory syndrome affecting the central nervous system in patients infected with HIV. *Brain*. 2011;134:928–946.
Meintjes G, Wilkinson RJ, Morroni C, et al. Randomized placebo-controlled trial of prednisone for paradoxical tuberculosis-associated immune reconstitution inflammatory syndrome. *AIDS*. 2010 Sep 24;24(15):2381–2390.
Mitjà O, Alemany A, Marks M; SHARE-NET writing group. Mpox in people with advanced HIV infection: a global case series. *Lancet*. 2023a;401(10380):939–949. Erratum in: *Lancet*. 2023b;401(10383):1158.
Mitjà O, Ogoina D, Titanji BK, et al. Monkeypox. *Lancet*. 2023c;401(10370):60–74.
Müller M, Wandel S, Colebunders R, et al. Immune reconstitution inflammatory syndrome in patients starting antiretroviral therapy for HIV infection: a systematic review and meta-analysis. *Lancet Infect Dis*. 2010;10:251–261.
Nahid P, Dorman SE, Alipanah N, et al. Official American Thoracic Society/Centers for Disease Control and Prevention/Infectious Diseases Society of America clinical practice guidelines: treatment of drug-susceptible tuberculosis. *Clin Infect Dis*. 2016;63(7) e147–e195.
NAMSAL ANRS 12313 Study Group. Dultegravir-based or low-dose efavirenz-based regimen for the treatment of HIV-1. *N Engl J Med*. 2019;381(9):816–826.
Novak RM, Richardson JT, Buchacz K, et al.; HIV Outpatient Study (HOPS) Investigators. Immune reconstitution inflammatory syndrome: incidence and implications for mortality. *AIDS*. March 27, 2012;26(6):721–730.
Oliver BG, Elliott JH, Price P, et al. Mediators of innate and adaptive immune responses differentially affect immune restoration disease associated with *Mycobacterium tuberculosis* in HIV patients beginning antiretroviral therapy. *J Infect Dis*. 2010;202:1728–1737.
Porter BO, Ouedraogo GL, Hodge JN, et al. d-Dimer and CRP levels are elevated prior to antiretroviral treatment in patients who develop IRIS. *Clin Immunol*. 2010 Jul;136(1):42–50.
Shelburne SA, Montes M, Hamill RJ. Immune reconstitution inflammatory syndrome: more answers, more questions. *J Antimicrob Chemother*. 2006;57(2):167.
Stek C, Allwood B, Walker NF, et al. The immune mechanisms of lung parenchymal damage in tuberculosis and the role of host-directed therapy. *Front Microbiol*. 2018;9:2603. doi:10.3389/fmicb.2018.02603
Tan K, Roda R, Ostrow L, et al. PML-IRIS in patients with HIV infection: clinical manifestations and treatment with steroids. *Neurology*. 2009;72(17):1458–1464.
U.S. Department of Health and Human Services (DHHS). Guidelines for the prevention and treatment of opportunistic infections in adults and adolescents with HIV. National Institutes of Health, Centers for Disease Control and Prevention, HIV Medicine Association, and Infectious Diseases Society of America. https://clinicalinfo.hiv.gov/en/guidelines/adult-and-adolescent-opportunistic-infection. Published 2024. Accessed August 21, 2024.
Wormser GP, Horowitz H, Dworkin B. Low-dose dexamethasone as adjunctive therapy for disseminated Mycobacterium avium complex infections in AIDS patients. *Antimicrob Agents Chemother*. 1994;38(9):2215–2217.
Zolopa AR, Anderson J, Komarow L, et al. Early antiretroviral therapy reduces AIDS progression/death in individuals with acute opportunistic infections: a multicenter randomized strategy trial. *PLoS One*. 2009;4(5):e5575.

21.

ANTIRETROVIRAL THERAPY FOR CHILDREN AND NEWBORNS

Karin Nielsen-Saines

CHAPTER GOALS

Upon completion of this chapter, the reader should be able to:

- Understand the basics regarding pathogenesis of perinatal HIV transmission and be aware of landmark studies targeting prevention of perinatal HIV transmission.
- Understand the concept of HIV exposure versus HIV infection.
- Comprehend the specific challenges of early HIV diagnosis of infants, understand the importance of timing of transmission for diagnosis and pathogenesis, and become familiar with new breastfeeding guidelines for mothers living with HIV.
- Be aware of the concept of HIV remission in early treated infants.
- Broadly describe the HIV disease course in children and surrogate markers of disease.
- Appreciate specific caveats guiding antiretroviral use in children, particularly in newborns receiving presumptive HIV therapy.

INTRODUCTION

In the absence of interventions to curtail perinatal HIV-1 transmission, HIV-1 infection in children parallels that of mothers of childbearing age. Perinatal transmission accounts for nearly all worldwide cases of pediatric HIV-1 infection today, with the exception of behavioral acquisition among adolescents. It was noted early in the HIV epidemic that perinatal transmission occurs in 25%–30% of cases when there is no maternal antiretroviral (ARV) treatment (Newell, 1991; Scott et al., 1989). When breastfeeding until 12 months of age by untreated mothers is included, transmission risk can be as high as 40%. Infection may be transmitted during pregnancy, at the time of labor and delivery, and via breastfeeding. According to recent global estimates, 84% of 1.2 million pregnant patients living with HIV in 2023 received antiretroviral therapy (ART) to prevent perinatal transmission (WHO, 2024). In the same year, 120,000 children aged 0–14 years were newly infected with HIV, bringing the total number of children aged 0–14 years living with HIV to 1.37 million worldwide (UNICEF, 2024). The annual number of new HIV infections in children has continued to decline. In 2021, the number of new cases in children was 160,000, reflecting a 25% decline over 2 years. The total number of cases in children also declined by 20% over the same period (UNICEF, 2024). Estimates of 120,000 new HIV infections in children in 2023 equate to 329 children infected per day per year.

Further progress was adversely impacted by the COVID-19 pandemic, which stalled preventive efforts across the globe. Although ART can reduce perinatal transmission to less than 1% (Dorenbaum et al., 2002; Flynn et al., 2018; Fowler et al., 2016), failure to diagnose HIV-1 infection in women and/or lack of treatment availability still contribute to ongoing transmissions worldwide. Additionally, management of HIV-1 in children has to include consideration of several factors. These include: early diagnosis of infection, the natural history of HIV-1 infection in children, surrogate markers of disease, suitable pediatric drug formulations, drug metabolism and pharmacokinetics of ARVs, and the general paucity of pediatric treatment data compared to adult data.

LEARNING OBJECTIVES

- Discuss advances in ART for prevention of perinatal HIV transmission, particularly for postexposure infant prophylaxis.
- Review pediatric-specific issues of early HIV diagnosis, timing and pathogenesis of HIV disease, and use of surrogate markers of HIV infection.
- Discuss current guidelines for management of ARVs in children within the context of what drugs to use, when to start, and when to change ART.

WHAT'S NEW?

- All newborns who were exposed perinatally to HIV should receive postpartum antiretroviral (ARV) drugs to reduce the risk of perinatal transmission of HIV.
- Newborn ARV regimens administered at doses that are appropriate for the infant's gestational age should

be initiated as close to the time of birth as possible, preferably within 6 hours of delivery.

- A newborn's ARV regimen should be determined based on maternal and infant factors that influence the risk of perinatal transmission of HIV. The uses of ARV regimens in newborns include the following:
- **ARV prophylaxis**: The administration of one or more ARV drugs to a newborn without documented HIV infection to reduce the risk of perinatal acquisition of HIV.
- **Presumptive HIV therapy**: The administration of a three-drug ARV regimen to newborns who are at highest risk of perinatal acquisition of HIV. Presumptive HIV therapy is intended to be preliminary treatment for a newborn who is later documented to have HIV, but it also serves as prophylaxis against HIV acquisition.
- **HIV therapy**: The administration of a three-drug ARV regimen at treatment doses (antiretroviral therapy [ART]) to newborns with documented HIV infection.
- For newborns at low-risk of perinatal HIV acquisition, U.S. guidelines recommend a 2-week zidovudine (ZDV) ARV regimen for prophylaxis if the newborn is ≥37 weeks gestation and born to a person with HIV who:
  - Is currently receiving and has received at least 10 consecutive weeks of ART during pregnancy; *and*
  - Has achieved and maintained *or* maintained viral suppression (defined as at least two consecutive tests with HIV RNA <50 copies/mL obtained at least 4 weeks apart) for the remainder of the pregnancy; *and*
  - Has a viral load <50 copies/mL at or after 36 weeks; *and*
  - Did not have acute HIV infection during pregnancy; *and*
  - Has reported good ART adherence, and adherence concerns have not been identified.
- Infants born to individuals who do not meet the criteria above or criteria for high risk below but who have a viral load <50 copies/mL at or after 36 weeks gestation should receive ZDV alone for 4–6 weeks.
- Newborns at high risk of perinatal acquisition of HIV should receive presumptive HIV therapy with three-drug regimens administered from birth for 2–6 weeks; if the duration of the three-drug regimen is shorter than 6 weeks, ZDV should be continued alone, to complete a total of 6 weeks of prophylaxis. Newborns at high risk of HIV acquisition include those born to people with HIV who:
  - Have not received antepartum ARV drugs, *or*
  - Have received only intrapartum ARV drugs, *or*
  - Have received antepartum ARV drugs but who did not achieve viral suppression (defined as at least two consecutive tests with HIV RNA level <50 copies/mL obtained at least 4 weeks apart) within 4 weeks of delivery, *or*
  - Had primary or acute HIV infection during pregnancy.
- All premature infants <37 weeks gestation who are not at high risk of perinatal acquisition of HIV should receive ZDV for 4–6 weeks.
- Infants of people who have primary or acute HIV infection while breastfeeding should be managed like infants at high risk of perinatal transmission with presumptive HIV therapy.
- The use of ARV drugs other than ZDV, lamivudine, and nevirapine cannot be recommended for any indication in premature newborns (<37 weeks gestational age) because of the lack of dosing and safety data.
- If an individual presents with unknown HIV status and has a positive expedited HIV test during labor or shortly after delivery, their infant should begin presumptive HIV therapy. If supplemental maternal testing is negative, the infant's ARV regimen should be discontinued.
- People with HIV should receive patient-centered, evidence-based counseling to support shared decision-making about infant feeding.
- Providers with questions about ARV management of perinatal HIV exposure should consult an expert in pediatric HIV infection or the National Perinatal HIV Hotline (1-888-448-8765), which provides free clinical consultation on all aspects of perinatal HIV, including newborn care.
- ART should be initiated immediately in all infants with confirmed HIV infection.
- Pre-pregnancy care should include testing of sexually active women for HIV. All pregnant women should be tested for HIV as early as possible during pregnancy. Partners of pregnant women should be encouraged to undergo HIV testing if their status is unknown.
- HIV testing is recommended for infants and children in foster care and adoptees for whom maternal HIV infection status is unknown.
- HIV antibody tests should not be used in children aged <18 months. For diagnosis of HIV in younger populations, virologic assays such as HIV RNA or HIV DNA nucleic acid tests are recommended. HIV RNA or HIV DNA nucleic acid tests are equally recommended.
- Assays that detect non-B subtype HIV or Group O HIV infections (HIV RNA NAT or a dual-target total DNA/RNA test) are recommended for use in infants born to mothers with known or suspected non-B subtype virus or Group O infections. If a mother of an infant acquired HIV outside of the United States and has had

repeated undetectable HIV RNA by standard testing, consultation with a clinical virologist on more sensitive HIV nucleic acid testing is suggested.

- Initial combination therapy for ARV treatment-naive children includes the use of integrase strand transfer inhibitor (INSTI)-based regimens which include two nucleoside analogue reverse transcriptase inhibitors (NRTIs). BIC/FTC/TAF is now recommended as a preferred INSTI-based regimen for children aged ≥2 years and weighing ≥14 kg who can swallow pills. Children who are unable to swallow pills should use DTG-based regimens with oral suspension formulations. In some circumstances, an ART regimen of two NRTIs plus a non-nucleoside reverse transcriptase inhibitor or a boosted protease inhibitor (PI) as the anchor drug may be indicated for the initial treatment of children. FTC/TAF is recommended as a preferred dual NRTI combination in children and adolescents weighing >14 kg when used with an INSTI or non-nuculeoside reverse transcriptase inhibitor (NNRTI). Abacavir (ABC) plus lamivudine (3TC) or FTC are the preferred dual NRTI combinations in children aged >3 months and is also approved for use in full-term children from the time of birth to 3 months of age. A negative test for the human leukocyte antigen (HLA) B5701 allele should be obtained before ABC initiation, regardless of age. Two-drug ART regimens and drugs such as fostemsavir and ibalizumab are not approved for treatment initiation in children.
- The long-acting injectable regimen CAB/RPV Suspension is recommended for treatment of HIV in children and adolescents aged ≥12 years and weighing ≥35 kg with HIV RNA levels <50 copies/mL on a stable ARV regimen, with no history of treatment failure, and no known or suspected resistance to CAB or RPV. Oral lead-in dosing of CAB and RPV is now an option, rather than a requirement, when starting CAB/RPV Suspension; patients may proceed to CAB/RPV Suspension directly from their current ARV regimen.
- DTG is recommended as a preferred ARV drug throughout pregnancy, and INSTI-based therapy continues to be the ART of choice during pregnancy.

KEY POINTS

- Infants and children with HIV have a different, more progressive disease course as compared to adults, given that early infection leads to sustained, high-magnitude viremia with significant seeding of reservoirs in the first months of life, prior to full maturation of the immune system.
- Early diagnosis of HIV infection is pivotal in the management of infants and prevention of HIV-associated morbidity and mortality.
- The availability of potent pediatric ARV formulations encompassing different classes of drugs for infants and young children with HIV is still limited and needs further development.
- Infant postexposure HIV prophylaxis varies according to the perinatal risk scenario; in some situations, presumptive therapy may be implemented.
- Early ARV treatment (i.e., at the time of diagnosis) is the mainstay of pediatric HIV infection, particularly for infants younger than 12 months of age, and is also highly recommended for older children.
- Early treatment of young infants diagnosed shortly after birth is the best approach to reduce the seeding of viral reservoirs and to potentially attain prolonged periods of HIV remission off ARVs, a strategy evaluated in prospective clinical trials.

ANTIRETROVIRALS FOR HIV-EXPOSED INFANTS

Advances in the delivery of ART in the antepartum, peripartum, and postpartum periods has led to a global decrease in perinatal HIV transmission rates. The U.S. Centers for Disease Control and Prevention (CDC) estimates that the number of infants born annually with HIV in the United States decreased from 1,650 in 1991 to 100–200 in 2004, with 91 cases of HIV diagnosed in children younger than 13 years of age in 2018 and 62 by 2022 (CDC, 2024). Although there has been a dramatic decline in pediatric HIV cases resulting from perinatal transmission in the past two decades, HIV infection of young adults is on the rise, with most new HIV diagnoses in the United States occurring in 25–34-year age group, with the third highest group of new infections occurring in individuals 13–24 years of age (CDC, 2022). These populations are the least likely of any age group to be aware of their infection status, retained in care, or have a suppressed virus load (CDC, 2022). For pediatric cases under 13 years of age, the provision of ARVs to infants born to women with HIV as prophylaxis has been standard of care in the Unites States since 1994, when the results of Pediatric AIDS Clinical Trials Group study 076 were published (Connor et al., 1994). That study demonstrated that zidovudine monotherapy given to the mother starting at 16 weeks gestation, accompanied by an intravenous zidovudine infusion during labor and delivery, followed by zidovudine given 4 times per day to the infant from birth to 6 weeks of age, was highly efficacious in preventing perinatal HIV transmission compared to placebo (8% vs. 25% respectively, p <0.001). In resource rich settings, 2–6 weeks of zidovudine given to the infant initiated at birth (administered at 2 mg/kg per dose 4 times a day or 4 mg/kg per dose twice a day) continues to be standard of care (Ruane et al., 2013). The major toxicities of zidovudine used as infant prophylaxis include anemia and neutropenia; however, these are dose-dependent and self-limiting, tend to occur toward the end of the course of treatment, and rarely require interruption of prophylaxis (Lahoz et al., 2010). In resource-limited settings, single-dose nevirapine to the infant (2 mg/kg) shortly after birth was used for many years as standard of care, following publication of HIVNET 012 (Guay et al., 1999), which documented the efficacy of this approach in reducing perinatal HIV transmission when associated with single-dose nevirapine given to the mother at the time of labor. Nevertheless, this approach induced a large wave of HIV drug resistance in infants who ultimately acquired HIV infection, rendering nevirapine use problematic for early infant treatment strategies in the developing world. Among infants with HIV whose mothers were not treated with ARVs throughout the course of pregnancy (and are therefore at higher risk of HIV acquisition), double ARV prophylaxis initiated within 48 hours of birth with 3 doses of nevirapine in the first week of life concurrently with 6 weeks of zidovudine was shown to be more efficacious for prevention of intrapartum infection than zidovudine alone (Nielsen-Saines et al., 2011). An alternative, equally efficacious regimen was the use of lamivudine and nelfinavir in the first 2 weeks of life concurrent with 6 weeks of zidovudine (Nielsen-Saines et al., 2011). Lopinavir/ritonavir suspension is currently not recommended by the U.S. Food and Drug Administration (FDA) for use in infants younger than 2 weeks of age; however, raltegravir has proven to be highly effective (Clarke et al., 2020). In resource-limited settings, the use of daily nevirapine prophylaxis to HIV-exposed infants up to 6 months of age was shown to be effective and safe in the prevention of postpartum HIV acquisition (Coovadia et al., 2012). Presently, however, most settings in sub-Saharan Africa transitioned to WHO Option B+, which recommends treatment with ART for all women with HIV during pregnancy, lactation, and onward with no further treatment interruption (WHO, 2021).

The selection of ART to reduce perinatal HIV transmission must include consideration of optimal treatment for pregnant women with HIV and balance potential for fetal harm. Maternal factors that should be considered include the mother's viral load, degree of immunosuppression, medications being used to treat comorbid conditions (e.g., tuberculosis, hepatitis C virus), and the potential for inducing HIV drug resistance. Transmission of resistant HIV to infants has been described but is generally an infrequent event (de Lourdes Teixeira et al., 2015; Yeganeh et al., 2018). Other considerations to prevent perinatal HIV transmission include a scheduled delivery to minimize prolonged rupture of membranes, including a recommendation from the American College of Obstetrics for scheduled cesarean section for women with viral loads exceeding HIV RNA levels of 1,000 copies/mL (Committee on Obstetric Practice ACOG, 2001). In a meta-analysis of 15 North American and European cohorts of pregnant women with HIV ($n = 100$), perinatal transmission rates differed by 5% for those with scheduled delivery by cesarean section (transmission rate, 2%) as compared with those with other delivery modes (transmission rate, 7.3%; International Perinatal HIV Group, 1999). Evaluation of the morbidity and mortality related to such scheduled cesarean sections suggests that pregnant women with HIV may have a higher incidence of postpartum hemorrhage with resultant transfusion, sepsis, pneumonia, and death than their pregnant peers without HIV undergoing the same scheduled procedure (odds ratio 1.6) (Louis et al., 2007). Pregnant women with HIV who do not have detectable viral loads should be informed preoperatively of their risk for having morbidity related to cesarean section performed to prevent perinatal HIV transmission. Although intravenous zidovudine was recommended in the past for use throughout labor and delivery, for women with HIV with an undetectable viral load during pregnancy, current recommendations advise continuation of oral ARV regimens throughout labor and delivery without the need for intravenous zidovudine.

DIAGNOSIS

Early diagnosis of HIV-1 infection is crucial for identification of at-risk infants and consequent initiation of treatment. All HIV-1 exposed infants carry maternal HIV-1 antibodies until approximately 15–18 months of age. Thus, early pediatric diagnosis relies on identification of the virus, usually via HIV-1 DNA or RNA PCR techniques. The former measures integrated virus in the host genome, and the latter measures circulating plasma virus. HIV-1 co-culture is not routinely performed because of cost and time, although it is also a reliable diagnostic method. Infants infected in utero usually have positive PCR results within the first 48 hours of birth, while infants infected at the time of labor and delivery may have a negative HIV DNA or RNA PCR result at birth, followed by a positive result 1 week to 2 months following birth (Bryson et al., 1992). Breastfed infants have continuing HIV exposure and thus can develop a positive HIV DNA or RNA PCR result at any time. The risk of transmission by breastfeeding from an untreated mother with HIV is approximately 16% (Fowler and Newell, 2002). After maternal ARV treatment in the postpartum period (regardless of CD4 cell count) became standard of care globally, several studies demonstrated a dramatic decline in the risk of postpartum transmission to around 2% to less than 1% currently (Flynn et al., 2018; Fowler et al., 2016; Marazzi et al., 2007; Marazzi et al., 2009; Marazzi et al., 2010). Repeat PCR testing in the first few months of life is critical for the determination of the timing of infection, with sensitivity of a PCR result reaching 96% by 4 weeks of life in the absence of breastfeeding (Dunn et al., 1992; Nielsen and Bryson, 2000). Infant HIV virologic diagnosis requires serial nucleic acid testing. In many settings, infants are tested within the first 48 hours of life to identify in utero infection. Current guidelines recommend that infants be tested between 14 and 21 days, 1 and 2 months, and 4 and 6 months of life (DHHS Pediatric Panel, 2024).

TIMING OF INFECTION

Acquisition of HIV infection may occur in utero, intrapartum, or through breastfeeding. Even before ARV treatment was recommended for all pregnant women, two-thirds of HIV-exposed infants escaped HIV infection. Approximately 30%–50% of infants who contract HIV infection will acquire it in utero, and 50%–70% will acquire the infection during the intrapartum period (Cao et al., 1997; Dickover et al., 1996; Mayaux et al., 1997). In order to characterize the timing of HIV infection, a working definition was created for acquisition of infection in utero and intrapartum (Bryson et al., 1992). An infant is considered to have in utero infection if virologic tests (HIV DNA or RNA PCR) are positive within 48 hours of life. Due to the risk of presence of maternal blood, umbilical cord blood samples should not be used for diagnostic evaluations. Infants are considered to have intrapartum HIV infection if diagnostic tests within the first 48 hours of life are negative but further virologic testing after 1 week of life is positive. There is evidence that HIV transmission occurs late in pregnancy or at delivery.

Postpartum transmission of HIV via breastfeeding has been an ongoing challenge for perinatal preventive HIV efforts worldwide. HIV can be transmitted as cell-associated or cell-free virus in breast milk (Lyimo et al., 2012). Mastitis, which triggers migration of inflammatory cells, is also a known risk factor for HIV breast-milk transmission (Semrau et al., 2013), as is nonexclusive breastfeeding (Coutsoudis et al., 1999) or the presence of oral thrush in the infant (Read et al., 2009). Longer duration of breastfeeding is also a well-known risk factor for transmission (Becquet et al., 2005), as is maternal primary infection during lactation (Morrison et al., 2015). In areas where safe alternatives to breastfeeding are not available, formula feeding has been shown to be associated with higher morbidity and mortality. Provision of combination ART to lactating people with HIV increases HIV-free survival in infants, with improved infant outcomes in terms of growth and reduced infections (Inter-agency Task Team on the Prevention and Treatment of HIV Infection in Pregnant Women Mothers and Children [IATT], CDC, WHO, and UNICEF, 2015; Marazzi et al., 2007; Marazzi et al., 2009; Marazzi et al., 2010). Successful screening during pregnancy with the availability of ART for pregnant and lactating patients with HIV through the WHO B+ program (WHO, 2021) has decreased early and late postpartum HIV transmission via breastfeeding over time. In patients with $CD4^+$ T-cell counts higher than 350 cells/mm^3 in sub-Saharan Africa, the PROMISE Study observed an in utero transmission rate of HIV at 1 week of age of 0.5% when patients received ART during pregnancy (Fowler et al., 2016). Further follow-up of the same infants revealed very low breastfeeding transmission rates (0.57%) when mothers received ART during lactation or infants received prophylactic infant nevirapine (0.58%) during the first 18 months of life or following cessation of breastfeeding, whichever occurred first (Flynn et al., 2018).

In the United States, the recommendation to completely abstain from breastfeeding by a person living with HIV has been revisited (DHHS Pediatric Panel, 2024). Current guidelines recommend that people with HIV should receive evidence-based, patient-centered counseling to support shared decision-making about infant feeding (DHHS Pediatric Panel, 2024). Counseling about infant feeding should begin prior to conception or as early as possible in pregnancy; information about and plans for infant feeding should be reviewed throughout pregnancy and again after delivery. During counseling, people should be informed that replacement feeding with properly prepared formula or pasteurized donor human milk from a milk bank eliminates the risk of postnatal HIV transmission to the infant. Achieving and maintaining viral suppression through ART use during pregnancy and postpartum decreases breastfeeding transmission risk to less than 1%, but not to zero (DHHS Pediatric Panel, 2024). Therefore, the premise that "U = U" (undetectable = untransmissible) does not apply to breastfeeding transmission. Replacement feeding with formula or banked pasteurized donor human milk is recommended to eliminate the risk of HIV transmission through breastfeeding when people with HIV are not on ART and/or do not have a suppressed viral load during pregnancy (at a minimum throughout the third trimester), as well as at delivery. Individuals with HIV who are on ART with a sustained undetectable viral load and who choose to breastfeed should be supported in this decision, and conversely, those living with HIV who choose to formula feed should also be supported in this decision. If breastfeeding is chosen by a parent living with HIV, exclusive breastfeeding up to 6 months of age is recommended over mixed feeding (i.e., breast milk and formula), acknowledging that there may be intermittent need to give formula (e.g., infant weight loss, milk supply not yet established, mother not having enough stored milk). Solids should be introduced as recommended at 6 months of age, but not before (DHHS Pediatric Panel, 2024). It is important to document sustained viral suppression before delivery and throughout breastfeeding. One approach is to monitor plasma viral load of the parent monthly or every 2 months during breastfeeding (Yusuf et al., 2022).

If a breastfeeding parent develops detectable viremia, guidelines recommend that breastfeeding be temporarily stopped. If a repeat viral load is undetectable, breastfeeding may resume. If the repeat viral load remains detectable, parents should be counseled about the risk of postnatal transmission conferred by ongoing breastfeeding, with guidelines recommending immediate cessation of breastfeeding. Infants with newly identified exposure to breastmilk from a person with viremia should be managed using the ARV prophylaxis approach of an infant identified at high risk of transmission (DHHS Pediatric Panel, 2024). There are no clear guidelines about the use of ARV prophylaxis to infants breastfed by parents with undetectable viremia. Some experts opt to maintain ARV prophylaxis to the infant while breastfeeding is ongoing; management of infants breastfed by individuals living with HIV has been the topic of recent reviews (Abuogi et al., 2024; Boyce et al., 2024).

The timing of HIV-1 infection (in utero vs. intrapartum) is somewhat predictive of the patient's subsequent clinical course (Dickover et al., 1994). Early onset of AIDS-defining conditions was historically more frequently observed in infants who acquired HIV in utero—and sustained early, prolonged elevated HIV RNA levels. However, after early initiation of ART to all infants at the time of diagnosis became standard, these differences in clinical course are no longer observed.

As in adults, prolonged periods of elevated HIV RNA levels are predictive of disease progression. Infants with HIV undergo primary infection, either in utero or shortly after birth. Therefore, they tend to have very elevated virus loads in the first months of life (Figure 21.1).

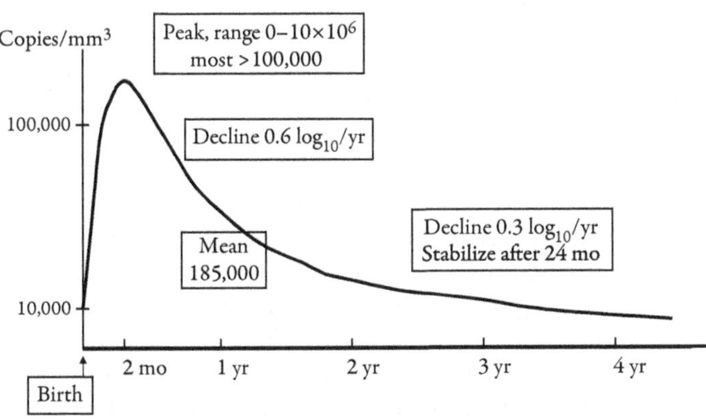

Figure 21.1 Natural course of HIV RNA viremia in children. SOURCE: Figure courtesy of Palumbo PE, based on work from Palumbo PE, et al. JAMA. 1998;279(10):756–761.

MATERNAL RISK FACTORS FOR HIV TRANSMISSION

Maternal risk factors associated with enhanced perinatal HIV transmission include untreated HIV disease; seroconversion during pregnancy or breastfeeding; substance use; heterosexual infection by sexual partners with risk factors for acquiring HIV disease; presence of maternal syphilis (Yeganeh et al., 2015) and other STIs (Adachi et al., 2015; Adachi et al., 2016; Adachi et al., 2018a); risk of CMV transmission (Adachi et al., 2017; Adachi et al., 2018b); and maternal transfusion before 1985. Prospective and retrospective evaluations of maternal predictors for perinatal HIV transmission have been the focus of multiple studies. Maternal transmission predictors identified to date include maternal viremia (measured as quantitative HIV RNA PCR or viral load) (Gabiano et al., 1992; Magder et al., 2005); maternal immunosuppression, inadequate immune response (measured by the $CD4^+$ T-cell count, neutralizing antibody production) (Magder et al., 2005); and viral characteristics (chemokine receptor tropism, HIV drug resistance patterns of maternal virus at delivery or infant virus at birth) (Scarlatti, 2004). Pregnancy and placental variables (e.g., delivery mode, duration of membrane rupture, and chorioamnionitis) may also influence the risk for perinatal HIV transmission (Mwanyumba et al., 2002; St Louis et al., 1993; International Perinatal HIV Group, 1999). Infant variables evaluated as transmission predictors include specific HLA markers and the infant cellular immune response (cytokine production, activated T-cell function) (European Collaborative Study, 1991; Luzuriaga et al., 1991; Magder et al., 2005; Polycarpou et al., 2002). In addition, immunogenetic factors (chemokine coreceptor expression) have been suggested to confer protection against progression of disease (Sei et al., 2001).

EARLY TREATMENT INITIATION AND HIV REMISSION IN HIV-EXPOSED INFANTS

ART given to infants and children suppresses viremia, reduces high infant mortality, and improves clinical outcome; however, children must continue lifelong ARV treatment. The major barrier to achieving HIV remission in children, as in adults, is the early establishment of long-lived latent cellular reservoirs in $CD4^+$ T cells and other sites, with continued low-level replication and rebound viremia once taken off ARTs (Persaud et al., 2012). It is postulated that, through treatment of very early HIV infection, the establishment, quantity, or even elimination of latent reservoirs could be achieved by reducing viral spread into memory $CD4^+$ T-cell reservoirs, which would potentially allow patients to thrive off ARTs without viral rebound, as evidenced by the "Mississippi baby" who remained in ARV-free viral remission for 27 months after early combination ART (Luzuriaga et al., 2015; Persaud et al., 2013; Siliciano and Silicano, 2014). Importantly, there are emerging data that very early therapy during acute HIV infection in both adults and children quantitatively modifies HIV persistence and may influence the rate of reservoir decay. This approach is presently being further evaluated in ongoing clinical trials such as IMPAACT P1115 (Persaud et al., 2024).

DISEASE COURSE

The natural history of pediatric HIV-1 infection is bimodal (Scott, 1991). Studies conducted in developed countries prior to ARV availability demonstrate that approximately 20% of children exhibit very rapid disease progression, with rapid loss of $CD4^+$ T-cell counts and development of AIDS-defining conditions before 2 years of age (Nielsen et al., 1997). The majority of children with HIV (approximately 60%–65%), however, will have intermediate disease progression, with the presence of AIDS-defining events by 7–8 years of age. There is a small subset of children (similar to adults), approximately 15%–20%, who have very slow to no disease progression by age 8 years, and an even smaller set of "elite controllers" (<5%). These children enter adolescence with minimal to no symptoms of HIV disease. Studies conducted in Africa have demonstrated an even faster pace of disease progression, with the majority of pediatric patients having AIDS-defining conditions by age 5 years (Newell et al., 2004). This might be due to the higher overall burden of disease and presence of multiple coinfections. ART makes it possible to alter the natural history of HIV disease and transform disease progressors into nonprogressors. This translates into improvements in quality of life and reductions in HIV-associated disease morbidity and mortality.

Infants with in utero infection appear to have a more rapid disease course when compared to infants who acquire HIV infection intrapartum, prior to the recommendation to initiate combination ART to all infants at the time of early diagnosis. Infants who acquire HIV in utero still have normal $CD4^+$ T-cell values at birth and are usually born with a low virus load (as measured by DNA or RNA PCR) (Dickover et al., 1996; Mayaux et al., 1996). In addition, even those who acquire HIV in utero are asymptomatic at birth. In utero infection appears to result from transplacental passage of virus or ascending viral infection in patients with prolonged rupture of membranes (Minkoff et al., 1995). In animal models, researchers have demonstrated that viral infection of the amniotic fluid with simian immunodeficiency virus resulted in infection of all offspring (Van Rompay et al., 1995). Intrapartum transmission of HIV infection is responsible for the majority of perinatal cases. In a prospective study of 271 infants with HIV using HIV DNA PCR, 38% of children were found to be positive within 48 hours of life; 93% were positive by 14 days of age; and 96% of all infected children were positive by 4 weeks of age (Dunn et al., 1992). There are infants who might not have detectable virus as late as 3 months following delivery in selected cases. Untreated infants tend to maintain a very high virus burden throughout their first year of life, and immunologic patterns of primary viremia in infants have long been described (Luzuriaga et al., 1997). High-level viremia might persist for a longer period of time in infants compared to adults undergoing primary infection; untreated early infection is associated with a high mortality risk (Violari et al., 2008). Prior to the advent of combination ART, discordant twin infections were reported, with the firstborn twin having a higher risk of infection (Duliege et al., 1995).

SURROGATE MARKERS OF DISEASE

The goal of ART is to reduce HIV-1 viral load as much as possible while restoring or preserving immune function. Viral load is generally measured by assays that detect or quantify free virus in plasma, with new-generation assays being able to identify virus isolates of different subtypes. Immune function is measured primarily by evaluating T-cell subsets, particularly $CD4^+$ T-cell absolute numbers and percentages. Declining counts parallel disease progression, with declines in $CD4^+$ T cells usually following peak HIV RNA viremia. One important caveat in the management of children with HIV is that $CD4^+$ T-cell numbers, particularly in infants, differ significantly from adults and do not achieve similar levels until after 5 years. Therefore, an infant with a $CD4^+$ T-cell count of 750 cells/mm^3 or less is at significant risk for the development of AIDS-defining conditions because normal values are generally greater than 2,000 cells/mm^3.

ANTIRETROVIRALS IN CHILDREN

One general principle in the use of ARV therapy is that continued viral replication in the presence of ART promotes development of HIV drug resistance. Resistance to one specific ARV agent may, in turn, confer resistance to other drugs within the same class. Current standard of practice is that, once therapy is started, long-term or lifelong treatment is warranted. In children, the efficacy of ART is often extrapolated from data obtained from adult clinical trials because of the lack of pediatric data. There are, however, significant age-related differences between children and adults. These encompass body composition, renal excretion, liver metabolism, and gastrointestinal function. This leads to differences in drug distribution and metabolism, drug clearance, drug dosing, and different toxicities for children. In addition, protein binding and drug clearance of some specific ARVs may differ by race/ethnicity, owing to the presence of genetic polymorphisms. Nevertheless, often therapeutic doses for infants and children are not available. Liquid or palatable formulations for children do not exist for many ARVs, and adherence depends on adult caretakers. It is crucial when initiating ART to take into consideration the presence of comorbidities and co-medications, and to avoid overlapping drug toxicities (e.g., coexisting tuberculosis or severe malnutrition). Studies have shown a significant benefit of not delaying ART in life-threatening situations such as childhood malnutrition (Buonomo, et al., 2012; Mmbaga et al., 2024; Moramarco et al., 2016). It is also important to consider ARV cross-resistance and future therapeutic options.

GUIDELINES

Treatment guidelines have been developed over the years to address critical concerns about the use of ART in children. Major concerns have always included: optimal timing of ART initiation, preferred ARV choices, efficacy and toxicity monitoring approaches, and when to change therapy. Over time, guidelines in resource-limited and resource-rich settings have converged somewhat. In the United States, traditionally, most children have been treated when identified as having HIV-1 infection, regardless of symptomatology. Given multiple therapeutic options and the general availability of viral load monitoring, guidelines in developed countries over the years have relied on virus load measures for predicting early switches in therapy (DHHS Panel on Antiretroviral Therapy and Medical Management of HIV-Infected Children, 2024). Randomized clinical trials, such as the CHER trial in South Africa, demonstrated that early ART for infants diagnosed before 12 months of age is clearly beneficial in reducing morbidity and mortality (Violari et al., 2008).

Currently, the U.S. pediatric ART guidelines panel has increased the strength of its recommendations for initiating ART in all children at the time of diagnosis, and considers prompt ART initiation a medical emergency (Panel on Antiretroviral Therapy and Medical Management, 2024). Thus, the panel recommends that all children receive ART, regardless of symptoms or $CD4^+$ T-cell count. WHO treatment guidelines for treatment of children with HIV infection also reflect the need for early treatment initiation (WHO, 2021).

TIMING OF INITIATION OF THERAPY

Early versus deferred ART initiation in children with HIV was previously a controversial matter, but this is no longer a subject of debate. It is currently universally accepted in both resource-limited and resource-rich settings that ART should be started at the time of HIV diagnosis in all children, regardless of age. Starting therapy early in asymptomatic children controls viral replication before genetic mutations develop, leading to fewer numbers of circulating viral strains. It also prevents immune system destruction and avoids disease progression, including prevention of establishment of viral reservoirs in the brain. With this strategy, viral seeding of latent cells or CD4⁺ T-cell reservoirs can often be circumvented. Given the significant repercussions to cognitive development when treatment is delayed, there is presently no justification to delay treatment for children with HIV.

CHANGE IN THERAPY

The decision to change ARVs varies slightly according to the pediatric guidelines employed, and variability is mostly due to the surrogate markers used. Nevertheless, most experts agree that indicators of treatment failure include progression of HIV disease, growth failure, development of opportunistic infections while on established therapy, decline in $CD4^+$ percentiles, development of or worsening HIV encephalopathy, and significant increases in virus load. Tolerability, palatability, and drug toxicities are also reasons that ARV regimens are switched in children, as in adults. ARV regimen simplification is recommended whenever possible, as the greatest predictor of achieving an undetectable plasma virus load is medication adherence.

SPECIFIC ANTIRETROVIRAL AGENTS

ARVs currently available for use in the United States are listed in Table 21.1. Optimal ARV combinations for children may differ slightly from that of adults. In infants, particularly those younger than 1 year of age, there is often a need to use very potent ARV regimens for the reduction of persistently elevated viral loads (Luzuriaga et al., 2004; Palumbo et al., 2010). The use of many ARVs is also limited in younger children (especially those younger than 4 years old) because of the lack of liquid formulations, as depicted in Table 21.1. Commonly used pediatric ART regimens include one PI such as ritonavir/lopinavir, or atazanavir or darunavir (in older children) in combination with a double NRTI backbone. The PIs may be substituted with NNRTIs such as nevirapine or efavirenz (EFV) (the latter in older children). Specific ARV regimens to be avoided include any type of mono or dual therapy, and atazanavir without boosting. Treatment guidelines recommend use of integrase inhibitors in children as preferred regimens, contingent on availability of pediatric formulations. Long-acting ARVs such as cabotegravir/rilpivirine have been shown to be very effective in adolescents living with HIV (Gaur et al., 2024; Lowenthal et al., 2024). In resource-limited settings, treatment studies have demonstrated greater durability of viral load suppression in children treated with ritonavir/lopinavir-based regimens versus nevirapine-based regimens, although, interestingly, nevirapine has been shown to be associated with improved growth in this population (Chadwick et al., 2011). Raltegravir and dolutegravir have been increasingly recommended for use in the pediatric population in WHO guidelines and the WHO-led Paediatric Antiretroviral Drug Optimization (PADO) group (Penazzato, 2022; WHO, 2021). Pediatric U.S. guidelines are extensively detailed in the following website: https://clinicalinfo.hiv.gov/en/guidelines/pediatric-arv.

Table 21.1 **ARVS AVAILABLE FOR TREATMENT IN THE UNITED STATES**

NRTIs:	**PIs:**
Zidovudine (ZDV/AZT)[a]	**Ritonavir (RTV)**[a]
Lamivudine (3TC)[a]	**Lopinavir/ritonavir (LPV/r)**[a]
Abacavir (ABC)[a]	**Atazanavir (ATV)**
Tenofovir disoproxil fumarate (TDF)	**Darunavir (DRV)**
Tenofovir alafenamide (TAF)	**Tipranavir (TPV)**
Emtricitabine (FTC)	**Fosamprenavir (FOS)**
NNRTIs:	**Fusion inhibitors:**
Nevirapine (NVP)[a]	**Enfuvirtide (ENF)**
Efavirenz (EFV)	**R-5 receptor inhibitors:**
Etravirine (ETR)	**Maraviroc (MVC)**
Rilpivirine (RPV)	**Attachment inhibitors:**
Doravirine (DOR)	**Fostemsavir (FTR)**
	Post-attachment inhibitors:
Combination ARVs[b]**:**	**Ibalizumab-uiyk (IBA)**
ZDV/3TC	
ZDV/3TC/ABC	**Integrase inhibitors:**
TDF/FTC or TAF/FTC	**Raltegravir (RAL)**
3TC/TDF	**Dolutegravir (DTG)**
ABC/3TC	**Elvitegravir (EVG)**
ABC/DTG/3TC	**Bictegravir (BIC)**
EFV/TDF/FTC	**Cabotegravir (long-acting injectable agent, CAB)**
EFV/3TC/TDF	
FTC/RPV/TDF (or TAF)	**Pharmacokinetic enhancers:**
ATV/cobi	**Ritonavir**
BIC/FTC/TAF	**Cobicistat**
DRV/cobi	
DRV/cobi/FTC/TAF	
DTG/3TC	
DTG/RPV	
DOR/3TC/TDF	
EVG/cobi/FTC/TDF (or TAF)	
LPV/r	
CAB/RPV	
Capsid inhibitors:	
Lenacapavir	

[a] Pediatric formulations available.

[b] Additional formulations such as NVP/ZDV/3TC and NVP/D4T/3TC are available to children in pediatric formulations as generic drugs in resource-limited settings.

TOXICITIES AND ADVERSE EFFECTS

The complications and side effects of specific ARVs are multiple. The most frequent toxicities of zidovudine are hematologic, particularly anemia and neutropenia. These may resolve with dose reduction. All NRTIs may cause some degree of mitochondrial toxicity. Zidovudine may cause myopathy, and peripheral neuropathy is seen with this drug and rarely with 3TC. Abacavir is uncommonly associated with a potentially fatal hypersensitivity reaction, which occurs in 1% of pediatric patients. It manifests as flu-like symptoms with or without a rash, abdominal pain, sore throat, and myalgias. If the drug has been interrupted in this scenario, shock will ensue when restarted. NNRTIs most commonly cause skin rashes (about 40%) and have rarely been associated with Steven-Johnsons syndrome. EFV can induce central nervous system symptoms such as dizziness, insomnia, and nightmares, which have been reported shortly after initiation of treatment with this drug. Previously there was concern about the use of nevirapine during pregnancy in women with $CD4^+$ T-cell counts greater than $250/mm^3$ because of an increased risk of hepatic failure (Hitti et al., 2004), but additional studies failed to demonstrate an association (De Lazzari et al., 2008).

PIs have multiple drug-drug interactions because of their cytochrome P450 metabolism in the liver. Their most common side effects are gastrointestinal symptoms. Hepatitis and hyperbilirubinemia are not uncommon. In adults, they have been shown to induce lipodystrophy, diabetes, and increased atherosclerosis because of lipid abnormalities. These findings are also recognized in children, although clinically significant complications are seen less frequently. There are also recent concerns about the potential for osteopenia and osteoporosis in children, either induced by ART (notably TDF) or HIV disease itself (Mora et al., 2004). With TAF increasingly replacing TDF use, it is likely that concerns for osteopenia in children with HIV will decline over time.

IMMUNE RECONSTITUTION INFLAMMATORY SYNDROME

One recognized potential complication of potent ART is the immune reconstitution inflammatory syndrome (IRIS). This is most frequently observed in people who initiate ART with low $CD4^+$ T-cell counts and is associated with a wide range of reactivation of previously latent pathogens, with tuberculosis being a common underlying condition. The underlying pathogenesis appears to start with unrecognized, low-level colonization of opportunistic pathogens in people who have moderate to severe immunosuppression. With ART initiation and subsequent recovery of immunity to the underlying organism, there is a paradoxical clinical deterioration owing to a dysregulated, overly exuberant immune response. This syndrome usually presents in the first 6 weeks after ART initiation and may resolve either with the use of steroids or temporary ART discontinuation. It is infrequently seen in pediatric HIV practice in developed countries, particularly because children are generally treated earlier. However, it is prevalent in the developing world and may carry high morbidity and mortality. As more children are treated early after diagnosis, it should become an increasingly rare complication of ART use in children.

BENEFITS OF THERAPY

Despite various complications and controversies, the benefits of ART in children with HIV are overwhelming. In the United States, the annual mortality in pediatric HIV patients decreased to less than 1% as of 1999 because of treatment availability (Gortmaker et al., 2001; Jeremy et al., 2005). ART effectively decreases virus load, preserves and restores immune function, decreases the risk of comorbidities, reduces hospitalizations, improves survival, improves quality of life, and restores hope to children and their families. Many perinatally infected children who initiated treatment early in life are now adults with families and children of their own. ART has also changed the AIDS paradigm. As one patient once said, "HIV is no longer a disease you die from, but a disease you live with."

REFERENCES

Abuogi L, Noble L, Smith C, et al.; American Academy of Pediatrics Committee on Pediatric and Adolescent HIV, Section on Breastfeeding. Infant feeding for persons living with and at risk for HIV in the United States: clinical report. *Pediatrics*. 2024;153(6): e2024066843

Adachi K, Klausner JD, Bristow CC, et al.; NICHD HPTN 040 Study Team. Chlamydia and gonorrhea in HIV-infected pregnant women and infant HIV transmission. *Sex Transm Dis*. 2015;42(10):554–565.

Adachi K, Klausner JD, Xu J, et al.; NICHD HPTN 040 Study Team. Chlamydia trachomatis and Neisseria gonorrhoeae in HIV-infected pregnant women and adverse infant outcomes. *Pediatr Infect Dis J*. 2016;35(8):894–900.

Adachi K, Xu J, Ank B, et al.; NICHD HPTN 040 Study Team. Congenital cytomegalovirus and HIV perinatal transmission. *Pediatr Infect Dis J*. 2018b;37(10):1016–1021.

Adachi K, Xu J, Ank B, et al.; NICHD HPTN 040 Study Team. Cytomegalovirus urinary shedding in HIV-infected pregnant women and congenital cytomegalovirus infection. *Clin Infect Dis*. 2017;65(3):405–413.

Adachi K, Xu J, Yeganeh N, et al.; NICHD HPTN 040 Study Team. Combined evaluation of sexually transmitted infections in HIV-infected pregnant women and infant HIV transmission. *PLoS One*. 2018a;13(1):e0189851.

Becquet R, Ekouevi DK, Viho I, et al. Acceptability of exclusive breast-feeding with early cessation to prevent HIV transmission through breast milk, ANRS 1201/1202 ditrame plus, abidjan, Cote d'Ivoire. *J AIDS*. 2005;40(5):600–608.

Boyce TG, Havens PL, Henderson SL, et al. From guidelines to practice: a programmatic model for implementation of the updated infant feeding recommendations for people living with HIV. *J Pediatric Infect Dis Soc*. 2024 Jul 20;13(7):381–385.

Buonomo E, De Luca S, Thembo D, et al. Nutritional rehabilitation of HIV-exposed infants in Malawi: results from the Drug Resources Enhancement Against AIDS and Malnutrition program. *Int J Environ Res Public Health*. **2012**;9(2):421–434.

Bryson YJ, Luzuriaga K, Sullivan JL, et al. Proposed definitions for in utero versus intrapartum transmission of HIV-1. *N Engl J Med*. 1992;327:1246–1247.

Cao Y, Krogstad P, Korber BT, et al. Maternal HIV-1 viral load and vertical transmission of infection: the Ariel Project for the prevention of HIV transmission from mother to infant. *Nat Med*. 1997;3(5):549–552.

Centers for Disease Control and Prevention (CDC). HIV surveillance report: diagnoses, deaths, and prevalence of HIV in the United States and 6 territories and freely associated states, 2022. https://stacks.cdc.

gov/view/cdc/156509. Published May 21, 2024. Accessed August 7, 2024.
CDC. HIV in the US by age. https://www.cdc.gov/hiv/data-research/facts-stats/age.html. Published April 22, 2024. Accessed August 7, 2024.
Chadwick EG, Yogev R, Alvero CG, et al.; International Pediatric Adolescent Clinical Trials Group (IMPAACT) P1030 Team. Long-term outcomes for HIV-infected infants less than 6 months of age at initiation of lopinavir/ritonavir combination antiretroviral therapy. *AIDS*. 2011;25:643–649.
Clarke D, Acost EP, Cababasay M, et al.; International Pediatric Adolescent Clinical Trials Group (IMPAACT) P1110 Team. Raltegravir (RAL) in neonates: dosing, pharmacokinetics (PK), and safety in HIV-1–exposed neonates at risk of infection (IMPAACT P1110). *JAIDS*. 2020; 84:70–77.
Committee on Obstetric Practice. ACOG committee opinion scheduled cesarean delivery and the prevention of vertical transmission of HIV infection: number 234, May 2000 (replaces number 219, August 1999). *Int J Gynaecol Obstet*. 2001;73:279–281.
Connor EM, Sperling RS, Gelber R, et al. Reduction of maternal-infant transmission of human immunodeficiency virus type 1 with zidovudine treatment. Pediatric AIDS Clinical Trials Group Protocol 076 Study Group. *N Engl J Med*. 1994;331(18):1173–1180.
Coovadia HM, Brown ER, Fowler MG, et al.; HPTN 046 Protocol Team. Efficacy and safety of an extended nevirapine regimen in infant children of breastfeeding mothers with HIV-1 infection for prevention of postnatal HIV-1 transmission (HPTN 046): a randomised, double-blind, placebo-controlled trial. *Lancet*. 2012; 379(9812):221–228.
Coutsoudis A, Pillay K, Spooner E, et al. Influence of infant-feeding patterns on early mother-to-child transmission of HIV-1 in Durban, South Africa: a prospective cohort study. South African Vitamin A Study Group. *Lancet*. 1999;354(9177):471–476.
De Lazzari E, León A, Arnaiz JA, et al. Hepatotoxicity of nevirapine in virologically suppressed patients according to gender and CD4 cell counts. *HIV Med*. 2008;9:221–226.
de Lourdes Teixeira M, Nafea S, Yeganeh N, et al. High rates of baseline antiretroviral resistance among HIV-infected pregnant women in an HIV referral centre in Rio de Janeiro, Brazil. *Int J STD AIDS*. 2015 Nov;26(13):922–928.
DHHS. Pediatric Panel on Antiretroviral Therapy and Medical Management of Children Living with HIV. Guidelines for the use of antiretroviral agents in pediatric HIV infection. Department of Health and Human Services. https://clinicalinfo.hiv.gov/en/guidelines/pediatric-arv. Published June 27, 2024. Accessed August 7, 2024.
Dickover RE, Dillon M, Gillette SG, et al. Rapid increases in load of human immunodeficiency virus correlate with early disease progression and loss of CD4 cells in vertically infected infants. *J Infect Dis*. 1994;170:1279–1284.
Dickover RE, Garratty EM, Herman SA, et al. Identification of levels of maternal HIV-1 RNA associated with risk of perinatal transmission. Effect of maternal zidovudine treatment on viral load. *JAMA*. 1996;275(8):599–605.
Dorenbaum A, Cunningham CK, Gelber RD, et al. Two-dose intrapartum/newborn nevirapine and standard antiretroviral therapy to reduce perinatal HIV transmission: a randomized trial. *JAMA*. 2002;288:189–198.
Duliege AM, Amos CI, Felton S, et al. Birth order, delivery route, and concordance in the transmission of human immunodeficiency virus type 1 from mothers to twins. International Registry of HIV-Exposed Twins. *J Pediatr*. 1995;126:625–632.
Dunn DT, Newell ML, Ades AE, et al. Risk of human immunodeficiency virus type 1 transmission through breastfeeding. *Lancet*. 1992;340:585–588.
European Collaborative Study. Children born to women with HIV-1 infection: natural history and risk of transmission. *Lancet*. 1991;337:253–260.
Flynn PM, Taha TE, Cababasay M, et al. Prevention of HIV-1 transmission through breastfeeding: efficacy and safety of maternal antiretroviral therapy versus infant nevirapine prophylaxis for duration of breastfeeding in HIV-1-infected women with high CD4 cell count (IMPAACT PROMISE): a randomized, open-label, clinical trial. *J AIDS*. April 1, 2018;77(4):383–392.
Fowler MG, Newell ML. Breastfeeding and HIV-1 transmission in resource-limited settings. *J AIDS*. 2002;30:230–239.
Fowler MG, Qin M, Fiscus SA, et al. Benefits and risks of antiretroviral therapy for perinatal HIV prevention. *N Engl J Med*. 2016;375(18):1726–1737.
Gabiano C, Tovo PA, de Martino M, et al. Mother-to-child transmission of human immunodeficiency virus type 1: risk of infection and correlates of transmission. *Pediatrics*. 1992;90:369–374.
Gaur AH, Capparelli EV, Calabrese K, et al. IMPAACT 2017 Collaborators; IMPAACT 2017 Team. Safety and pharmacokinetics of oral and long-acting injectable cabotegravir or long-acting injectable rilpivirine in virologically suppressed adolescents with HIV (IMPAACT 2017/MOCHA): a phase 1/2, multicentre, open-label, non-comparative, dose-finding study. *Lancet HIV*. 2024;11(4):e211–e221.
Gortmaker SL, Hughes M, Cervia J, et al.; Pediatric AIDS Clinical Trials Group Protocol 219 Team. Effect of combination therapy including protease inhibitors on mortality among children and adolescents infected with HIV-1. *N Engl J Med*. 2001;345(21):1522–1528.
Guay LA, Musoke P, Fleming T, et al. Intrapartum and neonatal single-dose nevirapine compared with zidovudine for prevention of mother-to-child transmission of HIV-1 in Kampala, Uganda: HIVNET 012 randomised trial. *Lancet*. 1999;354(9181):795–802.
Hitti J, Frenkel LM, Stek AM, et al.; PACTG 1022 Study Team. Maternal toxicity with continuous nevirapine in pregnancy: results from PACTG 1022. *J AIDS*. 2004;36:772–776.
Inter-agency Task Team on the Prevention and Treatment of HIV Infection in Pregnant Women Mothers and Children (IATT), CDC, WHO, and UNICEF. Monitoring and evaluation framework for antiretroviral treatment for pregnant and breastfeeding women living with HIV and their infants. https://www.childrenandaids.org/sites/default/files/2017-05/IATT-Framework-Monitoring-Evaluation-Framework-for-ART-Treat.pdf. Published 2015. Accessed February 2, 2025.
International Perinatal HIV Group. The mode of delivery and the risk of vertical transmission of human immunodeficiency virus type 1: a meta-analysis of 15 prospective cohort studies. *N Engl J Med*. 1999;340(13):977–987.
Jeremy RJ, Kim S, Nozyce M, et al.; Pediatric AIDS Clinical Trials Group (PACTG) 338 & 377 Study Teams. Neuropsychological functioning and viral load in stable antiretroviral therapy-experienced HIV-infected children. *Pediatrics*. 2005;115:380–387.
Lahoz R, Noguera A, Rovira N, et al. Antiretroviral-related hematologic short-term toxicity in healthy infants: implications of the new neonatal 4-week zidovudine regimen. *Ped Inf Dis J*. 2010;29(4):376–379.
Louis J, Landon MB, Gersnoviez RJ, et al. Perioperative morbidity and mortality among human immunodeficiency virus infected women undergoing cesarean delivery. *Obstet Gynecol*. 2007;110(2 Pt 1):385–390.
Lowenthal ED, Chapman J, Ohrenschall R, et al.; IMPAACT 2017 Collaborators; IMPAACT 2017 Team. Acceptability and tolerability of long-acting injectable cabotegravir or rilpivirine in the first cohort of virologically suppressed adolescents living with HIV (IMPAACT 2017/MOCHA): a secondary analysis of a phase 1/2, multicentre, open-label, non-comparative dose-finding study. *Lancet HIV*. 2024;11(4):e222–e232.
Luzuriaga K, Bryson Y, Krogstad P, et al. Combination treatment with zidovudine, didanosine, and nevirapine in infants with human immunodeficiency virus type 1 infection. *N Engl J Med*. 1997;336:1343–1349.
Luzuriaga K, Gay H, Ziemniak C, et al. Viremic relapse after HIV-1 remission in a perinatally infected child. *N Engl J Med*. 2015;372:786–788.
Luzuriaga K, Koup RA, Pikora CA, et al. Deficient human immunodeficiency virus type 1-specific cytotoxic T cell responses in vertically infected children. *J Pediatr*. 1991;119:230–236.

Luzuriaga K, McManus M, Mofenson L, et al.; PACTG 356 Investigators. A trial of three antiretroviral regimens in HIV-1-infected children. *N Engl J Med.* 2004; 350(24):2471–2480.

Lyimo MA, Mosi MN, Housman ML, et al. Breast milk from Tanzanian women has divergent effects on cell-free and cell-associated HIV-1 infection in vitro. *PLoS One.* 2012;7(8):e43815.

Magder LS, Mofenson L, Paul ME, et al. Risk factors for in utero and intrapartum transmission of HIV. *J AIDS.* 2005;38:87–95.

Marazzi CM, Germano P, Liotta G, et al. Implementing anti-retroviral triple therapy to prevent HIV mother-to-child transmission: a public health approach in resource-limited settings. *Eur J Pediatr.* 2007;166(12):1305–1307.

Marazzi MC, Liotta G, Nielsen-Saines K, et al. Extended antenatal antiretroviral use correlates with improved infant outcomes throughout the first year of life. *AIDS.* 2010;24(18):2819–2826.

Marazzi MC, Nielsen-Saines K, Buonomo E, et al. Increased infant human immunodeficiency virus-type one free survival at one year of age in sub-Saharan Africa with maternal use of highly active antiretroviral therapy during breast-feeding. *Ped Inf Dis J.* 2009;28(6):483–487.

Mayaux MJ, Burgard M, Teglas JP, et al. Neonatal characteristics in rapidly progressive perinatally acquired HIV-1 disease. The French Pediatric HIV Infection Study Group. *JAMA.* 1996;275:606–610.

Mayaux MJ, Dussaix E, Isopet J, et al. Maternal virus load during pregnancy and mother-to-child transmission of human immunodeficiency virus type 1: the French perinatal cohort studies. SEROGEST cohort group. *J Infect Dis.* 1997;175(1):172–175.

Minkoff H, Burns DN, Landesman S, et al. The relationship of the duration of ruptured membranes to vertical transmission of human immunodeficiency virus. *Am J Obstet Gynecol.* 1995;173:585–589.

Mmbaga BT, Ngocho JS, Tierney C, et al. Effects of combination antiretroviral therapy and nutritional rehabilitation on growth in children aged 6–36 months with severe acute malnutrition in IMPAACT protocol P1092. *J Pediatric Infect Dis Soc.* 2024;29:piae053.

Mora S, Zamproni I, Beccio S, et al. Longitudinal changes of bone mineral density and metabolism in antiretroviral-treated human immunodeficiency virus-infected children. *J Clin Endocrinol Metab.* 2004;89:24–28.

Moramarco S, Amerio G, Ciarlantini C, et al. Community-based management of child malnutrition in Zambia: HIV/AIDS infection and other risk factors on child survival. *Int J Environ Res Public Health.* **2016**;13(7):666. doi:10.3390/ijerph13070666

Morrison S, John-Stewart G, Egessa JJ, et al. Rapid antiretroviral therapy initiation for women in an HIV-1 prevention clinical trial experiencing primary HIV-1 infection during pregnancy or breastfeeding. *PLoS One.* 2015;10(10):e0140773.

Mwanyumba F, Gaillard P, Inion I, et al. Placental inflammation and perinatal transmission of HIV-1. *J AIDS.* 2002;29:262–269.

Newell ML. The natural history of vertically acquired HIV infection. The European Collaborative Study. *J Perinat Med.* 1991;19(Suppl 1):257–262.

Newell ML, Coovadia H, Cortina-Borja M, et al.; Ghent International AIDS Society (IAS) Working Group on HIV Infection in Women and Children. Mortality of infected and uninfected infants born to HIV-infected mothers in Africa: a pooled analysis. *Lancet.* 2004;364:1236–1243.

Nielsen K, Bryson YJ. Diagnosis of HIV infection in children. *Pediatr Clin N Am.* 2000;47:39–63.

Nielsen K, McSherry G, Petru A, et al. A descriptive survey of pediatric human immunodeficiency virus-infected long-term survivors. *Pediatrics.* 1997;99:pe4.

Nielsen-Saines K, Watts DH, Veloso VG, et al.; for the NICHD HPTN 040/ PACTG 1043 Protocol Team. Phase III randomized trial of the safety and efficacy of three neonatal antiretroviral regimens for prevention of intrapartum HIV-1 transmission (NICHD HPTN 040/ PACTG 1043). Late Breaker Abstract 124LB. Presented at the 18th Conference on Retroviruses and Opportunistic Infections. Boston, MA; February 27–March 2, 2011.

Palumbo P, Lindsey JC, Hughes MD, et al. Antiretroviral treatment for children with peripartum nevirapine exposure. *N Engl J Med.* 2010;363:1510–1520.

Palumbo PE, Raskino C, Fiscus S, et al. Predictive value of quantitative plasma HIV RNA and CD4\+ lymphocyte count in HIV-infected infants and children. *JAMA.* 1998;279:756–761.

Penazzato M, Townsend CL, Sam-Agudu NA, et al. Advancing the prevention and treatment of HIV in children: priorities for research and development. *Lancet HIV.* 2022;9(9):e658–e666.

Persaud D, Bryson Y, Nelson BS, et al. HIV-1 reservoir size after neonatal antiretroviral therapy and the potential to evaluate antiretroviral-therapy-free remission (IMPAACT P1115): a phase 1/2 proof-of-concept study. *Lancet HIV.* 2024 Jan;11(1):e20–e30.

Persaud D, Gay G, Ziemniak C, et al. Absence of detectable HIV-1 viremia after treatment cessation in an infant. *N Engl J Med.* 2013;369:1828–1835.

Persaud D, Palumbo PE, Ziemniak C, et al. Dynamics of the resting CD4\+ T cell latent HIV reservoir in infants initiating highly active antiretroviral therapy less than six months of age. *AIDS.* 2012 Jul 31;26(12):1483–1490.

Polycarpou A, Ntais C, Korber BT, et al. Association between maternal and infant class I and II HLA alleles and of their concordance with the risk of perinatal HIV type 1 transmission. *AIDS Res Hum Retroviruses.* 2002;18:741–746.

Read JS, Mwatha A, Richardson B, et al. Primary HIV-1 infection among infants in sub-Saharan Africa: HPTN 024. *J AIDS.* 2009;51(3):317–322.

Ruane PJ, DeJesus E, Berger D, et al. Antiviral activity, safety, and pharmacokinetics/pharmacodynamics of tenofovir alafenamide as 10-day monotherapy in HIV-1-positive adults. *J AIDS.* 2013;63(4):449–455.

Scarlatti G. Mother-to-child transmission of HIV-1: advances and controversies of the twentieth centuries. *AIDS Rev.* 2004;6:67–78.

Scott GB. HIV infection in children: clinical features and management. *J AIDS.* 1991;4:109–115.

Scott GB, Hutto C, Makuch RW, et al. Survival in children with perinatally acquired human immunodeficiency virus type 1 infection. *N Engl J Med.* 1989;321:1791–1796.

Sei S, Boler AM, Nguyen GT, et al. Protective effect of CCR5 delta 32 heterozygosity is restricted by SDF-1 genotype in children with HIV-1 infection. *AIDS.* 2001;15:1343–1352.

Semrau K, Kuhn L, Brooks DR, et al. Dynamics of breast milk HIV-1 RNA with unilateral mastitis or abscess. *J AIDS.* 2013;62(3):348–355.

Siliciano JD, Siliciano RF. Recent developments in the search for a cure for HIV-1 infections: targeting the latent reservoir for HIV-1. *J Allergy Clin Immunol.* 2014;134:12–19.

St Louis ME, Kamenga M, Brown C, et al. Risk for perinatal HIV-1 transmission according to maternal immunologic, virologic, and placental factors. *JAMA.* 1993;269:2853–2859.

UNICEF. HIV statistics: global and regional trends. https://data.unicef.org/topic/hivaids/global-regional-trends/. Published July 2024. Accessed August 7, 2024.

Van Rompay KK, Otsyula MG, Marthas ML, et al. Immediate zidovudine treatment protects simian immunodeficiency virus-infected newborn macaques against rapid onset of AIDS. *Antimicrob Agents Chemother.* 1995;39:125–131.

Violari A, Cotton MF, Gibb DM, et al.; CHER Study Team. Early antiretroviral therapy and mortality among HIV-infected infants. *N Engl J Med.* 2008;359:2233–2244.

World Health Organization (WHO). HIV: estimated percentage of pregnant women living with HIV who received antiretrovirals for preventing mother-to-child transmission. https://www.who.int/data/gho/data/indicators/indicator-details/GHO/estimated-percentage-of-pregnant-women-living-with-hiv-who-received-antiretrovirals-for-preventing-mother-to-child-transmission. Published July 22, 2024. Accessed August 7, 2024.

World Health Organization (WHO). Priorities for antiretroviral drug optimization in adults and children: report of a CADO, PADO and HIVResNeT joint meeting, 27 September–15 October 2021. https://iris.who.int/bitstream/handle/10665/360543/9789240053038-eng.pdf?sequence=1. Published 2021. Accessed August 7, 2024.

Yeganeh N, Kerin T, Ank B, et al. HIV antiretroviral resistance and transmission in mother-infant pairs enrolled in a large perinatal study. *Clin Inf Dis.* 2018;66(11):1770–1777.

Yeganeh N, Watts HD, Camarca M, et al. Syphilis in HIV-infected mothers and infants: results from the NICHD/HPTN 040 study. *Pediatr Infect Dis J.* 2015;34(3):e52–e57.

Yusuf HE, Knott-Grasso MA, Anderson J, et al. Experience and outcomes of breastfed infants of women living with HIV in the United States: findings from a single-center breastfeeding support initiative. *J Pediatric Infect Dis Soc.* 2022;11(1):24–27.

22.

SELECT TOPICS IN THE CARE OF CISGENDER WOMEN WITH HIV

Aasith Villavicencio Paz, Jillian T. Baron, Christina E. Maguire, and William R. Short

CONTRACEPTION AND PRE-PREGNANCY CARE

LEARNING OBJECTIVE

Discuss family planning and pre-pregnancy care considerations in serodifferent couples with HIV.

WHAT'S NEW?

- While this chapter is focused on the care of cisgender women, many of these topics, including contraception and pre-pregnancy care, relate to transgender and gender-diverse individuals. In recognition of that, gender-inclusive language is used as much as possible. When reviewing data, results are discussed using gender-specific terminology as used by the publications. More research is needed on epidemiologic trends and pre-pregnancy care specific to transgender and gender-diverse individuals.
- Infant feeding guidance has been updated to reflect the most recent U.S. Department of Health and Human Services (DHHS) guidelines and Clinical Reports from the American Academy of Pediatrics. Evidence-based, culturally sensitive, patient- and family-centered counseling on infant feeding is recommended for all people with HIV. All providers (adult and pediatric) should utilize a nonjudgmental, supportive, harm-reduction approach when caring for people with HIV without sustained viral suppression on ART who desire to breastfeed.

KEY POINTS

- Healthcare providers should be proactive in addressing issues related to pre-pregnancy care and contraception among individuals with HIV who are of childbearing potential.
- People with HIV (PWH) should strive to achieve long-term, maximal suppression of viral load prior to attempts at conception. New recommendations address situations in which maximal suppression has been achieved, has not been achieved, or is unknown in serodifferent couples.
- HIV infection does not preclude the use of any methods of hormonal contraception; however, providers must be aware of potential drug-drug interactions between hormonal contraceptive methods and ART.
- Emergency contraception should be offered to individuals with HIV when clinically appropriate. Drug-drug interactions must be considered when using hormonal emergency contraception in combination with ART.

Females (sex assigned at birth) account for approximately 22% of persons with HIV aged 13 years and older, and 19% of new HIV diagnoses in the United States in 2022 (CDC, 2024a). This supports continued emphasis on family planning and pre-pregnancy care. The goals of family planning and pre-pregnancy care are to promote conception planning, reduce unintended pregnancy, and support safer conception and pregnancy for the pregnant individual, fetus/infant, and partner. All individuals of childbearing age and potential with HIV should be offered comprehensive family planning and pre-pregnancy care as part of routine primary care (ACOG, 2019).

THE IMPORTANCE OF FAMILY PLANNING AND PRE-PREGNANCY CARE

It is increasingly important for all healthcare providers to be proactive in identifying and addressing issues related to pre-pregnancy care and contraception for PWH who are of childbearing age. In areas where ARVs are widely available and accessible, HIV has become a chronic disease with life expectancy comparable to that of persons without HIV (van Sighem et al., 2010). In the United States, perinatal transmission rates of HIV have been reduced to less than 1%, resulting in an overall rate of perinatally acquired HIV of 1.1 per 100,000 live births in 2022. Nevertheless, important disparities persist: among Black individuals with HIV, the rate is 5.5 per 100,000 (CDC, 2024b). Many studies demonstrate that fertility desires in women with HIV are very similar to those in women without HIV (Finocchario-Kessler et al., 2012; Loutfy et al., 2009; Nattabi et al., 2009; Squires et al., 2011). In the Women's Interagency HIV Study cohort, there was a 150% increase in live birth rates among women with HIV in the ART era when compared to the pre-ART era (Sharma et al., 2007). Current estimates indicate that 5,000 women with HIV give birth annually in the United States (Nesheim et al., 2018).

Studies among women with HIV suggest that unintended pregnancies are approximately 50% or higher (Loutfy et al., 2009; Massad et al., 2004; Sutton et al., 2018). Many pregnancies among women with HIV occur despite the use of contraception (Massad et al., 2004), implying that pregnancies may have been unintended; this highlights the importance of routine contraceptive counseling. Unplanned pregnancy rates among women with HIV have been reported to be as high as 78% (Sutton et al., 2018). Women with unplanned pregnancies are less likely to have received OB/GYN care in the past year (Sutton et al., 2018). Additionally, research shows that contraception is underused despite women with HIV often wishing to discuss their reproductive plans with healthcare providers (Hoyt et al., 2012).

PRE-PREGNANCY COUNSELING FOR PERSONS OF CHILDBEARING POTENTIAL WITH HIV

Childbearing desires and plans may change over time, including the preferred timing of pregnancy, and therefore these areas should be assessed throughout the course of a person's HIV care, including during initial evaluations and regularly thereafter. Providers should be the ones to start these conversations (DHHS, 2024b). A comprehensive HIV, medical, and OB/GYN history and an understanding of patient goals are important areas to focus counseling and assist in shared decision-making. Individuals who wish to prevent or delay pregnancy should receive information about contraception options and effectiveness, adverse effects, and other advantages or disadvantages (e.g., like non-contraceptive benefits as well as drug interactions with ART or other medications). Routine primary care, including promoting healthy weight and diet and screening for substance use, should also be addressed.

PWH should be given information about the risk, rates, and prevention of perinatal transmission and the potential effects of HIV and ART on pregnancy course and outcomes. For couples in serodifferent relationships, PWH should be counseled about the benefits of ART in reducing sexual HIV transmission (Cohen et al., 2016). Disclosure and knowledge of HIV status for both partners are particularly important when conception is planned and should be encouraged and supported if considered safe. It is also important to reinforce to patients that nondisclosure may have legal ramifications in certain jurisdictions. Knowledge of applicable HIV disclosure laws may therefore be particularly useful when counseling patients about these concerns.

CARE FOR INDIVIDUALS WISHING TO PREVENT OR DELAY PREGNANCY

PWH and those who may have frequent "high-risk" exposures to HIV should receive counseling and have access to all contraceptive methods, including emergency contraception (pills or IUD) when needed, as affirmed by an expert panel from the Centers for Disease Control and Prevention (CDC) adopting the 2019 World Health Organization (WHO) guidelines (Tepper et al., 2020; WHO, 2019). Special care must be taken to address any potential drug-drug interactions with ART (Robinson et al., 2012), which also applies to antiretrovirals (ARVs) used as pre- and postexposure prophylaxis (PrEP and PEP). The ECHO trial, which showed no significant difference in HIV acquisition risk among 7,715 women using intramuscular depot medroxyprogesterone acetate, copper intrauterine device (IUD), or levonorgestrel implants (ECHO Trial Consortium, 2019), was the most relevant data that informed 2019 WHO guidelines which recommended increased access to contraception in populations deemed at risk for HIV.

Both the copper IUD (Cu-IUD) and levonorgestrel-containing IUD can be initiated or continued in people with HIV who are clinically stable and doing well on ART. Pharmacokinetic interactions between hormonal contraceptives (primarily studied with combined estrogen-progestin oral contraceptives) and some protease inhibitors (PIs) and non-nucleoside reverse transcriptase inhibitors (NNRTIs) may potentially decrease contraceptive effectiveness or increase the risk of adverse effects, specifically efavirenz (Landolt et al., 2013; Patel et al., 2015) or darunavir/ritonavir (Sekar et al., 2008). Although the true clinical effect is not clear, an additional or alternative contraceptive method is generally advised if hormonal contraception is considered while on efavirenz or darunavir/ritonavir (DHHS 2024b). Oral contraceptives have also been linked to lower peak concentrations of the long-acting injectable cabotegravir (CAB-LA), which has not been deemed clinically relevant, as other pharmacokinetic parameters remain unchanged (Blairet al., 2020). For a detailed list of contraceptive drugs and their potential interactions with specific ARVs, current DHHS guidelines include a table labeled "Drug Interactions Between Antiretroviral Agents and Hormonal Contraceptives" in the section on "Prepregnancy Counseling and Care for People of Childbearing Age with HIV" (DHHS, 2024).

The WHO and CDC state that with the use of contraceptive methods involving spermicides containing nonoxynol-9, the risks generally outweigh the advantages because of the potential disruption of cervical mucosa, which may increase viral shedding and HIV transmission to the seronegative partners (Tepper et al., 2020; WHO, 2019).

Emergency contraception, including emergency oral contraceptives or the copper IUD, should be offered to individuals with HIV if clinically appropriate. When oral contraceptives (either combination or levonorgestrel only) are used with ARVs, the potential for drug interactions seems to be similar to when they are used for routine contraception (DHHS, 2024b). In PWH taking efavirenz, the emergency dose of levonorgestrel should be doubled to improve pharmacokinetics in the setting of that drug-drug interaction and increase the exposure time to levonorgestrel (Scarsi et al., 2023). Currently, although no clinical data are available on interactions between ART and ulipristal acetate, they are anticipated based on the metabolism of the latter through the CYP3A4 pathway (DHHS, 2024b; Krishna et al., 2020).

Regardless of which hormonal contraception choice is made, family planning conversations should include counseling on further HIV prevention with PrEP and PEP, condoms, as well as the prevention, testing, and treatment of sexually transmitted infections (STIs).

CARE FOR INDIVIDUALS WITH HIV WANTING TO BECOME PREGNANT

Interventions recommended by the DHHS guidelines for individuals who want to become pregnant include the following:

- Overall health should be optimized, with attention to standard primary care and optimal management of chronic diseases as well as substance (including tobacco and alcohol) use.
- Benefits of smoking cessation and the elimination of other drugs and alcohol for pregnant individuals and developing fetuses should be reviewed, and referrals to cessation/treatment services should be offered.
- All current medications, including prescription, over-the-counter, and complementary/alternative medications, should be reviewed, and potential adverse effects in pregnancy should be assessed.
- The need to initiate or modify an ART regimen should be evaluated for all individuals with HIV prior to conception. For individuals on ART, a stable and maximally suppressed viral load should be achieved prior to conception. ART selection should take into account current treatment guidelines, what is known about the use of specific drugs in pregnancy, and the risk of teratogenicity or other adverse effects. Regularly updated guidelines for HIV monitoring and ART management during conception and the prenatal period are available at https://clinicalinfo.hiv.gov/guidelines/perinatal.
- Both partners should be screened for genital tract infections, and these should be treated if present. Genital tract inflammation is associated with shedding of HIV, even in the setting of fully suppressed HIV viral load, and may additionally increase plasma viremia (Johnson and Lewis, 2008).
- Immunizations should be reviewed and updated, and folic acid supplementation should be started.
- Screening for anxiety, depression, and intimate partner violence should be conducted, and assistance should be offered to people experiencing these conditions.
- Multidisciplinary care is recommended, including expert consultation (specialists in HIV, OB/GYN, reproductive endocrinology, maternal/fetal medicine, and infertility experts when needed), as well as case management and peer and social support.

INFANT FEEDING COUNSELING

Pregnancy counseling should include discussions and counseling on infant feeding plans. Previous guidelines in the United States did not recommend breastfeeding for people with HIV because of the availability of sustainable and safe formula alternatives. Nevertheless, many individuals preferred and chose to breastfeed (Tuthill et al., 2019; Yusuf et al., 2022). Studies have shown that in the setting of undetectable HIV viral load among breastfeeding mothers on ART, the possibility of HIV transmission is very low (<1%) but not zero (Flynn et al., 2021). Updated guidelines acknowledge this risk and state that the only way to completely eliminate the risk of HIV transmission is by replacing breast milk with formula or donor milk. However, they also recommend evidence-based, culturally sensitive, and patient- and family-centered counseling for shared decision-making on infant feeding (Abuogi et al., 2024; DHHS, 2024b). People with HIV who opt to breastfeed should be supported and offered risk-mitigation strategies that include but are not limited to supporting maternal ART adherence, close monitoring to ensure maternal viral suppression before delivery and throughout breastfeeding, and consideration of infant ARV prophylaxis (Abuogi et al., 2024; DHHS, 2024b). The National Perinatal HIV Hotline (1-888-448-8765) is available for clinician consultation regarding infant feeding by individuals with HIV.

HIV SERO-POSITIVE COUPLES

In couples where both partners are living with HIV, a crucial aspect of the reproductive effort is ensuring that both partners have optimized their individual health. This should be accomplished from both the general and HIV-specific perspectives and involve regular visits to their primary care provider(s), gynecologist, and HIV specialist(s) for both partners, as applicable. For both partners, sustained optimal viral suppression (defined as at least two recorded measurements of HIV plasma viral load below the limits of detection, obtained at least 3 months apart) through ART is critical. Each partner should be evaluated and treated for STIs to avoid pregnancy complications, with rescreening as needed. Condomless intercourse should be timed to coincide with ovulation.

Along with discussions aimed at identifying potential fetal risks and benefits during pregnancy, it is also important to explore and address psychosocial issues to the fullest extent possible. While there have been advances to allow couples to conceive with a significantly lower risk of superinfection or viral mutation, other issues remain. Specifically, although ART has significantly extended the life expectancy of PWH (Marcus et al., 2020), it is unclear how well that correlates to life expectancy in uninfected control populations. This in and of itself is not enough to counsel against conception but should be a part of conversations on the risks and benefits of conception in PWH (American Society for Reproductive Medicine (ASRM), 2021).

HIV SERODIFFERENT COUPLES

In couples desiring natural conception where one partner is HIV-negative, the goal is to minimize the risk of HIV transmission to the HIV-negative partner and the baby. Two large studies found no occurrences of genetically linked HIV transmissions between heterosexual couples while the PWH was virally suppressed (Cohen et al., 2016; Rodger et al., 2016). In light of this, the partner with HIV should receive ART to achieve sustained, maximal viral suppression prior to attempting conception (DHHS, 2024b).

The PARTNERS 1 trial was conducted to investigate HIV transmission rates in serodifferent couples (both heterosexual and MSM) when maximal viral suppression (≤200 copies/mL) with ART was achieved in the partner with HIV; 1,166 couples in the trial engaged in regular, condomless sex. At the end of 1.3 years, no cases of HIV transmission to the HIV-negative partner were demonstrated (Rodger et al., 2016). The HTPN 052 trial followed 1,763 individuals with HIV to compare the rates of HIV-1 transmission with early versus delayed ART initiation; no transmission was seen with partners with stable viral suppression (defined as <400 copies/mL) (Cohen et al., 2016). Similar results were found in a study of 161 serodifferent couples attempting to conceive naturally: 144 were successful, 107 babies were born, and no cases of perinatal transmission or sexual transmission to the uninfected partner were noted (Del Romero et al., 2016; DHHS, 2024b). HIV treatment as a prevention strategy is further supported by a systematic review, which found no cases of HIV transmission with viral loads <600 copies/mL, and rare cases of possible transmission with viral loads 600–1,000 copies/mL (Broyles et al., 2023).

Based on the results of these trials, several recommendations have been made regarding natural conception between serodifferent partners:

1. Patients should be made aware that there is no risk of HIV transmission through condomless sex when the seropositive partner has sustained viral suppression (two viral load measurements of <200 copies/mL, at least 3 months apart) on ART. For serodifferent couples with sustained viral suppression seeking to conceive naturally, condomless intercourse in the peri-ovulatory period (2–3 days preceding ovulation) and the day of ovulation is advised.
2. For serodifferent couples seeking to conceive naturally through condomless intercourse when the PWH has *not* maintained viral suppression, regular use of PrEP is recommended to reduce the risk of HIV acquisition by the partner without HIV. Currently, daily oral tenofovir disoproxil fumarate (TDF)/emtricitabine (FTC) is preferred over other PrEP regimens, including CAB-LA, for the person planning to become pregnant due to its established safety and efficacy data. Condomless sex should be limited to days of peak fertility.
3. For serodifferent couples who wish to conceive naturally through condomless intercourse during peak fertility, it is unclear whether the use of PrEP for the partner without HIV further reduces the risk of sexual transmission when the PWH has already achieved viral suppression.

Providers may present the optional use of ovulation kits to couples to better predict peak fertility and assist in the timing of condomless intercourse.

In serodifferent couples who elect to use PrEP during the conception period, the CDC currently recommends that the partner without HIV begin daily TDF/FTC one month prior to attempting conception and continue for one month beyond the last vaginal exposure (DHHS, 2024b). As in people who are using PrEP for routine HIV prophylaxis, baseline HIV and pregnancy testing should be drawn and repeated at 3-month intervals (or more frequently as indicated), and renal function should be monitored carefully (DHHS, 2024b).

RECOMMENDED READING

Department of Health and Human Services (DHHS) on Treatment of HIV During Pregnancy and Prevention of Perinatal Transmission. Recommendations for the use of antiretroviral drugs during pregnancy and interventions to reduce perinatal HIV transmission in the United States. https://clinicalinfo.hiv.gov/en/guidelines/perinatal. Published 2024b. Accessed June 23, 2024b.

HPV, CERVICAL CANCER, AND ANAL CANCER PREVENTION

LEARNING OBJECTIVE

Discuss the clinical importance of HPV infection in women with HIV, the recommended frequency and screening methods for cervical cancer and anal cancer, including HPV testing, and the role of HPV vaccination.

WHATS NEW?

- The DHHS guidelines for individuals with HIV have new anal cancer screening and treatment guidelines

KEY POINTS

- Cervical cancer screening should begin at the time of diagnosis but not earlier than 21 years of age.
- Between the ages of 21 and 29 years, cervical cytology is used without HPV co-testing due to the high prevalence of HPV in this age group. If normal, the screening is repeated every 12 months. If the patient has three consecutive normal screenings, the testing interval should be increased to every three years.
- At age 30 years and older, cervical cancer screening is performed with either cytology alone or combined with HPV co-testing.
- Unlike the general population, women with HIV who are aged 65 years and older should continue cervical cancer screening.
- Anal cancer screening is now recommended for PWH, including use of high-resolution anoscopy (HRA) as indicated based on symptoms, exam findings, and anal cytology (with or without HPV co-testing).

CERVICAL HPV INFECTION IN WOMEN WITH HIV

In general, infection with HPV, the cause of cervical cancer, is quite common, with 50%–100% of women in the United States estimated to acquire HPV during their lifetime (Chesson et al., 2014). In 2018, around 6% of all cervical cancer cases worldwide were in women with HIV, with a total of 33,000 new cases (Stelzle et al., 2021). Compared with HIV-negative women, women with HIV have a higher prevalence and incidence of HPV (Ahdieh-Grant et al., 2004; Branca et al., 2004). Women with HIV show a longer persistence of HPV (Ahdieh-Grant et al., 2004; Sun et al., 1997), higher HPV levels (Jamieson et al., 2002), higher prevalence of multiple HPV subtypes (Firnhaber et al., 2010; Jamieson et al., 2002; Sahasrabuddhe et al., 2007) and of oncogenic subtypes (Lissouba et al., 2013). In addition, there is increased HPV prevalence and persistence of high-risk HPV with decreasing $CD4^+$ T-cell counts and increasing HIV RNA levels (Liu et al., 2018). Compared to women without HIV, women with HIV are more likely to have abnormal cervical cytology and precancerous lesions (Denny et al., 2012; Ellerbrock et al., 2000; Liu et al., 2018), and both frequency and severity of cervical dysplasia increase with declining $CD4^+$ T-cell counts (Davis et al., 2001; Massad et al., 2001; Massad et al., 2008). Recurrent cervical dysplasia after treatment is more common among women with HIV (Holcomb et al., 1999; Lima et al., 2009). Rates of cervical cancer are also significantly higher among women with HIV compared to women in the general population (Liu et al., 2018; Stelzle et al., 2021) and higher associated mortality (Coghill et al., 2015). Several HPV subtypes have been associated with the development of squamous intraepithelial lesions and cervical cancer, including most commonly HPV-16 (found in almost half of all cervical cancers) and HPV-18 (found in 10%–12% of cervical cancers) and less commonly HPV-31, -33, -35, -39, -45, -51, -52, -56, -58, -59, and -68 (each accounting for <5% of cervical cancers) (de Sanjose et al., 2010).

HPV also causes significant disease burden from many anogenital cancers (vulvar, vaginal, anal) and oropharyngeal cancers, as well as anogenital warts in cisgender women with HIV. However, there are no guidelines for universal screening for non-cervical HPV-associated cancers as there are for cervical cancer and now anal cancer. A vaginal cuff Pap test is recommended for select patients with a history of high-grade cervical intraepithelial neoplasia, adenocarcinoma in situ, or invasive cervical cancer (DHHS, 2024a).

CERVICAL CANCER SCREENING

Because of the high level of HPV infection and higher prevalence of oncogenic subtypes, women with HIV must be regularly screened for cervical dysplasia. Although a single Pap smear has historically been associated with high false-negative rates (10%–25%), regular screening can significantly improve accuracy (Stoler, 2000), and Pap smear screening programs have been associated with marked reductions in cervical cancer incidence (Yang et al., 2018).

In the setting of increased rates of cervical cancer among PWH, guidelines have typically recommended cervical cancer screening more frequently, at a younger age, and continued through older ages. More recently, data from the HIV/AIDS Cancer Match Study, including 164,084 women with HIV, found the highest incidence rates of invasive cervical cancer among 35–39-year-olds and 40–44-year-olds. No cases of invasive cervical cancer occurred among <25-year-olds (Stier et al., 2021). Given the rarity of invasive cervical cancer among PWH younger than 25 years old, the NIH-CDC-HIVMA/IDSA guidelines now recommend starting cervical cancer screening at age 21 years, which permits sufficient time to identify early dysplastic changes prior to age 25. After the age of 25 years, the risk of invasive cervical cancer among PWH consistently outpaces the general populations at all age groups. In light of higher-than-normal risk of cervical cancer, screening should continue throughout the PWH's lifetime and not end at age 65 years. However, after age 65, clinicians should assess the individual absolute risk of cervical cancer and the person's life expectancy to guide shared decision-making regarding ongoing screening.

Table 22.1 summarizes the cervical cancer screening recommendations from the NIH-CDC-HIVMA/IDSA. The recommendations are categorized into three groups: women with HIV aged younger than 21 years, between 21 and 29 years, and 30 years and older.

A potential new alternative to in-clinic screening with Pap smear and HPV testing for the general population is mailing HPV self-collection kits, which was successful in prior U.S. studies involving under-screened, underserved individuals, including randomized controlled trials (Pretsch et al., 2023; Smith et al., 2018; Winer et al., 2018). The Food and Drug Administration (FDA) recently approved the use of self-collected vaginal specimens for HPV testing when clinicians cannot collect samples in a healthcare setting (FDA, 2024). HPV self-collection is not recommended for PWH at this time, but further data are likely to come in the future as the National Cancer Institute conducts a nationwide clinical trial to further evaluate self-collected HPV testing (NCI, 2024).

HPV VACCINATION

HPV vaccination has been shown to reduce the rates of cervical cancer and precancerous lesions up to more than 90% (Ellingson et al., 2023; Lei et al., 2020), with one dose proven to be enough for immunogenicity in the general population (Baisley et al., 2024; Barnabas et al., 2022). The Advisory Committee on Immunization Practices (ACIP) recommends administering the nine-valent HPV vaccine between 9 and 12 years of age, with catch-up recommended for up to 26 years of age, and shared decision-making between 27 and 45 years of age, given increased effectiveness at younger ages (Egemen et al., 2022; Ellingson et al., 2023). DDHS guidelines recommend the same schedule for people with HIV but with three doses for all ages (0, 1–2, 6 months) due to concern for lower immunogenicity (DHHS, 2024a).

Table 22.1 CERVICAL CANCER SCREENING RECOMMENDATIONS FOR WOMEN WITH HIV

AGE	SCHEDULE	FOLLOW-UP RECOMMENDATIONS FOR ABNORMAL RESULTS
<21	• No screening recommended	
21–29 years	• Cytology at initial HIV diagnosis • Co-testing not recommended due to high prevalence of HPV in this age group • Repeat screening 12 months after HIV diagnosis if initial screen is normal • Increase screening interval to 3 years after 3 consecutive normal tests	• AS-CUS: Repeat cytology in 6–12 months • LSIL or greater: Colposcopy

≥30 years	OPTION 1: Cytology without HPV test at initial HIV diagnosis
	  • Repeat screen 12 months after HIV diagnosis if screen is normal
	  • Increase screening interval to 3 years after 3 consecutive normal tests
	
	OPTION 2: Cytology with high-risk HPV (hr-HPV) co-testing at HIV diagnosis
	  • Repeat in 3 years if both negative
	
	Do not discontinue screening for either option at 65 years; continue screening throughout lifetime for women with HIV.
		OPTION 1:
		• Repeat cytology in 6–12 months if cytology shows AS-CUS and HPV is negative or unavailable. Colposcopy if AS-CUS or greater on repeat cytology.
		• LSIL or greater: Colposcopy
		
		OPTION 2:
		• Normal cytology, positive HPV 16 or 18: Colposcopy
		• Normal cytology, positive hr-HPV not 16 or 18 or no typing: Repeat co-testing in 1 year
		• AS-CUS, hr-HPV negative: Repeat cytology in 6–12 months or co-testing in 1 year
		• AS-CUS, hr-HPV positive: Colposcopy
		• Colposcopy if cytology shows LSIL or greater regardless of HPV status
		• Colposcopy if ≥AS-CUS or positive hr-HPV on any repeat testing

Abbreviations: AS-CUS = atypical squamous cells of undetermined significance; hr-HPV = high-risk HPV; LSIL = low-grade squamous intraepithelial lesion.

Source: Department of Health and Human Services (DHHS). Guidelines for the prevention and treatment of opportunistic infections in adults and adolescents with HIV. https://clinicalinfo.hiv.gov/en/guidelines/hiv-clinical-guidelines-adult-and-adolescent-opportunistic-infections/. Published 2024. Accessed August 10, 2024.

ANAL CANCER SCREENING

Updated DHHS guidelines were released in 2024 regarding anal cancer screening (DHHS, 2024a), and now recommend that all adults with HIV are assessed at least once per year for anal symptoms regardless of anal intercourse history. Digital anorectal examination (DARE) and standard anoscopy are recommended for symptomatic transgender women, along with MSM younger than 35 and all other PWH younger than 45 years of age (which would include cisgender women). Previously, results from the Anal Cancer–HSIL Outcomes Research (ANCHOR) trial showed that PWH 35 years of age with biopsy-proven anal high-grade squamous intraepithelial lesion (HSIL) who received treatment primarily with office-based electrocautery had lower rates of progression to anal cancer compared with those randomized to active monitoring (Palefsky et al., 2022). Sixteen percent of participants in the ANCHOR trial were of female gender (Palefsky et al., 2022). These ANCHOR study results highlighted the need for screening of HPV-related squamous intraepithelial lesions (SIL) and scaling high-resolution anoscopy (HRA) services for people with abnormal results. The DHHS guidelines now recommend anal cancer screening with anal cytology alone or high-risk HPV (hr-HPV) for all PWH ages 45 and older, including cisgender women, and that screening should begin earlier (starting at 35 years) for transgender women and MSM with HIV. The management of screening results is outlined in Table 22.2, which includes indications for HRA. HRA is also recommended in PWH if abnormal DARE or anal symptoms are reported (DDHS, 2024a). Of note, the International Anal Neoplasia Society (IANS) guidelines accept hrHPV alone for anal cancer screening (Stier et al., 2024).

In settings where HRA is not available, assessment of anal symptoms and DARE without laboratory testing (anal cytology or hr-HPV co-testing) is advised (DHHS, 2024a). This is a key consideration, as expertise is needed to interpret screening results and to ensure access to ablative treatments and follow-up; however, recent estimates indicate that many PWH who are at the highest risk for anal cancer do not have access to HRA services (Rim et al., 2024).

Updated guidelines also recommend consideration of specific additional risk factors for anal cancer, namely screening with prompt referral to HRA for PWH with any of the following characteristics: older age, prolonged immune suppression and HIV infection duration, history of AIDS, smoking, positive HPV16 or 18 testing, and higher grade cytologic abnormalities (DHHS, 2024a). Other important risk factors identified from a recent meta-analysis include history of anogenital warts, HPV-related precancerous lesions, or cancer (cervical, vulvar, vaginal), which is particularly relevant for people assigned female at birth (Clifford et al., 2021).

Table 22.2 ASSESSMENT OF ANAL CYTOLOGY AND HPV RESULTS IN PEOPLE WITH HIV

HR-HPV CO-TESTING	CYTOLOGY	HPV TESTING	FOLLOW-UP RECOMMENDATIONS FOR RESULTS
Yes	Normal	hr-HPV positive HPV 16 or 18 positive	HRA
		hr-HPV positive No HPV typing	Repeat co-testing in 6 months
		hr-HPV positive HPV 16 and 18 negative	Repeat co-testing in 1 year
		hr-HPV negative	Repeat co-testing in 3 years
	ASC-US	hr-HPV positive	HRA
		hr-HPV negative	Repeat co-testing in 1 year
	≥ LSIL	any	HRA
No	≥ ASC-US	—	HRA
	Normal	—	Repeat screen 12 months after HIV diagnosis if screen is normal. Increase screening interval to 3 years after 3 consecutive (yearly) normal tests.

Abbreviations: ASC-US = atypical squamous cells of undetermined significance; hr-HPV = high-risk HPV; LSIL = low-grade squamous intraepithelial lesion.

Source: Department of Health and Human Services (DHHS). Guidelines for the prevention and treatment of opportunistic infections in adults and adolescents with HIV. https://clinicalinfo.hiv.gov/en/guidelines/hiv-clinical-guidelines-adult-and-adolescent-opportunistic-infections/. Published 2024. Accessed August 24, 2024.

CONSIDERATIONS FOR GENDER-DIVERSE PATIENTS

Transgender and gender-diverse individuals who have a cervix are at risk of HPV infection but are less likely than cisgender women to receive regular Pap tests (Hsiao, 2016). Transgender persons are also disproportionately affected by HIV (Clark et al., 2017). Transgender men and gender-diverse persons with HIV should receive cervical cancer screenings on the same schedule as cisgender women, as outlined above. Screening procedures should be performed in a supportive and culturally sensitive manner, and providers should be aware that exogenous testosterone use may increase the likelihood of unsatisfactory testing result (Badowski et al., 2021; Hsiao, 2016). More specific recommendations for Pap smears in transgender populations can be found at: https://transcare.ucsf.edu/guidelines/cervical-cancer.

RECOMMENDED READING

American College of Obstetricians and Gynecologists. ACOG Committee Opinion No. 762: Prepregnancy counseling. *Obstet Gynecol.* 2019 Jan;133(1):e78–e89. doi:10.1097/AOG.0000000000003013.

Bloomfield GS, Alenezi F, Barasa FA, et al. Human immunodeficiency virus and heart failure in low- and middle-income countries. *JACC Heart Fail.* 2015;3:579–590.

Carten ML, Kiser JJ, Kwara A, et al. Pharmacokinetic interactions between the hormonal emergency contraception, levonorgestrel (Plan B), and efavirenz. *Infect Dis Obstet Gynecol.* 2012;2012:137192. doi:10.1155/2012/137192

Department of Health and Human Services, Panel on Opportunistic Infections in HIV-Infected Adults and Adolescents. Guidelines for the prevention and treatment of opportunistic infections in HIV-infected adults and adolescents: recommendations from the Centers for Disease Control and Prevention, the National Institutes of Health, and the HIV Medicine Association of the Infectious Diseases Society of America. https://clinicalinfo.hiv.gov/en/guidelines/adult-and-adolescent-opportunistic-infection Published 2024. Accessed September 15, 2024.

ART IN PREGNANCY

GOAL

Upon completion of this section, the reader should be able to describe the appropriate management of antiretroviral (ARV) medications for pregnant individuals with HIV.

INTRODUCTION

Over time, research has demonstrated that proper prevention strategies and interventions during pregnancy, labor, and delivery can significantly reduce the rate of mother-to-child transmission (MTCT) of HIV. In 1994, a pivotal study of the Pediatric AIDS Clinical Trials Group 076 demonstrated that the use of zidovudine (ZDV) monotherapy during pregnancy substantially reduced the risk of HIV transmission to infants by 67% (Connor et al., 1994). The protocol consisted of oral administration of ZDV initiated between 14 and 34 weeks of gestation and continued throughout pregnancy, followed by intrapartum administration of intravenous ZDV and oral administration of ZDV to the newborn for 6 weeks after delivery. Additional studies have demonstrated the effectiveness of the use of combination ART, further decreasing the risk of HIV transmission to 1%–2% (Cooper et al., 2002). Based on recent data, there have been modifications to the original protocol, including a more selective use of intravenous ZDV based on maternal viral load and changing practices regarding postnatal administration of ART to the newborn. With increased emphasis on early testing for HIV and modernized protocols for antepartum management, perinatal transmission of HIV has decreased significantly. Only 32 infants were born with perinatally acquired HIV in the United States in 2019 (CDC, 2024). Pre-pregnancy ART, surgical delivery (when indicated), and infant ARV prophylaxis/presumptive therapy are additional key prevention strategies.

LEARNING OBJECTIVE

Review the clinical management of pregnant individuals with HIV, including recommendations for the use of ARVs and drug disposition.

WHAT'S NEW?

- Initiation of the combination regimen of long-acting injectable cabotegravir (CAB) and rilpivirine (RPV) is not recommended during pregnancy due to insufficient dosing, pharmacokinetics (PK), and safety data. For people who become pregnant while already receiving long-acting injectable CAB plus RPV, shared decision-making is recommended to decide whether this regimen should be continued or whether switching to a recommended oral regimen is preferred, noting that some women may have few alternative options. For people who are considering becoming pregnant in the near future, CAB and RPV injections should be stopped at least 1 year before conception, given the long half-life of the drug. If switching to a preferred alternative oral regimen, this should happen within 4 weeks of the last CAB and RPV doses. If CAB/RPV is continued during pregnancy, more frequent viral monitoring should be considered.
- For pregnant PWH who previously received long-acting injectable CAB as pre-exposure prophylaxis (PrEP), initial use of ritonavir-boosted darunavir (DRV/r) is preferred over integrase inhibitor (INSTI)-based regimens, pending baseline genotypic resistance testing for INSTI mutations. For pregnant PWH without prior use of long-acting injectable CAB, DRV/r is now an alternative ARV drug for pregnancy.
- Use of ritonavir-boosted protease inhibitors (PIs) may be associated with increased risk of preterm birth. However, if PIs are needed, darunavir (DRV) or atazanavir (ATV) is recommended over lopinavir (LPV). In pregnancy, DRV/r requires twice daily dosing, so some U.S. guidelines panel members prefer ritonavir-boosted ATV due to reduced pill burden. LPV/r is not recommended but may be needed in special cases (e.g., liquid formulation needed for G-tube administration). LPV/r warrants caution during pregnancy since the solution contains ethanol and propylene glycol.
- BIC (bictegravir)/TAF/FTC is now recommended as an alternative ART regimen in pregnancy by the DHHS guidelines, based on PK and safety data which showed lower drug levels in the second and third trimesters compared to nonpregnant or postpartum patients (however, levels were still above the EC95 [95% maximal effective concentration]), suggesting effective viral suppression. No safety concerns were seen.
- Information regarding the newest long-acting injectable agent, lenacapavir (LEN), was added, and changes were made to recommendations for fostemsavir (FTR) and ibalizumab (IBA). There are insufficient data on PK, efficacy, or safety for these newer medications. However, they can be continued in special circumstances (e.g., heavily ART-experienced pregnant PWH or people with no ART alternatives). More frequent viral load monitoring should be done in such cases. The same recommendation applies to etravirine (ETR), nevirapine (NVP), maraviroc (MVC), and enfuvirtide (T20).

KEY POINTS

- ART should be initiated in all pregnant PWH regardless of $CD4^+$ T-cell count or HIV-1 RNA level. ARVs should be given as combination therapy, similar to that prescribed for nonpregnant individuals with HIV, with the goal of complete and sustained virologic suppression.
- The goal of ART during pregnancy is to "achieve and maintain HIV viral suppression to undetectable levels (i.e., HIV RNA below the lower limits of detection of an ultrasensitive assay)" to maximize the health of the pregnant individual and decrease perinatal transmission risk (DHHS, 2024b, n.p.).
- ART changes during pregnancy have been associated with the loss of virologic control and are independently associated with perinatal transmission of HIV.
- All cases of prenatal antiretroviral exposure should be reported to the APR (www.apregistry.com).

PHYSIOLOGIC CHANGES DURING PREGNANCY

Physiologic changes that occur during pregnancy may alter drug disposition and lead to decreased drug exposure. These changes may be associated with incomplete virologic suppression, virologic failure, and/or the development of HIV drug resistance (Mirochnick and Capparelli., 2004). Therefore, an understanding of pharmacokinetic changes that can occur with ARVs during pregnancy is essential for making appropriate dose modifications to maintain efficacy and minimize toxicity. Box 22.1 summarizes some of the physiologic changes that occur during pregnancy that could affect drug disposition. Some pharmacokinetic changes during pregnancy can

Box 22.1 **EFFECT OF PREGNANCY ON DRUG DISPOSITION**

COMPONENTS OF DRUG DISPOSITION

ABSORPTION

- Decrease intestinal motility resulting in increased gastric emptying
- Reduced gastric acid secretion with gastric pH increase affecting absorption of weak acids and bases

NAUSEA AND VOMITING

- Changes in distribution
- Total body water increases
- Protein binding to albumin and α-1 acid glycoprotein decreases

METABOLISM

- Induction of hepatic metabolic pathways
- Estrogen and progesterone may compete for metabolic binding sites

EXCRETION

- Increased clearance of drugs eliminated by renal clearance

be overcome by maximizing dosing strategies of ARVs, such as twice-daily use of DRV and RAL. Another example of how physiologic changes can affect ARVs includes cobicistat-boosted regimens and the increased activity of hepatic cytochrome P450 3A enzymes during pregnancy. One phase 4 pharmacokinetic study evaluating 14 women in their third trimester who were on regimens containing EVG/c found that 77%–85% of women had troughs below the effective concentration needed to inhibit 90% of the virus. This is thought to be due to both increased clearance and shorter half-life of EVG as well as decreased cobicistat exposure (Bukkems et al., 2020). These results were echoed in the second trimester, as well as with other cobicistat-boosted regimens (Momper et al., 2018). DRV/c exposures were measured in six women, and 89%–92% (total DRV) and 32%–41% (unbound DRV) decreased trough concentrations compared to postpartum exposures were noted. Cobicistat similarly had a trough that was 83% lower than postpartum exposures (Crauwels et al., 2019). The median ATV trough in 11 pregnant women was 0.21 mcg/mL in the second trimester, 0.21 mcg/mL in the third trimester, and 0.61 mcg/mL postpartum (Momper et al., 2022).

TRANSPLACENTAL TRANSFER OF ANTIRETROVIRAL DRUGS

Although the risk of transmission involving PWH with undetectable viral load is very low (approximately 0.04%), the use of agents that cross the placenta and act as PrEP for the fetus is an important facet of care to prevent perinatal transmission (DHHS, 2024b; Warszawski et al., 2008). In general, nucleoside reverse transcriptase inhibitors (NRTIs), non-nucleoside reverse transcriptase inhibitors (NNRTIs), and integrase inhibitors (INSTIs) readily cross the placenta. Protease inhibitors (PIs) are highly protein bound and, therefore, only a small percentage of drug that is unbound is free to transfer. Newer agents such as fostemsavir and ibalizumab do not have available human data on placental transfer (DHHS, 2024b).

BASIC PRINCIPLES ON THE USE OF ANTIRETROVIRALS IN PREGNANCY

- Antiretrovirals (ARVs) should be initiated in all pregnant people with HIV regardless of $CD4^+$ T-cell count or HIV-1 viral load.
- The regimen should have optimal efficacy, safety, and tolerability.
- The regimen should contain at least one drug with good placental passage.
- The provider should consider multiple factors when selecting a regimen, including baseline ARV resistance (determined by HIV genotype and treatment history), comorbidities, convenience, adverse effects, drug interactions, pharmacokinetics, and experience in pregnancy.
- Individuals entering pregnancy on ARVs should continue their regimen if it is effective, well tolerated, and does not contain agents that are teratogenic.

RECOMMENDATIONS

ARV-Naive Individuals

All individuals with HIV should receive a potent ARV regimen to reduce the risk of perinatal transmission. For an updated list, U.S. DHHS guidelines provide detail on *preferred* and *alternate* regimens for women who have never received ART and are pregnant. Current preferred regimens include DTG plus TDF or tenofovir alafenamide (TAF) plus FTC or lamivudine (3TC); as well as DTG plus abacavir (ABC) plus 3TC (the person must be HLA-B*5701 negative, and not have hepatitis B coinfection) (Table 22.3). Ritonavir-boosted darunavir (DRV/r) is preferred over an INSTI-based regimen for pregnant individuals who have prior use of long-acting injectable cabotegravir as PrEP. BIC/TAF/FTC is now recommended as an alternative ART based on small studies describing its PK, safety, and efficacy. Lower drug levels were seen in the second and third trimesters compared to nonpregnant or postpartum patients. However, levels were still above the EC95 (95% maximal effective concentration), indicating effective viral suppression, which was seen with participant viral load monitoring (Zhang et al., 2024). Recently, a large multi-site cohort study of pregnant patients with HIV on

Table 22.3 ARV PRINCIPLES IN PREGNANCY, CONCEPTION, AND CONTRACEPTION

REGIMEN	USE IN ART- NAIVE PEOPLE	CONTINUING ART FOR PEOPLE WHO BECOME PREGNANT THAT ARE VIRALLY SUPPRESSED	ART FOR NON-PREGNANT PEOPLE WHO ARE TRYING TO CONCEIVE	OTHER COMMENTS	EFFECTS ON CONTRACEPTION
NRTI Backbones					
ABC/3TC	Preferred	Continue	Preferred	Testing for the HLA-B*5701 allele should be performed and documented as negative before starting ABC, and individuals should be educated about symptoms of ABC hypersensitivity reactions.	—
TAF/FTC	Preferred	Continue	Preferred	Associated with fewer adverse birth outcomes and higher gestational weight compared to TDF/FTC	No evidence of human teratogenicity with TAF (defined as 1.5-fold increase in birth defects)
TDF/FTC	Preferred	Continue	Preferred		Fetal bone and early-life growth abnormalities described with TDF, but it appears safe overall
INSTI					
BIC/TAF/FTC	Alternative	Continue	Alternative	PK and safety data in pregnancy are limited, but no safety concerns. Lower drug levels in the second and third trimesters, with BIC reduced more than DTG. Despite this, BIC levels remain above the EC95, suggesting effective viral load suppression.	-
CAB/RPV	Not recommended	Shared decision-making to continue with frequent vial load monitoring or switch	Insufficient data	Not recommended due to lack of data.	—
DTG	Preferred	Continue	Preferred	DTG is not preferred for initial treatment in people with newly diagnosed HIV infection if prior use of PrEP with long-acting injectable CAB (concern for INSTI resistance): DRV/r preferred.	—
EVG/c/TAF/FTC	Not recommended	Continue with frequent viral load monitoring or switch	Not recommended	Decreased levels of cobicistat in second and third trimesters with increased risk for virologic breakthrough	—
RAL	Alternative	Continue	Alternative	Must use 400 mg twice daily (no data available for 1,200 mg once daily extended-release tablets). Alternative use in pregnancy due to lower genetic barrier to resistance compared with DTG, and need for twice daily dosing	—

(*continued*)

Table 22.3 CONTINUED

REGIMEN	USE IN ART- NAIVE PEOPLE	CONTINUING ART FOR PEOPLE WHO BECOME PREGNANT THAT ARE VIRALLY SUPPRESSED	ART FOR NON-PREGNANT PEOPLE WHO ARE TRYING TO CONCEIVE	OTHER COMMENTS	EFFECTS ON CONTRACEPTION
NNRTI					
DOR	Insufficient data	Continue with frequent viral load monitoring or consider switching due to insufficient data	Insufficient data	No data on use in pregnancy.	—
EFV	Alternative	Continue	Alternative	—	Consider alternative or barrier contraception in addition to COC/P/R, POPs, etonogestrel implants.
ETV	Not recommended	Continue	Not recommended, except in special circumstances	Not recommended due to limited data	—
NVP	Not recommended	Continue	Not recommended, except in special circumstances	Not recommended due to high risk for adverse events, need for lead-in dosing, as well as low barrier to resistance	—
RPV	Alternative	Continue	Alternative	Little experience in pregnancy and PK suggests lower levels in second and third trimesters with increased risk of virologic rebound	—
Protease Inhibitors					
ATV/r	Alternative	Continue	Alternative	Consider neonatal bilirubin monitoring when given throughout pregnancy.	—
DRV/r	Alternative/ preferred in special circumstances	Continue	Alternative	Must use twice daily dosing strategy.	Consider alternative or barrier contraception in addition to COC/P/R, POPs, etonogestrel implants.
LPV/r	Not recommended except in special circumstances	Continue	Not recommended except in special circumstances	Must use twice daily dosing strategy. Some experts recommend higher dosing strategy during the second and third trimesters. Use of LPV/r is associated with increased risk of preterm delivery as well as more nausea.	—
ATV/c	Not recommended	Continue with frequent viral load monitoring or switch	Not recommended	Decreased levels of cobicistat in second and third trimester with increased risk for virologic breakthroughs	Contraindicated with drospirenone-containing hormonal contraceptives due to risk of hypokalemia

DRV/c	Not recommended	Continue with frequent viral load monitoring or switch	Not recommended	Decreased levels of cobicistat in second and third trimester with increased risk for virologic breakthroughs	Monitoring with drospirenone-containing hormonal contraceptives due to risk of hypokalemia
Entry, Attachment, and Fusion Inhibitors					
FTR	Not recommended	Continue	Not recommended except in special circumstances	No data on use in pregnancy	—
IBA	Not recommended	Continue	Not recommended except in special circumstances	No data on use in pregnancy	—
LEN	Not recommended	Continue	Not recommended except in special circumstances	Insufficient pharmacokinetic data.	—
MVC	Not recommended	Continue	Not recommended, except in special circumstances	Not recommended in non-pregnant patients given limited pharmacokinetic data in pregnancy	—
T-20	Not recommended	Continue	Not recommended, except in special circumstances	—	—

Abbreviations: ABC/3TC = abacavir/lamivudine; ATV/c = atazanavir/cobicistat; ATV/r = atazanavir/ritonavir; BIC/TAF/FTC = bictegravir/tenofovir alafenamide/emtricitabine; CAB/RPV = cabotegravir/rilpivirine; COC/P/R: combined oral contraceptives/patch/ring; DTG = dolutegravir; DOR = doravirine; DRV/c = darunavir/cobisistat; DRV/r = darunavir/ritonavir; EVG/c/TAF/FTC = elvitegravir/cobisistat/tenofovir alafenamide/emtricitabine; FTR = fostemsavir; IBA = ibalizumab; INSTI = integrase strand transfer inhibitor; LEN = Lenacapavir; LPV/r = lopinavir/ritonavir; MVC = maraviroc; NRTI = nucleoside reverse transcriptase inhibitor; POP = progrestin-only pill; RAL = raltegravir; T-20 = enfuvirtide; TAF/FTC = tenofovir alafenamide/emtricitabine; TDF/FTC = tenofovir disoproxil fumarate/emtricitabine.

Source: Department of Health and Human Services (DHHS). Panel on Treatment of HIV During Pregnancy and Prevention of Perinatal Transmission. Recommendations for the use of antiretroviral drugs during pregnancy and interventions to reduce perinatal HIV transmission in the United States. https://clinicalinfo.hiv.gov/en/guidelines/perinatal. Published 2024. Accessed June 23, 2024.

BIC/TAF/FTC was published: viral suppression was seen in 90% of the 147 individuals, including 96% among those who started ART preconception, and 85% in people who started ART while pregnant (Holt et al., 2024). There was one case of perinatal transmission, but this was presumed due to acute HIV seroconversion during pregnancy (Holt et al., 2024). Other advantages of BIC/TAF/FTC include a high barrier to resistance, no food requirement, and once daily dosing. The long-acting injectable combination of CAB plus RPV is not recommended to start during pregnancy due to insufficient data.

PREGNANCY WHILE ON ANTIRETROVIRAL THERAPY

Pregnant individuals with established HIV infection who present for care in the first trimester should be counseled about the risks and benefits of ART. If possible, they should be maintained on their current ART regimen, as discontinuations may lead to the loss of virologic control, which could adversely affect the health of the fetus, including increasing the risk of HIV transmission. In a prospective cohort of 937 mother–infant pairs, interruption of ART during the first and third trimesters was independently associated with perinatal transmission of HIV. The overall rate of HIV transmission was 1.3%, compared to the rate associated with first- and third-trimester interruptions of ART, which were 4.9% and 18.2%, respectively (Galli et al., 2009).

In the past, there had been concern over the teratogenic effects of EFV use in the first trimester of pregnancy. Specifically, preclinical primate data and retrospective reports raised concern about an increased risk of neural tube defects (NTDs) with EFV use in pregnancy. It is important to note that the neural tube closes at 36–39 days after the last menstrual period. Thus, the risk of NTDs is restricted to the first 5–6 weeks of pregnancy. A meta-analysis that included data on 1,437 first-trimester EFV exposures showed no overall increased risk of birth defects compared to women on other ARV drugs. There was one NTD, giving an incidence of 0.07% (Ford et al., 2011). Thus, the U.S. DHHS panel has updated its recommendation to note that EFV is an alternative NNRTI regimen, given extensive prior experience with use of this agent in pregnancy. Co-formulated EFV/TDF/FTC may be a useful regimen in women who require coadministration of drugs with significant interactions with otherwise preferred ART combinations, or in those who need the convenience of a single tablet combination and are not eligible for DTG. It is important to screen for antenatal and postpartum depression (DHHS, 2024b).

The Tsepamo birth outcome study is an ongoing observational study funded by the U.S. National Institutes of Health (NIH) in Botswana comparing birth outcomes among pregnant women taking EFV- versus DTG-based regimens. In 2018, an interim analysis was reported on women who were taking DTG-containing regimens before or during conception, which revealed that 4 out of 429 newborns (0.94%) had NTDs. In comparison, NTDs occurred in 14 out of 11,3000 (0.0012%) of infants born to women receiving non-DTG-based regimens at the time of conception, and 3 out of 5,787 (0.05%) of women on EFV-containing regimens (Zash et al., 2018). In an updated analysis, 9 of out of 5,680 deliveries (0.15%) resulted in NTDs (Zash et al., 2019). This rate is not dissimilar from other studies suggesting an NTD rate of 0.10% in non-DTG-based regimens, 0.06% in EFV-based regimens, and 0.07% in mothers without HIV (Zash et al., 2021). As a result of Tsepamo's updated findings, DTG is now recommended as a preferred agent in both pregnancy and women who are trying to conceive (DHHS, 2024b). Surveillance data from the United Kingdom and Ireland indicate that RAL use in pregnancy was not associated with any NTDs (Baxevanidi et al., 2021), and thus it is listed as an alternative ARV for initiation in pregnant women (for virologically suppressed women who become pregnant while taking RAL, it may be continued). As mentioned above, for ART-naive individuals, BIC/TAF/FTC is now an alternative regimen to continue when viral suppression was achieved prior to pregnancy.

Previous data raised the question of whether ritonavir-boosted PIs may increase the risk of preterm delivery (PTD), with the highest risk of PTD associated with lopinavir/ritonavir. Multiple studies have noted an association between PI regimens, with the risk of PTD at an adjusted odds ratio of 1.32 (95% CI: 1.04–1.6) (Mesfin et al., 2016); however, there are also multiple studies that suggest a lack of an effect. In one network meta-analysis, use of ZDV/3TC plus LPV/r was associated with the highest risk of PTD, as compared to ZDV and other regimens (relative risk ranging from 1.43 to 1.81) (Tshivuila-Matala et al., 2020). That finding was mirrored when comparing LPV/r to ATV/r (unadjusted risk ratio 1.97; 95% CI: 1.2–3.4) (Rough et al., 2018). Overall, the effect that boosted PIs have on PTD rates remains uncertain. However, some pregnant people require a PI-based regimen, in which case, DRV/r is preferred over LPV/r.

Historically, TDF was the only tenofovir product recommended for use in pregnancy. However, newer data suggest that use of TAF is safe, and TAF is now listed as a preferred option during pregnancy. When comparing initiation of DTG + TAF/FTC versus DTG + TDF/FTC starting between 14 and 28 weeks gestation, use of TAF was associated with lower adverse pregnancy outcomes (24% vs. 44%, 95% CI: −17.3, −0.3; $p = 0.043$) and no difference in infant adverse events, but was associated with higher maternal weight gain (0.378 kg/week vs. 0.319 kg/week, 95% CI: 0.013, 0.103; $p = 0.011$) (Lockman et al., 2021).

Multiple regimens are listed as recommended regimens for nonpregnant people who are virally suppressed that are not recommended in pregnancy because of a lack of sufficient data, including oral and injectable two-drug regimens such as DTG/3TC, DTG/RPV, and CAB/RPV. If patients have maintained viral suppression on a two-drug oral regimen, clinicians can consider continuing this regimen with increased frequency of viral load monitoring (every 1–2 months). For people who become pregnant while on CAB/RPV and are virally suppressed, shared decision-making is recommended regarding whether to continue this long-acting combination or switch to a different oral combination.

PREGNANCY WITHOUT VIRAL SUPPRESSION

In late pregnancy, lack of virologic suppression could be due to either inadequate time on ART, poor adherence, or virologic failure. Providers must consider several things when evaluating a pregnant PWH experiencing viremia; these include medication adherence, tolerability, correct dosing, drug interactions, and HIV drug resistance. If there is a concern for resistance, resistance testing should be obtained, and expert consultation is advised.

Case reports involving the use of RAL-containing regimens in late pregnancy describe rapid HIV viral decay, which has been demonstrated with INSTIs. Additionally, there are data demonstrating superior viral load suppression at the time of delivery in pregnant PWH receiving DTG-containing regimens versus EFV-based regimens (DHHS, 2024b). Thus, DTG-containing regimens are preferred in pregnant people if they are not tolerating their current regimen, or viral suppression has not been achieved.

INTRAPARTUM ZIDOVUDINE DURING LABOR

The DHHS guidelines recommend that PWH with HIV-1 RNA counts of greater than 1,000 copies/mL, an unknown viral load near delivery (within 4 weeks), or a known or suspected lack of medication adherence should receive intravenous ZDV prior to delivery. People with no prior known diagnosis of HIV who have a positive antigen/antibody screening result at the time of labor should also receive intravenous ZDV (DHHS 2024b). In the past, all women with HIV were given intravenous ZDV during labor regardless of viral load, as it was part of the PACTG 076 protocol noted earlier (Table 22.2).

The French Perinatal Cohort evaluated perinatal transmission in more than 11,000 pregnant women with HIV receiving ART. The overall rate of perinatal transmission was 0.9% in those who received intravenous ZDV and 1.8% without intravenous ZDV. Among women with HIV-1 RNA levels of more than 1,000 copies/mL, the risk of transmission without ZDV was 10.2% compared to 2.5% with intravenous ZDV if neonates received only ZDV for prophylaxis, but was no different without or with intrapartum ZDV if the neonate received intensified prophylaxis with two or more ARV drugs. Among women with HIV-1 RNA levels of less than 1,000 copies/mL at delivery, zero transmissions occurred among 369 women who did not receive intravenous ZDV, compared to 0.6% of those receiving intravenous ZDV (Briand et al., 2013). Based on these and other studies, intravenous ZDV should continue to be administered to women with HIV RNA counts of greater than 1,000 copies/mL near delivery regardless of intrapartum ART regimen. Intrapartum ZDV administration may be considered and assessed on a case-by-case basis in women with HIV-1 RNA levels in the range of 50 to 999 copies/mL, as the risk of transmission is slightly higher (1%–2% vs. 1% or less). Additionally, patients with HIV-1 RNA levels greater than 1,000 copies/mL should be scheduled for cesarean delivery at 38 weeks gestation to reduce the rate of perinatal transmission (ACOG, 2019).

ANTIRETROVIRAL PREGNANCY REGISTRY

Established in 1989, the Antiretroviral Pregnancy Registry (APR) is an international, observational, exposure registration and follow-up study which collects data on pregnant people with HIV taking ARVs, with the overall goal of detecting major teratogenic effects. Registration is voluntary and confidential; however, providers are strongly encouraged to enroll pregnant patients in the registry at the time of the initial evaluation of the pregnant woman. Reports have been received from 67 countries (predominantly the United States). More information is available at: www.APRegistry.com.

REFERENCES

Abuogi L, Noble L, Smith C, Committee on Pediatric and Adolescent HIV, Section on Breastfeeding. Infant feeding for persons living with and at Risk for HIV in the United States: clinical report. *Pediatrics.* 2024 Jun;153(6):e2024066843. 10.1542/peds.2024-066843

Ahdieh-Grant L, Li R, Levine AM et al. Highly active antiretroviral therapy and cervical squamous intraepithelial lesions in human immunodeficiency virus-positive women. *J Natl Cancer Inst.* 2004;96(14):1070–1076. doi:10.1093/jnci/djh192

American Society for Reproductive Medicine (ASRM) Ethics Committee. Human immunodeficiency virus and infertility treatment: an Ethics Committee opinion. https://www.asrm.org/practice-guidance/ethics-opinions/human-immunodeciency-virus-and-infertility-treatment-an-ethics-committee-opinion-2021/. Published 2021. Accessed June 24, 2024.

Badowski ME, Britt N, Huesgen EC, et al. Pharmacotherapy considerations in transgender individuals living with human immunodeficiency virus. *Pharmacotherapy.* 2021;41(3):299–314. doi:10.1002/phar.2499

Baisley K, Kemp TJ, Mugo NR, et al. Comparing one dose of HPV vaccine in girls aged 9–14 years in Tanzania (DoRIS) with one dose in young women aged 15–20 years in Kenya (KEN SHE): an immunobridging analysis of randomised controlled trials. *Lancet Glob Health.* 2024;12(3):e491–e499. doi:10.1016/S2214-109X(23)00586-7

Barnabas RV, Brown ER, Onono MA, et al. Efficacy of single-dose HPV vaccination among young African women. *NEJM Evid.* 2022;1(5):EVIDoa2100056. doi:10.1056/EVIDoa2100056. PMID: 35693874.

Baxevanidi E, Asif S, Qavi A, et al. Chronic Comorbidities in Pregnant Women with HIV. Conference on Retroviruses and Opportunistic Infections. March 6–11, 2021. Virtual. Abstract 572. https://www.croiconference.org/abstract/predicted-long-term-adverse-birth-and-child-health-outcomes-in-the-advance-trial/.

Blair CS, Li S, Chau G, et al.; HPTN 077 Study Team. Brief report: hormonal contraception use and cabotegravir pharmacokinetics in HIV-uninfected women enrolled in HPTN 077. *J Acquir Immune Defic Syndr.* 2020;85(1):93–97.

Branca M, Costa S, Mariani L. Assessment of risk factors and human papillomavirus (HPV) related pathogenetic mechanisms of CIN in HIV-positive and HIV-negative women: study design and baseline data of the HPV-PathogenISS study. *Eur J Gynaecol Oncol.* 2004;25(6):689–698.

Briand N, Jasseron C, Sibiude J, et al. Cesarean section for HIV-infected women in the combination antiretroviral therapies era, 2000–2010. *Am J Obstet Gynecol.* 2013;209(4):335.e1–335.e12.

Broyles LN, Luo R, Boeras D, Vojnov L. The risk of sexual transmission of HIV in individuals with low-level HIV viraemia: a systematic review. *Lancet.* 2023;402(10400):464–471. doi:10.1016/S0140-6736(23)00877-2

Bukkems V, Necsoi C, Tenorio CH, et al. Clinically significant lower elvitegravir exposure during the third trimester of pregnant patients living with human immunodeficiency virus: data from the pharmacokinetics of antiretroviral agents in HIV-infected pregnant women (PANNA) network. *Clin Infect Dis.* 2020;71(10):e714–e717.

Centers for Disease Control and Prevention (CDC). Estimated HIV incidence and prevalence in the United States, 2018–2022. *HIV Surveillance Supplemental Report* 2024;29(1). https://www.cdc.gov/hiv-data/nhss/estimated-hiv-incidence-and-prevalence.html. Published May 2024a. Accessed June 23, 2024.

CDC. Monitoring selected national HIV prevention and care objectives by using HIV surveillance data—United States and 6 territories and freely associated states, 2022. *HIV Surveillance Supplemental Report* 2024;29(2). https://www.cdc.gov/hiv-data/nhss/national-hiv-prevention-and-care-outcomes.html. Published May 2024b. Accessed June 23, 2024.

Chesson HW, Dunne EF, Hariri S, Markowitz LE. The estimated lifetime probability of acquiring human papillomavirus in the United States. *Sex Transm Dis.* 2014;41(11):660–664. https://doi.org/10.1097/olq.0000000000000193

Clark H, Babu AS, Wiewel EW, et al. Diagnosed HIV infection in transgender adults and adolescents: results from the National HIV Surveillance System, 2009–2014. *AIDS Behav.* 2017 Sep;21(9):2774–2783. https://doi.org/10.1007/s10461-016-1656-7

Clifford GM, Georges D, Shiels MS, et al. A meta-analysis of anal cancer incidence by risk group: Toward a unified anal cancer risk scale. *Int J Cancer.* 2021;148(1):38–47. doi:10.1002/ijc.33185.

Coghill AE, Shiels MS, Suneja G, Engels EA. Elevated cancer-specific mortality among HIV-infected patients in the United States. *J Clin Oncol.* 2015;33(21):2376–2383. doi:10.1200/JCO.2014.59.5967

Cohen MS, Chen YQ, McCauley M, et al. Antiretroviral therapy for the prevention of HIV-1 transmission. *N Engl J Med.* 2016;375(9):830–839. doi:10.1056/NEJMoa1600693

Connor EM, Sperling RS, Gelber R, et al. Reduction of maternal-infant transmission of human immunodeficiency virus type 1 with zidovudine treatment. Pediatric AIDS Clinical Trials Group Protocol 076 Study Group. *N Engl J Med.* 1994;331(18):1173–1180.

Cooper ER, Charurat M, Mofenson L, et al; Women and Infants' Transmission Study Group. Combination antiretroviral strategies for the treatment of pregnant HIV-1-infected women and prevention of perinatal HIV-1 transmission. *J Acquir Immune Defic Syndr.* 2002;29(5):484–94.

Crauwels HM, Osiyemi O, Zorrilla C, et al. Reduced exposure to darunavir and cobicistat in HIV-1-infected pregnant women receiving a darunavir/cobicistat-based regimen. *HIV Med.* 2019;20(5):337–343. doi:10.1111/hiv.12721

Davis AT, Chakraborty H, Flowers L, Mosunjac MB. Cervical dysplasia in women infected with the human immunodeficiency virus (HIV): a correlation with HIV viral load and CD4+ count. *Gynecol Oncol.* 2001;80(3):350–4.

de Sanjose S, Quint WG, Alemany L, et al. Human papillomavirus genotype attribution in invasive cervical cancer: a retrospective cross-sectional worldwide study. *Lancet Oncol.* 2010;11(11):1048–1056. doi:10.1016/S1470-2045(10)70230-8

Denny LA, Franceschi S, de Sanjosé S, et al. Human papillomavirus, human immunodeficiency virus and immunosuppression. *Vaccine.* 2012;30(Suppl 5):F168–F174.

Del Romero J, Baza MB, Río I, et al. Natural conception in HIV-serodiscordant couples with the infected partner in suppressive antiretroviral therapy: a prospective cohort study. *Medicine (Baltimore).* 2016;95(30):e4398. doi:10.1097/MD.0000000000004398

Department of Health and Human Services (DHHS). Guidelines for the prevention and treatment of opportunistic infections in adults and adolescents with HIV. https://clinicalinfo.hiv.gov/en/guidelines/hiv-clinical-guidelines-adult-and-adolescent-opportunistic-infections/. Published 2024a. Accessed June 23, 2024.

Department of Health and Human Services (DHHS). Panel on Treatment of HIV During Pregnancy and Prevention of Perinatal Transmission. Recommendations for the use of antiretroviral drugs during pregnancy and interventions to reduce perinatal HIV transmission in the United States. https://clinicalinfo.hiv.gov/en/guidelines/perinatal. Published 2024b. Accessed June 23, 2024.

Egemen D, Katki HA, Chaturvedi AK, Landy R, Cheung LC. Variation in human papillomavirus vaccination effectiveness in the US by age at vaccination. *JAMA Network Open.* 2022;5(10):e2238041. https://doi.org/10.1001/jamanetworkopen.2022.38041

Ellerbrock TV, Chiasson MA, Bush TJ, et al. Incidence of cervical squamous intraepithelial lesions in HIV-infected women. *JAMA.* 2000;283(8):1031–1037. https://doi.org/10.1001/jama.283.8.1031

Ellingson MK, Sheikha H, Nyhan K, et al. Human papillomavirus vaccine effectiveness by age at vaccination: a systematic review. *Hum Vaccin Immunother.* 2023;19(2):2239085. doi:10.1080/21645515.2023.2239085

Evidence for Contraceptive Options and HIV Outcomes (ECHO) Trial Consortium. HIV incidence among women using intramuscular depot medroxyprogesterone acetate, a copper intrauterine device, or a levonorgestrel implant for contraception: a randomised, multicentre, open-label trial *Lancet.* 2019;394(10195):303–313. doi:10.1016/S0140-6736(19)31288-7. Published correction appears in *Lancet.* 2019 Jul 27;394(10195):302. doi:10.1016/S0140-6736(19)31408-4.

FDA Roundup: May 17, 2024. https://www.fda.gov/news-events/press-announcements/fda-roundup-may-17-2024. Published May 17, 2024. Accessed September 9, 2024.

Finocchario-Kessler S, Bastos FI, Malta M, et al. Discussing childbearing with HIV-infected women of reproductive age in clinical care: a comparison of Brazil and the US. *AIDS Behav.* 2012;16(1):99–107. doi:10.1007/s10461-011-9906-1

Flynn PM, Taha TE, Cababasay M; PROMISE Study Team. Association of maternal viral load and CD4 count with perinatal HIV-1 transmission risk during breastfeeding in the PROMISE postpartum component. *J Acquir Immune Defic Syndr.* 2021;88(2):206–213.

Ford N, Calmy A, Mofenson L. Safety of efavirenz in the first trimester of pregnancy: an updated systematic review and meta-analysis. *AIDS.* 2011;25(18):2301–2304.

Galli L, Puliti D, Chiappini E, et al; Italian Register for HIV Infection in Children. Is the interruption of antiretroviral treatment during pregnancy an additional major risk factor for mother-to-child transmission of HIV type 1? *Clin Infect Dis.* 2009;48(9):1310–1317.

Firnhaber C, Van Le H, Pettifor A. et al. Association between cervical dysplasia and human papillomavirus in HIV seropositive women from Johannesburg South Africa. *Cancer Causes Control.* 2010;21(3):433–443. https://doi.org/10.1007/s10552-009-9475-z

Holcomb K, Matthews RP, Chapman JE, et al. The efficacy of cervical conization in the treatment of cervical intraepithelial neoplasia in HIV-positive women. *Gynecol Oncol.* 1999;74(3):428–431. https://doi.org/10.1006/gyno.1999.5479

Holt LM, Short WR, Momplaisir F, et al. Bictegravir use during pregnancy: a multi-center retrospective analysis evaluating HIV viral suppression and perinatal outcomes. *Clin Infect Dis.* 2024:ciae218. doi:10.1093/cid/ciae218

Hoyt MJ, Storm DS, Aaron E, Anderson J. Preconception and contraceptive care for women living with HIV. *Infect Dis Obstet Gynecol.* 2012;2012:604183. doi:10.1155/2012/604183

Hsiao KT. Screening for cervical cancer in transgender men. UCSF Transgender Care. Published 2016. https://transcare.ucsf.edu/guidelines/cervical-cancer. Accessed June 17, 2016.

Jamieson DJ, Duerr A, Burk R, et al. Characterization of genital human papillomavirus infection in women who have or who are at risk of having HIV infection. *Am J Obstet Gynecol.* 2002;186(1):21–27. https://doi.org/https://doi.org/10.1067/mob.2002.119776

Johnson LF, Lewis DA. The effect of genital tract infections on HIV-1 shedding in the genital tract: a systematic review and meta-analysis. *Sex Transm Dis.* 2008;35(11):946–959. doi:10.1097/OLQ.0b013e3181812d15

Krishna GR, Haddad LB. Interactions between hormonal contraception and anti-retroviral therapy: an updated review. *Curr Obstet Gynecol Rep.* 2020;9(3):98–104. doi:10.1007/s13669-020-00289-7

Landolt NK, Phanuphak N, Ubolyam S, et al. Efavirenz, in contrast to nevirapine, is associated with unfavorable progesterone and antiretroviral levels when coadministered with combined oral contraceptives.

J Acquir Immune Defic Syndr. 2013;62(5):534–539. doi:10.1097/QAI.0b013e31827e8f98

Lei J, Ploner A, Elfström KM, et al. HPV vaccination and the risk of invasive cervical cancer. *N Engl J Med*. 2020;383(14):1340–1348.

Lima MI, Tafuri A, Araújo AC, de Miranda Lima L, Melo VH. Cervical intraepithelial neoplasia recurrence after conization in HIV-positive and HIV-negative women. *Int J Gynecol Obstet*. 2009;104(2):100–104. https://doi.org/https://doi.org/10.1016/j.ijgo.2008.10.009

Lissouba P, Van de Perre P, Auvert B. Association of genital human papillomavirus infection with HIV acquisition: a systematic review and meta-analysis. *Sex Transm Infect*. 2013;89(5):350–356. https://doi.org/10.1136/sextrans-2011-050346

Liu G, Sharma M, Tan N, Barnabas RV. HIV-positive women have higher risk of human papilloma virus infection, precancerous lesions, and cervical cancer. *AIDS*. 2018;32(6):795–808.

Lockman S, Brummel SS, Ziemba L; IMPAACT 2010/VESTED Study Team and Investigators. Efficacy and safety of dolutegravir with emtricitabine and tenofovir alafenamide fumarate or tenofovir disoproxil fumarate, and efavirenz, emtricitabine, and tenofovir disoproxil fumarate HIV antiretroviral therapy regimens started in pregnancy (IMPAACT 2010/VESTED): a multicentre, open-label, randomised, controlled, phase 3 trial. *Lancet*. 2021;397(10281):1276–1292.

Loutfy MR, Hart TA, Mohammed SS, et al. Fertility desires and intentions of HIV-positive women of reproductive age in Ontario, Canada: a cross-sectional study. *PLoS One*. 2009;4(12):e7925. doi:10.1371/journal.pone.0007925

Marcus JL, Leyden WA, Alexeeff SE, et al. Comparison of overall and comorbidity-free life expectancy between insured adults with and without HIV infection, 2000–2016. *JAMA Netw Open*. 2020;3(6):e207954. doi:10.1001/jamanetworkopen.2020.7954

Massad LS, Ahdieh L, Benning L, et al. Evolution of cervical abnormalities among women with HIV-1: evidence from surveillance cytology in the women's interagency HIV study. *J Acquir Immune Defic Syndr*. 2001;27(5):432–442.

Massad LS, Seaberg EC, Wright RL, et al. Squamous cervical lesions in women with human immunodeficiency virus: long-term follow-up. *Obstet Gynecol*. 2008;111(6):1388–1393.

Massad LS, Springer G, Jacobson L, et al. Pregnancy rates and predictors of conception, miscarriage and abortion in US women with HIV. *AIDS*. 2004;18(2):281–286. doi:10.1097/00002030-200401230-00018

Mesfin YM, Kibret KT, Taye A. Is protease inhibitors based antiretroviral therapy during pregnancy associated with an increased risk of preterm birth? Systematic review and a meta-analysis. *Reprod Health*. 2016;13:30. doi:10.1186/s12978-016-0149-5

Mirochnick M, Capparelli E. Pharmacokinetics of antiretrovirals in pregnant women. *Clin Pharmacokinet*. 2004;43(15):1071–1087.

Momper JD, Best BM, Wang J, et al.; IMPAACT P1026s Protocol Team. Elvitegravir/cobicistat pharmacokinetics in pregnant and postpartum women with HIV. *AIDS*. 2018;32(17):2507–2516.

Momper JD, Wang J, Stek A, et al.; IMPAACT P1026s Protocol Team. Pharmacokinetics of atazanavir boosted with cobicistat in pregnant and postpartum women with HIV. *J Acquir Immune Defic Syndr*. 2022;89(3):303–309.

Nattabi B, Li J, Thompson SC, et al. A systematic review of factors influencing fertility desires and intentions among people living with HIV/AIDS: implications for policy and service delivery. *AIDS Behav*. 2009;13(5):949–968. doi:10.1007/s10461-009-9537-y

NCI launches network to study self-collection for HPV testing to prevent cervical cancer. 2024. https://prevention.cancer.gov/news-and-events/blog/nci-launches-network-study-self-collection-hpv-testing-prevent-cervical-cancer

Nesheim SR, Linley L, Gray KM, et al. Country of birth of children with diagnosed HIV infection in the United States, 2008–2014. *J Acquir Immune Defic Syndr*. 2018;77(1):23–30. doi:10.1097/QAI.0000000000001572

Palefsky JM, Lee JY, Jay N, et al. Treatment of anal high-grade squamous intraepithelial lesions to prevent anal cancer. *N Engl J Med*. 2022 Jun 16;386(24):2273–2282. doi:10.1056/NEJMoa2201048

Patel RC, Onono M, Gandhi M, et al. Pregnancy rates in HIV-positive women using contraceptives and efavirenz-based or nevirapine-based antiretroviral therapy in Kenya: a retrospective cohort study. *Lancet HIV*. 2015;2(11):e474–e482. doi:10.1016/S2352-3018(15)00184-8

Pretsch PK, Spees LP, Brewer NT, et al. Effect of HPV self-collection kits on cervical cancer screening uptake among under-screened women from low-income US backgrounds (MBMT-3): a phase 3, open-label, randomised controlled trial. *Lancet Public Health*. 2023;8(6):e411–e421. doi:10.1016/S2468-2667(23)00076-2. Erratum in: *Lancet Public Health*. 2023;8(11):e838. doi:10.1016/S2468-2667(23)00253-0.

Rim SH, Saraiya M, Beer L, Tie Y, Yuan X, Weiser J. Access to high-resolution anoscopy among persons with HIV and abnormal anal cytology results. *JAMA Network Open*. 2024;7(3):e240068. doi:10.1001/jamanetworkopen.2024.0068

Robinson JA, Jamshidi R, Burke AE. Contraception for the HIV-positive woman: a review of interactions between hormonal contraception and antiretroviral therapy. *Infect Dis Obstet Gynecol*. 2012;2012:890160. doi:10.1155/2012/890160

Rodger AJ, Cambiano V, Bruun T, et al. Sexual activity without condoms and risk of HIV transmission in serodifferent couples when the HIV-positive partner is using suppressive antiretroviral therapy. JAMA. 2016 Aug 9;316(6):667. doi:10.1001/jama.2016.10914. Published correction appears in *JAMA*. 2016;316(2):171–181. doi:10.1001/jama.2016.5148

Rough K, Seage GR 3rd, Williams PL; PHACS and the IMPAACT P1025 Study Teams. Birth outcomes for pregnant women with HIV using tenofovir-emtricitabine. *N Engl J Med*. 2018;378(17):1593–1603.

Sahasrabuddhe VV, Mwanahamuntu MH, Vermund SH, et al. Prevalence and distribution of HPV genotypes among HIV-infected women in Zambia. *Br J Cancer*. 2007;96(9):1480–1483.

Scarsi KK, Smeaton LM, Podany AT, et al. Pharmacokinetics of dose-adjusted levonorgestrel emergency contraception combined with efavirenz-based antiretroviral therapy or rifampicin-containing tuberculosis regimens. *Contraception*. 2023;121:109951. doi:10.1016/j.contraception.2023.109951

Sekar VJ, Lefebvre E, Guzman SS, et al. Pharmacokinetic interaction between ethinyl estradiol, norethindrone and darunavir with low-dose ritonavir in healthy women. *Antivir Ther*. 2008;13(4):563–569.

Sharma A, Feldman JG, Golub ET, et al. Live birth patterns among human immunodeficiency virus-infected women before and after the availability of highly active antiretroviral therapy. *Am J Obstet Gynecol*. 2007;196(6):541.e1–541.e5416. doi:10.1016/j.ajog.2007.01.005

Smith JS, Des Marais AC, Deal AM, et al. Mailed human papillomavirus self-collection with Papanicolaou test referral for infrequently screened women in the United States. *Sex Transm Dis*. 2018;45(1):42–48.

Squires KE, Hodder SL, Feinberg J, et al. Health needs of HIV-infected women in the United States: insights from the women living positive survey. *AIDS Patient Care STDS*. 2011;25(5):279–285. doi:10.1089/apc.2010.0228

Stelzle D, Tanaka LF, Lee KK, et al. Estimates of the global burden of cervical cancer associated with HIV. *Lancet Glob Health*. 2021;9(2):e161–e169.

Stier EA, Clarke MA, Deshmukh AA, et al. International Anal Neoplasia Society's consensus guidelines for anal cancer screening. *Int J Cancer*. 2024;154(10):1694–1702. doi:10.1002/ijc.34850

Stier EA, Engels E, Horner MJ, et al. Cervical cancer incidence stratified by age in women with HIV compared with the general population in the United States, 2002–2016. *AIDS*. 2021;35(11):1851–1856. Stoler MH. Advances in cervical screening technology. *Mod Pathol*. 2000;13(3):275–84.

Sun XW, Kuhn L, Ellerbrock TV, et al. Human papillomavirus infection in women infected with the human immunodeficiency virus. *N Engl J Med*. 1997;337(19):1343–1349. doi:10.1056/NEJM199711063371903

Sutton MY, Zhou W, Frazier EL. Unplanned pregnancies and contraceptive use among HIV- positive women in care. *PLoS One*. 2018;13(5):e0197216. doi:10.1371/journal.pone.0197216

Tepper NK, Curtis KM, Cox S, Whiteman MK. Update to U.S. medical eligibility criteria for contraceptive use, 2016: updated recommendations for the use of contraception among women at high risk for HIV infection. *MMWR*. 2020;69(14):405–410. doi:10.15585/mmwr.mm6914a3

Tshivuila-Matala COO, Honeyman S, Nesbitt C, et al. Adverse perinatal outcomes associated with antiretroviral therapy regimens: systematic review and network meta-analysis. *AIDS*. 2020;34(11):1643–1656.

Tuthill EL, Tomori C, Van Natta M, Coleman JS. "In the United States, we say, 'No breastfeeding,' but that is no longer realistic": provider perspectives towards infant feeding among women living with HIV in the United States. *J Int AIDS Soc*. 2019;22(1):e25224. doi:10.1002/jia2.25224.

van Sighem AI, Gras LA, Reiss P; ATHENA National Observational Cohort Study. Life expectancy of recently diagnosed asymptomatic HIV-infected patients approaches that of uninfected individuals. *AIDS*. 2010;24(10):1527–1535. doi:10.1097/QAD.0b013e32833a3946

Warszawski J, Tubiana R, Le Chenadec J, et; ANRS French Perinatal Cohort. Mother-to-child HIV transmission despite antiretroviral therapy in the ANRS French Perinatal Cohort. *AIDS*. 2008;22(2):289–299.

Winer RL, Tiro JA, Miglioretti DL, et al. Rationale and design of the HOME trial: a pragmatic randomized controlled trial of home-based human papillomavirus (HPV) self-sampling for increasing cervical cancer screening uptake and effectiveness in a U.S. healthcare system. *Contemp Clin Trials*. 2018;64:77–87. doi:10.1016/j.cct.2017.11.004. Erratum in: *Contemp Clin Trials*. 2019;84:105811. doi:10.1016/j.cct.2019.07.003

World Health Organization. *Contraceptive Eligibility for Women at High Risk of HIV: Guidance Statement: Recommendations on Contraceptive Methods Used by Women at High Risk of HIV*. Geneva: World Health Organization; 2019. https://www.who.int/reproductivehealth/publications/contraceptive-eligibility-women-at-high-risk-of-HIV/en/

Yang DX, Soulos PR, Davis B, et al. Impact of widespread cervical cancer screening: number of cancers prevented and changes in race-specific incidence. *Am J Clin Oncol*. 2018;41(3):289–294. https://doi.org/10.1097/coc.0000000000000264

Yusuf HE, Knott-Grasso MA, Anderson J, Livingston A, et al. Experience and outcomes of breastfed infants of women living with HIV in the United States: findings from a single-center breastfeeding support initiative. *J Pediatric Infect Dis Soc*. 2022;11(1):24–27. doi:10.1093/jpids/piab116. Erratum in: *J Pediatric Infect Dis Soc*. 2022;11(5):240. doi:10.1093/jpids/piab134

Zash R, Caniglia EC, Diseko M, et al. Maternal weight and birth outcomes among women on antiretroviral treatment from conception in a birth surveillance study in Botswana. *J Int AIDS Soc*. 2021;24(6):e25763.

Zash R, Holmes L, Diseko M, et al. Neural-tube defects and antiretroviral treatment regimens in Botswana. *N Engl J Med*. 2019;381(9):827–840.

Zash R, Makhema J, Shapiro RL. Neural-tube defects with dolutegravir treatment from the time of conception. *N Engl J Med*. 2018;379(10):979–981.

Zhang H, Hindman JT, Lin L, et al. A study of the pharmacokinetics, safety, and efficacy of bictegravir/emtricitabine/tenofovir alafenamide in virologically suppressed pregnant women with HIV. *AIDS*. 2024;38(1):F1–F9. https://doi.org/10.1097/qad.0000000000003783

23.

AGING AND HIV

Aroonsiri Howell, John D. Zeuli, and Anchalee Avihingsanon

LEARNING OBJECTIVES

- Describe how HIV care and management for older people with HIV (PWH) differs from the care and management for younger PWH.
- Understand how to conduct a Comprehensive Geriatric Assessment to assess function, mobility/fall risk, frailty, cognition, mood, and issues related to polypharmacy.
- Discuss a comprehensive medication assessment, nutrition and weight changes, social and monetary issues impacting care, symptom burdens and pain, and advanced planning.
- Review specific coexisting conditions common to aging that are impacted by HIV, including diabetes mellitus, hypertension, bone disease, peripheral neuropathy, certain cancers, and recommended vaccinations.

WHAT'S NEW

- Some society guidelines (for example, the latest European AIDS Clinical Society recommendations) now provide specific information regarding the care of older people living with HIV (EACS, 2023).

KEY POINTS

- Each older PWH has unique and complex individualized needs, and disease-centric guidelines should not be applied the same way for every patient.
- Disease management in older PWH should be individualized based on aging phenotypes, interactions with multimorbidity, and patient preferences.
- The Veterans Aging Cohort Study (VACS) index 2.0 may be used to identify aging phenotypes and can provide prognostic information to help prioritize interventions and guide shared decision-making with PWH and caregivers.

INTRODUCTION

There are increasing proportions of older PWH. It is estimated that at year-end 2022, persons aged 55–64 years made up the largest percentage of PWH (27%) (CDC, 2024). Part of this group consisted of individuals who have aged with chronic HIV infection, but a large proportion also represent cases of new HIV diagnoses, with 11% of all new HIV transmissions in 2022 diagnosed in PWH aged 55 years and older.

Although many recommendations on the management of people with HIV infection are not age specific, PWH over the age of 50 years differ from their younger counterparts in many aspects, including diagnostic considerations, immune response to ART, and multimorbidity. In this chapter, we outline these differences, offer a strategy on how to care for this unique population, provide a practical guide on how to perform a Comprehensive Geriatric Assessment (CGA), and describe special considerations for problem-based management of PWH over the age of 50.

DIFFERENCES IN OLDER PWH COMPARED TO YOUNGER PWH

The most common mode of HIV transmission among adults aged 50 years and older is through sexual contact. Among men, male-to-male sexual contact is the most common transmission risk, while heterosexual contact is the most common among women (CDC, 2018). This may be due to a false sense of security among older adults who view sexually transmitted infections (STI) as a condition of the young, and who may forgo safer sex practices based on this perception (Pilowsky and Wu, 2015). They may also forgo use of barrier contraceptives when unintended pregnancy is no longer a concern. Even though sexual exposure is the most common mode of HIV transmission among PWH aged 50 years and older, prior research has found that healthcare professionals often underestimate the level of sexual activity among older adults and their risk of STI exposure (Lindau et al., 2007; Pilowsky and Wu, 2015).

Moreover, many symptoms of acute HIV infection mimic those of other conditions that are common among older adults and may be difficult for clinicians to tease apart. Headache, loss of energy, loss of appetite, flu-like symptoms, and weight loss are common in older adults and can be caused by a myriad of conditions associated with older age, such as malignancy, frailty, or seasonal respiratory infections.

With inaccurate perception of HIV exposure risk and symptom mimicry, underdiagnoses and late diagnoses of HIV transmissions are common among older adults (Dai et al., 2015; Pilowsky and Wu, 2015). Late diagnosis is associated with delayed treatment, impaired response to (and decreased tolerability of) ART, increased morbidity and mortality, lost opportunity to prevent onward transmission, and increased cost of health care (British HIV Association, 2023). As a result, it is essential that clinicians maintain a high suspicion and routinely screen older adults for HIV, regardless of risk perception. Although guidelines from the Centers for Disease Control and Prevention (CDC) recommends routine screening up to the age of 64 years (CDC, 2006), the rationale or research evidence for this age cutoff was not included, and the authors recommend routine screening for all older adults, as risk perception may be inaccurate in this population.

Despite successful viral suppression with ART, older adults have less robust immunologic recovery compared to their younger counterparts, with associated increase in mortality (Mpondo et al., 2016; Semeere et al., 2014; Vinikoor et al., 2014). Consequently, early HIV diagnosis and treatment are of great importance.

MULTIMORBIDITY

Older PWH are at increased risk of *multimorbidity* (Guaraldi et al., 2014), defined as the development of multiple chronic conditions that do not simply coexist, but together interact to worsen health outcomes. Compared to people without HIV, older PWH have higher burdens of cardiovascular, metabolic, pulmonary, renal, bone, and malignant diseases (Schouten et al., 2014). Multimorbidity is likely contributed by both lifestyle risk factors as well as chronic HIV infection, with a longer duration of severe immunodeficiency ($CD4^+$ counts <200 cells/μL) correlating with higher comorbidity burden (Schouten et al., 2014).

Multimorbidity has important ramifications on health outcomes. It is associated with self-reported poor health, declines in self-rated health status, and increased mortality (adjusted odds ratio 11.87; 95% CI: 5.72–24.62) (Koroukian et al., 2015). With increasing disease burden, PWH with multimorbidity are also at risk of fragmentation in care because of the involvement of multiple clinicians in multiple settings. Guidelines for one disease may conflict with another, as most are disease-centric recommendations based on the "ideal" patient without multimorbidity (Tinetti et al., 2012). Treatments for one disease may inadvertently worsen other conditions, and increased treatment burden stemming from efforts to adhere to all relevant disease-centric guidelines without prioritization may not bring improvement in mortality or quality of life.

MANAGEMENT STRATEGY FOR THE CARE OF OLDER PWH

Each older PWH has unique and complex, individualized needs. Older PWH cannot be described fully by one-dimensional classifications, such as chronological age or single disease entities. Aging occurs at different rates in different individuals, and within the same individual in different organs, resulting in different aging phenotypes that cannot be predicted by chronological age alone. Additionally, viewing PWH by a single disease entity ignores the importance of multimorbidity and the often multifactorial nature of their diseases. Most importantly, different PWH have different goals and preferences. Consequently, applying disease-centric guidelines uniformly to every patient without considering aging phenotypes, multimorbidity, or individual preference ignores the unique care needs of each patient and likely will not lead to desirable patient-centered outcomes.

Understanding that not all PWH aged 50 years and older should be approached the same way, clinicians may utilize the Veterans Aging Cohort Study (VACS) index (Justice et al., 2013b) to distinguish between those who are aging well and those who may appear phenotypically older than their chronological age. The VACS index has been shown to correlate with functional status (John et al., 2014), provide insight to clinician assessment of severity of illness (Justice et al., 2013b), and predict cause-specific (Justice et al., 2012) as well as all-cause mortality (Justice et al., 2013a). Based on prognosis predicted by the VACS index, clinicians can elicit patient preferences, identify diseases and risk factors that affect these goals, calculate the likely effects and lag time to benefit (Lee et al., 2013) of various disease-centric guidelines on these goals, and use this information to prioritize interventions and guide shared decision-making with patients and caregivers. The recently updated VACS index 2.0 is freely accessible on MDCalc (https://www.mdcalc.com/calc/10402/veterans-aging-cohort-study-vacs-2.0-index), and utilizes the following information:

- Age, sex
- BMI
- CD4 count, HIV-1 RNA level
- Estimated glomerular filtration rate (GFR)
- ALT/AST
- Hemoglobin, WBC, platelet count
- Albumin
- Hepatitis C coinfection.

COMPREHENSIVE GERIATRIC ASSESSMENT

Comprehensive Geriatric Assessment (CGA) is a multidisciplinary diagnostic and treatment process that evaluates medical, psychosocial, and functional needs in order to develop a coordinated intervention/plan to maximize overall health with aging (Stuck et al., 1993). CGA is based on the idea that a systematic evaluation of an older patient may lead to early detection of geriatric concerns, help prevent complications, and aid the formation of comprehensive treatment plans (Bellera et al., 2012).

There is no peer-reviewed literature to demonstrate the efficacy of CGA in older PWH, although, owing to increased risks of geriatric syndromes in older PWH, many studies advocate for CGA in this population. In people without HIV, CGA in the home may improve functional status, prevent institutionalization, and reduce mortality (Huss et al., 2008). CGA in the hospital, especially in dedicated units, may improve survival (Ellis et al., 2017). However, CGA in outpatient settings has not been found to consistently show benefits (Stuck et al., 1993), possibly because of the variability in adherence to the recommendations in CGA. CGA as part of inpatient geriatric consultation (except for specific conditions such as hip fracture) have shown little benefit (Ellis et al., 2017; Stuck et al., 1993). Studies have shown that more complex CGA programs that address adherence or target patients at higher risk of admission may improve outcomes including physical functioning, social functioning, pain, mental/physical/emotional health, and overall well-being (Reuben et al., 1999).

PERFORMING A COMPREHENSIVE GERIATRIC ASSESSMENT

Consider avoiding assessing all domains of CGA in a single visit—this could be overwhelming and tiring for some patients, as well as their family members or other caregivers. It may make sense to prioritize domains that are most likely to be abnormal or clinically urgent (i.e., likely to cause complications or catastrophic outcomes). Once the most urgent domains have been identified and managed, the remaining nonurgent domains may be completed at subsequent visits. Various care team members may be designated to manage certain domains of the CGA based on their expertise or availability. For example, it may make sense for a pharmacist to assess patients for polypharmacy, instead of a physician.

There is no consensus on selection criteria for patients who may benefit from CGA. However, prior programs have used criteria such as age, medical comorbidities/complexity, specific geriatric syndromes such as falls/dementia, previous or predicted high healthcare utilization rates, or at times of transition, such as from hospital to home, or from home to nursing homes/long-term care facilities.

Additionally, there is no consensus on what domains should be included in CGA and what tools are appropriate for each domain. However, most programs include some or all of the following domains. Except when noted, corresponding interventions are described in more details in the European AIDS Clinical Society guideline, accessible through website or mobile app (https://www.eacsociety.org/guidelines/eacs-guidelines/) (EACS, 2023).

FUNCTIONAL STATUS

The Activity of Daily Living (ADL) and Instrumental Activity of Daily Living (IADL) assessment tools have been utilized in PWH, are simple to perform, and can readily identify essential deficits that may guide interventions. To assess functional status, providers may ask about ADLs/IADLs and determine who does them (patient or others). ADLs consist of bathing, dressing, grooming, toileting, transferring, and eating. IADLs consist of cooking, shopping, managing medications, using the phone, doing housework, doing laundry, driving or using public transportation, and managing finances (Katz et al., 1963).

MOBILITY/FALLS

Subjective information may be elicited by asking PWH if they had a *fall* in the past 12 months, defined as unexpectedly dropping to the floor or ground from a standing, walking, or bending position (Erlandson et al., 2012; Erlandson et al., 2016; Ruiz et al., 2013). Objective information may be obtained through provider-administered measures such as the Timed Get-Up-and-Go (TUG) test (Podsiadlo and Richardson, 1991), in which the patient is timed while he/she/they rises from a chair, walks 3 meters, turns, walks back, and sits down again. The TUG has been used in prior HIV studies (Grinspoon et al., 1996; Grinspoon et al., 1998) and explores multiple components of mobility, including gait speed, balance, and proximal muscle strength. The TUG has also been shown to correlate with functional capacity and more formal tests on balance and gait speed (Podsiadlo and Richardson, 1991). Although various cutoffs have been used in prior studies, the CDC recommends that an older adult who takes ≥12 seconds to complete TUG should be considered at risk of falling (CDC, 2017).

FRAILTY

There is no consensus on the best tools to assess for frailty in older PWH (Conroy, 2009; Brothers and Rockwood, 2019). The Fried frailty phenotype (Fried et al., 2001) is commonly used in HIV research and has been operationalized for clinical practice (Rockwood et al., 2007) to consist of five components (no items = robust; 1–2 = prefrail; 3–5 = frail):

1. *Weight loss*: defined as loss of either ≥10 pounds or ≥5% of body weight in the past year.
2. *Exhaustion* (poor endurance and energy): defined as self-reporting of feeling "tired all the time."
3. *Low physical activity levels and energy expenditure*: defined as needing assistance with walking to being unable to walk.
4. *Slowness*: defined as a time of ≥19 seconds on TUG test.
5. *Weakness*: defined as abnormal strength on physical examination.

The VACS index is another frailty tool specifically validated in PWH, with more details described below. An online calculator is accessible on MDCalc at: (https://www.mdcalc.com/calc/10402/veterans-aging-cohort-study-vacs-2.0-index). Prior HIV studies have also used the Frailty Index. Because it follows the cumulative deficit approach and assesses for at least 30 and up to 75 health variables (Searle et al., 2008), this may prove cumbersome in clinical practice.

COGNITION/SAFETY CONCERNS

Age is a risk factor for cognitive impairment associated with HIV as well as other causes (Chan and Brew, 2014). In the general population, the U.S. Preventive Services Task

Force (USPSTF) recommends that the current evidence is insufficient (Grade I) to assess the balance of benefits and harms of screening for cognitive impairment in older adults (USPSTF, 2020). In PWH, the IAS-USA recommends periodic assessment of cognitive function using a validated instrument in those >60 years old (Gandhi et al., 2023). It should be noted that many studies of cognitive impairment screening in PWH focus on the entity of HIV-associated neurocognitive disorder (HAND), although in clinical practice, providers would likely need to screen for cognitive impairment from all causes, as older PWH may also develop non-HIV-specific conditions such as Alzheimer disease or vascular dementia. Providers may consider using the Montreal Cognitive Assessment (MoCA, https://mocacognition.com/), since it has been studied extensively in PWH (Rosca et al., 2019; Sangarlangkarn et al., 2019), and it is commonly used to screen for other causes of cognitive impairment. The HIV Dementia Scale (Power et al., 1995) and the International HIV Dementia Scale (Sacktor et al., 2005) were developed to screen for HAND, but their effectiveness in screening for other causes of dementia is unclear. Even though the Mini-Mental Status Exam is regularly used in HIV-negative individuals, it does not assess for executive function, which may be especially impaired in HAND (Valcour et al., 2011). Neuropsychological testing may be inaccessible or cumbersome for older PWH to complete, although may be helpful in some scenarios.

MOOD

Depression and post-traumatic stress disorder (PTSD) are common in older PWH, especially women and men who have sex with men (Gallagher et al., 2008). Screening for depression and assessment of its severity is important since depression may affect quality of life, engagement in care, and adherence to medications. Social isolation may also have a negative impact on mental health (Reuda et al., 2014). Multiple tools have been used in PWH to screen for depression, including a screening Patient Health Questionnaire (PHQ-2) with subsequent diagnostic PHQ-9 (Chibanda et al., 2016; EACS, 2023); the Beck Depression Inventory II (BDI-II) (Rodkjaer et al., 2016); or the Center for Epidemiological Studies (CES-D) (Mueses-Marin et al., 2019). Although as many as 14 tools have been used to screen for PTSD in PWH (Gallagher et al., 2008), the post-traumatic stress disorder checklist (PCL-5) was validated for use in HIV primary care (Verhey et al., 2018). Because the understanding and perception of depression or other mental health conditions can be affected by culture, it is important to use tools that have been validated locally if available (Sangarlangkarn et al., 2019).

POLYPHARMACY

Older PWH face a unique challenge of managing the burden of HIV disease in the context of chronic multidrug antiretroviral therapy (ART), increased risk of polypharmacy owing to multimorbidity, decreasing end organ function, and physiologic pharmacodynamic changes resulting in a narrower therapeutic index for many drug therapies. HIV providers need to be aware of polypharmacy in older PWH and take steps to optimize medication safety and effective medication use (King et al., 2024).

The term *polypharmacy* has been variably defined in the literature, usually meaning that a patient medication profile has reached a threshold number of medications (often 6 or more) with the degree of polypharmacy correlated to a larger number of absolute medications. It has also been associated with duration of time on multiple medications, and characterized as to whether or not multiple medications were appropriate for a given condition (appropriate vs. inappropriate polypharmacy) (Masnoon et al., 2017). The nature of chronic combined ART for PWH in an aging population already at risk of higher medication burden predisposes for potential drug therapy issues (e.g., drug interactions, additive adverse effects/toxicities, pharmacodynamic sensitivity, pill burden, and medication errors). Consequently, it has been shown that the burden of polypharmacy is greater in older PWH than older patients in the general population (Kong et al., 2019) and greater than in younger PWH (Holtzman et al., 2013; Marzolini, 2011).

ART-SPECIFIC CLINICAL CONSIDERATIONS

Multiple factors (e.g., ART history, HIV drug resistance, history of adverse effects, drug interactions, and comorbid conditions) will dictate the selection of appropriate ART and are covered in detail elsewhere in this volume, but special considerations can be employed to mitigate age-related concerns in older PWH. Table 23.1 lists relevant class and drug-specific considerations for older PWH.

ADVERSE-EFFECT CONSIDERATIONS

Data remain limited on the prevalence of specific adverse-effect rates of ART in older PWH, since these patients are often excluded from clinical trials on the basis of confounding illness/multimorbidity, decreased drug clearance, drug-drug interactions that may affect primary outcomes, discontinuation rates, or adverse effect assessment. Although more data evaluating antiretroviral therapy in older PWH are being published (Ramgopal et al., 2020), clinicians still need a heightened awareness of adverse effects of ART, taking into account the extended duration of therapy, potential additive adverse effects from other drug therapy, historical toxicities from older ART, and increased risk of complications owing to certain disease states (i.e., cardiovascular disease, diabetes, and osteopenia/osteoporosis).

MEDICATION CLEARANCE CONSIDERATIONS

Aging is associated with loss of function in both the kidney and liver, which can lead to reduced drug metabolism and excretion, increased drug exposure, and predisposition for

Table 23.1 CLASS AND DRUG-SPECIFIC CONSIDERATIONS FOR THE SELECTION OF ART IN OLDER PEOPLE WITH HIV

INSTIs	Often INSTIs are preferred agents given limited drug interactions (except for EVG/c) and favorable adverse effect profile. Potential association with weight gain. Possible neuropsychiatric adverse effects (e.g., dizziness, depression, and insomnia), though rare. Polyvalent mineral supplements (e.g., calcium, iron) should be spaced accordingly to avoid chelation. BIC and DTG inhibit tubular secretion of creatinine and may cause a stable 0.1–0.2 mg/dL increase in serum creatinine without effect on GFR. BIC and DTG have been associated with weight gain.
NNRTIs	EFZ may be a concern in older PWH because of the high incidence of neuropsychiatric adverse effects (e.g., dizziness, altered sensorium, worsening depression, and vivid dreams/nightmares), notable drug interactions (CYP2B6/3A4 inducer), and association with metabolic abnormalities (e.g., glucose and lipid abnormalities). Acid suppression decreases RPV absorption (PPIs are contraindicated with use), and the food requirement for RPV administration may be inconvenient for older patients. RPV has been associated with QT prolongation, which may be more relevant in older PWH. DOR has less clinical data but may be a favorable option given minimal AEs.
PIs	Notable drug interactions must be accounted for with the PI and boosting agent combinations. PIs as a class have both inhibition and induction effects on cytochrome P450 enzymes. The PI class is also associated with lipid abnormalities, metabolic abnormalities, and CV events. Both DRV and ATV require food for administration. ATV has been shown to have a lower association with CV events than DRV, but ATV absorption is reduced with acid suppression therapy. ATV inhibits UGT and leads to increased indirect serum bilirubin. Skin yellowing, scleral icterus, and bile salt deposition of the skin/consequent pruritis can occur in some patients. Risk is higher based on UGT1A1 genotype.
Boosting agents (i.e., ritonavir and cobicistat)	Both agents pose noteworthy drug interactions as potent CYP3A4 and 2D6 inhibitors. Cobicistat lacks any relevant CYP induction (RTV induces several CYP enzymes) and may afford lower gastrointestinal adverse effects. Cobicistat may also have a lower risk of lipid effect given the independent association of ritonavir with hypertriglyceridemia. Cobicistat also inhibits tubular secretion of creatinine and may cause a stable 0.1–0.2 mg/dL increase in serum creatinine without effect on GFR.
NRTIs	Older NRTIs (DDI, D4T) should not be used given their high risk of mitochondrial toxicity (lactic acidosis, hepatotoxicity, and lipodystrophy) and availability of alternatives. AZT can contribute to macrocytic anemia and peripheral neuropathy and should generally be avoided in older PWH. Tenofovir is associated with nephrotoxicity, Fanconi syndrome, and bone mineral density decreases. TAF affords a lower systemic exposure of tenofovir versus TDF, and TAF has demonstrated less effect on serum creatinine and lower bone mineral density changes during treatment, but it may increase lipids. TAF has been associated with weight gain. ABC has been associated with CV disease and CV-associated mortality in some studies, though its role as a risk factor is unclear.

ABC = abacavir; AEs = adverse events; ATV = atazanavir; AZT = zidovudine; BIC = bictegravir; CV = cardiovascular; D4T = stavudine; DDI = didanosine; DOR = doravirine; DRV = darunavir; DTG = dolutegravir; EFZ = efavirenz; EVG/c = elvitegravir/cobicistat; GFR = glomerular filtration rate; PI = protease inhibitor; RPV = rilpivirine; RTV = ritonavir; TAF = tenofovir alafenamide; TDF = tenofovir disoproxil fumarate; UGT = UDP-glucuronosyltransferase.

potentially more drug toxicity (Knobel et al., 2001; Lindeman et al., 1985; Schmucker, 2001; Wellons et al., 2002). Declining drug clearance with age highlights the need to monitor glomerular filtration rate (GFR) and dose-adjust ART as well as other drug therapies accordingly. The CKD-EPI equation has been postulated in a small subset of people with HIV on stable ART to best predict GFR (Vrouenraets et al., 2012), but the Cockcroft-Gault estimated creatinine clearance remains the standard in clinical trial evaluation and should be used for medication dosing where renal adjustments are required (Abrass et al., 2012). The Childs Pugh score should be calculated for people with chronic liver disease. The DHHS guideline provides a summary table (Appendix B, Table 12, Antiretroviral Dosing Recommendations in Adults with Renal or Hepatic Insufficiency) for dosing adjustments of ART based on estimated creatinine clearance and liver compromise (DHHS, 2024).

COMPREHENSIVE MEDICATION ASSESSMENT

A defined systematic approach to routine medication review will enable identification of medication concerns, guide intervention to address medication issues, optimize prescribing practices, and mitigate or prevent complications arising from polypharmacy in older PWH. Routine and regular medication review should be performed at every care visit, and detailed medication reconciliation should occur at least annually.

We recommend the following systematic approach to medication review in older PWH:

1. Obtain a comprehensive, accurate medication list to perform medication reconciliation.
2. Discontinue unnecessary medication therapy or supplements and optimize nonpharmacologic approaches to aid disease management.
3. Consider new medication therapy for needed indications.
4. Screen for drug interactions.
5. Confirm dosing appropriateness based on renal and liver function and relevant drug interactions.
6. Optimize and simplify the dosing regimen.

The "brown bag review" (Weiss et al., 2016) is a helpful approach to medication reconciliation, where patients are encouraged to bring all medications, herbal medications/supplements, creams/ointments, inhalers, and eye drops (essentially any item that they use regularly to optimize their health) in a brown bag to their appointment for discussion and review. An advantage to the brown bag approach is that patients can physically point out specific medications and describe how they physically take them, which is particularly helpful when actual administration differs from instructions printed on the prescription label. Other helpful ways to garner the medication list can be: (1) to obtain a medication profile and dispensing history from their pharmacy for the last 3–6 months, and (2) screen health information networks (i.e., Surescripts) to garner medication-dispensing histories (this can be viewed/pulled in by certain electronic health record systems).

After confirming an up-to-date medication list, providers need to align each medication with an indication for therapy, enabling assessment of appropriateness for the indication. Further, each indication for drug therapy can be assessed for nonpharmacologic measures to reduce medication need. The BEERS criteria (AGS, 2023), medication appropriateness index (Hanlon and Schmader, 2013; Hanlon et al., 1992), and Screening Tool of Older Persons' Prescriptions (STOPP)/Screening Tool to Alert to Right Treatment (START) (Gallagher et al., 2008) can be utilized to effectively determine inappropriate medications in older PWH that can be discontinued or changed to safer alternatives. The BEERS criteria help provide guidance on inappropriate medication selection in older patients, while the medication appropriateness index utilizes a 10-item assessment to determine degree of medication appropriateness. The STOPP helps identify inappropriate medications in the setting of specific diseases, and START advocates for utilizing appropriate, effective therapy for a given condition. While inappropriate or harmful medications should be removed, appropriate and indicated medications (e.g., aspirin for prophylaxis of cardiovascular stent thrombosis) should be added where appropriate.

Medication interaction screening will assess for additive toxicity of multiple therapies, determine if increased/decreased exposure of drugs is expected, or identify if efficacy concerns may arise from the medication profile. Electronic drug database platforms (Micromedex, Lexi-Comp, and iFacts) often have drug-interaction screening tools to assist clinicians, although reviewing the metabolic pathways and enzyme inhibitor/inducer status of profile medications will also help identify potential problems (see Mechanisms of Antiretroviral-Associated Drug Interactions table of the DHHS guidelines). The DHHS guidelines, as well as the University of Liverpool website (www.hiv-druginteractions.org/), offer in-depth interaction details and recommendations for antiretroviral therapy (DHHS 2024).

Finally, medications need to be dosed appropriately for medication clearance (using estimated creatinine clearance and Child-Pugh scores where appropriate) with medication regimens simplified to reduce regimen complexity. Simplification may mean consolidating administration times to reduce the number of times in the day the patient takes medication and/or offering co-formulated tablets to reduce pill burden.

The drug therapy evaluation will need to continually screen for adverse effects, toxicity, and barriers to adherence to maximize safe medication use, ensure efficacy of therapy, and reduce complications related to polypharmacy. This requires providers to:

1. Screen for any new clinical signs/symptoms as a potential adverse drug effect.
2. Monitor for changes in renal and liver function and dose-adjust medication(s) appropriately.
3. Monitor for socioeconomic barriers (i.e., job loss, insurance, or income) to appropriate medication therapy, engaging social services/case management as able.
4. Continue to discuss goals of care and perceived treatment burden, adjusting or stopping medication therapy that may no longer be congruent with the patient's wishes.

Clinically trained HIV pharmacists are key care team members who can aid in providing optimal care to older PWH (Schafer et al., 2016). Pharmacists are poised to assist in medication therapy management services and are optimal providers to comprehensively reconcile patient medication profiles, screen for drug interaction, and assist with screening of antiretroviral and other drug-related toxicities. When HIV clinical pharmacy services are available, we recommend integrating pharmacists into the care team to aid with the comprehensive and systemic medication review in older PWH. Additional information on the role of pharmacists in HIV care can be found in Chapter 12.

SOCIAL/FINANCIAL ISSUES

A complete social history should be taken. At the initial visit, providers should ask with whom the patient lives and what types of help/services (e.g., nursing, physical therapy, and home health aides) he/she/they have in the home and their community to determine the types of support that are currently available and what additional services may be needed. Caregivers should be screened periodically for caregiver burnout (Adelman et al., 2014). Elder mistreatment or abuse should be evaluated when there are worrisome signs such as bruises, burn or bite marks, pressure ulcers, or malnutrition without clinical explanation (NCEA, 2023). A financial history should include determination of health insurance and identification of financial power of attorney in case patients become too ill to manage their finances.

NUTRITION/WEIGHT CHANGES

There is no consensus on an appropriate nutritional screening tool in older PWH since there are few studies in this area (Ruiz and Kammerman, 2010). The Rapid Nutrition Screening for HIV disease (RNS-H) is the only validated tool in PWH (Wright and Epps, 2020). It has seven questions, takes 10 minutes to administer, and includes important outcomes such as food security, anthropometric measures, and nutritional complications such as dysphagia or diarrhea.

SYMPTOM BURDEN/PAIN

The HIV Symptom Index (Justice et al., 2001) assesses bothersome HIV symptoms (Kilbourne et al., 2002; Ruiz and Kamerman, 2010; Whalen et al., 1994) and has demonstrated strong associations with disease severity and physical and mental health (Justice et al., 2001). This scale can help providers determine which symptoms are present, evaluate the overall symptom burden, and track the severity of symptoms over time.

For older people with HIV experiencing pain (such as that which accompanies chronic peripheral neuropathy), the first step in pain management involves assessing the characteristics of the pain and conducting biopsychosocial diagnostic evaluation of the pain, including assessing for associated conditions such as depression and anxiety or substance use. The Infectious Disease Society of America recommends using the Brief Pain Inventory-Short Form (BPI-SF) (Goodin et al., 2018) or the PEG (average **P**ain intensity, interference with **E**njoyment of life, and interference with **G**eneral activity) (Merlin et al., 2018) to understand the functional impact of pain. Using this information, providers can develop treatment plans that improve not only pain, but also acknowledge and address physical as well as emotional functions.

ADVANCE CARE PLANNING

Advance care planning, which is also discussed in Chapter 38, "Legal Issues," is defined as a process of communication between individuals and their healthcare agents to understand, reflect on, discuss, and plan for future healthcare decisions for a time when individuals may not be able to make their own healthcare decisions, to help maximize patient autonomy. With the increased risk of neurocognitive impairment and debility from multimorbidity, advance care planning is essential among older PWH. Without clear documentation of a surrogate decision-maker for health care and finances, decisions regarding emergent or end-of-life care may be legally deferred to estranged family members who are unaware of the patient's preferences or HIV status (Sangarlangkarn et al., 2016). Although there are no specific guidelines for PWH, the National Institute of Aging recommends advance care planning in all patients with chronic life-limiting illness or anyone older than 55 years old regardless of health status (National Institute on Aging, 2022).

There are no formal guidelines on the optimal time to initiate advance care planning in PWH. However, it is important to keep in mind that a conversation that is too early may result in changing patient preferences over time or the discussion becoming too abstract/far off in the future, while a conversation that is too late may result in patients being too sick or cognitively impaired to communicate preferences, leading to care that does not match patient preferences. With the lack of validated tools in PWH, providers may use the well-established "Respecting Choices" (Pecanac et al., 2014) paradigm, detailing three stages of planning based on the patient's state of health. It should be noted that in cases of late diagnosis with advanced HIV disease at the time of ART initiation, short-term prognosis depends on the severity of the acute illness (such as opportunistic infections), while longer-term prognosis depends on the patient's adherence to ART and their retention in HIV primary care. As a result, advance care planning in this setting needs to balance the optimism surrounding the effectiveness of ART against the severity of acute illness and the long-term challenges of retention in care.

If a patient appears to have cognitive impairment, either from baseline dementia or delirium related to other comorbid disease, capacity should be assessed. It should be noted that patients with cognitive impairment/delirium/dementia should not be dismissed as not having capacity. *Capacity* is treatment and scenario specific, and is defined as the ability to use information regarding a proposed intervention to make a choice that is congruent with the patient's values and preferences. Despite cognitive impairment, if patients can demonstrate understanding, expressing a choice, appreciation, and reasoning, then they are deemed to have capacity to make medical decisions. Any provider can determine capacity, not only psychiatrists or geriatricians.

SPECIAL CONSIDERATIONS FOR PROBLEM-BASED MANAGEMENT OF OLDER PWH

DIABETES

Although primary care guidelines for the management of PWH by the Infectious Disease Society of America (IDSA) did not include age-specific glycemic goals for PWH, AAVHIM recommends a target hemoglobin A1C of 8% for older PWH with frailty, less than 5-year life-expectancy, high risk for hypoglycemia, or high risk for polypharmacy (AAHIVM, 2023). This recommendation mirrors the guideline on standards of medical care in diabetes from the American Diabetes Association (ADA, 2024; Thompson et al., 2021). This topic is also discussed further in Chapter 32, "Endocrine Disorders and Metabolic Complications in HIV."

HYPERTENSION

Goal blood pressure for people with hypertension in the general population remains controversial and presents a challenge for clinicians, with even less evidence to guide management among the people with HIV. This topic is also discussed further in Chapter 29, "Cardiovascular Disease." The Systolic Blood Pressure Intervention Trial (SPRINT) was halted early in September 2015 because of the benefits of lowering systolic blood pressure to below 120 mmHg (Ambrosius et al., 2014), and results of SPRINT have affected a change in guidelines in the United States and other countries. The American College of Cardiology and the American Heart Association guideline currently recommends a blood pressure cutoff of 130/80 mmHg (Whelton et al., 2018). The 2018 Canadian Hypertension Education Program Guidelines recommend a target systolic blood pressure ranging from <120 to 140 mmHg based on risk stratification, with no specific guidelines on older adults or PWH (Hypertension Canada, 2022). However, the Eighth Joint National Committee (JNC8) recommendation has not been updated since SPRINT, and the goal remains <150/90 mmHg in hypertensive adults aged 60 years and older, and <140/90 mmHg for all hypertensive adults with diabetes or nondiabetic chronic kidney disease (James et al., 2014). Current gaps include lack of specific recommendations for people with HIV and lack of consensus among varying guidelines. A sensible approach may include promotion of lifestyle changes (e.g., exercise and careful weight management) and careful up-titration of blood pressure medications to achieve a goal blood pressure of 125/90 mmHg, as long as the patient does not experience medication side effects such as dizziness or falls.

BONE

Certain lifestyle and HIV-related factors put PWH at higher risk of osteoporosis, including smoking, alcohol use, chronic glucocorticoid therapy, low consumption of calcium and vitamin D, low physical activity, immune dysfunction, persistent inflammation, and side effects of antiretroviral medications (Castronuovo et al., 2015). Modifiable risk factors should be addressed, and viral suppression should be achieved with ART. The IDSA recommends baseline bone densitometry (DXA) screening for osteoporosis in HIV-positive postmenopausal women and men aged ≥50 years (Thompson et al., 2021). If osteoporosis is detected, bisphosphonates may be considered as initial therapy. This topic is also discussed further in Chapter 33, "HIV and Bone Health."

AGE-RELATED SEXUAL CHANGES

Age-related sexual changes in PWH include menopause in women and hypogonadism in men.

IDSA guidelines advise that although hormone replacement therapy may be considered in patients with severe menopausal symptoms, it should be used only for a limited period of time at the lowest effective dose. This is because hormone replacement therapy has been associated with a small increased risk of breast cancer, cardiovascular disease, and thromboembolic morbidity in the general population (Thompson et al., 2021). Morning serum testosterone level may be assessed in older men with HIV who are experiencing decreased libido, erectile dysfunction, reduced bone mass or low trauma fractures, hot flashes, or sweats. Low testosterone levels should be confirmed with repeat testing. Full recommendations are included in the IDSA guidelines (Thompson et al., 2021).

MALIGNANCY

As with the general population, age is a risk factor for multiple types of malignancies among PWH. According to the IDSA, mammography should be performed annually in women with HIV ≥50 years, and colorectal cancer screening should be performed beginning at age 45 years in asymptomatic PWH with average risk (Thompson et al., 2021). The U.S. Preventive Services Task Force recommends annual screening for lung cancer with low-dose computed tomography (CT) in adults aged 50–80 years who have a 20 pack-year smoking history and currently smoke or have quit within the past 15 years. The screening should be discontinued once the patient has not smoked for 15 years or develops a health problem that limits life expectancy or the ability/willingness to have curative lung surgery (Jonas et al., 2021). Although there was concern that PWH will have a higher false positive rate from chronic lung changes related to immunosuppression-related pulmonary infections, one study has shown this may not be true (Sigel et al., 2014). There was a similar likelihood of pulmonary nodules meeting National Lung Screening Trial criteria for a positive CT scan among PWH and people without HIV. There were also similar patterns of clinical evaluation triggered by the CT scan, suggesting that the follow-up may not be more aggressive among PWH (Sigel et al., 2014).

SELECT IMMUNIZATIONS

Live-attenuated varicella vaccination can be given to adult PWH without evidence of immunity with $CD4^+$ T-cell counts ≥200 cells/μL (Grohskopf et al., 2019), as no transmission of vaccine strain varicella-zoster virus has been documented in PWH with $CD4^+$ T-cell counts above this threshold (Shafran, 2016).

Regarding zoster prevention, recombinant zoster vaccine (RZV) has higher and more long-lasting efficacy against herpes zoster and postherpetic neuralgia than herpes zoster live-attenuated vaccine, and the CDC preferentially recommends RZV in all persons aged ≥50 years. However, initial efficacy studies did not include immunocompromised persons, and the CDC does not make recommendations regarding use of RZV in this population, although it may be reasonable to vaccinate PWH aged 50 years and older with $CD4^+$ T-cell counts ≥200 cells/μL (Thompson et al., 2021).

One study showed superior immunogenicity in adults 65 years and older who received high-dose inactivated influenza vaccine (IIV) (Fluzone High-Dose HD-IIV3) compared to standard dosing (Fluzone SD-IIV3). Similar results were shown in a small clinical trial among PWH aged 18 years and older (McKittrick et al., 2013). Currently, the CDC recommends any IIV formulation (standard dose or high dose, trivalent or quadrivalent, unadjuvanted or adjuvanted) for patients aged 65 years and older, regardless of HIV status (Grohskopf et al., 2019). We recommend high-dose IIV in older PWH because of its superior immunogenicity.

PWH aged 50 years and older should receive COVID-19 vaccine, including seasonal boosters.

CONCLUSION

There is an increasing proportion of older PWH, and they differ from their younger counterparts in many ways, including the risk for late diagnoses or underdiagnoses, decreased immunologic recovery, and increased multimorbidity. However, each older PWH is a unique and complex individual, and disease-centric guidelines should not be applied the same way in every patient. The management of diseases in older PWH should be individualized based on aging phenotypes, multimorbidity interactions, and patient preferences. The VACS index may identify aging phenotypes and provide useful prognostic information to help prioritize interventions and guide shared decision-making with patients and caregivers.

REFERENCES

Abrass C, Appelbaum J, Boyd C, et al. Summary report from the human immunodeficiency virus and aging consensus project: treatment strategies for clinicians managing older individuals with the human immunodeficiency virus. *J Am Geriatr Soc.* 2012;60(5):974–979.

Adelman RD, Tmanova LL, Delgado D, et al. Caregiver burden: a clinical review. *JAMA.* 2014;311(10):1052–1060. http://doi:10.1001/jama.2014.304

Ambrosius WT, Sink KM, Foy CG, et al. The design and rationale of a multicenter clinical trial comparing two strategies for control of systolic blood pressure: the Systolic Blood Pressure Intervention Trial (SPRINT). *Clin Trials.* 2014;11(5):532–546.

American Academy of HIV Medicine (AAHIVM). Recommended treatment strategies for clinicians managing older patients with HIV. https://education.aahivm.org/courses/55527. Published August 25, 2023. Accessed August 30, 2024.

American Diabetes Association Professional Practice Committee; Summary of Revisions: *Standards of Care in Diabetes—2024. Diabetes Care.* 2024;47 (Suppl 1): S5–S10. https://doi.org/10.2337/dc24-SREV

American Geriatrics Society (AGS). American Geriatrics Society 2023 updated AGS updated Beers Criteria® for potentially inappropriate medication use in older adults. *J Am Geriatr Soc.* 2023;71(7):2052–2081.

Bellera CA, Rainfray M, Mathoulin-Pelissier S, et al. Screening older cancer patients: first evaluation of the G-8 geriatric screening tool. *Ann Oncol.* 2012;23:2166–2172.

Brothers TD, Rockwood K. Frailty: a new vulnerability indicator in people aging with HIV. *Eur Geriatr Med.* 2019;10(2):219–226. http://doi:10.1007/s41999-018-0143-2

Castronuovo D, Pinzone MR, Moreno S, et al. HIV infection and bone disease: a review of the literature. *Infect Dis Trop Med.* 2015;1(2):e116.

Centers for Disease Control and Prevention (CDC). Assessment timed up and go (TUG). https:// www.cdc.gov/steadi/media/pdfs/steadi-assessment-tug-508.pdf. Published 2017. Accessed August 30, 2024.

CDC. Diagnoses, deaths, and prevalence of HIV in the United States and 6 territories and freely associated states, 2022. HIV Surveillance Report, 2022;35. http://www.cdc.gov/hiv-data/nhss/hiv-diagnoses-deaths-prevalence.html. Published May 2024. Accessed July 18, 2024.

CDC. Diagnoses of HIV infection among adults aged 50 years and older in the United States and dependent areas, 2011–2016. HIV Surveillance Supplemental Report 2018;23(5). http://www.cdc.gov/hiv/library/reports/hivsurveillance.html. Published August 2018. Accessed August 30, 2024.

CDC. Revised recommendations for HIV testing of adults, adolescents, and pregnant women in health-care settings. www.cdc.gov/mmwr/preview/mmwrhtml/rr5514a1.htm. Published September 22, 2006. Accessed August 30, 2024.

Chan P, Brew BJ. HIV associated neurocognitive disorders in the modern antiviral treatment era: prevalence, characteristics, biomarkers, and effects of treatment. *Curr HIV/AIDS Rep.* 2014;11(3):317–324. http://doi:10.1007/s11904-014-0221-0

Chibanda D, Verhey R, Gibson LJ, et al. Validation of screening tools for depression and anxiety disorders in a primary care population with high HIV prevalence in Zimbabwe. *J Affect Disord.* 2016;198:50–55. http://doi:10.1016/j.jad.2016.03.006

Conroy S. Defining frailty—the holy grail of geriatric medicine. *J Nutr Heal Aging.* 2009;13(4):389. http://doi:10.1007/s12603-009-0050-9

Dai SY, Liu JJ, Fan YG, et al. Prevalence and factors associated with late HIV diagnosis. *J Med Virol.* 2015;87(6):970–977. http://doi:10.1002/jmv.24066

Ellis G, Gardner M, Tsiachristas A, et al. Comprehensive geriatric assessment for older adults admitted to hospital. *Cochrane Database Syst Rev.* 2017;9(9):CD006211. http://doi:10.1002/14651858.CD006211.pub3

Erlandson KM, Allshouse AA, Jankowski CM, et al. Risk factors for falls in HIV-infected persons. *J Acquir Immune Defic Syndr.* 2012;61:484–489.

Erlandson KM, Plankey MW, Springer G, et al. Fall frequency and associated factors among men and women with or at risk for HIV infection. *HIV Med.* 2016;17:740–748.

European AIDS Clinical Society. Guidelines version 12.0. https://www.eacsociety.org/guidelines/eacs-guidelines/. Published October 2023. Accessed May 30, 2024.

Fried LP, Tangen CM, Walston J, et al. Frailty in older adults: evidence for a phenotype. *J Gerontol A Biol Sci Med Sci.* 2001;56(3):M146–M157.

Gallagher P, Ryan C, Byrne S, et al. STOPP (Screening Tool of Older Person's Prescriptions) and START (Screening Tool to Alert doctors to Right Treatment): consensus validation. *Int J Clin Pharmacol Ther.* 2008;46(2):72–83.

Gandhi RT, Bedimo R, Hoy JF, et al. Antiretroviral drugs for treatment and prevention of HIV infection in adults: 2022 recommendations of the International Antiviral Society–USA Panel. *JAMA.* 2023;329(1):63–84.

Goodin BR, Owens MA, White DM, et al. Intersectional health-related stigma in persons living with HIV and chronic pain: implications for depressive symptoms. *AIDS Care.* 2018;30(Suppl 2):66–73. http://doi:10.1080/09540121.2018.1468012

Grinspoon S, Corcoran C, Askari H, et al. Effects of androgen administration in men with the AIDS wasting syndrome: a randomized, double-blind, placebo-controlled trial. *Ann Intern Med.* 1998;129:18–26.

Grinspoon S, Corcoran C, Lee K, et al. Loss of lean body and muscle mass correlates with androgen levels in hypogonadal men with acquired immunodeficiency syndrome and wasting. *J Clin Endocrinol Metab.* 1996;81:4051–4058.

Grohskopf LA, Alyanak E, Broder KR, et al. Prevention and control of seasonal influenza with vaccines: recommendations of the Advisory Committee on Immunization Practices—United States, 2019–20 influenza season. *MMWR Recomm Rep.* 2019;68(RR-3):1–21.

Guaraldi G, Silva AR, Stentarelli C. Multimorbidity and functional status assessment. *Curr Opin HIV AIDS.* 2014;9(4):386–397.

Hanlon JT, Schmader KE. The medication appropriateness index at 20: where it started, where it has been, and where it may be going. *Drugs Aging.* 2013;30(11):893–900.

Hanlon JT, Schmader KE, Samsa GP, et al. A method for assessing drug therapy appropriateness. *J Clin Epidemiol.* 1992;45(10):1045–1051.

Holtzman C, Armon C, Tedaldi E, et al. Polypharmacy and risk of antiretroviral drug interactions among the aging HIV-infected population. *J Gen Intern Med.* 2013;28(10):1302–1310.

Huss A, Stuck AE, Rubenstein LZ, et al. Multidimensional preventive home visit programs for community-dwelling older adults: a systematic review and meta-analysis of randomized controlled trials. *J Gerontol A Biol Sci Med Sci.* 2008;63(3):298.

Hypertension Canada. 2020–2022 hypertension highlights. https://hypertension.ca/wp-content/uploads/2020/10/2020-22-HT-Guidelines-E-WEB_v3b.pdf. Published 2020. Accessed August 30, 2024.

James PA, Oparil S, Carter BL, et al. 2014 Evidence-based guideline for the management of high blood pressure in adults: report from the panel members appointed to the eighth Joint National Committee (JNC 8). *JAMA.* 2014;311(5):507–520. http://doi:10.1001/jama.2013.284427

John M, Hessol N, Hare CB, et al. 1607: Veterans Aging Cohort Study (VACS) index, functional status, and other patient reported outcomes in older HIV-positive (HIV+) adults. *Open Forum Infect Dis.* 2014;1(Suppl 1):S428–S429. http://doi:10.1093/ofid/ofu052.1153

Jonas DE, Reuland DS, Reddy SM, et al. *Screening for Lung Cancer with Low-Dose Computed Tomography: An Evidence Review for the U.S. Preventive Services Task Force.* Rockville, MD: Agency for Healthcare Research and Quality; 2021 Mar. Evidence Synthesis, No. 198. https://www.ncbi.nlm.nih.gov/books/NBK568573/. Accessed July 17, 2024.

Justice A, Tate J, Brown S, et al. Can the Veterans Aging Cohort Study Index improve clinical judgment for both HIV infected and uninfected veterans? *J Gen Intern Med.* 2013b;28:S39–S39.

Justice AC, Holmes H, Gifford AL, et al., Development and validation of a self-completed HIV symptom index. *J Clin Epidemiol.* 2001;54(12):S77–S90.

Justice AC, Modur SP, Tate JP, et al. Predictive accuracy of the Veterans Aging Cohort Study index for mortality with HIV infection: a North American cross cohort analysis. *J Acquir Immune Defic Syndr.* 2013a;62(2):149–163. http://doi:10.1097/QAI.0b013e31827df36c

Justice AC, Tate J, Freiberg M, et al. Reply to Chow et al. *Clin Infect Dis.* 2012;55(5)751–752.

Katz S, Ford AB, Moskowitz RW, et al. Studies of illness in the aged. The index of ADL: a standardized measure of biological and psychosocial function. *JAMA.* 1963;185:914–919.

Kilbourne AM, Justice AC, Rollman BL, et al. Clinical importance of HIV and depressive symptoms among veterans with HIV infection. *JGIM.* 2002;17(7):512–520.

King EM, Tkachuk S, Tseng A. Aging on antiretrovirals: reviewing the need for pharmacologic data in elderly people with HIV. *AIDS.* 2024;38(11):1609–1616.

Knobel H, Guelar A, Valldecillo G, et al. Response to highly active antiretroviral therapy in HIV-infected patients aged 60 years or older after 24 months follow-up. *AIDS.* 2001;15(12):1591–1593.

Kong AM, Pozen A, Anastos K, et al. Non-HIV comorbid conditions and polypharmacy among people living with HIV age 65 or older compared with HIV-negative individuals age 65 or older in the United States: a retrospective claims-based analysis. *AIDS Patient Care STDS.* 2019;33(3):93–103.

Koroukian SM, Warner DF, Owusu C, Given CW. Multimorbidity redefined: prospective health outcomes and the cumulative effect of co-occurring conditions. *Prev Chronic Dis.* 2015;12:E55.

Lee SJ, Leipzig RM, Walter LC. Incorporating lag time to benefit into prevention decisions for older adults. *JAMA.* 2013;310(24):2609–2610.

Lindau ST, Schumm LP, Laumann EO, et al. A study of sexuality and health among older adults in the United States. *N Engl J Med.* 2007;357(8):762–774.

Lindeman RD, Tobin J, Shock NW. Longitudinal studies on the rate of decline in renal function with age. *J Am Geriatr Soc.* 1985;33(4):278–285.

Marzolini C, Back D, Weber R, et al. Ageing with HIV: medication use and risk for potential drug-drug interactions. *J Antimicrob Chemother.* 2011;66(9):2107–2111.

Masnoon N, Shakib S, Kalisch-Ellett L, et al. What is polypharmacy? A systematic review of definitions. *BMC Geriatr.* 2017;17(1):230.

McKittrick N, Frank I, Jacobson JM, et al. Improved immunogenicity with high-dose seasonal influenza vaccine in HIV-infected persons: a single-center, parallel, randomized trial. *Ann Intern Med.* 2013;158(1):19–26.

Merlin JS, Westfall AO, Long D, et al. A randomized pilot trial of a novel behavioral intervention for chronic pain tailored to individuals with HIV. *AIDS Behav.* 2018;22(8):2733–2742.

Mpondo BC, Gunda DW, Kilonzo SB, et al. Immunological and clinical responses following the use of antiretroviral therapy among elderly HIV-positive individuals attending care and treatment clinic in Northwestern Tanzania: a retrospective cohort study. *J Sex Transm Dis.* 2016;2016:5235269.

Mueses-Marín H, Montaño D, Galindo J, et al. Psychometric properties and validity of the Center for Epidemiological Studies Depression Scale (CES-D) in a population attending an HIV clinic in Cali, Colombia. *Biomedica.* 2019;39(1):33–45. http://doi:10.7705/biomedica.v39i1.3843

National Center on Elder Abuse (NCEA). NCEA website. https://ncea.acl.gov/. Published December 13, 2023. Accessed August 30, 2024.

National Institute on Aging. Advance care planning. httpss:// www.nia.nih.gov/health/advance-care-planning/advance-care-planning-advance-directives-health-care. Published 2022. Accessed August 30, 2024.

Panel on Antiretroviral Guidelines for Adults and Adolescents. Guidelines for the use of antiretroviral agents in adults and adolescents with HIV. Appendix B, Table 12. Department of Health and Human Services. https://clinicalinfo.hiv.gov/en/guidelines/adult-and-adolescent-arv. Published February 27, 2024. Accessed July 20, 2024.

Pecanac KE, Repenshek MF, Tennenbaum D, et al. Respecting Choices® and advance directives in a diverse community. *J Palliat Med.* 2014;17(3):282–287. http://doi:10.1089/jpm.2013.0047

Pilowsky D, Wu L-T. Sexual risk behaviors and HIV risk among Americans aged 50 years or older: a review. *Subst Abuse Rehabil.* 2015;6:51. http://doi:10.2147/sar.s78808

Podsiadlo D, Richardson S. The timed "Up and Go": a test of basic functional mobility for frail elderly persons. *J Am Geriatr Soc.* 1991;39:142–148.

Power C, Selnes OA, Grim JA, et al. HIV dementia scale: a rapid screening test. *J Acquir Immune Defic Syndr Hum Retrovirology.* 1995;8(3):273–278. http://doi:10.1097/00042560-199503010-00008

Ramgopal M, Maggiolo F, Ward D, et al. Pooled analysis of 4 international trials of bictegravir/emtricitabine/tenofovir alafenamide (B/F/Taf) in adults aged 65 or older demonstrating safety and efficacy: week 48 results. *J Int AIDS Soc.* 2020;23(Suppl 4):e25547.

Reuben DB, Frank JC, Hirsch SH, et al. A randomized clinical trial of outpatient comprehensive geriatric assessment coupled with an intervention to increase adherence to recommendations. *J Am Geriatr Soc.* 1999;47(3):269.

Rockwood K, Andrew M, Mitnitski A. A comparison of two approaches to measuring frailty in elderly people. *J Gerontol A Biol Sci Med Sci.* 2007;62(7):738–743. http://doi:10.1093/gerona/62.7.738

Rodkjaer L, Gabel C, Laursen T, et al. Simple and practical screening approach to identify HIV-infected individuals with depression or at risk of developing depression. *HIV Med.* 2016;17(10):749–757.

Rosca EC, Albarqouni L, Simu M. Montreal Cognitive Assessment (MoCA) for HIV-associated neurocognitive disorders. *Neuropsychol Rev.* 2019;29(3):313–327.

Rueda S, Law S, Rourke SB. Psychosocial, mental health, and behavioral issues of aging with HIV. *Curr Opin HIV AIDS.* 2014;9(4):325–331.

Ruiz M, Kamerman LA. Nutritional screening tools for HIV-infected patients: implications for elderly patients. *J Int Assoc Physicians AIDS Care.* 2010;9:362–367.

Ruiz MA, Reske T, Cefalu C, et al. Falls in HIV-infected patients: a geriatric syndrome in a susceptible population. *J Int Assoc Provid AIDS Care.* 2013;12:266–269.

Sacktor NC, Wong M, Nakasujja N, et al. The International HIV Dementia Scale: a new rapid screening test for HIV dementia. *AIDS.* 2005;19(13):1367–1374.

Sangarlangkarn A, Apornpong T, Justice AC, et al. Screening tools for targeted comprehensive geriatric assessment in HIV-infected patients 50 years and older. *Int J STD AIDS.* 2019;30(10):1009–1017.

Sangarlangkarn A, Merlin JS, Tucker RO, et al. Advance care planning and HIV infection in the era of antiretroviral therapy: a review. *Top Antivir Med*. 2016;23(5):174–180.

Schafer JJ, Gill TK, Sherman EM, et al. ASHP guidelines on pharmacist involvement in HIV care. *Am J Health Syst Pharm*. 2016;73(7):468–494.

Schmucker, D. L. Liver function and phase I drug metabolism in the elderly: a paradox. *Drugs Aging*. 2001;18(11):837–851.

Schouten J, Wit FW, Stolte IG, et al. Cross-sectional comparison of the prevalence of age-associated comorbidities and their risk factors between HIV-infected and uninfected individuals: the AGEHIV cohort study. *Clin Infect Dis*. 2014;59(12):1787–1797.

Searle SD, Mitnitski A, Gahbauer EA, et al. A standard procedure for creating a frailty index. *BMC Geriatr*. 2008;8:24.

Semeere AS, Lwanga I, Sempa J, et al. Mortality and immunological recovery among older adults on antiretroviral therapy at a large urban HIV clinic in Kampala, Uganda. *J Acquir Immune Defic Syndr*. 2014;67(4):382–389.

Shafran SD. Live attenuated herpes zoster vaccine for HIV-infected adults. *HIV Med*. 2016:17(4):305–310.

Sigel K, Wisnivesky J, Shahrir S, et al. Findings in asymptomatic HIV infected patients undergoing chest computed tomography testing: implications for lung cancer screening. *AIDS*. 2014;28(7):1007–1014.

StuckAE,SiuAL,WielandGD,etal.Comprehensivegeriatricassessment:a meta-analysisofcontrolledtrials.*Lancet*.1993;342(8878):1032–1036. http://doi:10.1016/0140-6736(93)92884-V

Thompson MA, Horgerg MA, Agwu AL et al. Primary care guidelines for the management of persons infected with human immunodeficiency virus: 2020 update by the HIV Medicine Association of the Infectious Diseases Society of America. *Clin Infect Dis*. 2021;73(11):e3572–e3605.

Tinetti ME, Fried TR, Boyd CM. Designing health care for the most common chronic condition: multimorbidity. *JAMA*. 2012;307(23):2493–2494. Published correction appears in *JAMA*. 2012 Jul 18;308(3):238.

U.S. Preventive Services Task Force. Screening for cognitive impairment in older adults: US Preventive Services Task Force Recommendation Statement. *JAMA*. 2020;323(8):757–763. doi:10.1001/jama.2020.0435

Valcour V, Paul R, Chiao S, et al. Screening for cognitive impairment in human immunodeficiency virus. *Clin Infect Dis*. 2011;53(8):836–842. http://doi:10.1093/cid/cir524

Verhey R, Chibanda D, Gibson L, et al. Validation of the posttraumatic stress disorder checklist–5 (PCL-5) in a primary care population with high HIV prevalence in Zimbabwe. *BMC Psychiatry*. 2018;18(1):109. http://doi:10.1186/s12888-018-1688-9

Vinikoor MJ, Joseph J, Mwale J, et al. Age at antiretroviral therapy initiation predicts immune recovery, death, and loss to follow-up among HIV-infected adults in urban Zambia. *AIDS Res Hum Retroviruses*. 2014;30(10):949–955. http://doi:10.1089/AID.2014.0046

Vrouenraets SM, Fux CA, Wit FW, et al. A comparison of measured and estimated glomerular filtration rate in successfully treated HIV-patients with preserved renal function. *Clin Nephrol*. 2012;77(4):311–320.

Weiss BD, Brega AG, LeBlanc WG, et al. Improving the effectiveness of medication review: guidance from the Health Literacy Universal Precautions Toolkit. *J Am Board Fam Med*. 2016;29(1):18–23.

Wellons, MF, Sanders L, Edwards LJ, et al. HIV infection: treatment outcomes in older and younger adults. *J Am Geriatr Soc*. 2002;50(4):603–607.

Whalen CC, Antani M, Carey J, et al. An index of symptoms for infection with human immunodeficiency virus: reliability and validity. *J Clin Epidemiol*. 1994;47(5):537–546.

Whelton PK, Carey RM, Aronow WS, et al. ACC/AHA/AAPA/ABC/ACPM/AGS/APhA/ASH/ASPC/NMA/PCNA guideline for the prevention, detection, evaluation, and management of high blood pressure in adults. *J Am Coll Cardiol*. 2018;71:e127–e248.

Wright L, Epps JB. Development and validation of a HIV disease–specific nutrition screening tool. *Top Clin Nutr*. 2020;35(3):264–269.

24.

SOLID ORGAN TRANSPLANTATION IN PEOPLE WITH HIV

Christine M. Durand

INTRODUCTION

The advent of effective combination antiretroviral therapy (ART) has resulted in increased life expectancy for people with HIV (PWH). With declining opportunistic infections, end-organ disease—both directly and indirectly associated with HIV—has become a major cause of morbidity and mortality in this population. Solid organ transplantation, once considered contraindicated for individuals with HIV, has demonstrated success and is now considered the standard of care for end-stage organ disease in this population.

LEARNING OBJECTIVES

- Discuss the evaluation and management of the transplant candidate with HIV and clinical outcomes for solid organ transplant recipients with HIV.
- Explain key drug-drug interactions between immunosuppressive agents and ART in transplant recipients with HIV.

WHAT'S NEW?

- In the era of effective hepatitis C virus (HCV) treatment, studies have found that patient and graft survival rates in liver transplant recipients with HIV have improved and are now equivalent to those without HIV.
- Emerging evidence from registry studies shows that patient and graft survival rates in heart and lung transplant recipients with HIV are similar to recipients without HIV.
- The HIV Organ Policy Equity (HOPE) Act, signed into U.S. law in 2013, allows the use of organs from donors with HIV to be used for transplant for recipients with HIV under research protocols. Early studies of HIV donor to HIV recipient (HIV D+/R+) kidney and liver transplantation are encouraging.

KEY POINTS

- End-organ disease has become a major cause of morbidity and mortality in PWH because of increased life expectancy, thus increasing the demand for organ transplantation in this population.
- The care of transplant recipients with HIV warrants a multidisciplinary team approach, including the specific organ transplant team, pharmacists, infectious disease/HIV specialists, nurses, patients, and their families.
- Transplant-related immunosuppression for recipients with HIV has not been associated with loss of virologic control or increased opportunistic infections.
- To avoid drug-drug interactions between antiretroviral therapy (ART) and post-transplant immunosuppression for recipients with HIV, integrase strand transfer inhibitor-based ART regimens are preferred.
- Kidney transplant recipients with HIV face an increased risk of allograft rejection after transplant.
- HCV treatment is essential to improve outcomes among liver and kidney transplant recipients with HIV-HCV coinfection.

PRETRANSPLANT EVALUATION

CRITERIA FOR TRANSPLANTATION

Many of the following recommendations are based on the National Institutes of Health (NIH)–funded Solid Organ Transplantation in HIV: Multi-site Study (HIVTR Study), which was a prospective observational study of kidney and liver transplantation in PWH conducted across 26 transplant centers in the United States between 2002 and 2013 (Roland et al., 2016; Stock et al., 2010; Terrault et al., 2012).

- Any opportunistic infections or malignancies should be completely treated prior to transplant. There are limited data on outcomes of transplant recipients who have a history of progressive multifocal leukoencephalopathy, visceral Kaposi's sarcoma, chronic cryptosporidiosis, or primary central nervous system lymphoma, as these individuals were excluded from clinical trials of kidney and liver transplantation for PWH.
- Transplant candidates with HIV should meet standard criteria for transplantation.
- Transplant candidates with HIV should be on a stable ART regimen.

Kidney, Heart, and Lung Transplant Candidate Criteria

- $CD4^+$ T-cell count should generally be ≥200 cells/mm^3 prior to transplant.
- HIV RNA should be suppressed to below the assay's limit of detection (excluding viral "blips" of 20–200 copies/mL, which are common and unlikely to be clinically significant) (Nettles et al., 2005).

Liver Transplant Candidate Criteria

- $CD4^+$ T-cell count should generally be ≥100 cells/mm^3. A lower $CD4^+$ T-cell count criteria has been allowed for liver transplant candidates because of the impact of portal hypertension and splenomegaly on lowering overall lymphocyte counts.
- HIV RNA should be suppressed to below the limit of detection of the assay (excluding viral "blips" of 20–200 copies/mL, which are common and unlikely to be clinically significant) (Nettles et al., 2005).

PRETRANSPLANT INFECTION SCREENING AND VACCINATIONS

Latent Tuberculosis

- All candidates should be screened for latent tuberculosis (TB) prior to transplantation, with either a tuberculin skin test or interferon-gamma release assay (Blumberg and Roger, 2019; DHHS, 2024). Patients should be treated if they have evidence of latent TB. The preferred regimen is isoniazid (INH) ± vitamin B_6 for 9 months, completing at least 6 of the 9 months prior to transplantation. For liver transplantation, when prophylactic treatment cannot be completed prior to transplant, or if the risk of toxicity is too high, treatment should be completed when possible after transplant.

Syphilis

- Test for and treat syphilis prior to transplant.

Other Infectious Conditions

- Test for cytomegalovirus (CMV), Epstein–Barr virus, herpes simplex virus, varicella zoster virus (VZV), and viral hepatitis serologies in all candidates. In addition, coccidioides and strongyloides serologies should be tested if the recipient has exposure to endemic areas.

Vaccinations

Prior to transplant, people with HIV should receive all standard vaccinations per Advisory Committee on Immunization Practices (ACIP)/Centers for Disease Control and Prevention (CDC) and other professional society guidelines. Select vaccine recommendations are summarized here; providers should review current ACIP/CDC guidelines for the most up-to-date and complete guidance. Live vaccines such as varicella and mumps/measles/rubella (MMR) vaccines should not be given pretransplant if $CD4^+$ T-cell count is less than 300 cells/mm^3 (Miro et al., 2014). No live vaccines should be given post-transplant. In general, live vaccines should be avoided within 4 weeks of transplant.

- All candidates should be vaccinated against hepatitis A and B if not already immune.
- Seasonal influenza vaccine and SARS-CoV-2 vaccines should be given yearly. The high-dose influenza vaccine has demonstrated better immunogenicity and is safe in solid organ transplant recipients (Mombelli et al., 2018).
- Vaccination against *S. pneumoniae* should be given per ACIP/CDC recommendations.
- Tdap vaccine should be given if not received in the past 10 years.
- HPV vaccine should be given to persons aged 9–45 years.
- Meningococcal conjugate vaccine (MenACWY) should be given to all candidates, and the serogroup B meningococcal vaccine should be given to candidates between 16 and 23 years of age.
- Varicella vaccine should be given to those who are VZV seronegative (and have CD4 ≥300 cells/mm^3) prior to transplant.
- Recombinant zoster vaccine (RSV, Shingrix) has shown safety and immunogenicity in immunocompromised populations (Berkowitz et al., 2015; Stadtmauer et al., 2014) and should be considered to prevent zoster reactivation, which is common among PWH and transplant recipients.

WHEN TO REFER

- For all organ types, referral should occur at the same level of organ dysfunction that would prompt referral for people without HIV.

POST-TRANSPLANT MANAGEMENT AND CARE

All pre-, peri-, and post-transplant care should be coordinated among a multidisciplinary team consisting of the transplant surgeon, an infectious disease (ID) or HIV specialist, an organ specialist (e.g., nephrologist, hepatologist, cardiologist, pulmonologist), a primary care provider, a transplant coordinator, a transplant pharmacist, a social worker, and nursing staff.

IMMUNOSUPPRESSION THERAPY

Induction Immunosuppression for Kidney Transplantation

For kidney transplantation, induction immunosuppression at the time of transplant typically includes a lymphocyte-depleting regimen with antithymocyte globulin (ATG) or a non-lymphocyte-depleting regimen with an interleukin 2 receptor antagonist (anti-IL2R), a less potent monoclonal antibody that blocks early T-cell activation (Gabardi et al., 2011). There remains debate about which agent is optimal for transplant recipients with HIV. The HIVTR study suggested that the use of antithymocyte globulin was associated with a higher risk of graft loss and hospitalizations owing to infections (Stock et al., 2010). However, subsequent studies found a 2.6-fold lower risk of acute rejection and equivalent graft survival in transplant recipients with HIV who received ATG induction (Locke et al., 2014). A subsequent study of 830 renal transplant recipients with HIV found a 40% lower rate of rejection among those who received ATG for induction compared to either no induction or anti-IL-2R induction without evidence of increased infections (Kucirka et al., 2016). The choice of induction therapy should be made on a case-by-case basis, accounting for the individual's risk of rejection, although recent evidence suggests that ATG is generally safe in PWH undergoing kidney transplantation.

Maintenance Immunosuppression

Maintenance immunosuppression generally consists of triple therapy including calcineurin inhibitors (CNIs) (e.g., cyclosporine and tacrolimus) with an antimetabolite (e.g., mycophenolate mofetil) and corticosteroids. A mammalian target of rapamycin (mTOR) inhibitor (e.g., sirolimus and everolimus) may be substituted if a patient is unable to tolerate CNIs or antimetabolites. The HIVTR study found an increased risk of rejection with the use of cyclosporine compared to tacrolimus (Stock et al., 2010), and sirolimus was found to be associated with a higher rate of rejection (Locke et al., 2014). Early steroid withdrawal has also been associated with a 60% higher risk of allograft rejection in kidney transplant recipients with HIV (Werbel et al., 2021).

ANTIRETROVIRAL THERAPY MANAGEMENT AMONG TRANSPLANT RECIPIENTS

Managing interactions between immunosuppressive agents and ART can be challenging. In ambulatory settings, clinicians will most frequently encounter maintenance immunosuppressive regimens consisting of a combination of a calcineurin inhibitor, antimetabolite, and corticosteroids, as described above. In some individuals, an mTOR inhibitor will be used in place of one of these agents or as adjunctive therapy. Understanding the pharmacokinetics of each of these drug classes is crucial to safely manage transplant recipients with HIV. Calcineurin inhibitors are substrates, as well as weak inhibitors of cytochrome P450 3A4 (CYP3A4), and therefore have potential for significant interaction with antiretroviral agents that are CYP3A4 inhibitors or inducers. mTOR inhibitors are substrates of CYP3A4, and dosing must be adjusted in the presence of CYP3A4 inhibitors or inducers. The antimetabolites mycophenolate mofetil and azathioprine are not substrates for CYP3A4 and therefore have no expected or documented interactions with ART.

ART should not be interrupted in the post-transplant period. The optimal regimen for individual patients varies based on the person's ART resistance pattern and prior ART exposures as well as overall clinical profile. As indicated above, drug-drug interactions between CNIs, mTOR inhibitors, and some antiretroviral medications (i.e., protease inhibitors and some non-nucleoside reverse transcriptase inhibitors) may affect metabolism of immunosuppressant medications and potentially contribute to drug toxicity or rejection (Frasetto et al., 2007; Trullas et al., 2011; van Maarseveen et al., 2012). General guidelines by class are provided below. There are no absolute contraindications, as dosing modifications based on therapeutic drug monitoring of the immunosuppressants can compensate for the altered metabolism of these drugs.

Integrase Strand Transfer Inhibitors (INSTIs)

INSTIs have no or only minimal effects on CYP3A metabolism; thus, there are few potential drug interactions with immunosuppressants, making this class of ART optimal for use in PWH after solid organ transplantation. Although experience is greatest with raltegravir (Barau et al., 2014; Bickel et al., 2010; Di Biago et al., 2009; Miro et al., 2010), the absence of interaction and stability of immunosuppressant dosing are likely to be similar for other INSTIs, including dolutegravir and bictegravir. Because dolutegravir and bictegravir interfere with tubular secretion of creatinine, mild elevations of creatinine may be observed after dolutegravir (or bictegravir) initiation: these do not represent a decline in glomerular filtration rate (Lee et al., 2016). However, when INSTIs such as elvitegravir are given in combination with the pharmacoenhancer cobicistat, this will cause potent CYP3A4 inhibition (see "Protease Inhibitors (PIs) and Pharmacoenhancers," below). Thus, cobicistat should be avoided, if possible, for the reasons discussed above.

Nucleoside Reverse Transcriptase Inhibitors (NRTIs)

NRTIs are not expected to have significant drug-drug interactions with post-transplant immunosuppression and are often included in post-transplant ART regimens. Older NRTIs with significant mitochondrial toxicity, such as zidovudine, should be avoided because antagonism when used with mycophenolate and zidovudine may exacerbate bone marrow suppression. Tenofovir disoproxil fumarate can be nephrotoxic and should be replaced with its newer formulation, tenofovir alafenamide.

Non-Nucleoside Reverse Transcriptase Inhibitors (NNRTIs)

Older NNRTIs such as efavirenz, nevirapine, and etravirine are strong CYP3A4 inducers, thus increasing the metabolism of CNIs and decreasing their serum levels (mTOR levels may be similarly affected). The dose of these immunosuppressive agents frequently needs to be increased with close monitoring of drug levels. Newer NNRTIs such as rilpivirine and doravirine are not potent inducers and are not expected to impact CNI levels significantly (Spagnuolo et al., 2019). For transplant recipients taking proton pump inhibitors, rilpivirine should not be used.

Protease Inhibitors (PIs) and Pharmacoenhancers

Protease inhibitors (PIs) given in combination with low-dose ritonavir or cobicistat, known as "boosted PIs," act both as strong CYP3A4 inhibitors (and sometimes also weak inducers) and decrease the metabolism of CNIs and mTOR inhibitors, resulting in higher levels of these agents. Thus, it is imperative that if boosted PIs or cobicistat must be used, the dosages of both CNIs and mTOR inhibitors commonly must be decreased and the dosing interval increased, with close monitoring of drug levels, to avoid toxicity *and* maintain therapeutic immunosuppressive drug levels. Additionally, the use of boosted PIs in kidney transplant recipients has been linked to an increased risk of graft loss and death in one recent study, while in another study it was found to actually be associated with reduced graft failure rates (Sawinski et al., 2017; Sparkes et al., 2018). This suggests that PIs should be used sparingly and with careful monitoring.

Boosted PIs also decrease the clearance of glucocorticoids, which may cause a Cushing-like syndrome. In addition, they may exacerbate hyperlipidemia post-transplant and potentiate CNI-induced impaired glucose tolerance.

CCR5 Antagonists

The CCR5 antagonist maraviroc does not have significant drug interactions with immunosuppressants and represent a good option for individuals with R5 tropic virus. Notably, blockade of CCR5 expression leads to a reduction in lymphocyte chemotaxis and has been hypothesized to reduce inflammation and potentially allograft rejection. It has been shown to reduce severe graft-versus-host-disease after bone marrow transplantation (Reshef et al., 2012) and is currently under study to reduce rejection among kidney transplant recipients with HIV (clinicaltrials.gov; NCT02741323).

Newer ART Agents and Formulations (Including Long-Acting Agents)

Ibalizumab is a monoclonal antibody for the CD4 T-cell receptor, which does not have drug-drug interactions with immunosuppressants. Fostemsavir is an HIV attachment inhibitor that blocks the interaction between the CD4 T-cell receptor and the HIV envelope protein gp120. Neither of these antiretroviral medications is expected to have problematic drug interactions with immunosuppressants, although there is limited experience with their use in transplant recipients at this time. Lenacapavir (an HIV-1 capsid inhibitor administered subcutaneously every 6 months) is a moderate inhibitor of CYP3A4 and may increase concentrations of tacrolimus; therefore monitoring is recommended.

The combination regimen of long-acting injectable cabotegravir and long-acting injectable rilpivirine can be given every 4–8 weeks to people with HIV who are virologically suppressed for at least 6 months. Data is limited in the peritransplant setting, but no problematic drug-drug interactions are anticipated.

POST-TRANSPLANT INFECTION PROPHYLAXIS

In addition to standard post-transplant CMV prophylaxis, kidney and liver transplant recipients with HIV should receive the following prophylaxis:

- *Pneumocystis jiroveci*
  - Prophylaxis with trimethoprim/sulfamethoxazole (TMP/SMX) or dapsone (if sulfa allergic or bone marrow suppression is an issue, provided glucose-6-phosphate dehydrogenase (G-6PD) levels are normal). Atovaquone can also be used as a secondary alternative to TMP/SMX.
  - Prophylaxis is recommended for at least one year (Blumberg and Roger, 2019) although some centers used shorter regimens, stopping once CD4 counts recover >200 cells/mm^3.
- *Mycobacterium avium* complex (MAC)
  - Some experts recommend primary prophylaxis against MAC with azithromycin for persons with CD4+ T-cell count less than 50 cells/mm3 (Blumberg and Roger, 2019). However, recent opportunistic infection guidelines have eliminated CD4$^+$-directed prophylaxis for MAC generally for PWH, owing to low incidence (i.e., primary prophylaxis is no longer recommended for persons who immediately initiate ART, and may be discontinued in persons who are continuing on a fully suppressive ART regimen) (DHHS, 2024; Gandhi et al., 2023). Thus, some experts do not use MAC prophylaxis post-transplant even with CD4 counts <50 cells/mm^3.
- Toxoplasmosis
  - TMP/SMX should be used if CD4+ T-cell count is less than 100 cells/mm3 and if either the recipient or the donor carries IgG antibodies against *Toxoplasma gondii*. Atovaquone can be used if a patient cannot tolerate TMP/SMX or dapsone (Blumberg and Roger, 2019).
- Prior opportunistic infections (OIs)
  - Continue secondary prophylaxis for OIs such as cryptococcus or coccidioidomycosis until CD4$^+$ T-cell counts are above the discontinuation threshold (i.e., CD4$^+$ >200 cells/mm^3) for approximately three to six months, although some providers may prefer lifelong secondary prophylaxis as data are limited (Blumberg and Roger, 2019).

OUTCOMES

PATIENT AND GRAFT SURVIVAL AND REJECTION

Kidney Transplantation

A review of over 1,400 individuals with HIV listed for kidney transplant showed a 79% reduction in the risk of death at 5 years for those who received a transplant, compared with those who remained on dialysis (Locke et al., 2017). Several studies have shown patient and graft survival rates for kidney transplant recipients with HIV that are largely comparable to the transplant population as a whole. The HIVTR study included 150 kidney transplant recipients with well-controlled HIV and demonstrated excellent 1- and 3-year patient and graft survival rates that were above the rates for recipients aged older than 65 years (Stock et al., 2010). The overall patient and graft survival rates of kidney transplant recipients with HIV in the HIVTR study were between the rates observed in HIV-uninfected, older recipients and all recipients, with rates of 94.6% ± 2% and 90.4% at 1 year, and 88.2% ± 3.8% and 73.7% at 3 years, respectively. Kidneys from living donors were associated with improved survival; and the use of ATG, HCV coinfection, and older age were associated with decreased survival (Stock et al., 2010). Subsequently, the use of ATG induction was found to be associated with patient and graft survival rates equivalent to a cohort without HIV (Locke et al., 2014).

The HIVTR study also found the rate of acute rejection to be 2- to 3-fold higher, with a rate of 31% at 1 year and 41% at 3 years in kidney transplant recipients with HIV compared to rates in recipients without HIV (Stock et al., 2010). ATG induction has been associated with a 2.6-fold decrease in the rate of acute rejection compared to that of patients who did not receive any induction (Locke et al., 2014), and a 40% lower rate of rejection compared to those who received either no induction or anti-IL-2R induction (Kucirka et al., 2016).

A study utilizing national data from the U.S. Scientific Registry of Transplant Recipients (SRTR) that included 510 kidney transplant recipients with HIV showed that, in the absence of HCV coinfection, 5- and 10-year patient and graft survival for recipients with and without HIV was similar (Locke et al., 2015).

Liver Transplantation

Data also support liver transplantation in individuals with HIV. The HIVTR study included 125 liver transplant recipients with HIV and demonstrated a survival benefit of liver transplantation for individuals with end-stage liver disease (ESLD) and Model for End-Stage Liver Disease (MELD) score greater than 15 (Roland et al., 2016). In this study, overall survival was acceptable; however, it was lower for liver transplant recipients with HIV and HCV, with a 3-year survival of 60% versus 79% for those with HIV-HCV coinfection versus HCV mono-infection, respectively (Terrault et al., 2012). More recent studies from both Europe and the United States in the era of direct-acting antivirals (DAAs) for HCV have shown that liver transplant outcomes are similar in recipients with and without HIV (Campos-Varela et al., 2021; Campos-Varela et al., 2020).

Heart and Lung Transplantation

The NIH-funded multicenter HIVTR study did not study heart and lung transplantation in PWH; however, accumulating real-world data suggest that outcomes of thoracic transplantation in this population are good. These data include both international case series (Koval et al., 2019; Rouzaud et al., 2022) as well as larger, retrospective registry-based studies that included matched controls without HIV (Chen et al., 2019; Doberne et al., 2021; Donohue et al., 2024). Overall, studies demonstrate equivalent post-transplant patient survival and graft survival. Findings with regard to acute rejection are mixed; some studies demonstrate similar rates (Chen et al., 2019; Donohue et al., 2024) and others finding slightly higher rates among heart and/or lung recipients with HIV (Koval et al., 2019; Donohue et al., 2024; Rouzaud et al., 2022), similar to what has been reported for kidney transplantation in PWH (Locke et al., 2014; Stock et al., 2010).

PERSONS WITH HIV/HCV COINFECTION

Kidney Transplantation

Studies prior to the advent of HCV curative therapies showed that kidney transplant recipients with HIV and HCV had lower 3-year patient survival and graft survival rates (73% and 60%, respectively) compared to recipients without either infection (90% and 86%, respectively), with HIV infection only (89% and 81%, respectively), and with HCV infection only (84% and 78%, respectively) (Sawinski et al., 2015a; Sawinski et al., 2015b). Recipients with coinfection are also at a higher risk of acute rejection at 1 year, and the use of induction in this population confers a survival benefit (Vivanco et al., 2013). More recent studies have shown that these disparities are not present in the era of DAA therapy (Zarinsefat et al., 2022).

Liver Transplantation

As discussed above, prior to the era of curative HCV therapy, liver transplant recipients with both HIV and HCV had worse outcomes compared to recipients with either virus alone. Initial studies of liver transplantation in recipients with HIV showed that the 3-year patient and graft survival rates for patients with HIV/HCV coinfection were lower (53% and 74%, respectively) than those for recipients with HCV mono-infection (60% and 79%, respectively) (Terrault et al., 2012). More recent studies on temporal trends in liver transplant recipients with HIV have demonstrated improvement (Campos-Varela et al., 2020; Zarinsefat et al., 2022).

RISK OF INFECTION, IMMUNE RECOVERY, AND MALIGNANCY

Overall, 38% of kidney recipients had infections post-transplant in the HIVTR study. These infections consisted of predominantly genitourinary infections (26%), respiratory tract infections (20%), and bacteremia (19%) (Stock et al., 2010). This study also reported five cases of new opportunistic infections, including two cases of cutaneous Kaposi's sarcoma, one case of cryptosporidiosis, one presumed case of *P. jiroveci*, and one case of candida esophagitis. Despite an initial decline in $CD4^+$ T-cell count post-transplant, which was more pronounced with ATG induction, there was no increase in complications associated with HIV disease or progression of HIV (Stock et al., 2010).

Another study found that individuals with pretransplant $CD4^+$ T-cell counts of less than 350 cells/mm^3 had a lower $CD4^+$ T-cell nadir 4-weeks post-transplant, which was associated with prolonged $CD4^+$ T-cell lymphopenia, and increased risk for serious infections (Suarez et al., 2016). Induction with ATG is associated with a more significant $CD4^+$ T-cell nadir post-transplant; however, larger observational studies have not identified an independent increased risk in infections with ATG use (Kucirka et al., 2016).

Based on limited available data, the incidence of new or recurrent cancer after transplantation in recipients with HIV is not significantly different from recipients without HIV. In the HIVTR study, 9% of patients (11.2% of liver recipients and 8.7% of kidney recipients) developed post-transplant malignancies (including skin cancer, cutaneous Kaposi's sarcoma, penile squamous cell cancer, head and neck cancer, renal cell cancer, lymphoma, recurrence of pretransplant hepatocellular carcinoma, and cholangiocarcinoma), and 3% of patients died from a cancer-related cause (Stock et al., 2010). The same study showed an increased risk of developing high-grade squamous intraepithelial lesions after transplantation in 89 patients followed for anal cytology; this requires further study (Nissen et al., 2012).

DONORS WITH HIV: THE HOPE ACT

With recognition of major advances in HIV and transplantation medicine, the HOPE Act of 2013 lifted the federal ban on the use of organs from donors with HIV in the United States. This legislation was also based on promising data from a cohort of HIV D+/R+ kidney transplant recipients in South Africa who had had good outcomes (Muller et al., 2015). The HOPE Act allows HIV D+/R+ transplantation within research protocols and was implemented in 2015. The HOPE in Action Multicenter Consortium is a multicenter transplant collaborative including more than 30 transplant centers performing HIV D+/R+ within research studies to explore the safety and feasibility of this practice.

The HOPE Act has received widespread support among the community of people living with HIV, with high rates of willingness both to donate (Nguyen et al., 2018) and to receive organs from donors with HIV (Seaman et al., 2020). The first HIV D+/R+ deceased donor kidney and liver transplants were performed in 2016 (Malani, 2016). The HOPE in Action kidney pilot study compared outcomes between recipients with HIV who received kidneys from donors with and without HIV and reported excellent survival (100% in both arms) and no increased risk of graft failure, HIV viremia, opportunistic infections, or serious adverse events between groups (Durand et al., 2021). The HOPE in Action liver pilot study similarly compared outcomes between recipients with HIV who received livers from donors with and without HIV and found no significant differences in 1-year graft survival (96% vs. 100%), rejection (10.8% vs. 18.2%), HIV breakthrough (8% vs. 10%), or serious adverse events (Durand et al., 2022). Overall patient survival was good (83% vs. 100%); however, there was a higher rate of viral infections (i.e., CMV, HHV8) and cancer in the recipients of livers from donors with HIV, which translated to a higher mortality. Results of larger NIH-funded studies from the HOPE in Action Multicenter Consortium are anticipated (clinicaltrials.gov NCT03500315 and NCT0374393).

CONCLUSION

People with HIV and end-stage organ disease can experience a survival benefit from transplantation. Post-transplant immunosuppression does not appear to advance HIV disease or increase the risk of opportunistic infection. Prior to the advent of DAAs, recipients with HCV had worse clinical outcomes, partially owing to a more aggressive post-transplant HCV recurrence, but these disparities have improved with HCV cure. Anticipation and careful management of drug-drug interactions are crucial. Care of transplant recipients with HIV should include an integrated and coordinated group of providers, including the transplant team, pharmacists, infectious disease/HIV specialists, and nurses, in addition to patients and caregivers.

ACKNOWLEDGMENTS

This chapter is an extension of previous work and contributions made by authors involved with prior editions of this content: Jennifer Husson, Eurides Lopes, Carolyn Kramer, and Emily Blumberg.

REFERENCES

Barau C, Braun J, Vincent C, et al. Pharmacokinetic study of raltegravir in HIV-infected patients with end-stage liver disease: the LIVERAL-ANRS 148 study. *Clin Infect Dis*. 2014;59(8):1177–1184.

Berkowitz EM, Moyle G, Stellbrink H-J, et al. Safety and immunogenicity of an adjuvanted herpes zoster subunit candidate vaccine in HIV-positive adults: a phase 1/2a randomized, placebo-controlled study. *J Infect Dis*. 2015;211(8):1279–1287.

Bickel M, Anadol E, Vogel M, et al. Daily dosing of tacrolimus in patients treated with HIV-1 therapy containing a ritonavir-boosted protease inhibitor or raltegravir. *J Antimicrob Chemother*. 2010;65(5):999–1004.

Blumberg EA, Roger CC. Solid organ transplantation in the HIV-infected patient: guidelines from the American Society of Transplantation Infectious Diseases Community of Practice. *Clin Transplant.* 2019; 33:e13499.

Campos-Varela I, Dodge JL, Berenguer M et al. Temporal trends and outcomes in liver transplantation for recipients with human immunodeficiency virus infection in Europe and United States. *Transplantation.* 2020 Oct;104(10):2078–2086.

Campos-Varela I, Dodge JL, Terrault NA, et al. Nonviral liver disease is the leading indication for liver transplant in the United States in persons living with human immunodeficiency virus. *Am J Transplant.* 2021;21(9):3148–3156.

Chen C, Wen X, Yadav A, et al. Outcomes in human immunodeficiency virus-infected recipients of heart transplants. *Clin Transplant.* 2019;33(1):e13440.

Clinical Trials.gov. NCT02741323.

Di Biagio A, Rosso R, Siccardi M, et al. Lack of interaction between raltegravir and cyclosporine in an HIV-infected liver transplant recipient. *J Antimicrob Chemother.* 2009;64(4):874–875.

Doberne JW, Jawitz OK, Raman V, et al. Heart transplantation survival outcomes of HIV positive and negative recipients. *Ann Thorac Surg.* 2021;111:1465–1471.

Donohue JK, Chan EG, Clifford S, et al. Lung transplantation in HIV seropositive recipients: an analysis of the UNOS registry. *Clin Transplant.* 2024;38:e15246.

Durand CM, Florman S, Motter JD, et al. HOPE in action: a prospective multicenter pilot study of liver transplantation from donors with HIV to recipients with HIV. *Am J Transplant.* 2022 Mar;22(3):853–864.

Durand CM, Zhang W, Brown DM, et al. A prospective multicenter pilot study of HIV-positive deceased donor to HIV-positive recipient kidney transplantation: HOPE in action. *Am J Transplant.* 2021 May;21(5):1754–1764.Frasetto LA, Browne M, Cheng A, et al. Immunosuppressant pharmacokinetics and dosing modifications in HIV-1 infected liver and kidney transplant recipients. *Am J Transplant.* 2007 Dec;7(12):2816–2820. https://www.ncbi.nlm.nih.gov/pubmed/17949460

Gabardi S, Martin ST, Roberts KL, Grafals M. Induction immunosuppressive therapies in renal transplantation. *Am J Health Syst Pharm.* 2011;68:211–218.

Gandhi RT, Bedimo R, Hoy JF, et al. Antiretroviral drugs for treatment and prevention of HIV infection in adults: 2022 recommendations of the International Antiviral Society-USA Panel. *JAMA.* 2023;329(1):63–84.

Koval CE, Farr J, Krisl J, et al. Heart or lung transplant outcomes in HIV-infected recipients. *J Heart Lung Transplant.* 2019 Dec;38(12):1296–1305.

Kucirka LM, Durand CM, Bae S, et al. Induction immunosuppression and clinical outcomes in kidney transplant recipients infected with human immunodeficiency virus. *Am J Transplant.* 2016;16(8):2368–2376.

Lee DH, Malat GE, Bias TE, et al. Serum creatinine elevation after switch to dolutegravir in a human immunodeficiency virus-positive kidney transplant recipient. *Trans Inf Disease.* 2016;18(4):625–627.

Locke JE, Gustafson MD, Mehta S, et al. Survival benefit of kidney transplantation in HIV-infected patients. *Ann Surg.* 2017;265(3):604–608.

Locke JE, James NT, Mannon RB, et al. Immunosuppression regimen and the risk of acute rejection in HIV-positive kidney transplant recipients. *Transplantation.* 2014;97(4):446–450.

Locke JE, Mehta S, Reed RD, et al. A national study of outcomes among HIV-infected kidney transplant recipients. *J Am Soc Nephrol.* 2015;265:2222–2229.

Malani P. HIV and transplantation: new reasons for HOPE. *JAMA.* 2016;316(2):136–138.

Miro JM, Agüero F, Duclos-Vallée JC, et al. Infections in solid organ transplant HIV-positive patients. *Clin Microbiol Infect.* 2014;20:119–130.

Miro JM, Ricart MJ, Trullas JC, et al. Simultaneous pancreas–kidney transplantation in HIV-infected patients: a case report and literature review. *Transplant Proc.* 2010;42(9):3887–3891.

Mombelli M, Rettby N, Perreau M, et al. Immunogenicity and safety of double versus standard dose of the seasonal influenza vaccine in solid-organ transplant recipients: a randomized controlled trial. *Vaccine.* 2018;36(41):6163–6169.

Muller E, Barday Z, Kahn D. HIV-positive-to-HIV-positive kidney transplantation: results at 3 and 5 years. *N Engl J Med.* 2015;372:613–620.

Nettles RE, Kieffer TL, Kwon P, et al. Intermittent HIV-1 viremia (Blips) and drug resistance in patients receiving HAART. *JAMA.* 2005;293(7):817–829.

Nguyen AQ, Anjum SK, Halpern SE, et al. Willingness to donate organs among people living with HIV. *J Acquir Immune Defic Syndr.* 2018;79(1):e30–e36.

Nissen NN, Barin B, Stock PG. Malignancy in the HIV-positive patients undergoing liver and kidney transplantation. *Curr Opin Oncol.* 2012;24:517–521.

Panel on Opportunistic Infections in Adults and Adolescents with HIV. Guidelines for the prevention and treatment of opportunistic infections in adults and adolescents with HIV: recommendations from the Centers for Disease Control and Prevention, the National Institutes of Health, and the HIV Medicine Association of the Infectious Diseases Society of America. https://clinicalinfo.hiv.gov/en/guidelines/hiv-clinical-guidelines-adult-and-adolescent-opportunistic-infections/whats-new2024. Published 2024. Accessed July 15, 2024.

Reshef R, Luger SM, Hexner E, et al. Blockade of lymphocyte chemotaxis in visceral graft-versus-host disease. *N Engl J Med.* 2012;367(2):135–145.

Roland ME, Barin B, Huprikar S, et al.; HIVTR Study Team. Survival in HIV-positive transplant recipients compared with transplant candidates and with HIV-negative controls. *AIDS.* 2016;30(3):435–444.

Rouzaud C, Berastegui, Picard C, et al. Lung transplantation in HIV-positive patients: a European retrospective cohort study. *Eur Resp J.* 2022;60:2200189.

Sawinski D, Forde KA, Eddinger K, et al. Superior outcomes in HIV-positive kidney transplant patients compared with HCV-infected or HIV/HCV co-infected recipients. *Kidney Int.* 2015a;88:341–349.

Sawinski D, Goldberg DS, Blumberg E, et al. Beyond the NIH multicenter HIV transplant trial experience: outcomes of HIV$^{\backslash+}$ liver transplant recipients compared to HCV$^{\backslash+}$ or HIV\+/HCV$^{\backslash+}$ co-infected recipients in the United States. *Clin Infect Dis.* 2015b;61(7):1054–1062.

Sawinski D, Shelton BA, Mehta S, et al. Impact of protease inhibitor-based anti-retroviral therapy on outcomes for HIV\+ kidney transplant recipients. *Am J Transplant.* 2017;17(12):3114–3122.

Seaman SM, Van Pilsum Rasmussen SE, Nguyen AQ, et al. Brief report: willingness to accept HIV-infected and increased infectious risk donor organs among transplant candidates living with HIV. *J Acquir Immune Defic Syndr.* 2020;85(1):88–92.

Spagnuolo V, Uberti-Foppa C, Castagna A. Pharmacotherapeutic management of HIV in transplant patients. *Expert Opin Pharmacother.* 2019;20(10):1235–1250.

Sparkes T, Manitpisitkul W, Masters B, et al. Impact of antiretroviral regimen on renal transplant outcomes in HIV-positive recipients. *Transpl Infect Dis.* 2018;e12992.

Stadtmauer EA, Sullivan KM, Marty FM, et al. A phase 1/2 study of an adjuvanted varicella-zoster virus subunit vaccine in autologous hematopoietic cell transplant recipients. *Blood.* 2014;124(19):2921–2929.

Stock P, Barin B, Murphy B, et al. Outcomes of kidney transplantation in HIV-positive recipients. *N Engl J Med.* 2010;363:2001–2014.

Suarez JF, Rosa R, Lorio MA, et al. Pretransplant CD4 count influences immune reconstitution and risk of infectious complications in human immunodeficiency virus-infected kidney allograft recipients. *Am J Transpl.* 2016;16(8):2463–2472.

Terrault N, Roland ME, Schiano T, et al. Outcomes of liver transplant recipients with hepatitis C and human immunodeficiency virus coinfection. *Liver Transpl.* 2012;18(6):716–726.

Trullas JC, Cofan F, Tuset M, et al. Renal transplantation in HIV-positive patients: 2010 update. *Kidney Int.* 2011 Apr;79(8):825–842.

van Maarseveen EM, Rogers CC, Trofe-Clark J, et al. Drug-drug interactions between antiretroviral and immunosuppressive agents in HIV-positive patients after solid organ transplantation: a review. *AIDS Patient Care STDs*. 2012;26(10):568–581.

Vivanco M, Friedmann P, Zia Y, et al. Campath induction in HCV and HCV/HIV-seropositive kidney transplant recipients. *Transpl Int*. 2013;26(10):1016–1026.

Werbel WA, Bae S, Yu S, et al. Early steroid withdrawal in HIV-infected kidney transplant recipients: utilization and outcomes. *Am J Transplant*. 2021;21(2):717–726.

Zarinsefat A, Gulati A, Shui A, et al. Long-term outcomes following kidney and liver transplant in recipients with HIV. *JAMA Surg*. 2022;157(3):240–247.

25.

MALIGNANCIES IN HIV

Eva H. Clark and Elizabeth Y. Chiao

CHAPTER GOALS

- Review the epidemiology and role of antiretroviral therapy (ART) on the impact of malignancies in people with HIV (PWH).
- Discuss the role of human herpes virus-8 (HHV-8) in the development of Kaposi's sarcoma (KS), which remains the most common tumor associated with HIV infection.
- Discuss the role of Epstein–Barr virus (EBV) in primary central nervous system lymphoma (PCNSL) and other HIV-associated lymphomas.
- Review the role of human papillomavirus (HPV) in virally mediated anogenital, oropharyngeal, and squamous cell cancers.
- Discuss additional relatively common malignancies in PWH, including lung, prostate, and colorectal cancer.
- Emphasize that antiretroviral therapy (ART) initiation is of utmost importance for all malignancies in PWH and summarize National Comprehensive Cancer Center Network (NCCN) guidelines for malignancies in PWH.

INTRODUCTION

LEARNING OBJECTIVE

Discuss the epidemiology and risk factors of virally mediated and non-virally mediated malignancies in PWH.

WHAT'S NEW?

Strategies for implementation of cancer prevention tools are gaining prominence.

KEY POINTS

- Malignancies in people with HIV (PWH) remain a major health concern and are among the leading causes of death among PWH.
- Antiretroviral therapy (ART) continues to contribute to decreasing malignancy rates overall.
- PWH tend to be diagnosed with cancer at younger ages.
- Most PWH diagnosed with either virally associated or non-virally associated cancer should receive standard of care treatments recommended for people without HIV
- HIV testing should be standard for individuals with newly diagnosed malignant disease.

Malignancies were one of the earliest recognized manifestations of the AIDS epidemic. Kaposi sarcoma (KS) became one of the first entities associated with AIDS (Ziegler et al., 1984). Subsequently, intermediate-grade and high-grade non-Hodgkin's lymphoma (NHL), invasive cervical cancer, and primary central nervous system lymphoma (PCNSL) were defined by the U.S. Centers for Disease Control and Prevention (CDC) as "AIDS-defining conditions" (CDC, 2008); recent expert consensus supports retiring this phrase because it does not capture all cancers associated with immunodeficiency (Engels et al., 2024). Since the advent of combination ART, other cancers with an increased incidence in PWH have been identified to include Hodgkin's disease and anal, liver, lung, oropharyngeal, colorectal, and renal cancers (Patel et al., 2008). The increasing longevity of PWH, as well as concurrent modifiable risk factors such as tobacco use, may also influence the epidemiology of these malignancies.

The introduction of combination ART in the mid-1990s significantly improved outcomes of PWH. ART has dramatically decreased the incidence of virally mediated HIV-associated malignancies, such as KS and PCNSL (Silverberg et al., 2015). However, with longer survival, it has become evident that PWH are at increased risk for many cancer types, including those not traditionally associated with immunodeficiency. Multiple risk factors include degree and duration of viremia, low $CD4^{+}$ T-cell count nadir, coinfection with oncogenic viruses (e.g., HPV, EBV, HHV-8, HCV, and HBV), and personal carcinogenic exposure, which should be considered when implementing risk-mitigation strategies (Kowalkowski et al., 2014; Riedel et al., 2015b; Vallet-Prichard & Pol, 2004). Most recent studies of cancer treatment outcomes demonstrate that PWH have outcomes similar to people without HIV. Because of the benefit of ART on cancer outcomes in PWH, it is recommended that most patients be treated similarly to those without HIV, and that ART should be administered concurrently with appropriate chemotherapy, radiotherapy, or immunotherapy (Chiao et al., 2010; Reid et al., 2018).

A large U.S. registry study during the post-ART era included 448,258 PWH from 1996 to 2012 and found an elevated risk for development of cancer overall (standardized incidence ratio [SIR] 1.69, 95% confidence interval [CI]: 1.67–1.72), KS (SIR 498.11, 95% CI: 477.82–519.03), NHL (SIR 11.51, 95% CI: 11.14–11.89), cervical cancer (SIR 3.24, 95% CI: 2.94–3.56), most other virus-related cancers (e.g., anal [SIR 19.06, 95% CI: 18.13–20.03], liver [SIR 3.21, 95% CI: 3.02–3.41], and Hodgkin's lymphoma [SIR 7.70, 95% CI: 7.20–8.23]), as well as several cancers unrelated to viruses (e.g., lung [SIR 1.97, 95% CI: 1.89–2.05]) (Hernández-Ramírez et al., 2017). However, their SIRs significantly decreased over the study period for KS, two subtypes of NHL, and cancers of the anus, liver, and lung, although they remained elevated compared to the general population. SIRs did not increase over time for any cancer. Additionally, older PWH seem to have a higher risk for most cancer types. When this same dataset was stratified by age, PWH older than 50 years were more likely to develop KS (SIR, 103.34), NHL (3.05), Hodgkin's lymphoma (7.61), cervical (2.02), anal (14.00), lung (1.71), liver (2.91), and oral cavity/pharyngeal (1.66) cancers, but were less likely to develop breast (0.61), prostate (0.47), and colon (0.63) cancers (Mahale et al., 2018) compared to the general population. The South African HIV Cancer Match Study, a study of more than 5 million PWH, found that the most common cancers in PWH during 2004–2014 were cervical cancer, KS, and breast cancer (Ruffieux et al., 2023). More recent studies indicate that PWH have an increased risk not only for these initial cancers, but also for developing a second primary cancer (Hessol et al., 2018; Mahale et al., 2020).

PWH also may be at higher risk for certain malignancies at younger ages. Shiels and colleagues (2010c) used the national U.S. HIV/AIDS Cancer Match Study to demonstrate that PWH are *not* at increased risk for colon, prostate, or breast cancer at younger ages, but they were significantly (p <0.001) younger at the time of diagnosis of lung (50 vs. 54 years) and anal cancer (42 vs. 45 years). They also found that the age of diagnosis of Hodgkin's lymphoma was significantly older than that of the general population (42 vs. 40 years; p <0.001). A study using data from the HIV/AIDS Cancer Match Study found that PWH with cancer tended to be younger than age 50 years compared to their counterparts without HIV, whose cancer occurred more often after age 60 years. This study also found that PWH presented with more advanced-stage cancers with distant disease (32.2%) compared to people without HIV (17.7%), and experienced higher cancer-specific mortality (Coghill et al., 2015). By comparing data from both the North American AIDS Cohort Collaboration on Research and Design (NA-ACCORD) and the U.S. Cancer Statistics Surveillance, Epidemiology, and End Results (SEER) program, Shiels and colleagues (2017) found that PWH were diagnosed with lung cancer, anal cancer, head and neck cancer, kidney cancer, and myeloma at earlier ages than their counterparts without HIV. However, in a recent metanalysis from studies of women with breast cancer in North America and sub-Saharan Africa, women with HIV (WWH) from both continents were more likely to be diagnosed with advanced-stage (3 and 4) disease and have poorer survival (Brandão et al., 2021).

Cancer outcomes tend to be worse in PWH compared to the general population. A study utilizing data from the HIV/AIDS Cancer Match Study during 2001–2019 found that PWH were more likely to *not* receive treatment for cervical cancer, diffuse large B-cell lymphoma (DLBCL), HL, lung cancer, prostate cancer, colon cancer, and breast cancer; importantly, this association decreased over time for breast, colon, and prostate cancer (McGee-Avila et al., 2024). A U.S. retrospective study found that cancer-related mortality among PWH compared to people without HIV (1996–2010) was significantly elevated for colorectal, pancreatic, lung, breast, and prostate cancer as well as melanoma (Coghill et al., 2015). Although cancer mortality remains high in PWH, it has declined over time. One U.S. population-based registry study found cancer-attributed mortality for PWH was 386.9 per 100,000 person-years (Horner et al., 2021); most cancer deaths were due to NHL (3.5%), lung cancer (2.4%), KS (1.3%), liver cancer (1.1%), and anal cancer (0.6%), and cancer mortality was highest among PWH 60 years or older. Previous evidence suggested that treatment of PWH and cancer could be more difficult than that of the general population, that PWH presented with more advanced disease, and that PWH may not tolerate cancer therapies as well as people without HIV (Bower et al., 2003). However, most of these studies were published before widespread use of integrase inhibitors and other recent ART advances. Given the higher incidence, incidence at an earlier age, and potentially poor outcomes for PWH, screening for early signs of malignancy when possible helps facilitate earlier diagnosis. Further research is needed to examine recommendations for optimal screening practices for specific cancers (beyond existing specific recommendation for cervical cancer) among PWH.

Management of malignancies in PWH presents many challenges, including the risk of further compromise to the immune system with chemotherapy, toxicities of treatment, pharmacologic interactions between ART and chemotherapy drugs, and the risk of intercurrent opportunistic infections (Mandell et al., 2010; Reid et al., 2018). The safety profile and feasibility of ART administration with concurrent chemotherapy have improved with recent use of integrase inhibitors. Guidelines for managing cancer in PWH were released in 2018 by the National Comprehensive Cancer Network (NCCN, 2024d; Reid, 2018). They advise that PWH who develop cancer should be cared for by both an oncologist and an HIV specialist and should receive cancer therapy according to standard guidelines developed for the general population. The patient's ART may need to be modified if there are potential interactions with the proposed cancer therapy, but generally ART should be continued during cancer therapy.

RECOMMENDED READING

Engles EA, Shiels MS, Barnabas RV, et al. State of the science and future directions for research on HIV and cancer: Summary of a joint workshop sponsored by IARC and NCI. *Int J Cancer.* 2024;154(4):596–606.

Horner MJ, Shiels MS, Pfeiffer RM, et al. Deaths attributable to cancer in the United States HIV population during 2001–2015. *Clin Infect Dis*. 2021;72(9):e224–e231. http://doi:10.1093/cid/ciaa1016
McGee-Avila JK, Suneja G, Engels EA, et al. Cancer treatment disparities in people with HIV in the United States, 2001–2019. *J Clin Oncol*. 2024 May 20;42(15):1810–1820.
Reid E, Suneja G, Ambinder RF, et al. Cancer in people living with HIV, Version 1.2018, NCCN clinical practice guidelines in oncology. *J Natl Compr Canc Netw*. 2018;16(8):986–1017.
Shiels MS, Islam JY, Rosenberg PS, et al. Projected cancer incidence rates and burden of incident cancer cases in HIV-infected adults in the United States through 2030. *Ann Intern Med*. 2018 Jun 19;168(12):866–873. http://doi:10.7326/M17-2499
Silverberg MJ, Lau B, Achenbach CJ, et al. Cumulative incidence of cancer among persons with HIV in North America. *Ann Intern Med*. 2015;163(7):507–518.
Silverberg MJ, Leyden W, Hernandez-Ramirez RU, et al. Timing of antiretroviral therapy initiation and risk of cancer among persons living with HIV. *Clin Infect Dis*. 2021 Jun 1; 72(11): 1900–1909.

KAPOSI'S SARCOMA

LEARNING OBJECTIVES

- Discuss the epidemiology of Kaposi's sarcoma (KS).
- Discuss the pathogenesis and clinical manifestations.
- Review the treatments for KS, including local and systemic therapies.

WHAT'S NEW?

The incidence of KS continues to decline with the use of ART, but it remains significantly elevated in areas with endemic disease, such as sub-Saharan Africa. Novel therapies are emerging for HIV-related KS.

KEY POINTS

- The presence of human herpes virus-8 (HHV-8) and advanced immunosuppression are both associated with risk of KS development and other lymphoproliferative states, such as multicentric Castleman's disease (MCD) and primary effusion lymphoma (PEL).
- Treatment for KS includes ART, local therapy, and systemic therapy.
- The goals of treatment are palliative and generally noncurative.
- Chemotherapy and radiotherapy have relatively high response rates for KS.
- In general, treatment decisions and referrals to oncology should be based on evidence of symptomatic or systemic disease.
- Radiotherapy should be avoided in the pelvis and lower extremities because of damage to the lymphatics and the potential for lymphedema and skin breakdown.

EPIDEMIOLOGY

KS was first described in 1872 by Moritz Kaposi, a Hungarian dermatologist. Four types of KS have been described: classic, endemic, transplant-associated, and AIDS-associated or epidemic KS. Classic KS is typically seen in elderly men of Mediterranean or Eastern European descent and is characterized by cutaneous lesions of the lower extremities (Iscovich et al., 2000). The endemic form, found primarily in sub-Saharan Africa, is often more aggressive and morbid, with visceral involvement (Friedman-Kien and Saltzman, 1990). Transplant-associated KS was first described in the 1970s and is seen in immunosuppressed allograft recipients. Although cutaneous disease is the most common presentation, visceral disease has been described in multiple organs (Penn, 1979).

AIDS-associated KS was first described in men who have sex with men (MSM) in the early 1980s, at the advent of the HIV epidemic (Friedman-Kien, 1981). This malignancy disproportionately affected MSM with AIDS, who were estimated to have a 20-fold higher risk of developing KS compared to other HIV transmission risk groups (Beral et al., 1990; Hoover et al., 1993). KS is rarely reported in people who inject drugs or other HIV risk groups (Mitsuyasu et al., 1984; Safai, 1987).

The incidence of KS in high-income countries has declined markedly with widespread use of ART. Of 85,922 overall cases of KS in the United States between 1990 and 2007, the proportion of KS in persons with AIDS declined from 89% in 1990–1995 to 67% in 2001–2007 ($p < 0.001$) (Shiels et al., 2011b). Cumulative incidence of KS by age 75 years was among the highest compared to other cancers (lung, anal, colorectal, Hodgkin's lymphoma, liver, and oropharyngeal) from 1995 to 2009 at 4.1%. However, KS incidence decreased by 4% per year from 2005 to 2009 compared to 1996–1999 rates ($p < 0.01$) (Silverberg et al., 2015). Similarly, the Swiss HIV Cohort Study showed that the KS incidence was 33.3 per 1,000 patient-years (py) in 1984–1986 and did not change significantly in the subsequent periods until 1996–1998, when it declined to 5.1 per 1,000 py (95% CI: 3.9–6.5) and then further decreased to 1.4 per 1,000 py in 1999–2001 (Franceschi et al., 2008). A Brazilian retrospective cohort also described a decreased incidence of KS from 1998 to 2010, with an incidence rate ratio per year of 0.89 (95% CI: 0.83–0.97) (Castilho et al., 2015). In 2010, KS accounted for approximately 12% of cancers diagnosed in PWH (Robbins et al., 2015). Despite the overall decline in KS, there remain concerning differences in improvement in traditionally underserved racial and geographic groups. Between 2001 and 2013, Royse and colleagues evaluated 4,455 KS cases in U.S. men and determined that the annual percent change (APC) for KS incidence significantly decreased for white men between 2001 and 2013 (APC −4.52, $p = 0.02$) (Royse et al., 2017). In contrast, the APC for Black men was not significant (APC −1.84, $p = 0.09$), and the APC among Southern Black men significantly increased (+3.0, $p = 0.03$). Similarly, re-evaluation of this data for 20–34-year-old men between 2001 and 2018 indicated that the U.S. KS incidence rate increased by 1.5%

per year in non-Hispanic Black men but decreased by 3.5% per year in non-Hispanic white men (Suk et al., 2022); this difference was most evident among young Black men living in the South. Taken together, these epidemiologic studies suggest that rising KS in young Black men is likely related to the relatively high incidence of advanced HIV disease in this population.

In areas of southern Africa where KS is endemic, this cancer reached epidemic proportions during the initial AIDS epidemic owing to lack of ART. For instance, in Zimbabwe, KS was reported to represent 40% of all cancers in men (Chokunonga et al., 2000). A prospective cohort from 2004 to 2010 found that the incidence in Zimbabwe, Botswana, South Africa, and Zambia reached 413 per 100,000 py (95% CI: 342–497), with higher rates among groups aged older than 60 years (Rohner et al., 2014). Despite the increased availability of ART in these countries, estimates of KS have minimally decreased in PWH on ART, with the incidence of KS remaining high at 164 per 100,000 py (95% CI: 151–178) (Rohner et al., 2014). KS remains the leading cause of cancer incidence and death in men in several sub-Saharan African countries (Sung et al., 2021). In 2020, the global estimated age-standardized incidence rate of KS was 0.39 per 100,000, with an estimated 34,270 newly diagnosed cases and 15,086 deaths due to KS (age-standardized mortality rate of 0.18 per 100,000) (Fu et al., 2023). In the same year, Africa accounted for 73% of KS incidence and 87% of KS deaths.

PATHOGENESIS

In 1994, Chang and Moore (Chang et al., 1994) discovered a new herpesvirus, HHV-8 or KS herpes virus (KSHV), in more than 90% of AIDS-KS tissue samples. Although the KS types vary in epidemiology and clinical presentation, all are associated with HHV-8. In 2003, HHV-8 viremia was shown to be an early marker of KS, and the risk of developing disease was demonstrated to increase with HHV-8 antibody titers (Engels et al., 2003; Newton et al., 2003). HHV-8 also is associated with rare lymphoproliferative diseases most often seen in PWH, including multicentric Castleman's disease (MCD) and a rare form of NHL called primary effusion lymphoma (PEL). Although HHV-8 infection is necessary for developing HHV-8-associated disease, it is not sufficient; in fact, HHV-8 viremia is prevalent only in a subset of cases. In an analysis of 335 people with HIV-associated KS, only 130 (39%) were viremic, with a mean HHV-8 viral load of 6,630 DNA copies/mL (Haq et al., 2016). Among PWH, immunosuppression confers the greatest risk and is most predictive of development of KS (Jacobson et al., 2000; Renwick et al., 1998).

The pathogenesis of KS is complex and involves viral processes and dysregulation of cytokine pathways. The HHV-8 genome encodes many homologues of human cellular gene products involved in inflammation, cell cycle regulation, and angiogenesis, such as viral cyclin-D1, vascular endothelial growth factor (VEGF), basic fibroblast growth factor, and interleukin-6 (IL-6) (Cannon, 2000). Much work has been done on the tumorigenesis of KS. HHV-8 infection leads to upregulation of Toll-like receptor 4 (TLR4), its adaptor MyD88, and coreceptors CD14 and MD2 (Gruffaz et al., 2018). The TLR4 pathway seems to be activated constitutively in HHV-8-transformed cells, resulting in chronic induction of IL-6, IL-1β, and IL-18. IL-6 production in turn results in activation of the STAT3 pathway, an essential event for uncontrolled cellular proliferation and transformation. Gruffaz and colleagues have shown that TLR4 stimulation with lipopolysaccharides or live bacteria enhanced tumorigenesis, while TLR4 antagonist CLI095 inhibited it. A regulatory transactivating (Tat) protein of HIV is released by infected cells and guards KS cells from apoptosis (Deregibus et al., 2002), stimulates growth and angiogenesis (Barillari and Ensoli, 2002; Ensoli et al., 1990), and increases the production and release of matrix metalloproteinases (MMPs) from endothelial and inflammatory cells. MMPs contribute to the angiogenesis found in KS lesions (Impola et al., 2003; Lafrenie et al., 1996). Clinically, HHV-8-mediated systemic inflammation that develops in people with HHV-8 but without MCD is recognized as KSHV-inflammatory cytokine syndrome (KICS) (Polizzotto et al., 2016).

The mechanism of HHV-8 transmission remains unclear. HHV-8 has been detected in semen, prostate tissue (Monini et al., 1996), and breast milk (Dedicoat et al., 2004). The virus is often shed from the oropharynx of both immunocompetent and immunocompromised people in areas where HHV-8 is endemic (Casper et al., 2004; Casper et al., 2007). Behaviors associated with exposure to saliva are correlated with a higher risk of HHV-8 infection, implicating both sexual and horizontal transmission (Casper et al., 2006; Plancoulaine et al., 2000). A relatively high HHV-8 seroprevalence has been described among people who inject drugs, and an increased incidence of HHV-8 infection has been noted among transfusion recipients in areas where HHV-8 is endemic, suggesting that parenteral transmission may be possible (Cannon et al., 2001; Hladik et al., 2006). Transmission of HHV-8 from donors of solid organs has also been described (Barozzi et al., 2003; Luppi et al., 2000).

CLINICAL MANIFESTATIONS

HHV-8 is associated with four specific conditions: KS, multicentric Castleman's disease (MCD), primary effusion lymphoma (PEL), and KSHV-associated inflammatory cytokine syndrome (KICS). Patients may have one or multiple of these HHV-8-related conditions and may present with a wide range of symptoms related to cytokine dysregulation. Only KS will be discussed here.

KS is an angioproliferative disease varying from an indolent to fulminant disease with potential for significant morbidity and mortality. The disease can occur in individuals with a wide range of $CD4^+$ T-cell counts but becomes increasingly common as immune function declines. The progression of disease may be rapid or slow. PWH with limited disease and controlled HIV infection usually do reasonably well. However, in the setting of uncontrolled HIV, viral replication, and low $CD4^+$ T-cell counts, KS progresses rapidly.

The skin is the most common site of presentation. Visceral involvement occurs less commonly, although with disease progression KS frequently involves the gastrointestinal (GI) tract (see below). At autopsy, almost every organ system can show involvement. Visceral disease is rare in the absence of extensive cutaneous disease.

The cutaneous presentation of KS occurs in 95% of cases. Lesions may occur anywhere on the skin. Common sites include the face (particularly the periorbital area and tip of the nose), external ear, mouth, torso, and lower extremities. They can evolve from macules or nodular tumors to large plaque-like tumor masses that involve extensive cutaneous surfaces and eventually evolve into ulcerating tumors. Lesion color may vary from violaceous in light-skinned individuals to brownish-black in dark-skinned individuals. Lesions are generally nonblanching and nonpruritic, and may occasionally be associated with some pain, particularly in the setting of immune reconstitution inflammatory syndrome (IRIS).

Lymphedema associated with KS usually appears in people with visible cutaneous lesions, and edema may be out of proportion to the extent of visible lesions. Lymphedema also may occur in people with no visible skin lesions. Common sites include the face, neck, external genitals, and lower extremities. A contiguous area of skin usually is involved as well.

Oral cavity involvement is seen in approximately one-third of people with KS and is the initial site of diagnosis 15% of the time (Dezube et al., 2004). These lesions may be flat or nodular and are red or purplish. They usually appear on the hard palate, but they may develop on the soft palate, gingival areas, and tongue. Oral lesions, if extensive, may cause tooth loss, pain, and ulceration. Involvement of the oral cavity correlates with KS in the GI tract.

Gastrointestinal (GI) KS has been reported in 40% of cases at initial diagnosis (Dezube et al., 2004) and any segment of the GI tract may be involved. Visceral spread of KS that involves the GI tract is rarely symptomatic. However, with disease progression, patients may experience symptoms of abdominal pain, nausea, vomiting, or GI bleeding (Danzig et al., 1991). Rare cases of obstruction, perforation, or protein-losing enteropathy have been reported (Friedman, 1988). In PWH with advanced immunosuppression ($CD4^+$ T-cell count <100 cells/mm^3), GI KS may be more severe with complications. Some believe that screening endoscopy to detect occult disease may be warranted in these scenarios (Nagata et al., 2012).

Pulmonary KS also occurs; however, in contrast to KS at other visceral sites, lung involvement is generally symptomatic. Common symptoms include cough, bronchospasm, dyspnea, and hemoptysis. This complication tends to occur in the setting of advanced AIDS, with most individuals having $CD4^+$ T-cell counts of less than 100 cells/mm^3 (Gill et al., 1989) and in people with more extensive cutaneous disease (e.g., with >50 lesions). Of note, it can occur in people with minimal and absent cutaneous KS. The disease is often rapidly progressive when it involves the lungs; median survival time was 2–6 months in the pre-ART era (Kaplan et al., 1988). Respiratory failure is often the cause of death. Radiographic appearance is variable, with the characteristic reticulonodular pattern seen in approximately one-third of patients (Kaplan et al., 1988). Otherwise, diffuse interstitial infiltrates, pleural effusions, and hilar adenopathy may be seen (Levine and Tulpule, 2001).

Once KS is clinically suspected, diagnosis is made by biopsy and histologic examination or by presumptive diagnosis based on the endoscopic appearance of a visceral lesion (Aboulafia, 2001). A histologic confirmation is essential to exclude other conditions that can mimic KS. Endoscopically, the classic appearance of small submucosal vascular nodules establishes the diagnosis of GI KS. It may be difficult to establish a diagnosis of GI KS by biopsy because many lesions are submucosal (Hengge et al., 2002). In people with suspected pulmonary KS, violaceous endobronchial lesions typically are observed on bronchoscopic examination. A presumptive diagnosis of pulmonary KS can be made based on characteristic radiographic and endobronchial findings in people who have had KS at other sites (Kaplan et al., 1988). Endobronchial biopsy is discouraged because of the risk of hemorrhage. Gallium scanning may be helpful in differentiating KS from pulmonary infection because KS is not gallium-avid (Kaplan et al., 1988). In resource-limited and endemic settings, treatment is often initiated without biopsy given the high prevalence of disease and limited access to pathology resources.

In the pre-ART era, the Advancing Clinical Therapeutics Globally (ACTG) network developed a staging system based on tumor extent (T), severity of immunosuppression (I), and presence of systemic illness (S) (Krown et al., 1997). Two different risk categories were noted based on this staging system: a *good risk*, defined as T0I0S0; and a *poor risk*, defined as T1I1S1 (Table 25.1).

Based on epidemiological, clinical, staging, and survival data of patients in two Italian prospective cohort studies (n = 211), Nasti and colleagues concluded that, in the ART era, a refinement of the ACTG staging system is needed (Nasti et al., 2003b). $CD4^+$ T-cell counts in this study did not provide prognostic information, and only the combination of T1S1 identified people with unfavorable prognosis. The 3-year survival rate for people with T1S1 was 53%, which was significantly lower compared to the 3-year survival rates of people with T0S0, T1S0, and T0S1, which were 88%, 80%, and 81%, respectively. Several studies have found other prognostic markers for KS. Another study developed a prognostic index predicting poor survival, including not having KS as the AIDS-defining illness, decreasing $CD4^+$ T-cell count, being aged 50 years or older, and having a concurrent AIDS-associated illness (Stebbing et al., 2006). Other variables, including $CD8^+$ T-cell count (Stebbing et al., 2007) and detectable HHV-8 DNA in plasma at the time of diagnosis (El Amari et al., 2008), have also been associated with poor KS prognosis.

TREATMENT

Impact of Antiretroviral Therapy

ART is a key component in the treatment of KS and should be initiated or optimized to achieve complete HIV RNA suppression in all PWH with AIDS-associated KS. The inhibition of HIV replication, decreased production of the Tat protein, restored immunity to HHV-8, and the direct antiangiogenic

Table 25.1 AIDS CLINICAL TRIALS GROUP (ACTG) TUMOR STAGING SYSTEM

CHARACTERISTIC	GOOD RISK (0)	POOR RISK (1)
	All of the following:	*Any of the following:*
Tumor (T)	Tumor confined to skin and/or lymph nodes and/or minimal oral disease[a]	Tumor-associated edema or ulceration; extensive oral KS; GI KS; other visceral KS
Immune system (I)	CD4 count ≥150 cells/mm^3	CD4$^+$ T-cell count <150 cells/mm^3
Systemic illness (S)	No history of OI or thrush; no systemic symptoms; Karnofsky performance status ≥70	History of OI and/or thrush; systemic symptoms; Karnofsky performance status <70; other HIV-related illnesses

[a] Nonnodular KS confined to the palate.

GI = gastrointestinal; KS = Kaposi's sarcoma; OI = opportunistic infection.

Adapted from Krown SE, et al. *J Clin Oncol.* 1989;7(9):1201–1207 and incorporating revision by Krown SE, et al. *J Clin Oncol.* 1997;15(9):3085–3092, with permission from the American Society of Clinical Oncology.

activity of some protease inhibitors (PIs) are among the many benefits of ART (Dubrow et al., 2017; Noy, 2003). Some older data suggested that PIs have an anti-KS effect (Sgadari et al., 2003); however, non-PI-containing ART regimens also lead to KS regression.

Combination ART has been associated with a lengthening of time to KS treatment failure with either local or systemic therapy for KS. A retrospective study found a median time of 20.4 months from the initiation of ART plus chemotherapy versus 6 months with just chemotherapy to detect treatment failure among PWH with KS (Bower et al., 1999). PWH who were receiving ART at KS diagnosis have a less aggressive presentation versus individuals who were ART-naive at the time of KS diagnosis (Nasti et al., 2003a). Another retrospective analysis from 1990 to 1999 found an 81% reduction in the risk of death among PWH with KS after the initiation of ART (Tam et al., 2002).

KS-associated IRIS has been well described. Some PWH may experience painful enlarged lesions or progression of KS lesions during the first months of ART. In a prospective study of 69 PWH and HHV-8 coinfection, approximately 12% of patients experienced IRIS-KS after initiation of ART (Letang et al., 2010).

Local Treatment

Local treatment should be reserved for people with minimal or locally symptomatic disease, or for people who are not responding to or cannot tolerate systemic therapy. These people should concurrently receive ART. Current options for local treatment include the following:

- Radiotherapy has been the mainstay of local therapy for KS. It is best suited for individuals with a single or a few locally symptomatic areas (not in the lower extremities) or for symptomatic disease that requires rapid tumor reduction. Electron beam radiation applied to the entire face is highly effective in relief of facial edema. Radiotherapy also can be useful for treatment of dysphagia caused by pharyngeal lesions and tumor masses of the eye or the extremities (Hill, 1987). Radiotherapy, whether given as whole-body electron beam therapy, fractionated focal radiation therapy, or single treatments, has produced complete remissions in 50%–80% of cases (Cooper and Steinfeld, 1991; Pluda et al., 1992). Complications such as severe mucositis, radiotherapy fibrosis, loss of skin compliance, and chronic lymphedema may occur with these treatments. Radiotherapy is not recommended for the lower extremities because of potential skin changes and the high risk for cellulitis.
- With intralesional chemotherapy, vinblastine has been most commonly used, with a reported response rate of 70% in older studies (Boudreaux et al., 1993). Small cutaneous lesions can be treated with intralesional chemotherapy for cosmetic purposes. Repeated treatments may be necessary. Intralesional chemotherapy can cause significant pain and areas of hyperpigmentation after treatment.
- Alitretinoin gel is a topical treatment that may be used for relatively asymptomatic people with KS lesions that do not respond to ART alone and for whom the KS is predominantly an issue of cosmesis. A response rate of 49% (n = 184) in a phase 3 study was reported (Walmsley et al., 1999). Adverse effects include dry skin and light hypersensitivity.
- Cryotherapy with liquid nitrogen and laser therapy have been used successfully for isolated small KS lesions. Given the significant mucosal toxicity associated with radiotherapy in the treatment of oral lesions, laser surgery may be substituted for radiation.
- There are several new therapies being explored for treatment of local KS, including a phase 1 trial of intralesional nivolumab, which is an immune check point inhibitor (NCT03316274) (Bender-Ignacio et al., 2018).

Systemic Treatment

Treatment of KS is generally not considered curative and was not shown to have a significant impact on survival in the pre-ART era. A South African randomized trial of ART alone versus ART plus chemotherapy demonstrated a significant difference in KS response but no difference in survival between the two arms (Mosam et al., 2012), although it should be emphasized that only second-line chemotherapy (noon-Taxol or -Doxil regimens) was studied. Another study demonstrated that immediate treatment with oral etoposide resulted in early clinical benefits that were no longer observed 48 weeks post therapy. A post hoc analysis of that study evaluated the effect of oral etoposide on the development of KS-IRIS and early progressive disease (KS-PD) after starting ART and found that etoposide decreased the development of KS-IRIS and KS-PD after ART initiation.

Importantly, these studies need to be reinterpreted in the context of a more recent landmark three-arm randomized clinical trial conducted by the ACTG/AIDS Malignancy Consortium (AMC) in 11 sites in Brazil, Kenya, Malawi, South Africa, Uganda, and Zimbabwe, which compared oral etoposide plus ART and bleomycin plus vincristine plus ART to paclitaxel plus ART. The study was stopped early because the paclitaxel arm demonstrated superior progression-free survival at week 48 compared to the other two arms (Krown et al., 2020). The most significant side effects of paclitaxel are hypersensitivity, myelosuppression, peripheral neuropathy, alopecia, and drug interactions with ART. Thus, paclitaxel is currently recommended as first-line therapy in resource-limited settings.

Systemic intravenous chemotherapy is used for people with symptomatic, poor-risk, visceral disease, extensive skin involvement, significant edema, or rapidly progressive KS. As described previously, the goal of systemic chemotherapy is mainly palliation of symptoms. In the United States and other resource-rich settings, large randomized studies have established liposomal anthracyclines (doxorubicin and daunorubicin) as first-line single-agent chemotherapy agents compared to combination chemotherapy treatment (Gill et al., 1996; Northfelt et al., 1998; Stewart et al., 1998). Liposomal anthracyclines alone can achieve response rates equal to or better than combination chemotherapy, with a lower incidence of toxicity such as nausea, fatigue, alopecia, and neuropathy. Neutropenia, however, occurred as frequently with the liposomal agent as with the standard combination regimen. Prognosis is favorable; in one study of 140 patients with T1 disease who were treated with ART and liposomal anthracycline chemotherapy, the 5-year overall survival was 85% (Bower et al., 2014).

In resource-rich settings, paclitaxel is a highly active agent often used as second-line therapy. It has significant anti-tumor activity in people with previously untreated (Gill et al., 1995) and refractory KS (Saville et al., 1995). Because liposomal doxorubicin is not available in many low- and middle-income countries (LMICs), other regimens, including bleomycin and vincristine, have been utilized for KS treatment. Regarding comparison of liposomal anthracyclines versus taxanes, a small randomized trial of paclitaxel compared to liposomal doxorubicin showed that both therapies improved symptoms such as pain and swelling in PWH with advanced KS (Cianfrocca et al., 2010). Additionally, they demonstrated comparable response rates, progression-free survival, and median survival, though a slightly higher rate of grade 3 to 5 toxicity occurred in the paclitaxel arm (Cianfrocca et al., 2010). A 2014 Cochrane review indicated no observed difference between liposomal doxorubicin, liposomal daunorubicin, and paclitaxel for PWH on ART (Gbabe et al., 2014).

In the United States, because a long-term cure of KS is difficult to measure given that hyperpigmented inactive lesions often persist, the primary goals of treatment for patients with KS are palliation of symptoms and improved cosmesis. Consultation with a KS-experienced oncologist or dermatologist should be considered for most PWH diagnosed with this malignancy.

Several newer therapies are currently being studied for severe KS. Inhibition of the KS-activated mammalian target of rapamycin (mTOR) signaling pathway has been examined in an AMC study and has shown promising results (Krown et al., 2012). Imatinib, a platelet-derived growth factor receptor/c-kit inhibitor, induced responses in 10 of 30 participants with KS when given up to 1 year in a multicenter phase 2 trial (Koon et al., 2014). The VEGF-A inhibitor, bevacizumab, was shown in another phase 2 trial to produce complete and partial responses in 3 and 2 of 16 participants, respectively (Uldrick et al., 2012). Two immunomodulatory agents with antiangiogenic effects, pomalidomide (oral) and lenalidomide (intravenous), have been evaluated in clinical trials. Pomalidomide was found to be well tolerated and active in KS regardless of HIV status (NCT02659930) (Polizzotto et al., 2016; Ramaswami et al., 2022). Lenalidomide was well tolerated in ART-experienced PWH with progressive KS previously treated with chemotherapy, but its phase 2 trial was halted due to lack of responses in this study population (Pourcher et al., 2017). Combining nivolumab with ipilimumab was promising in a phase 2 clinical trial of participants with previously treated progressive KS (Zer et al., 2022). Several other targeted therapies for KS are under evaluation in clinical trials (Bender-Ignacio et al., 2018).

Treatment for KS may need to be modified if an additional HHV-8 related condition is present simultaneously, such as multicentric Castelman's disease (MCD), primary effusion lymphoma (PEL), or KSHV-associated inflammatory cytokine syndrome (KICS) (Patel et al., 2023).

RECOMMENDED READING

Cianfrocca M, Lee S, Von Roenn J, et al. Randomized trial of paclitaxel vs. pegylated liposomal doxorubicin for advanced human immunodeficiency virus-associated Kaposi sarcoma: evidence of symptom palliation from chemotherapy. *Cancer*. 2010;116(16):3969–3677.

Fu L, Tian T, Wang B, et al. Global patterns and trends in Kaposi sarcoma incidence: a population-based study. *Lancet Glob Health*. 2023 Oct;11(10):e1566–e1575.

Hosseinipour MC, Kang M, Krown SE, Bukuru A, et al. As-needed vs immediate etoposide chemotherapy in combination with antiretroviral therapy for mild-to-moderate AIDS-associated Kaposi sarcoma in resource-limited settings: A5264/AMC-067 randomized clinical trial. *Clin Infect Dis*. 2018;67(2):251–260.

Krown SE, Moser CB, MacPhail P, et al. Treatment of advanced AIDS-associated Kaposi sarcoma in resource-limited settings: a three-arm, open-label, randomised, non-inferiority trial. *Lancet*. 2020;395(10231):1195–1207. http://doi:10.1016/S0140-6736(19)33222-2

Luo Q, Johnson AS, Hall HI, et al. Kaposi sarcoma rates among persons living with human immunodeficiency virus in the United States: 2008–2016. *Clin Infect Dis*. 2021;73(7):e2226–e2233.

Patel R, Lurain K, Yarchoan R, et al. Clinical management of Kaposi sarcoma herpesvirus-associated diseases: an update on disease manifestations and treatment strategies. *Expert Rev Anti Infect Ther*. 2023;21(9):929–941.

Polizzotto MN, Uldrick TS, Wyvill KM, et al. Clinical features and outcomes of patients with symptomatic Kaposi sarcoma herpesvirus (KSHV)-associated inflammation: prospective characterization of KSHV inflammatory cytokine syndrome (KICS). *Clin Infect Dis*. 2016 Mar 15;62(6):730–738. https://doi.org/10.1093/cid/civ996

Ramaswami R, Polizzotto MN, Lurain K, et al. Safety, activity, and long-term outcomes of pomalidomide in the treatment of Kaposi sarcoma among individuals with or without HIV infection. *Clin Cancer Res*. 2022;28(5):840–850.

Reid E, Suneja G, Ambinder RF, et al. Cancer in people living with HIV, Version 1.2018, NCCN clinical practice guidelines in oncology. *J Natl Compr Canc Netw*. 2018;16(8):986–1017.

Shiels MS, Pfeiffer RM, Hall HI, et al. Proportions of Kaposi sarcoma, selected non-Hodgkin lymphomas, and cervical cancer in the United States occurring in persons with AIDS, 1980–2007. *JAMA*. 2011;305(14):1450–1459.

Suk R, White DL, Knights S, et al. Incidence trends of Kaposi sarcoma among young non-Hispanic Black men by US regions, 2001–2018. *JNCI Cancer Spectr*. 2022;6(6):pkac078.

Zer A, Icht O, Yosef L, et al. Phase II single-arm study of nivolumab and ipilimumab (Nivo/Ipi) in previously treated classical Kaposi sarcoma (cKS). *Ann Oncol*. 2022;33(7):720–727.

HIV-RELATED PRIMARY CENTRAL NERVOUS SYSTEM LYMPHOMA

LEARNING OBJECTIVES

- Review the epidemiology of primary central nervous system lymphoma (PCNSL) in PWH.
- Review the pathophysiology and clinical presentation of PCNSL in PWH.
- Review chemotherapeutic strategies for treatment PCNSL in PWH.
- Discuss survival among PWH with PCNSL.

WHAT'S NEW?

Fluorodeoxyglucose–positron emission tomography (FDG-PET) and magnetic resonance spectroscopy provide less invasive strategies to characterize severity of disease and distinguish it from other pathologies.

KEY POINTS

- Epstein–Barr virus (EBV) mediated oncogenesis in the setting of advanced immunosuppression is largely responsible for PCNSL.
- Treatment with ART should be initiated and maintained for all PWH with PCNSL.
- Despite improved survival in the ART era, overall survival remains poor.

Primary CNS lymphoma (PCNSL) is a rare type of NHL, accounting for 1%–2% of all NHLs and less than 5% of all primary brain tumors (Lister et al., 2002). PCNSL has been diagnosed in 1.6%–9.0% of people with AIDS and represents the second most common intracranial mass lesion in this population (Rosenblum et al., 1988; Welch et al., 1984). The vast majority of PCNSL has been linked to EBV-infected B cells that reach the CNS during advanced immunodeficiency (Cingolani et al., 2005). MacMahon and colleagues (1991) noted that EBV genes important for oncogenesis are abundant in patients with PCNSL, suggesting a pathogenic role of EBV in this setting. This association suggests that the pathogenesis of PCNSL might differ from systemic NHL, which has a 40%–50% association with EBV (Ballerini et al., 1993; Hamilton-Dutoit et al., 1989).

EPIDEMIOLOGY

Prior to effective ART, the relative risk of PCNSL was approximately 1,000-fold and as high as 3,600-fold in people with AIDS compared to the general population (Cote et al., 1996). The age-adjusted incidence of PCNSL in the United States had increased substantially since the 1970s, from 0.16 per 100,000 py in 1973–1984 to 0.48 per 100,000 py in 1985–1997 (Olson et al., 2002). However, with the introduction of ART in the mid- to late 1990s, the incidence of PCNSL in PWH significantly decreased (Hoffman et al., 2001; Wolf et al., 2005). In the Multicenter AIDS Cohort Study (MACS), the incidence rate in 2,734 men with HIV declined from 4.3 to 0.4 per 100,000 py (Sacktor et al., 2001). In another study, PCNSL accounted for only 1% of lymphoma diagnoses in PWH in the period 2006–2015 (Gopal et al., 2013). Despite this dramatic decrease in incidence, survival rates have not significantly improved, especially compared to those of people without HIV (Bayraktar et al., 2011; Conti et al., 2000).

CLINICAL PRESENTATION

The clinical presentation of PCNSL does not vary significantly by HIV status. Symptoms may include headaches, confusion, lethargy, memory loss, personality changes, and seizures. On examination, people may present with hemiparesis, aphasia, and cranial nerve palsies. Lesions are most common in the cerebrum, basal ganglia, and brainstem. More diffuse and multifocal involvement is seen in HIV-related PCNSL (Gage et al., 2000). These lesions are contrast-enhancing on computed tomography (CT) and magnetic resonance imaging (MRI). Before ART, the median CD4$^+$ T-cell count at presentation was less than 50 cells/mm^3 (Levine et al., 1991).

Polymerase chain reaction (PCR) to detect EBV DNA in the cerebrospinal fluid is useful for diagnosing AIDS-associated PCNSL. Identification of EBV by PCR can detect most cases of AIDS-related PCNSL with a sensitivity of 80%–100% and specificity for lymphoma of 93%–100% (Bossolasco et al., 2002). Cerebrospinal fluid cytology alone has limited utility because of poor sensitivity and specificity (Ekstein et al., 2006).

Single-photon emission CT has been suggested as a less-invasive technique for diagnosis. However, due to conflicting data regarding sensitivity and specificity, its role in the diagnosis of PCNSL remains limited (Licho et al., 2002; Ruiz et al., 1994). FDG-PET and magnetic resonance spectroscopy are two other imaging modalities that can aid in distinguishing cerebral PCNSL lesions from other infectious CNS pathologies such as toxoplasmosis. Magnetic resonance spectroscopy typically shows decreased *N*-acetylaspartate and increased choline, which reflects neoplastic cell proliferation (Westwood et al., 2013). FDG-PET can also help identify extracerebral systemic disease involvement (Lewitschnig et al., 2013). Currently, the gold standard for diagnosis of PCNSL is stereotactic brain biopsy. In patients in whom a brain biopsy is unobtainable, the combination of imaging, negative toxoplasma serology, previous toxoplasmosis prophylaxis, and positive EBV cerebrospinal fluid by PCR may be sufficient to make a presumptive diagnosis.

TREATMENT AND SURVIVAL

The relative rarity of PCNSL precludes large-scale randomized trials; therefore, the optimal treatment for PCNSL has not been determined. Norden et al. showed that HIV infection significantly reduced median overall survival to 2 months versus 12 months in people without HIV (Norden et al., 2011). Despite good initial response rates to treatment, median survival times with treatment remain only 2–5.5 months (Baumgartner et al., 1990). The previous standard treatment of PWH with AIDS-related PCNSL was palliative corticosteroids and whole-brain radiation that achieved a complete response in 20%–50% of patients (Cote et al., 1996). Radiation alone can improve symptoms and extend median survival, but this is likely affected by a person's baseline functional status and not the dose of radiation received (Goldstein et al., 1991).

Regarding chemotherapy for AIDS-related PCNSL, high-dose methotrexate is currently recommended for first-line therapy. An early pilot study used high-dose intravenous methotrexate in 15 patients, including 10 with histologically confirmed PCNSL (mean $CD4^+$ T-cell count was 30 cells/mm^3) (Jacomet et al., 1997). *Complete responses*, defined as clinical improvement and disappearance of contrast-enhancing brain abnormalities on CT or MRI, were obtained in 7 of 15 patients (3 of 10 with histological diagnosis and 4 of 5 patients without histological confirmation). Six patients failed to respond, one patient relapsed at 6 months, and two patients died of severe sepsis. The median survival time was 290 days for the 10 patients with histological diagnosis and 347 days for the 5 patients without histological confirmation. Corticosteroids were also administered, and individuals ultimately received ART including a PI. In a retrospective study, 20 PWH were treated with methotrexate-based regimens: some received high-dose methotrexate alone, some received high-dose methotrexate and rituximab, and others received a variety of other regimens (Gupta et al., 2017). The median survival in people treated before ART and without high-dose methotrexate was 2 months, whereas with ART and high-dose methotrexate-based regimens the median survival had not yet been reached with a median follow-up of 27 months. In people without HIV and PCNSL, high-dose intravenous methotrexate remains the standard of care for those who can tolerate the therapy, and available evidence supports this strategy combined with ART in PWH. In 2016, the IELSG32 trial provided a high level of evidence supporting the use of matrix combination (methotrexate, cytarabine, and rituximab with or without thiotepa) as the new standard chemoimmunotherapy for patients aged up to 70 years with newly diagnosed PCNSL (Ferreri et al., 2016). A phase 2 trial is underway evaluating induction with rituximab, high-dose methotrexate, and leucovorin every 2 weeks for six cycles, followed by consolidation with high-dose methotrexate alone (NCT00267865). Whole-brain radiation is traditionally reserved for people with poor performance status (NCCN 2024e); however, in the second randomization of the IELSG32 trial, both whole-brain radiotherapy and autologous stem cell transplantation were found to be feasible and effective as consolidation therapies after high-dose methotrexate-based chemoimmunotherapy (Ferreri et al., 2017). Finally, a small prospective series from investigators at the National Cancer Institute demonstrated that 8 of 12 PWH and PCNSL who received ART, rituximab, and high-dose methotrexate (R-HD-MTX) had sustained complete response (67%), including 3 who received second-line therapy without relapse at 2 years. The estimated 60-month overall survival was 67% (95% CI: 32–86), and, with median potential follow-up of 82 months, the median overall survival was not reached. They concluded that treatment with ART and R-HD-MTX is associated with a high response rate, $CD4^+$ T-lymphocyte reconstitution, and long-term survival with preservation or improvement of neurocognitive function. In addition, the regimen was tolerable, even for people with advanced HIV, significant comorbidities, and CNS infections (Lurain et al., 2020).

ROLE OF ANTIRETROVIRAL THERAPY

Combination ART should be initiated in all individuals with AIDS-related PCNSL who are undertaking treatment because it is associated with significant improvement in survival. In the pre-ART era, radiotherapy prolonged survival for 2–5.5 months compared to palliative care (Donahue et al., 1995). McGowan and Shaw (1998) were the first to describe a case of remission maintained for more than 2 years after treatment with ART alone in an individual who had PCNSL. Other case reports have also reported similar PCNSL response to ART (Aboulafia and Puswella, 2007; Travi et al., 2012). In a retrospective analysis, Hoffman and colleagues (2001) showed that survival times of individuals receiving ART in addition to radiotherapy differed significantly from those of people receiving radiotherapy or palliative care alone. Four of the six persons receiving ART survived for more than 1.5 years. In another retrospective analysis, Skiest and Crosby (2003) demonstrated a prolonged median survival of 667 days in individuals who received ART. These findings strongly suggest that immune recovery contributes to longer remission in PWH and PCNSL.

RECOMMENDED READING

Cingolani A, Fratino L, Scoppettuolo G, et al. Changing pattern of primary cerebral lymphoma in the highly active antiretroviral therapy era. *J Neurovirol.* 2005;11(Suppl 3):38–44.

Ferreri AJM, Cwynarski K, Pulczynski E, et al. Whole-brain radiotherapy or autologous stem-cell transplantation as consolidation strategies after high-dose methotrexate-based chemoimmunotherapy in patients with primary CNS lymphoma: results of the second randomisation of the International Extranodal Lymphoma Study Group-32 phase 2 trial. *Lancet Haematol.* 2017 Nov;4(11):e510–e523.

Gupta NK, Nolan A, Omuro A, et al. Long-term survival in AIDS-related primary central nervous system lymphoma. *Neuro Oncol.* 2017;19:99–108

Westwood TD, Hogan C, Julyan PJ, et al. Utility of FDG-PETCT and magnetic resonance spectroscopy in differentiating between cerebral lymphoma and non-malignant CNS lesions in HIV-infected patients. *Eur J Radiol.* 2013;82(8):e374–e379.

SYSTEMIC LYMPHOMA

LEARNING OBJECTIVES

- Review the epidemiology of non-Hodgkin's lymphoma (NHL).
- Review the pathophysiology and clinical manifestations of NHL.
- Review the treatment of NHL and survival outcomes.

WHAT'S NEW?

- Survival for PWH and NHL continues to improve in the ART era; however, incidence remains significantly higher compared to that of people without HIV.
- Intensive chemotherapy and autologous hematopoietic cell transplantation (HCT) are safe in PWH and are associated with improved outcomes.
- CAR T-cell therapy is emerging as a safe and effective therapy for PWH and chemotherapy refractory NHL.

KEY POINTS

- NHL development is likely a multifactorial interplay among host immune factors as well as the presence of viral mediators including EBV and HHV-8. Disease can occur in a variety of nodal and extranodal sites, and some forms of NHL are more aggressive than others, such as PEL.
- Prognostic factors include host immunity, the presence of injection drug use, performance status, and the degree of tumor burden.
- Treatment with ART and intensive chemotherapy with consideration of HCT are cornerstones of NHL treatment. Allogeneic stem cell transplantation using cells from CCR5delta2/delta32 donors appears to have resulted in HIV cure.

The first cases of AIDS-related NHL were described in 1982 (Ziegler et al., 1982). In 1985, NHL was added to the list of AIDS-defining malignancies. Before the ART era, it was estimated to occur in approximately 8% of all HIV cases (Kaplan et al., 1989), and it is currently the second most common neoplasm occurring among PWH (Knowles, 2001).

The World Health Organization has divided AIDS-related lymphomas (ARLs) into three categories (Box 25.1):

1. Lymphomas also occurring in immunocompetent patients, such as Burkitt's lymphoma (BL) and diffuse large B-cell lymphoma (DLBCL).
2. Lymphomas occurring specifically in PWH, such as PEL and plasmablastic lymphoma.
3. Lymphomas also occurring in other immunodeficiency states, such as polymorphic or post-transplant lymphoproliferative disorder-like B-cell lymphoma.

DLBCL and BL are the most common ARLs, representing approximately 90% of these malignancies (Besson et al., 2001). Only intermediate-grade or high-grade lymphomas are considered AIDS-defining.

EPIDEMIOLOGY

There are more than 30 types of NHLs, including DLBCL and BL. Individuals with impaired cell-mediated immunity show a marked increase in the incidence of NHL. This has been best described in immunosuppressed allograft recipients. Similar trends were seen in PWH in the pre-ART era.

Box 25.1 AIDS-RELATED LYMPHOMAS: WORLD HEALTH ORGANIZATION CLASSIFICATION

Lymphomas also occurring in immunocompetent people with HIV:
Burkitt's lymphoma
Diffuse large B-cell lymphoma: centroblastic, immunoblastic, and anaplastic variants
Lymphomas occurring specifically in PWH:
Primary effusion lymphoma
Plasmablastic lymphoma
Lymphomas also occurring in other immunodeficiency states:
Polymorphic or post-transplant lymphoproliferative disorder-like B-cell lymphoma

Source: Adapted from Raphael M, Said J, Dorisch B et al., Lymphomas associated with HIV infection. In: Swerdlow SH, Campo E, Harris NL et al., eds., *World Health Organization Classification of Tumours of Haematopoietic and Lymphoid Tissue.* 4th ed. Lyon, France: IARC Press; 2008.

The CDC examined data of 2,824 NHL cases occurring in 97,258 PLWH between 1981 and 1989 in the United States, and estimated that risk was 60 times greater in PWH (Beral et al., 1991). Variability by histologic subtype has also been noted, with up to 600-fold excess risk for immunoblastic lymphoma (IBL) (Cote et al., 1997). In a study evaluating the cumulative incidence of NHL in PWH living in the United States and Canada (n = 86,620), the incidence of NHL from 1996 to 2009 was 4.5% by age 75 years compared to only 0.7% in persons without HIV (n = 196,987) (Silverberg et al., 2015). Data from the U.S. Centers for AIDS Research network including 23,050 PWH diagnosed between 1996 and 2011 indicated that lymphomas developed in 2.1% (Gopal et al., 2013). Most of these were DLBCL (42.2%), followed by Hodgkin's lymphoma (HL; 16.6%), Burkitt's lymphoma (BL; 11.8%), PCNSL (11.3%), and other NHLs (18.1%). A study of 4,312 patients including 1,514 (35%) PWH found that, in months 3–60 from time of BL diagnosis, PWH had a 55% increase in risk of death compared to people without HIV (95% CI: 1.38–1.75, $p < 0.0001$) (Wieland et al., 2024). A multicenter retrospective analysis from Brazil involving 276 PWH and lymphoma diagnosed during 2000–2019 found that the factors associated with poor survival included performance status, lymphoma subtype and stage including CNS penetration, and beta-2-microglobulin level (Cordova-Vargas et al., 2023).

PATHOGENESIS

The pathogenesis of HIV-related NHL is most likely multifactorial, involving HIV, immune dysfunction, cytokine dysregulation, and other viral antigens, including EBV and HHV-8 (Gates et al., 2003). EBV is present in approximately 40%–50% of cases of AIDS-related systemic NHL (Hamilton-Dutoit et al., 1989). This contrasts with a report by Ballerini and colleagues (1993), who reported 100% EBV coinfection in the immunoblastic lymphoma variant of DLBCL. Expression of the latent EBV transforming proteins EBNA-2 and LMP-1 is known to play a central role in the initiation and maintenance of EBV-induced B-cell growth and proliferation (Liebowitz and Kieff, 1989). Both EBNA-2 and LMP-1 can serve as targets for cytotoxic T-cells; thus, their expression induces T-cell immune surveillance and regulates lymphomagenesis in individuals who are immunocompetent. With immunodeficiency states such as late-stage HIV, EBNA-2 and LMP-1 expression may become unregulated and subsequently lead to uncontrolled proliferation of EBV-infected cells (Gaidano and Dalla-Favera, 1995). Genetic alterations involving oncogenes and tumor suppressor genes may also occur, and often *MYC* and *BCL6* translocations are implicated in neoplastic development (Chadburn et al., 2013).

Expression of HHV-8 also is associated with PEL, which presents malignant pleural, peritoneal, or pericardial effusions with a paucity of nodal masses. It is aggressive and often refractory to chemotherapy. HHV-8 has been universally found in malignant cells, often in conjunction with EBV (Komanduri et al., 1996). Neoplastic cells have an immunoblastic to plasmablastic appearance. Most PELs have lymphocyte activation markers (CD30 and CD38) without normal B-cell markers (CD19 and CD20).

CLINICAL CHARACTERISTICS

Approximately two-thirds of ARLs are classified as DLBCL (Navarro and Kaplan, 2006). AIDS-related systemic NHL usually presented as widespread disease involving extranodal sites in the pre-ART era (Knowles et al., 1988). The most common sites of extranodal disease are the gastrointestinal tract, CNS, bone marrow, and liver. It has been reported that 95% of patients from several institutions had evidence of extranodal disease, including 42% with CNS involvement and 33% with bone marrow involvement (Ziegler et al., 1984). In a multicenter retrospective review of pooled data from 886 PWH with DLBCL, CNS involvement was found in 13% of patients and was not associated with reduced overall survival (Barta et al., 2016). However, CNS relapse was associated with a median overall survival of only 1.6 months. GI NHL occurs in approximately 30% of PWH with NHL. Most of these cases involve the stomach, but virtually any site in the GI tract or hepatobiliary tree can be involved (Burkes et al., 1986). Interestingly, most cases of plasmablastic lymphomas are associated with characteristic development of oral cavity lesions and predominate in mucosal sites (Chadburn et al., 2013). In the ART era, among PWH with virologic suppression, Gerard and colleagues found that NHL occurred at a median $CD4^+$ T-cell count of 297 cells/mm^3. In addition, they found that 65% of the cases occurred within 18 months of initiating ART (Gerard et al., 2009). Other studies have shown that PEL and immunoblastic NHL are seen in PWH with lower $CD4^+$ T-cell counts, of older age, and with a prior diagnosis of AIDS, whereas Burkitt's NHL tends to occur in PWH with more preserved immune function (Knowles, 1996). In a more recent study of 23,050 PWH diagnosed between 1996 and 2011, individuals with Hodgkin's lymphoma and Burkitt's NHL had the highest $CD4^+$ T-cell counts, while people with PCNSL had the lowest (Gopal et al., 2013). In 2010, NHL accounted for approximately 21% of cancers diagnosed in PWH (Robbins et al., 2015).

PROGNOSTIC FEATURES

Historically, poor prognostic factors for people with HIV-related NHL have included age older than 35 years, $CD4^+$ T-cell count of less than 100 cells/mm^3, history of injection drug use, history of AIDS-defining condition, poor performance status, elevated lactate dehydrogenase, tumor bulk or stage of disease, and International Prognostic Index (IPI) (Straus et al., 1998). The IPI includes clinical features that reflect tumor growth and invasive potential (tumor stage, serum lactate dehydrogenase [LDH] level, and number of extranodal disease sites), the patient's response to the tumor (performance status), and the patient's ability to tolerate intensive therapy (age and performance status). The simplified model for younger patients (age-adjusted IPI) uses a subgroup of these clinical features (i.e., tumor stage, LDH level, and performance status). Lim and colleagues (2005) compared prognostic factors for survival and use of the IPI in pre- and post-ART PWH with DLBCL. In groups with low-, low-intermediate-, and high-intermediate-risk IPI disease, the 3-year overall survival rates were 20%, 22%, and 5% in the pre-ART era and improved to 64%, 64%, and 50% in the post-ART era.

Of note, PEL and extra-cavity PEL are known to be aggressive malignancies with a traditionally dismal prognosis. An early study found a median survival time of 6 months and few survivors beyond 12 months. Poor performance status and lack of ART portend worse prognosis (Boulanger et al., 2005). However, PEL prognosis may be improving. A more recent single-center retrospective study of 15 patients found that complete remission was achieved in 14 (93.3%); 4 of these patients later relapsed, and 2 patients died (Cattaneo et al., 2015). Overall survival rate at 3 years was 66.7%.

Barta and colleagues (2014) developed an AIDS-related lymphoma IPI that combines the age-adjusted IPI with an HIV severity score including $CD4^+$ T-cell count, HIV RNA levels, and prior history of AIDS to risk-stratify HIV-related lymphomas. Using this scoring system, this group evaluated patients enrolled in HIV-associated lymphoma trials between 2005 and 2010 and found that individual HIV-related factors such as low $CD4^+$ T-cell counts (<50 cells/mm^3) and prior history of AIDS were no longer associated with poorer outcomes (Barta et al., 2015).

TREATMENT

The treatment for AIDS-related lymphoma is similar to that of people without HIV, with some exceptions (Reid et al., 2018). Intrathecal chemotherapy prophylaxis is necessary because PWH are at an increased risk for CNS involvement. Those cases include lymphomas with aggressive pathologic features, including BL, plasmablastic lymphoma, and presentations consistent with possible CNS involvement. The use of hematopoietic stimulants such as granulocyte colony-stimulating factor (G-CSF) may aid in reducing chemotherapy-induced cytopenic complications. *Pneumocystis jirovecii* pneumonia prophylaxis is administered with standard-dose chemotherapy, irrespective of $CD4^+$ T-cell count.

Chemotherapy in the Pre-ART and Current ART Eras

In the pre-ART era, PWH with NHL had a poor prognosis, were managed on low-dose chemotherapy regimens because of concern for toxicity, and had a median survival of 5–8 months (Kaplan et al., 1997; Sandler and Kaplan, 1996). In addition to persistent neoplasia contributing to death, many patients in this era died because of the infectious complications of opportunistic diseases (Lowenthal et al., 1988).

With current HIV treatments, standard combination chemotherapy regimens are used successfully to treat NHL without excessive toxicity. The AMC reported on 65 patients given reduced doses of cyclophosphamide and doxorubicin combined with vincristine and prednisone (modified CHOP) or full doses of CHOP combined with G-CSF with concomitant ART. Complete response rates were 30% and 48% in the reduced- and full-dose groups, respectively (Ratner et al., 2001). Other studies of CHOP-based chemotherapy and concurrent ART describe median survival times of approximately 2 years. In patients with BL, a particularly aggressive form of NHL, intensive chemotherapy with cyclophosphamide, doxorubicin, high-dose methotrexate/ifosfamide, etoposide, and high-dose cytarabine (CODOX-M/IVAC) resulted in rates of event-free survival and remission similar to those of their counterparts without HIV (Wang et al., 2003).

Risk-adaptive chemotherapy has also been studied comparing the post- to pre-ART era. One study randomly assigned 485 PWH to chemotherapy after risk stratification based on an HIV score (comprising performance status, prior AIDS, and $CD4^+$ T-cell counts <100 cells/mm^3): 218 "good-risk" patients (HIV score 0) received doxorubicin, cyclophosphamide, vindesine, bleomycin, and prednisone (ACVBP) or CHOP; 177 "intermediate-risk" patients (HIV score 1) received CHOP or low-dose CHP; and 90 "poor-risk" patients (HIV score 2 or 3) received low-dose CHOP or vincristine and steroids. Five-year overall survival in the good-risk group was 51% for ACVBP versus 47% for CHOP ($p = 0.85$); that in the intermediate-risk group was 28% for CHOP versus 24% for low-dose CHOP ($p = 0.19$); and that in the poor-risk group was 11% for low-dose CHOP versus 3% for vincristine and steroids ($p = 0.14$). Factors which significantly improved overall survival were ART (relative risk [RR] 1.6; $p = 0.0002$), HIV score (RR 1.7; $p = 0.0001$), and IPI score (RR 1.5; $p = 0.0012$) but not chemotherapy intensity (Mounier et al., 2006).

A regimen of cyclophosphamide, doxorubicin, and etoposide with or without ART (only didanosine) resulted in a complete response rate of 45% and median overall survival of 12.8 months. At the time of the analysis, 30% in the pre-ART group were alive, compared with 47% in the ART group. Further, patients in the ART group experienced less nonhematologic toxicity (22% vs. 42%), thrombocytopenia (31% vs. 52%), and anemia (9% vs. 27%) (Sparano et al., 2004). A similar regimen, etoposide, prednisone, vincristine, and doxorubicin (EPOCH), has been used more commonly and with perhaps even more success. In two retrospective pooled analyses, Barta and colleagues (2012, 2013) concluded that EPOCH is superior to CHOP; however, these studies were limited by the potential confounder that experience with CHOP occurred in earlier time periods than that with EPOCH.

For treatment of PEL, a 2012 multicenter retrospective study found no survival benefit from regimens that were more intensive than CHOP (Castillo et al., 2012). A 2015 single-institution retrospective study of 15 patients treated with CHOP or CHOP-like regimens found that complete remission was achieved in 14 (93.3%); 4 of these subsequently relapsed (Cattaneo et al., 2015).

Regimens That Include Rituximab

In the early 2000s, uncertainty existed around the use of rituximab in PWH with low CD4+ T-cell counts because of concern for increased infection risk (Gates and Kaplan, 2003; Avivi et al., 2003). However, with subsequent experience, there is now a general consensus that outcomes are improved when rituximab is added to the chemotherapy regimens discussed earlier; thus, rituximab should be regarded as the standard of care for both DLBCL and BL. Two multicenter retrospective analyses of DLBCL patients with and without HIV treated with rituximab plus CHOP (R-CHOP) completed in the early 2000s showed conflicting results. Coutinho and colleagues (2014) evaluated patients treated between 2003 and 2011 and found that HIV positivity was associated with an improved 5-year overall survival rate (78% compared with 64% in patients without HIV). In contrast, Baptista and colleagues (2015) evaluated patients treated between 2001 and 2011 and found that HIV positivity was associated with a worse 5-year survival rate (56% compared with 74% in patients without HIV). However, in the latter study PWH had a worse performance status and higher Ann Arbor stages than did patients without HIV, and, when complete response rates were compared among patients with high tumor burdens, there was no difference between the two groups. The safety and feasibility of R-CHOP in populations of LMICs is being established by studies such as a phase 2 trial of R-CHOP in patients with and without HIV and DLBCL in Malawi (Kimani et al., 2021) (NCT02660710).

Other regimens for NHL have also been examined in PWH. Sparano and colleagues examined rituximab plus infusional etoposide, vincristine, doxorubicin, cyclophosphamide, and prednisone (R-EPOCH) given either concurrently or sequentially. In the concurrent arm, 35 of 48 evaluable patients (73%; 95% CI: 58–85) had a complete response, whereas 29 of 53 evaluable patients in the sequential arm (55%; 95% CI: 41–68) had a complete response. Toxicity was comparable, although PWH with a baseline CD4+ T-cell count of less than 50 cells/mm^3 had a high infectious death rate in the concurrent arm (Sparano et al., 2010). A prospective, uncontrolled phase 2 trial of short-course R-EPOCH in PWH with untreated NHL indicated that low-intensity regimens can be effective (NCT00006436). A phase 2 trial of ibrutinib (a small molecule drug that binds permanently to Bruton's tyrosine kinase) in combination with R-EPOCH in stage II–IV DLBCL is ongoing (NCT03220022). Evidence remains unclear whether R-CHOP or R-EPOCH is best for patients with ARLs. A large multicenter trial addressed this question in the population without HIV and showed no difference between R-CHOP and dose-adjusted R-EPOCH in event-free survival or overall survival (Wilson et al., 2016). Despite a paucity of large studies in PWH, treatment with either R-CHOP or R-EPOCH is usually effective at achieving remission in PWH with DLBCL, and most patients who achieve remission remain lymphoma-free.

Regarding BL, a 2012 study examined CODOX-M, followed by IVAC with or without rituximab (Rodrigo et al., 2012). Most patients were on ART and had a median CD4+ T-cell count of 375 cells/mm^3. Of the 14 patients who received ART and had intensive chemotherapy and rituximab, 10 survived to the follow-up period of nearly 12 months. Complications included late neutropenia, which responded well to G-CSF. Because of the predilection of herpesvirus reactivation with rituximab, study participants received prophylaxis for herpes simplex and varicella zoster and preemptive monitoring of cytomegalovirus. Similarly, a prospective multicenter trial showed that modified CODOX-M/IVAC with rituximab was safe and effective in PWH receiving ART, and the 2-year overall survival rate for 34 patients with HIV-related Burkitt's lymphoma (BL) was 69% (Noy et al., 2015). A study of short-course low-intensity R-EPOCH in 13 patients with BL including 11 PWH found that the overall survival at a median follow-up of 73 months was even better, 90% (Dunleavy et al., 2013). A multicenter retrospective analysis of 41 PWH and BL in China found similar overall response rates for patients receiving R-EPOCH and R-Hyper-CVAD (59% and 58.2%, respectively) (Zhao et al., 2023). They also found that patients given rituximab-containing regimens had similar complete remission rates (25% vs. 23.5%) and overall survival time (45.69 ± 11.58 vs. 47.79 ± 11.72 months, $p = 0.907$) compared to patients not given rituximab, but more patients not given rituximab progressed (33.3% vs. 47.1%). In contrast, a study in Singapore of 34 patients with adult BL, including seven PWH, who received rituximab with standard first-line chemotherapy (mostly R-EPOCH) had excellent outcomes with 100% CR and no relapses (Tan et al., 2023). No randomized data are available to determine which regimen is best in PWH with BL.

Intrathecal Chemotherapy for AIDS-Related NHL

CNS involvement by systemic DLBCL has long been recognized as a problem, especially in PWH. To date there have not been any formal studies to evaluate the role of intrathecal prophylaxis in PWH and DLBCL. In the absence of definitive data, clinicians routinely administer intrathecal prophylaxis to people with the following characteristics: extranodal involvement of two or more sites, elevated lactate dehydrogenase levels, or bone marrow or testicular involvement.

Alternative Therapies for AIDS-Related NHL

Targeted anticancer therapies are increasingly used for several types of uncommon but aggressive ARLs, but data remain sparse. A 2017 systematic review evaluated the use of bortezomib (a 26S proteasome inhibitor that is used for multiple myeloma) in 21 patients with plasmablastic lymphoma, of whom 11 received bortezomib as initial treatment and 10 received bortezomib for relapsed disease. The study included 11 participants with and 10 without HIV. The overall response rate to bortezomib-containing regimens was 100% as initial therapy and 90% in the relapsed setting, and 2-year survival of patients treated with bortezomib initially was 55% (Guerrero-Garcia et al., 2017). Daratumumab, a CD38-directed human IgG1κ monoclonal antibody also used for multiple myeloma, has been shown to be effective in controlling a case of refractory PEL (Shah et al., 2018). The biologic agent pembrolizumab has undergone phase 1 trials for patients with advanced NHL and seems to have an acceptable safety profile (Uldrick et al., 2019) (NCT02595866). Pembrolizumab has also been evaluated with and without pomalidomide in a retrospective review of stage IV relapsed and/or primary refractory HIV-associated NHL, demonstrating a response rate of 50% in that setting (Lurain, et al., 2021).

A retrospective review of 23 PWH with classic Hodgkin lymphoma treated with nivolumab or pembrolizumab showed favorable outcomes, including a median progression-free survival of 21.2 months that did not differ between PWH with <200 versus ≥200 CD4+ cells/mm^3 (Lurain et al., 2021). Brentuximab vedotin plus doxorubicin, vinblastine, and dacarbazine (AVD) was found to be safe in a phase 2 trial of 41 PWH and stage III–IV classic Hodgkin's lymphoma and 7 PWH with stage II classic Hodgkin's lymphoma (NCT01771107; Rubinstein et al., 2023). All patients who completed treatment achieved a complete response, and 2-year progression-free survival was 87% (95% CI: 71–94).

Chimeric antigen receptor (CAR) T-cell therapy is increasingly used for treatment of refractory lymphomas in the general population and is emerging as an effective treatment for PWH as well. Abramson and colleagues (2019) reported two PWH and high-grade B-cell lymphoma successfully treated with commercially available anti-CD19 CAR T-cells. A review of six cases of PWH and DLBCL treated with CAR T-cell therapy showed complete remissions in three and partial remission in one (Hattenhauer et al., 2023). Further, such therapies are being developed as potential cures for HIV (NCT03617198) (Rust et al., 2020).

Hematopoietic Cell Transplantation for AIDS-Related NHL

Autologous hematopoietic cell transplantation (HCT) has long been the optimal therapy for high-risk and refractory NHL in patients without HIV, and now a sufficient number of PWH have undergone autologous HCT to determine that it is a safe and feasible approach for patients with ARLs who meet criteria for transplantation (Navarro and Kaplan, 2006). A multicenter study to evaluate the safety and efficacy of autologous HCT for PWH and lymphoma evaluated 40 patients with persistent or recurrent ARLs (DLBCL, plasmablastic lymphoma, Burkitt's or Burkitt-like lymphoma, or classical Hodgkin's lymphoma) (Alvarnas et al., 2016). Overall survival and time to progression were similar for PWH when compared with matched controls without HIV. Uninterrupted ART should be continued in these patients during the peritransplant period, when feasible, to maintain virological suppression and avoid untoward effects of acute virological rebound, including opportunistic infections (Woolfrey et al., 2008). Administration of ART is generally considered safe, with minimal effect on the transplantation course, including adverse drug-drug interactions or other significant adverse events (Johnston et al., 2016).

One study showed that low CD4$^+$ T-cell count, marrow involvement, and poor performance status independently affected survival with HCT (Re et al., 2009). Overall survival has been reported to be 50%–55% at 9 months (Gabarre et al., 2000; Re et al., 2003); 71% at 21 months (Diez-Martin et al., 2003); and 85% at 32 months (Krishnan et al., 2005). Most published studies (one exception is a French series, Diez-Martin et al., 2003) have required HIV disease to be under control for HCT, either by low to undetectable HIV RNA levels or by CD4$^+$ T-cell counts of more than 100 cells/mm^3. One study showed a similar incidence of relapse, overall survival, and progression-free survival in cohorts of people with and without HIV and lymphoma who received HCT (Diez-Martin et al., 2009). Long-term survival of autologous HCT for relapsed/refractory lymphoma was examined in a retrospective review of survivors with HIV (Zanet et al., 2015). This study found a survival of 65% at 5 years for 37 patients. Among 26 patients who achieved complete remission, overall survival at 10 years was 91%, and event-free survival was 36%. Nine patients developed opportunistic infections at a median of 0.4 years post HCT.

Regarding allogeneic bone marrow transplant (alloBMT), one famous case reported in 2009 demonstrated that allogeneic HCT with donor cells that are resistant to HIV infection (in this case, because of a homozygous deletion polymorphism in the donor's CCR5 gene) can cure HIV infection (Hutter et al., 2009). Although fascinating, this outcome is the exception rather than the rule with allogeneic HCT. Importantly, caution must be observed because, in typical alloBMTs, the HIV reservoir disappears along with the patient's T-cells but can aggressively rebound if ART is discontinued (Henrich et al., 2014; Sugarman et al., 2016). A prospective multicenter trial of matched related or unrelated allogeneic HCT in PWH included 17 patients with acute leukemias, myelodysplasia, Hodgkin's lymphomas, and NHLs (Ambinder et al., 2017). No deaths occurred by 100 days post-transplant, and the overall survival rate at 1 year was 57%. Subsequent deaths were due to relapsed or progressive disease in five patients, acute graft-versus-host disease, adult respiratory distress syndrome, and liver failure. The overall conclusion from this trial was that allogeneic HCT should be considered the standard of care for PWH who meet usual transplant eligibility criteria. Other studies are currently being conducted to explore gene-modified autologous and allo-HSCT with HIV-resistant cells (Bender-Ignacio et al., 2018; DiGiusto et al., 2016; Lederman et al., 2016). Other recent studies have contributed important observations on the latent HIV reservoir dynamics post stem cell transplant. Eberhard and colleagues (2020) found strong CD4$^+$ and CD8$^+$ T-cell activation following allo-HSCT that peaked between months 2 and 3 after HSCT, demonstrating that there is a period of high immune activation and a potential window of vulnerability for HIV reservoir re-seeding during that time. In another small study of allogeneic transplant where post-transplant cyclophosphamide was used for graft-versus-host disease prophylaxis to expand donor options, Durant and colleagues demonstrated that among 6 patients with available follow-up, the HIV latent reservoir was not detected post-allo-HSCT in 4 patients with more than 95% donor chimerism, consistent with a 2.06–2.54 $\log_{10}$ reduction in the HIV latent reservoir. However, the HIV latent reservoir remained stable in the 2 patients with less than 95% donor chimerism. Although 3 of the 6 patients ultimately died after allo-HSCT, this study supports the use of allo-HSCT for PWH and reinforces the observation that allo-HSCT alone diminishes but does not completely eliminate the HIV latent reservoir (Durand et al., 2020).

Chemotherapy: ART Interactions

ART interruption during cancer treatment should generally be avoided because it increases the risk of severe consequences (including immunologic compromise, opportunistic infection, and death) (El-Sadr et al., 2006) and it improves tolerance and outcomes of cancer treatment. However, interactions between ART and proposed anticancer therapeutic options must always be checked, as many medications used for chemotherapy (e.g., cyclophosphamide and vincristine) and immunotherapy are metabolized via the CYP3A4 isoenzyme. PIs (including ritonavir), non-nucleoside reverse transcriptase inhibitors (NNRTIs), and pharmacokinetic boosters such as cobicistat inhibit and induce CYP3A4, with the potential for altered chemotherapeutic and cytotoxic effects. Thus, chemotherapy without antiretroviral drugs has been studied because of concerns of drug interactions with chemotherapy and nonadherence to ART resulting in increased HIV drug resistance (Powles et al., 2000). Further, PIs have been associated with increased incidence of neutropenia with concomitant chemotherapy (Bower et al., 2004a).

Many currently used ARV agents are unlikely to lead to problematic drug-drug interactions with chemotherapeutic agents. Those with the fewest potential interactions include integrase strand transfer inhibitors (INSTIs) (e.g., raltegravir, dolutegravir, bictegravir, and cabotegravir). Raltegravir, an INSTI metabolized via glucuronidation, has been given simultaneously with CHOP and with other antimetabolites such as gemcitabine and methotrexate, as well as with monoclonal antibodies rituximab and trastuzumab, with good tolerability and durable viral suppression (Bañon et al., 2014). ART regimens that include an INSTI improve virologic and immunologic responses in ART-naive patients and are considered in the U.S. Department of Health and Human Services (US DHHS, 2024a) ART guidelines for HIV disease as an acceptable first-line therapy; thus, ART regimens containing an INSTI should be leveraged for PWH undergoing cancer treatment (Fulco et al., 2010).

Impact of ART

Most studies have shown that the incidence of HIV-related NHL, like that for most other cancers associated with immunodeficiency in PWH, has declined over time. In a meta-analysis by Appleby and colleagues (2000) that included 47,936 PWH with NHL (including PCNSL), the incidence declined from 6.2 cases per 1,000 py in the pre-ART era to 3.6 cases per 1,000 py in the post-ART era (p <0.0001).

In a population-based, record-linkage study of cancer in 472,378 people with AIDS from 1980 to 2006, the cumulative incidence of NHL declined from 3.8% during 1990–1995 to 2.2% during 1996–2006. Of note, NHL was the most common AIDS-defining cancer during the pre-ART era (53%) (Simard et al., 2011). In addition, the Swiss Cohort study examined 429 NHL cases of 12,959 PWH from 1993 to 2006. NHL incidence reached 13.6 per 1,000 py in 1993–1995 and declined to 1.8 in 2002–2006. Combination ART use was associated with a decline in NHL incidence (hazard ratio [HR] 0.26; 95% CI: 0.20–0.33) (Polesel et al., 2008).

A retrospective study using U.S. and Canadian data from 1996 to 2009 showed a significant decline in the annual hazard rate of NHL (−8%) in PWH compared to that of people without HIV, signifying a narrowing of the gap of NHL burden between people with and without HIV (Silverberg et al., 2015). This reduction also represents the benefit of immunological recovery and viral control.

RECOMMENDED READING

Abramson JS, Irwin KE, Frigault MJ, et al. Successful anti-CD19 CAR T-cell therapy in HIV-infected patients with refractory high-grade B-cell lymphoma. *Cancer.* 2019;125:3692–3698

Alvarnas JC, Le Rademacher J, Wang Y, et al. Autologous hematopoietic cell transplantation for HIV-related lymphoma: results of the BMT CTN 0803/AMC 071 trial. *Blood.* 2016;128:1050–1058.

Bañon S, Machuca I, Araujo S, et al. Efficacy, safety, and lack of interactions with the use of raltegravir in HIV-infected patients undergoing antineoplastic chemotherapy. *J Intern AIDS Soc.* 2014;17(4 Suppl 3):19590.

Cordova-Vargas J, de Oliveira Marque M, Pereira J, et al. Factors associated with survival in patients with lymphoma and HIV. *AIDS.* 2023;37(8):1217–1226.

Hattenhauer ST, Mispelbaum R, Hentrich M, et al. Enabling CAR T-cell therapies for HIV-positive lymphoma patients: a call for action. *HIV Med.* 2023;24(9):957–964.

Kimani S, Painschab MS, Kaimila B, et al. Safety and efficacy of rituximab in patients with diffuse large B-cell lymphoma in Malawi: a prospective, single-arm, non-randomised phase 1/2 clinical trial. *Lancet Glob Health.* 2021;9(7):e1008–e1016. http://doi:10.1016/S2214-109X(21)00181-9

Lurain K, Ramaswami R, Mangusan R, et al. Use of pembrolizumab with or without pomalidomide in HIV-associated non-Hodgkin's lymphoma. *J Immunother Cancer.* 2021;9(2):e002097. http://doi: 10.1136/jitc-2020-002097. PMID: 33608378; PMCID: PMC7898875.

Rubinstein PG, Moore PC, Bimali M, et al. Brentuximab vedotin with AVD for stage II–IV HIV-related Hodgkin lymphoma (AMC 085): phase 2 results from an open-label, single arm, multicentre phase 1/2 trial. *Lancet Haematol.* 2023;10(8):e624–e632.

Rust B, Kiem HP, Uldrick T. CAR T-cell therapy for cancer and HIV through novel approaches to HIV-associated haematological malignancies. *Lancet Haematol.* 2020;7(9):e690–e696. http://doi:10.1016/S2352-3026(20)30142-3

Tan JY, Qiu TY, Chiang J, et al. Burkitt lymphoma: no impact of HIV status on outcomes with rituximab-based chemoimmunotherapy. *Leuk Lymphoma.* 2023;64(3):586–596.

Uldrick TS, Gonçalves PH, Abdul-Hay M, et al. Assessment of the safety of pembrolizumab in patients with HIV and advanced cancer: a phase 1 study. *JAMA Oncol.* 2019;5(9):1332–1339. http://doi:10.1001/jamaoncol.2019.2244

Wieland CL, Tuin AM, Dort EJ, et al. Long-term survival rates and treatment trends of Burkitt lymphoma in patients with HIV: a National Cancer Database (NCDB) study. *Cancers (Basel).* 2024;16(7):1397.

Zanet E, Taborelli M, Rupolo M, et al. Postautologous stem cell transplantation long-term outcomes in 26 PLWH affected by relapsed/refractory lymphoma. *AIDS.* 2015;29(17):2303–2308.

Zhao J, Min H, Huang Y, et al. Clinical characteristics and outcomes of newly diagnosed patients with human immunodeficiency virus-associated Burkitt lymphoma: the Central and Western China AIDS lymphoma league 002 study (CALL-002 study). *Infect Agent Cancer.* 2023;18(1):79.

ANOGENITAL NEOPLASIA

LEARNING OBJECTIVES

- Review the risk factors and epidemiology of anogenital neoplasias.
- Review the impact of anogenital neoplasias and squamous cell cancer of the anus (SCCA).
- Discuss treatment of anogenital neoplasias and SCCA, including the role of ART.

WHAT'S NEW?

- Molecular HPV testing is the cervical cancer screening modality recommended by the WHO.
- Women are recognized as a high-risk group for SCCA, and predisposing factors include positivity for high-risk human papilloma virus (HPV) serotypes. Some experts recommend screening all women with HIV ≥35 years old for HPV-related anal disease regardless of cervical cytology results.
- HPV vaccination in women with HIV (WWH) has demonstrated durable immunogenicity and safety.
- HPV vaccination for men with HIV beyond recommended ages may be beneficial and cost-effective in preventing invasive neoplasia.

KEY POINTS

- Screening with either cervical Papanicolaou (Pap) smear or high-risk HPV molecular testing in women is a key surveillance measure for detecting precancerous lesions. Screening with anal Pap smear in men and women with risk factors is also recommended, although uptake of this practice may be contingent on the availability of high-resolution anoscopy.
- HPV vaccination for PWH is safe and efficacious.

Anogenital neoplasia refers to anal and cervical carcinomas and their precursor lesions. One of the most important risk factors associated with anogenital neoplasia is HPV infection. HPV is a DNA virus that generally infects stratified squamous epithelium. More than 100 HPV serotypes have been identified to date, and at least 30 of these have a high predilection for the anogenital tract. HPV serotypes 6 and 11 have been associated with benign disease, whereas serotypes including 16, 18, 31, 33, 45, 52, and 58 are associated with high-grade cervical or anal squamous intraepithelial lesions (SILs) or cervical and anal carcinomas.

For PWH, HPV infection has a well-established relationship with the increased risk of developing anogenital neoplasia (Bjorge et al., 2002; Palefsky et al., 1991). Invasive and in situ forms of not only cervical and anal cancer but also vulvar/vaginal and penile cancers are reported among PWH (Frisch et al., 2000a; Frish and Goodman, 2000b; Smith et al., 2019).

PATHOGENESIS OF HPV IN HIV INFECTION

The increased prevalence of HPV disease associated with HIV infection may be mediated by impaired T-cell and antigen-presenting cell function. However, local effects of HIV infection may also upregulate HPV replication and oncogenesis. The HPV viral oncogenes E6 and E7 can immortalize primary keratinocytes and transform cells in culture (Barbosa et al., 1989; Munger et al., 1989). In an animal model of estrogen-stimulated HPV-induced cervical cancer, expression of E7 alone resulted in precancers and cancer, whereas the expression of E6 and E7 together resulted in larger cancers (Riley et al., 2003). Although the exact mechanisms of HIV-related immunosuppression and HPV coinfection have not been determined, several in vitro studies have shown that the HIV Tat protein can drive replication of HPV-16 and HPV-18 through the overexpression of E7 and other genes in the early region (Tornesello et al., 1993; Vernone et al., 1993).

EPIDEMIOLOGY OF HIV-ASSOCIATED CERVICAL INTRAEPITHELIAL NEOPLASIA

The relationship between HIV infection and cervical intraepithelial neoplasia (CIN) has been shown in many studies. Mandelblatt and colleagues (1999) performed a meta-analysis of 15 cross-sectional studies published during 1986–1998 that evaluated the prevalence of cervical neoplasia, HPV infection, and HIV infection. They found that among women with HPV infection, WWH were significantly more likely to develop cervical neoplasia, and this effect was related to the degree of immunodeficiency. Several other studies have also shown that WWH are at higher risk for CIN, including that by Ahdieh and colleagues (2000), who found that 13% of WWH versus 2% of women without HIV had abnormal cytological findings. They also found that WWH had a much lower rate of HPV clearance and that, in a multivariate model, the increased rate of CIN among WWH was fully accounted for by HPV persistence (Ahdieh et al., 2000). A 2016 study from Kaiser found that WWH had 2-fold higher odds of cervical intraepithelial neoplasia grade 2^+ ($CIN2^+$) and $CIN3^+$, but this was only in women with a recent $CD4^+$ T-cell count of less than 500 cells/mm^3 (Silverberg et al., 2016).

EPIDEMIOLOGY OF HIV-ASSOCIATED CERVICAL CARCINOMA

Since 1993, invasive cervical cancer has been listed by the CDC as an "AIDS-defining" condition. Globally, the risk of cervical cancer is higher in WWH (RR 6.07, 95% CI: 4.40–8.37) (Stelzle, 2021). In the United States, where the incidence of cervical cancer in general is relatively low, the incidence in WWH is 66% higher than in women without HIV (Brickman et al., 2015). However, in some areas of Africa, cervical cancer incidence is much higher, nearly 168 per 100,000 women (Lince-Deroche, 2015). A recent systemic review and meta-analysis found that 63.8% (95% CI: 58.9–68.1) of women in southern Africa and 27.4% (95% CI: 23.7–31.7) of women in eastern Africa with cervical cancer were living with HIV (Stelzle et al., 2021). The same study demonstrated age-standardized incidence rates of HIV-attributable cervical cancer to be >20 per 100,000 in six countries, all in southern or eastern Africa. These data were supported by the South African HIV Cancer Match Study, which found that the most common cancer in WWH was cervical cancer (Ruffieux et al. 2023). Cervical cancer incidence and mortality remain higher in WWH than in women without HIV, especially in resource-limited settings (Rohner, 2020).

Quantifying the contribution of HIV infection to cervical cancer development among WWH was challenging in the pre-ART era. A 1996 study that evaluated the relationship between HIV and cervical cancer found no conclusive evidence that HIV per se increased the risk of cervical cancer among WWH (International Agency for Research on Cancer, 1996). In LMICs with access to ART, several studies have shown an increased risk of cervical cancer. Using a national AIDS–cancer linked registry database of cases through 1998, researchers found a RR of 5.4 for invasive cervical cancer among WWH compared to the general population (Frisch et al., 2001). In a study of the Global Burden of Disease dataset of 1990–2019, in 2019, the greatest burden of cervical cancer occurred in eastern and southern Africa, with an age standardized rate of 254.44 per 100,000 population (95% CI: 168.86–329.28) (Wan et al., 2023).

Unfortunately, widespread utilization of ART has not been consistently associated with a decreased incidence of AIDS-related cervical cancer. Researchers showed an increasing proportion of cervical cancers in persons with AIDS from 0.11% in 1980–1989 (95% CI: 0.08–0.13) to 0.69% in 2001–2007 (95% CI: 0.49–0.89) (Shiels et al., 2011a). Even in the post-ART era, WWH and cervical cancer seem to have worse outcomes. For instance, a Nigerian study of 239 women with cervical cancer, including 47 WWH, demonstrated that WWH and cervical cancer were younger (median age 46 versus 57 years), were diagnosed at more advanced stages, and had significantly worse overall survival (12-month overall survival of 67.6% versus 84.1%) (Musa et al., 2023).

EFFECT OF ART ON HIV-ASSOCIATED CERVICAL DYSPLASIA

Although ART has significantly improved the survival of PWH through immune reconstitution and has decreased the incidence of opportunistic infections, the effects of ART on HPV infection and CIN among WWH remain unclear. Whereas three older studies did not find a significant reduction in risk of cervical dysplasia among women on ART (Lillo et al., 2001; Moore et al., 2002; Orlando et al., 1999), a more recent prospective study did find a reduction in cervical dysplasia risk related to ART (Minkoff et al., 2010).

In the United States, a large retrospective analysis performed by the Women's Interagency HIV Study (WIHS) group found that, among 741 WWH, those on ART were 40% (95% CI: 4–81) more likely to exhibit a regression of cervical lesions and were also significantly less likely to have progression of CIN (odds ratio [OR] 0.68) (Minkoff et al., 2001). The same group prospectively evaluated 286 WWH who initiated ART (Minkoff et al., 2010). They were assessed semiannually for HPV infection (by PCR) and SILs. Combination ART initiation among adherent women was associated with a significant reduction in HPV prevalence, incident detection of oncogenic HPV infection, and decreased prevalence and more rapid clearance of oncogenic HPV-positive SILs (Minkoff et al., 2010). More recently, a large systematic review involving studies from resource-limited settings evaluated WWH with high-grade cervical lesions (high-grade squamous intraepithelial lesions [HSIL]-CIN2\+) and found that WWH on ART had lower prevalence of high-risk HPV compared to women not on ART (Kelly et al., 2018). ART was also associated with a decreased risk of HSIL-CIN2+ incidence, SIL progression, and increased likelihood of SIL or CIN regression. Further, three of the included studies indicated that ART was associated with a reduction in invasive cervical cancer incidence. Collectively, the data suggest that treating HIV infection with ART has a beneficial effect on progression of HPV-related cervical disease, but there has not been a substantial decrease in cervical cancer incidence, and both incidence and mortality among WWH remain unacceptably high in LMICs (Greene et al., 2019).

SCREENING, TREATMENT, AND PREVENTION OF HIV-ASSOCIATED CERVICAL DYSPLASIA

Screening

World Health Organization guidelines (WHO) favor cervical cancer screening strategies utilizing molecular HPV tests (Hall et al., 2023). They state that: women should be screened for cervical cancer every 5–10 years starting at age 30. Women living with HIV should be screened every 3 years starting at age 25. The global strategy encourages a minimum of two lifetime screens with a high-performance HPV test by age 35 and again by age 45 years. Globally, cervical cancer screening utilizing molecular HPV screening for WWH has scaled up dramatically since 2020 (Kalamya et al., 2024; WHO, 2024).

Current U.S. Public Health Service and Infectious Diseases Society of America guidelines recommend that WWH undergo a complete history and a physical examination that includes a pelvic exam and cervical Pap test at the time of initial evaluation. Screening for WWH should commence within 1 year of the onset of sexual activity regardless of mode of HIV transmission (e.g., sexual activity or perinatal exposure) but no later than age 21 years. Young women (i.e., those aged 21–29 years) should have only a Pap test at the time of initial diagnosis with HIV. Co-testing (Pap test and high-risk HPV molecular test) is not recommended for women with HIV younger than 30 years. If the initial Pap test for young (or newly diagnosed) WWH is normal, the next one should be performed in 12 months (although some experts still recommend a repeat Pap test at 6 months after baseline testing). If results of three consecutive Pap tests are normal, follow-up Pap tests can be done every 3 years. For women aged 30 years or older, either Pap testing alone or co-testing with both Pap and HPV are acceptable screening strategies. For women who undergo Pap testing alone, the protocol is identical to that described for women younger than 30. For women who undergo co-testing, Pap and HPV testing should be done at the time of HIV diagnosis (or starting at age 30 years). If the Pap is normal and the HPV screening test is negative, repeat screening can be done in 3 years. Women who have a normal Pap test but are positive for high-risk HPV should have repeat co-testing in 1 year (unless genotype testing for 16 or 16/18 is positive, in which case the patient should be referred for colposcopy). If either of the co-tests at 1 year is abnormal (i.e., abnormal cytology or positive HPV), referral to colposcopy is recommended. Any WWH with an abnormal Pap smear that shows atypical squamous cell of undetermined significance (ASCUS) or higher-grade lesions should undergo colposcopy. Cervical cancer screening in WWH should continue throughout their lifetime and not end at age 65 years, as in the general population.

Treatment

Treatment options for CIN are similar for women with and without HIV and include cryotherapy, loop electrosurgical excision procedure (LEEP), and cold knife conization (Santesso et al., 2016). These options are generally safe and effective. Cryotherapy is an especially important option for women living in resource-limited settings. A recent South African study evaluated 220 WWH who were randomly assigned to cryotherapy or no treatment (Firnhaber et al., 2017). Among participants, 94% were receiving ART (median $CD4^+$ T-cell count was 499 cells/mm^3) and 59% were high-risk HPV-positive. Cryotherapy reduced progression to HSIL, with 2 of 99 (2%) progressing in the cryotherapy group vs. 15 of 103 (15%) in the no-treatment group, translating to an 86% reduction (95% CI: 41–97; $p = 0.002$). Participants in the cryotherapy arm experienced greater regression to normal histology and improved cytologic outcomes.

Of note, endocervical extension is more frequent among WWH (Foulot et al., 2008). Therefore, LEEP is thought to be less effective and recurrence rates are higher in WWH than in women without HIV, although another recent South African study found that rates of cumulative $CIN2^+$ were lower after LEEP than cryotherapy treatment at 6 months (Smith et al., 2017). Importantly, in this study, both treatments appeared effective in reducing $CIN2^+$ by more than 70% at 12 months. Most recently, a randomized trial conducted in Kenya demonstrated that 60 (30%) of WWH randomized to cryotherapy had recurrent CIN grade 2 or higher compared to 37 (19%) in the LEEP group (relative risk [RR], 1.71 [95% CI: 1.12–2.65]; risk difference, 7.9% [95% CI: 1.9%–14.0%]; $p = .01$).

Invasive cervical cancer diagnosed in WWH is treated using the same criteria and protocols as those for women without HIV if no other contraindications for treatment exist (Reid et al., 2018). Limited data exist on the treatment of cervical cancer in WWH (Ntekim et al., 2015). One prospective cohort of 348 patients with cervical cancer in Botswana compared outcomes between women with and without HIV (Dryden-Peterson et al., 2016). The WWH group had a median $CD4^+$ T-cell count of 397 cells/mm^3, and HIV infection was significantly associated with an increased risk of death among all women (HR 1.95; 95% CI: 1.20–3.17) as well as among the subset of women who received guideline-concordant curative therapy (HR 2.63; 95% CI: 1.05–6.55). These results suggest that HIV infection has an adverse effect on cervical cancer survival. The effect was greater for women with a lower $CD4^+$ T-cell count, suggesting that immune suppression plays a significant role. It is unknown whether findings of this study may be extrapolated to resource-rich environments, as survival of both women with and without HIV and cervical cancer was lower in this study than would be expected in many resource-rich countries. A prospective cohort study of 1,131 Botswanan women with stage IB–IVB cervical cancer, including 789 WWH, found that HIV status was not significantly associated with overall survival for patients receiving curative chemoradiation, but was associated with overall survival for patients receiving definitive radiation alone (in the unadjusted analysis only) (Meghani et al., 2024).

Regarding newer therapies, a phase 3 trial that includes WWH in South Africa indicates that standard chemoradiotherapy with modulated electrohyperthermia (a noninvasive intervention using 13.56 MHz radiofrequency treatment) is effective for disease control of locally advanced cervical cancer and 6-month local disease-free survival (Minaar et al., 2019).

Primary Prevention

Currently there are three U.S. Food and Drug Administration (FDA)–approved HPV vaccines: bivalent, quadrivalent, and nine-valent. All three prevent HPV-16 and HPV-18 infections and prevent precancers (and likely cancers) caused by HPV-16 and HPV-18. In addition, the quadrivalent and nine-valent HPV vaccines prevent HPV-6 and HPV-11 infections and genital warts attributed to these types. The nine-valent vaccine also prevents infection and precancers attributed to five additional types (31, 33, 45, 52, and 58). The WHO supports a two-dose schedule (two doses 6–12 months apart) for girls and women with HIV aged 9–20 years, and two doses 6 months apart for WWH older than 21 years; they stress vaccinating PWH as a priority population (WHO, 2022). The CDC continues to recommend the three-dose schedule (at 0, 1–2, and 6 months) for PWH 9–26 years old. Although the CDC has not yet released recommendations for older individuals, the FDA has approved the HPV vaccine for individuals aged up to 45 years old; older individuals should also receive the three-dose series (0, 1–2, and 6 months) (CDC, 2021). Data are emerging supporting the immunogenicity of an alternative two-dose, nine-valent HPV vaccine strategy for PWH (McClymont, 2023; Rungmaitree et al., 2022; WHO, 2022). Additionally, starting ART early likely reduces the risk of high-risk HPV infection and cervical cancer.

EPIDEMIOLOGY OF HIV-ASSOCIATED ANAL INTRAEPITHELIAL NEOPLASIA

Unlike cervical HPV infection, which peaks in the third decade in women, anal HPV infection is highly prevalent throughout adult life among MSM well into the sixth decade (Chin-Hong et al., 2004; Schiffman and Kjaer, 2003). HPV-16 is the most common type of high-risk HPV among people with or without HIV (Lin and Chen, 2018). In one meta-analysis of 31 studies, the pooled prevalence of anal HPV detected by PCR was 89% versus 53.6% in men with and without HIV ($p = 0.047$) (Machalek et al., 2012). In addition, the prevalence of HPV-16 and HPV-18, associated with high-grade neoplasia and malignancy, was also significantly higher in men with HIV.

Several studies report increasing prevalence of anal intraepithelial neoplasia (AIN) among men and women with HIV (Hessol et al., 2013; Islami et al., 2017; Palefsky, 2017). A population-based cancer-HIV registry linkage study between 1996 and 2019 found average annual increases in AIN grade III of 15% per year for women and 12% per year for men with HIV (compared to 8% for women and men without HIV) (Haas et al., 2024). The five-year cumulative incidence of anal cancer post-AIN III for PWH with a prior AIDS diagnosis was greater than 3%. A multicenter trial reported a 27% prevalence of anal HSIL among women with HIV (Stier et al., 2020). A study in which 114 WWH without anal HSIL were followed for 2 years found that positive anal high-risk HPV testing or abnormal anal cytology was associated with an increased risk of anal HSIL and that the presence of anal high-risk HPV with abnormal cytology was associated with a 2-year cumulative risk of anal HSIL of 65.6% (Stier et al., 2024). Palefsky and colleagues (2001) found that the RR of developing HSIL was 3.7 for MSM with HIV compared to MSM without HIV. Several studies indicate that between 41% and 97% of men with HIV have anal dysplasia on anal Pap smear screening (Kiviat et al., 2002; Palefsky et al., 2001; Piketty et al.,2008). A study of 93 PWH (mostly MSM) in an acute HIV cohort found that the baseline prevalence of anal HSIL was 19.7 per 100 person-years (py) and that risk factors for anal HSIL were anal HPV 16 (adjusted hazards ratio [aHR] 4.33; 95% CI: 1.03–18.18), anal HPV 18/45 (aHR 6.82; 95% CI: 1.57–29.51), other anal high-risk HPV (aHR 4.23; 95% CI: 1.27–14.14), syphilis infection (aHR 4.67; 95% CI: 1.10–19.90) and CD4 count <350 cells/mm^3 (aHR 3.09; 95% CI 1.28–7.48) (Thitipatarakorn et al., 2024).

EPIDEMIOLOGY OF HIV-ASSOCIATED SQUAMOUS CELL CANCER OF THE ANUS

HIV seropositivity is associated with an increased incidence of anal cancer in both men (HR 20.73; 95% CI: 15.60–27.56) and women (HR 12.88; 95% CI: 8.69–19.07) (Michaud et al., 2020). Even before the HIV epidemic, anal cancer incidence among MSM was estimated to be as high as approximately 35 cases per 100,000 py. This rate is comparable to the incidence of cervical cancer in the United States before the advent of routine cervical cytology (Daling et al., 1987; Melbye et al., 1994). In the 1960s, the annual incidence of SCCA among men in the United States was relatively low and stable, with approximately 0.5 cases per 100,000 persons. Since then, studies have shown a steady increase. A U.S. population-based analysis of the SEER program data found that the incidence of SCCA in the United States among men increased from 1.06 per 100,000 persons during 1973–1979 to 2.04 per 100,000 persons during 1996–2004 (Johnson et al., 2004).

Many studies have shown that the incidence of SCCA is higher in PWH. In a meta-analysis, researchers examined nine studies published before November 2011 reporting anal cancer incidence in MSM (Machalek et al., 2012). The incidence of anal cancer was significantly higher in men with than without HIV ($p = 0.011$). This result has been mirrored in several studies in the United States and Europe, which show that the incidence of anal cancer among PWH ranges from 42 to 137 cases per 100,000 py, a rate 30–100 times higher than that of the general population (D'Souza et al., 2008; Patel et al., 2008; Piketty et al., 2008). Anal cancer incidence may be higher in Black MSM with HIV; one multicenter study found a weighted HR of 2.37 (95% CI: 1.17–4.82) compared to non-Black MSM (McNeil et al., 2022).

SCCA may be overlooked in the female population; however, the rate of HPV-related anal cancers among women appears to be higher than that in men (1.8 vs. 1.2 per 100,000 persons) (CDC, 2012). Other publications have found incidence rates as high as 18–30 per 100,000 persons (Piketty et al., 2012; Silverberg et al., 2012). Incidence of anal cancer in WWH in higher income countries is also high (3.9–30 per 100,000 persons) (Stier et al., 2015). Women with CD4$^+$ T-cell counts of less than 200 cells/mm^3 have a nearly 15-fold higher risk of developing invasive SCCA compared to the general population (SIR 14.5; 95% CI: 8.8–22.4) (Chaturvedi et al., 2009). Like the effects of HPV on cervical endothelium, the virus can lead to high-grade precancerous lesions and anal cancer. A systematic review of SCCA in women revealed higher prevalence of HPV in the anus versus cervix in most studies reviewed (16%–85% vs. 17%–70%, respectively), and that concordant HPV genotypes were found in 9%–16% of women. Risk factors for anal HPV included cervical HPV, low CD4$^+$ T-cell count, smoking, and perianal warts (Stier et al., 2015).

Machalek and colleagues found that the incidence of anal cancer was higher in the ART era: from 1996 onward, the annual incidence of SCCA was 78 per 100,000 persons compared to 22 per 100,000 persons prior to this time (Machalek et al., 2012). The reason for this increase is unclear, although improved survival associated with ART may have allowed sufficient time for men with chronic HPV infection to develop anal cancer. More recently, a study using the North American AIDS Cohort Collaboration on Research and Design during 2001–2016 found that age standardized anal cancer incidence declined by 2.2% per year (95% CI: −4.4–0.1%) in the United States but remained stable in Canada (Deshmukh et al., 2024). The same study found that anal cancer risk was inversely proportional to CD4$^+$ count, supporting prior studies indicating that risk factors associated with SCCA are associated with greater immunosuppression, including nadir CD4⁺ T-cell count and HIV RNA levels greater than 500,000 copies/mL (Guiguet et al., 2009). A recent meta-analysis of evidence published over the last two decades indicates that, although PWH have higher anal cancer-related mortality than people without HIV, the overall survival and anal cancer–specific survival HRs were not significantly different between the two groups (Sumner et al., 2022). In contrast, a retrospective cohort study using data from the HIV/AIDS Cancer Match Study over a similar time period found that HIV was associated with an increase in all-cause mortality in both men (1.35 times; 95% CI: 1.24–1.47) and women (2.47 times; 95% CI: 2.10–2.90) (Shing et al., 2024). Groups with worse all-cause mortality included non-Hispanic Black PWH and those with CD4 <200 cells/mm^3.

SCREENING, TREATMENT, AND PREVENTION OF HIV-ASSOCIATED ANAL DYSPLASIA

As discussed previously, PWH are at an increased risk for SCCA and AIN. SCCA shares many biologic similarities with cervical cancer, including detectable dysplastic precursor lesions and high-risk HPV infection. In women, abnormal cervical cytology results are a risk factor for abnormal anal cytology results, although women may have anal dysplasia without concomitant cervical disease. Some studies show a higher prevalence of HPV-related anal disease than HPV-related cervical disease in women (Gaisa et al., 2017; Kojic et al., 2011; Liu et al., 2020). Consequently, many have recommended annual anal Pap screening for PWH (Bosch et al., 1995).

The New York State Department of Health AIDS Institute published anal dysplasia and cancer screening guidelines in 2022, recommending annual screening for all PWH ≥35 years old for HPV-related anal disease (Hirsch et al., 2022). The European AIDS Clinical Society (EACS) guidelines recommend digital rectal exam (DRE) with or without an anal Pap smear every 1–3 years in MSM (EACS, 2023). The International Anal Neoplasia Society (IANS) recommends starting screening at age 35 years for MSM and transgender women with HIV using anal cytology, high-risk HPV testing, or high-risk HPV-cytology co-testing (Stier et al., 2024). In July 2024, the U.S. Department of Health and Human Services released new guidance for anal cancer screening among PWH, recommending that all adults with HIV be assessed at least once yearly for anal abnormalities and undergo digital anorectal examination (DARE). If HRA is available, MSM and transgender women with HIV ≥35 years, and all PWH ≥45 years, should undergo additional lab-based screening (i.e., anal cytology with or without HPV co-testing) (US DHHS, 2024b). Unfortunately, rates of anal cancer screening via cytology remain low (Rim et al., 2024). Further, despite evolving guidelines (especially across resource-rich settings), there is a lack of consensus and rigorous evidence regarding recommendations for performing annual DARE in patients at risk for SCCA. A phase 2 clinical trial assessed the feasibility of teaching MSM to recognize palpable masses in the anal canal using self or partner exams (Nyitray et al., 2018). Results indicated that tumors 3 mm or larger may be detectable by self or partner exams, which is significant as there is a high cure rate for tumors 10 mm or smaller.

Anal Pap smears have a similar sensitivity and specificity as cervical Pap smears, and can be performed by randomly obtaining squamous cells from the anal canal using a Dacron swab. They are then fixed in liquid cytology media. Like cervical cytology protocols, abnormal anal cytologic findings are confirmed by high-resolution anoscopy-directed biopsy of visualized lesions (Figure 25.1). Screening via HPV molecular testing remains controversial because of the high prevalence of high-risk HPV infection in PWH (Benevolo et al., 2016; Berry et al., 2009). However, presence of high-risk HPV genotype 16 is associated with concurrent high-grade anal lesions in WWH (Heard et al., 2015, 2016). One study in which high-resolution anoscopy was performed on 156 PWH who tested negative for high-risk HPV by anal

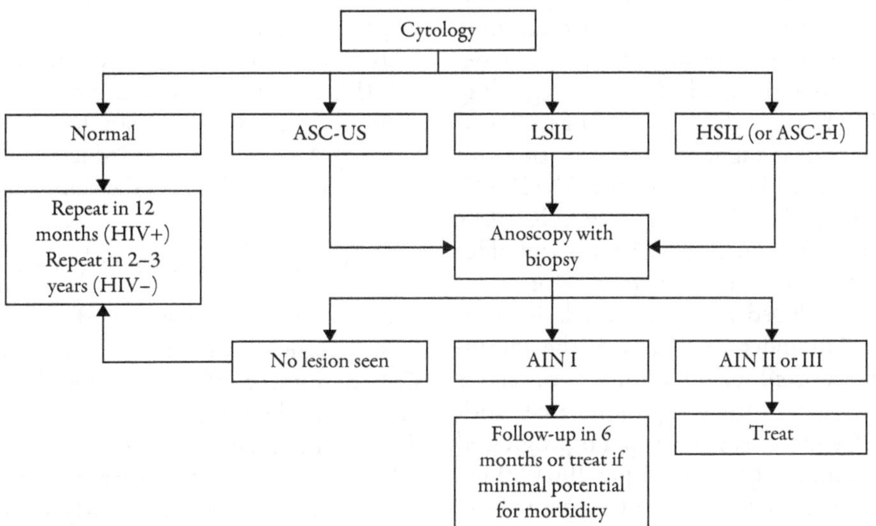

Figure 25.1 Screening protocol for anal intraepithelial neoplasia (AIN). SOURCE: From Park IU, et al. *Curr Infect Dis Rep.* 2010 March;12(2):126–133.

swab found that an approximately 8% risk of anal precancer remains for PWH who test high-risk HPV negative by swab (Wang et al., 2020). Anal cytology is categorized according to the Bethesda system for cervical cytology: ASCUS, low-grade squamous intraepithelial lesion, and HSIL. The New York State Health Department AIDS Institute recommends HPV testing only for PWH with anal cytology results of ASCUS (Hirsch et al., 2022); if HPV testing is negative, then anal cytology should be repeated in 1 year, and if HPV testing is positive for high-risk HPV, then the patient should be referred for high-resolution anoscopy. The new DHHS recommendations for PWH delineate different pathways to follow based on whether high-risk HPV co-testing was performed with initial cytology (DHHS, 2024b).

Note that there are no definitive clinical studies showing that anal Pap smears decrease SCCA-related morbidity and mortality among PWH, though studies evaluating this and related questions, such as the Anal Cancer/HSIL Outcomes Research (ANCHOR) study, have been underway (Lee et al., 2022). Further, anal cytology should not be performed if evaluation with high-resolution anoscopy is not available. Women with a history of cervical or vulvar neoplasias are more likely to have anal HPV infection and abnormal anal cytology (Stier et al., 2015). The presence of anal warts or condyloma acuminata may also be an indicator for HPV infection of the anal canal and may warrant further screening. High-risk patients should be followed every 6 months for at least 5 years, ideally with periodic photographic documentation of the perianal region. There should be a low threshold to repeat biopsies of any changing lesion. Per the New York State Health Department AIDS Institute recommendations, anal cancer screening may be stopped for PWH with life expectancy less than 10 years and for non–sexually active PWH with two consecutive negative anal cytology specimens (Hirsch et al., 2022).

Treatment

The surveillance of patients with AIN II and III is predominantly aimed at the identification of early invasive carcinoma that can be treated by local excision or localized chemo-/immune-therapy and/or radiation. Little data exist regarding the management of AIN, but it is thought that, like CIN, if AIN can be eradicated, then malignant transformation can be prevented. This is supported by results of the ANCHOR study (Palefsky et al., 2022) (NCT02135419). The ANCHOR study assigned more than 4,000 men aged 35 years and older with HIV and biopsy-proven anal HSIL to receive either HSIL treatment (which included office-based ablative procedures, ablation or excision under anesthesia, or the administration of topical fluorouracil or imiquimod) or active monitoring without treatment. This study found that, with a median follow-up of 25.8 months, 9 participants progressed to anal cancer in the treatment group (173 per 100,000 py; 95% CI: 90–332) and 21 in the active-monitoring group (402 per 100,000 py; 95% CI: 262–616). Targeted biopsies using high-resolution anoscopy and 3% acetic acid to the anal canal mucosa (like colposcopy) can help identify areas of AIN.

Treatment options for anal dysplasia are similar for people with and without HIV. These include topical trichloroacetic acid, liquid nitrogen, imiquimod, fluorouracil, infrared coagulation, electrocautery, carbon dioxide (CO_2) laser, and surgical excision. One randomized trial of 156 MSM with HIV showed that electrocautery is better than imiquimod and fluorouracil in the treatment of AIN but recognized that recurrence rates were substantial (Richel et al., 2013). Of note, several new therapies are being evaluated for PWH with anal dysplasia. These include two Australian studies: a phase 2 trial evaluating the immunomodulator pomalidomide in anal HSIL (NCT03113942) and a phase 1 study evaluating a new topical drug with direct anti-HPV activity, ABI-1968 (NCT03202992).

The recommended treatment for PWH with anal cancer is the same as that recommended for the general population (Reid et al., 2018). In the general population, concurrent chemoradiotherapy with 5-fluorouracil (5-FU) infusion and mitomycin (or cisplatin) has been established as the standard-of-care regimen for nonmetastatic anal cancer (Leiker et al., 2020). In the ART era, reports on clinical outcomes of PWH with anal cancer have been conflicting. Some studies have shown that people with and without HIV had comparable disease control and survival (Blazy et al., 2005; Chiao et al., 2008; Fraunholz et al., 2011), whereas others have suggested that PWH (particularly those with increased time between anal cancer diagnosis and treatment and those with lower post-treatment $CD4^+$ T-cell counts) may do worse in terms of treatment-related toxicity and/or an increased risk for local relapse (Grew et al., 2015; Oehler-Janne, 2008; Susko et al., 2020). Existing evidence is limited by mostly retrospective data as well as small numbers of patients studied; thus further investigation into this question is needed.

Prevention

Routine vaccination with quadrivalent HPV or the nine-valent HPV vaccine is now available for all individuals aged 9–45 years to prevent genital warts and the development of precancerous and cancerous HPV-mediated lesions. The CDC's Advisory Committee on Immunization Practices (ACIP), however, still does not recommend routine vaccination of persons older than 26 years (Murthy et al., 2022). Starting ART early likely reduces the risk of high-risk HPV infection and anal cancer development (Kelly et al., 2020).

EFFECT OF ART ON ANAL DYSPLASIA

Like studies evaluating the effect of ART on cervical dysplasia, studies evaluating the effect of ART on anal dysplasia have found conflicting results. This may be related to the significant design and methodological differences among these studies. Two small case series described outcomes of HIV-associated SCCA, with 5-year survival rates of 47%–60% (Jephcott et al., 2004; Myerson et al., 2001). In studies that specifically compared survival among patients with SCCA in the pre-ART versus ART eras, there was a nonsignificant trend toward improved survival, better tolerability of chemoradiotherapy, and improved local tumor control in the ART era (Bower et al., 2004b; Cleator et al., 2000; Stadler et al., 2004).

Palefsky and colleagues (2001) compared the rates of progression and regression of anal dysplasia after 6 months of ART. They found that the overall likelihood of lesion progression or regression was not affected by ART initiation. However, among individuals starting ART at higher $CD4^+$ T-cell counts, ART demonstrated a nonsignificant benefit on anal dysplasia lesions. In contrast, Wilkin and colleagues (2004) conducted a cross-sectional study evaluating anal HPV infection and anal dysplasia in 98 men with HIV. In multivariate analyses, they found that ART and higher nadir $CD4^+$ T-cell count were significantly protective for anal dysplasia by histology but were not protective of anal HPV infection. A Canadian study retrospectively evaluated 1,691 MSM with HIV and found that immunosuppression with nadir $CD4^+$ T-cell count of less than 100 cells/mm^3 was a risk factor for anal cancer (OR 3.08; $p = 0.01$). They also found that men treated during the pre-ART era had a higher incidence (370 vs. 93 per 100,000 py) and shorter lead time to development of anal cancer compared to those in the post-ART era (Duncan et al., 2015). Therefore, although it is unclear if ART initiation influences the natural history of AIN in PWH, ART is beneficial for men undergoing treatment for HPV-related disease.

RECOMMENDED READING

Brandão M, Bruzzone M, Franzoi MA, et al. Impact of HIV infection on baseline characteristics and survival of women with breast cancer. *AIDS*. 2021;35(4):605–618. http://doi:10.1097/QAD.0000000000002810. PMID: 33394680.

Deshmukh AA, Lun YY, Damgacioglu H, et al. Recent and projected incidence trends and risk of anal cancer among people with HIV in North America. *J Natl Cancer Inst*. 2024;116(9):1450–1458. doi:10.1093/jnci/djae096

Greene SA, De Vuyst H, John-Stewart GC, et al. Effect of cryotherapy vs loop electrosurgical excision procedure on cervical disease recurrence among women with HIV and high-grade cervical lesions in Kenya: a randomized clinical trial. *JAMA*. 2019;322(16):1570–1579.

Haas CB, Engels EA, Palefsky JM, et al. Severe anal intraepithelial neoplasia trends and subsequent invasive anal cancer in the United States. *J Natl Cancer Inst*. 2024;116(1):97–104.

Hall MT, Simms KT, Murray JM, et al. Benefits and harms of cervical screening, triage and treatment strategies in women living with HIV. *Nat Med*. 2023;29(12):3059–3066.

Hirsch BE, McGowan JP, Fine SM, et al. *Screening for anal dysplasia and cancer in adults with HIV*. Baltimore, MD: Johns Hopkins University Press; 2022. PMID: 32369310.

Kojic EM, Kang M, Cespedes MS, et al. Immunogenicity and safety of the quadrivalent human papillomavirus vaccine in HIV-1-infected women. *Clin Infect Dis*. 2014;59(1):127–135.

Lee JY, Lensing SY, Berry-Lawhorn JM, et al. Design of the Anal Cancer/HSIL Outcomes Research study (ANCHOR study): a randomized study to prevent anal cancer among persons living with HIV. *Contemp Clin Trials*. 2022 Feb;113:106679. http://doi:10.1016/j.cct.2022.106679

Leiker AJ, Wang CJ, Sanford NN, et al. Feasibility and outcome of routine use of concurrent chemoradiation in PLWH with squamous cell anal cancer. *Am J Clin Oncol*. 2020;43(10):701–708. http://doi:10.1097/COC.0000000000000736

McClymont E, Money D. The shift to one-dose HPV vaccination: where does this leave women living with HIV? *Int J Gynaecol Obstet*. 2023;162(1):4–5.

McNeil CJ, Lee JS, Cole SR, et al. Anal cancer incidence in men with HIV who have sex with men: are Black men at higher risk? *AIDS*. 2022 Apr 1;36(5):657–664. http://doi:10.1097/QAD.0000000000003151

Meghani K, Puri P, Bazzett-Matabele L, et al. Significance of HIV status in cervical cancer patients receiving curative chemoradiation therapy, definitive radiation alone, or palliative radiation in Botswana. *Cancer*. 2024;130(14):2462–2471. doi:10.1002/cncr.35289.

Musa J, Kocherginsky M, Magaji FA, et al. Epidemiology and survival outcomes of HIV-associated cervical cancer in Nigeria. *Infect Agent Cancer*. 2023;18(1):68.

Palefsky JM, Lee JY, Jay N, et al. Treatment of anal high-grade squamous intraepithelial lesions to prevent anal cancer. *N Engl J Med*. 2022 Jun 16;386(24):2273–2282. http://doi:10.1056/NEJMoa2201048

Piketty C, Selinger-Leneman H, Grabar S, et al. Marked increase in the incidence of invasive anal cancer among HIV-infected patients despite treatment with combination antiretroviral therapy. *AIDS (London)*. 2008;22(10):1203–1211.

Rim SH, Beer L, Saraiya M, et al. Prevalence of anal cytology screening among persons with HIV and lack of access to high-resolution anoscopy at HIV care facilities. *J Natl Cancer Inst*. 2024; 116(8):1319–1332. doi:10.1093/jnci/djae094ae094.

Rohner E, Bütikofer L, Schmidlin K, et al. Cervical cancer risk in women living with HIV across four continents: a multicohort study. *Int J Cancer*. 2020;146(3):601–609. http://doi:10.1002/ijc.32260

Ruffieux Y, muchengeti M, Olago V, et al. Age and cancer incidence in 5.2 million people with human immunodeficiency virus (HIV): the South African HIV Cancer Match Study. *Clin Infect Dis*. 2023;76(8):1440–1448.

Rungmaitree S, Thepthai C, Toh ZQ, et al. Immunogenicity of a two-dose human papillomavirus vaccine schedule in HIV-infected adolescents with immune reconstitution. *Vaccines (Basel)*. 2022;10(1):118.

Shing JZ, Engels EA, Austin AA, et al. Survival by sex and HIV status in patients with anal cancer in the USA between 2001 and 2019: a retrospective cohort study. *Lancet HIV*. 2024;11(1):e31–e41.

Smith AJB, Varma S, Rositch AF, et al. Gynecologic cancer in HIV-positive women: a systematic review and meta-analysis. *Am J Obstet Gynecol*. 2019;221(3):194–207. http://doi:10.1016/j.ajog.2019.02.022

Stelzle D, Tanaka LF, Lee KK, et al. Estimates of the global burden of cervical cancer associated with HIV. *Lancet Glob Health*. 2021;9(2):e161–e169. http://doi:10.1016/S2214-109X(20)30459-9

Stier EA, Clarke MA, Deshmukh AA, et al. International Anal Neoplasia Society's consensus guidelines for anal cancer screening. *Int J Cancer*. 2024;154(10):1694–1702.

Stier EA, Jain M, Joshi H, et al. Two-year incidence and cumulative risk and predictors of anal high-grade squamous intraepithelial lesions (anal precancer) among women with human immunodeficiency virus. *Clin Infect Dis*. 2024;78(3):681–689.

Stier EA, Sebring MC, Mendez AE, et al. Prevalence of anal human papillomavirus infection and anal HPV-related disorders in women: a systematic review. *Am J Ob Gyn*. 2015;213(3):278–309.

Sumner L, Kamitani E, Chase S, Wang Y. A systematic review and meta-analysis of mortality in anal cancer patients by HIV status. *Cancer Epidemiol*. 2022;76:102069. http://doi:10.1016/j.canep.2021.102069

Thitipatarakorn S, Teeratakulpisarn N, Nonenoy S, et al. Prevalence and incidence of anal high-grade squamous intraepithelial lesions in a cohort of cisgender men and transgender women who have sex with men diagnosed and treated during acute HIV acquisition in Bangkok, Thailand. *J Int AIDS Soc*. 2024;27(5):e26242.

Wan Z, Zhao J, Xu L, et al. Global and regional estimates of cervical cancer burden associated with human immunodeficiency virus infection from 1990 to 2019. *J Med Virol*. 2023;95(6):e28891.

LUNG CANCER

LEARNING OBJECTIVES

- Review the epidemiology and risks of lung cancer in PWH.
- Review the pathogenesis of lung cancer.
- Discuss the treatment of lung cancer.
- Discuss the treatment outcomes and mortality associated with lung cancer in PWH.

WHAT'S NEW?

- Lung cancer incidence in PWH has increased during the ART era.
- Surgery, chemotherapy, and radiation are mainstays of standard treatment for PWH.
- Treatment disparities between people with and without HIV may contribute to poor survival of those with lung cancer.

KEY POINTS

- Tobacco cessation is of utmost importance in preventing lung cancers in PWH.
- PWH have a higher incidence of lung cancer than the general population, although a predominant histology of non–small cell lung cancer (NSCLC) is common in both groups.
- PWH have worse survival, which may be due to frequent presentation with advanced disease.
- No specific guidelines for treating PWH and lung cancer exist, and more rigorous studies evaluating standards of care are needed.

Lung cancer is the leading cause of death attributed to cancer in the general U.S. population and is common in PWH as well (Frisch et al., 2001). Lung cancers in HIV are primarily NSCLC types, including adenocarcinoma and squamous cell carcinoma. This largely reflects the trend of histology types among the general population in Western settings (Cadranel et al., 2006). Mortality from lung cancer remains high in PWH compared to the general population, especially for patients presenting at advanced stages (Coghill et al., 2015; Shiels et al., 2010a).

The incidence of lung cancer has increased for several reasons, including increased life expectancy with contemporary ART and longer cumulative exposure to carcinogens known to be associated with lung cancer development, namely tobacco smoke. Notably, tobacco exposure in PWH remains a significant health problem, with disproportionate use compared to the general population (Altekruse et al., 2018; Clifford et al., 2012; Rahmanian et al., 2011). Because of this increased risk, smoking cessation is of utmost importance (Shepherd et al., 2018). Immunosuppression may also be a contributing factor; however, this relationship has not been clearly elucidated.

The U.S. Preventive Services Task Force (USPSTF) recommends screening for lung cancer using chest CT in individuals aged 50–80 years with a ≥20-pack-year smoking history. Optimal screening criteria for PWH are unknown, but healthcare providers should follow the general USPSTF recommendations while this is studied further (Sellers et al., 2022).

EPIDEMIOLOGY OF LUNG CANCER IN HIV

Data from large HIV and cancer registries in the United States estimated the incidence of lung cancer in PWH to be 59 per 100,000 py from 1991 to 2002 (Engels et al., 2008). This same study found that the incidence of lung cancer increased from 51 per 100,000 py to 126 per 100,000 py between people with HIV versus advanced HIV/AIDS (Engels et al., 2008). In another study including Canadian data, researchers found that, from 1996 to 2009, the incidence of lung cancer in PWH was 129 per 100,000 py compared to 45.4 per 100,000 py in people without HIV. The incidence of lung cancer was higher for persons aged 75 years than for those aged 65 years (3.4% vs. 2.2%), which supports the increased risk of cancer development attributable to aging (Silverberg et al., 2015). Researchers evaluated a Californian cohort between 1996 and 2011 and found that the lung cancer rate was 66 per 100,000 py for PWH and 33 per 100,000 py for people without HIV (rate ratio 2.0; 95% CI: 1.7–2.2) (Marcus et al., 2017). A Ugandan study evaluating overall cancer incidence in PWH from 1988 to 2002 found the incidence of lung cancer over time to be increased, with a SIR of 5 (Mbulaiteye et al., 2006). Another study using the Swiss HIV Cohort Study and Swiss Cancer Registries found that cancers of the trachea, lung, and bronchus were significantly elevated in PWH compared to the general population (SIR 3.2) (Clifford et al., 2005).

The impact of ART on the incidence and risk of lung cancer remains unclear. Studies attempting to evaluate the incidence of lung cancer during the pre-ART and ART eras have found mixed results, with increased incidence in both eras. The previously cited study by Silverberg and colleagues (2015) showed that cumulative incidence of lung cancer in North America continued to increase in the ART era, with a cumulative incidence of 3.7% from 2005 to 2009 compared to 1.8% from 1996 to 2009. Another study examining data from 34 states showed similar results, with a steady increase in the number of lung cancers (35 to 283 cases) from 1991 to 2005, which largely occurred in persons older than 50 years (Shiels et al., 2011a).

RISK FACTORS ASSOCIATED WITH LUNG CANCER IN HIV

Risk factors for lung cancer are multiple and include tobacco exposure, injection drug use, and possibly HIV infection itself. Other comorbid pulmonary diseases, such as chronic obstructive pulmonary disease and bacterial pneumonia, are more common in people with than without HIV and may place PWH at higher risk for cancer due to persistent states of inflammation (Crothers et al., 2011; Shebl et al., 2010). Inflammatory markers circulating in the blood have been associated with theoretical risk of lung cancer; these include C-reactive protein, serum amyloid, soluble tumor necrosis factor receptor-2 (sTNFR2), lymphoid differentiation cytokine interleukin-7 (IL-7), and various leukocyte-derived chemokines (Shiels, 2013). However, it remains to be determined exactly how these inflammatory states that are not confounded by smoking or other traditional risk factors like pneumonia impact the risk of lung cancer.

Cigarette smoking has repeatedly been implicated as a major risk factor for lung cancer in the general population as well as in PWH (Altekruse et al., 2018; Shepherd et al., 2018). Prevalence of cigarette smoking among PWH is estimated to be between 42% and 59%, greatly exceeding that of the general population by 2- to 3-fold (Altekruse et al., 2018; Mdodo et al., 2015; Tesoriero, 2010). In a Swiss study, all persons with cancer of the respiratory tract were smokers, and there was a 3-fold higher excess risk of these cancers (Clifford et al., 2005). A similar finding was demonstrated in a U.S. study which showed that PWH and lung cancer were 1.3 times more likely to be current or former smokers and to have greater pack-year tobacco consumption history compared to those with HIV but without cancer (D'Jaen et al., 2010). Shiels and colleagues found that PWH who smoked more than 1.43 packs per day had twice the risk of lung cancer compared to PWH who smoked less. Compared to people without HIV who smoked less than 1.43 packs per day, those with HIV and who smoked more than 1.43 packs per day had a 7.2 times higher risk of developing lung cancer (Shiels et al., 2010a). A more recent study of the NA-ACCORD consortium found that PWH diagnosed with cancer were more likely to have been smokers (79%) compared to those without cancer (73%) (Altekruse et al., 2018). Smoking was associated with increased risk of cancer overall (HR 1.33; 95% CI: 1.18–1.49), smoking-related cancers (HR 2.31; CI: 1.80–2.98), and lung cancer (HR 17.80; CI: 5.60–56.63). Researchers recently used an HIV microsimulation model to evaluate cumulative lung cancer mortality by smoking exposure and found that PWH who continue to smoke have a 16.6%–29.8% estimated mortality depending on sex and smoking intensity, while estimated mortality decreased to 3.7%–7.9% for those who quit smoking and to 1.2%–1.6% for never smokers (Reddy et al., 2017). Even PWH who were adherent to ART were 6–13 times more likely to die from lung cancer than from traditional AIDS-related causes. When the authors applied this model to the current U.S. population with HIV, they found that 9.3% could die from lung cancer if their smoking habits do not change.

Other studies have not found the same association with smoking. In one, researchers studied 5,238 PWH and found that the overall smoking-adjusted SIR for lung cancer was 2.5 times higher than that of the general population (95% CI: 1.6–3.5) (Engels et al., 2006). However, in an analysis that assumed all participants smoked, the smoking-adjusted SIR was only 1.7. This suggests that smoking did not account for all excess risk of lung cancer in HIV (Engels et al., 2006). In a mortality analysis it was found that, after adjusting for smoking and other patient characteristics, the risk of death was 3.8 times higher for people with versus without HIV (Shiels et al., 2010a). A large Veterans Administration study found that the incidence rate ratio (1.7) of lung cancer in PWH remained significantly elevated after multivariable adjustment for confounders, including smoking, compared to persons without HIV (Sigel et al., 2012). These studies suggest that, independent of smoking, HIV positivity portends a higher incidence and mortality risk for lung cancer.

Injection drug use (IDU) among PWH has also been associated with an increased risk of lung cancer in some studies. One analysis demonstrated that people with IDU, with or without HIV, had an increased risk of lung cancer, with SIRs of 14.3 and 6.2, respectively (Serraino et al., 2000). Other studies have found little evidence to support this association. In a study that included 2,086 participants (the AIDS Link to the Intravenous Experience Study), IDU was not associated with increased risk of lung cancer (Kirk et al., 2007).

HIV itself may also be associated with the development of lung cancer because of directly acting oncogenic effects. HIV-1 replication depends on Tat protein expression, which can upregulate expression of proto-oncogenes *c-myc*, *c-fos*, and *c-jun* to enhance cellular proliferation, including human adenocarcinoma cell lines (El-Solh et al., 1997). Allelic loss and changes in microsatellites, which are short tandem repeat DNA sequences, have also been described in other malignancies, such as KS, NHL, and SCCA, and have been found in lung cancers of PWH (Wistuba et al., 1998). These genetic alterations may lead to activation of oncogenes and loss of tumor suppressor genes. However, the lack of HIV viral integration into cellular DNA of somatic neoplastic cells challenges this hypothesis of oncogenesis because cancer cells can have background genetic alterations, and immunosuppression can also be associated with microsatellite changes (Bedi et al., 1995). Poor control of HIV also could contribute to the development of lung cancer. A study of PWH included in the U.S. VACS found that increased risk of lung cancer was associated with low $CD4^+$ T-cell count, low CD4/CD8 ratio, high HIV RNA levels, and more cumulative episodes of bacterial pneumonia (Sigel et al., 2017). Another recent study similarly noted that a $CD4^+$ T-cell count of less than 200 cells/mm^3 was associated with a younger age at lung cancer diagnosis (Shiels et al., 2017). In contrast, a large Californian cohort study did not find an association between increased development of lung cancer and $CD4^+$ T-cell count of less than 200 cells/mm^3 (Marcus et al., 2017).

Although men historically have been considered at higher risk for lung cancer, women also share a significant proportion of lung cancer diagnoses. This may be due to the increase in women tobacco smokers in the population or the increase in the number of WWH. The WIHS compared data from the National Health and Nutritional Examination (NHANES) II and SEER. Researchers found that WWH have higher lifetime cigarette consumption as well as an elevated SIR of 3 (95% CI: 1.7–5.1) compared to the general population with an SIR of 2.11 (95% CI: 0.25–7.61). Further, these data did not vary by pre-ART versus ART era (Levine et al., 2010). A French study evaluating cancer in PWH in the pre-ART and ART eras found that the SIR of women was 3 times higher than that of men in the ART era (6.28 vs. 2.12) (Herida et al., 2003). Several additional studies have shown greater incidence in women with SIR ranging from 1.6 to 16.7 (Calabresi et al., 2013; Clifford et al., 2005; Ramirez-Marrero et al., 2010).

DIAGNOSIS AND CLINICAL PRESENTATION OF LUNG CANCER IN HIV

Despite the increased risk of cancer with aging, PWH and lung cancer tend to be younger. In several studies, age at presentation ranged from 38 to 57 years. This is far below the age of presentation among the general population, which is closer to the seventh decade of life (Winstone et al., 2013). A large South African study of 1,805 patients with lung cancer, including 133 PWH, found that PWH were younger (mean age 54.6 years) compared to patients without HIV (60.3 years) (Bhikoo et al., 2024). Stage at presentation also tends to be advanced in PWH, with a majority presenting with stages III or IV. In the Bhikoo et al. study, only 7 of 133 PWH and lung cancer presented with potentially curable NSCLC compared to 240 of 1,292 patients without HIV. This likely contributes to the poor survivability of these patients (Sigel et al., 2012; Winstone et al., 2013).

The majority of histological types mirror those of the general population, with greater than 50% consisting of NSCLC. Adenocarcinoma is the predominant NSCLC (36%), followed by squamous cell carcinoma (30%) (Sigel et al., 2012). Many patients present with advanced disease and have symptoms of persistent cough and chest pain (Karp et al., 1993). Early diagnosis of lung cancer improves prognosis; however, screening with plain chest radiography at any interval has not been shown to be effective and is not recommended. Use of low-dose chest CT (LDCT) may be beneficial. The U.S. Preventive Services Task Force (USPSTF) recommendation to screen high-risk patients for lung cancer with LDCT was based on findings from the National Lung Screening Trial (National Lung Screening Trial Research Team, 2011). This was a large, randomized trial that found a 20% reduction in lung cancer mortality after implementing annual screening by LDCT in patients aged 55–74 years with at least a 30-pack-year smoking history. Because of improved mortality benefit, current USPSTF guidelines recommend lung cancer screening with LDCT for people aged 55–80 in the general population with at least a 30-pack-year smoking history and who currently smoke or who have quit within 15 years (Moyer, 2014). Of note, a handful of studies evaluating LDCT in PWH have suggested that, especially in people with low $CD4^+$ T-cell counts, false-positive LDCT findings may be more likely owing to prior lung infections (Sigel et al., 2014; Ronit et al., 2017). A recent modeling study evaluating patients with HIV with $CD4^+$ T-cell counts of at least 500 cells/mm^3 found that screening using the Centers for Medicare & Medicaid Services (CMS) criteria (i.e., age 55–77, 30-pack-years of smoking, and current smoker or quit within 15 years of screening) would reduce lung cancer mortality by 18.9%, similar to the mortality reduction of people without HIV (Kong, 2018). Thus, the benefit and cost-effectiveness of LDCT in patients with HIV remain unknown, but following the USPSTF and NCCN guidelines for the general population is reasonable after discussing risks (e.g., false positives and radiation exposure) and benefits (e.g., early detection and better prognosis) (Reid et al., 2018). Currently, a French multicenter prospective pilot study (ANRS EP48 HIV-CHEST cohort) is evaluating the utility of LDCT in PWH (NCT01207986) (Makinson et al., 2015).

Understanding the mechanisms underlying the development of lung cancer in PWH could lead to improved lung cancer screening methodologies. Researchers recently studied the molecular mechanisms underlying the gene expression profiles of lung cancer in PWH and identified 758 differentially expressed genes in HIV-associated lung cancer (Zheng et al., 2018). Specifically, they found that the expression levels of SIX1 and TFAP2A mRNA are increased in HIV-associated lung cancer and that expression levels of ADH1B, INMT, and SYNPO2 mRNA are decreased.

TREATMENT OF LUNG CANCER

There are no alternative or specific treatment guidelines for lung cancer in PWH. Most randomized trials for lung cancer have historically excluded PWH because of concerns regarding immune suppression, toxicity, and drug interactions with ART (Persad et al., 2008). Current treatment strategies mainly involve protocols for patients without HIV and depend on tumor histology, stage of disease, and underlying host factors such as comorbidities and pulmonary function. Patients with NSCLC are staged (I–IV) based on the tumor node metastasis system, with stage I disease confined to localized tumor without invasion into the chest wall, diaphragm, mediastinum, or surrounding structures and stage IV indicating metastatic disease (Shepherd et al., 2007). MRI of the brain should also be pursued for stage II or higher to identify intracranial metastasis. For localized, nonmetastatic disease, surgical resection is the preferred strategy with the intent to cure those patients able to undergo surgery. Surgery (i.e., lobectomy, sublobular resection, and video-assisted thoracoscopy) may be followed by adjuvant chemotherapy or radiation for those with more advanced stages or invasion (NCCN, 2024b). For nonsurgical candidates, ablation with radiotherapy can be considered. Studies evaluating surgery in PWH have been described mainly in small case-control series and case reports. Patients undergoing surgery for localized disease (stage I or stage II) tolerated surgery well with minimal complications (Cadranel et al., 2006).

For patients with advanced NSCLC or recurrence after initial definitive therapy, the goals of therapy are largely palliative. For patients with solitary metastasis or recurrence, curative intention with additional surgery or radiotherapy may be indicated and beneficial to help prolong survival. However, risks and benefits must be weighed in advanced disease to avoid undue adverse events and toxicities. Systemic therapy with combination chemotherapy using a platinum-based regimen is the mainstay agent with or without additional agents, such as the VEGF inhibitor bevacizumab (NCCN, 2024b).

While HIV infection is often an exclusion criterion in lung cancer clinical trials, the use of immunotherapy and chemotherapy for lung cancer treatment in PWH is feasible, and it has been used in patients to treat metastatic disease and as adjuvant therapy and in combination with radiation for locally advanced disease. One large retrospective study found similar rates of treatment modality between people with and without HIV (Sigel et al., 2013). Limited data from case series have provided heterogeneous results regarding the use of chemotherapeutic agents, efficacy, and drug toxicities in people with HIV and lung cancer (Bower et al., 2003; Powles et al., 2003; Spano et al., 2004). Recently a French phase 2 trial of PWH with advanced nonsquamous NSCLC showed that first-line four-cycle induction with carboplatin plus pemetrexed, followed by pemetrexed maintenance, was effective and reasonably well tolerated (Lavole et al., 2020). Additional studies to evaluate the efficacy, tolerability, and safety of chemotherapy in patients with HIV are needed.

Additional molecular and genetic mutation analysis for potential genetic-directed therapy targets has been explored. These should be performed when possible in patients with advanced-stage NSCLC, namely for the presence of epidermal growth factor receptor (EGFR) and anaplasmic lymphoma kinase (NCCN, 2024b). Other targets include RAS family oncogenes, the mTOR signaling pathway, and the MEK signaling pathway. Treatment with EGFR tyrosine kinase inhibitors such as erlotinib may also be considered for patients with this specific EGFR mutation in the tumor. However, long-term survival has yet to be established with the use of these agents (Okuma et al., 2014). Several novel treatment regimens are being studied in PWH with advanced lung cancer. Immunotherapies such as nivolumab, ipilimumab, and durvalumab are being evaluated in PWH and advanced solid tumors, including NSCLC (NCT03304093 and NCT02408861) (Rasmussen et al., 2021) (Bender-Ignacio et al., 2018; Gonzalez-Cao, 2020) (NCT03094286). Nivolumab as second- or third-line treatment for PWH and NSCLC appears to be well tolerated (Lavole et al., 2021).

SURVIVAL OF LUNG CANCER IN HIV

Survival among PWH and lung cancer is worse compared to that of their counterparts without HIV. Researchers analyzed data from 1996 to 2010 and found that all-cause mortality and cancer-specific mortality risk were respectively 85% and 28% higher for PWH with lung cancer compared to patients without HIV (Coghill et al., 2015). For patients with local-stage NSCLC receiving standard cancer therapy, PWH continued to have greater cancer-related deaths compared to patients without HIV (HR 1.8; 95% CI: 1.21–2.7) (Coghill et al., 2015). Another large study utilizing SEER registry data compared 267 PWH to 1,428 patients without HIV with similar cancer stage and histology of NSCLC (Sigel et al., 2013). Both groups with stage I to IIIA disease received surgery, chemotherapy, and radiotherapy at similar rates. Among the PWH group, 82% died during follow-up compared to 66% of the group without HIV ($p < 0.001$). Median overall survival for PWH was only 6 months compared to 20 months for the cohort without HIV. Overall, 5-year survival was also poor for PWH at 9% compared to 23% for the group without HIV. PWH and advanced disease (stage IIIB to IV) had the worst survival, with 9–20 times greater risk of death compared to PWH with only localized disease. Moreover, a major proportion of PWH also died from non-cancer-related causes (31% vs. 9%; $p < 0.001$).

Such disparities may be explained by several hypotheses, including the fact that PWH experienced overall greater mortality than the general population. It may be that tumors behave more aggressively in PWH due to tumor effect or poor immunological surveillance due to a lack of fully intact cellular immunity. Evaluation of the NA-ACCORD dataset found that PWH with a history of an AIDS-defining illness at lung cancer diagnosis had higher mortality and poorer survival after diagnosis compared to those without (Grover et al., 2018). Poor tolerability of surgery and chemotherapy may also contribute to worse outcomes. More studies are needed. Lastly, health disparities in treatment between PWH and populations without HIV may contribute to poor survival. Data from the Texas Cancer Registry from 1995 to 2009 showed that PWH and NSCLC received any cancer treatments less frequently despite greater numbers presenting at younger ages and with distant-stage disease (Suneja et al., 2013). PWH and local-stage NSCLC were less likely to receive surgery (45.5% vs. 62.5%; $p = 0.04$) than patients without HIV. PWH with regional disease were less likely to receive systemic chemotherapy. For distant disease, PWH received less chemotherapy or radiation (31.1% vs. 45.5%; $p = 0.0009$) (Suneja et al., 2013).

RECOMMENDED READING

Bhikoo R, Allwood BW, Irusen EM, et al. Lung cancer presents at a younger age and is less likely to be curable in people living with HIV. *Respiration.* 2024;103(1):47–50.

Coghill AE, Shiels MS, Suneja G, et al. Elevated cancer-specific mortality among HIV-infected patients in the United States. *J Clin Oncol.* 2015;33(21):2376–2383.

Gonzalez-Cao M, Morán T, Dalmau J, et al. Assessment of the feasibility and safety of durvalumab for treatment of solid tumors in patients with HIV-1 infection: the phase 2 DURVAST study. *JAMA Oncol.* 2020;7:1063–1067. http://doi:10.1001/jamaoncol.2020.0465

Grover S, Desir F, Jing Y, et al. Reduced cancer survival among adults with HIV and AIDS-defining illnesses despite no difference in cancer stage at diagnosis. *J Acquir Immune Defic Syndr.* 2018;79(4):421–429.

Lavole A, Greillier L, Mazieres J, et al. First-line carboplatin plus pemetrexed with pemetrexed maintenance in HIV+ patients with advanced non-squamous non-small cell lung cancer: the phase II IFCT-1001 CHIVA trial. *Eur Respir J.* 2020;56(2):1902066. http://doi:10.1183/13993003.02066-2019

Lavole A, Mazieres J, Schneider S, et al. Assessment of nivolumab in HIV-Infected patients with advanced non-small cell lung cancer after prior chemotherapy: the IFCT-1602 CHIVA2 phase 2 clinical trial. *Lung Cancer.* 2021;158:146–150. http://doi:10.1016/j.lungcan.2021.05.031

Rasmussen TA, Rajdev L, Rhodes A, et al. Impact of anti-PD-1 and anti-CTLA-4 on the human immunodeficiency virus (HIV) reservoir in people living with HIV with cancer on antiretroviral therapy: the AIDS Malignancy Consortium 095 study. *Clin Infect Dis.* 2021;73(7):e1973–e1981. http://doi:10.1093/cid/ciaa1530

Sellers SA, Edmonds A, Ramirez C, et al. Optimal lung cancer screening criteria among persons living with HIV. *J Acquir Immune Defic Syndr.* 2022;90(2):184–192. http://doi:10.1097/QAI.0000000000002930

Sigel K, Crothers K, Dubrow R, et al. Prognosis in HIV-infected patients with non-small cell lung cancer. *Br J Cancer.* 2013;109:1974–1980.
Suneja G, Shiels MS, Melville SK. Disparities in the treatment and outcomes of lung cancer among HIV-infected Individuals. *AIDS.* 2013;27(3):459–468.

PROSTATE CANCER

LEARNING OBJECTIVES

- Review the epidemiology and risk factors for prostate cancer in men with HIV.
- Review the current screening recommendations for prostate cancer.
- Discuss the treatment options for prostate cancer in men with HIV.

WHAT'S NEW?

- Since the advent of prostate-specific antigen (PSA) testing, the incidence of prostate cancer has increased in men with HIV. However, the true incidence may be similar to that of men without HIV.
- Routine prostate cancer screening with PSA testing is not recommended.

KEY POINTS

- Prostate cancer represents a significant burden of neoplastic disease and mortality in men with and without HIV.
- Prostate cancer appears to be associated with states of immunological control.
- Screening with serum PSA testing should not routinely be implemented, having a "D" recommendation by the U.S. Preventive Services Task Force.
- Decision to treat early-stage cancer versus watchful waiting should be carefully considered because evidence of long-term mortality benefits remains unclear.
- First-line therapies include radical prostatectomy and radiation.

Prostate cancer remains the leading cancer diagnosis among men in the United States and other high-income countries. It is the second leading cause of cancer deaths after lung cancer. Increased screening efforts in the United States led to increased incidence after the PSA test became widely available in 1992. However, screening and treatment are controversial because of the occult and often indolent nature of untreated prostate cancer, especially in older men with limited life expectancy. The mortality benefit of diagnosis and treatment of early-stage prostate cancer remains unproven; thus, emphasis on screening and early detection has waned in recent years. Compared to other malignancies, such as lung or anal cancer, some studies have demonstrated HIV infection to be associated with a reduced risk of prostate cancer (Sun et al., 2021). Regardless, diagnosis of prostate cancer carries a significant clinical impact on patients' sexual, genitourinary, and overall health.

EPIDEMIOLOGY OF PROSTATE CANCER IN HIV

Men with HIV in the United States experienced an increased incidence of prostate cancer after 1990 compared to the preceding decade, from 0.2% to 2.2% of all cancers in a retrospective study of population-based registry data (Engels et al., 2006). In the same study, the incidence increased during the pre-ART and post-ART eras, which may be explained by the introduction of the PSA screening test. Another large retrospective review also found that prostate cancer in men with HIV increased from 1992 to 2003 (Patel et al., 2008). However, the group with HIV had significantly lower rates of cancer compared to the general population in the pre-ART era (15 vs. 47 per 100,000 py) and the ART era (38 vs. 61 per 100,000 py) (Patel et al., 2008). Another study that examined the PSA testing era (1992 to 2007) found an incidence of 28 per 100,000 py in men with HIV. However, the incidence in men with HIV compared to the expected rate in the general population during this same time period was significantly reduced, with an SIR of only 0.5 (95% CI: 0.44–0.57) (Shiels et al., 2010b). A study of the VACS between 2000 and 2015 found lower rates of PSA screening and prostate biopsies among PWH compared to the HIV-negative group (Leapman et al., 2022). Prostate cancer incidence was similar in both groups (IRR 0.93; 95% CI: 0.86–1.01). The South African HIV Cancer Match Study found that prostate cancer was the most frequent cancer type in older men (Ruffieux et al. 2023). A South Africa study of insured men found no difference in prostate cancer diagnosis rates between men with and without HIV when they adjusted their model for confounders (Ruffieux et al., 2024).

Of note, some disparity remains when prostate cancer diagnoses are compared among races. One study that evaluated men enrolled in the MACS from 1996 to 2010 found an incidence of 169 per 100,000 py among all men 40–70 years old compared to 276 per 100,000 py among African American men with HIV (Dutta et al., 2017). In this study, prostate cancer risk was similar by HIV status (IRR 1.0; 95% CI: 0.55–1.82), but nearly 3-fold higher in African Americans compared to non-African Americans in adjusted models (IRRs 2.66 and 3.22; 95% CI: 1.36–5.18 and 1.27–8.16 for all or men with HIV, respectively).

RISK FACTORS FOR PROSTATE CANCER

Postulated risk factors that promote development of prostate cancer in men with HIV include exposure to carcinogens and use of androgen supplementation to treat hypogonadism. Coinfection with oncogenic viruses may also promote neoplasia (Montgomery et al., 2006). Chronic inflammatory states promoted by HIV systemically and localized to the prostate, as well as chronic prostatitis, may contribute to cancer development (Leport et al., 1989; Smith et al., 2004).

Prostate cancer and risk of death have been associated with tobacco exposure in several studies. However, other studies have demonstrated conflicting data. Two large meta-analyses found similar results (Huncharek et al., 2010; Islami et al., 2014). Huncharek and colleagues found a dose-dependent relationship with incidence of prostate cancer in patients without HIV, with the heaviest smokers having a 13% increased risk of cancer. Islami and colleagues (2014) found smoking to be associated with an increased risk of death (RR 1.24) from prostate cancer, which was dose-dependent. The incidence of prostate cancer, however, was not statistically significant overall. In fact, baseline cigarette smoking was inversely associated with incidence of prostate cancer.

Unlike other malignancies in HIV, immunological control with increasing $CD4^+$ T-cell count has been associated with increased risk of prostate cancer, with a RR that is 3-fold greater in the ART era (Shiels et al., 2010b). In several studies, men with HIV and prostate cancer had robust $CD4^+$ T-cell counts of greater than 300 cells/mm^3 (Hsiao et al., 2009; Marcus et al., 2014; Pantanowitz et al., 2008). A systematic review found that most patients were on ART at the time of diagnosis (Vaziri et al., 2022). Overall, data from numerous studies suggest that variations in prostate cancer deficits in men with HIV are due to differential PSA screening in this population and not to immunologic status.

PROSTATE CANCER SCREENING

The primary tools for diagnosis of prostate cancer include serum PSA measurement, DRE, and, ultimately, prostate biopsy for definitive histologic diagnosis. Both European and U.S. guidelines have recommended against routine screening with PSA in men regardless of HIV status (Heidenreich et al., 2014; Moyer et al., 2012). Rather, whether to perform individual screening with PSA for early detection should be a well-informed, mutual decision between provider and patient, based on possible benefits and harms of a positive PSA test. Optimal interval of PSA screening has also not been established. DRE alone has limited sensitivity (6%–8%) of detecting prostate cancer (Gosselaar et al., 2009; Okotie et al., 2007). The combination of an abnormal DRE versus normal DRE with PSA level of higher than 3 ng/mL may enhance positive predictive value of cancer detection at 48% versus 22% (Gosselaar et al., 2008).

CLINICAL PRESENTATION

Prostate cancer diagnosis in HIV often occurs in the fifth and sixth decades of life, and patients often have a family history of prostate cancer (Hsiao et al., 2009; Ong et al., 2015; Shiels et al., 2010b). Limited data suggest that men with HIV may present more often with late-stage disease compared to the general population (Shiels et al., 2015). A large California cohort found more localized cancer compared to regional or distant disease among men with HIV (88% vs. 7%), which was similar to the pattern found in men without HIV (Marcus et al., 2014). Other studies have found no difference in presentation with early or advanced disease (Hsiao et al., 2009; Riedel et al., 2015a). African Americans without HIV have a greater likelihood of presenting with advanced-stage prostate cancer in the general population (Siegel et al., 2012). Among PWH, African Americans may represent a higher risk group for prostate cancer because they are generally overrepresented among PWH in the United States.

TREATMENT AND TREATMENT OUTCOMES OF PROSTATE CANCER

Treatment of prostate cancer in men with HIV is similar to that of men without HIV and is based on stage and grade of disease with use of the Gleason score (ranging from 2 to 10). For localized disease (stage I and stage II) not spread to lymph nodes or distant sites, strategies include active surveillance (PSA monitoring and/or repeat biopsy), radical prostatectomy, or radiation therapy (external beam radiation therapy [EBRT] and/or brachytherapy) with or without androgen deprivation. For locally advanced disease (stage III) that has spread outside the prostate gland, surgery or radiation with androgen deprivation therapy are alternatives. A Gleason score greater than 8 represents high-risk neoplasia, even if disease is localized. The optimal choice between surgical intervention and radiation is unclear for these patients, and careful consideration of individual risks and benefits should be discussed on a case-by-case basis (Grimm et al., 2012).

Treatment of disseminated disease, which often involves osteoblastic lesions, typically involves androgen deprivation therapy, castration (medical or surgical), and systemic chemotherapy. Two phase 3 trials examining the use of abiraterone and enzalutamide for treatment of metastatic, castration-resistant prostate cancer have shown clinical benefit with these agents, which target the androgen-synthesis pathway (Loriot et al., 2015; Ryan et al., 2015). Chemotherapy with taxane-based regimens has also shown success in prolonging survival in men with castration-resistant prostate cancer. Docetaxel plus prednisone is currently the standard, initial cytotoxic chemotherapy used in metastatic, castration-resistant disease (Berthold et al., 2008).

Few studies have evaluated the safety, tolerability, and efficacy of treatments for prostate cancer in men with HIV. Most studies have been small and limited to the evaluation of EBRT with the heterogeneity of dosing. One Veterans Administration study described outcomes of 15 patients who received an EBRT dose-escalation approach (75.6 Gy to 79.2 Gy) for localized disease: 13 were treated with concomitant ART, and the 5-year event-free survival was 92.3% (Schreiber et al., 2014). Toxicities included urinary frequency and rectal bleeding. Another study evaluating EBRT (72 Gy to 81 Gy) for localized prostate cancer in men with HIV compared to men without HIV found that 26% of men with HIV had biochemical failure compared to 12% of matched controls without HIV. At a mean of 36 months, there were no deaths in the HIV group. Genitourinary and anal adverse events were overall mild (Kahn et al., 2012). A systematic review of nine studies including 187 patients with HIV and prostate cancer found that most were treated with either EBRT (59%) or brachytherapy (20.5%). The 4–5-year biochemical failure-free rate was 87%–97%, and the 5-year cancer-specific survival was 84%–97% (Vaziri et al., 2022).

The risk of death from prostate cancer is associated with advanced disease compared to local or regional prostate cancer (Shiels et al., 2010b). In a large retrospective study of HIV and cancer registries from 1996 to 2010, mortality of prostate cancer was significantly higher for men with HIV compared to that of men without HIV (HR 1.57; 95% CI: 1.02–2.41) even after adjusting for patient characteristics and cancer stage (Coghill et al., 2015). Cancer deaths were also greater in men with HIV after adjusting for treatment, but this was not significant (HR 1.64; 95% CI: 0.93–2.89). One study that used data from 1996 to 2002 found a 2.1-fold increased risk of death from prostate cancer in men with HIV compared to men without HIV (Marcus et al., 2014).

RECOMMENDED READING

Coghill AE, Shiels MS, Suneja G, et al. Elevated cancer-specific mortality among HIV-infected patients in the United States. *J Clin Oncol.* 2015;33(21):2376–2383.

Leapman MS, Stone K, Wadia R, et al. Prostate cancer screening and incidence among aging persons living with HIV. *J Urol.* 2022;207(2):324–332.

Marcus JL, Chao CR, Leyden WA, et al. Prostate cancer incidence and prostate-specific antigen testing among HIV-positive and HIV-negative men. *J Acquir Immune Defic Syndr.* 2014;66:495–502.

Moyer VA. Screening for prostate cancer: US Preventive Services Task Force recommendation statement. *Ann Intern Med.* 2012;157(2):120–135.

Ruffieux Y, Fernandez Villalobos NV, Didden C, et al. Prostate cancer diagnosis rates among insured men with and without HIV in South Africa: a cohort study. *Cancer Epidemiol Biomarkers Prev.* 2024;33(8):1057–1064.

Shiels MS, Goedert JJ, Moore RD, et al. Risk of prostate cancer in U.S. men with AIDS. *Cancer Epidemiol Biomarkers Prev.* 2010;19(11):2910–2915.

Sun D, Cao M, Li H, et al. Risk of prostate cancer in men with HIV/AIDS: a systematic review and meta-analysis. *Prostate Cancer Prostatic Dis.* 2021;24(1):24–34.

Vaziri T, Rao YJ, Whalen M, et al. Prostate cancer outcomes in patients living with HIV/AIDS treated with radiation therapy: a systematic review. *Adv Radiat Oncol.* 2022;8(1):101074

COLORECTAL ADENOCARCINOMA

LEARNING OBJECTIVES

- Review the epidemiology of colorectal cancer in the HIV population.
- Discuss the screening methods for colorectal cancer.
- Review treatment modalities and outcomes in patients with HIV and colorectal cancer.

WHAT'S NEW?

- The incidence of colon cancer has increased in the population with HIV compared to the general population in the ART era, and mortality remains high compared to that of the population without HIV.
- Patients with HIV disproportionately receive less colorectal cancer screening than the general population.
- Standard chemoradiation and surgical approaches for treating colorectal cancer appear to be well tolerated in PWH, although more research is needed in this area.

KEY POINTS

- Colorectal cancer presents a major health and mortality burden in the population with HIV.
- Colorectal cancer presentation occurs often in younger patients and with more advanced disease compared to the general population.
- Significant disparities exist in screening PWH for colorectal cancer compared to patients without HIV.
- Standard treatment includes surgery and neoadjuvant and/or adjuvant chemoradiation.
- Survival is significantly worse compared to that of patients without HIV and colorectal cancer.

In the United States, colorectal cancer (CRC) is the third leading cause of cancer death in the general population for both men and women. It has been the focus of large-scale primary prevention screening efforts to identify patients with early disease (Siegel et al., 2014). Vigilance for neoplastic processes such as colorectal cancer must be maintained in PWH because they are often diagnosed at advanced stages and can be overlooked because of presentation at a younger age and lack of traditional risk factors such as family history (Chapman et al., 2009; Yegüez et al., 2003). This phenomenon was characterized by early case reports of colorectal adenocarcinoma in PWH. Patients were often males, aged in their 20s to 40s, and with advanced immunosuppression (Cappell et al., 1988; Klugman et al., 1994; Ravalli et al., 1989).

PWH who are considered "average" risk are offered screening less frequently than the general population (Nayudu et al., 2012). Further, disparities in cancer treatment between individuals with and without HIV are also prevalent. PWH are less likely to receive treatment for colon cancer than their counterparts without HIV (Suneja et al., 2013). The lack of screening and treatment is likely to contribute to poorer outcomes and excess mortality in PWH.

EPIDEMIOLOGY OF COLON CANCER IN HIV

PWH have a higher incidence of CRC than the general population. A large U.S. study that examined cancer incidence in PWH compared to the general population from 1992 to 2003 found an increased SIR during the early time period of 1992–1995 (39.9 per 100,000 py) compared to the later time period of 2000–2003 (66.2 per 100,000 py). During both time periods, the rates were greater than those of the general population (20.4 and 21.1 per 100,000 py, respectively) (Patel et al., 2008). In a more recent study using U.S. and Canadian data from 2006–2009, the incidence rate of CRC in PWH was 36.4 per 100,000 py compared to 27.7 per 100,000 py in people without HIV. During this study period, the cumulative incidence declined by 6% per year for patients without HIV but increased in those with HIV by 5% per year. This may reflect the declining death rate among PWH (Silverberg et al., 2015).

A large Taiwanese study that used the National Health Insurance Research Database from 1998 to 2009 found that, among 1,282 PWH and cancer, the incidence of CRC, excluding anal cancer, was 51 per 100,000 py with an SIR of 5.9 (95% CI: 4.15–8.37). Interestingly, colon cancer was relatively common in women, with an incidence of 156 per 100,000 py (Chen et al., 2014). In the U.S. surveillance study using the HIV/AIDS Cancer Match Study registry data from 1991 to 2002, the incidence of CRC, excluding anal cancer, was 15 per 100,000 py (Engels et al., 2008).

Immunosuppression likely plays a role in the epidemiology of CRC. A study by Silverberg et al. stratified groups by $CD4^+$ T-cell count and found that those with HIV and less than 200 cells/mm^3 had an 80% higher RR compared to a protective effect of higher $CD4^+$ T-cell counts (Silverberg et al., 2011). Another study found that patients with duration of HIV of greater than 10 years and $CD4^+$ T-cell counts of less than 200 cells/mm^3 had greater odds of having distal colon neoplastic lesions compared to those with higher $CD4^+$ T-cell counts (Bini et al., 2006). On the contrary, many other studies have not shown significant differences in rates among PWH or reduction of CRC in the ART era. Several studies support increases in CRC in the ART era. The lack of reporting of CRC in advanced immunosuppression, coupled with the increase in CRC in the ART era, may be explained by increased longevity of the population with HIV as well as an increase in screening measures, allowing for more diagnoses.

COLORECTAL CANCER SCREENING IN THE HIV POPULATION

Screening for CRC in PWH reflects that recommended for the general population with normal cancer risk. *Normal cancer risk* is defined as no personal history of CRC, adenomatous polyps, or inflammatory bowel disease and no first-degree relative with a history of CRC. The U.S. Preventive Services Task Force recommends that for adults with an average risk of CRC, screening with fecal occult blood testing, flexible sigmoidoscopy, or colonoscopy should begin at age 45 years and continue until age 75 years. The current screening interval for colonoscopy is 10 years. For those with increased risk, such as an immediate family member with a history of CRC, screening should begin at age 40 years or 10 years prior to the relative's age at onset of CRC, whichever occurs first (Whitlock et al., 2008). Unfortunately, overall screening rates are suboptimal, and one study found that only 64.5% of screening-eligible people aged 50–75 years surveyed in the Behavioral Risk Factor Surveillance System reported having one of the recommended tests (Joseph et al., 2012).

Screening PWH based on standard guidelines has been more challenging, with significant disparity compared to the general population. A retrospective study in New York identified 565 screening-eligible PWH with average risk and found that only 25% underwent screening colonoscopy within 10 years. The median age was 58 years, and most of these patients had well-controlled HIV compared to those who did not have colonoscopy. Among those who had colonoscopy and biopsy, 32% of biopsies were of tubular adenomas, which exceeds the detection rate of tubular adenomas in the general population for men (34%) and women (27%) (Nayudu et al., 2012). A prospective study performed among New York veterans from 1998 to 2003 included 2,217 controls without HIV and 165 PWH (85.5% on ART and 45.5% with undetectable HIV RNA levels) (Bini et al., 2006). Among the PWH eligible for CRC screening, 91.9% underwent flexible sigmoidoscopy, which was similar to the percentage who underwent it in the cohort without HIV. More polyps were identified in the group with HIV (30.9% vs. 23%; $p = 0.2$), and polyps in the group with HIV were more likely to have neoplastic features compared to those of the controls (25.5% vs. 13.1%; $p < 0.001$; OR 2.27; 95% CI: 1.57–3.29). The study found that duration of HIV over 10 years and lower $CD4^+$ T-cell count were significantly associated with having distal neoplasias. Colonoscopy showed a higher prevalence of proximal colon neoplastic lesions in the group with HIV compared to the controls without HIV (61.2% vs. 47.8%; $p = 0.07$) (Bini et al., 2006). Although not statistically significant, it appears that PWH are at high risk for malignant potential compared to their counterparts without HIV. Another study comparing CRC screening in PWH and controls demonstrated similar results as those obtained in the New York veterans study. This study compared 302 PWH to 302 patients without HIV and found that PWH were significantly less likely to have any type of screening modality (55.6% vs. 77.8%; $p < 0.0001$). Undetectable HIV RNA levels, older age, and a family history were variables associated with having at least one CRC screening (Reinhold et al., 2005).

Appropriate use of screening for eligible persons is of utmost importance for PWH because polyps may have more high-risk features than those of the general population. Barriers to colonoscopy referral and screening should be identified and managed. One pilot study randomizing screening-eligible PWH to receive educational material and in-person decision-making support showed increased screening colonoscopy uptake (Ferron et al., 2015). Based on this, efforts to increase on-time screening in eligible PWH should be undertaken.

CLINICAL PRESENTATION

With regard to early presentations of CRC, one recent study compared the prevalence, type, and location of neoplastic lesions found on colonoscopy in 263 PWH matched with 657 patients without HIV and found that PWH were less likely to have any neoplastic lesions (21.3% vs. 27.7%, $p < 0.05$), adenoma (20.5% vs. 27.1%, $p = 0.04$), tubular adenomas greater than 10 mm (0.4% vs. 2.9%, $p = 0.02$), and serrated adenomas (0.0% vs. 2.6%, $p < 0.01$) (Fantry et al., 2016). They also found a nonsignificant increased prevalence of adenocarcinoma in PWH compared with people without HIV (1.5% vs. 0.8%, $p = 0.29$). However, at the time of diagnosis in PWH,

CRC is often advanced and occurs in younger patients compared to the general population. Researchers from the Italian Cooperative Group AIDS and Tumors evaluated 27 PWH and 54 matched patients without HIV who were diagnosed with CRC between 1985 and 2003 (Berretta et al., 2009). The majority were diagnosed in the ART era, with a median age of 48 years in both groups. Median $CD4^+$ T-cell count at the time of diagnosis was 325 cells/mm^3. In PWH, the stage was predominantly Dukes's stage D (distant metastasis) compared to those without HIV (74% vs. 35%; $p = 0.002$). Histopathology showed poorly differentiated adenocarcinoma in 66% of the cohort with HIV compared to 26% in the matched controls without HIV (Berretta et al., 2009).

A case-control study from Southern California also found that CRC of PWH occurred mainly in those younger than 50 years (72%) and with advanced disease (stages III and IV). PWH had a younger to older age ratio of 3:1 compared to the population controls, whose ratio was 1.33. In most patients, biopsy findings revealed poorly differentiated adenocarcinoma (64%). Of note, the mean $CD4^+$ T-cell count at time of diagnosis was robust at 467 cells/mm^3 (Wasserberg et al., 2007).

One multicenter retrospective study of 17 PWH and confirmed CRC from 1988 to 2003 reported a mean age of 43 years at diagnosis and most with $CD4^+$ T-cell counts of less than 500 cells/mm^3 (not specified further) (Chapman et al., 2009). Most tumors arose in the right side of the colon (57%) and with advanced-stage IV disease (47%) and histopathology with grade 2 or 3 adenocarcinomas (79%). Most metastatic sites were to the liver but also included lung, peritoneum, and subcutaneous sites (Chapman et al., 2009). Sigel and colleagues subsequently evaluated 184 patients with CRC (38 PWH and 146 patients without HIV) and found that PWH were more likely to have smoked ($p = 0.001$), have right-sided colorectal cancer (37% vs. 14%; $p = 0.003$), and tumor-infiltrating lymphocytes above 50/10 high-power fields (21% vs. 7%). They also evaluated mismatch repair protein (MMR) expression levels between the two groups (as MMR is a marker for microsatellite instability) but found no difference between the two groups ($p = 0.6$) (Sigel et al., 2016). Given the presence of right-sided colonic tumors, colonoscopy in PWH may have a greater diagnostic yield compared to flexible sigmoidoscopy. Further prospective studies should be performed to evaluate the various screening techniques.

TREATMENT FOR COLORECTAL CANCER IN HIV

Treatment for CRC in PWH is the same as that for those without HIV and primarily depends on clinical staging, which is determined by physical exam and radiographic imaging. CT scanning is mandatory for determining regional extension, nodal involvement, or distant metastasis in the tumor, nodal, and metastatic staging system. Stages range from stage I to stage IV as the disease advances from confined disease to the colonic mucosa, regional lymph node involvement, and involvement of one or more distant organs including peritoneal seeding. For patients with stage II to IV disease, imaging with CT scan of the chest, abdomen, and pelvis is recommended (NCCN, 2024c). Further imaging with MRI may be useful for better characterization of the liver for metastatic disease, especially in the setting of background steatosis (Shahani et al., 2014). Testing with the tumor marker carcinoembryonic antigen (CEA) should be performed prior to treatment to help serve as a guide in the post-treatment follow-up. This test has not been validated for use specifically in PWH, nor has there been robust evidence supporting survival benefit in the general population. Still, CEA remains a standard pre- and post-treatment test for its prognostic utility (Locker, 2006).

Treatment for localized disease can be curative with endoscopic resection of a carcinomatous polyp or surgical resection with simple colectomy and anastomosis. Surgery remains the cornerstone of therapy for localized disease, and margins should be free of cancer. Locally advanced disease or poorly differentiated polypoid lesions may warrant more invasive or radical surgery. If invasion involves surrounding structures, larger resection of contiguous, multivisceral structures is indicated to ensure negative margins in the affected noncolonic organs (NCCN, 2024c). This approach has yielded improved prognosis and outcomes in patients with locally advanced disease (Govindarajan et al., 2006; Lehnert et al., 2002). Tumor location is also an important aspect in consideration of surgical approach because management of CRC involving the rectum (especially the lower rectum) may compromise anal sphincter tone and genitourinary function. If the anus is involved, sphincter-sparing surgery may be considered with adjuvant or neoadjuvant chemotherapy and radiation (NCCN, 2024a; Sauer et al., 2012).

Colorectal adenocarcinoma typically metastasizes to the liver, lung, lymph nodes, and peritoneum. With limited metastatic disease, curative surgery remains an option to improve survival; however, recurrence of disease is a reality for some patients (Neef et al., 2009; Shah et al., 2006).

Chemoradiotherapy in CRC

Neoadjuvant and adjuvant chemotherapies are generally considered for patients with advanced or metastatic disease when the expectation of noncurative surgery is present. Neoadjuvant chemoradiotherapy (CRT) is a standard approach to therapy in locally advanced rectal cancer (T3 or N1-2) prior to surgery or rectal cancer that is unresectable or medically inoperable. This consists of fractionated radiation therapy, usually with a 5-fluorouracil (5-FU)-based regimen in combination with other agents, such as capecitabine or oxaliplatin and leucovorin (NCCN, 2024c; Sauer et al., 2012). Adjuvant CRT following resection to eliminate microscopic foci of tumors and promote recurrence-free survival has been most beneficial in patients with nodal involvement (stage III) (Smith et al., 2004). Typical regimens include 5-FU/leucovorin- or capecitabine-based regimens (NCCN, 2024c). Other adjuvant therapies in metastatic disease include the vascular endothelial and epidermal growth factor inhibitor bevacizumab and cetuximab, respectively. Overall survival benefit of these agents remains controversial, and they may cause excess adverse events (da Gramont et al., 2012; Taieb et al., 2014).

TREATMENT OUTCOMES AND SURVIVAL OF PATIENTS WITH HIV AND CRC

There is a paucity of data on the efficacy, tolerability, and treatment outcomes of CRC for PWH. As previously discussed, PWH tend to present with more advanced disease, which may require both surgery and chemoradiation. In one case series, 10 PWH with stage III or IV disease underwent segmental colon or rectal resection. One patient underwent complete pelvic exenteration (Wasserberg et al., 2007). All patients also received first-line adjuvant chemotherapy with 5-FU/leucovorin. Four patients received additional CPT-11 or irinotecan for metastatic disease. Of the patients with rectal involvement, 1 received neoadjuvant 5-FU/leucovorin-based chemoradiation, and 3 received adjuvant radiation. Overall, chemotherapy was tolerated well, but some did experience grade 3 adverse events with neutropenia and anemia (Wasserberg et al., 2007).

Another case series from Italy reported on 27 PWH, the majority with metastatic CRC (Berretta et al., 2009). Of those with metastatic disease, 3 received neoadjuvant oxaliplatin-based chemotherapy for liver metastasis, 7 underwent palliative chemotherapy, and 2 were treated with 5-FU chemoradiation. The remaining patients with metastatic disease underwent palliation. One patient who received radiation incurred hemorrhagic proctitis, which prompted treatment cessation (Berretta et al., 2009). Overall, chemotherapy was tolerated well in the group, with few grade 3 neutropenic events.

Surgical resection provides the best curative treatment for localized colon cancer, and this has been demonstrated with SEER data (2005–2011) showing 5-year survival rates of 90% for localized disease. However, survival declines steeply with regional or nodal involvement (70%) and with distant metastasis (13%) (Howlader et al., 2015). PWH may not receive surgery when indicated, giving them a survival disadvantage. This disparity was highlighted in a follow-up study, with the group releasing a brief report on its experience treating 14 PWH and CRC-related liver metastasis (Berretta et al., 2010). Only 3 PWH initially had unresectable liver metastasis as determined by a multidisciplinary team; however, the other 11 underwent FOLFOX-4 treatment. Three people in the group that underwent surgery received neoadjuvant chemotherapy with FOLFOX-4 or FOLFIRI, followed by liver segmentectomy (n = 2) or liver segmentectomy plus radiofrequency ablation (n = 1). These 3 PWH tolerated the treatments well, remained on ART without any grade 3 or 4 toxicities, and 2 of the 3 PWH remained disease-free at 21-month follow-up. This study suggests that an aggressive surgical approach for metastatic CRC can be successfully performed in PWH. Narrowing the treatment gap between the population with HIV and the general population remains an important goal to help improve survival outcomes for PWH.

Mortality for PWH and CRC remains high compared to that for the general population. A large retrospective study estimated that PWH and CRC have a 50% higher risk of mortality compared to patients without HIV (Coghill et al., 2015). Smaller case control studies have shown markedly poorer survival for PWH compared to controls without HIV, with 4-year survival of 15% and 49%, respectively (Berretta et al., 2009). A more recent study found that PWH and CRC had reduced overall survival (p = 0.02) when compared to their counterparts without HIV, but no difference in progression-free survival (Sigel et al., 2016). It has been hypothesized that PWH are less likely to receive therapy and, therefore, on a population level, will have poorer survival. HIV positivity should not preclude delivery of the standard of care. Further studies are needed to rigorously evaluate the standard of care delivered to these patients. Disparities in screening and treatment of PWH and CRC are likely to perpetuate their less-than-optimal survival outcomes.

RECOMMENDED READING

Berretta M, Cappellani A, Di Benedetto F, et al. Clinical presentation and outcome of colorectal cancer in PLWH: a clinical case–control study. *Onkologie*. 2009;32:319–324.

Bini EJ, Park J, Francois F. Use of flexible sigmoidoscopy to screen for colorectal cancer in HIV-infected patients 50 years of age or older. *JAMA Intern Med*. 2006;166(15):1626–1631.

IMMUNE CHECK POINT INHIBITOR THERAPY FOR MALIGNANCIES IN PEOPLE WITH HIV

LEARNING OBJECTIVES

Review the mechanism and proposed use of immune check point inhibitor (ICPI) therapy for PWH and cancer.

WHAT'S NEW?

ICPI therapy is currently being evaluated in PWH and in patients with well-controlled HIV infection is thought to be just as efficacious for the treatment of various cancers in PWH as for the general population.

KEY POINTS

- ICPIs target key immune regulatory pathways and thus can untether T-cell-mediated anti-tumor responses, which could help target certain cancers in PWH.
- ICPIs like PD-1 inhibitors may also be able to help eliminate the cells that carry integrated HIV DNA, thus contributing to elimination of the patient's HIV reservoir.
- PD-1/PD-L1 inhibitors have been approved for melanoma, NSCLC and other lung cancers, renal cell carcinoma, Hodgkin's lymphoma, head and neck squamous cell cancers, several types of breast cancers, gastric cancer, urothelial cancer, and colorectal cancer in the general population; studies evaluating their use in PWH are ongoing.

ICPIs are a relatively new class of immunotherapy medications that inhibit suppression of effector T-cell responses. In other words, they help to turn on the cancer or infectious agent-suppressed cell-medicated immune again. Most of these are monoclonal antibodies directed against immune check points that block the interaction between the immune check point and their respective check point ligands. One type of immune check point is programmed cell death-1 (PD-1), which is predominantly expressed on T-cells. The interaction of PD-1 with its ligands (PD-L1 and -L2) expressed on antigen-presenting cells and tumors sends a negative signal to T-cells, which can lead to T-cell exhaustion or dysfunction. T-cell exhaustion is now recognized as a key mechanism contributing to impaired T-cell responses against tumors and some pathogens.

ICPI therapies are an appealing treatment option for many cancers that express PD-1 because they have broad activity with good response rates, they frequently induce long-term disease control, and they are relatively nontoxic. So far, six monoclonal antibodies that target PD-1 or PD-L1 have been approved by the FDA. The first, a PD-1 inhibitor, pembrolizumab, was approved in September 2014 for the treatment of advanced or unresectable melanoma in patients failing other treatments and was so successful it later became the first-line treatment (Robert et al., 2014). It is now approved for NSCLC (Garon et al., 2015), head and neck squamous cell cancers, refractory Hodgkin's lymphoma, primary mediastinal large B-cell lymphoma, advanced urothelial carcinoma, advanced gastric cancer, some types of colorectal cancers, and advanced cervical cancer. A second PD-1 inhibitor, nivolumab, was subsequently approved in 2015 for the treatment of melanoma and is now also approved for NSCLC, renal cell carcinoma, Hodgkin's lymphoma, head and neck squamous cell cancers, advanced urothelial carcinomas, certain colorectal cancers, and hepatocellular carcinoma. The third, fourth, and fifth approvals were for PD-L1 inhibitors (atezolizumab, durvalumab, and avelumab) for the treatment of various malignancies including bladder cancer, NSCLC, SCLC, breast cancer, melanoma, hepatocellular carcinoma, Merkel cell carcinoma, and renal cell carcinoma. The sixth approval (2018) was for cemiplimab, another PD-1 monoclonal antibody, for patients with metastatic or locally advanced cutaneous squamous cell carcinoma, and later for NSCLC and basal cell carcinoma (2021). Most recently, dostarlimab was approved in 2021 for the treatment of endometrial carcinoma and mismatch repair deficient (dMMR) solid cancers. Many more are in the pipeline.

Therapies with ICPIs are an exciting prospect for PWH because they have the potential to not only treat the patient's cancer but also eliminate or reduce the HIV reservoirs that persist despite ART (Day et al., 2006; Trautmann et al., 2006). The concept behind this latter theoretical use is that HIV persistence is thought to stem primarily from the presence of integrated copies of the proviral genome within long-lived cells. Because active viral gene expression causes cell death due to viral cytopathic effects and the immune response, long-lived cells likely harbor transcriptionally silent, latent provirus, which is the remaining major barrier to finding a cure for HIV. Several studies offer evidence as to why PD-1 may be an important part of this process. PD-1 has been found to be upregulated on HIV-specific $CD8^+$ T-cells and has been correlated with disease progression (Day et al., 2006). Blockade of PD-L1 was shown to enhance IFN-γ secretion by HIV-specific $CD8^+$ T-cells, suggesting that PD-1 signaling might play a role in limiting T-cell responses against HIV (Petrovas et al., 2006; Zhang et al., 2007). Check points that are considered markers of T-cell exhaustion, such as PD-1, TIM-3, and LAG-3, have been used to predict time of viremia rebound after treatment interruption (Hurst et al., 2015). Another study suggested a role for the immune check point TIGIT in limiting antiviral T-cell responses in PWH (Chew et al., 2016). This study also showed that TIGIT expression was coexpressed with PD-1 and upregulated on T-cells from both PWH and simian immunodeficiency virus (SIV)-infected macaques. The AIDS Clinical Trials 5326 Study Team recently demonstrated that treatment with an anti-PD-L1 antibody enhanced HIV-specific $CD8^+$ T-cell response in 2 of 8 PWH on ART (Gay et al., 2017). Further, a recent sub-analysis of the AMC 095, "Nivolumab and Ipilimumab in Treating Patients with HIV-Associated Relapsed or Refractory Classical Hodgkin Lymphoma or Solid Tumors That Are Metastatic or Cannot Be Removed by Surgery," evaluated the frequency of replication-competent HIV in participants before cycle 1 and after at least one dose of therapy (for all samples available) among participants who had suppressed HIV RNA levels. This study demonstrated that among 33 participants who received nivolumab alone, there was no effect on HIV latency or the latent HIV reservoir. However, in 7 participants, a modest increase in cell-associated unspliced RNA was induced (CA-US HIV RNA) and may potentially eliminate cells containing replication-competent HIV (Rasmussen et al., 2021). A trial of IV pembrolizumab, given every 3 weeks to 32 PWH and cancer, demonstrated an increase in CA-US HIV RNA (NCT02595866; Uldrick et al., 2022). Although these studies suggest that immune check points may limit T-cell responses during HIV infection and that immune check point blockade might be beneficial in PWH, larger studies are required to determine the therapeutic benefit of immune check point blockade in PWH on ART.

With regard to cancer therapy, treatment with PD-1/PD-L1 inhibitors may be even more useful in people with cancer with than without HIV because at least one study recently observed that, while PD-L1 expression is high in tumor cells from both people with and without HIV and NSCLC, it was associated with poor prognosis only in PWH (Okuma et al., 2018). However, to date, only a handful of case reports and small case series offer data about PWH treated with these new medications (Guihot et al., 2018; Heppt et al., 2017; Le Garff et al., 2017; Wightman et al., 2015, Lurain et al., 2024). Many of the PD-1/PDL-1 inhibitor therapies currently in use or being tested in PWH have been mentioned throughout this chapter. A large retrospective study from the Cancer Therapy Using Checkpoint Inhibitors in People Living with HIV-International (CATCH-IT) Consortium evaluated 390 PWH who received anti-PD-1/PD-L1 therapies for a variety of cancers, including NSCLC, HCC, and head and neck squamous cell carcinoma, and concluded that immune check point inhibitors are safe for PWH (El Zarif et al., 2023). In addition, there are several larger clinical trials underway (Bender-Ignacio et al., 2018). The Cancer Immunotherapy Trials Network conducted a trial of pembrolizumab in PWH with solid tumors and Hodgkin's lymphoma (NCT02595866). They accrued 30 PWH and multiple different types of both cancers and found that pembrolizumab had acceptable safety in patients with cancer, treated with ART and a $CD4^{+}$ T-cell count of greater than 100 cells/mm^3. Despite the report of a treatment-emergent episode of B-cell clonal proliferation in a patient with KS, there was a clinical benefit to participants with lung cancer, NHL, and KS (Uldrick et al., 2019). Other trials are still pending, including one that will evaluate pembrolizumab in PWH and advanced cancers (NCT02595866). Nivolumab has been used safely in PWH and KS as well as a variety of solid tumors (Rajdev et al., 2024). A French trial will evaluate therapy with nivolumab in PWH with NSCLC (NCT03304093). Another French study is following PWH who receive ICPIs as part of routine cancer care to evaluate their safety and effects on the HIV reservoir (NCT03354936). Pending the results of these trials, HIV positivity is not thought to be a contraindication to treatment with PD-1 inhibitors, although PWH with low $CD4^{+}$ T-cell counts should be monitored closely both for treatment response and for IRIS.

REFERENCES

Abramson JS, Irwin KE, Frigault MJ, et al. Successful anti-CD19 CAR T-cell therapy in HIV-infected patients with refractory high-grade B-cell lymphoma. *Cancer.* 2019;125: 3692–3698.

Aboulafia DM. Kaposi's sarcoma. *Clinics Derm.* 2001;19(3):269–283.

Aboulafia DM, Puswella AL. Highly active antiretroviral therapy as the sole treatment for AIDS-related primary central nervous system lymphoma: a case report with implications for treatment. *AIDS Patient Care STDs.* 2007;21(12):900–907.

Ahdieh L, Munoz A, Vlahov D, et al. Cervical neoplasia and repeated positivity of human papillomavirus infection in human immunodeficiency virus-seropositive and -seronegative women. *Am J Epidemiol.* 2000;151(12):1148–1157.

Altekruse SF, Shiels MS, Modur SP, et al. Cancer burden attributable to cigarette smoking among HIV-infected people in North America. *AIDS.* 2018;32(4):513–521.

Alvarnas JC, Le Rademacher J, Wang Y, et al. Autologous hematopoietic cell transplantation for HIV-related lymphoma: results of the BMT CTN 0803/AMC 071 trial. *Blood.* 2016;128:1050–1058.

Ambinder RF, Wu J, Logan B, et al. Allogeneic hematopoietic cell transplant (alloHCT) for hematologic malignancies in human immunodeficiency virus infected (HIV) patients (pts): Blood and Marrow Transplant Clinical Trials Network (BMT CTN 0903)/ AIDS Malignancy Consortium (AMC-080) trial. *J Clin Oncol.* 2017;35(Suppl 15):abstr 7006.

Appleby P, Beral V, Newton R, et al. Highly active antiretroviral therapy and incidence of cancer in human immunodeficiency virus-infected adults. *Cancer Inst.* 2000;92:1823–1830.

Avivi I, Robinson S, Goldstone A. Clinical use of rituximab in hematological malignancies. *Br J Cancer.* 2003;89(8):1389–1394.

Ballerini P, Gaidano G, Gong JZ, et al. Multiple genetic lesions in acquired immunodeficiency syndrome-related non-Hodgkin's lymphoma. *Blood.* 1993;81(1):166–176.

Barillari G, Ensoli B. Angiogenic effects of extracellular human immunodeficiency virus type 1 Tat protein and its role in the pathogenesis of AIDS-associated Kaposi's sarcoma. *Clin Microbiol Rev.* 2002;15(2):310–326.

Bañon S, Machuca I, Araujo S, et al. Efficacy, safety, and lack of interactions with the use of raltegravir in HIV-infected patients undergoing antineoplastic chemotherapy. *J Intern AIDS Soc.* 2014;17(4 Suppl 3):19590.

Baptista MJ, Garcia O, Morgades M, et al. HIV-infection impact on clinical-biological features and outcome of diffuse large B-cell lymphoma treated with R-CHOP in the combination antiretroviral therapy era. *AIDS.* 2015;29:811–818.

Barbosa MS, Schlegel R. The E6 and E7 genes of HPV-18 are sufficient for inducing two-stage in vitro transformation of human keratinocytes. *Oncogene.* 1989;4(12):1529–1532.

Barozzi P, Luppi M, Facchetti F, et al. Post-transplant Kaposi sarcoma originates from the seeding of donor-derived progenitors. *Nature Med.* 2003;9(5):554–561.

Barta SK, Joshi J, Mounier N, et al. Central nervous system involvement in AIDS-related lymphomas. *Br J Haematol.* 2016;173:857–866.

Barta SK, Lee JY, Kaplan LD, et al. Pooled analysis of AIDS malignancy consortium trials evaluating rituximab plus CHOP or infusional EPOCH chemotherapy in HIV-associated non-Hodgkin lymphoma. *Cancer.* 2012;118:3977–3983.

Barta SK, Samuel MS, Xue X, et al. Changes in the influence of lymphoma- and HIV-specific factors on outcomes in AIDS-related non-Hodgkin lymphoma. *Ann Oncol.* 2015;26:958–966.

Barta SK, Xue X, Wang D, et al. A new prognostic score for AIDS-related lymphomas in the rituximab-era. *Haematologica.* 2014;99:1731–1737.

Barta SK, Xue X, Wang D, et al. Treatment factors affecting outcomes in HIV-associated non-Hodgkin lymphomas: a pooled analysis of 1546 patients. *Blood.* 2013;122:3251–3262.

Baumgartner JE, Rachlin JR, Beckstead JH, et al. Primary central nervous system lymphomas: natural history and response to radiation therapy in 55 patients with acquired immunodeficiency syndrome. *J Neurosurg.* 1990;73(2):206–211.

Bayraktar S, Bayraktar UD, Ramos JC, et al. Primary CNS lymphoma in HIV positive and negative patients: comparison of clinical characteristics, outcome and prognostic factors. *J Neurooncol.* 2011;101:257–265.

Bedi GC, Westra WH, Farzedegan H, et al. Microsatellite instability in primary neoplasms from HIV\+ patients. *Nature Med.* 1995;1(1):65–68.

Bender-Ignacio R, Lin LL, Rajdev L, et al. Evolving paradigms in HIV malignancies: review of ongoing clinical trials. *J Natl Compr Canc Netw.* 2018;16(8):1018–1026.

Benevolo M, Donà MG, Ravenda PS, et al. Anal human papillomavirus infection: prevalence, diagnosis and treatment of related lesions. *Expert Rev Anti Infect Ther.* 2016;14(5):465–477.

Beral V, Peterman T, Berkelman R, et al. AIDS-associated non-Hodgkin lymphoma. *Lancet.* 1991;337(8745):805–809.

Beral V, Peterman TA, Berkelman RL, et al. Kaposi's sarcoma among persons with AIDS: a sexually transmitted infection? *Lancet.* 1990;335(8682):123–128.

Berretta M, Cappellani A, Di Benedetto F, et al. Clinical presentation and outcome of colorectal cancer in PLWH: a clinical case–control study. *Onkologie.* 2009;32:319–324.

Berretta M, Zanet E, Basile F, et al. HIV positive patients with liver metastasis from colorectal cancer deserve the same therapeutic approach as the general population. *Onkkologie.* 2010;33:203–204.

Berry JM, Palefsky JM, Jay N, et al. Performance characteristics of anal cytology and human papillomavirus testing in patients with high-resolution anoscopy-guided biopsy of high-grade anal intraepithelial neoplasia. *Dis Colon Rectum.* 2009;52(2):239–247.

Berthold DR, Pond GR, Soban F, et al. Docetaxel plus prednisone or mitoxantrone plus prednisone for advanced prostate cancer: updated survival in the TAX 327 study. *J Clin Oncol.* 2008;26(2):242–245.

Besson C, Goubar A, Gabarre J, et al. Changes in AIDS-related lymphoma since the era of highly active antiretroviral therapy. *Blood.* 2001;98(8):2339–2344.

Bhikoo R, Allwood BW, Irusen EM, et al. Lung cancer presents at a younger age and is less likely to be curable in people living with HIV. *Respiration*. 2024;103(1):47–50.

Bini EJ, Park J, Francois F. Use of flexible sigmoidoscopy to screen for colorectal cancer in HIV-infected patients 50 years of age or older. *JAMA Intern Med*. 2006;166(15):1626–1631.

Bjorge T, Engeland A, Luostarinen T, et al. Human papillomavirus infection as a risk factor for anal and perianal skin cancer in a prospective study. *Br J Cancer*. 2002;87(1):61–64.

Blazy A, Hennequin C, Gornet JM, et al. Anal carcinomas in PLWH: high-dose chemoradiotherapy is feasible in the era of highly active antiretroviral therapy. *Dis Colon Rectum*. 2005;48(6):1176–1181.

Bosch FX, Manos MM, Munoz N, et al. Prevalence of human papillomavirus in cervical cancer: a worldwide perspective. *J Natl Cancer Inst*. 1995;87(11):796–802.

Bossolasco S, Cinque P, Ponzoni M, et al. Epstein–Barr virus DNA load in cerebrospinal fluid and plasma of patients with AIDS-related lymphoma. *J Neurovirol*. 2002;8(5):432–438.

Boudreaux AA, Smith LL, Cosby CD, et al. Intralesional vinblastine for cutaneous Kaposi's sarcoma associated with acquired immunodeficiency syndrome: a clinical trial to evaluate efficacy and discomfort associated with infection. *J Am Acad Derm*. 1993;28(1):61–65.

Boulanger E, Gerard L, Gabarre J, et al. Prognostic factors and outcome of human herpesvirus 8-associated primary effusion lymphoma in patients with AIDS. *J Clin Oncol*. 2005;23(19):4372–4380.

Bower M, Dalla Pria A, Coyle C, et al. Prospective stage-stratified approach to AIDS-related Kaposi's sarcoma. *J Clin Oncol*. 2014;32:409–414.

Bower M, Fox P, Fife K, et al. Highly active anti-retroviral therapy (HAART) prolongs time to treatment failure in Kaposi's sarcoma. *AIDS*. 1999;13(15):2105–2111.

Bower M, McCall-Peat N, Ryan N, et al. Protease inhibitors potentiate chemotherapy-induced neutropenia. *Blood*. 2004a;104(9): 2943–2946.

Bower M, Powles T, Nelson M, et al. HIV-related lung cancer in the era of highly active antiretroviral therapy. *AIDS (London)*. 2003;17(3):371–375.

Bower M, Powles T, Newsom-Davis T, et al. HIV-associated anal cancer: has highly active antiretroviral therapy reduced the incidence or improved the outcome? *J Acquir Immune Defic Syndr*. 2004b;37(5):1563–1565.

Brandão M, Bruzzone M, Franzoi MA, et al. Impact of HIV infection on baseline characteristics and survival of women with breast cancer. *AIDS*. 2021;35(4):605–618. http://doi:10.1097/QAD.0000000000002810. PMID: 33394680.

Brickman C, Palefsky JM. Review: human papillomavirus in the HIV-infected host: epidemiology and pathogenesis in the antiretroviral era. *Curr HIV/AIDS Rep*. 2015;12(1):6–15.

Burkes RL, Meyer PR, Gill PS, et al. Rectal lymphoma in homosexual men. *Arch Intern Med*. 1986;146(5):913–915.

Cadranel J, Garfield D, Lavole A, et al. Lung cancer in HIV infected patients: facts, questions, and challenges. *Thorax*. 2006;61:1000–1008.

Calabresi A, Ferraresi A, Festa A, et al. Incidence of AIDS-defining cancers and virus-related and non-virus-related non-AIDS-defining cancers among HIV-infected patients compared with the general population in a large health district of northern Italy, 1999–2000. *HIV Med*. 2013;14(8):481–490.

Cannon MJ. Kaposi's sarcoma-associated herpesvirus and acquired immunodeficiency syndrome-related malignancy. *Semin Oncol*. 2000;27:408–419.

Cannon MJ, Dollard SC, Smith DK, et al. Blood-borne and sexual transmission of human herpesvirus 8 in women with or at risk for human immunodeficiency virus infection. *N Engl J Med*. 2001;344(9):637–643.

Cappell MS, Yao F, Cho KC. Colonic adenocarcinoma associated with the acquired immune deficiency syndrome. *Cancer*. 1988:62:616–619.

Casper C, Carrell D, Miller KG, et al. HIV serodiscordant sex partners and the prevalence of human herpesvirus 8 infection among HIV negative men who have sex with men: baseline data from the EXPLORE study. *Sex Transm Infect*. 2006;82(3):229–235.

Casper C, Krantz E, Selke S, et al. Frequent and asymptomatic oropharyngeal shedding of human herpesvirus 8 among immunocompetent men. *J Infect Dis*. 2007;195(1):30–36.

Casper C, Redman M, Huang ML, et al. HIV infection and human herpesvirus-8 oral shedding among men who have sex with men. *J Acquir Immune Defic Syndr*. 2004;35(3):233–238.

Castilho JL, Luz PM, Shepherd BE, et al. HIV and cancer: a comparative retrospective study of Brazilian and US clinical cohorts. *Infect Agent Cancer*. 2015;10(4):1–10.

Castillo JJ, Furman M, Beltrán BE, et al. Human immunodeficiency virus–associated plasmablastic lymphoma. *Cancer*. 2012;118:5270–5277.

Cattaneo C, Re A, Ungari M, et al. Plasmablastic lymphoma among human immunodeficiency virus-positive patients: results of a single center's experience. *Leuk Lymphoma*. 2015;56:267–269.

Centers for Disease Control and Prevention (CDC). AIDS-defining conditions. https://www.cdc.gov/mmwr/preview/mmwrhtml/rr5710a2.htm. Published 2008. Accessed October 8, 2022.

CDC. Human papillomavirus-associated cancers—United States, 2004–2008. *MMWR*. 2012;61(15):258–261.

CDC. Human papilloma virus (HPV): administering HPV vaccine. https://www.cdc.gov/vaccines/vpd/hpv/hcp/administration.html#:~:text=Dosage%20and%20Schedule,-CDC%20recommends%20routine&text=HPV%20vaccination%20is%20administered%20as,years%2C%20and%20for%20immunocompromised%20persons. Published November 16, 2021. Accessed August 13, 2024.

Chadburn A, Abdul-Nabi AM, Teruya BS, et al. Lymphoid proliferations associated with human immunodeficiency virus infection. *Arch Path Lab Med*. 2013;137(3):360–370.

Chang Y, Cesarman E, Pessin MS, et al. Identification of herpesvirus-like DNA sequences in AIDS-associated Kaposi's sarcoma. *Science*. 1994;266(5192):1865–1869.

Chapman C, Aboulafia DM, Dezube BJ, et al. Human immunodeficiency virus-associated adenocarcinoma of the colon: clinicopathologic findings and outcome. *Clin Colorectal Cancer*. 2009;8(4):215–219.

Chaturvedi AK, Madeleine MM, Biggar RJ, et al. Risk of human papillomavirus-associated cancers among persons with AIDS. *J Natl Cancer Inst*. 2009;101(16):1120–1130.

Chen YH, Lin MW, Bhatia K, et al. Cancer incidence in a nationwide HIV/AIDS patient cohort in Taiwan in 1998–2000. *J Acquir Immune Defic Syndr*. 2014;65(4):463–472.

Chew GM, Fujita T, Webb GM, et al. TIGIT marks exhausted T cells, correlates with disease progression, and serves as a target for immune restoration in HIV and SIV infection. *PLoS Pathog*. 2016;12:e1005349.

Chiao EY, Dezube BJ, Krown SE, et al. Time for oncologists to opt in for routine opt-out HIV testing? *JAMA*. 2010;304(3):334–339.

Chiao EY, Giordano TP, Richardson P, et al. Human immunodeficiency virus-associated squamous cell cancer of the anus: epidemiology and outcomes in the highly active antiretroviral therapy era. *J Clin Oncol*. 2008;26(3):474–479.

Chin-Hong PV, Vittinghoff E, Cranston RD, et al. Age-specific prevalence of anal human papillomavirus infection in HIV-negative sexually active men who have sex with men: the EXPLORE study. *J Infect Dis*. 2004;190(12):2070–2076.

Chokunonga E, Levy LM, Bassett MT, et al. Cancer incidence in the African population of Harare, Zimbabwe: second results from the cancer registry 1993–1995. *Int J Cancer*. 2000;85(1):54–59.

Cianfrocca M, Lee S, Von Roenn J, et al. Randomized trial of paclitaxel vs. pegylated liposomal doxorubicin for advanced human immunodeficiency virus-associated Kaposi sarcoma: evidence of symptom palliation from chemotherapy. *Cancer*. 2010;116(16):3969–3977.

Cingolani A, Fratino L, Scoppettuolo G, et al. Changing pattern of primary cerebral lymphoma in the highly active antiretroviral therapy era. *J Neurovirol*. 2005; 11(Suppl 3):38–44.

Cleator S, Fife K, Nelson M, et al. Treatment of HIV-associated invasive anal cancer with combined chemoradiation. *Eur J Cancer (Oxford: 1990)*. 2000;36(6):754–758.
Clifford GM, Lise M, Franceschi S, et al. Lung cancer in the Swiss HIV Cohort Study: role of smoking, immunodeficiency, and pulmonary infection. *Br J Cancer*. 2012;106:448–452.
Clifford GM, Polesel J, Richenbach M, et al. Cancer risk in the Swiss HIV Cohort Study: associations with immunodeficiency, smoking, and highly active antiretroviral therapy. *J Natl Cancer Inst*. 2005;97(6):425–432.
Coghill AE, Shiels MS, Suneja G, et al. Elevated cancer-specific mortality among HIV-infected patients in the United States. *J Clin Oncol*. 2015;33(21):2376–2383.
Conti S, Masocco M, Pezzotti P, et al. Differential impact of combined antiretroviral therapy on the survival of Italian patients with specific AIDS-defining illnesses. *J Acquir Immune Defic Syndr*. 2000;25(5):451–458.
Cooper JS, Steinfeld AD, Lerch I. Intentions and outcomes in the radiotherapeutic management of epidemic Kaposi's sarcoma. *Int J Radiat Oncol Biol Phys*. 1991;20(3):419–422.
Corales R, Taege A, Rehm S, et al. Regression of AIDS-related CNS lymphoma with HAART. Abstract MoPpB1086. Proceedings of the XIII International AIDS Conference. Durban, South Africa; 2000.
Cote TR, Biggar RJ, Rosenberg PS, et al. Non-Hodgkin's lymphoma among people with AIDS: incidence, presentation and public health burden. *Int J Cancer*. 1997;73(5):645–650.
Cote TR, Manns A, Hardy CR, et al.; AIDS/Cancer Study Group. Epidemiology of brain lymphoma among people with or without acquired immunodeficiency syndrome. *J Natl Cancer Inst*. 1996;88(10):675–679.
Coutinho R, Pria AD, Gandhi S, et al. HIV status does not impair the outcome of patients diagnosed with diffuse large B-cell lymphoma treated with R-CHOP in the cART era. *AIDS*. 2014;28:689–697.
Crothers K, Huang, L, Goulet JL, et al. HIV infection and risk for incident pulmonary diseases in the combination antiretroviral therapy era. *Am J Respir Crit Care Med*. 2011;183(3):388–395.
Da Gramont A, Van Cutsem E, Schmoll HJ, et al. Bevacizumab plus oxaliplatin-based chemotherapy as adjuvant treatment for colon cancer (AVANT): a phase 3 randomised controlled trial. *Lancet Oncol*. 2012;13(12):1225–1233.
Daling JR, Weiss NS, Hislop TG, et al. Sexual practices, sexually transmitted diseases, and the incidence of anal cancer. *N Engl J Med*. 1987;317(16):973–977.
Danzig JB, Brandt LJ, Reinus JF, et al. Gastrointestinal malignancy in patients with AIDS. *Am J Gastroenterol*. 1991;86(6):715–718.
Day CL, Kaufmann DE, Kiepiela P, et al. PD-1 expression on HIV-specific T cells is associated with T-cell exhaustion and disease progression. *Nature*. 2006;443:350–354.
Dedicoat M, Newton R, Alkharsah KR, et al. Mother-to-child transmission of human herpesvirus-8 in South Africa. *J Infect Dis*. 2004;190(6):1068–1075.
Deregibus M, Cantalupp IV, Doublier S, et al. HIV-1-Tat protein activates phosphatidylinositol 3-kinase/AKT-dependent survival pathways in Kaposi's sarcoma cells. *J Biol Chem*. 2002;277(28):25195–25202.
Dezube BJ, Pantanowitz L, Aboulafia DM. Management of AIDS-related Kaposi sarcoma: advances in target discovery and treatment. *AIDS Reader*. 2004;14(5):236–238, 243.
Diez-Martin J, Balsalobre P, Carrion R. et al. Long-term survival after autologous stem cell transplant (ASCT) in AIDS related lymphoma patients (Abstract 868). *Blood*. 2003;247a:102.
Diez-Martin JL, Balsalobre P, Re A, et al. Comparable survival between HIV\+ and HIV–non-Hodgkin and Hodgkin lymphoma patients undergoing autologous peripheral blood stem cell transplantation. *Blood*. 2009;113(23):6011–6014.
DiGiusto DL, Cannon PM, Holmes MC, et al. Preclinical development and qualification of ZFN-mediated CCR5 disruption in human hematopoietic stem/progenitor cells. *Mol Ther Methods Clin Dev*. 2016;3:16067.
D'Jaen GA, Pantanowitz L, Bower M, et al. Human immunodeficiency virus-associated primary lung cancer in the era of highly active antiretroviral therapy: a multi-institutional collaboration. *Clin Lung Cancer*. 2010;11(6):396–404.
Donahue BR, Sullivan JW, Cooper JS. Additional experience with empiric radiotherapy for presumed human immunodeficiency virus-associated primary central nervous system lymphoma. *Cancer*. 1995;76(2):328–332.
Dryden-Peterson S, Bvochora-Nsingo M, Suneja G, et al. HIV infection and survival among women with cervical cancer. *J Clin Oncol*. 2016;34:3749–3757.
D'Souza G, Wiley D, Li X, et al. Incidence and epidemiology of anal cancer in the multicenter AIDS cohort study. *J Acquir Immune Defic Syndr*. 2008;48:491–499.
Dubrow R, Qin L, Lin H, et al. Association of CD4\+ T-cell count, HIV-1 RNA viral load, and antiretroviral therapy with Kaposi sarcoma risk among HIV-infected persons in the United States and Canada. *J Acquir Immune Defic Syndr*. 2017;75(4):382–390.
Duncan KC, Chan KJ, Chiu CG, et al. HAART slows progression to anal cancer in HIV-infected MSM. *AIDS*. 2015;29:305–311.
Dunleavy K, Pittaluga S, Shovlin M, et al. Low-intensity therapy in adults with Burkitt's lymphoma. *N Engl J Med*. 2013;369:1915–1925.
Durand CM, Capoferri AA, Redd AD, et al. Allogeneic bone marrow transplantation with post-transplant cyclophosphamide for patients with HIV and haematological malignancies: a feasibility study. *Lancet HIV*. 2020;7(9):e602–e610.
Dutta A, Uno H, Holman A, et al. Racial differences in prostate cancer risk in young HIV-positive and HIV-negative men: a prospective cohort study. *Cancer Causes Control*. 2017;28(7):767–777.
Eberhard JM, Angin M, Passaes C, et al. Vulnerability to reservoir reseeding due to high immune activation after allogeneic hematopoietic stem cell transplantation in individuals with HIV-1. *Sci Transl Med*. 2020;12(542):eaay9355.
Ekstein D, Ben-Yehuda D, Slyusarevsky E, et al. CSF analysis of IgH gene rearrangement in CNS lymphoma: relationship to the disease course. *J Neurol Sci*. 2006;247:39–46.
El Amari EB, Toutous-Trellu L, Gayet-Ageron A, et al. Predicting the evolution of Kaposi sarcoma in the highly active antiretroviral therapy era. *AIDS*. 2008;22(9):1019–1028.
El-Sadr WM, Lundgren J, Neaton JD, et al. CD4\+ count-guided interruption of antiretroviral treatment. *N Engl J Med*. 2006;355:2283–2296.
El-Solh A, Kumar NM, Nair MP, et al. An RDG-containing peptide from HIV-1 TAT-(65–80) modulates protooncogene expression in human bronchoalveolar carcinoma cell line, A549. *Immunol Invest*. 1997;26(3):351–370.
El Zarif T, Nassar AH, Adib E, et al. Safety and activity of immune checkpoint inhibitors in people living with HIV and cancer: a real-world report from the Cancer Therapy Using Checkpoint Inhibitors in People Living with HIV-International (CATCH-IT) Consortium. *J Clin Oncol*. 2023;41(21):3712–3723.
Engels EA, Biggar RJ, Hall I, et al. Cancer risk in people infected with human immunodeficiency virus in the United States. *Intern J Cancer*. 2008;123:187–194.
Engels EA, Biggar RJ, Marshall VA, et al. Detection and quantification of Kaposi's sarcoma-associated herpesvirus to predict AIDS-associated Kaposi's sarcoma. *AIDS (London)*. 2003;17(12):1847–1851.
Engels EA, Brock MV, Chen J, et al. Elevated incidence of lung cancer among HIV-infected individuals. *J Clin Oncol*. 2006;24(9):1383–1388.
Engels EA, Shiels MS, Barnabas RV, et al. State of the science and future directions for research on HIV and cancer: summary of a joint workshop sponsored by IARC and NCI. *Int J Cancer*. 2024;154(4):596–606. doi:10.1002/ijc.34727
Ensoli B, Barillari G, Salahuddin S, et al. Tat protein of HIV-1 stimulates growth of cells derived from Kaposi's sarcoma lesions of AIDS patients. *Nature*. 1990;345(6270):84–86.
European AIDS Clinical Society (EACS). Guidelines version 12.0. https:// eacs.sanfordguide.com. Published October 2023. Accessed August 13, 2024.

Fantry LE, Nowak RG, Fisher LH, et al. Colonoscopy findings in HIV-infected men and women from an urban US cohort compared with non-HIV-infected men and women. *AIDS Res Hum Retroviruses.* 2016;32(9):860–867

Ferreri AJM, Cwynarski K, Pulczynski E, et al. Chemoimmunotherapy with methotrexate, cytarabine, thiotepa, and rituximab (MATRix regimen) in patients with primary CNS lymphoma: results of the first randomisation of the International Extranodal Lymphoma Study Group-32 (IELSG32) phase 2 trial. *Lancet Haematol.* 2016;3(5):e217–e227.

Ferreri AJM, Cwynarski K, Pulczynski E, et al. Whole-brain radiotherapy or autologous stem-cell transplantation as consolidation strategies after high-dose methotrexate-based chemoimmunotherapy in patients with primary CNS lymphoma: results of the second randomisation of the International Extranodal Lymphoma Study Group-32 phase 2 trial. *Lancet Haematol.* 2017;4(11):e510–e523.

Ferron P, Asfour SS, Metsch LR, et al. Impact of a multifaceted intervention on promoting adherence to screening colonoscopy among persons in HIV primary care: a pilot study. *Clin Transi Sci.* 2015;8(4):290–297.

Firnhaber C, Swarts A, Goeieman B, et al. Cryotherapy reduces progression of cervical intraepithelial neoplasia grade 1 in South African HIV-infected women: a randomized, controlled trial. *J Acquir Immune Defic Syndr.* 2017;76(5):532–538.

Foulot H, Heard I, Potard V, et al. Surgical management of cervical intraepithelial neoplasia in HIV-infected women. *Eur J Obstet Gynecol Reprod Biol.* 2008;141:153–157.

Franceschi S, Dal Maso L, Rickenbach M, et al. Kaposi sarcoma incidence in the Swiss HIV Cohort Study before and after highly active antiretroviral therapy. *Br J Cancer.* 2008;99(5):800–804.

Fraunholz I, Rabeneck D, Gerstein J, et al. Concurrent chemoradiotherapy with 5-fluorouracil and mitomycin C for anal carcinoma: are there differences between HIV-positive and HIV-negative patients in the era of highly active antiretroviral therapy? *Radiother Oncol.* 2011;98(1):99–104.

Friedman SL. Gastrointestinal and hepatobiliary neoplasms in AIDS. *Gastroenterol Clin North Am.* 1988;17(3):465–486.

Friedman-Kien AE. Disseminated Kaposi's sarcoma syndrome in young homosexual men. *J Am Acad Dermatol.* 1981;5(4):468–471.

Friedman-Kien AE, Saltzman BR. Clinical manifestations of classical, endemic African, and epidemic AIDS-associated Kaposi's sarcoma. *J Am Acad Dermatol.* 1990; 22(6 Pt 2):1237–1250.

Frisch M, Biggar RJ, Engels EA, et al.; AIDS–Cancer Match Registry Study Group. Association of cancer with AIDS-related immunosuppression in adults. *JAMA.* 2001;285(13):1736–1745.

Frisch M, Biggar RJ, Goedert JJ. Human papillomavirus-associated cancers in patients with human immunodeficiency virus infection and acquired immunodeficiency syndrome. *J Nat Cancer Institute.* 2000a;92(18):1500–1510.

Frisch M, Goodman MT. Human papillomavirus-associated carcinomas in Hawaii and the mainland U.S. *Cancer.* 2000b;88(6):1464–1469.

Fulco PP, Hynicka L, Rackley D. Raltegravir-based HAART regimen in a patient with large B-cell lymphoma. *Ann Pharmacother.* 2010;44(2):377–382.

Gabarre J, Azar N, Autran B, et al. High-dose therapy and autologous haematopoietic stem-cell transplantation for HIV-1-associated lymphoma. *Lancet.* 2000;355(9209):1071–1072.

Gage JT, Vance EA, Hildenbrand PG, et al. Brain lesion and AIDS. *Proc Baylor Univ Medical Center.* 2000;13(4):424–429.

Gaidano G, Dalla-Favera R. Molecular pathogenesis of AIDS-related lymphomas. *Adv Cancer Res.* 1995;67:113–153.

Gaisa M, Ita-Nagy F, Sigel K, et al. High rates of anal high-grade squamous intraepitelial lesions in HIV-infected women who do not meet screening guidelines. *Clin Infect Dis.* 2017;64(3)289–294.

Garon EB, Rizvi NA, Hui R, et al. Pembrolizumab for the treatment of non-small-cell lung cancer. *N Engl J Med.* 2015;372:2018–2028.

Gates AE, Kaplan LD. Biology and management of AIDS-associated non-Hodgkin's lymphoma. *Hematol Oncol Clin North Am.* 2003;17(3):821–841.

Gay CL, Bosch RJ, Ritz J, et al. Clinical trial of the anti-PD-L1 antibody BMS-936559 in HIV-1 infected participants on suppressive antiretroviral therapy. *J Infect Dis.* 2017 Jun 1;215(11):1725–1733.

Gbabe OF, Okwundu CI: Dedicoat M, et al. Treatment of severe or progressive Kaposi's sarcoma in HIV-infected adults. *Cochrane Database Syst Rev.* 2014;9:CD003256.

Gerard L, Meignin V, Galicier L, et al. Characteristics of non-Hodgkin lymphoma arising in HIV-infected patients with suppressed HIV replication. *AIDS.* 2009;23(17):2301–2308.

Gill ON, Weinberg JR, Fisher IS, et al. Meta-surveillance: safer cyber-surveillance. *Lancet.* 1995;346(8977):776.

Gill PS, Akil B, Colletti P, et al. Pulmonary Kaposi's sarcoma: clinical findings and results of therapy. *Am J Med.* 1989;87(1):57–61.

Gill PS, Wernz J, Scadden DT, et al. Randomized phase III trial of liposomal daunorubicin vs. doxorubicin, bleomycin, and vincristine in AIDS-related Kaposi's sarcoma. *J Clin Oncol.* 1996;14(8):2353–2364.

Goldstein JD, Dickson DW, Moser FG, et al. Primary central nervous system lymphoma in acquired immune deficiency syndrome: a clinical and pathologic study with results of treatment with radiation. *Cancer.* 1991;67(11):2756–2765.

Gopal S, Patel MR, Yanik EL, et al. Temporal trends in presentation and survival for HIV-associated lymphoma in the antiretroviral therapy era. *J Natl Cancer Inst.* 2013;105:1221–1229.

Gosselaar C, Roobol MJ, Roemeling S, et al. The role of the digital rectal examination in subsequent screening visits in the European Randomized Study of Screening for Prostate Cancer (ERSPC), Rotterdam. *Eur Urol.* 2008;54:581–588.

Gosselaar C, Roobol MJ, van den Bergh RC, et al. Digital rectal examination and the diagnosis of prostate cancer—a study based on 8 years and three screenings within the European Randomized Study of Screening for Prostate Cancer (ERSPC), Rotterdam. *Eur Urol.* 2009;55(1):139–146.

Govindarajan A, Coburn NH, Kiss A, et al. Population-based assessment of the surgical management of locally advanced colorectal cancer. *J Natl Cancer Inst.* 2006;98(20):1474–1481.

Grew D, Bitterman D, Leichman CG, et al. HIV infection is associated with poor outcomes for patients with anal cancer in the highly active antiretroviral therapy era. *Dis Colon Rectum.* 2015;58(12):1130–1136.

Grimm P, Billiet I, Bostwick D, et al. Comparative analysis of prostate specific antigen free survival outcomes for patients with low, intermediate, and high risk prostate cancer treatment by radical therapy: results from the Prostate Cancer Results Study Group. *Br J Urol Int.* 2012;109(Suppl 1):22–29.

Grover S, Desir F, Jing Y, et al. Reduced cancer survival among adults with HIV and AIDS-defining illnesses despite no difference in cancer stage at diagnosis. *J Acquir Immune Defic Syndr.* 2018;79(4):421–429.

Gruffaz M, Vasan K, Tan B, et al. TLR4-mediated inflammation promotes KSHV-induced cellular transformation and tumorigenesis by activating the STAT3 pathway. *Cancer Res.* 2018 Dec 15;77(24):7094–7108.

Guerrero-Garcia TA, Mogollon RJ, Castillo JJ. Bortezomib in plasmablastic lymphoma: a glimpse of hope for a hard-to-treat disease. *Leuk Res.* 2017;62:12–16.

Guiguet M, Boue F, Cadranel J, et al. Effect of immunodeficiency, HIV viral load, and antiretroviral therapy on the risk of individual malignancies (FHDH-ANRS CO4): a prospective cohort study. *Lancet Oncol.* 2009;10(12):1152–1159.

Guihot A, Marcelin, AG, Massiani MA, et al. Drastic decrease of the HIV reservoir in a patient treated with nivolumab for lung cancer. *Ann Oncol.* 2018;29(2):517–518.

Gupta NK, Nolan A, Omuro A, et al. Long-term survival in AIDS-related primary central nervous system lymphoma. *Neuro Oncol.* 2017;19:99–108.

Hamilton-Dutoit SJ, Pallesen G, Karkov J, et al. Identification of EBV-DNA in tumour cells of AIDS-related lymphomas by in-situ hybridisation. *Lancet.* 1989;1(8637):554–552.

Haq IU, Dalla Pria A, Papanastasopoulos P, et al. The clinical application of plasma Kaposi sarcoma herpesvirus viral load as a tumour biomarker: results from 704 patients. *HIV Med.* 2016;17:56–61.

Heard I, Etienney I, Potard V, et al. High prevalence of anal human papillomavirus-associated cancer precursors in a contemporary cohort of asymptomatic HIV-infected women. *Clin Infect Dis.* 2015;60(10):1559–1568.

Heard I, Pizot-Martin I, Potard V, et al. Prevalence of and risk factors for anal oncogenic human papillomavirus infection among HIV-infected women in France in the combination antiretroviral therapy era. *J Infect Dis.* 2016;213(9):1455–1461.

Heidenreich A, Bastian PJ, Bellmunt J, et al. European Association of Urology (EAU) guidelines on prostate cancer: part 1. Screening, diagnosis, and local treatment with curative intent—update 2013. *Eur Urol.* 2014;65(1):124–137.

Hengge UR, Ruzicka T, Tyring SK, et al. Update on Kaposi's sarcoma and other HHV8 associated diseases: part 1. Epidemiology, environmental predispositions, clinical manifestations, and therapy. *Lancet Infect Dis.* 2002;2(5):281–292.

Henrich TJ, Hanhauser E, Marty FM, et al. Antiretroviral-free HIV-1 remission and viral rebound after allogeneic stem cell transplantation: report of 2 cases. *Ann Intern Med.* 2014;161:319–327.

Heppt MV, Schlaak M, Eigenlter TK et al. Checkpoint blockade for metastatic melanoma and Merkel cell carcinoma in PLWH. *Ann Oncol.* 2017;28(12):3104–3106.

Herida M, Mary-Krause M, Kaphan R, et al. Incidence of non-AIDS defining cancers before and during the highly active antiretroviral therapy era in a cohort of human immunodeficiency virus-infected patients. *J Clin Oncol.* 2003;21;3447–3453.

Hernández-Ramírez RU, Shiels MS, Dubrow R, et al. Cancer risk in HIV-infected people in the USA from 1996 to 2012: a population-based, registry-linkage study. *Lancet HIV.* 2017;4(11):e495–e504.

Hessol NA, Whittemore H, Vittinghoff E, et al. Incidence of first and second primary cancers diagnosed among people with HIV, 1985–2013: a population-based, registry linkage study. *Lancet HIV.* 2018;5(11):e647–e655.

Hill DR. The role of radiotherapy for epidemic Kaposi's sarcoma. *Semin Oncol.* 1987;14:1207.

Hirsch B, Fine SM, Vail R, et al. *Screening for Anal Dysplasia and Cancer in Adults with HIV.* Baltimore, MD: Johns Hopkins University Press; 2022 Aug. PMID: 32369310.

Hladik W, Dollard SC, Mermin J, et al. Transmission of human herpesvirus 8 by blood transfusion. *N Engl J Med.* 2006;355(13):1331–1338.

Hoffmann C, Tabrizian S, Wolf E, et al. Survival of AIDS patients with primary central nervous system lymphoma is dramatically improved by HAART-induced immune recovery. *AIDS.* 2001;15(16):2119–2127.

Hoover DR, Black C, Jacobson LP, et al. Epidemiologic analysis of Kaposi's sarcoma as an early and later AIDS outcome in homosexual men. *Am J Epidemiol.* 1993;138(4):266–278.

Horner MJ, Shiels MS, Pfeiffer RM, et al. Deaths attributable to cancer in the United States HIV population during 2001–2015. *Clin Infect Dis.* 2021;72(9):e224–e231.

Hosseinipour MC, Kang M, Krown SE, Bukuru A, et al. As-needed vs immediate etoposide NCT03094286chemotherapy in combination with antiretroviral therapy for mild-to-moderate AIDS-associated Kaposi sarcoma in resource-limited settings: A5264/AMC-067 Randomized clinical trial. *Clin Infect Dis.* 2018;67(2):251–260.

Howlader N, Noone AM, Krapcho M, et al. *SEER Statistics Review, 1975–2012.* Bethesda, MD: National Cancer Institute; 2015. http://seer.cancer.gov/archive/csr/1975_2012

Hsiao W, Anastasia K, Hall J, et al. Association between HIV status and positive prostate biopsy in a study of US veterans. *Scientific World J.* 2009;9:102–108.

Huncharek M, Haddock KS, Reid R, et al. Smoking as a risk factor for prostate cancer: a meta-analysis of 24 prospective cohort studies. *Am J Pub Health.* 2010;100(4):693–701.

Hurst J, Hoffmann M, Pace M, et al. Immunological biomarkers predict HIV-1 viral rebound after treatment interruption. *Nat Commun.* 2015;6:8495.

Hutter G, Nowak D, Mossner M, et al. Long-term control of HIV by CCR5 Delta32/Delta32 stem-cell transplantation. *N Engl J Med.* 2009;360:692–698.

Impola U, Cuccuru MA, Masala MV, et al. Preliminary communication: matrix metalloproteinases in Kaposi's sarcoma. *Br J Dermatol.* 2003;149(4):905–907.

International Agency for Research on Cancer. *Human Immunodeficiency Viruses and Human T-Cell Lymphotropic Viruses.* Geneva: World Health Organization; 1996.

Iscovich J, Boffetta P, Franceschi S, et al. Classic Kaposi sarcoma: epidemiology and risk factors. *Cancer.* 2000;88(3):500–517.

Islami F, Ferlay J, Lortet-Tieulent J, et al. International trends in anal cancer incidence rates. *Int J Epidemiol.* 2017;46(3):924–938. doi:10.1093/ije/dyw276

Islami F, Moreira DM, Boffetta P, et al. A systematic review and meta-analysis of tobacco use and prostate cancer mortality and incidence in prospective cohort-studies. *Eur Urol.* 2014;66(6):1054–1064.

Jacobson LP, Jenkins FJ, Springer G, et al. Interaction of human immunodeficiency virus type 1 and human herpesvirus type 8 infections on the incidence of Kaposi's sarcoma. *J Infect Dis.* 2000;181(6):1940–1949.

Jacomet C, Girard PM, Lebrette MG, et al. Intravenous methotrexate for primary central nervous system non-Hodgkin's lymphoma in AIDS. *AIDS.* 1997;11(14):1725–1730.

Jephcott CR, Paltiel C, Hay J. Quality of life after non-surgical treatment of anal carcinoma: a case–control study of long-term survivors. *Clin Oncol.* 2004;16(8):530–535.

Johnson LG, Madeleine MM, Newcomer LM, et al. Anal cancer incidence and survival: the surveillance, epidemiology, and end results experience, 1973–2000. *Cancer.* 2004;101(2):281–288.

Johnston C, Harrington R, Jain R, et al. Safety and efficacy of combination antiretroviral therapy in human immunodeficiency virus-infected adults undergoing autologous or allogeneic hematopoietic cell transplantation for hematologic malignancies. *Biol Blood Marrow Transplant.* 2016;22:149–156.

Joseph DA, King JB, Miller JW, et al. Prevalence of colorectal cancer screening among adults—behavioral risk factor surveillance system, United States, 2010. *MMWR.* 2012;61(2):51–56.

Kahn S, Jani A, Edelman S, et al. Matched cohort analysis of outcomes of definitive radiotherapy for prostate cancer in human immunodeficiency virus-positive patients. *Int Radiat Oncol Biol Physics.* 2012;83(1):16–21.

Kalamya JN, DeCuir J, Alger SX, et al. Provision of cervical cancer services for women living with HIV, Uganda. *Bull World Health Organ.* 2024;102(6):382–388.

Kaplan LD, Abrams DI, Feigal E, et al. AIDS-associated non-Hodgkin's lymphoma in San Francisco. *JAMA.* 1989;261(5):719–724.

Kaplan LD, Hopewell PC, Jaffe H, et al. Kaposi's sarcoma involving the lung in patients with the acquired immunodeficiency syndrome. *J Acquir Immune Defic Syndr.* 1988;1(1):23–30.

Kaplan LD, Straus DJ, Testa MA, et al. Low-dose compared with standard-dose m-BACOD chemotherapy for non-Hodgkin's lymphoma associated with human immunodeficiency virus infection. National Institute of Allergy and Infectious Diseases AIDS Clinical Trials Group. *N Engl J Med.* 1997;336(23):1641–1648.

Karp J, Profeta G, Marantz PR, et al. Lung cancer in patients with immunodeficiency syndrome. *Chest.* 1993;103(2):410–413.

Kelly H, Chikandiwa A, Vilches LA, et al. Association of antiretroviral therapy with anal high-risk human papillomavirus, anal intraepithelial neoplasia, and anal cancer in people living with HIV: a systematic review and meta-analysis. *Lancet HIV.* 2020;7(4):e262–e278.

Kelly H, Weiss HA, Benavente Y, et al. Association of antiretroviral therapy with high-risk human papillomavirus, cervical intraepithelial neoplasia, and invasive cervical cancer in women living with HIV: a systematic review and meta-analysis. *Lancet HIV.* 2018;5(1):e45–e58. doi:10.1016/S2352-3018(17)30149-2

Kimani S, Painschab MS, Kaimila B, et al. Safety and efficacy of rituximab in patients with diffuse large B-cell lymphoma in Malawi: a prospective, single-arm, non-randomized phase ½ clinical trial. *Lancet Glob Health.* 2021;9(7):e1008–e1016.

Kirk GD, Merlo C, O'Driscoll P, et al. HIV infection is associated with an increased risk for lung cancer, independent of smoking. *Clin Infect Dis.* 2007;45(1):103–110.

Kiviat NB, Hawes S, Lampinen T, et al. The effect of HAART on detection of anal HPV and squamous intraepithelial lesions among HIV infected homosexual men. Paper presented at the 6th International Conference on Malignancies in AIDS and Other Immunodeficiencies. Bethesda, MD; 2002.

Klugman AD, Schaffner J. Colon adenocarcinoma in HIV infection: a case report and review. *Am J Gastroenterol.* 1994;89(2):254–256.

Knowles DM. Etiology and pathogenesis of AIDS-related non-Hodgkin's lymphoma. *Hematol Oncol Clin North Am.* 1996;10(5):1081–1109.

Knowles DM. *Neoplastic Hematopathology.* Philadelphia: Lippincott Williams & Wilkins; 2001.

Knowles DM, Chamulak GA, Subar M, et al. Lymphoid neoplasia associated with the acquired immunodeficiency syndrome (AIDS): the New York University Medical Center experience with 105 patients (1981–1986). *Ann Intern Med.* 1988;108(5):744–753.

Kojic EM, Cu-Uvin S, Conley L, et al. Human papillomavirus infection and cytologic abnormalities of the anus and cervix among HIV-infected women in the study to understand the natural history of HIV/AIDS in the era of effective therapy (the SUN study). *Sex Transm Dis.* 2011;38(4):253–259.

Komanduri KV, Luce JA, McGrath MS, et al. The natural history and molecular heterogeneity of HIV-associated primary malignant lymphomatous effusions. *J Acquir Immune Defic Syndr.* 1996;13(3):215–226.

Kong CY, Sigel K, Criss SD, et al. Benefits and harms of lung cancer screening in HIV-infected individuals with CD4\+ cell count at least 500 cells/μl. *AIDS.* 2018;32(10):1333–1342.

Koon HB, Krown SE, Lee JY, et al. Phase II trial of imatinib in AIDS-associated Kaposi's sarcoma: AIDS Malignancy Consortium Protocol 042. *J Clin Oncol.* 2014;32(5):402–408.

Kowalkowski MA, Day RS, Chan W, et al. Cumulative HIV viremia and non-AIDs-defining malignancies among a sample of HIV-infected male veterans. *J Acquir Immune Defic Syndr.* 2014;62(2):204–211.

Krishnan A, Molina A, Zaia J, et al. Durable remissions with autologous stem cell transplantation for high-risk HIV-associated lymphomas. *Blood.* 2005;105(2):874–878.

Krown SE, Metroka C, Wernz JC. Kaposi's sarcoma in the acquired immune deficiency syndrome: a proposal for uniform evaluation, response, and staging criteria. AIDS Clinical Trials Group Oncology Committee. *J Clin Oncol.* 1989;7(9):1201–1207. doi:10.1200/JCO.1989.7.9.1201

Krown SE, Moser CB, MacPhail P, et al. Treatment of advanced AIDS-associated Kaposi sarcoma in resource-limited settings: a three-arm, open-label, randomised, non-inferiority trial. *Lancet.* 2020;395(10231):1195–1207.

Krown SE, Roy D, Lee JY, et al. Rapamycin with antiretroviral therapy in AIDS-associated Kaposi sarcoma: an AIDS Malignancy Consortium study. *J Acquir Immune Defic Syndr.* 2012;59(5):447–454.

Krown SE, Testa MA, Huang J. AIDS-related Kaposi's sarcoma: prospective validation of the AIDS Clinical Trials Group staging classification. AIDS Clinical Trials Group Oncology Committee. *J Clin Oncol.* 1997;15(9):3085–3092.

Lafrenie RM, Wahl LM, Epstein JS, et al. HIV-1-Tat modulates the function of monocytes and alters their interactions with microvessel endothelial cells: a mechanism of HIV pathogenesis. *J Immunol.* 1996;156(4):1638–1645.

Lavole A, Greillier L, Mazieres J, et al. First-Line carboplatin plus pemetrexed with pemetrexed maintenance in HIV+ patients with advanced non-squamous non-small cell lung cancer: the phase II IFCT-1001 CHIVA trial. *Eur Respir J.* 2020;56(2):1902066.

Leapman MS, Stone K, Wadia R, et al. Prostate cancer screening and incidence among aging persons living with HIV. *J Urol.* 2022;207(2):324–332.

Lederman MM, Cannon PM, Currier JS, et al. A cure for HIV infection: "not in my lifetime" or "just around the corner"? *Pathog Immun.* 2016;1:154–164.

Lee JY, Lensing SY, Berry-Lawhorn JM, et al. Design of the Anal Cancer/HSIL Outcomes Research study (ANCHOR study): a randomized study to prevent anal cancer among persons living with HIV. *Contemp Clin Trials.* 2022;113:106679.

Le Garff G, Samri A, Lambert-Niclot S, et al. Transient HIV-specific T cells increase inflammation in an HIV-infected patient treated with nivolumab. *AIDS.* 2017;31(7):1048–1051.

Lehnert T, Methner M, Pollok A, et al. Multivisceral resection for locally advanced primary colon and rectal cancer: an analysis of prognostic factors in 201 patients. *Ann Surg.* 2002;235(2):217–225.

Leiker AJ, Wang CJ, Sanford NN, et al. Feasibility and outcome of routine use of concurrent chemoradiation in PLWH with squamous cell anal cancer. *Am J Clin Oncol.* 2020;43(10):701–708.

Leport C, Rousseau F, Perronne C, et al. Bacterial prostatitis in patients infected with the human immunodeficiency virus. *J Urol.* 1989;141(2):334–336.

Letang E, Almeida J, Miró J, et al. Predictors of immune reconstitution inflammatory syndrome-associated with Kaposi sarcoma in Mozambique: a prospective study. *J Acquir Immune Defic Syndr.* 2010;53(5):589–597.

Levine AM, Seaberg EC, Hessol NA, et al. HIV as a risk factor for lung cancer in women: data from the Women's Interagency HIV study. *J Clin Oncol.* 2010;28(9):1514–1519.

Levine AM, Sullivan-Halley J, Pike MC, et al. Human immunodeficiency virus-related lymphoma: prognostic factors predictive of survival. *Cancer.* 1991;68(11):2466–2472.

Levine AM, Tulpule A. Clinical aspects and management of AIDS-related Kaposi's sarcoma. *Eur J Cancer.* 2001;37(10):1288–1295.

Lewitschnig S, Gedela K, Toby M, et al. 18F-FDG PET/CT in HIV-related central nervous system pathology. *Eur J Nucl Mol Imaging.* 2013;40(9):1420–1427.

Licho R, Litofsky NS, Senitko M, et al. Inaccuracy of Tl-201 brain SPECT in distinguishing cerebral infections from lymphoma in patients with AIDS. *Clin Nuclear Med.* 2002;27(2):81–86.

Liebowitz D, Kieff E. Epstein–Barr virus latent membrane protein: induction of B-cell activation antigens and membrane patch formation does not require vimentin. *J Virol.* 1989;63(9):4051–4054.

Lillo FB, Ferrari D, Veglia F, et al. Human papillomavirus infection and associated cervical disease in human immunodeficiency virus-infected women: effect of highly active antiretroviral therapy. *J Infect Dis.* 2001;184(5):547–551.

Lim S-T, Karim R, Tulpule A, et al. Prognostic factors in HIV-related diffuse large-cell lymphoma: before versus after highly active antiretroviral therapy. *J Clin Oncol.* 2005;23(33):8477–8482.

Lin W, Chen S. Checkpoint kinase 1 is overexpressed during hPV16-induced cervical carcinogenesis. *Gynecol Obstet Invest.* 2018;83(3):2990395.

Lince-Deroche N, Phiri J, Michelow P, et al. Costs and cost effectiveness of three approaches for cervical cancer screening among HIV-positive women in Johannesburg, South Africa. *PLoS One.* 2015;10(11):e0141969.

Lister A, Abrey LE, Sandlund JT. Central nervous system lymphoma. *Am Soc Hematol. Educ Prog.* 2002:283–296. doi:10.1182/asheducation-2002.1.283

Liu Y, Sigel KM, Westra W, et al. HIV-infected patients with anal cancer precursors: clinicopathological characteristics and human papillomavirus subtype distribution. *Dis Colon Rectum.* 2020;63(7):890–896.

Locker GY, Hamilton S, Harris J, et al. ASCO 2006 update of recommendations for the use of tumor markers in gastrointestinal cancer. *J Clin Oncol.* 2006:24(33):5313.

Loriot Y, Miler K, Sternberg CN, et al. Effect of enzalutamide on health-related quality of life, pain, and skeletal-related events in asymptomatic and minimally symptomatic, chemotherapy-naive patients with metastatic castration-resistant prostate cancer (PREVAIL): results from a randomised, phase 3 trial. *Lancet Oncol.* 2015;16(5):509–521.

Lowenthal DA, Straus DJ, Wise Campbell S, et al. AIDS-related lymphoid neoplasia: the Memorial Hospital experience. *Cancer.* 1988;61(11):2325–2337.

Luppi M, Barozzi P, Santagostino G, et al. Molecular evidence of organ-related transmission of Kaposi sarcoma-associated herpesvirus or human herpesvirus-8 in transplant patients. *Blood.* 2000;96(9):3279–3281.

Lurain K, Ramaswami R, Mangusan R, et al. Use of pembrolizumab with or without pomalidomide in HIV-associated non-Hodgkin's lymphoma. *J Immunother Cancer.* 2021 Feb;9(2):e002097.

Lurain K, Uldrick TS, Ramaswami R, et al. Treatment of HIV-associated primary CNS lymphoma with antiretroviral therapy, rituximab, and high-dose methotrexate. *Blood.* 2020;136(19):2229–2232.

Lurain K, Zarif TE, Ramaswami R, et al. Real-world multicenter study of PD-1 blockade in HIV-associated classical hodgkin lymphoma across the United States. *Clin Lymphoma Myeloma Leuk.* 2024;24(12):873. doi:10.1016/j.clml.2024.10.011. *Clin Lymphoma Myeloma Leuk.* 2024;24(8):523–530. doi:10.1016/j.clml.2024.03.011

Machalek DA, Poynten M, Jin F, et al. Anal human papillomavirus infection and associated neoplastic lesions in men who have sex with men: a systematic review and meta-analysis. *Lancet Oncol.* 2012;13(5):487–500.

MacMahon EM, Glass JD, Hayward SD, et al. Epstein–Barr virus in AIDS-related primary central nervous system lymphoma. *Lancet.* 1991;338(8773):969–973.

Mahale P, Engels EA, Coghill AE, et al. Cancer risk in older persons living with human immunodeficiency virus infection in the United States. *Clin Infect Dis.* 2018;67(1):50–57.

Mahale P, Ugoji C, Engles EA, et al. Cancer risk following lymphoid malignancies among HIV-infected people. *AIDS.* 2020;34(8):1237–1245.

Makinson A, Cheret A, Abgrall S, et al. *Early Lung Cancer Diagnosis in HIV Infected Population with an Important Smoking History with Low-Dose Ct: A Pilot Study (EP48 HIV CHEST).* Bethesda, MD: National Library of Medicine; 2015. https://www.clinicaltrials.gov/ct2/show/NCT01207986?term=NCT01207986&rank=1.

Mandelblatt JS, Kanetsky P, Eggert L, et al. Is HIV infection a cofactor for cervical squamous cell neoplasia? *Cancer Epidemiol.* 1999;8(1):97–106.

Mandell SP, Mack CD, Bulger EM. Motor vehicle mismatch: a national perspective. *Injury Prev.* 2010;16(5):309–314.

Marcus JL, Chao CR, Leyden WA, et al. Prostate cancer incidence and prostate-specific antigen testing among HIV-positive and HIV-negative men. *J Acquir Immune Defic Syndr.* 2014;66:495–502.

Marcus JL, Leyden WA, Chao CR, et al. Immunodeficiency, AIDS-related pneumonia, and risk of lung cancer among HIV-infected individuals. *AIDS.* 2017;31(7):989–993.

Mbulaiteye SM, Katabira ET, Wabinga H, et al. Spectrum of cancers among HIV-infected persons in Africa: the Uganda AIDS-Center Registry Match Study. *Int J Cancer.* 2006;118(4):985–990.

McGowan JP, Shah S. Long-term remission of AIDS-related primary central nervous system lymphoma associated with highly active antiretroviral therapy. *AIDS (London).* 1998;12(8):952–954.

McNeil CJ, Lee JS, Cole SR, et al. Anal cancer incidence in men with HIV who have sex with men: are Black men at higher risk? *AIDS.* 2022;36(5):657–664.

Mdodo R, Frazier EL, Dube SR, et al. Cigarette smoking prevalence among adults with HIV compared with the general adult population in the United States: cross-sectional surveys. *Ann Intern Med.* 2015;162(5):335–344.

Melbye M, Rabkin C, Frisch M, et al. Changing patterns of anal cancer incidence in the United States, 1940–1989. *Am J Epidemiol.* 1994;139(8):772–780.

Michaud JM, Zhang T, Shireman TI, et al. Hazard of cervical, oropharyngeal, and anal cancers in HIV-infected and HIV-uninfected Medicaid beneficiaries. *Cancer Epidemiol Biomarkers Prev.* 2020;29(7):1447–1457.

Minaar CA, Baeyens A, Akinwale Ayeni O, et al. Defining characteristics of nodal disease on PET/CT scans in patients with HIV-positive and -negative locally advanced cervical cancer in South Africa. *Tomography.* 2019;5(4):339–345.

Minkoff H, Ahdieh L, Massad, LS et al. The effect of highly active antiretroviral therapy on cervical cytologic changes associated with oncogenic HPV among HIV-infected women. *J Acquir Immune Defic Syndr.* 2001;15(16):2157–2164.

Minkoff H, Zhong Y, Burk RD, et al. Influence of adherent and effective antiretroviral therapy use on human papillomavirus infection and squamous intraepithelial lesions in human immunodeficiency virus-positive women. *J Infect Dis.* 2010;201(5):681–690.

Mitsuyasu RT, Groopman JE. Biology and therapy of Kaposi's sarcoma. *Semin Oncol.* 1984;11(1):53–59.

Monini P, de Lellis L, Fabris M, et al. Kaposi's sarcoma-associated herpesvirus DNA sequences in prostate tissue and human semen. *N Engl J Med.* 1996;334(18):1168–1172.

Montgomery JD, Jacobson LP, Dhir R, Jenkins FJ. Detection of human herpesvirus 8 (HHV-8) in normal prostates. *Prostate.* 2006;66(12):1302–1310.

Moore AL, Sabin CA, Madge S, et al. Highly active antiretroviral therapy and cervical intraepithelial neoplasia. *AIDS.* 2002;16(6):927–929.

Mosam A, Shaik F, Uldrick TS, et al. A randomized controlled trial of HAART versus HAART and chemotherapy in therapy-naive patients with HIV-associated Kaposi sarcoma in South Africa. *J Acquir Immune Defic Syndr.* 2012;60(2):150.

Mounier N, Spina M, Gabarre J, et al. AIDS-related non-Hodgkin lymphoma: final analysis of 485 patients treated with risk-adapted intensive chemotherapy. *Blood.* 2006;107(10):3832–3840.

Moyer VA. Screening for prostate cancer: US Preventive Services Task Force recommendation statement. *Ann Intern Med.* 2012;157(2):120–135.

Moyer VA. Screening for lung cancer: US Preventative Services Task Force recommendation statement. *Ann Intern Med.* 2014;160(5):330–338.

Munger K, Phelps WC, Bubb V, et al. The E6 and E7 genes of the human papillomavirus type 16 together are necessary and sufficient for transformation of primary human keratinocytes. *J Virol.* 1989;63(10):4417–4421.

Murthy N, Wodi AP, Bernstein H, et al. Advisory Committee on Immunization Practices recommended immunization schedule for adults aged 19 years or older—United States, 2022. *MMWR.* 2022;71:229–233.

Myerson RJ, Kong F, Birnbaum EH, et al. Radiation therapy for epidermoid carcinoma of the anal canal: clinical and treatment factors associated with outcome. *Radiother Oncol.* 2001;61(1):15–22.

Nagata N, Shimbo T, Yazaki H, et al. Predictive clinical factors in the diagnosis of gastrointestinal Kaposi's sarcoma and its endoscopic severity. *PLoS One.* 2012;7(11):1–7.

Nasti G, Martellotta F, Berretta M, et al. Impact of highly active antiretroviral therapy on the presenting features and outcome of patients with acquired immunodeficiency syndrome-related Kaposi sarcoma. *Cancer.* 2003a;98(11):2440–2446.

Nasti G, Talamini R, Antinori A, et al. AIDS-related Kaposi's sarcoma: evaluation of potential new prognostic factors and assessment of the AIDS Clinical Trial Group Staging System in the HAART Era—the Italian Cooperative Group on AIDS and Tumors and the Italian Cohort of Patients Naive from Antiretrovirals. *J Clin Oncol.* 2003b;21(15):2876–2882.

National Comprehensive Cancer Network NCCN. NCCN clinical practice guidelines in oncology. Rectal cancer, version 3.2024. https://www.nccn.org/guidelines/guidelines-detail?category=1&id=1461. Published March 2024a. Accessed August 13, 2024.

NCCN. NCCN clinical practice guidelines in oncology. Non-small cell lung cancer, version 7.2024. https://www.nccn.org/guidelines/guidelines-detail?category=1&id=1450. Published July 2024b. Accessed August 13, 2024.

NCCN. NCCN clinical practice guidelines in oncology. Colon cancer, version 4.2024. https://www.nccn.org/guidelines/guidelines-detail?category=1&id=1428. Published April 2024c. Accessed August 14, 2024.

NCCN. NCCN clinical practice guidelines in oncology. Cancer in people with HIV, version 2.2024. https://www.nccn.org/guidelines/guidelines-detail?category=4&id=1487. Published February 2024d. Accessed August 13, 2024.

NCCN. NCCN clinical practice guidelines in oncology. Central nervous system cancers, version 2.2024. https://www.nccn.org/guideli

nes/guidelines-detail?category=1&id=1425. Published February 2024e. Accessed August 13, 2024.

National Lung Screening Trial Research Team. Reduced lung-cancer mortality with low-dose computed tomographic screening. *N Engl J Med*. 2011;365(5):395–409.

Navarro WH, Kaplan LD. AIDS-related lymphoproliferative disease. *Blood*. 2006;107(1):13–20.

Nayudu SK, Balar B. Colorectal cancer screening in human immunodeficiency virus populations: are they at average risk? *World J Gastrointestinal Oncol*. 2012;4(12):259–264.

NCT00006436. Clinicaltrials.gov. EPOCH and rituximab to treat non-Hodgkin's lymphoma in patients with HIV infection.

NCT00267865. Clinicaltrials.gov. Chemotherapy and HAART to treat AIDS-related primary brain lymphoma.

NCT01207986. Clinicaltrials.gov. Early lung cancer diagnosis in HIV infected population with an important smoking history with low dose CT: a pilot study.

NCT02135419. Clinicaltrials.gov. Topical or ablative treatment in preventing anal cancer in patients with HIV and anal high-grade squamous intraepithelial lesions.

NCT02408861. Clinicaltrials.gov. Nivolumab and ipilimumab in treating patients with a HIV associated relapsed or refractory classical Hodgkin lymphoma or solid tumors that are metastatic or cannot be removed by surgery.

NCT02595866. Clinicaltrials.gov. Testing the addition of an experimental medication MK-3475 (pembrolizumab) to usual antiretroviral medications in patients with HIV and cancer.

NCT02659930. Clinicaltrials.gov. Pomalidomide in combination with liposomal doxorubicin in people with advanced or refractory Kaposi sarcoma.

NCT02660710. Clinicaltrials.gov. Rituximab plus CHOP chemotherapy for diffuse large B-cell lymphoma.

NCT03094286. Clinicaltrials.gov. Durvalumab in solid tumors.

NCT03113942. Clinicaltrials.gov. Study of pomalidomide in anal cancer precursors.

NCT03202992. Clinicaltrals.gov. Study of topical ABI-1968 in subjects with precancerous anal lesions resulting from human papillomavirus (HPV) infection.

NCT03304093. Clinicaltrials.gov. Immunotherapy by nivolumab for HIV+ patients.

NCT03316274. Clinicaltrials.gov. Intra-lesional nivolumab therapy for limited cutaneous Kaposi sarcoma.

NCT03354936. Clinicaltrials.gov. ANRS CO24 OncoVIHAC (onco VIH anti checkpoint).

NCT03617198. Clinicaltrials.gov. CD4 CAR+ ZFN-modified T cells in HIV therapy.

Neef H, Horth W, Makowiec F, et al. Outcome after resection of hepatic and pulmonary metastasis of colorectal cancer. *J Gastrointest Surg*. 2009;13(10):1813–1820.

Newton R, Ziegler J, Bourboulia D, et al. Infection with Kaposi's sarcoma-associated herpesvirus (KSHV) and human immunodeficiency virus (HIV) in relation to the risk and clinical presentation of Kaposi's sarcoma in Uganda. *Br J Cancer*. 2003;89(3):502–504.

Norden AD, Drappatz J, Wen PY, et al. Survival among patients with primary central nervous system lymphoma, 1973–2004. *J Neuro-Oncol*. 2011;101(3):487–493.

Northfelt DW, Dezube BJ, Thommes JA, et al. Pegylated-liposomal doxorubicin versus doxorubicin, bleomycin, and vincristine in the treatment of AIDS-related Kaposi's sarcoma: results of a randomized phase III clinical trial. *J Clin Oncol*. 1998;16(7):2445–2451.

Noy A. Update in Kaposi sarcoma. *Curr Opin Oncol*. 2003;15(5):379–381.

Noy A, Lee JY, Cesarman E, et al. AMC 048: modified CODOX-M/IVAC-rituximab is safe and effective for HIV-associated Burkitt lymphoma. *Blood*. 2015;126:160–166.

Ntekim A, Campbell O, Rothenbacher D. Optimal management of cervical cancer in PLWH: a systematic review. *Cancer Med*. 2015;4:1381–1393.

Nyitray AG, Hicks JT, Hwang LY, et al. A phase II clinical study to assess the feasibility of self and partner anal examinations to detect anal canal abnormalities including anal cancer. *Sex Transm Infect*. 2018 Mar;94(2):124–130.

Oehler-Janne C, Huguet F, Provencher S, et al. HIV-specific differences in outcome of squamous cell carcinoma of the anal canal: a multicentric cohort study of PLWH receiving highly active antiretroviral therapy. *J Clin Oncol*. 2008;26(15):2550–2557.

Okotie OT, Roehl KA, Han M, et al. Characteristics of prostate cancer detected by digital rectal examination only. *Urology*. 2007;70(6):1117–1120.

Okuma Y, Hishima T, Kashima J, et al. High PD-L1 expression indicates poor prognosis of HIV-infected patients with non-small cell lung cancer. *Cancer Immunol Immunother*. March 2018;67(3):495–505.

Okuma Y, Hosomi Y, Imamura A. Lung cancer patients harboring epidermal growth factor receptor mutation among those infected by human immunodeficiency virus. *Onco Targets Ther*. 2014;31:111–115.

Olson JE, Janney CA, Rao RD, et al. The continuing increase in the incidence of primary central nervous system non-Hodgkin lymphoma: a surveillance, epidemiology, and end results analysis. *Cancer*. 2002;95(7):1504–1510.

Ong WL, Manohar P, Millar J, et al. Clinicopathological characteristics and management of prostate cancer in the human immunodeficiency virus (HIV)-positive population: experience in an Australian major HIV center. *Br J Urol Int*. 2015;116(Suppl 3):5–10.

Orlando G, Fasolo MM, Schiavini M, et al. Role of highly active antiretroviral therapy in human papillomavirus-induced genital dysplasia in HIV-1-infected patients. *AIDS (London)*. 1999;13(3):424–425.

Palefsky JM. Human papillomavirus-associated anal and cervical cancers in HIV-infected individuals: incidence and prevention in the antiretroviral era. *Curr Opin HIV AIDS*. 2017;12(1):26–30.

Palefsky JM, Holly EA, Gonzales J, et al. Detection of human papillomavirus DNA in anal intraepithelial neoplasia and anal cancer. *Cancer Res*. 1991;51(3):1014–1019.

Palefsky JM, Holly EA, Ralston ML, et al. Effect of highly active antiretroviral therapy on the natural history of anal squamous intraepithelial lesions and anal human papillomavirus infection. *J Acquir Immune Defic Syndr*. 2001;28(5):422–428.

Palefsky JM, Lee JY, Jay N, et al. Treatment of anal high-grade squamous intraepithelial lesion to prevent anal cancer. *N Engl J Med*. 2022;386(24):227302282.

Pantanowitz L, Bohac G, Cooley T, et al. Human immunodeficiency virus-associated prostate cancer: clinicopathological findings and outcome in a multi-institutional study. *Br J Urol Int*. 2008;101:1519–1523.

Penn I. Kaposi's sarcoma in organ transplant recipients: report of 20 cases. *Transplantation*. 1979;27(1):8–11.

Persad GC, Little RF, Grady C. Including persons with HIV infection in cancer clinical trials. *J Clin Oncol*. 2008;26(7):1027–1032.

Petrovas C, Casazza JP, Brenchley JM, et al. PD-1 is a regulator of virus-specific CD8\+ T-cell survival in HIV infection. *J Exp Med*. 2006;203:2281–2292.

Piketty C, Seliger-Leneman H, Bouvier AM. Incidence of HIV-related anal cancer remains increased despite long-term combined antiretroviral treatment: results from the French Hospital Database on HIV. *J Clin Oncol*. 2012;30(35):4360–4366.

Piketty C, Selinger-Leneman H, Grabar S, et al. Marked increase in the incidence of invasive anal cancer among HIV-infected patients despite treatment with combination antiretroviral therapy. *AIDS*. 2008;22(10):1203–1211.

Plancoulaine S, Abel L, van Beveren M, et al. Human herpesvirus 8 transmission from mother to child and between siblings in an endemic population. *Lancet*. 2000;356(9235):1062–1065.

Pluda J, Broder S, Yarchoan R. Therapy of AIDS and AIDS-associated neoplasms. *Cancer Chemother Biol Response Modif*. 1992;13:404–439.

Polesel J, Clifford GM, Rickenbach M, et al. Non-Hodgkin lymphoma incidence in the Swiss HIV Cohort Study before and after highly active antiretroviral therapy. *AIDS (London)*. 2008;22(2):301–306.

Polizzotto MN, Uldrick TS, Wyvill KM, et al. Clinical features and outcomes of patients with symptomatic Kaposi sarcoma herpesvirus (KSHV)-associated Inflammation: prospective characterization of KSHV inflammatory cytokine syndrome (KICS). *Clin Infect Dis*. 2016;62(6):730–738. http://doi: 10.1093/cid/civ996

Pourcher V, Desnoyer A, Assoumou L et al. Phase II trial of lenalidomide in HIV-infected patients with previously treated Kaposi's sarcoma: results of the ANRS 154 Lenakap Trial. *AIDS Res Hum Retroviruses*. 2017;33(1):1–10.

Powles T, Matthews G, Bower M. AIDS related systemic non-Hodgkin's lymphoma. *Sex Transm Infect*. 2000;76(5):335–341.

Powles T, Thirwell C, Newsom-Davis T, et al. Does HIV adversely influence the outcome in advanced non-small-cell lung cancer in the era of HAART? *Br J Cancer*. 2003;89:457–459.

Rahmanian S, Wewers ME, Koletar S, et al. Cigarette smoking in the HIV-infected population. *Proc Am Thorac Soc*. 2011;8(3):313–319.

Rajdev L, Wang CJ, Joshi H, et al. Assessment of the safety of nivolumab in people living with HIV with advanced cancer on antiretroviral therapy: the AIDS Malignancy Consortium 095 Study. *Cancer*. 2024;130(6):985–994.

Ramaswami R, Polizzotto MN, Lurain K, et al. Safety, activity, and long-term outcomes of pomalidomide in the treatment of Kaposi sarcoma among individuals with or without HIV infection. *Clin Cancer Res*. 2022;28(5):840–850.

Ramirez-Marrero FA, Smit E, de la Torre-Feliciano T, et al. Risk of cancer among Hispanics with AIDS compared with the general population in Puerto Rico: 1987–2003. *Puerto Rico Health Sci J*. 2010;29(3):256–264.

Rasmussen TA, Rajdev L, Rhodes A, et al. Impact of anti-PD-1 and anti-CTLA-4 on the human immunodeficiency virus (HIV) reservoir in people living with HIV with cancer on antiretroviral therapy: the AIDS Malignancy Consortium 095 study. *Clin Infect Dis*. 2021;73(7):e1973–e1981.

Ratner L, Lee J, Tang S, et al. Chemotherapy for human immunodeficiency virus-associated non-Hodgkin's lymphoma in combination with highly active antiretroviral therapy. *J Clin Oncol*. 2001;19(8):2171–2178.

Ravalli S, Chabon A, Khan A. Gastrointestinal neoplasia in young HIV antibody-positive patients. *Am J Clin Pathol*. 1989;91:458–461.

Re A, Cattaneo C, Michieli M, et al. High-dose therapy and autologous peripheral-blood stem-cell transplantation as salvage treatment for HIV-associated lymphoma in patients receiving highly active antiretroviral therapy. *J Clin Oncol*. 2003;21(23):4423–4427.

Re A, Michieli M, Casari S, et al. High-dose therapy and autologous peripheral blood stem cell transplantation as salvage treatment for AIDS-related lymphoma: long-term results of the Italian Cooperative Group on AIDS and Tumors (GICAT) study with analysis of prognostic factors. *Blood*. 2009;114(7):1306–1313.

Reddy KP, Kong CY, Hyle EP, et al. Lung cancer mortality associated with smoking and smoking cessation among people living with HIV in the United States. *JAMA Intern Med*. 2017 Nov 1;177(11):1613–1621.

Reid E, Suneja G, Ambinder RF, et al. Cancer in people living with HIV, version 1.2018, NCCN clinical practice guidelines in oncology. *J Natl Compr Canc Netw*. 2018;16(8):986–1017.

Reinhold JP, Moon M, Tenner CT, et al. Colorectal cancer screening in HIV-infected patients 50 years of age and older: missed opportunities for prevention. *Am J Gastroenterol*. 2005;100:1805–1812.

Renwick N, Halaby T, Weverling GJ, et al. Seroconversion for human herpesvirus 8 during HIV infection is highly predictive of Kaposi's sarcoma. *AIDS*. 1998;12(18):2481–2488.

Richel O, de Vries HJ, van Noesel CJ, et al. Comparison of imiquimod, topical fluorouracil, and electrocautery for the treatment of anal intraepithelial neoplasia in HIV-positive men who have sex with men: an open-label, randomised controlled trial. *Lancet Oncol*. 2013;14:346–353.

Riedel DJ, Cox ER, Stafford KA, et al. Clinical presentation and outcomes of prostate cancer in an urban cohort of predominantly African American, human immunodeficiency virus-infected patients. *Urology*. 2015;85(2):415–421.

Riedel DJ, Rositch AF, Redfield RR. Patterns of HIV viremia and viral suppression before diagnosis of non-AIDS-defining cancers in HIV-infected individuals. *Infect Agent Cancer*. 2015b;38(10):1–7.

Riley RR, Duensing S, Brake T, et al. Dissection of human papillomavirus E6 and E7 function in transgenic mouse models of cervical carcinogenesis. *Cancer Res*. 2003;63(16):4862–4871.

Robbins HA, Pfeiffer RM, Shiels MS, et al. Excess cancers among HIV-infected people in the United States. *J Natl Cancer Inst*. 2015;107:pii: dju503.

Robert C, Ribas A, Wolchok JD, et al. Anti-programmed-death-receptor-1 treatment with pembrolizumab in ipilimumab-refractory advanced melanoma: a randomised dose-comparison cohort of a phase 1 trial. *Lancet*. 2014;384:1109–1117.

Rodrigo JA, Hicks LK, Cheung MC, et al. HIV-associated Burkitt lymphoma: good efficacy and tolerance of intensive chemotherapy including CODOX-M/IVAC with or without rituximab in the HAART era. *Adv Hematol*. 2012;2012:1–9.

Rohner E, Bütikofer L, Schmidlin K, et al. Cervical cancer risk in women living with HIV across four continents: A multicohort study. *Int J Cancer*. 2020;146(3):601–609.

Rohner E, Valeri F, Maskew M, et al. Incidence rate of Kaposi sarcoma in HIV-infected patients on antiretroviral therapy in southern Africa: a prospective multicohort study. *J Acquir Immune Defic Syndr*. 2014;67(5):547–554.

Ronit A, Kristensen T, Klitbo DM, et al. Incidental lung cancers and positive computed tomography images in people living with HIV. *AIDS*. 2017;31:1973–1977.

Rosenblum ML, Levy RM, Bredesen DE, et al. Primary central nervous system lymphomas in patients with AIDS. *Ann Neurol*. 1988;23:S13–S16.

Royse K, El Chaer F, Amirian ES, et al. Disparities in Kaposi sarcoma incidence and survival in the United States: 2000–2013. *PLoS One*. 2017;12(8):e0182750.

Ruiz A, Ganz WI, Post MJ, et al. Use of thallium-201 brain SPECT to differentiate cerebral lymphoma from toxoplasma encephalitis in AIDS patients. *Am J Neuroradiol*. 1994;15(10):1885–1894.

Rust B, Kiem HP, and Uldrick T. CAR T-cell therapy for cancer and HIV through novel approaches to HIV-associated haematological malignancies. *Lancet Haematol*. 2020;7(9):e690–e696.

Ryan CJ, Smith MR, Fizazi K, et al. Abiraterone acetate plus prednisone versus placebo plus prednisone in chemotherapy-naive men with metastatic castration-resistant prostate cancer (COU-AA-302): final overall survival analysis of a randomised, double-blind, placebo-controlled phase 3 study. *Lancet Oncol*. 2015;16(2):152–160.

Sacktor N, Lyles RH, Skolasky R, et al. HIV-associated neurologic disease incidence changes: Multicenter AIDS Cohort Study, 1990–1998. *Neurology*. 2001;56(2):257–260.

Safai B. Pathophysiology and epidemiology of epidemic Kaposi's sarcoma. *Semin Oncol*. 1987;2:7–12.

Sandler AS, Kaplan LD. Diagnosis and management of systemic non-Hodgkin's lymphoma in HIV disease. *Hematol Oncol Clin North Am*. 1996;10(5):1111–1124.

Santesso N, Mustafa RA, Schunemann HJ, et al. World Health Organization guidelines for treatment of cervical intraepithelial neoplasia 2-3 and screen-and-treat strategies to prevent cervical cancer. *Int J Gynaecol Obstet*. 2016;132:252–258

Sauer R, Liersch T, Merkel S, et al. Preoperative versus postoperative chemoradiotherapy for locally advanced rectal cancer: results of the German CAO/ARO/AIO-94 randomized phase III trial after a median follow-up of 11 years. *J Clin Oncol*. 2012;20(16):1926–1933.

Saville M, Lietzau J, Pluda J, et al. Activity of placlitaxel (Taxol) as therapy for HIV-associated Kaposi's sarcoma. *Lancet*. 1995;346:26–28.

Schiffman M, Kjaer SK. Natural history of anogenital human papillomavirus infection and neoplasia. *JNCI Monographs*. 2003;2003(31):14–19.

Schreiber D, Chhabra A, Rineer J, et al. Outcomes and tolerance of human immunodeficiency virus-positive veterans undergoing dose-escalated external beam radiotherapy for localized prostate cancer. *Clin Genitourinary Cancer*. 2014;12(2):94–99.

Sellers SA, Edmonds A, Ramirez C, et al. Optimal lung cancer screening criteria among persons living with HIV. *J Acquir Immune Defic Syndr*. 2022;90(2):184–192.
Serraino D, Boschini A, Carrieri P, et al. Cancer risk among men with, or at risk of, HIV infection in southern Europe. *AIDS*. 2000;14(5):553–559.
Sgadari C, Monini P, Barillari G, et al. Use of HIV protease inhibitors to block Kaposi's sarcoma and tumour growth. *Lancet Oncol*. 2003;4(9):537–547.
Shah NN, Singavi AK, Harrington A. Daratumumab in primary effusion lymphoma. *N Engl J Med*. 2018;379(7):689–690.
Shah R, Al-Sukhni W, Kim RD, et al. Resection of hepatic and pulmonary metastasis from colorectal carcinoma. *JACS*. 2006;202(3):468–475.
Shahani AJ, Gulsoy EB, Gibbs JW, et al. Integrated approach to the data processing of four-dimensional datasets from phase-contrast x-ray tomography. *Opt Express*. 2014;22(20):24606–24621.
Shebl FM, Engels EA, Goedert JJ, et al. Pulmonary infections and risk of lung cancer among persons with AIDS. *J Acquir Immune Defic Syndr*. 2010;55:375–379.
Shepherd FA, Crowley J, van Houtte P, et al.; the IASLC Lung Cancer Staging Project. Clinical staging of small cell lung cancer in the forthcoming (seventh) edition of the Tumor, Node, Metastasis Classification for Lung Cancer. *J Thoracic Oncol*. 2007;2(12):1067–1077.
Shepherd L, Ryom L, Law M, et al. Cessation of cigarette smoking and the impact on cancer incidence in HIV-positive persons: the D:A:D study. *Clin Infect Dis*. 2018;68(4):650–657. http://doi:10.1093/cid/ciy508
Shiels MS, Althoff KN, Pfeiffer RM, et al. HIV infection, immunosuppression, and age at diagnosis of non-AIDS-defining cancers. *Clin Infect Dis*. 2017;64(4):468–475.
Shiels, MS, Cole SR, Mehta SH, et al. Lung cancer incidence and mortality among HIV-infected and HIV-uninfected injection drug users. *J Acquir Immune Defic Syndr*. 2010a;55(4):510–515.
Shiels MS, Copeland G, Goodman M, et al. Cancer stage at diagnosis in patients infected with the human immunodeficiency virus and transplant recipients. *Cancer*. 2015;121(12):1063–2071.
Shiels MS, Goedert JJ, Moore RD, et al. Reduced risk of prostate cancer in US men with AIDS. *Cancer Epidemiol Biomarkers Prev*. 2010b;19(11):2910–2915.
Shiels MS, Pfeiffer RM, Engels EA. Age at cancer diagnosis among persons with AIDS in the United States. *Ann Intern Med*. 2010c;153(7):452–460.
Shiels MS, Pfeiffer RM, Gail MH, et al. Cancer burden in the HIV-infected population in the United States. *J Nat Cancer Institute*. 2011a;103:753–762.
Shiels MS, Pfeiffer RM, Hall HI, et al. Proportions of Kaposi sarcoma, selected non-Hodgkin lymphomas, and cervical cancer in the United States occurring in persons with AIDS, 1980–2007. *JAMA*. 2011b;305(14):1450–1459.
Shiels MS, Pfeiffer RM, Hildesheim A, et al. Circulating inflammation markers and prospective risk for lung cancer. *J Nat Cancer Inst*. 2013;105(24):1871–1880.
Siegel R, DeSantis C, Jemal A. Colorectal cancer statistics, 2014. *CA Cancer J Clinicians*. 2014;64(2):104–117.
Siegel R, Naishadham D, Jemal A. Cancer statistics, 2012. *CA Cancer J Clinicians*. 2012;62(1):10–29.
Sigel C, Cavalcanti MS, Daniel T, et al. Clinicopathologic features of colorectal carcinoma in PLWH. *Cancer Epidemiol Biomarkers Prev*. 2016;25:1098–1104.
Sigel K, Crothers K, Dubrow R, et al. Prognosis in HIV-infected patients with non-small cell lung cancer. *Br J Cancer*. 2013;109:1974–1980.
Sigel K, Wisnivesky J, Crothers K, et al. Immunological and infectious risk factors for lung cancer in US veterans with HIV: a longitudinal cohort study. *Lancet HIV*. 2017;4(2):e67–e73.
Sigel K, Wisnevesky J, Gordon K, et al. HIV as an independent risk factor for incident lung cancer. *AIDS*. 2012;26:1017–1025.
Sigel K, Wisnivesky J, Shahrir S, et al. Findings in asymptomatic HIV-infected patients undergoing chest computed tomography testing: implications for lung cancer screening. *AIDS*. 2014;28(7):1007–1014.
Silverberg MJ, Chao C, Leyden WA, et al. HIV infection, immunodeficiency, viral replication, and the risk of cancer. *Cancer Epidemiol Biomarkers Prev*. 2011;20(12):2551–2559.
Silverberg MJ, Lau B, Achenbach CJ, et al. Cumulative incidence of cancer among persons with HIV in North America. *Ann Intern Med*. 2015;163(7):507–518.
Silverberg MJ, Lau B, Justic AC, et al. Risk of anal cancer in HIV-infected and HIV-uninfected individuals in North America. *Clin Infect Dis*. 2012;54(17):1026–1034.
Silverberg MJ, Leyden W, Steven Gregorich S, et al. Is intensive cervical cancer screening justified in immunosuppressed women? Abstract 162. Paper presented at the Conference on Retroviruses and Opportunistic Infections (CROI). Boston, MA; February 22–25, 2016.
Simard EP, Pfeiffer RM, Engels EA. Cumulative incidence of cancer among individuals with acquired immunodeficiency syndrome in the United States. *Cancer*. 2011;117(5):1089–1096.
Simard EP, Pfeiffer RM, Engels EA. Spectrum of cancer risk late after AIDS onset in the United States. *Arch Intern Med*. 2010;170(15):1337–1345.
Skiest DJ, Crosby C. Survival is prolonged by highly active antiretroviral therapy in AIDS patients with primary central nervous system lymphoma. *AIDS*. 2003;17(12):1787–1793.
Smith AJB, Varma S, Rositch AF, et al. Gynecologic cancer in HIV-positive women: a systematic review and meta-analysis. *Am J Obstet Gynecol*. 2019;221(3):194–207. http://doi:10.1016/j.ajog.2019.02.022
Smith DM, Kingery JD, Wong JK, et al. The prostate as a reservoir for HIV-1. *AIDS*. 2004;18(11):1600–1602.
Smith JS, Sanusi B, Swarts A, et al. A randomized clinical trial comparing cervical dysplasia treatment with cryotherapy vs loop electrosurgical excision procedure in HIV-seropositive women from Johannesburg, South Africa. *Am J Obstet Gynecol*. 2017;217(2):183.e1–183.e11.
Smith RE, Colangelo L, Wieand HS, et al. Randomized trial of adjuvant therapy in colon carcinoma: 10-Year results of NSABP Protocol C-01. *J Natl Cancer Inst*. 2004;96(15):1128–1132.
Spano JP, Massiani MA, Bentata M, et al. Lung cancer in patients with HIV infection and review of the literature. *Med Oncol*. 2004;21:109–115.
Sparano JA, Lee S, Chen MG, et al. Phase II trial of infusional cyclophosphamide, doxorubicin, and etoposide in patients with HIV-associated non-Hodgkin's lymphoma: an Eastern Cooperative Oncology Group Trial (E1494). *J Clin Oncol*. 2004;22(8):1491–1500.
Sparano JA, Lee JY, Kaplan LD, et al. Rituximab plus concurrent infusional EPOCH chemotherapy is highly effective in HIV-associated B-cell non-Hodgkin lymphoma. *Blood*. 2010;115(15):3008–3016.
Stadler RF, Gregorcyk SG, Euhus DM, et al. Outcome of HIV-infected patients with invasive squamous-cell carcinoma of the anal canal in the era of highly active antiretroviral therapy. *Dis Colon Rectum*. 2004;47(8):1305–1309.
Stebbing J, Sanitt A, Nelson M, et al. A prognostic index for AIDS-associated Kaposi's sarcoma in the era of highly active antiretroviral therapy. *Lancet*. 2006;367(9521):1495–1502.
Stebbing J, Sanitt A, Teague A, et al. Prognostic significance of immune subset measurement in individuals with AIDS-associated Kaposi's sarcoma. *J Clin Oncol*. 2007;25(16):2230–2235.
Stelzle D, Tanaka LF, Lee KK, et al. Estimates of the global burden of cervical cancer associated with HIV. *Lancet Glob Health*. 2021;9(2):e161–e169.
Stewart S, Jablonowski H, Goebel FD, et al. Randomized comparative trial of pegylated liposomal doxorubicin versus bleomycin and vincristine in the treatment of AIDS-related Kaposi's sarcoma: International Pegylated Liposomal Doxorubicin Study Group. *J Clin Oncol*. 1998;16(2):683–691.

Stier EA, Abbasi W, Agyemang AF, et al. Brief report: recurrence of anal high-grade squamous intraepithelial lesions among women living with HIV. *J Acquir Immune Defic Syndr*. 2020;84(1):66–69.
Stier EA, Sebring MC, Mendez AE, et al. Prevalence of anal human papillomavirus infection and anal HPV-related disorders in women: a systematic review. *Am J Ob Gyn*. 2015;213(3):278–309.
Straus DJ, Huang J, Testa MA, et al. Prognostic factors in the treatment of human immunodeficiency virus-associated non-Hodgkin's lymphoma: analysis of AIDS Clinical Trials Group protocol 142—low-dose versus standard-dose m-BACOD plus granulocyte-macrophage colony-stimulating factor; National Institute of Allergy and Infectious Diseases. *J Clin Oncol*. 1998;16(11):3601–3606.
Sugarman J, Lewin SR, Henrich TJ, et al. Ethics of ART interruption after stem-cell transplantation. *Lancet HIV*. 2016;3:e8–e10.
Sumner L, Kamitani E, Chase S, et al. A systematic review and meta-analysis of mortality in anal cancer patients by HIV status. *Cancer Epidemiol*. 2022;76:102069.
Sun D, Cao M, Li H, et al. Risk of prostate cancer in men with HIV/AIDS: a systematic review and meta-analysis. *Prostate Cancer Prostatic Dis*. 2021;24(1):24–34.
Suneja G, Shiels MS, Melville SK. Disparities in the treatment and outcomes of lung cancer among HIV-infected individuals. *AIDS*. 2013;27(3):459–468.
Sung H, Ferlay J, Siegel RL, et al. Global Cancer Statistics 2020: GLOBOCAN estimates of incidence and mortality worldwide for 36 cancers in 185 countries. *CA Cancer J Clin*. 2021;71(3):209–249.
Susko M, Wang, CJ, Lazar AA, et al. Factors impacting differential outcomes in the definitive radiation treatment of anal cancer between HIV-positive and HIV-negative patients. *Oncologist*. 2020;25(9):772–779.
Taieb J, Tabernero J, Mini E, et al. Oxaliplatin, fluorouracil, and leucovorin with or without cetuximab in patients with resected stage III colon cancer (PETACC-8): an open-label, randomised phase III trial. *Lancet Oncol*. 2014;15(8):862–873.
Tam HK, Zhang Z-F, Jacobson LP, et al. Effect of highly active antiretroviral therapy on survival among HIV-infected men with Kaposi sarcoma or non-Hodgkin lymphoma. *Int J Cancer*. 2002;98(6):916–922.
Tesoriero JM, Gieryic SM, Carrascal A, et al. Smoking among HIV-positive New Yorkers: prevalence, frequency, and opportunities for cessation. *AIDS Behav*. 2010;14(4):824–835.
Tornesello ML, Buonaguro FM, Beth-Giraldo E, et al. Human immunodeficiency virus type 1 Tat gene enhances human papillomavirus early gene expression. *Intervirology*. 1993;36(2):57–64.
Trautmann L, Janbazian L, Chomont N, et al. Upregulation of PD-1 expression on HIV-specific CD8\+ T cells leads to reversible immune dysfunction. *Nat Med*. 2006;12:1198–1202.
Travi G, Ferreri A, Cinque P, et al. Long term remission of HIV-associated primary CNS lymphoma achieved with highly active antiretroviral therapy alone. *J Clin Oncol*. 2012;30(10):e119–e121.
Uldrick TS, Adams SV, Fromentin R, et al. Pembrolizumab induces HIV latency reversal in people living with HIV and cancer on antiretroviral therapy. *Sci Transl Med*. 2022 Jan 26;14(629):eabl3836.
Uldrick TS, Gonçalves PH, Abdul-Hay M, et al. Assessment of the safety of pembrolizumab in patients with HIV and advanced cancer: a phase 1 study. *JAMA Oncol*. 2019;5(9):1332–1339.
Uldrick TS, Polizzotto MN, Yarchoan R. Recent advances in Kaposi sarcoma herpesvirus-associated multicentric Castleman disease. *Curr Opin Oncol*. 2012;24(5):495–505.
U.S. Department of Health and Human Services (DHHS). Panel on Antiretroviral Guidelines for Adults and Adolescents. Guidelines for the use of antiretroviral agents in adults and adolescents with HIV. Department of Health and Human Services. https://clinicalinfo.hiv.gov/en/guidelines/adult-and-adolescent-arv. Published February 27, 2024a. Accessed August 13, 2024.
U.S. Department of Health and Human Services (DHHS). Panel on Guidelines for the Prevention and Treatment of Opportunistic Infections in Adults and Adolescents with HIV. Guidelines for the prevention and treatment of opportunistic infections in HIV-infected adults and adolescents: recommendations from the Centers for Disease Control and Prevention, the National Institutes of Health, and the HIV Medicine Association of the Infectious Diseases Society of America. https://clinicalinfo.hiv.gov/en/guidelines/hiv-clinical-guidelines-adult-and-adolescent-opportunistic-infections/human-0. Published July 29, 2024b. Accessed August 13, 2024.
Vallet-Pichard A, Pol S. Hepatitis viruses and human immunodeficiency virus co-infection: pathogenesis and treatment. *J Hepatol*. 2004;41(1):156–166.
Vernone SD, Hart CE, Reeves WC, et al. The HIV-1 Tat protein enhances E2-dependent human papillomavirus 16 transcription. *Virus Res*. 1993;27(2):133–145.
Walmsley S, Northfelt DW, Melosky B, et al. Treatment of AIDS-related cutaneous Kaposi's sarcoma with topical alitretinoin (9-cis-retinoic acid) gel: Panretin Gel North American Study Group. *J Acquir Immune Defic Syndr*. 1999;22(3):235–246.
Wang ES, Straus DJ, Teruya-Felstein J, et al. Intensive chemotherapy with cyclophosphamide, doxorubicine, high-dose methotrexade/ifosfamide, etoposide, and high-dose cytarabine (CODOX-M/IVAC) for human immunodeficiency virus-associated Burkett lymphoma. *Cancer*. 2003;98(3):1196–1205.
Wang Y, Wang Y, Gaisa MM, et al. Negative predictive value of human papillomavirus testing: implications for anal cancer screening in people living with HIV/AIDS. *J Oncol*. 2020;2020:6352315. doi:10.1155/2020/6352315
Wasserberg N, Nunoo-Mensah JW, Gonzalez Ruiz C, et al. Colorectal cancer in HIV-infected patients: a case control study. *Colorectal Dis*. 2007;22(10):1217–1221.
Welch K, Finkbeiner W, Alpers CE, et al. Autopsy findings in the acquired immune deficiency syndrome. *JAMA*. 1984;252(9):1152–1159.
Westwood TD, Hogan C, Julyan PJ, et al. Utility of FDG-PETCT and magnetic resonance spectroscopy in differentiating between cerebral lymphoma and non-malignant CNS lesions in HIV-infected patients. *Eur J Radiol*. 2013;82(8):e374–e379.
Whitlock EP, Lin JS, Liles E, et al. Screening for colorectal cancer: a targeted, updated systematic review for the US Preventive Services Task Force. *Ann Intern Med*. 2008:149(9):638–658.
Wightman F, Solomon A, Kumar SS, et al. Effect of ipilimumab on the HIV reservoir in an HIV-infected individual with metastatic melanoma. *AIDS*. 2015;29(4):504–506.
Wilkin TJ, Palmer S, Brudney KF, et al. Anal intraepithelial neoplasia in heterosexual and homosexual HIV-positive men with access to antiretroviral therapy. *J Infect Dis*. 2004;190(9):1685–1691.
Wilson WH, Sin-Ho J, Pitcher BN, et al. Phase III randomized study of R-CHOP versus DA-EPOCH-R and molecular analysis of untreated diffuse large B-cell lymphoma: CALGB/Alliance 50303. *Blood*. 2016;128:469.
Winstone, TA, Man SF, Hull M, et al. Epidemic of lung cancer in patients with HIV infection. *Chest*. 2013;143(2):305–314.
Wistuba IL, Behrens C, Milchgrub S, et al. Comparison of molecular changes in lung cancers in HIV-positive and HIV-indeterminate subjects. *JAMA*. 1998;279(19):1554–1559.
Wolf T, Brodt H-R, Fichtlscherer S, et al. Changing incidence and prognostic factors of survival in AIDS-related non-Hodgkin's lymphoma in the era of highly active antiretroviral therapy (HAART). *Leuk Lymphoma*. 2005;46(2):207–215.
Woolfrey AE, Malhotra U, Harrington RD, et al. Generation of HIV-1-specific CD8\+ cell responses following allogeneic hematopoietic cell transplantation. *Blood*. 2008;112(8):3484–3487.
World Health Organization. Fact sheets: cervical cancer. https://www.who.int/news-room/fact-sheets/detail/cervical-cancer. Published March 5, 2024. Accessed August 14, 2024.
World Health Organization. Human papillomavirus vaccines: WHO position paper (2022 update) *Weekly Epid Record*. 2022;(50)97:645–672.

Yegüez JF, Martinez SA, Sands DR, et al. Colorectal malignancies in PLWH. *Am Surg.* 2003;69(11):981–987.
Zanet E, Taborelli M, Rupolo M, et al. Postautologous stem cell transplantation long-term outcomes in 26 PLWH affected by relapsed/refractory lymphoma. *AIDS.* 2015;29(17): 2303–2308.
Zhang JY, Zhang Z, Wang X, et al. PD-1 up-regulation is correlated with HIV-specific memory CD8\+ T-cell exhaustion in typical progressors but not in long-term nonprogressors. *Blood.* 2007;109:4671–4678.
Zheng J, Wang L, Cheng Z, et al. Molecular changes of lung malignancy in HIV infection. *Sci Rep.* 2018;8(1):13128.
Ziegler JL, Drew WL, Miner RC, et al. Outbreak of Burkitt's-like lymphoma in homosexual men. *Lancet.* 1982;2(8299): 631–633.
Ziegler JL, Templeton AC, Vogel CL. Kaposi's sarcoma: a comparison of classical, endemic, and epidemic forms. *Semin Oncol.* 1984;11(1):47–52.

26.

UNDERSTANDING AND MANAGING ANTINEOPLASTIC AND ANTIRETROVIRAL THERAPY

Elizabeth M. Sherman and Taylor K. Gill

LEARNING OBJECTIVE

To review concepts regarding the safe and effective use of antineoplastic and antiretroviral therapy (ART) in people with HIV (PWH) and cancer.

WHAT'S NEW?

The disease states of HIV and cancer are constantly evolving. New therapies are regularly introduced, and frequently published data continue to advance each area. New oral agents and long-acting ART for HIV and immunotherapy for cancer treatment bring exciting advancements.

KEY POINTS

- The use of combination ART in people with HIV (PWH) and malignancies is associated with improved HIV- and cancer-related outcomes.
- Combining ART and antineoplastic therapy is often complicated by significant drug-drug interactions, drug–disease state monitoring interactions, and overlapping toxicities.
- Definitive studies including both antineoplastics and antiretrovirals (ARVs) are uncommon, and clinical judgment must often be used to determine the appropriate course of treatment.
- Adjusting ART in response to significant drug interactions or overlapping toxicities is often more feasible than modifying antineoplastic protocols.
- A multidisciplinary care team that includes primary care providers, infectious disease clinicians, hematologists/oncologists, social workers/case managers, and clinical pharmacists should be utilized to address the challenges of combining HIV and cancer treatment.

INTRODUCTION

The incidence of many common cancers among persons with HIV (PWH) is higher than in the general population (National Comprehensive Cancer Network [NCCN] Guidelines, 2024). The elevated risk of cancer in PWH is multifactorial and likely due to a combination of underlying immune deficiency, chronic inflammation, coinfection with oncogenic viruses, and a higher prevalence of other cancer-related risk factors such as the use of tobacco and alcohol products.

Before the widespread use of ART, AIDS-defining malignancies (ADMs) such as Kaposi's sarcoma, non-Hodgkin's lymphoma, and invasive cervical cancer accounted for the largest burden of cancer in PWH (Rubinstein et al., 2014). These occurred most commonly in people with advanced HIV, and all are associated with oncogenic viruses. Following widespread use of ART in the mid-1990s, there was a substantial decline in the number of new AIDS diagnoses and AIDS-related deaths (Rubinstein et al., 2014). ART-mediated immune reconstitution then led to a decrease in ADMs. At the same time, the occurrence of non-AIDS-defining malignancies (NADMs) increased. These include Hodgkin's lymphoma, leukemia, and cancers of the head, neck, lung, kidney, liver, gastrointestinal tract, anus, and skin. Currently, NADMs cause more cancer-related morbidity and mortality than ADMs and will remain common among PWH, with lung and prostate cancer expected to emerge as the most prevalent cancer types in the next decade (Shiels et al., 2018).

Although ADMs most commonly occur in people with severe immune suppression, low $CD4^+$ T-cell count (<500 cells/mm^3) has been identified as a risk factor for both ADMs and NADMs (Torres and Mulanovich, 2014). This suggests that initiating ART to suppress HIV replication and reconstituting $CD4^+$ T-cell counts may reduce the overall risk of malignancies in PWH. Recently, viral suppression, particularly long-term suppression with ART, has been linked with ADM and NADM prevention. Despite this, cancer risk can remain elevated even in virally suppressed PWH in comparison to persons without HIV infection (Park et al., 2018).

In people with both HIV and cancer, the use of ART alongside chemotherapy is routinely recommended to improve overall survival. The administration of chemotherapy and ART concurrently can be complicated by a number of factors (Rudek et al., 2011), including limited data regarding safe and effective therapy combinations; significant drug-drug interactions among ART, antineoplastics, and supportive-care medications; drug–disease state monitoring interactions; and overlapping drug toxicities. The introduction of immunotherapy for cancer treatment advanced the treatment of many NADMs, including use of immune check point inhibitors and chimeric antigen receptor T-cell therapy.

GENERAL CONSIDERATIONS FOR COMBINING ANTINEOPLASTIC AND ANTIRETROVIRAL THERAPY

DRUG INTERACTIONS: CYP450

Drug interactions between ART and antineoplastic agents may occur via several different mechanisms. The most common are interactions that occur during the metabolism of medications from active to inactive substances via the cytochrome P450 enzyme system (CYP450). Medications may be substrates of CYP450, meaning that they use this system for metabolism, and their concentrations may be altered by concurrent administration with other agents. In addition, medications may be inducers or inhibitors of individual CYP450 isoenzymes, such as 3A4. CYP450 inducers will increase the metabolism of CYP450 substrates, thus decreasing the concentration of medication, which may lead to subtherapeutic medication levels. Conversely, CYP450 inhibitors will decrease the metabolism of CYP450 substrates, thus increasing the medication concentration, which may lead to toxicity. The timing of CYP450 interactions may also vary as enzyme inhibition occurs rapidly, with the maximum effect occurring when a medication is at steady state and enzyme induction occurring more slowly because of the need for enzyme synthesis (Di Francia et al., 2014). Many antiretroviral, antineoplastic, and supportive-care medications utilize the CYP450 system for metabolism, and drug interactions are expected to be a challenge in this context.

Several antineoplastic and supportive-care agents are substrates, inducers, or inhibitors of CYP3A4. The result is complex bidirectional interactions with ART (Rudek et al., 2011). Interacting chemotherapy agents include vinblastine, vincristine, paclitaxel, docetaxel, iphosphamide (ifosfamide), cyclophosphamide, tyrosine kinase inhibitors, and corticosteroids that are metabolized by CYP3A4 (Rubinstein et al., 2014). However, anthracyclines, antimetabolite agents, anti-tumor antibiotics, and platinum agents undergo non-CYP450 routes of metabolism and are unlikely to be altered by ART (Berretta et al., 2023). The greatest concern for drug-drug interactions is with ART regimens containing the pharmacokinetic enhancers, ritonavir or cobicistat, and protease inhibitors. These drugs inhibit CYP3A4 and thus may significantly interact, causing an increase in exposure and toxicity, particularly with anti-cancer agents metabolized by this pathway. Most first-generation non-nucleoside reverse transcriptase inhibitors induce CYP3A, which may decrease exposure and efficacy of cancer agents metabolized by this pathway. However, nucleoside reverse transcriptase inhibitors, the second-generation non-nucleoside reverse transcriptase inhibitors rilpivirine and doravirine, and integrase inhibitors have the least likelihood of causing significant interactions with chemotherapy (Navarro et al., 2021). Likewise, the HIV entry inhibitors enfuvirtide and ibalizumab are not metabolized by the CYP enzyme system, while maraviroc and fostemsavir are P450 substrates. The HIV capsid inhibitor, lenacapavir, moderately inhibits CYP3A. Thus, ART regimens containing oral integrase inhibitors without pharmacologic boosters are favored in the setting of malignancy, owing to a lower potential for drug interactions (NCCN guidelines 2024).

DRUG INTERACTIONS: P-GLYCOPROTEIN

To add to the complexity of interactions that occur with medication metabolism, there may also be absorption interactions with the p-glycoprotein efflux pump in the gastrointestinal tract. Like the CYP450 interactions, medications may be p-glycoprotein substrates, inducers, or inhibitors. P-glycoprotein inducers stimulate the efflux of medications back into the gastrointestinal lumen, thus decreasing the absorption and plasma concentrations of these medications. Likewise, p-glycoprotein inhibitors will increase the absorption of medication and increase plasma concentrations of substrates, which could lead to toxicities. Antiretrovirals that affect, and are affected by, p-glycoprotein include maraviroc, fostemsavir, lenacapavir, tenofovir, integrase inhibitors, and protease inhibitors. Long-acting injectable antiretroviral formulations do not rely on the gastrointestinal tract for absorption. Drug interactions with the injectable formulations of cabotegravir and rilpivirine may differ from oral formulations, and these differences should be considered when combining these agents with chemotherapy (Nhean et al., 2021). Literature has shown that p-glycoprotein is highly expressed in HIV-associated malignancies such as non-Hodgkin's lymphoma and plays a significant role in the effectiveness of both ART and antineoplastic therapy (Klibanov and Clark-Vetril, 2007). Therefore clinicians should be aware of ARV, antineoplastic, and supportive care agents that affect p-glycoprotein and should realize the potential for drug interactions with medications that influence, or are influenced by, this mechanism.

MEDICATION TOXICITIES

Overlapping toxicities of medication classes should also be carefully considered. Some ART and antineoplastic agents are known for causing severe adverse effects that may become additive when used in combination. For example, nucleoside reverse transcriptase inhibitors may cause neutropenia (e.g., zidovudine), peripheral neuropathy (e.g., didanosine), or nephrotoxicity (e.g., tenofovir). Peripheral neuropathy may also be associated with many cancer drugs, including platinum agents, taxanes, vinca alkaloids, brentuximab, bortezomib, and proteosome inhibitors (Berretta et al., 2023; Marino et al., 2024; NCCN Guidelines 2024). Utilizing newer nucleoside reverse transcriptase inhibitor formulations, such as tenofovir alafenamide, may minimize nephrotoxicity, especially in combination with nephrotoxic chemotherapy agents such as methotrexate and cisplatin (Navarro et al., 2021). Various non-nucleoside reverse transcriptase inhibitors are associated with rash and hepatic transaminase elevations, and the entry inhibitor maraviroc may cause hepatotoxicity. Molecularly targeted anticancer agents may have side effects as hepatotoxicity, rash, and cardiac toxicity (Marino et al., 2024). Hepatotoxicity may also be induced by taxanes, tamoxifen, and ribociclib (Marino et al., 2024). Protease inhibitors may lead to greater gastrointestinal upset, including nausea, vomiting, and diarrhea, and may potentiate the myelosuppressive effects of certain chemotherapy (Torres and Mulanovich, 2014). QT prolongation may occur with use of atazanavir or with supratherapeutic doses of rilpivirine or fostemsavir, and is also increasingly common with newer molecularly targeted anticancer agents, including tyrosine kinase inhibitors (Berretta et al., 2023; Marino et al., 2024). Integrase inhibitors, by contrast, are generally well-tolerated, and overlapping toxicities with antineoplastic agents are not projected to be a major concern. It is vitally important when devising medication regimens that serious adverse effects of all agents be identified and overlapping toxicities minimized when possible.

DRUG-DISEASE INTERACTIONS

Care team members should also remain cognizant of drug-disease interactions when combining ARV and antineoplastic agents. Disease-monitoring interactions are a concern because there are certain antiretroviral medications that increase oncologic disease markers such as bilirubin. Bilirubin is often used as a means for determining dosage adjustments for a number of chemotherapeutic agents, such as docetaxel, paclitaxel, doxorubicin, etoposide, irinotecan, imatinib, sorafenib, and vincristine (Beumer et al., 2014; Berretta et al., 2023). Atazanavir may cause unconjugated hyperbilirubinemia secondary to UGT1A1 inhibition, leading to possible inaccuracies in chemotherapy dosage determinations.

Conversely, there are also concerns that antineoplastic agents may affect the level of $CD4^+$ T cells, rendering the monitoring parameters of both disease states inaccurate (Klibanov and Clark-Vetril, 2007). This has especially been a concern with cancer immunotherapy, as this strategy utilizes a patient's immune system to detect and destroy cancer cells. While data are still evolving, cancer immunotherapy likely has similar effectiveness in PWH and causes no significant impact on plasma HIV RNA or CD4 count (Abu Khalaf et al., 2022). Additionally, cancer immunotherapy may be more efficient in PWH compared to persons without HIV because of HIV infection upregulating immunotherapy targets (Bressan et al., 2021). When antineoplastic agents are combined with ARV agents, there may also be medication absorption concerns because of the presence of disease complications such as gastrointestinal tumors, mucositis, and graft-versus-host disease (Torres and Mulanovich, 2014). HIV providers may need to adapt medication-selection practices in these situations, for example utilizing formulations such as liquids, capsules that may be opened, tablets that may be crushed, or injectable ART.

The key concepts of drug interactions, overlapping toxicities, and drug-disease interactions are just a few examples of the complexity of utilizing a combination ART and antineoplastic therapy. Specific literature and guideline recommendations to assist in the selection, dosing, and monitoring of these agents when used in combination are scarce. Thus, these concepts should be considered on a case-by-case basis and explored thoroughly when crafting a care plan that includes treatment of both HIV and oncologic diseases.

STRATEGIES FOR CLINICAL MANAGEMENT OF PEOPLE WITH CANCER AND HIV

Treatment of PWH and cancer is complex, and a variety of management strategies should be considered. Examples of management strategies include alterations to the ART or chemotherapy regimens, changes in monitoring frequency, and optimization of opportunistic infection prophylaxis and supportive care medications. Additionally, ensuring transportation, food, housing, and social/case management support is necessary. To address such challenges, people with HIV and cancer should be supported by a multidisciplinary team, including primary care providers, infectious disease clinicians, hematologists/oncologists, social workers/case managers, and clinical pharmacists. Communication among these professionals is essential.

In combining ART and anticancer drug therapy, drug interactions and overlapping toxicities can be minimized or avoided by altering either the ART regimen or chemotherapy regimen. With continued development of new ART, effective alternatives are often available when current ART is expected to affect the metabolism or share overlapping toxicities with systemic cancer therapies. In many instances, it is often simpler to substitute one or more components of a person's ART regimen to avoid the risk of drug interactions or additive toxicity. Continuation of long-acting antiretroviral agents may require careful consideration and monitoring because of residual concentrations that may remain after stopping. When determining interaction potential, drug-interaction resources such be consulted. Two examples of dedicated resources for the care of PWH and cancer include: the Toronto General Hospital Immunodeficiency Clinic (https://hivclinic.ca/drug-information/antiretroviral-interactions-with-chemotherapy-regimens/) and University of Liverpool HIV drug interaction website (http://www.hiv-druginteractions.org), including their cancer therapies treatment selector (www.hiv-druginteractions.org/prescribing_resources/hiv-ts-cancer). ART regimen changes should always be carried out in conjunction with an HIV specialist utilizing the person's complete ARV treatment history, past adverse events, and HIV drug resistance test results. Interruption of ART or a delay in ART initiation is not recommended due to increased mortality risk. Modifications to medications in an antineoplastic regimen or their doses may also be considered based on a person's tolerance and response. Regardless, both ART and chemotherapy should be individualized.

Increased monitoring for efficacy and toxicity is recommended when coadministering any ART regimen with chemotherapy. If an ARV regimen is modified, more intensive monitoring of tolerability, viral suppression, adherence, and laboratory changes is recommended after a regimen switch (e.g., once a month for the first 3 months and then every 3 months throughout cancer treatment) (NCCN Guidelines, 2024). Identification and enhanced monitoring for toxicities are also recommended and should be assessed individually.

Lastly, in PWH and cancer, opportunistic infection prophylaxis should be tailored and expanded with antimicrobials required for specific chemotherapy regimens or hematopoietic stem cell transplantation. Notably, medications used to prevent and/or treat opportunistic infections in PWH may also interact with cancer therapies, including rifamycins (via induction of hepatic metabolism), clarithromycin (via inhibition of CYP3A4), azole antifungals (via inhibition of various hepatic metabolic processes), and trimethoprim/sulfamethoxazole with methotrexate (via inhibition of methotrexate renal excretion and overlapping risk of bone marrow suppression) (NCCN Guidelines, 2024) The need for opportunistic infection prophylaxis should be re-evaluated on a regular basis and adjusted as indicated via coordination among both the HIV/infectious disease and oncology providers. Prophylaxis may need to be modified as a person's $CD4^+$ T-cell count decreases with many cytotoxic cancer therapies and radiation therapy, or increases after completion of therapy.

REFERENCES

Abu Khalaf S, Dandachi D, Granwehr BP, et al. Cancer immunotherapy in adult patients with HIV. *J Investig Med.* 2022 Apr;70(4):883–891.

Berretta M, Facchini BA, Colpani A, et al. New treatment strategies for HIV-positive cancer patients undergoing anticancer medical treatment: update of the literature. *Eur Rev Med Pharmacol Sci.* 2023;27(9):4185–4201.

Beumer JH, Venkataramanan R, Rudek MA. Pharmacotherapy in cancer patients with HIV/AIDS. *Clin Pharmcol Ther.* 2014;95(4):370–372.

Bressan S, Pierantoni A, Sharifi S, et al. Chemotherapy-induced hepatotoxicity in HIV patients. *Cells.* 2021 Oct 25;10(11):2871.

Di Francia R, Di Paolo M, Valente D, et al. Pharmacogenetic based drug-drug interactions between highly active antiretroviral therapy (HAART) and antiblastic chemotherapy. *WCRJ.* 2014;1(2): e386.

Klibanov OM, Clark-Vetril R. Oncologic complications of human immunodeficiency virus infection: changing epidemiology, treatments, and special considerations in the era of highly active antiretroviral therapy. *Pharmacotherapy.* 2007;27(1):122–136.

Marino A, Pavone G, Martorana F, et al. Navigating the nexus: HIV and breast cancer—a critical review. *Int J Mol Sci.* 2024;25(6):3222.

National Comprehensive Cancer Network (NCCN). Clinical practice guidelines in oncology. Cancer in people with HIV, version 2. https://www.nccn.org/guidelines/category_4. Published 2024. Accessed May 23, 2024.

Navarro JT, Moltó J, Tapia G, et al. Hodgkin lymphoma in people living with HIV. *Cancers.* 2021 Aug 29;13(17):4366.

Nhean S, Tseng A, Back D. The intersection of drug interactions and adverse reactions in contemporary antiretroviral therapy. *Curr Opin HIV AIDS.* 2021 Nov 1;16(6):292–302.

Park LS, Tate JP, Sigel K, et al. Association of viral suppression with lower AIDS-defining and non-AIDS-defining cancer incidence in HIV-infected veterans: a prospective cohort study. *Ann Intern Med.* 2018;169(2):87–96.

Rubinstein PG, Aboulafia DM, Zloza A. Malignancies in HIV/AIDS: from epidemiology to therapeutic challenges. *AIDS.* 2014;28(4):453–465.

Rudek MA, Flexner C, Ambinder RF. Use of antineoplastic agents in patients with cancer who have HIV/AIDS. *Lancet Oncol.* 2011;12(9):905–912.

Shiels MS, Islam JY, Rosengerg PS, et al. Projected cancer incidence rates and burden of incident cancer cases in HIV-infected adults in the United States through 2030. *Ann Intern Med.* 2018;168(12):866–873.

Torres HA, Mulanovich V. Management of HIV infection in patients with cancer receiving chemotherapy. *Clin Infect Dis.* 2014;59(1):106–114.

27.

DERMATOLOGIC COMPLICATIONS OF HIV

Craig Weeks

OVERVIEW OF CUTANEOUS FINDINGS IN HIV INFECTION

LEARNING OBJECTIVE

Upon completion of this chapter, the reader should be able to:

- Describe the dermatologic complications of HIV infection and their treatment.
- Review the approach to skin findings in the context of acute and chronic HIV infection.

WHAT'S NEW?

Multiple biopsies increase diagnostic yield for identification of cutaneous complications of HIV.

KEY POINTS

- Dermatoses that are rare in the general population but common in people with HIV (PWH) should prompt testing for HIV when there is no existing diagnosis.
- Correct diagnosis and management of skin concerns can improve the quality of life of PWH who have increased longevity with antiretroviral therapy (ART).
- The appearance of AIDS-defining cutaneous illnesses in previously immune-reconstituted PWH on ART should prompt a reassessment of $CD4^+$ T-cell count and HIV RNA levels.
- In people who have been on ART for less than 24 weeks, the appearance or worsening of dermatoses may be due to immune reconstitution inflammatory syndrome (IRIS).

The hallmark of HIV infection is immune dysregulation and immunosuppression. As the immune system deteriorates, inflammatory dermatoses, metabolic dysregulation, adverse drug reactions, opportunistic infections, and cutaneous malignancies become more common, atypical in presentation, and recalcitrant to therapy. Both acute and chronic skin concerns contribute significantly to reduced quality of life for PWH (Mirmirani et al., 2002).

The U.S. Centers for Disease Control and Prevention (CDC) recommends that individuals aged 13–64 years be tested for HIV at least once in their lifetime, with increased screening of high-risk individuals and testing based on symptoms. The presence of dermatoses uncommon in the general population but more frequently seen in PWH, or dermatoses strikingly recalcitrant to therapy, should warrant suspicion and testing for HIV. In people with known HIV, there is a correlation between $CD4^+$ count and the occurrence of characteristic dermatoses (Goldstein et al., 1997; Rigopoulos et al., 2004). If $CD4^+$ testing availability is limited, the World Health Organization's (WHO) clinical staging provides guidelines regarding skin findings that should raise suspicion for immune deterioration (Baveewo et al., 2011; Weinberg and Kovarik, 2010). Similarly, the occurrence of AIDS-defining illnesses such as Kaposi's sarcoma or acute systemic illnesses and infections in PWH previously well controlled on ART should prompt an assessment of $CD4^+$ count and HIV RNA levels to evaluate for immune deterioration. In PWH who have been on ART for less than 24 weeks, acute systemic illnesses may be due to IRIS or treatment toxicity and, during this period, do not follow the WHO clinical staging guidelines as closely (Ratnam et al., 2006). With these caveats, the dermatoses discussed in this chapter are presented along with the corresponding $CD4^+$ count at which they typically occur (Zancanaro et al., 2006).

HIV providers can competently diagnose many of the dermatological conditions described, as well as perform diagnostic biopsies and minor cosmetic procedures. Clinics often maintain a supply of liquid nitrogen to treat warts and an electrocautery machine known as a hyfrecator to electrodessicate lesions such as molluscum contagiosum. Referral to a dermatologist is recommended in settings of diagnostic or management uncertainty, scenarios involving acutely ill PWH, common or chronic dermatoses recalcitrant to therapies familiar to the HIV provider, and for optimal tissue procurement when the clinician is uncertain of appropriate biopsy site or method.

It is important for HIV providers to be aware that several serious disseminated opportunistic infections, some of which may be fatal, may first manifest as an acute cutaneous eruption. Therefore, it is important to perform skin biopsy in an acutely febrile immunocompromised PWH with a newly developed skin eruption. The biopsy should be accompanied with a request for urgent processing with special stains for bacteria, atypical mycobacteria, fungi, and viruses as appropriate. Tissue is placed in 10% formalin for routine processing, but a portion should be placed in normal saline so that cultures for microorganisms can be performed to aid in definitive diagnosis.

In general, when sampling a lesion, especially one that is papular or pustular, an early, new lesion that is not excoriated is most likely to yield tissue with changes that afford the

***Box 27.1* INDICATIONS FOR REFERRAL TO A DERMATOLOGIST**

Diagnostic uncertainty
Management uncertainty
Life-threatening differential diagnoses
Rapid progression
Persistence or recurrence despite therapy
Requires specialized medications
Requires specialized procedures
Suspected skin cancer
Indications for skin cancer screening
Pigmented lesions
Support to improve engagement in care, adherence
Patient request

dermatopathologist the best opportunity to make an accurate diagnosis (Altman et al., 2015). A notable exception is biopsy of suspected Kaposi's sarcoma because early lesions can present a confusing picture histologically. An older, more mature lesion, if present, will have greater diagnostic yield (Maurer, 2005). When in doubt, one should consider taking multiple biopsies from the lesion in different stages of evolution and from different cutaneous sites. If the clinician is uncomfortable performing a good skin biopsy, dermatological referral for evaluation and biopsy determination should be made. Box 27.1 provides guidelines for referral.

RECOMMENDED READING

Altman K, Vanness E, Westergaard RP. Cutaneous manifestations of human immunodeficiency virus: a clinical update. *Curr Infect Dis Rep.* 2015;17(3):464.

Mirmirani P, Maurer TA, Berger TG, et al. Skin-related quality of life in HIV-infected patients on highly active antiretroviral therapy. *J Cutan Med Surg.* 2002;6(1):10–15.

INFLAMMATORY DERMATOSES AND HIV

LEARNING OBJECTIVE

Discuss the incidence, presentation, and management of inflammatory dermatoses in HIV.

WHAT'S NEW?

Traditional immunosuppressants and newer biologic therapies have been used safely in controlled settings and for short courses in PWH with refractory psoriasis and debilitating psoriatic arthritis who are on concurrent ART.

KEY POINTS

- Initiation of ART, ultraviolet B (UVB), and oral retinoids are good initial therapies for PWH with psoriatic arthritis.
- Topical tacrolimus inhibitors and UV light have both been used safely in PWH.
- PWH receiving systemic biologics for debilitating psoriatic arthritis should be carefully selected and closely monitored.
- Papular pruritic eruption of AIDS and HIV-associated eosinophilic pustular folliculitis are HIV/AIDS-associated dermatologic illnesses that should prompt testing for HIV in a previously undiagnosed person.

SEBORRHEIC DERMATITIS

Seborrheic dermatitis is a common skin disorder, with a prevalence of approximately 5% in the general population. It is the most common dermatosis in PWH, with a prevalence of greater than 83% in people with HIV/AIDS in the pre-ART era (Sadick et al., 1990), and is seen at all clinical stages of the disease. *Malassezia* species are causative organisms. The typical presentation is of episodic, variably pruritic, thin, erythematous plaques with branny (small, husk-like) or greasy yellow-white scale involving the scalp and central face, particularly the eyebrows, forehead, and nasolabial folds. Scalp involvement ranges from light "dandruff" to crusted plaques. Involvement of the anterior chest and groin areas is common. HIV should be considered in rapid or exaggerated presentations with thick, extensive plaques and also in cases recalcitrant to advanced therapeutic interventions. The clinical differential for facial seborrheic dermatitis includes rosacea; an overlapping presentation with psoriasis called sebopsoriasis that is often more difficult to treat than standard seborrheic dermatitis; contact dermatitis; *tinea faciei*; and connective tissue disease. In *tinea faciei*, a potassium hydroxide (KOH) preparation can identify dermatophytes exhibiting characteristic hyphae. In contrast, seborrheic dermatitis is thought to be an inflammatory response to the commensal yeast *Malassezia* species where KOH evaluation is not helpful. The increased frequency and intensity of seborrheic dermatitis seen in PWH is thought to be due to a more vigorous inflammatory response as the yeast proliferate in the setting of $CD4^+$ lymphopenia (Oble et al., 2005; Pedrosa et al., 2014). Seborrheic dermatitis is a clinical diagnosis; thus, biopsy is infrequently performed. When it is needed, histology reveals psoriasiform hyperplasia, neutrophilic spongiosis, perifollicular mound parakeratosis with necrotic keratinocytes, and occasionally plasma cells (Soeprono et al., 1986). Treatment does not differ between PWH and HIV-negative persons; first-line therapy involves low- to mid-potency topical steroids for the face and trunk, respectively, topical antifungals such as ketoconazole, or combinations thereof (Osborne et al., 2003). More refractory cases can be treated with oral itraconazole 200 mg once daily, although attention must be paid to interactions with antiretroviral agents. ART improves HIV-associated seborrheic dermatitis, although PWH may continue to have episodic flares even on ART.

PSORIASIS

Psoriasis also presents at all clinical stages of HIV, but more frequently at $CD4^+$ counts of less than 350 cells/mm^3 (Bartlett et al., 2007). Psoriasis has a prevalence of approximately 2%–3% in the general population, with various series suggesting a similar or higher incidence in PWH (Mallon and Bunker, 2000; Obuch et al., 1992). The prevalence of psoriatic arthritis in the general population has previously been underestimated and is now thought to be approximately 11% among people with psoriasis in the United States, and it is more concentrated in PWH (Dover and Johnson, 1991; Gelfand et al., 2005). Psoriasis characteristically presents as variably pruritic, episodic, well-demarcated plaques with silvery white scale anywhere on the body but with a predilection for the scalp, elbows, lower back, gluteal folds, external genitalia, and acral sites. Preexisting psoriasis can worsen with HIV infection and immune deterioration, and psoriasis can develop de novo with HIV infection. De novo psoriasis in HIV often involves palmar-plantar locations with pustules, nail dystrophy, and psoriatic arthritis that can be debilitating. Inverse psoriasis (involving intertriginous areas), generalized pustular psoriasis, and erythrodermic psoriasis also occur more frequently in HIV (Obuch et al., 1992). Erythrodermic psoriasis can be difficult to distinguish from other causes of erythroderma, including atopic dermatitis, drug-induced erythroderma, pityriasis rubra pilaris, Sézary syndrome, and a paraneoplastic presentation or acute HIV infection; thus, it typically warrants a biopsy. Histology reveals parakeratosis, collections of neutrophils in the stratum corneum and epidermis, and a diminished granular layer. Whereas increased defensins and canthelicidins in the skin of people with psoriasis in the general population have been associated with their relatively low frequency of bacterial superinfection compared to other chronic dermatoses that also result in a compromised skin barrier (e.g., atopic dermatitis), there is an increased frequency of bacterial superinfection in PWH with psoriasis (Mallon and Bunker, 2000; Zheng et al., 2007). Theories regarding the increased incidence and severity of psoriasis in HIV include the fact that overexpression of tumor necrosis factor (TNF) occurs in both psoriasis and HIV. Furthermore, $CD4^+$ depletion in HIV skews the T-cell population to $CD8^+$ T-cells, the effector cells in psoriasis, and the HIV tat gene directly induces epidermal proliferation (Duvic, 1990; Kim et al., 1992).

In treating psoriasis, exacerbating medications should be discontinued. Of note, systemic steroids exacerbate psoriasis. Topical steroids, vitamin D analogues, and calcineurin inhibitors such as tacrolimus are first-line therapies for mild to moderate plaque psoriasis. A black box warning on tacrolimus and malignancy risk has not identified a causal relationship, and studies have shown that topical calcineurin inhibitors can be safely used in immunosuppressed PWH (de Moraes et al., 2007; Toutous-Trellu et al., 2005). Randomized controlled studies have not been conducted to evaluate the efficacy and safety of systemic treatments for psoriasis in the setting of HIV infection; thus, much of the following data are derived from case reports and case series.

Systemic therapies can be used in combination with each other and with topical treatments to optimize efficacy. ART and UV light are effective, first-line treatments for moderate to severe psoriasis and psoriatic arthritis (Duvic et al., 1994; Menon et al., 2010; Meola et al., 1993). UVB is preferentially used over psoralens plus UVA (PUVA) given its more favorable side effect profile. Although in vitro studies have shown that UVB light can activate latent HIV in chronically infected monocytes, it has not been associated with short-term changes in immune function in vivo or changes in HIV RNA levels in PWH receiving concomitant suppressive ART therapy (Breuer-McHam et al., 1999; Meola et al., 1993; Stanley et al., 1989). Oral retinoids, particularly acitretin, are an attractive second-line therapy because they are non-immunosuppressants with efficacy for moderate to severe psoriasis and psoriatic arthritis. Acitretin use is limited by hypertriglyceridemia; liver function test (LFT) elevation, particularly in combination with some antiretroviral medications; and an extended 3-year teratogenicity period in women of childbearing age due to re-esterification to etretinate (Dogra and Yadav, 2014).

PWH with refractory or debilitating psoriatic arthritis are candidates for immunosuppressant therapies, including low-dose methotrexate and brief courses of cyclosporine and TNF-α inhibitors. In one case report, dramatic improvement of HIV-associated psoriatic arthritis was achieved, but frequent polymicrobial infections were experienced on etanercept (Aboulafia et al., 2000). In a 2018 Cochrane review of 25 reported cases of systemic immunosuppressives used to treat psoriatic disease in PWH, including methotrexate, cyclosporine, etanercept, adalimumab, infliximab, and ustekinumab, evidence suggests that these biologic therapies may be effective for refractory psoriasis and may actually have a positive effect on $CD4^+$ counts and HIV viral load when used in combination with ART (Nakamura et al., 2018). Rigorous patient selection, concomitant ART, strict prophylaxis against opportunistic infections, and close monitoring of $CD4^+$ counts, HIV RNA, and clinical status are advised when treating HIV-associated psoriasis with immunosuppressant therapy.

ATOPIC DERMATITIS AND XEROSIS

The prevalence of eczema in the U.S. adult population is estimated at 10.7%, with approximately 17% experiencing at least one of four eczematous symptoms (Hanifin et al., 2007). An atopic dermatitis-like condition occurs frequently in PWH, often despite never having had a history of atopic dermatitis in childhood. One series reported a prevalence of 29% among PWH who attended an urban HIV clinic in the pre-ART era (Lin et al., 1995). Cases are generally characterized by pruritus and a spectrum of generalized scaling from xerosis to ichthyosis, with variable plaques and lichenification involving extremities and flexural areas (Singh and Rudikoff, 2003). Often, the xerotic condition initially presents when the $CD4^+$ count is still higher than 400 cells/mm^3 and is thus an early clinical sign of HIV infection, typically preceding other HIV-related papulosquamous disorders. Conversely, the generalized ichthyotic form typically occurs with $CD4^+$ counts less than 50 cells/mm^3 (Sadick et al., 1990). Decreased cellular immunity and a switch to the TH2-like cytokine profile, resulting in polyclonal activation of B cells with increased IgE production, are thought to contribute to the increased prevalence of atopic conditions in HIV (Nissen et al., 1999). Additionally, nutritional deficits and autonomic nervous dysfunction causing alterations in sweating, sebaceous gland secretion, and reduction in natural moisturizing factor secretion are thought to contribute to xerosis and ichthyosis (Cockerell and Calame, 2013). Decreased lipids and increased water are found in the dermis of PWH compared to HIV-negative reference groups, as well as excessive levels of epidermal carotenoids (mainly lycopene), potentially leading to these adverse effects and premature skin aging (Mischo et al., 2014). Biopsy, which is not regularly performed for this diagnosis, shows variable hyperkeratosis and parakeratosis, spongiosis, and superficial perivascular lymphocytic infiltrate. The clinical differential diagnosis includes scabies, psoriasis, and contact dermatitis. For erythematous plaques, topical steroid preparations, preferably ointments, and topical calcineurin inhibitors are appropriate first-line therapies. Topical keratolytics such as urea and lactic acid formulations are useful for areas of lichenification. Widespread flares may require short courses of systemic steroids, bridging to phototherapy for more sustained flares. Oral antihistamines and a dry skin care regimen of short lukewarm showers, frequent use of nonallergic emollients, and avoidance of allergens should be used in conjunction. Bacterial superinfection is common and should be managed with antibiotics.

PAPULAR PRURITIC ERUPTION OF AIDS

Papular pruritic eruption (PPE) is a markedly pruritic papulosquamous eruption characterized by symmetric crops of nonfollicular, often urticarial erythematous papules involving the extensor extremities. Excoriations and prurigo nodularis are frequently associated with secondary changes because of marked pruritus in this condition. PPE is uncommon in the general adult population but has a prevalence of 11%–46% in people with advanced HIV/AIDS, hence the designation "PPE of AIDS" (Eisman, 2006). It has a greater prevalence in people with HIV/AIDS in sub-Saharan Africa than in the United States. Among other theories, PPE is hypothesized to be due to an exaggerated response to arthropod antigens that occurs in the setting of immune dysregulation (Resneck et al., 2004). PPE can develop well before other symptoms and serologic diagnosis of HIV is made; however, its occurrence has historically been correlated with lower CD4$^+$ counts, particularly less than 100 cells/mm^3 (Boonchai et al., 1999; Cockerell and Calame, 2013). Of note, studies from India found otherwise, where one-third of cases occurred in PWH with CD4$^+$ counts above 350 cells/mm^3 (Farsani et al., 2013) and 86% above 200 cells/mm^3 (Mohammed et al., 2019). This difference is yet unexplained but highlights that PPE can be seen at any CD4$^+$ count.

The clinical differential of PPE includes eosinophilic folliculitis, which, in contrast, affects the face and upper trunk, and prurigo nodularis, which also may also be pruritic. The diagnosis is typically made clinically, based on the distribution of lesions. Early lesions without secondary changes carry the highest histologic diagnostic yield; they may show a dense perivascular and interstitial infiltrate of lymphocytes and some eosinophils and neutrophils, which may extend deeply around adnexa and vessels, although nonspecific findings occur (Calonje et al., 2012). The condition has a chronic waxing and waning course and is associated with decreased quality of life due to pruritus (Hevia et al., 1991; Liu et al., 2013). Given its association with low CD4$^+$ T-cell counts, ART initiation may improve disease course, although it can also flare with immune reconstitution. UVB has been shown to decrease both papules and pruritus, and may have greater efficacy when combined with other modalities, including oral antihistamines, pentoxifylline, topical steroids, topical tacrolimus, and topical anti-itch preparations (Bellavista et al., 2013). Reducing exposure to bites by wearing clothing that covers the skin and application of insect repellant is also recommended.

HIV-ASSOCIATED EOSINOPHILIC PUSTULAR FOLLICULITIS

Eosinophilic pustular folliculitis (EPF, or Ofugi's disease) is rare in the general adult population but common in people with HIV/AIDS, particularly at CD4$^+$ counts below 250 cells/mm^3. HIV-associated eosinophilic folliculitis is characterized by persistent, markedly pruritic erythematous, mostly follicular papules and occasional pustules on the face, trunk, and upper extremities. Urticarial plaques and nonfollicular erythematous papules are also described. Peripheral eosinophilia can also be common, along with elevated IgE levels (Rosenthal et al., 1991). It is thought to be an exaggerated cutaneous reaction to *Malassezia* yeast or other microorganisms colonizing the follicular infundibulum and reflects TH1/2 immune dysregulation. CD163$^+$ macrophages have been implicated in pathogenesis (Okada et al., 2013). Additional theories include autoimmune activation against antigens in sebocytes in PWH (Fearfield et al., 1999). The clinical differential includes PPE as well as acne, molluscum, and drug reactions. Biopsy may be useful, with erythematous nonexcoriated follicular lesions carrying the highest diagnostic yield. Spongiosis involving the follicular epithelium and intra- and perifollicular mixed infiltrate is typically seen, with eosinophilic abscess formation in long-standing lesions. Treatment is often difficult, with pruritus contributing to reduced quality of life. Phototherapy (UVB or UVA), oral antihistamines, itraconazole, isotretinoin, and metronidazole have all been used as treatment; however, no controlled clinical trials have been performed. Whereas classic EPF is preferentially treated with oral indomethacin, topical steroids are preferred for HIV-related EPF (Nomura et al., 2016), and other potential therapeutic modalities include UVB phototherapy and oral antihistamines.

RECOMMENDED READING

Cockerell CC, Calame A. *Cutaneous manifestations of HIV disease.* London: Manson; 2013.

Nomura T, Katoh M, Yamamoto Y, et al. Eosinophilic pustular folliculitis: A published work-based comprehensive analysis of therapeutic responsiveness. *J Dermatol.* 2016;43(8):919–927. http://doi: 10.1111/1346-8138.13287

ART DRUG REACTIONS AND INTERACTIONS

LEARNING OBJECTIVE

Describe common and important cutaneous adverse drug reactions in PWH and pertinent factors in their management.

WHAT'S NEW?

Several adverse drug reactions to ART medications have been identified that were not observed or were underrepresented in preapproval trials.

KEY POINTS

- Non-nucleoside reverse transcriptase inhibitors (NNRTIs) are the most common antiretroviral drugs that cause morbilliform skin eruptions.
- Abacavir hypersensitivity reaction can be fatal, and predisposed individuals can be identified by testing for the HLA-B5701 allele prior to commencing abacavir therapy.
- Ritonavir, a CYP34A inhibitor often used to boost other antiretroviral drugs, increases the levels of corticosteroids, which can result in hypothalamic–pituitary–adrenal (HPA) axis dysfunction and Cushing's syndrome. This should be considered when offering corticosteroid injections or using topical steroids over a large body surface area.

Historically, the incidence of medication-related skin rashes in PWH was approximately 50% (Davis and Shearer, 2008), although literature is lacking on the incidence with newer antiretrovirals. Drug hypersensitivity reactions are classified into two categories: those secondary to ART regimens, and those secondary to other medications taken by PWH. Since its inception, ART has revolutionized the management of HIV/AIDS, with new drug classes and single-tablet combination formulations designed to decrease pill burden. However, ART has been complicated by adverse drug reactions, including reactions that may not have been recognized or that were underrepresented in preapproval clinical trials (Introcaso et al., 2010). Thus, recognition of known reactions and identification of previously unreported drug reactions are extremely important in the management of antiretroviral-related drug hypersensitivity reactions. It can be particularly challenging to differentiate between drug hypersensitivity reactions, IRIS, and worsening HIV infection when people are commencing ART. Some adverse drug reactions are mediated through genetic and immunologic factors via the major histocompatibility complex (Chaponda and Pirmohamed, 2011). IgE levels increase with progression of HIV, and altered cytokine profiles are also believed to play a role (Davis and Shearer, 2008). Immune dysregulation in HIV is also thought to make PWH more susceptible to reactions to non-ART medications. In addition, antiretroviral drugs can result in alterations in the metabolism of other medications, particularly through the cytochrome P450 pathway, thus increasing their toxicity.

NON-NUCLEASE REVERSE TRANSCRIPTASE INHIBITORS

Although used far less commonly than in years past, awareness of NNRTI-related cutaneous syndromes remains important. NNRTIs are the most common antiretroviral agents to cause morbilliform skin eruptions, which are usually distributed over the face, trunk, and extremities. Nevirapine is well known for its role in causing rashes, particularly within the first 6 weeks of use. According to the manufacturer, 13% of patients taking nevirapine develop some degree of morbilliform eruption during early treatment; this has been reported to be as high as 28% in some populations (Introcaso et al., 2010). Many people with mild or moderate rash can continue therapy with close monitoring, and the rash will spontaneously resolve. Severe rash is seen in at least 8% of people, and development of concomitant hepatitis in the drug hypersensitivity syndrome is an indication for immediate discontinuation of nevirapine given the potential for fatal hepatitis. Risk factors for the development of morbilliform eruption with nevirapine use include higher $CD4^+$ count (>250 cells/mm^3 in women and >400 cells/mm^3 in men), lower HIV-1 RNA levels, Chinese ethnicity, and female gender (Davis and Shearer, 2008). In addition, nevirapine can cause the mucocutaneous Stevens–Johnson syndrome at a rate of 0.5%–1%, although PWH with $CD4^+$ counts of less than 200 cells/mm^3 (i.e., with AIDS) have a higher risk (Warren et al., 1998). Stevens–Johnson syndrome is characterized by flat, atypical targets or pruritic papules that are widespread or distributed on the trunk first and then spread to the neck, face, and proximal upper extremities. The palms and soles may be early sites of involvement. Bullae developing on the conjunctivae and mucous membranes of the nares, mouth, anorectal junction, vulvovaginal region, and urethral meatus are characteristic, with toxic epidermal necrolysis diagnosed when there is more than 30% body surface area skin detachment (Bolognia et al., 2012). In several studies, the use of prednisone and/or a 2-week lead-in dose of nevirapine 200 mg once daily failed to decrease the occurrence of the nevirapine-associated rash (Knobel et al., 2001); nevertheless, a dose-escalation protocol is recommended, starting with nevirapine 200 mg/day for 2 weeks, followed by an increase to the standard 400 mg/day dose only if there is no rash or no worsening rash after the trial 2-week period (Anton et al., 1999). Efavirenz and the second-generation etravirine, rilpivirine, and doravirine are also observed to cause similar hypersensitivity reactions, though much less commonly (Figure 27.1). This remains an

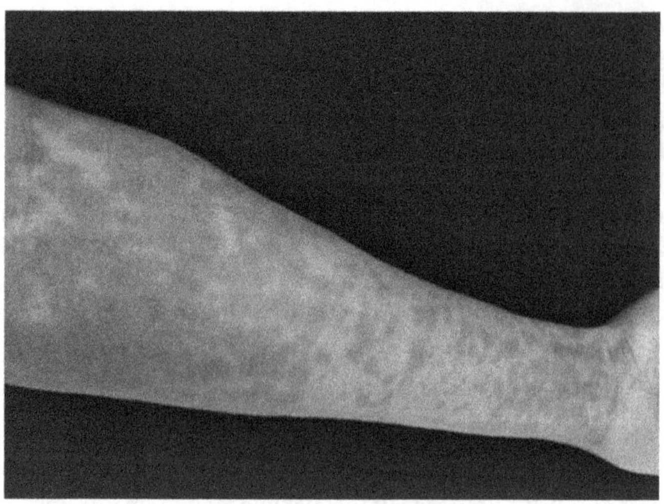

Figure 27.1 Cutaneous drug eruption caused by efavirenz. SOURCE: Spach, D. Cutaneous drug eruption caused by efavirenz: basic HIV primary care, cutaneous manifestations. In: Spach DH, et al. *National HIV Curriculum*. University of Washington Infectious Diseases Education & Assessment Program. Accessed June 30, 2024. https://www.hiv.uw.edu/go/basic-primary-care/cutaneous-manifestations/core-concept/all#cutaneous-drug-eruptions.

important consideration when assessing dermatitis, particularly during initiation of ART or modification or switch of a drug regimen (Yunihastuti et al., 2014).

NUCLEOSIDE REVERSE TRANSCRIPTASE INHIBITOR

Abacavir, a nucleoside reverse transcriptase inhibitor, can cause a multiorgan, potentially life-threatening hypersensitivity reaction (AHR), seen in 5%–8% of PWH on treatment. Symptoms consist of fever, rash, malaise, fatigue, tachypnea, pharyngitis, cough, wheezing, nausea, vomiting, and diarrhea that commence 9–11 days after initiating therapy. Symptoms that worsen with each subsequent dose are a classic characteristic of AHR. Symptoms of AHR recur within 24 hours of rechallenge and can be fatal. Therefore, continued use of abacavir in any person suspected to have AHR is contraindicated. Pre-ART genetic testing has shown that the absence of the HLA-B5701 allele dramatically decreases (by 99.9%) the likelihood of developing abacavir hypersensitivity (Mallal et al., 2008). For this reason, both the U.S. Department of Health and Human Services and International Antiviral Society USA guidelines recommend screening for the HLA-B5701 allele prior to initiation of any abacavir-containing regimen. Older NRTIs such as stavudine, didanosine and zidovudine were associated with peripheral and facial lipoatrophy, which will be discussed below.

PROTEASE INHIBITORS

Protease inhibitors (PIs) are generally associated with lipodystrophy, encompassing peripheral lipoatrophy and central adiposity, which can be an indication for discontinuation. The injectable fillers poly-l-lactic acid and calcium hydroxyapatite are approved for facial fat loss treatment associated with HIV treatment (Jagdeo et al., 2015), although the need for this has been dramatically reduced with avoidance of older PIs and NRTIs. Indinavir, no longer available in the United States, had the greatest variety of cutaneous side effects among PIs, including acute porphyria, Stevens–Johnson syndrome, hypersensitivity syndrome, morbilliform drug eruptions, gynecomastia, alopecia, pyogenic granuloma-like lesions, and paronychia (Ward et al., 2002). Approximately 6% of persons taking atazanavir report a mild rash not requiring treatment cessation. Although most PWH on atazanavir develop benign unconjugated hyperbilirubinemia, in some, it is severe enough to cause visible jaundice. Ritonavir and cobicistat are potent CYP34A inhibitors and decrease clearance of several corticosteroids, thus increasing their levels and the risk of hypothalamic–pituitary–adrenal axis dysfunction and Cushing's syndrome (Hyle et al., 2013). This should be considered when prescribing systemic steroids, inhaled corticosteroids such as fluticasone, or topical steroids when applied to a large body surface area.

OTHER ANTIRETROVIRAL THERAPIES

Few other antiretroviral drugs have a strong association with severe adverse drug reactions. Hypersensitivity to the fusion inhibitor enfuvirtide was seen in fewer than 1% of people taking it. However, 98% of users experience injection site reactions, which are frequently symptomatic (Ball et al., 2003). The enfuvirtide injection site reaction is characterized by tender erythema, induration, and nodule or cyst formation. On histology, a palisaded granulomatous response may be seen, with multinucleated cells aggregated around altered collagen, and surrounding eosinophils, histiocytes, lymphocytes, plasma cells, and variable fibrosis. The package insert for raltegravir, an integrase inhibitor, was updated to include dermatological side effects including Stevens–Johnson syndrome and toxic epidermal necrolysis following post-marketing case reports. Lenacapavir, a first-in-class capsid inhibitor, is administered via subcutaneous injection and, as such, may cause local injection site reactions (ISRs); in the CAPELLA trial, 65% of individuals on treatment reported ISRs; 61% were classified as Grade 1 (mild to moderate) including dermatologic symptoms of erythema, nodule formation, and pruritic, and no Grade 4 reactions were observed (Segal-Maurer et al., 2022). Injection site reactions are also commonly observed with the long-acting ART combination of cabotegravir plus rilpivirine, which is administered as two separate intramuscular injections (Teichner et al., 2024).

ANTIBIOTICS

Antibiotic drug reactions are seen at a higher rate in PWH than in the general population. Trimethoprim–sulfamethoxazole (TMP-SMX) is a commonly used antibiotic among PWH, especially for the prophylaxis and treatment of *Pneumocystis jirovecii* pneumonia (PJP). Reactions to TMP-SMX in individuals with known sulfa allergies are common and can be severe, including Stevens–Johnson Syndrome. Given its importance in the prevention and treatment of PJP, a desensitization schedule has been developed for people who have had reactions in the past and would benefit from its use. Desensitization has been successful using the following dosing schedule: an initial dose of trimethoprim 0.4 mg and sulfamethoxazole 2 mg, followed by doubling the dose daily over days 2–9, and at 10 days administering the full-strength dose (trimethoprim 160 mg/sulfamethoxazole 800 mg). Alternatives in individuals unable to tolerate TMP-SMX include decreased strength or less frequent dosing of TMP-SMX, dapsone with or without pyrimethamine/leucovorin, and atovaquone (Gompels et al., 1999).

RECOMMENDED READING

Hyle EP, Wood BR, Backman ES, et al. High frequency of hypothalamic–pituitary–adrenal axis dysfunction after local corticosteroid injection in HIV-infected patients on protease inhibitor therapy. *J AIDS*. 2013;63(5):602–608.

Introcaso CE, Hines JM, Kovarik CL. Cutaneous toxicities of antiretroviral therapy for HIV: part II. Nonnucleoside reverse transcriptase inhibitors, entry and fusion inhibitors, integrase inhibitors, and immune reconstitution syndrome. *J Am Acad Dermatol.* 2010;63(4):563–569; quiz 569–570.

CUTANEOUS OPPORTUNISTIC INFECTIONS

LEARNING OBJECTIVE

Discuss the diagnosis and management of viral, fungal, bacterial, and parasitic opportunistic infections in PWH.

WHAT'S NEW?

In 2024, the DHHS issued recommendations for anal cancer screening for some PWH, namely MSM and transgender women ≥35 years old and all others ≥45 years old; this includes anal symptom assessment and annual visual and digital rectal exam alone if no high-resolution anoscopy (HRA) referral resource is available, and with anal cytology + high-risk HPV testing if HRA is available.

KEY POINTS

- Cutaneous *Cryptococcus* may manifest before systemic symptoms; therefore, prompt diagnosis and management can prevent fatal outcomes.
- Molluscum, histoplasmosis, and *Cryptococcus* may all present with umbilicated papulonodules; however, there is a central white core to the molluscum lesion and most people appear well, as opposed to systemically ill presentations seen with cryptococcosis and histoplasmosis.
- Postherpetic neuralgia is common in herpes zoster infection, and initiation of gabapentin along with antiviral therapy at diagnosis may mitigate long-term neuralgia.
- The prozone effect may result in a false-negative syphilis test in PWH, and dilution of the assay should be requested when acute syphilis is suspected.
- The CDC recommends an intensive regimen for the management of crusted scabies: ivermectin dosed at 200 μg/kg taken on days 1, 2, 8, 9, and 15, and, for severe disease, also days 22 and 29, in combination with topical permethrin daily for 7 days and then twice a week until cure.

ONYCHOMYCOSIS

Onychomycosis is reported to affect approximately 2%–13% of the general population (Rosen et al., 2015) and is very common in PWH. Dermatophytes *Trichophyton mentagrophytes* and *T. rubrum* are responsible for most infections. Proximal subungual onychomycosis, seen as a solid white crescent extending from the nail bed, is seen in some PWH, especially those with a $CD4^{+}$ count of less than 450 cells/mm^3. Although it is not considered an AIDS-defining condition, it is highly suspicious for HIV infection and should prompt testing. *T. rubrum* is often the offending dermatophyte, although it also can be caused by *T. megninii*. In the general population, superficial white onychomycosis is typically caused by *T. mentagrophytes*, whereas in PWH, *T. rubrum* is the causative agent. The clinical differential includes psoriasis, lichen planus, trauma, and periungual squamous cell carcinoma. Most topical antifungals do not penetrate the thick nail keratin and thus are ineffective. Efinaconazole is a topical triazole solution for the treatment of onychomycosis; it is applied daily for 48 weeks to affected nails. Localized dermatitis is a potential side effect. In preapproval trials, a modest 15.2%–17.8% of patients achieved complete cure of onychomycosis. Tavorabole, a boron-based agent that was FDA-approved for onychomycosis in 2014, had even lower efficacy, with 6.5%–9.1% of patients achieving clearance (Zeichner, 2015). Terbinafine is considered first-line systemic therapy, dosed at 250 mg/day for 3 or 4 months for toenails and 6 weeks for fingernails (~50% cure rate). Itraconazole may also be effective at 200 mg/day for 3 months for toenails and 6 weeks for fingernails, or at 200 mg twice daily for 1 week per month for 3 months for toenails and 2 months for fingernails. The efficacy of fluconazole is lower than that of terbinafine and itraconazole. Patients with active liver disease should not receive terbinafine, and testing of LFTs at baseline and every 4–6 weeks is recommended given the risk of hepatotoxicity. Congestive heart disease is a contraindication to itraconazole use. In addition, itraconazole interacts with more medications compared to terbinafine (de Berker, 2009), particularly with the ART-boosting agents ritonavir and cobicistat. Finally, the etiologic agent of onychomycosis plays an important role in the choice of therapy. Nondermatophyte molds, such as *Scytalidium*, *Aspergillus*, and *Fusarium*, and yeast such as *Candida* are seen more commonly in PWH than in the general population. Much higher cure rates are achieved with itraconazole than with terbinafine for these organisms, whereas the reverse is true for dermatophytes (Cambuim et al., 2011; Warshaw et al., 2005). For these reasons, and given the potential side effects of systemic therapies, some dermatologists recommend culture of nail clippings before initiating therapy.

CANDIDIASIS

Angular cheilitis is typically caused by *Candida albicans* and presents as fissured white plaques at the angles of the lips. It occurs with some frequency in the elderly, but it may suggest HIV infection in young adults and warrants testing if there is no other known reason for immunosuppression. Topical antifungal creams are effective and avoid systemic circulation for this focal disease. Oropharyngeal involvement typically presents with painless atrophic or removable yellow-white pseudomembranous or hyperplastic plaques on the tongue, buccal mucosa, palate, and posterior mucosa (see Figure 27.2). Oral candidiasis is often a harbinger of immunologic failure in people on ART, although it can also be caused by steroids and antibiotics (Cockerell and Calame, 2013). The presence of oropharyngeal candidiasis should prompt consideration of esophageal involvement, particularly if there is associated retrosternal burning discomfort and/or odynophagia. Preferred treatment for oropharyngeal disease is a 1–2-week course of oral fluconazole, whereas a 2–3-week course of oral fluconazole or itraconazole oral solution is appropriate for suspected or confirmed esophageal disease.

Candida intertrigo is common in PWH, and can appear as eroded glistening erythematous plaques or as pustules with scale over a macerated erythematous surface within and extending from skin folds. While smaller lesions may be treated with topical antifungals, oral fluconazole or ketoconazole is recommended for larger or extensive plaques.

Vulvovaginal candidiasis can generally be treated with standard courses of oral fluconazole or topical azole antifungal agents. Longer courses of oral treatment can be used in cases of severe or recurrent disease.

CUTANEOUS CRYPTOCOCCOSIS

Cryptococcus neoformans causes an AIDS-defining systemic infection, with skin lesions preceding the more common central nervous system (CNS) and pulmonary involvement in only 10% of cases. The patient is typically febrile and very ill. Lesions can present as papules that may be umbilicated, nodules, pustules, ulcers, and plaques (Figure 27.3). A skin biopsy is necessary for diagnosis, revealing round yeast with narrow-based budding and a slimy capsule in a granulomatous or gelatinous background, highlighted by fungal stains. Serum and cerebrospinal fluid (CSF) cryptococcal antigen are both highly sensitive and specific. Culture is definitively diagnostic, and treatment is with amphotericin B, preferably liposomal given its more favorable renal side effect profile, plus flucytosine. Renal function should be closely monitored during treatment, as impairment would warrant flucytosine dose adjustment. After completion of induction and consolidation therapy, maintenance therapy with fluconazole 200 mg daily is indicated for at least 1 year. Discontinuation of maintenance therapy can be considered after 1 year if the patient is asymptomatic with virologic suppression on ART and a restored $CD4^+$ count ≥100 cells/mm^3. Maintenance therapy should be restarted if the $CD4^+$ count drops below 100 cells/mm^3. Failure to complete the entire course of maintenance therapy is the most common reason for recurrence of cryptococcal disease.

Initiation of ART is generally delayed in the setting of cryptococcosis: for non-CNS associated disease, the optimal time to begin ART and antifungal therapy is less clear. Many experts therefore recommend delaying ART initiation until 2–10 weeks of antifungal treatment have been completed to reduce the risk of IRIS. While IRIS is most often seen with CNS disease, primary/isolated cutaneous disease is rare, and initiation of ART prior to induction therapy could lead to unmasking of existing subclinical cryptococcal meningoencephalitis (Rhein et al., 2018). Confirming CNS culture sterility prior to initiation of ART helps mitigate the risk of IRIS.

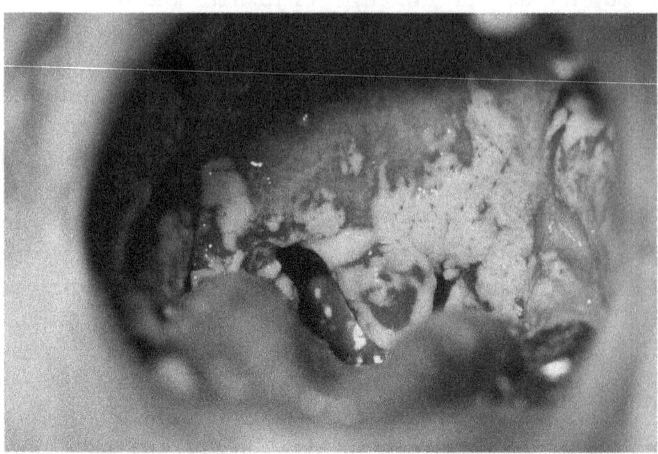

Figure 27.2 Oral thrush. SOURCE: CDC Public Health Image Library. Image ID 1217. https://phil.cdc.gov//PHIL_Images/1217/1217.tif. Accessed June 28, 2024.

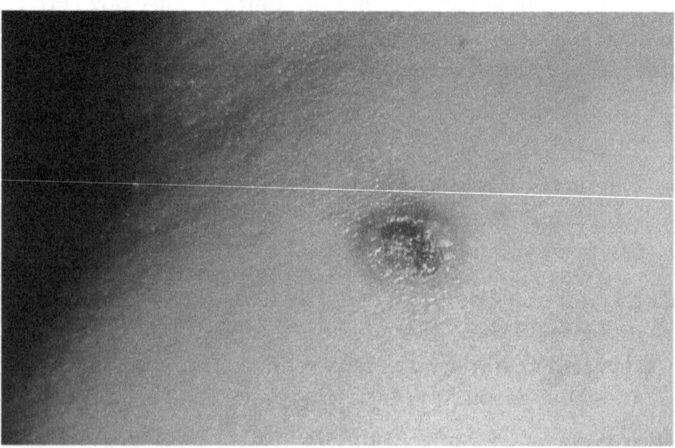

Figure 27.3 Cutaneous cryptococcosis. A skin lesion in a case of a disseminated fungal infection known as cryptococcosis, caused by a member of the genus *Cryptococcus*. Note the ovoid, crusty, central region of the lesion, which was surrounded by a raised, erythematous border. SOURCE: CDC Public Health Image Library. Image ID 14388. https://phil.cdc.gov/Details.aspx?pid=14388 Accessed June 26, 2024.

CUTANEOUS HISTOPLASMOSIS

Histoplasmosis is a common mycosis caused by the fungus *Histoplasma capsulatum*, endemic to the Ohio and Mississippi River basins. Primary cutaneous disease is rare and usually represents dissemination of pulmonary histoplasmosis. It manifests as a nonspecific rash characterized by diffuse erythematous macules, papules that may be umbilicated, pustules, crusted ulcers, or psoriasiform papules. The face is most often involved, followed by truncal and extremity involvement (Cockerell and Calame, 2013). The differential diagnosis includes molluscum contagiosum and cryptococcosis. While individuals with cutaneous histoplasmosis may be well appearing on initial presentation, the risk of rapid progression to severe disease with pulmonary, CNS, and gastrointestinal involvement warrants close monitoring (Wheat et al., 1990). Diagnosis of cutaneous histoplasmosis requires tissue biopsy, which reveals spores with a pseudo-capsule (the fungal wall) parasitizing macrophages. Blood or urine histoplasma antigen is a useful diagnostic tool in acute and disseminated histoplasmosis, but not as sensitive in chronic pulmonary disease. A positive blood or specimen culture confirms diagnosis. Treatment of histoplasmosis is universally recommended in PWH, including cutaneous involvement, regardless of disease severity, and consists of induction therapy, then more extended maintenance therapy. Less severe disease can be managed with 3 days of thrice daily oral itraconazole induction, followed by twice daily oral itraconazole maintenance for at least 12 months. More severe disease including meningitis requires, preferably, IV liposomal amphotericin B for upwards of 4–6 weeks, transitioned to oral itraconazole maintenance therapy when clinical improvement has been achieved. Similar to cryptococcosis, relapses can occur, and secondary prophylaxis with itraconazole is recommended in individuals with advanced HIV, especially those with $CD4^+$ <150 cells/mm^3 (DHHS, 2024b).

MOLLUSCUM CONTAGIOSUM

Molluscum (Figure 27.4) is a common viral infection in children and their caregivers, but it warrants testing for HIV in adults with limited exposure to children. Skin-colored discrete umbilicated papules are typical, although giant facial molluscum and extensive beard involvement occur with advanced immunosuppression. While many molluscum lesions will self-resolve with ART, giant molluscum can persist even after immune reconstitution, is extremely difficult to treat, and is stigmatizing. Molluscum is differentiated from cryptococcosis and histoplasmosis, which can also have umbilicated papules, by the presence of a central core in molluscum lesions. Also, individuals appear well with molluscum infection, whereas people with cryptococcal and histoplasma infection are systemically ill. Treatment options include cryotherapy or pulsed dye therapy for smaller lesions and curettage and excision for larger lesions; immune-modulating agents such as topical imiquimod, interferon-alpha and cimetidine; chemical agents (e.g., cantharidin, potassium hydroxide, podophyllotoxin, benzoyl peroxide, tretinoin, trichloroacetic acid, lactic acid, glycolic acid, and salicylic acid); antivirals (cidofovir); and photodynamic therapy with 5-aminolevulinic acid, which have all shown efficacy in case reports (Drain et al., 2014; Foissac et al., 2014; Leung et al., 2017), although high-quality clinical trial data are lacking.

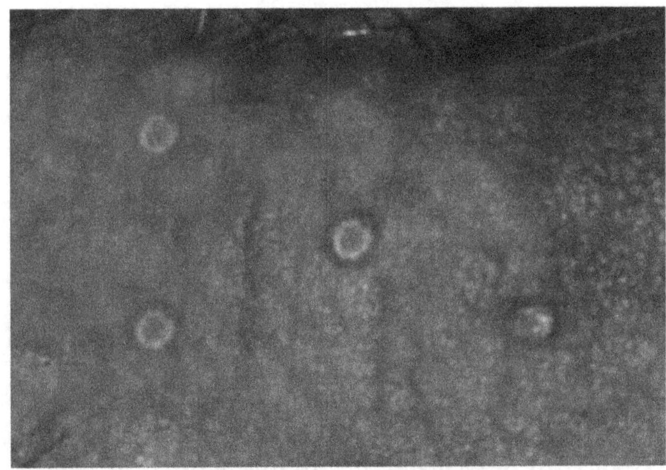

Figure 27.4 Molluscum contagiosum. SOURCE: Spach, D. Cutaneous drug eruption caused by efavirenz: basic HIV primary care, cutaneous manifestations. In: Spach DH, et al. *National HIV Curriculum*. University of Washington Infectious Diseases Education & Assessment Program. https://www.hiv.uw.edu/custom/primary-care/cutaneous-manifestations/8. Accessed June 30, 2024.

CONDYLOMA ACUMINATUM

Condyloma acuminatum (anogenital warts) (Figure 27.5), caused by the human papillomavirus (HPV), is the most common sexually transmitted infection in the United States. Warts appear as flesh-colored to gray, rounded to pointy papules, frequently on a short peduncle. Podophyllin, trichloroacetic acid, and cryotherapy are three of the most commonly

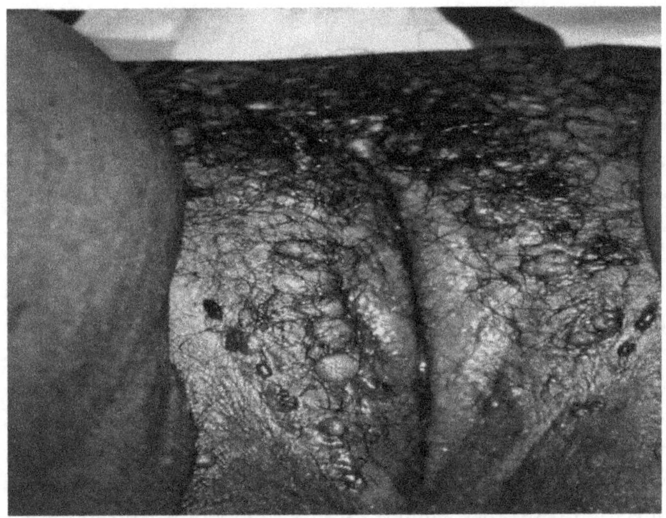

Figure 27.5 Condyloma acuminatum. This image depicts a close view of the exterior vaginal region of a female's perineum. It revealed the presence of numerous Condyloma acuminatum (genital warts), located primarily on the labia majora, which, in this woman's case, were long-standing, and remained after repeated attempts at their removal. SOURCE: CDC Public Health Image Library, Rein MF. Image ID 17418. https://phil.cdc.gov//PHIL_Images/17418/17418.tif. Accessed June 28, 2024.

used treatments for genital warts. Cryotherapy and trichloroacetic acid yield a treatment success rate of 75%, whereas that of podophyllin is reported to be 20%–50% (Murray et al., 2015). Therapies for recalcitrant anogenital warts include topical 5-fluoracil, cidofovir, intralesional interferon-α and surgical excision (Nambudiri et al., 2013).

Approximately 5% of MSM and 15% of MSM with HIV have a history of perianal warts. Anogenital warts are more common in women, and women with HIV are 5 times more likely than their uninfected counterparts to have these warts (Hagensee et al., 2004). In addition, squamous epithelial lesions occur in 79% of women with HIV with anal HPV infection compared to 43% of women without HIV. The frequency of intraepithelial neoplasia within anogenital warts warrants close surveillance after treatment (McCloskey et al., 2007). The ANCHOR study enrolled PWH aged ≥35 years with biopsy-proven anal HSIL to receive either treatment or active monitoring of these high-grade lesions. The trial was halted ahead of schedule when an interim analysis showed significantly lower risk of anal cancer in the treatment group when compared to active monitoring (Palefsky et al., 2022). Subsequently, in 2024, DHHS issued recommendations for anal cancer screening in MSM and transgender women ≥35 years old living with HIV and all other PWH ≥45 years old; screening involves anal symptom assessment and annual visual and digital rectal exam alone if no high-resolution anoscopy (HRA) referral resource is available, and with anal cytology + high-risk HPV testing if HRA is available. The disproportionate burden and consequence of HPV-associated disease highlights the paramount importance of HPV vaccination of all PWH 11–26 years old, according to Advisory Committee on Immunization Practices (ACIP) guidelines, and for unvaccinated PWH 27–45 years old with shared decision-making (DHHS, 2024a).

HERPES SIMPLEX

Herpes simplex virus (HSV) infection (Figures 27.6a and 27.6b) is caused by either HSV-1 or HSV-2 and is a common viral infection in the general population. In PWH, outbreaks occur more frequently and are less likely to self-resolve; at $CD4^+$ counts below 100 cells/mm^3, the incidence of HSV outbreaks reaches 27% (Severson and Tyring, 1999). Mucocutaneous lesions present as grouped vesicles on an erythematous base in the orolabial or genital tissue and can cause extensive and painful ulceration. HSV is also an important cause of proctitis in MSM and can be seen in the absence of anal ulcers (Klausner et al., 2004). Outbreaks are treated with valacyclovir 1 g by mouth twice daily for 5–10 days; acyclovir 400 mg 3 times a day is alternative therapy. Failure of lesions to improve within 7–10 days of therapy should prompt consideration of acyclovir resistance; such resistance in PWH is 10-fold higher than that in immunocompetent counterparts—6% and 0.6%, respectively (Lolis et al., 2008). Treatment requires intravenous foscarnet (preferred) or cidofovir (alternative), as resistance to acyclovir also implies resistance to valacyclovir, and, in many cases, famciclovir. Topical cidofovir and foscarnet have also been used with success (Strick et al., 2006).

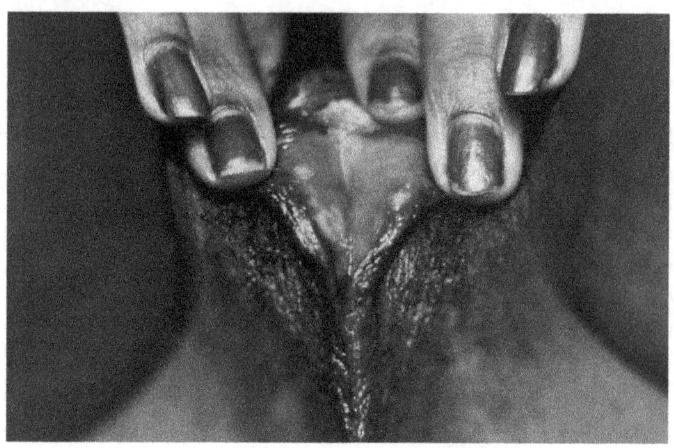

Figure 27.6a HSV-2 on female perineum. This image depicts a close view of a female's perineum, revealing what had been an outbreak of herpes genitalis, which had manifested as blistering around the vaginal introitus due to the herpes simplex 2 (HSV-2) virus, otherwise referred to as genital herpes. Sexually transmitted herpes simplex HSV-2 typically causes one or more blisters to form on or around the genitals or rectum, which break, leaving tender ulcers that may take 2–4 weeks to heal after making their initial appearance. SOURCE: CDC Public Health Image Library, Lindsley S. Image ID 15820. https://phil.cdc.gov//PHIL_Images/15820/15820.tif. Accessed June 28, 2024.

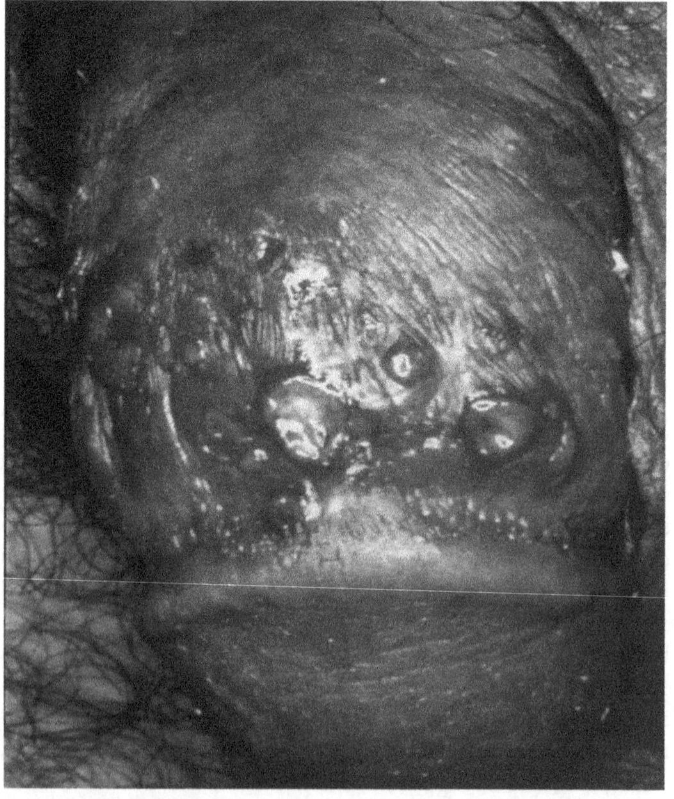

Figure 27.6b HSV-2 on male penis. This image depicts a close anterior view of a male patient's penis, which revealed the presence of a maculopapular herpetic rash on the penile shaft and corona of the glans penis. When signs of genital herpes do occur, they typically appear as one or more blisters, on or around the genitals or rectum. The blisters break, leaving tender ulcers (sores) that may take 2–4 weeks to heal the first time they appear. SOURCE: CDC Public Health Image Library, Flumara NJ, et al. Image ID 6471. https://phil.cdc.gov/Details.aspx?pid=6471. Accessed June 28, 2024.

HERPES ZOSTER

Varicella-zoster virus (VZV) (Figure 27.7) is a ubiquitous human herpesvirus (HHV-3) known to cause two unique cutaneous eruptions. Primary infection causes varicella (chickenpox), seen primarily in childhood, followed by immune control. Reactivation of latent VZV leads to herpes zoster infection (shingles); this can occur at any age, though it is strongly associated with waning immunity and increased age (Andrei and Snoeck, 2021). Immunosuppression is another important risk factor in VZV reactivation, making it an important cause of morbidity in PWH. Herpes zoster classically presents with clusters of painful vesicles on an erythematous base in a unilateral dermatomal distribution, most often in the thoracic area. The infection is usually limited to one dermatome in immunocompetent individuals, though multidermatomal involvement is common in PWH. Extensive cutaneous disease or disease recalcitrant to usual treatment warrants consideration of HIV testing. A prodrome of constitutional symptoms including fever, malaise, and headache may precede the eruptive phase.

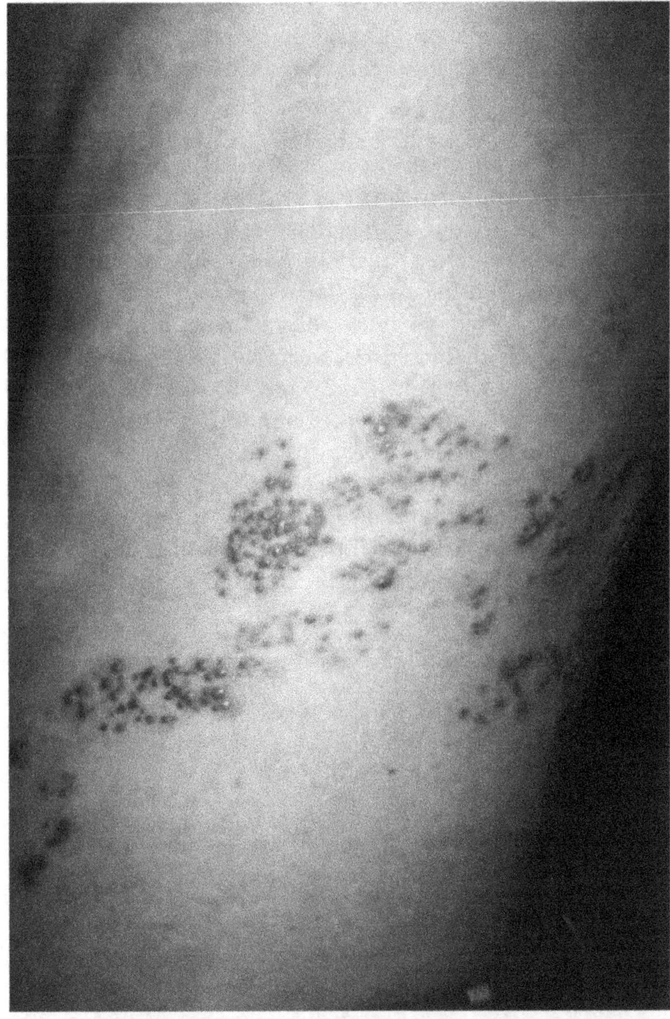

Figure 27.7 Varicella zoster virus (VZV, HHV-3). This view of a patient's skin revealed a maculopapular rash, which had been due to an outbreak of shingles, caused by the varicella zoster virus (VZV), also known as *Human herpesvirus 3* (HHV-3). The outbreak had taken place along the dermatomal innervation of the T10–T11 thoracic nerves emanating from the spinal cord at these two levels. SOURCE: CDC Public Health Image Library, Herrmann KL. Image ID 21506. https://phil.cdc.gov//PHIL_Images/21506/21506.tif. Accessed June 28, 2024.

Preferred therapy for acute localized herpes zoster is with oral valacyclovir 1,000 mg 3 times a day or famciclovir 500 mg 3 times a day for 7–10 days; acyclovir 800 mg 5 times a day is alternative therapy. Extensive cutaneous disease or other visceral involvement warrants intravenous acyclovir. Foscarnet 40 mg/kg 3 times a day is used for treatment of acyclovir-resistant VZV (Cockerell and Calame, 2013). Continual pain, referred to as postherpetic neuralgia (PHN), can occur and last months to years. Immunocompromised patients are at a higher risk of developing PHN, and effective, early treatment of pain with gabapentin and/or opioids at presentation, along with antivirals, can reduce the risk of PHN.

While no study has specifically evaluated vaccination in VZV-susceptible adolescents and adults with HIV, it is assumed to be safe and effective. The ACIP recommends consideration of vaccination for the prevention of primary varicella infection with the live-attenuated varicella vaccine (Varivax) in PWH without serologic evidence of immunity, provided their $CD4^+$ count is >200 cells/mm^3 (CDC, 2024d). Two vaccines for the prevention of herpes zoster (shingles) have been approved, but as of June 2020, the live-attenuated Zostavax (ZVL) is no longer available in the United States. The newer RZV is more immunogenic than its predecessor. It is not a live virus vaccine and as such it may be safe to give to PWH regardless of $CD4^+$ count, but this has yet to be determined in clinical trials. Nevertheless, in January 2022, the ACIP updated its recommendations for zoster vaccination, advising a two-dose RZV vaccination series in PWH aged 19 years and older without respect to $CD4^+$ count. PWH who already received ZVL should undergo revaccination with RZV (CDC, 2024d).

METHICILLIN-RESISTANT *STAPHYLOCOCCUS AUREUS*

Acquisition of the mecA gene by *Staphylococcus aureus* made it less sensitive to many of the antibiotics typically used to treat skin and soft-tissue infections, causing this form of community-acquired methicillin-resistant *S. aureus* (MRSA) to grow to epidemic proportions during the first decade of the twenty-first century. One study reported that the prevalence of MRSA was 18 times higher in PWH compared to the general population (Crum-Cianflone et al., 2007). More recent data have shown a reduction in MRSA-driven skin and soft-tissue infections in PWH from its peak in the later years of the decade (Hemmige et al., 2020).

Incision and drainage are the most important component of treatment for localized skin infections. Many cutaneous, community-acquired MRSA infections are generally sensitive to trimethoprim–sulfamethoxazole, doxycycline, clindamycin, and linezolid, and in refractory cases, culture and sensitivity data are helpful in guiding treatment. Both skin and nasal colonization are potential reservoirs for reinfection. Studies have indicated that mupirocin can be used to eradicate nasal colonization, whereas chlorhexidine can be used for the skin (Kuehnert et al., 2006).

BARTONELLOSIS

A genus of Gram-negative bacteria with a mammalian reservoir (cats and humans) and primarily arthropod transmission, *Bartonella* species cause a variety of clinical manifestations collectively known as bartonelloses. Of the over 30 species identified, *B. henselae* and *B. quintana* are an infrequent but important cause of opportunistic infection in PWH, namely bacillary angiomatosis (BA) (Akram et al., 2023). Stoler et al. identified BA early in the HIV pandemic in populations of individuals experiencing homelessness with HIV and advanced immunosuppression with CD4$^+$ counts <100 cells/mm^3 (1983). BA presents most commonly with cutaneous vascular lesions that evolve slowly, with or without systemic symptoms (see Figure 27.8). Lesion morphology varies, ranging from superficial purple "grape-like" papules in a focal or widespread distribution that gradually increase in size to larger, possibly ulcerated nodules. An important differential diagnosis includes Kaposi's sarcoma (KS), which can be difficult to distinguish due to potential atypical presentations (Hoffman et al., 2002; Koehler and Tappero, 1993). In contrast to KS, BA rarely manifest as patches or plaques and can be distinguished from KS on histology; BA shows a lobular capillary proliferation with an edematous stroma and clusters of neutrophils seen throughout the lesion, whereas KS shows uniform sheets of spindle cells and endothelial proliferation and stains positive for HHV-8 (Cockerell and Calame, 2013). There is often an amorphous material that represents colonies of bacteria, and culture for *Bartonella* speciation has clinical significance given that *Bartonella quintana* is more frequently associated with neurologic sequelae compared to *B. henselae* (Gasquet et al., 1998). Universal antibiotic treatment is indicated for PWH with BA; preferred treatment is doxycycline 100 mg twice daily, either oral or intravenous, depending on severity and presence of organ involvement. Treatment with either erythromycin or azithromycin is preferred in pregnancy. Rifampin is added for CNS involvement, multifocal disease, or bartonella endocarditis. Therapy is continued for at least 3 months until clinical resolution, and long-term suppressive therapy may be indicated if recurrent.

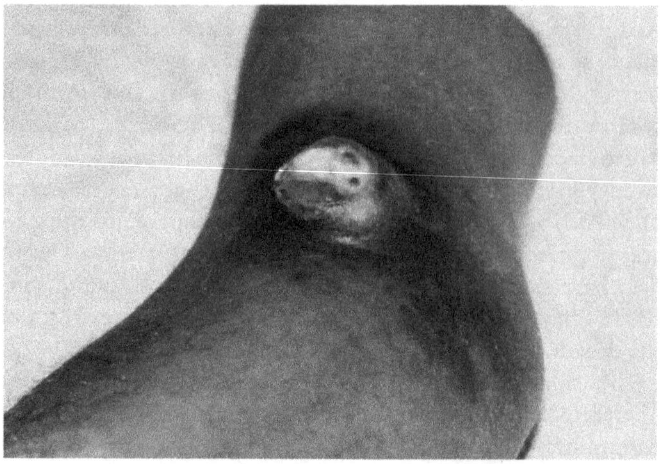

Figure 27.8 Nodular bacillary angiomatosis lesion in right antecubital fossa. SOURCE: Spach, D. Nodular bacillary angiomatosis lesion in right antecubital fossa: basic HIV Primary care, cutaneous manifestations. In: Spach DH, et al. *National HIV Curriculum*. University of Washington Infectious Diseases Education & Assessment Program. Accessed June 30, 2024. https://www.hiv.uw.edu/go/basic-primary-care/cutaneous-manifestations/core-concept/all#bacillary-angiomatosis.

SYPHILIS

Syphilis (Figures 27.9a and 27.9b) is a bacterial infection caused by the spirochete *Treponema pallidum* and progresses through characteristic stages and symptomatology. CDC data show that between 2018 and 2022, rates of syphilis increased nearly 80% and congenital syphilis increased by over 180% (CDC, 2024e). Cutaneous symptoms predominate in early syphilis and may be accompanied by constitutional symptoms, while dermatologic manifestations are typically absent in latent infection. Whereas tertiary syphilis develops after years to decades of untreated syphilis, neurosyphilis can occur during any stage of syphilis, and it is important to main a high degree of clinical suspicion and pursue diagnostic evaluation in the appropriate setting.

Primary syphilis typically presents with an asymptomatic orogenital chancre at the site of exposure that resolves within 4–6 weeks. While there can be overlap in primary and secondary syphilis in PWH, a generalized rash generally develops after resolution of the chancre in response to dissemination of spirochetes, causing a maculopapular to papulosquamous to psoriasiform rash which can mimic many other dermatoses. The color is characteristic, resembling a "clean-cut ham" or having a coppery tint. Palms and soles may have classic coppery-colored scaly plaques. Temporal, irregular, "moth-eaten" alopecia of the beard, scalp, and eyebrows may occur. Of concern, syphilis has an accelerated rate of progression in PWH and can have atypical presentations including multiple chancres and syphilitic vasculitis (Peeling et al., 2017). With a classic presentation, clinical suspicion often leads to diagnosis,

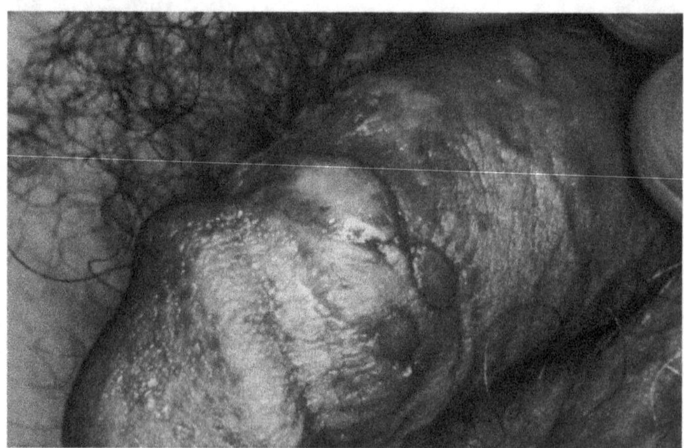

Figure 27.9a Primary syphilis. This photograph depicts a close view of a patient's penis, highlighting the presence of two lesions that were determined to be due to a case of primary syphilis, caused by the bacterial spirochete *Treponema pallidum*. SOURCE: CDC Public Health Image Library, Fiumara NJ. 1976. Image ID 17855. Accessed July 13, 2024. https://phil.cdc.gov/Details.aspx?pid=17855.

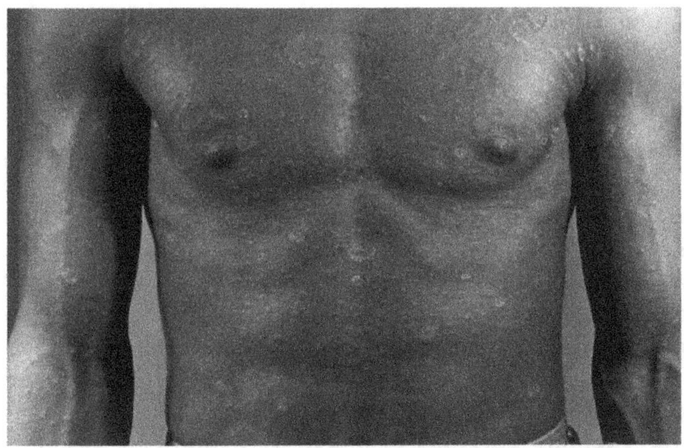

Figure 27.9b Secondary syphilis. This photograph depicted an anterior view of a male patient's torso and upper arms, which exhibited a flattened, pigmented macular rash, that was determined to be due to a secondary syphilis infection, caused by the bacterial spirochete *Treponema pallidum*. In this case, the characteristic secondary syphilitic rash also showed signs of scaling, or flaking. SOURCE: CDC Public Health Image Library. Image ID 17833. https://phil.cdc.gov/Details.aspx?pid=17833. Accessed July 13, 2024.

which is then confirmed with serologic or PCR testing of mucocutaneous sites. Serologic testing consists of a two-step algorithm involving treponemal and nontreponemal tests. The traditional algorithm first screens with a nontreponemal test (e.g., RPR, VDRL), which is then confirmed with a treponemal test (e.g., FTA, TPPA). A newer approach is the reverse algorithm, which first screens with a treponemal test and then confirms with a nontreponemal test. Diagnosis can be complicated by the prozone effect, in which a false-negative Rapid Plasma Reagin or Venereal Disease Research Laboratory result occurs in acute infection due to overwhelming antibody titers interfering with formation of an antigen-antibody lattice network in the test. Dilution of the assay overcomes this false-negative result, and should be requested when syphilis is suspected and there is a negative initial test result (Smith and Holman, 2004). Treatment of primary, secondary, and early latent syphilis is with penicillin G 2.4 million units once via intramuscular injection. Late latent syphilis (duration >1 year) is treated with penicillin G 2.4 million units intramuscular weekly for 3 doses. Neurosyphilis requires 10–14 days of intravenous penicillin. RPR should be followed at regular intervals, with a 4-fold decline in titer indicating appropriate treatment response, which can take up to 12 months in PWH (Ghanem et al., 2007). If an adequate response is not achieved and re-exposure has been ruled out as a possibility, consideration should be given for lumbar puncture to rule out an occult CNS infection/reservoir.

SCABIES

Scabies is caused by an infestation of the skin by the *Sarcoptes scabiei* mite. The first symptom of scabies is usually pruritus, especially at night. Scabies is a very common infection, with an approximate prevalence of 200 million annual cases (Global Burden of Disease, 2015). Scabies mites cannot jump or fly and therefore require skin-to-skin contact for infection to occur. Scabies mites have not demonstrated the ability to transmit HIV. Diagnosis is made through clinical examination. Burrow scrapings can be examined under a microscope for scabies mites, eggs, and feces; however, the absence of these on microscopic evaluation does not eliminate the possibility of infection. Dermoscopy has been shown to be a valuable tool in the diagnosis of scabies, with a characteristic "delta wing jet" appearance of burrows identified on dermoscopy (Suh et al., 2014).

"Norwegian" or "crusted" scabies (Figure 27.10) is a more florid infection leading to proliferation of heaped up, crusted burrows teeming with scabies mites. These crusted lesions typically occur in the web spaces of the hands and feet, over the elbows, and on the ears or temples. This typically occurs in highly immunocompromised patients, including PWH with low $CD4^+$ counts. Norwegian scabies is highly infectious and can be easily spread to healthcare workers by skin-to-skin contact.

Per CDC guidelines, first-line treatment of scabies is either topical permethrin cream or oral ivermectin (Workowski et al., 2021). Permethrin cream is applied below the neck (and above the neck if lesions are evident) and washed off after 8–14 hours on days 1 and 14, or ivermectin 200 μg/kg given on days 1 and 14. The CDC recommendation for treatment of crusted scabies to avoid treatment failure is an intensive regimen of ivermectin dosed at 200 μg/kg taken on days 1, 2, 8, 9, and 15, and, for severe disease, also on days 22 and 29, in combination with topical permethrin daily for 7 days

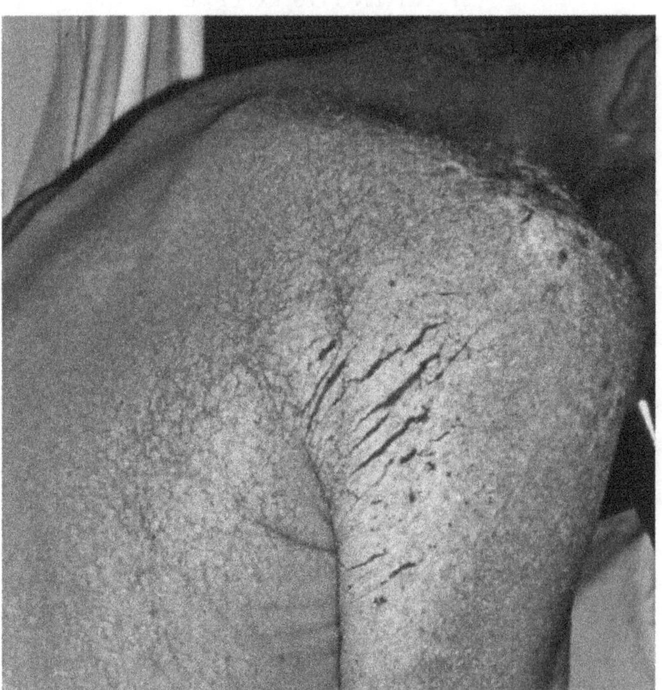

Figure 27.10 Crusted (Norwegian) scabies. This image of a patient with AIDS and a $CD4^+$ count less than 100 cells/mm^3 shows a diffuse erythematous rash, with plaque-like lesions in the shoulder region. SOURCE: Spach, D. Crusted scabies in a man with advanced immunosuppression: basic HIV primary care, cutaneous manifestations. In: Spach DH, et al. *National HIV Curriculum*. University of Washington Infectious Diseases Education & Assessment Program. Accessed June 30, 2024. https://www.hiv.uw.edu/go/basic-primary-care/cutaneous-manifestations/core-concept/all#scabies.

and then twice a week until cure (Ortega-Loayza et al., 2013). Treatment adherence may be difficult.

AMOEBA

Naegleria fowleri, *Balamuthia mandrillaris*, and *Acanthamoeba* are free-living protozoa that cause a rapidly progressive fatal infection in the immunocompromised host. *Acanthamoeba* is a recognized pathogen in immunocompromised individuals and has been cultured from the cornea, nasal and sinus cavities, ears, throat, lungs, and skin. *Acanthamoeba* can infect the skin directly or can spread to the skin by hematogenous dissemination from primary foci in the lungs or sinuses (Chandrasekar et al., 1997). More frequent sites of cutaneous involvement include the face, trunk, and extremities. The lesions typically present as nonspecific necrotic ulcers or nodules that may be quite tender or asymptomatic. Evaluations should include biopsy with histology showing trophozoites and culture for speciation. The survival rate is poor. Optimal treatment has not been determined; thus, combination therapy is recommended with miltefosine, fluconazole, and pentamidine. Trimethoprim–sulfamethoxazole, metronidazole, and a macrolide can be added to this regimen in people failing initial therapy (Mayer et al., 2011).

MPOX DISEASE (FORMERLY KNOWN AS MONKEY POX)

LEARNING OBJECTIVE

Discuss the demographics, presentation, diagnosis, treatment, and prevention of mpox.

KEY POINTS

- On July 23, 2022, and August 4, 2022, the WHO and U.S. DHHS, respectively, declared the mpox virus outbreak a public health emergency. The initial public health emergency was ended in mid-2023, though low-level community transmission is expected to persist. In August 2024, the WHO declared another public health emergency of international concern related to emergence of a new clade.
- Clinical disease is characterized by a viral prodrome followed by painful lesions, often anogenital, that can be severe and lead to disfiguring scarring.
- Vaccination with a two-dose series of Modified Vaccinia Ankara (MVA)-based vaccine (JYNNEOS) is currently recommended for PWH, given the risk for severe disease.

Monkeypox virus (MPV, MPX, MPXV) is one of the four *orthopoxvirus* known to cause human disease, along with *variola virus*, which causes smallpox, *cowpox virus*, and *vaccinia virus* (Bennett et al., 2020). Mpox, the clinical disease caused by MPV, has been an endemic zoonosis since the 1950s in parts of Africa, namely the Congo basin in central/western Africa; although sporadic outbreaks in nonendemic countries occur, sustained transmission had not been observed (Sklenovská and Van Ranst, 2018). In May 2022, a cluster of mpox first identified in the United Kingdom began to spread worldwide, leading the WHO to declare a public health emergency in July 2022, followed shortly thereafter by the DHHS in August 2022 (DHHS, 2024a). The WHO and DHHS public health emergencies were ended in the spring of 2023 after strategies to reduce transmission led to significant decline in incidence. Initial cases were associated with high-risk sexual behavior including having multiple and/or anonymous sexual partners, often in the presence of other co-occurring sexually transmitted infections. While a disproportionate burden of disease was seen in gay, bisexual, and other MSM, ongoing monitoring continues to support that any direct skin-to-skin contact can lead to transmission, including among household contacts. Demographic data also show that while most cases have occurred in white persons, Black and Hispanic persons, who make up 34% of the general population, account for more than one-half of mpox cases (Philpott et al., 2022). Further, 40% of those testing positive for mpox also have HIV. Whether this increased risk is due to viral, host, or other behavioral factors remains a subject of ongoing investigation; however, data do support that more severe mpox has been associated with lower $CD4^+$ count (Tarín-Vincente, 2022; Mitjà et al., 2023). Regardless of the reasons for these findings, it continues to highlight healthcare disparities and the importance of health equity.

Clinically, mpox manifests with a 1–2-week incubation period, followed by a systemic illness and rash. Systemic symptoms include a prodrome of fever, myalgias, malaise, headaches, predominant lymphadenopathy, or chills occurring as first symptom, not accompanied by a rash. Unique to the 2022 outbreak, a significant minority (42%) of those with mpox had a rash, typically anogenital and/or oral, as the first sign of illness; classic "prodromal" symptoms presented later in the disease course. The rash appears within 1–3 days of systemic illness, progressing through stages from maculopapular to vesicular to pustular over the course of 5–7 days. Lesions are characteristically painful and are generally but not always in the same stage of maturation; they can be few in number, first at the site of inoculation with subsequent spread more diffusely over time (Iñigo Martinez et al., 2022). Over the next 1–3 weeks, lesions scab over and heal. Individuals should be considered infectious until all lesions have scabbed over completely. Keeping lesions covered until this occurs can greatly reduce transmission (CDC, 2023; Philpott et al., 2022; Tarín-Vincente et al., 2022).

Diagnostic testing for mpox is via PCR testing for orthopoxvirus DNA, by swabbing lesions with a synthetic/noncotton swab, submitted in viral transport medium. Lesions need not be unroofed to obtain adequate genetic material for testing (CDC, 2024b). After diagnostic confirmation, many individuals will have a mild, self-limiting disease course requiring only supportive care; severe disease is uncommon. When it occurs, severe disease most often manifests as intense pain or secondary bacterial cellulitis of lesions, though bronchopneumonia, sepsis, encephalitis, myocarditis, and ocular lesions have been observed (Thornhill et al., 2022).

Treatment with oral or intravenous tecovirimat, developed for smallpox, is available via an expanded access Investigational

New Drug protocol for people who are at increased risk of severe disease and are exposed to or diagnosed with mpox (DHHS, 2024a). Two vaccines may be used for the prevention of mpox: MVA vaccine (JYNNEOS) and ACAM2000. MVA vaccine is made from attenuated, nonreplicating vaccinia virus, suitable for use in immunocompromised individuals (including PWH) and people with skin disorders, given as two doses (either subcutaneous or intradermal) 4 weeks apart. ACAM2000 is a replication-competent smallpox vaccine that should be avoided in immunocompromised people and those with certain skin conditions (CDC, 2024a). The two-dose mpox vaccination is also indicated as postexposure prophylaxis for individuals that have known close contact within the last 14 days with someone who tested positive for mpox (CDC, 2024c). Guidance published in October 2023 recommends vaccination with the two-dose JYNNEOS vaccine series for persons aged 18 years and older at risk for mpox (CDC, 2024a). Currently, there are no specific, different recommendations for mpox vaccination in PWH.

A significant increase in mpox cases in the Democratic Republic of the Congo (DRC) and surrounding countries in July–August 2024 involving a more severe clade (clade I, as opposed to clade II, which predominated in 2022) has caused the World Health Organization to declare the outbreak a public health emergency of international concern. Transmission has been noted not only through intimate contact, as with clade II, but also through household and fomite contact.

RECOMMENDED READING

Drain PK, Mosam A, Gounder L, et al. Recurrent giant molluscum contagiosum immune reconstitution inflammatory syndrome (IRIS) after initiation of antiretroviral therapy in an HIV-infected man. *Int J STD AIDS*. 2014;25(3):235–238.

McCloskey JC, Metcalf C, French MA, et al. The frequency of high-grade intraepithelial neoplasia in anal/perianal warts is higher than previously recognized. *Int J STD AIDS*. 2007;18(8):538–542.

Smith G, Holman RP. The prozone phenomenon with syphilis and HIV-1 co-infection. *South Med J*. 2004;97(4):379–382.

CUTANEOUS MALIGNANCIES IN HIV

LEARNING OBJECTIVE

Review the status of cutaneous malignancies in PWH.

WHAT'S NEW?

As life expectancy of PWH has increased, non-AIDS-defining cutaneous cancers have become a more prevalent cause of morbidity and mortality than classic conditions such as Kaposi's sarcoma.

KEY POINTS

- In the United States, first-line treatment for HIV-associated Kaposi's sarcoma (KS) remains antiretroviral therapy (ART), with chemotherapy indicated for progressive cutaneous disease or visceral involvement and radiation therapy for bulky obstructive tumors.
- There is an increased risk of metastatic disease in PWH with invasive melanoma, with worse outcomes associated with lower $CD4^+$ counts.
- There is a 3- to 5-fold increased risk of developing nonmelanoma skin cancer in HIV, and basal and squamous cell cancers are more aggressive in PWH.

KAPOSI'S SARCOMA

Prior to the HIV epidemic, Kaposi's sarcoma (KS) (Figures 27.11a and 27.11b) was rare in the United States. It was seen mostly in elderly men from the Mediterranean or recipients of solid organ transplants on immunosuppressive agents. An increasing prevalence of KS in the early HIV epidemic led to the discovery of human herpesvirus-8 (HHV-8), the causative agent of KS. KS most commonly presents with violaceous cutaneous patches, plaques, or nodules. While visceral lesions are less common, they are most frequently observed in the oral cavity at the gums/palate, gastrointestinal tract, and respiratory system. Biopsy reveals a vascular proliferation on histology with confirmatory HHV-8 immunostaining. First-line treatment for HIV-associated KS is ART. IRIS can result in KS progression during the initiation of ART, and patients on ART can still develop KS (Krown et al., 2008). Chemotherapy, typically with liposomal doxorubicin, is indicated for rapidly progressive cutaneous KS and when there is visceral involvement; radiation may be helpful when bulky plaques cause pain or lymphatic blockage (Murphy et al., 1997; Reid et al., 2019). There have been reports of HHV-8 reactivation and development of KS in patients exposed to topical and systemic steroids (Boudhir et al., 2013).

MELANOMA AND NONMELANOMA SKIN CANCERS

The non-AIDS-defining skin cancers include basal cell cancers, squamous cell cancers, and melanomas. Case reports

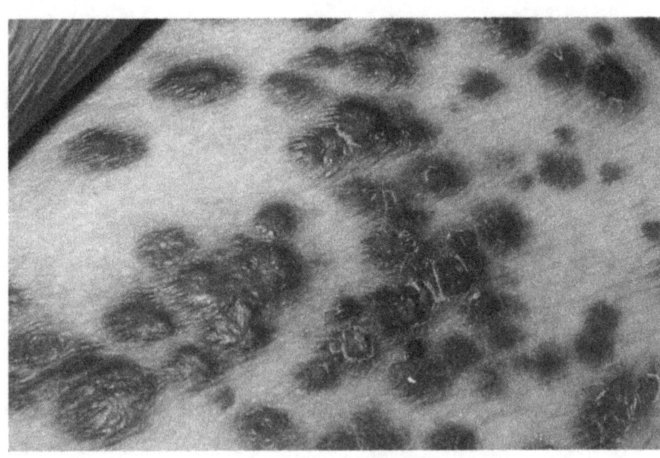

Figure 27.11a Kaposi's sarcoma on the skin of PWH. SOURCE: The website of the National Cancer Institute (https://www.cancer.gov). Image ID 2168. Accessed July 13, 2024.

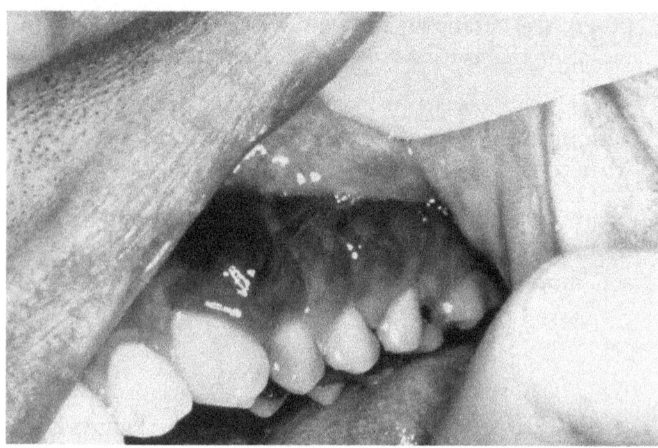

Figure 27.11b Kaposi's sarcoma in the mouth on the upper gums of PWH. SOURCE: The website of the National Cancer Institute (https://www.cancer.gov). Image ID 2166. Accessed July 13, 2024.

suggest an increased incidence of melanoma in PWH (Wilkins et al., 2006). In addition, PWH are more likely to develop metastases with invasive melanoma, and lower CD4$^+$ count is predictive of worse prognosis (Rodrigues et al., 2002). In addition, there is a 3- to 5-fold increased risk of developing nonmelanoma skin cancer in HIV. Basal cell carcinomas are more common than squamous cell carcinomas (SCCs), as is the case in the general population, but in contrast to immunocompromised transplant patients, in whom SCCs are more common. Both basal cell carcinomas and SCCs are more aggressive in PWH (Wilkins et al., 2006). Despite this, screening guidelines for melanoma, BCC, and SCC are the same for PWH as those for the general population.

ACKNOWLEDGMENTS

The author acknowledges John M. Curtain, Kudakwashe Mutyambizi, and Philip Bolduc, authors of this chapter in previous editions.

RECOMMENDED READING

Wilkins K, Turner R, Dolev JC, et al. Cutaneous malignancy and human immunodeficiency virus disease. *J Am Acad Dermatol.* 2006;54(2):189–206;quiz 207–110.

REFERENCES

Aboulafia D M, Bundow D, Wilske K, Ochs UI. Etanercept for the treatment of human immunodeficiency virus-associated psoriatic arthritis. *Mayo Clin Proc.* 2000;75(10):1093–1098.

Akram SM, Anwar MY, Thandra KC, Rawla P. Bacillary angiomatosis. In *StatPearls.* StatPearls https://www.ncbi.nlm.nih.gov/books/NBK448092/. Publishing; 2023. Accessed June 30, 2024.

Altman K, Vanness E, Westergaard RP. Cutaneous manifestations of human immunodeficiency virus: a clinical update. *Curr Infect Dis Rep.* 2015;17(3):464.

Andrei G, Snoeck R. Advances and perspectives in the management of varicella-zoster virus infections. *Molecules.* 2021 Feb 20;26(4):1132. https://doi.org/10.3390/molecules26041132

Anton P, Soriano V, Jimenez-Nacher I, et al. Incidence of rash and discontinuation of nevirapine using two different escalating initial doses. *AIDS.* 1999;13(4):524–525.

Ball RA, Kinchelow T; ISR Substudy Group. Injection site reactions with the HIV-1 fusion inhibitor enfuvirtide. *J Am Acad Dermatol.* 2003;49(5):826–831.

Bartlett BL, Khambaty M, Mendoza N, et al. Dermatological management of human immunodeficiency virus (HIV). *Skin Therapy Lett.* 2007;12(8):1–3.

Baveewo S, Ssali F, Karamagi C, et al. Validation of World Health Organisation HIV/AIDS clinical staging in predicting initiation of antiretroviral therapy and clinical predictors of low CD4^{++} T cell count in Uganda. *PLoS One.* 2011;6(5):e19089.

Bellavista S, D'Antuono A, Infusino SD, et al. Pruritic papular eruption in HIV: a case successfully treated with NB-UVB. *Dermatol Ther.* 2013;26(2):173–175.

Bennett JE, Dolin R, Blaser MJ, et al. In *Mandell, Douglas, and Bennett's Principles and Practice of Infectious Diseases*, vol. 2. New York: Elsevier; 2020:1809–1817.

Bolognia JL, Jorizzo JL, Schaffer J. *Dermatology.* 3rd ed. New York: Elsevier; 2012.

Boonchai W, Laohasrisakul R, Manonukul J, Kulthanan K. Pruritic papular eruption in HIV seropositive patients: a cutaneous marker for immunosuppression. *Int J Dermatol.* 1999;38(5):348–350.

Boudhir H, Mael-Ainin M, Senouci K, et al. Kaposi's disease: an unusual side-effect of topical corticosteroids. *Ann Dermatol Venereol.* 2013;140(6–7):459–461.

Breuer-McHam J, Marshall G, Adu-Oppong A, et al. Alterations in HIV expression in AIDS patients with psoriasis or pruritus treated with phototherapy. *J Am Acad Dermatol.* 1999;40(1):48–60.

Calonje E, Brenn T, Lazar A, Mckee P. *McKee's Pathology of the Skin.* 4th ed. St. Louis, MO: Saunders; 2012:901.

Cambuim II, Macedo DP, Delgado M, et al. Clinical and mycological evaluation of onychomycosis among Brazilian HIV/AIDS patients [in Portuguese]. *Rev Soc Bras Med Trop.* 2011;44(1):40–42.

Centers for Disease Control and Prevention (CDC). Interim clinical considerations for use of JYNNEOS and ACAM2000 vaccines during the 2022 U.S. monkeypox outbreak. https://www.cdc.gov/poxvirus/mpox/clinicians/vaccines/vaccine-considerations.html?CDC_AA_refVal=https%3A%2F%2Fwww.cdc.gov%2Fpoxvirus%2Fmpox%2Fhealth-departments%2Fvaccine-considerations.html. Published August 26, 2024a. Accessed August 29, 2024.

CDC. Monkeypox: clinical recognition, https://www.cdc.gov/poxvirus/monkeypox/clinicians/clinical-recognition.html. Published August 30, 2023. Accessed August 29, 2024.

CDC. Monkeypox: preparation and collection of specimens. https://www.cdc.gov/poxvirus/mpox/clinicians/prep-collection-specimens.html. Published April 29, 2024b. Accessed August 29, 2024.

CDC. Vaccination strategies. https:// www.cdc.gov/poxvirus/mpox/interim-considerations/overview.html. Published April 22, 2024c. Accessed August 29, 2024.

CDC. Sexually transmitted infections surveillance, 2023. https://www.cdc.gov/sti-statistics/annual/summary.html. Published November 12, 2024e. Accessed February 6, 2025.

CDC. Adult immunization schedule by age. 2024. https://www.cdc.gov/vaccines/hcp/imz-schedules/adult-age.html. Published November 21, 2024d. Accessed February 6, 2025.

Chandrasekar PH, Nandi PS, Fairfax MR, Crane LR. Cutaneous infections due to *Acanthamoeba* in patients with acquired immunodeficiency syndrome. *Arch Intern Med.* 1997;157(5):569–572.

Chaponda M, Pirmohamed M. Hypersensitivity reactions to HIV therapy. *Br J Clin Pharmacol.* 2011;71(5):659–671.

Cockerell C, Calame A. *Cutaneous Manifestations of HIV Disease.* London: Manson; 2013.

Crum-Cianflone NF, Burgi AA, Hale BR. Increasing rates of community-acquired methicillin-resistant *Staphylococcus aureus* infections among HIV-infected persons. *Int J STD AIDS*. 2007;18(8):521–526.

Davis CM, Shearer WT. Diagnosis and management of HIV drug hypersensitivity. *J Allergy Clin Immunol*. 2008;121(4):826–832, e825.

de Berker D. Clinical practice: fungal nail disease. *N Engl J Med*. 2009;360(20):2108–2116.

de Moraes AP, de Arruda EA, Vitoriano MA, et al. An open-label efficacy pilot study with pimecrolimus cream 1% in adults with facial seborrhoeic dermatitis infected with HIV. *J Eur Acad Dermatol Venereol*. 2007;21(5):596–601.

DHHS, Panel on Antiretroviral Guidelines for Adults and Adolescents. Guidelines for the use of antiretroviral agents in adults and adolescents with HIV. Department of Health and Human Services. https://clinicalinfo.hiv.gov/en/guidelines/adult-and-adolescent-arv. Published February 27, 2024a. Accessed August 29, 2024.

DHHS Panel on Guidelines for the Prevention and Treatment of Opportunistic Infections in Adults and Adolescents with HIV. Guidelines for the prevention and treatment of opportunistic infections in adults and adolescents with HIV. National Institutes of Health, Centers for Disease Control and Prevention, HIV Medicine Association, and Infectious Diseases Society of America. https://clinicalinfo.hiv.gov/en/guidelines/adult-and-adolescent-opportunistic-infection. Published August 15, 2024b. Accessed August 29, 2024.

Dogra S, Yadav S. Acitretin in psoriasis: an evolving scenario. *Int J Dermatol*. 2014;53(5):525–538.

Dover JS, Johnson RA. Cutaneous manifestations of human immunodeficiency virus infection: part II. *Arch Dermatol*. 1991;127(10):1549–1558.

Drain PK, Mosam A, Gounder L, et al. Recurrent giant molluscum contagiosum immune reconstitution inflammatory syndrome (IRIS) after initiation of antiretroviral therapy in an HIV-infected man. *Int J STD AIDS*. 2014;25(3):235–238.

Duvic M. Immunology of AIDS related to psoriasis. *J Invest Dermatol*. 1990;95(5):38S–40S.

Duvic M, Crane MM, Conant M, et al. Zidovudine improves psoriasis in human immunodeficiency virus-positive males. *Arch Dermatol*. 1994;130(4):447–451.

Eisman S. Pruritic papular eruption in HIV. *Dermatol Clin*. 2006;24(4):449–457, vi.

Farsani TT, Kore S, Nadol P, et al Etiology and risk factors associated with a pruritic papular eruption in people living with HIV in India. *J Int AIDS Soc*. 2013 Sep 3;16(1):17325. http://doi:10.7448/IAS.16.1.17325. PMID: 24004854; PMCID: PMC3763046.

Fearfield LA, Rowe A, Francis N, et al. Itchy folliculitis and human immunodeficiency virus infection: clinicopathological and immunological features, pathogenesis and treatment. *Br J Dermatol*. 1999;141(1):3–11.

Foissac M, Goehringer F, Ranaivo IM, et al. Efficacy and safety of intravenous cidofovir in the treatment of giant molluscum contagiosum in an immunosuppressed patient [in French]. *Ann Dermatol Venereol*. 2014;141(10):620–622.

Gasquet S, Maurin M, Brouqui P, et al. Bacillary angiomatosis in immunocompromised patients. *AIDS*. 1998;12(14):1793–1803.

Gelfand JM, Gladman DD, Mease PJ, et al. Epidemiology of psoriatic arthritis in the population of the United States. *J Am Acad Dermatol*. 2005;53(4):573.

Ghanem KG, Erbelding EJ, Wiener ZS, Rompalo AM. Serological response to syphilis treatment in HIV-positive and HIV-negative patients attending sexually transmitted diseases clinics. *Sex Transm Infect*. 2007;83(2):97–101.

Global Burden of Disease 2015 Disease and Injury Incidence and Prevalence Collaborators. Global, regional, and national incidence, prevalence and years lived with disability for 310 diseases and injuries, 1990–2015; a systematic analysis for the Global Burden of Disease Study 2015. *Lancet*. 2016;388(10053):1545.

Goldstein B, Berman B, Sukenik E, Frankel SJ. Correlation of skin disorders with CD4+ T cell lymphocyte counts in patients with HIV/AIDS. *J Am Acad Dermatol*. 1997;36(2 Pt 1):262–264.

Gompels MM, Simpson N, Snow M, et al. Desensitization to co-trimoxazole (trimethoprim-sulphamethoxazole) in HIV-infected patients: is patch testing a useful predictor of reaction? *J Infect*. 1999;38:111–115.

Hagensee ME, Cameron JE, Leigh JE, Clark RA. Human papillomavirus infection and disease in HIV-infected individuals. *Am J Med Sci*. 2004;328(1):57–63.

Hanifin JM, Reed ML, Eczema P, et al.; Impact Working Group. A population-based survey of eczema prevalence in the United States. *Dermatitis*. 2007;18(2):82–91.

Hemmige V, Arias CA, Pasalar S, Giordano TP. Skin and soft tissue infection in people living with human immunodeficiency virus in a large, urban, public healthcare system in Houston, Texas, 2009–2014. *Clin Infect Dis*. 2020;70(9):1985–1992. http://doi:10.1093/cid/ciz509

Hevia O, Jimenez-Acosta F, Ceballos PI, et al. Pruritic papular eruption of the acquired immunodeficiency syndrome: a clinicopathologic study. *J Am Acad Dermatol*. 1991;24(2 Pt 1):231–235.

Hoffman CF, Papadopoulos D, Palmer DM, et al. A case report of bacillary angiomatosis in a patient infected with human immunodeficiency virus. *Cutis*. 2002;69(3):175–178.

Hyle EP, Wood BR, Backman ES, et al. High frequency of hypothalamic–pituitary–adrenal axis dysfunction after local corticosteroid injection in HIV-infected patients on protease inhibitor therapy. *J AIDS*. 2013;63(5):602–608.

Iñigo Martínez J. Gil Montalbán E, Jiménez Bueno S, et al. Monkeypox outbreak predominantly affecting men who have sex with men, Madrid, Spain, 26 April to 16 June 2022. *Euro Surveill*. 2022;27(27):200471. https://doi.org/10.2807/1560-7917.ES.2022.27.27.2200471

Introcaso CE, Hines JM, Kovarik CL. Cutaneous toxicities of antiretroviral therapy for HIV: part II. Nonnucleoside reverse transcriptase inhibitors, entry and fusion inhibitors, integrase inhibitors, and immune reconstitution syndrome. *J Am Acad Dermatol*. 2010;63(4):563–569; quiz 569–570.

Jagdeo J, Ho D, Lo A, Carruthers A. A systematic review of filler agents for aesthetic treatment of HIV facial lipoatrophy (FLA). *J Am Acad Dermatol*. 2015; 73(6):1040–1054, e1014.

Kim CM, Vogel J, Jay G, Rhim JS. The HIV tat gene transforms human keratinocytes. *Oncogene*. 1992;7(8):1525–1529.

Klausner JD, Kohn R, Kent C. Etiology of clinical proctitis among men who have sex with men. *Clin Infect Dis*. 2004;38(2):300–2.

Knobel H, Miro JM, Domingo P, et al. Failure of a short-term prednisone regimen to prevent nevirapine-associated rash: a double-blind placebo-controlled trial: the GESIDA 09/99 study. *J AIDS*. 2001;28(1):14–18.

Koehler JE, Tappero JW. Bacillary angiomatosis and bacillary peliosis in patients infected with human immunodeficiency virus. *Clin Infect Dis*. 1993;17(4):612–624. doi:10.1093/clinids/17.4.612

Krown SE, Lee JY, Dittmer DP; AIDS Malignancy Consortium. More on HIV-associated Kaposi's sarcoma. *N Engl J Med*. 2008;358(5):535–536; author reply 536.

Kuehnert MJ, Kruszon-Moran D, Hill HA, et al. Prevalence of *Staphylococcus aureus* nasal colonization in the United States, 2001–2002. *J Infect Dis*. 2006;193(2):172–179.

Leung AKC, Barankin B, Hon KLE. Molluscum contagiosum: an update. *Recent Pat Inflamm Allergy Drug Discov*. 2017;11(1):22–31. http://doi:10.2174/1872213X11666170518114456

Lin RY, Lazarus TS. Asthma and related atopic disorders in outpatients attending an urban HIV clinic. *Ann Allergy Asthma Immunol*. 1995;74(6):510–515.

Liu Z, Xie Z, Zhang L, et al. Reliability and validity of dermatology life quality index: assessment of quality of life in human immunodeficiency virus/acquired immunodeficiency syndrome patients with pruritic papular eruption. *J Tradit Chin Med*. 2013;33(5):580–583.

Lolis MS, Gonzalez L, Cohen PJ, Schwartz RA. Drug-resistant herpes simplex virus in HIV infected patients. *Acta Dermatovenerol Croat*. 2008;16(4):204–208.

Mallal S, Phillips E, Carosi G, et al. HLA-B*5701 screening for hypersensitivity to abacavir. *N Engl J Med*. 2008;358(6):568–579.

Mallon E, Bunker CB. HIV-associated psoriasis. *AIDS Patient Care STDs*. 2000;14(5):239–246.

Maurer TA. Dermatologic manifestations of HIV infection. *Top HIV Med*. 2005; 13(5):149–154.

Mayer PL, Larkin JA, Hennessy JM. Amebic encephalitis. *Surg Neurol Int*. 2011;2:50.

McCloskey JC, Metcalf C, French MA, et al. The frequency of high-grade intraepithelial neoplasia in anal/perianal warts is higher than previously recognized. *Int J STD AIDS*. 2007;18(8):538–542.

Menon K, Van Voorhees AS, Bebo BF, et al. Psoriasis in patients with HIV infection: from the medical board of the National Psoriasis Foundation. *J Am Acad Dermatol*. 2010;62(2):291–299.

Meola T, Soter NA, Ostreicher R, Sanchez M, Moy JA. The safety of UVB phototherapy in patients with HIV infection. *J Am Acad Dermatol*. 1993;29(2 Pt 1):216–220.

Mirmirani P, Maurer TA, Berger TG, et al. Skin-related quality of life in HIV-infected patients on highly active antiretroviral therapy. *J Cutan Med Surg*. 2002;6(1):10–15.

Mischo M, von Kobyletzki LB, Bründermann E, et al. Similar appearance, different mechanisms: xerosis in HIV, atopic dermatitis and ageing. *Exp Dermatol*. 2014;23(6):446–448. http://doi:10.1111/exd.12425. PMID: 24758518.

Mitjà O, Alemany A, Marks M, et al. Mpox in people with advanced HIV infection: a global case series. *Lancet*. 2023;401(10370):60–74.

Mohammed S, Vellaisamy SG, Gopalan K, et al. Prevalence of pruritic papular eruption among HIV patients: a cross-sectional study. *Indian J Sex Transm Dis AIDS*. 2019;40(2):146–151. http://doi:10.4103/ijstd.IJSTD_69_18. PMID: 31922105; PMCID: PMC6896392.

Murphy M, Armstrong D, Sepkowitz KA, et al. Regression of AIDS-related Kaposi's sarcoma following treatment with an HIV-1 protease inhibitor. *AIDS*. 1997;11(2):261–262.

Murray H, Barber CJ, Foreman RM, et al.; GBD 2013 DALYs and HALE Collaborators. Global, regional, and national disability-adjusted life years (DALYs) for 306 diseases and injuries and healthy life expectancy (HALE) for 188 countries, 1990–2013: quantifying the epidemiological transition. *Lancet*. 2015;386:2145–2191.

Nakamura M, Abrouk M, Farahnik B, et al. Psoriasis treatment in HIV-positive patients: a systematic review of systemic immunosuppressive therapies. *Cutis*. 2018;101(1):38, 42, 56.

Nambudiri VE, Mutyambizi K, Walls AC, et al. Successful treatment of perianal giant condyloma acuminatum in an immunocompromised host with systemic interleukin 2 and topical cidofovir. *JAMA Dermatol*. 2013;149(9):1068–1070.

Nissen D, Nolte H, Permin H, et al. Evaluation of IgE-sensitization to fungi in HIV-positive patients with eczematous skin reactions. *Ann Allergy Asthma Immunol*. 1999;83(2):153–159.

Nomura T, Katoh M, Yamamoto Y, et al. Eosinophilic pustular folliculitis: A published work-based comprehensive analysis of therapeutic responsiveness. *J Dermatol*. 2016;43(8):919–927. http://doi: 10.1111/1346-8138.13287

Oble DA, Collett E, Hsieh M, et al. A novel T cell receptor transgenic animal model of seborrheic dermatitis-like skin disease. *J Invest Dermatol*. 2005;124(1):151–159.

Obuch ML, Maurer TA, Becker B, Berger TG. Psoriasis and human immunodeficiency virus infection. *J Am Acad Dermatol*. 1992;27(5 Pt 1):667–673.

Okada S, Fujimura T, Furudate S, et al. Immunosuppression-associated eosinophilic pustular folliculitis (IS-EPF) developing after highly active anti-retroviral therapy (HAART): the possible mechanisms through CD163⁺ M2 macrophages. *Eur J Dermatol*. 2013;23(5):713–714.

Ortega-Loayza AG, McCall CO, Nunley JR. Crusted scabies and multiple dosages of ivermectin. *J Drugs Dermatol*. 2013;12(5):584–585.

Osborne GE, Taylor C, Fuller LC. The management of HIV-related skin disease. Part II: neoplasms and inflammatory disorders. *Int J STD AIDS*. 2003;14:235.

Palefsky JM, Lee JY, Jay N; ANCHOR Investigators Group. Treatment of anal high-grade squamous intraepithelial lesions to prevent anal cancer. *N Engl J Med*. 2022;386(24):2273–2282. https://doi.org/10.1056/NEJMoa2201048

Pedrosa AF, Lisboa C, Goncalves Rodrigues A. Malassezia infections: a medical conundrum. *J Am Acad Dermatol*. 2014;71(1):170–176.

Peeling RW, Mabey D, Kamb ML, et al. Syphilis. *Nat Rev Dis Primers*. 2017;3:17073.

Philpott D, Hughes CM, Alroy KA, et al. Epidemiologic and clinical characteristics of monkeypox cases—United States, May 17–July 22, 2022. *MMWR*. 2022;71:1018–1022. http://dx.doi.org/10.15585/mmwr.mm7132e3

Ratnam I, Chiu C, Kandala NB, Easterbrook PJ. Incidence and risk factors for immune reconstitution inflammatory syndrome in an ethnically diverse HIV type 1-infected cohort. *Clin Infect Dis*. 2006;42(3):418–427.

Reid E, Suneja G, Ambinder R, et al. AIDS-related Kaposi sarcoma, version 2.2019, NCCN Clinical Practice Guidelines in Oncology. *J Natl Compr Canc Netw*. 2019 Feb;17(2):171–189.

Resneck JS Jr, Van Beek M, Furmanski L, et al. Etiology of pruritic papular eruption with HIV infection in Uganda. *JAMA*. 2004;292(21):2614–2621.

Rhein J, Hullsiek KH, Evans EE, et al. Detrimental outcomes of unmasking cryptococcal meningitis with recent ART initiation. *Open Forum Infect Dis*. 2018;5(8):ofy122.

Rigopoulos D, Paparizos V, Katsambas A. Cutaneous markers of HIV infection. *Clin Dermatol*. 2004;22(6):487–498.

Rodrigues LK, Klencke BJ, Vin-Christian K, et al. Altered clinical course of malignant melanoma in HIV-positive patients. *Arch Dermatol*. 2002;138(6):765–770.

Rosen T, Friedlander SF, Kircik L. Onychomycosis: epidemiology, diagnosis, and treatment in a changing landscape. *J Drugs Dermatol*. 2015;14(3):223–233.

Rosenthal D, LeBoit PE, Klumpp L, Berger TG. Human immunodeficiency virus-associated eosinophilic folliculitis: a unique dermatosis associated with advanced human immunodeficiency virus infection. *Arch Dermatol*. 1991;127(2):206–209.

Sadick NS, McNutt NS, Kaplan MH. Papulosquamous dermatoses of AIDS. *J Am Acad Dermatol*. 1990;22(6 Pt 2):1270–1277.

Segal-Maurer S, DeJesus E, Stellbrink H, et al. Capsid inhibition with lenacapavir in multidrug-resistant HIV-1 infection. *N Engl J Med*. 2022;386(19):1793–1803.

Severson JL, Tyring SK. Relation between herpes simplex viruses and human immunodeficiency virus infections. *Arch Dermatol*. 1999;135(11):1393–1397.

Singh F, Rudikoff D. HIV-associated pruritus: etiology and management. *Am J Clin Dermatol*. 2003;4(3):177–188.

Sklenovská N, Van Ranst M. Emergence of monkeypox as the most important orthopoxvirus infection in humans. *Front Public Health*. 2018;6:241. https://doi.org/10.3389/fpubh.2018.00241

Smith G, Holman RP. The prozone phenomenon with syphilis and HIV-1 co-infection. *South Med J*. 2004;97(4):379–382.

Soeprono FF, Schinella RA, Cockerell CJ, Comite SL. Seborrheic-like dermatitis of acquired immunodeficiency syndrome: a clinicopathologic study. *J Am Acad Dermatol*. 1986;14(2 Pt 1):242–248.

Stanley SK, Folks TM, Fauci AS. Induction of expression of human immunodeficiency virus in a chronically infected promonocytic cell line by ultraviolet irradiation. *AIDS Res Hum Retroviruses*. 1989;5(4):375–384.

Stoler MH, Bonfiglio TA, Steigbigel RT, et al. An atypical subcutaneous infection associated with acquired immune deficiency syndrome. *Am J Clin Pathol*. 1983;80:714–718.

Strick LB, Wald A, Celum C. Management of herpes simplex virus type 2 infection in HIV type 1-infected persons. *Clin Infect Dis*. 2006;43(3):347–356.

Suh KS, Han SH, Lee KH, et al. Mites and burrows are frequently found in nodular scabies by dermoscopy and histopathology. *J Am Acad Dermatol*. 2014; 71(5):1022–1023.

Tarín-Vicente EJ, Alemany A, Agud-Dios M, et al. Clinical presentation and virological assessment of confirmed human monkeypox virus cases in Spain: a prospective observational cohort study.

Lancet. 2022;400(10353):661–669. https://doi.org/10.1016/S0140-6736(22)01436-2
Teichner P, Chamay N, Elliot E, et al. Cabotegravir + rilpivirine long-acting: overview of injection guidance, injection site reactions, and best practices for intramuscular injection. *Open Forum Infect Dis*. 2024;11(6):ofae282.
Thornhill JP, Barkati S, Walmsley S, et al. Monkeypox virus infection in humans across 16 countries: April–June 2022. *N Engl J Med*. 2022;387(8):679–691. https://doi.org/10.1056/NEJMoa2207323
Toutous-Trellu L, Abraham S, Pechere M, et al. Topical tacrolimus for effective treatment of eosinophilic folliculitis associated with human immunodeficiency virus infection. *Arch Dermatol*. 2005;141(10):1203–1208.
Ward HA, Russo GG, Shrum J. Cutaneous manifestations of antiretroviral therapy. *J Am Acad Dermatol*. 2002;46(2):284–293.
Warren KJ, Boxwell DE, Kim NY, Drolet BA. Nevirapine-associated Stevens–Johnson syndrome. *Lancet*. 1998;351(9102):567.
Warshaw EM, Nelson D, Carver SM, et al. A pilot evaluation of pulse itraconazole vs. terbinafine for treatment of *Candida* toenail onychomycosis. *Int J Dermatol*. 2005;44(9):785–788.
Weinberg JL, Kovarik CL. The WHO clinical staging system for HIV/AIDS. *Virtual Mentor*. 2010;12(3):202–206.
Wheat LJ, Connolly-Stringfield PA, Baker RL, et al. Disseminated histoplasmosis in the acquired immune deficiency syndrome: clinical findings, diagnosis and treatment, and review of the literature. *Medicine*. 1990;69(6):361–374.
Wilkins K, Turner R, Dolev JC, et al. Cutaneous malignancy and human immunodeficiency virus disease. *J Am Acad Dermatol*. 2006;54(2):189–206; quiz 207–210.
Workowski KA, Backham LH, Chan PA, et al. Sexually transmitted diseases treatment guidelines, 2021. *MMWR Recomm Rep*. 2021;70(4):1–187.
Yunihastuti E, Widhani A, Karjadi TH. Drug hypersensitivity in human immunodeficiency virus-infected patient: challenging diagnosis and management. *Asia Pac Allergy*. 2014;4(1):54–67.
Zancanaro PC, McGirt LY, Mamelak AJ, et al. Cutaneous manifestations of HIV in the era of highly active antiretroviral therapy: an institutional urban clinic experience. *J Am Acad Dermatol*. 2006;54(4):581–588.
Zeichner JA. New topical therapeutic options in the management of superficial fungal infections. *J Drugs Dermatol*. 2015;14(10):s35–s41.
Zheng Y, Niyonsaba F, Ushio H, et al. Cathelicidin LL-37 induces the generation of reactive oxygen species and release of human alpha-efensins from neutrophils. *Br J Dermatol*. 2007;157(6):1124–1131.

28.

NEUROLOGICAL COMPLICATIONS OF HIV INFECTION

Rodrigo Hasbun and Joseph S. Kass

LEARNING OBJECTIVE

Discuss the clinical features, differential diagnosis, and management of HIV-associated neurocognitive disorders (HAND).

HIV-ASSOCIATED NEUROCOGNITIVE DISORDER

Rodrigo Hasbun

WHAT'S NEW?

- Four distinctive biotypes of HIV-associated neurocognitive disorders (HAND) have been described based on viral and immune pathogenesis (T-cell-mediated HIV encephalitis, central nervous system [CNS] viral escape, HIV protein-associated encephalopathy, and macrophage-mediated HIV encephalitis).
- Neurocognitive impairment has been associated with lack of retention in care in older adults, virologic failure, and, when coupled with frailty, it is associated with greater risk for falls, disability, and death.
- CNS-targeted antiretroviral therapy (ART) for HAND has shown no benefit in eight clinical trials.

KEY POINTS

- There is a high prevalence of HAND in PWH who are ART-naive, as well as PWH on ART with virologic suppression.
- Rapid screening tools such as the Montreal Cognitive Assessment test and the Frontal Assessment Battery test have been evaluated for their use in diagnosing HAND in the clinic.
- HAND is associated with significant cognitive, behavioral, and motor abnormalities that can impact ART adherence, virologic success, retention in care in older individuals, and quality of life.
- A recent meta-analysis of eight clinical trials of CNS-targeted ART did not show benefit in HAND; for PWH with CD8$^+$ T-cell encephalitis, corticosteroids should be considered.

Despite the use of combination ART with virologic suppression, up to 39% of PWH currently have neurocognitive impairment (Métral et al., 2020), and up to 42% of patients have at least 1 copy/mL of HIV-1 RNA in the cerebrospinal fluid (CSF) (Anderson et al., 2017). It is unclear if inadequate CSF penetration by some antiretrovirals (ARVs) accounts for this high prevalence and whether CNS-active ART improves cognitive impairment. However, higher CSF penetration scores have been correlated with a lower probability of detectable CSF HIV RNA levels (Anderson et al., 2017). One study of 1,063 PWH documented that CSF viral escape (i.e., detectable CSF RNA levels) occurred in 7.2%, with the most important predictor being a regimen composed of protease inhibitors (PIs) (especially atazanavir) and nucleoside reverse transcriptase inhibitors (NRTIs) (Mukerji et al., 2018). Another study showed that 10% of patients with virologic suppression in the serum had viral escape (Edén et al., 2010). CSF viral escape may be either symptomatic or asymptomatic (Patel et al., 2018). Newer medications, particularly the integrase strand transfer inhibitors (INSTIs) such as bictegravir, attain adequate CSF levels and could account for the paucity of symptomatic CSF viral escape cases that have more recently been reported (Tiraboshi et al., 2019).

Recently, it has been proposed to divide HAND into four distinct biotypes based on viral and immune pathogenesis (Johnson and Nath, 2022):

1. **T-cell-mediated HIV encephalitis**: A severe manifestation of symptomatic CSF viral escape called CD8$^+$ T-cell encephalitis has been described in PWH receiving ART with good immunological response (Lescure et al., 2013). Patients can present with neurocognitive impairment, headache, focal neurological deficits, and seizures, with magnetic resonance imaging (MRI) of the brain showing bilateral white matter lesions. CSF usually shows lymphocytic pleocytosis with CD8$^+$ T-cells greater than 65%. A brain biopsy, if performed, shows pronounced CD8$^+$ T-cell infiltration with the presence of scant HIV antigens (Figure 28.1) (Johnson et al., 2013). Patients improve dramatically with corticosteroids and with improved CNS penetration of their ART regimen. In the largest case series to date, the use of corticosteroids decreased mortality from 69% to 30% in patients with CD8$^+$ T-cell encephalitis (Lucas et al., 2021). The optimal dose and duration of corticosteroids are currently unknown.

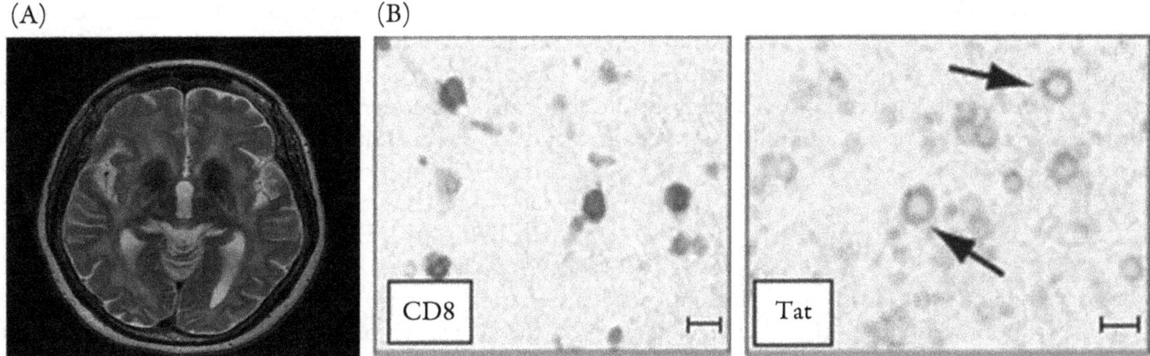

Figure 28.1 (A) Magnetic resonance imaging of a PWH with virological suppression for 4 years with biopsy-proven CD8+ T-cell encephalitis. (B) The presence of CD8+ T cells and HIV Tat antigens on brain biopsy and arrows point to stained HIV Tat antigens. SOURCE: Johnson TP, et al. *Proc Natl Acad Sci USA*. 2013;110:13588–13593.

2. **CNS viral escape**: PWH receiving ART regimens with low CNS penetration, complicated by poor medication adherence or HIV drug-resistant viral mutations, can have detectable CSF HIV RNA levels despite virological suppression in the blood. These individuals may experience headaches, tremors, memory impairment, or even focal neurological deficits or seizures. MRI of the brain can show white matter changes in the deep brain nuclei. Although unproven, switching ART regimens to enhance CNS penetration should be considered. This entity is now seen less frequently in clinical practice, as INSTIs have excellent CNS penetration in contrast to PIs.
3. **HIV protein-associated encephalopathy**: This syndrome is observed in PWH on ART with undetectable plasma and CSF HIV RNA levels, but with detectable HIV proteins such as Tat in the CSF. The HIV viral proteins Tat, Nef, gp120, Vpr, and Gag have been associated with slowly progressive cognitive and psychomotor impairments with neuroimaging findings of cerebral atrophy. If brain biopsy (or autopsy) is performed, neuronal loss, Aβ, and Tau are found. Unfortunately, there are no known treatments at this time for this condition.
4. **Macrophage-mediated HIV encephalitis**: HIV causes a chronic form of encephalitis (HIVE) that is clinically characterized by either dementia or mild neurocognitive impairment. Since the introduction of combination ART in 1996, the incidence of HIV-associated dementia (HAD) has decreased by 50% (McArthur et al., 2005), but the prevalence of mild neurocognitive disorder (MND) has increased up to 39% (Robertson et al., 2007). HIVE is the result of direct microglial infection, interruption of trophic factors, or inflammatory cytokines (Boisse et al., 2008). HIV enters the brain primarily by the "Trojan horse mechanism": it is carried by monocytes and lymphocytes that cross the blood–brain barrier. HIV has a predilection for the basal ganglia, deep white matter, and hippocampus, resulting in subcortical dementia. Brain computed tomography (CT) scanning or MRI typically shows cerebral atrophy and symmetrical white matter lesions. HIV-associated dementia (HAD) is a diagnosis of exclusion; other coinfections (e.g., JC virus-associated progressive multifocal leukoencephalopathy [PML], hepatitis C, neurosyphilis, and cryptococcal meningitis), cerebrovascular disease, malnutrition, and substance use/other toxic exposure should be ruled out before establishing the diagnosis.

Neuropsychological impairment is a surrogate marker for the presence of HIVE on autopsy (Cherner et al., 2002). Cognitive impairment has also been associated with poor adherence to ART (Maggiolo et al., 2007), lack of retention in care in older adults (Jacks et al., 2015), and a negative impact on quality of life. In the pre-ART era, it was shown to be an independent predictor of death (Ellis et al., 1997). Further, CSF HIV RNA levels are increased in PWH with neurocognitive impairment, as are several CSF biomarker levels, such as tumor necrosis-α, neurofilament light, neopterin, β2 microglobulin, and monocyte chemotactic protein-1 (Boisse et al., 2008). A clinical model identified the following variables as associated with detectable CSF viral load: detectable serum HIV-1 RNA on polymerase chain reaction (PCR); a CNS penetration score lower than 9; non-Caucasian race; less than 95% ART adherence; depression; and less than 36 months of ART duration (Hammond et al., 2014).

CLINICAL MANIFESTATIONS OF HAND

The clinical manifestations of HAND are related to involvement of HIV in the subcortical structures. The following findings may be observed: slowing of neurocognitive processing speed; motor and psychomotor abnormalities; and executive, planning, or multitasking dysfunction (Valcour, 2011c). HAND affects the following three domains:

- Cognitive: memory, concentration, mental processing speed, and comprehension;
- Behavioral: apathy, depression, agitation, and sometimes mania;
- Motor function: unsteady gait, poor coordination, abnormal tone, and tremors.

In addition, PWH with CD8+ T-cell encephalitis can present with new-onset seizures, *status epilepticus*, and altered mental status. Further, HAND is associated with virologic failure (Shahani et al., 2018), and when combined with frailty, it is associated with a greater risk of falls, disability, and death (Erlandson et al., 2019).

RISK FACTORS

Several studies have documented host genetic factors (polymorphisms in apolipoprotein E4, chemokine receptor CCR2, and monocyte chemoattractant protein-1), HIV-specific disease factors (history of AIDS-defining illness or low CD4+ T-cell nadir, particular HIV variants, HIV RNA levels in CSF, duration of HIV infection, and older age at seroconversion), age >50 years old, and comorbidities (e.g., anemia, vascular disease, metabolic abnormalities, and hepatitis C coinfection) associated with HAND (Alfahad and Nath, 2013).

SCREENING TOOLS FOR COGNITIVE IMPAIRMENT

Despite the high prevalence of HAND reported from HIV clinics, it has not become routine to screen all PWH for cognitive impairment or to consider more CNS-active ART for people experiencing associated symptoms, even though recommendations to do so have been made from an international consortium (Mind Exchange Working Group, 2013). Screening tools under evaluation for HAND include several versions of the HIV-associated dementia (HAD) scale, the Mini Mental Status Exam (MMSE), standardized questionnaires that assess symptoms such as the Medical Outcomes survey, and the Montreal Cognitive Assessment (MoCA) and Frontal Assessment Battery test. The dementia scales are reliable but only in severe cases of HAND; the MMSE is not sensitive enough to detect HAND; and the subjective reporting of cognitive symptoms will miss some cases because of limited patient insight or mood disturbances (Valcour, 2011a, 2011b). The MMSE is now proprietary. Studies have shown that the MoCA is a rapid, reliable, and sensitive test to detect cognitive impairment in PWH (Hasbun et al., 2012, Rosca et al., 2019). A large study comparing different screening tools for HAND showed the Frontal Assessment Battery test had the highest correct classification rate (Triunfo et al., 2018).

DEFINITIONS OF NEUROCOGNITIVE DISORDERS

In 2007, the diagnostic criteria for HAND were revised (Antinori, 2007). Three classifications of HAND were defined using these new criteria: asymptomatic neurocognitive impairment (ANI), MND, and HIV-associated dementia (HAD). ANI was defined as having a combination of the following: (1) an acquired mild-to-moderate impairment in cognitive function, documented by a score of at least one standard deviation below demographically corrected norms on tests on at least two different cognitive domains; (2) the functional impairment has been seen for more than 1 month; (3) the impairment does not meet criteria for delirium or dementia; and (4) the cognitive impairment is not fully explained by comorbid conditions. The definition of MND is identical to that of ANI, but it also includes interference with activities of daily living. The diagnosis of HAD includes a marked cognitive impairment.

Another approach to defining neurocognitive impairment is the utilization of the Global Deficit Score, which considers both the number and severity of the individual's performance on a battery of standardized tests (Jacks et al., 2015). More recently, experts in the field have proposed modifying the 2007 HAND definition to exclude ANI (Nightingale et al., 2021). They propose a new framework that relies more heavily on clinical observations than neurocognitive testing.

CEREBROSPINAL FLUID ACTIVITY OF ANTIRETROVIRALS

There are currently more than 30 U.S. Food and Drug Administration (FDA)–approved ARVs or combinations in eight mechanistic classes for the treatment of HIV infection, but only some have adequate CSF penetration (U.S. Department of Health and Human Services [USDHHS], 2024a). The CNS penetration-effectiveness (CPE) score was designed to classify different ARVs on the basis of their capability to lower CSF RNA levels (Letendre, 2011). ARVs were assigned a score from 1 to 4 based on their chemical properties, CSF penetration, and/or effectiveness in CNS studies (Table 28.1). A higher CNS penetration score was associated with higher virologic suppression in the CSF (Letendre et al., 2010). In addition, a higher CSF penetration score is associated with a lower rate of neurocognitive impairment (Carvalhal et al., 2016).

Eight randomized studies in the current era have evaluated the impact of CNS-active ARVs in HAND. A meta-analysis of 3,303 PWH with 13,103 person-years of follow-up showed no benefit of ART with high CNS penetration on HIV-associated cognitive impairment (Webb et al., 2023). Furthermore, multiple clinical trials have shown no effective therapy for PWH with HAND (Ellis et al., 2023).

RECOMMENDED READING

Johnson TP, Nath A. Biotypes of HIV-associated neurocognitive disorders based on viral and immune pathogenesis. *Curr Opin Infect Dis.* 2022 Jun 12;35(3):223–230.

Nightingale S, Dreyer AJ, Saylor D, Gisslén M, Winston A, Joska JA. Moving on from HAND: why we need new criteria for cognitive impairment in persons living with human immunodeficiency virus and a proposed way forward. *Clin Infect Dis.* 2021 Sep 15;73(6):1113–1118.

Webb AJ, Borrelli EP, Vyas A, Taylor LE, Buchanan AL. The effect of antiretroviral therapy with high central nervous system penetration on HIV-related cognitive impairment: a systematic review and meta-analysis. *AIDS Care.* 2023;35(11):1635–1646.

Table 28.1 CNS PENETRATION-EFFECTIVENESS (CPE) SCORE OF DIFFERENT ARVS

DRUG CLASS	4	3	2	1
NRTIs	Zidovudine	Abacavir Emtricitabine	Didanosine Lamivudine Stavudine	Tenofovir Zalcitabine
NNRTIs	Nevirapine	Delavirdine Efavirenz	Etravirine	
Protease inhibitors	Indinavir	Darunavir/ritonavir Fosamprenavir/ritonavir Indinavir Lopinavir/ritonavir	Atazanavir Atazanavir/ritonavir Fosamprenavir	Nelfinavir Ritonavir Saquinavir Saquinavir/ritonavir
Entry/fusion inhibitors		Maraviroc		Enfuvirtide
Integrase strand transfer inhibitors		Raltegravir Dolutegravir		

NRTI = nucleoside reverse transcriptase inhibitor; NNRTI = non-nucleoside reverse transcriptase inhibitor.

Adapted from Letendre S. *Top Antivir Med*. 2011;19(4):137–142.

MENINGITIS

Rodrigo Hasbun

LEARNING OBJECTIVE

Review the differential diagnosis and clinical management of meningitis in people with HIV (PWH).

WHAT'S NEW?

- In contrast with many other opportunistic infections, ART initiation should be deferred in cryptococcal meningitis (generally, it is deferred for 4–6 weeks after antifungal agents are initiated).
- A clinical trial showed that one dose of liposomal amphotericin B in combination with oral flucytosine and oral fluconazole in patients with cryptococcal meningitis in Africa was as effective as the standard of care (Jarvis et al., 2022). This new regimen is now advocated by the World Health Organization (WHO) as first-line therapy.
- Although the U.S. Centers for Disease Control and Prevention (CDC) recommends universal HIV screening/testing, it is done in only 50% of CNS infection cases.
- Meningococcal A vaccine has decreased the burden of meningococcal meningitis serogroup A in Africa, but outbreaks remain with non-A serogroup meningococcal or nonmeningococcal meningitis isolates.

KEY POINTS

- The differential diagnosis of meningitis in PWH is broad (e.g., viral, bacterial, fungal, mycobacterial, and lymphomatous) (Table 28.2).
- All adults with meningitis should be tested for HIV.
- Meningitis in PWH is usually treatable, and the underlying cause should be thoroughly investigated.

Table 28.2 CAUSES OF MENINGITIS IN PWH

Viral	Acute HIV infection, $CD8^+$ T-cell encephalitis, enterovirus, herpes simplex virus, arboviruses (West Nile virus, St. Louis encephalitis), cytomegalovirus, varicella zoster virus, influenza virus, Epstein–Barr virus, lymphocytic choriomeningitis virus, mumps
Bacterial	Bacterial meningitis, endocarditis, parameningeal focus (e.g., epidural abscess and mastoiditis), syphilis, Lyme disease, *Mycoplasma pneumoniae*, *Bartonella henselae*, *Brucella* species, *Ehrlichia*, *Rickettsia*, leptospirosis, *Mycobacterium tuberculosis*
Fungal	*Cryptococcus neoformans*, *Coccidioides immitis*, *Histoplasma capsulatum*, *Aspergillus species*, zygomycosis
Parasitic	*Naegleria/Acanthamoeba*, *Taenia solium*, *Angiostrongylus cantonensis*, *Toxoplasma gondii*
Noninfectious	Medications (e.g., antibiotics and nonsteroidal anti-inflammatory drugs), meningeal carcinomatosis (lymphoma and leukemia), vasculitis, chemical meningitis (intrathecal injections and spinal anesthesia), seizures

- A meta-analysis of studies of meningitis in PWH in Africa documented that the three most common causes were *C. neoformans*, *M. tuberculosis*, and bacterial meningitis.

NEUROLOGIC EVENTS IN EARLY-STAGE HIV INFECTION

Acute HIV infection may manifest as an "aseptic meningitis" presentation, but this is most likely underdiagnosed, as <50% of adults with meningitis are tested for HIV, and only 1% are tested for HIV RNA levels to rule out HIV seroconversion syndrome (Ma et al., 2020). Individuals with HIV exposure and acute HIV infection may present with severe headache, stiff neck, diffuse macular rash, photophobia, and lymphocytic pleocytosis in the CSF. Patients with acute HIV infection typically have positive plasma HIV RNA levels with or without a positive HIV p24 antigen in very early stage of the infection (Fiebig I).

Approximately one-third of PWH who present with meningitis do so during early stages of HIV disease (i.e., $CD4^+$ T-cell count >200 cells/mm^3) (Vigil et al., 2018). The most common causes of meningitis in these patients are herpes simplex type 2 (HSV-2), varicella zoster virus (VZV), and arboviruses (e.g., West Nile, St. Louis encephalitis). HSV-2 can present with the initial genital outbreak of herpes or in patients with recurrent episodes of aseptic meningitis (Mollaret's meningitis). Arboviruses should be suspected in the summer and fall in patients with fever and recent mosquito bites. Unfortunately, viral PCR and arboviral serologies are obtained in the minority of meningitis cases (Nesher et al., 2016; Shukla et al., 2017). Other less common causes of meningitis in PWH include VZV, syphilis, and bacterial meningitis.

VZV can present with a dermatomal vesicular rash and an aseptic meningitis, and the diagnosis of VZV meningitis should prompt screening for HIV. In more advanced stages of HIV infection, VZV can present as disseminated disease. It can also present without a rash (zoster sine herpete), with the Ramsay–Hunt syndrome, or with stroke, myelopathy, retinitis, or encephalitis. The diagnosis is made by CSF VZV PCR or by CSF anti-VZV antibody, or presumptively from VZV PCR from a vesicular lesion in someone presenting with a CNS-involving infection. CSF VZV PCR has a specificity of greater than 95% but a sensitivity of only 30%. A positive VZV PCR confirms the diagnosis, but a negative test does not rule out the diagnosis. CSF anti-VZV antibody is the more sensitive test, with a 98% sensitivity (Aberle et al., 2005; DeBiasi and Tyler, 2004; Nagel, 2007; Osiro and Salomon, 2017). Treatment is with high-dose intravenous acyclovir.

Syphilis can also present as an aseptic meningitis syndrome and should be considered in people with a diffuse rash involving the palms and soles. A serum rapid plasma reagin of *greater than 1:32* and a $CD4^+$ T-cell count of less than 350 cells/mm^3 are associated with neurosyphilis and should prompt the performance of a lumbar puncture (Marra et al., 2004).

Bacterial meningitis represents a diagnostic consideration in all stages of HIV, but its incidence has decreased with the advent of conjugate vaccines (Lopez Castelblanco et al., 2014). If bacterial meningitis is suspected, intravenous dexamethasone and antibiotic therapy with vancomycin, ceftriaxone, and ampicillin should be initiated to cover for *Streptococcus pneumoniae*, *Neisseria meningitides*, and *Listeria monocytogenes* until CSF cultures are negative (Tunkel et al., 2004). If the patient has *Listeria monocytogenes* or *Cryptococcus neoformans* meningitis, dexamethasone should be discontinued, as its use has been associated with higher mortality or morbidity, respectively (Beardsley, et al., 2016; Charlier et al., 2017). Of note, one multicenter study observed delayed cerebral injury in 4% of patients with bacterial meningitis, and this was associated with the use of adjunctive steroids (Gallegos et al., 2018). Despite this, dexamethasone should continue to be used in pneumococcal meningitis, where it is associated with a decrease in mortality (Hasbun et al., 2017).

NEUROLOGIC EVENTS IN LATE-STAGE, ADVANCED HIV INFECTION ($CD4^+$ T-CELL COUNT <200 CELLS/MM^3)

The most common cause of meningitis in people with advanced immunosuppression is *Cryptococcus neoformans*, *M. tuberculosis* (TB), cytomegalovirus (CMV), and toxoplasmosis. In cryptococcal meningitis, the CSF examination typically shows lymphocytic pleocytosis, but inflammation may be absent. CSF India ink examination is positive in up to 50% of cases, and the CSF cryptococcal antigen test is positive in approximately 90% of cases. The film array multiplex meningitis encephalitis PCR panel that includes *Cryptococcus neoformans* or *gattii* can be falsely negative in up to 50% of cryptococcal isolates, and testing should be combined with a cryptococcal antigen (Leisman et al., 2018). An opening pressure should be documented since elevated opening pressure is associated with higher CSF fungal burden and higher neurological morbidity and mortality (Gambarin and Hamill, 2002). The preferred therapy for cryptococcal meningitis is a combination of liposomal amphotericin B 3–4 mg/kg IV once daily plus flucytosine 25 mg/kg by mouth 4 times a day, or amphotericin B deoxycholate at 0.7–1 mg/kg IV once daily plus flucytosine 25 mg/kg 4 times a day for 2 weeks, followed by consolidation therapy with fluconazole 800 mg/day by mouth or a dose reduction to 400 mg by mouth once daily in clinically stable patients with negative CSF cultures. This regimen is followed by maintenance therapy with fluconazole 200 mg by mouth once daily for ≥1 year from initiation of antifungal therapy.

Among patients with ongoing symptoms of elevated intracranial pressure, daily therapeutic CSF drainage is necessary to decrease intracranial hypertension (i.e., >25 cm of H_2O) by repeat lumbar punctures. Temporary percutaneous lumbar drains or ventriculostomy may be required if persistent elevations in intracranial pressure occur, as measured by lumbar puncture (Perfect et al., 2012). If flucytosine is not available or the patient experiences drug toxicity, the treatment regimen can be switched to a combination of amphotericin B with fluconazole either 800 mg or 1,200 mg once daily for 14 days. A repeat lumbar puncture should be done at the end of the 2-week period to document a negative CSF fungal culture. Intravenous amphotericin B should be continued if the patient has persistently positive CSF cultures, is clinically deteriorating or comatose, or has persistently elevated and symptomatic intracranial pressures (Perfect et al., 2012). A therapeutic lumbar puncture to decrease intracranial pressure was associated with a reduced risk of death in a study performed in Africa (Rolfes et al., 2014). The same study also documented that ART should be delayed until 4–6 weeks after initial presentation to avoid an increase in mortality (Boulware et al., 2014).

In resource-limited countries, Molloy and colleagues (2018) demonstrated that 1 week of intravenous amphotericin B plus oral flucytosine and 2 weeks of fluconazole plus flucytosine were both effective as induction therapy for cryptococcal meningitis. A more recent clinical trial conducted in Africa concluded that a single dose of liposomal amphotericin B plus 2 weeks of oral flucytosine and oral fluconazole was as effective in treating cryptococcal meningitis as the WHO-recommended treatment at that time (1 week of amphotericin B plus oral flucytosine for 7 days, followed by oral fluconazole for 7 days) (Jarvis et al., 2022). Subsequently, the WHO updated its recommendation, and its June 2022 guidelines advocate for a single dose of liposomal amphotericin B plus oral flucytosine and fluconazole as the preferred regimen (WHO, 2022). A recent clinical trial showed that one single dose of liposomal amphotericin B in combination with oral flucytosine and oral fluconazole in patients with cryptococcal meningitis in Africa was as effective as the WHO-recommended induction therapy with 1 week regimen of amphotericin B deoxycholate and flucytosine standard of care (Jarvis et al., 2022). This new regimen of one single IV dose of liposomal amphotericin B is now advocated by the WHO as the first-line therapy as of April 2022.

CMV can cause meningitis, ventriculitis, polyradiculitis, polyradiculomyelopathy, retinitis, esophagitis, and colitis in people with advanced HIV disease ($CD4^+$ T-cell count <50 cells/mm^3), and is associated with adverse clinical outcomes in approximately two-thirds of patients (Handley et al., 2021). CMV infection of the nervous system accounts for fewer than 1% of CMV infections in PWH (McCutchan, 1995) and often develops concurrently with other, more common CMV extraneural disease manifestations such as retinitis or gastrointestinal involvement even while individuals are on treatment with ganciclovir for extra-CNS disease (Bermann and Kim, 1994). CMV encephalitis is the most common manifestation of CNS infection owing to CMV. CSF examination typically shows low or absent pleocytosis in up to 22% of patients, with CSF protein levels <100 mg/ml in 60% of patients. CMV encephalitis can have typical MRI findings of periventricular enhancement in up to one-third of patients.

Clinically, infection can present as diffuse encephalitis, ventriculoencephalitis, or focal encephalitis. Diffuse encephalitis develops over several weeks and thus presents subacutely with memory loss, attention and concentration difficulties, and delirium. Focal neurological deficits may also be seen. Pathologically, microglial nodules may be found in the cortex, brainstem, cerebellum, and basal ganglia, occurring most commonly in gray matter (Morgello et al., 1987). On neuroimaging, MRI may show a variety of patterns. The brain may appear normal, or it may show hyperintense T2 lesions in the areas described previously and nodular lesions with or without enhancement on T1 postcontrast images (Maschke et al., 2002). Ventriculoencephalitis presents with lethargy, confusion, cranial nerve deficits, ataxia, and focal neurological deficits, and it sometimes occurs concomitantly with CMV polyradiculitis. Ventriculoencephalitis may be more insidious in onset and has a poorer prognosis (Maschke et al., 2002). Pathologically, necrotizing lesions are seen in the ventricular system, and imaging shows periventricular enhancement with or without ventriculomegaly. The third and least common type of CMV encephalitis, focal encephalitis, presents with focal neurological deficits corresponding to a cerebral mass lesion. MRI will show ring-enhancing lesions with surrounding edema.

CSF PCR for CMV DNA confirms the diagnosis of CMV encephalitis. The detection of other viruses often confounds the diagnosis; thus, the index of suspicion must be based on the presentation and imaging findings in the context of profound immunosuppression. The differential diagnosis for CMV encephalitis must include HIV encephalitis, PML, and neurosyphilis. When CMV encephalitis presents as a ring-enhancing lesion, the differential diagnosis expands to other etiologies known to present similarly, such as toxoplasmosis, primary CNS lymphoma, and tuberculous meningitis with tuberculomas (Offiah and Turnbull, 2006).

CMV is treated initially with intravenous ganciclovir 5 mg/kg every 12 hours and then switched to oral valganciclovir once patients are determined to be clinically stable (U.S. Department of Health and Human Services [USDHHS], 2024b). Occasionally, in cases of severe encephalitis, combination treatment with both ganciclovir and foscarnet has been used (Portegies et al., 2004; Silva et al., 2010). Cidofovir can be used as an alternate treatment option. Empiric treatment of CMV infection is often advised because CSF results may be delayed.

Mycobacterial TB can occur at any stage of HIV infection, but extrapulmonary disease (e.g., meningitis, lymphadenitis, pleuritis, and pericarditis) occurs more frequently in PWH with $CD4^+$ T-cell counts of less than 200 cells/mm^3. The overall incidence of TB has declined in the United States, and there are fewer than 1,000 cases of coinfection reported annually (USDHHS, 2024b). TB and HIV must be treated together rather than sequentially, particularly in people with $CD4^+$ T-cell counts less than 50 cells/mm^3. Tuberculous meningitis usually has a subacute to chronic presentation, lymphocytic pleocytosis, a low CSF glucose, and basilar involvement with cranial nerve palsies and altered mental status. A Thwaites's diagnostic score less than 4 (which covers five parameters: age, duration of illness, white blood cell count, total CSF white blood cell count, and percentage of CSF neutrophils) or a Lancet consensus score of greater than 6 (including 20 parameters divided in four categories: clinical,

CSF, CNS imaging, and evidence of TB elsewhere) indicate possible TB meningitis, and patients with these scores should be considered for empiric therapy. The CSF acid-fast bacilli smear is insensitive, and CSF cultures are positive in only 38%–88% of cases (Thwaites, 2012). Caution should be used, however, as neuro brucellosis and fungal meningitis may also have high scores for TB meningitis (Erdem et al., 2015; Sulaiman et al., 2020). A CSF *M. tuberculosis* PCR and an adenosine deaminase level can also aid in the diagnosis. The duration of treatment is 1 year. The mortality is higher for PWH than those without HIV and TB meningitis (51.3% vs. 23%) (Thao et al., 2018). Prognostic factors for death in people with HIV-TB coinfection include severity of illness, lower CSF pleocytosis, lower weight, lower CD4$^+$ T-cell counts, and abnormal sodium levels (Thao et al., 2018).

Finally, toxoplasmosis may also present with a meningitis/encephalitis presentation in PWH with advanced AIDS (Opintan et al., 2017). Toxoplasmosis classically presents with fever, focal neurological signs, seizures, and headaches, with MRI of the brain showing multiple ring-enhancing lesions. Toxoplasmosis is a very unlikely cause of disease if the serum anti-toxoplasma IgG is negative (Rosenow and Hirschfield, 2007). If the serology is negative or the neuroimaging is not suggestive of toxoplasmosis, an early brain biopsy is advocated (Rosenow and Hirschfield, 2007).

MENINGITIS IN PWH VERSUS PERSONS WITHOUT HIV

A study of 549 adults with community-acquired meningitis who were tested for HIV revealed that 25% had HIV infection (Vigi et al., 2018). PWH presented with fewer meningeal symptoms (e.g., headache, neck stiffness, and Kernig's sign) but with higher rates of hypoglycorrhachia, elevated CSF protein, and abnormal cranial imaging. PWH were also more likely to have cryptococcal meningitis, neurosyphilis, and VZV than people without HIV. PWH were also more likely to have a pathogen identified (57%) compared to people without HIV (31%). An adverse clinical outcome was seen in approximately 25% of patients, with abnormal neurological exams and hypoglycorrhachia being identified as predictors. HIV coinfection was not associated with an adverse outcome. Another study comparing adults with and without HIV and encephalitis showed that up to 30% of PWH had more than one causative organism, were less likely to have unknown etiologies, and had a higher 1-year mortality (Reimer-McAtee et al., 2023).

IMMUNE RECONSTITUTION INFLAMMATORY SYNDROME IN HIV

Immune reconstitution inflammatory syndrome (IRIS) occurs after the initiation of combination ART and either "unmasks" a previous subclinical infection or worsens a known infection despite appropriate therapy (paradoxical reaction). In the CNS, IRIS can develop with many opportunistic processes, most commonly cryptococcal meningitis, TB meningitis, and PML (Huis in't Veld et al., 2012). The two most common and serious CNS IRIS events are cryptococcal and tuberculous meningitis. TB IRIS usually presents between a few weeks to 3 months after the initiation of ART, and it can present with meningitis or tuberculomas, or both. Risk factors include low CD4$^+$ T-cell counts, disseminated TB, and extrapulmonary TB. Treatment should consist of adjunctive steroids. CSF acid-fast bacilli cultures are typically negative. Cryptococcal IRIS can develop between 1 and 10 months after initiating ART and can present as culture-negative meningitis, cryptococcomas, pneumonitis, and/or lymphadenopathy. A brief course of adjunctive steroids should be considered.

Additionally, CD8$^+$ T-cell encephalitis syndrome has been described in patients receiving ART with low or undetectable serum HIV RNA levels (Lucas et al., 2021). These patients usually have a low CD4$^+$ T-cell count nadir and a history of opportunistic infections, and they usually present with high CD4$^+$ T-cell counts. As described previously, symptoms include memory disturbances, headaches, diplopia, ataxia, and sometimes seizures. MRI shows bilateral white matter lesions, and CSF shows lymphocytic pleocytosis with detectable CSF HIV RNA. Treatment involves corticosteroids and optimizing CNS penetration of ART.

MENINGITIS IN RESOURCE-LIMITED COUNTRIES

The majority of patients with meningitis in Africa have unknown etiologies and higher rates of death and neurological sequelae due to delays in care (Barichello et al., 2023). A recent study of 1,501 patients with meningitis in Mozambique showed that only ~10% had an etiologic diagnosis (61% bacterial meningitis and 39% cryptococcal meningitis) (Nhantumbo et al., 2022). A review of 1,303 episodes of meningitis with confirmed etiologies among PWH in sub-Saharan Africa showed that 52% had cryptococcal meningitis; 19.6% had TB meningitis; 14.2% had bacterial meningitis; and 14.2% had other etiologies (Veltman et al., 2014). Mortality rates were high, ranging from 25% to 68% across studies.

MYELOPATHY

Joseph S. Kass

LEARNING OBJECTIVE

Discuss the clinical presentation, differential diagnosis, and management of HIV-associated vacuolar myelopathy in PWH.

WHAT'S NEW?

HIV-associated vacuolar myelopathy (VM) remains rare in the current era of early ART initiation for all PWH. However, in people who have been diagnosed with VM, symptoms may be very debilitating, leading to poor quality of life and disability as some PWH age with this condition.

KEY POINTS

- Vacuolar myelopathy (VM is an uncommon complication that tends to occur in the late stages of HIV infection.
- Acute transverse myelitis and inflammatory CSF are unlikely to be VM.
- Human T-cell lymphotropic virus type 1 (HTLV-1) infection is another infectious cause of myelopathy, and it should be considered in endemic geographic areas and in cases of coinfection with HIV.
- Both HIV and HTLV-1 can cause chronic myelopathy involving dorsal and lateral columns.
- The workup for a PWH with myelopathy includes MRI of the spine with and without contrast and may include CSF analysis and investigations for nutritional deficiencies and toxic agents.

HIV-ASSOCIATED VACUOLAR MYELOPATHY

PWH may develop myelopathy for many reasons. At the time of acute HIV infection, acute transverse myelitis may develop, whereas severe immunosuppression puts individuals at risk of developing HIV-associated VM as well as opportunistic processes that either invade or compress the spinal cord. PWH may also develop myelopathy from causes typical among the general population without HIV, such as spondylosis with spinal stenosis.

Primary HIV-associated acute transverse myelitis is a rare inflammatory myelopathy resulting from immune activation and typically develops within days to weeks of acute HIV infection. Individuals present with acute myelopathy in the thoracic region, experiencing lower extremity weakness, a thoracic sensory deficit with numbness below the sensory level, sphincter dysfunction, and eventually hyperreflexia and spasticity. CSF is typically inflammatory with lymphocytic pleocytosis. This acute transverse myelitis tends to respond well to steroids, intravenous immunoglobulin (IVIG), and ART (Hamada et al., 2011).

In contrast, VM is a chronic myelopathy seen in the late stages of HIV infection and affects 10%–15% of untreated people with advanced HIV/AIDS. VM unfolds as a slow, painless progression of neurologic symptoms over several months, most commonly lower extremity weakness and spasticity (Di Rocco, 1999). Patients typically report progressive weakness or clumsiness in the lower extremities, as well as leg cramps and difficulty walking. Urinary symptoms such as frequency and urgency, along with erectile dysfunction, are also common. Sensation in the legs, particularly proprioception and vibratory sense, is usually impaired, but a clear sensory level on the trunk is unusual. Arms are typically spared until advanced-stage disease. Localized back pain is not a common feature. Individuals are also typically hyperreflexic in the lower extremities (hyperreflexia may spread to the upper extremities if the cervical cord is involved) and exhibit extensor plantar responses. There is no effective treatment for VM. Patients with VM often have coexisting HAD and peripheral neuropathy. Rehabilitation is helpful in maximizing physical capacity. ART does not appear to alter the natural history of the disease (Banks et al., 2002). Antispasmodic agents such as baclofen, tizanidine, or botulinum toxin can be used for symptomatic relief of spasticity.

VM is the result of a chronic inflammatory degeneration with vacuolization and myelin pallor of the lateral and posterior tracts, typically affecting the thoracic cord most severely. On histologic examination, the lateral and dorsal columns demonstrate axonal injury and macrophage infiltration with lipid-laden macrophages and microglia infected with HIV (Dal Pan et al., 1997; Petito et al., 1994; Tyor et al., 1993). As many as 20%–50% of individuals with AIDS may have pathological evidence of VM at autopsy (Dal Pan et al., 1994; Di Rocco and Simpson, 1998; McArthur et al., 2005), yet only 6.5%–10% of individuals with AIDS manifest clinical VM (Cho and Vaitkevicius, 2012). MRI of the spinal cord in VM lacks pathognomonic features to differentiate it from non-HIV-related spinal cord disease. Although the spinal cord may appear normal, most affected spinal cords appear atrophic with or without hyperintensities on T2-weighted images (Chong et al., 1999; Yousem and Grossman, 2010).

The differential diagnosis for myelopathy in PWH is broad and includes the following categories: (1) infections, including HTLV-1-associated myelopathy/tropical spastic paraparesis (HAM/TSP; discussed later), tuberculosis (TB) spondylitis or meningomyelitis, cytomegalovirus (CMV) radiculomyelitis, varicella zoster myelitis, *Toxoplasma* myelopathy, neurosyphilis with tabes dorsalis, and bacterial epidural abscess (particularly among people who inject drugs); (2) neoplastic diseases, especially lymphoma and spinal metastases from systemic neoplasms; (3) nutritional deficiencies such as B_{12}, folate, copper, thiamine (presenting as beriberi), and vitamin E; and (4) toxic etiologies such as lathyrism (Di Rocco and Simpson, 1998). Thus, an MRI of the spinal cord with and without contrast, lumbar puncture with CSF analysis, and serum analysis for vitamin and mineral deficiencies are needed to evaluate for these etiologies (Chong et al., 1999).

Clinicians should initially consider common infectious causes. One study from Cape Town, South Africa—an area known for a high prevalence of TB and HIV—reviewed 216 cases of myelopathy and cauda equina syndrome in PWH (median $CD4^+$ T-cell count 185 cell/mm^3). Investigators found that 68% of myelopathy cases were due to TB (Candy et al., 2014). This large number of TB-related myelopathy in PWH has also been seen in other small studies in Africa (Bhigjee et al., 2001; Modi et al., 2011). TB spondylitis could be diagnosed radiographically with a high degree of certainty using MRI, and the diagnosis was confirmed with either CSF analysis or open biopsy.

MRI IN HIV-ASSOCIATED VACUOLAR MYELOPATHY

MRI of the spinal cord in VM is nonspecific and lacks pathognomonic features to differentiate it from non-HIV-related spinal cord disease. The spinal cord may appear normal, but the most affected spinal cords appear atrophic with or without hyperintensities on T2-weighted images (Chong et al., 1999; Yousem and Grossman, 2010).

HTLV-1-ASSOCIATED MYELOPATHY (HAM)/ TROPICAL SPASTIC PARAPARESIS (TSP)

HTLV-1 is a retrovirus that is T-cell tropic and causes a proliferation of T-cells (Manns et al., 1999). Although its full disease spectrum remains unknown, the virus is associated with adult T-cell leukemia/lymphoma, uveitis, and HAM, which is also referred to as tropical spastic paraparesis (TSP). The prevalence of HTLV-1 infection increases with age, and it is more common in women than men. It is also geographically clustered, with high rates in southern Japan, the Caribbean, areas of Africa, the Middle East, South America, the Pacific Melanesian Islands, and Papua New Guinea. Among low-risk groups in the United States and Europe, seroprevalence is approximately 1%, with the majority of individuals remaining asymptomatic. Approximately 1% of HTLV-1-positive individuals develop myelopathy (Pillat et al., 2011). Given the overlapping risk factors for both HIV and HTLV-1 infection, HIV and HTLV-1 coinfection should be considered in PWH presenting with a slowly progressive myelopathy.

Patients with HAM present with progressive muscle weakness in the legs, hyperreflexia, clonus, extensor plantar responses, sensory disturbances, urinary incontinence, and lower back pain. HTLV-1 antibodies are present in both plasma and the CSF, as well as in brain and spinal cord tissue. The diagnostic approach to HAM/TSP is similar to that outlined previously for VM, including MRI of the spine with and without contrast, lumbar puncture, and an investigation for nutritional deficiencies and toxic exposures. Definitive diagnosis requires an assay to detect HTLV-1 antibodies in plasma and CSF, including an assay capable of distinguishing between HTLV-1 and HTLV-2.

HAM/TSP is thought to arise from chronic inflammation of the spinal cord attributable to a brisk activation of cytotoxic T lymphocytes against HTLV-1 within the central nervous system (Yamauchi et al., 2021). No antiretroviral or immune-modulating therapy has proven curative. INF-α is the only medication that has been tested for the treatment of HAM/TSP in a randomized controlled trial, and it demonstrated improved neurological symptoms after 4 weeks of therapy (Izumo et al., 1996). Corticosteroids remain the most commonly used disease-modifying agent despite observational studies that offer conflicting data about their benefit in the treatment of HTLV-1 myelopathy. Research is underway to develop new therapies in addition to preventive and therapeutic vaccines for HTLV-1 (Martin and Taylor, 2011), but currently, prevention education, particularly regarding breastfeeding and sexual transmission, is the only known method of reducing incidence.

RECOMMENDED READING

Di Rocco A. Diseases of the spinal cord in human immunodeficiency virus infection. *Semin Neurol.* 1999;19:151–155.

Izumo S, Goto I, Itoyama Y, et al. Interferon-alpha is effective in HTLV-I-associated myelopathy: a multicenter, randomized, double-blind, controlled trial. *Neurology.* 1996;46:1016–1021.

Manns A, Hisada M, La Grenade L. Human T-lymphotropic virus type I infection. *Lancet.* 1999;353:1951–1958.

Yamauchi J, Araya N, Yagishita N, et al. An update on human T-cell leukemia virus type I (HTLV-1)-associated myelopathy/tropical spastic paraparesis (HAM/TSP) focusing on clinical and laboratory biomarkers. *Pharmacol Ther.* 2021;218:107669.

DISTAL SYMMETRICAL POLYNEUROPATHY

Joseph S. Kass

WHAT'S NEW?

In a recent study of virologically suppressed PWH, peripheral neurology was independently associated with increasing age, a history of dideoxynucleoside drug use such as the nucleoside reverse transcriptase inhibitors (NRTIs) didanosine (ddI), stavudine (d4T), and zalcitabine (ddC) (even after many years of drug exposure, since these drugs are no longer used), nadir $CD4^+$ T-cell count, and metabolic syndrome.

KEY POINTS

- Distal symmetrical polyneuropathy (DSPN) is the most common neurologic complication of HIV infection, occurring in 30%–67% of PWH.
- Antiretroviral (ARV) toxic neuropathy is associated with use of dideoxynucleoside drugs, even many years after drug exposure has ceased.
- Metabolic syndrome is an independent risk factor for peripheral neuropathy.
- Treatment includes removal of neurotoxins and management of pain and discomfort.

DSPN occurs in 30%–67% of PWH, making it the most common neurologic complication in HIV disease (Ellis et al., 2010; Evans et al., 2011, Schuldt et al., 2023). Its incidence increases in advanced HIV (Schifitto et al., 2002; Simpson et al., 2006). DSPN may develop at any time after the onset of HIV infection, with a mean time to developing neuropathy of 9.5 years after HIV diagnosis (Robinson-Papp and Simpson, 2009b). However, one small study suggested that signs of neuropathy may be detected in as many as 35% of PWH at a median of only 3.5 months after HIV transmission (Wang et al., 2014). Although the etiology of DSPN is still under investigation, it is most likely an indirect result of HIV infection, probably through immune-mediated mechanisms (Pardo et al., 2001).

Advanced immunosuppression was the major risk factor for developing DSPN before the advent of ART; it remains a risk factor for untreated PWH (Childs et al., 1999; Vecchio et al., 2020). Risk factors for developing DSPN among PWH on ART include older age, Caucasian race, lower hemoglobin levels, hypertriglyceridemia, lower $CD4^+$ T-cell count nadir, current combination ART use, and past use of the dideoxynucleoside drugs (didanosine, stavudine, and zalcitabine) (Banerjee et al., 2011; Ellis et al., 2010; Simpson et al., 2006; Tagliati et al., 1999). Although the prevalence of DSPN appears to decline with ART initiation (Ellis et al., 2010; Vecchio et al., 2020), ART-treated PWH with undetectable viral loads and higher CD4⁺ T-cell counts may still develop this condition (Verma et al., 2004). Virologically suppressed PWH who initiated ART after CD4⁺ T-cell counts fall below 350/μL appear to be at increased risk of DSPN compared to those who never achieved that degree of immunosuppression. This correlation holds true even after adjusting for age, duration of HIV infection, and use of dideoxynucleoside drugs (didanosine, stavudine, and zalcitabine) ("d-drugs"). It also suggests that earlier initiation of ART may help reduce the risk of DSPN; however, the elevated risk of DSPN in PWH who experience a low CD4⁺ nadir is independent of the eventual success of ART in achieving virologic suppression (Ellis et al., 2010).

Neuropathy associated with d-drugs, such as didanosine, stavudine, and zalcitabine, is the only neurologic complication of HIV that has increased since the introduction of ART (Keswani et al., 2002). The risk of ARV toxic neuropathy (ATN) was substantially higher when didanosine and stavudine were used together, especially when combined with hydroxyurea (Moore et al., 2000). DSPN and ATN are clinically very similar, although ATN often has a more acute onset with more rapid progression (Pardo et al., 2001; Price et al., 1999). One hypothesis is that mitochondrial dysfunction mediates NRTI toxicity (Kallianpur and Hulgan, 2009). D-drugs are no longer recommended for use as HIV treatment because of their unacceptable toxicities, and the commercialization of zalcitabine was discontinued in the United States in 2006.

A recent study examining factors associated with peripheral neuropathy in effectively virologically suppressed adults with HIV analyzed all individuals in the PIVOT (Protease Inhibitor Monotherapy Versus Ongoing Triple Therapy) trial with data on peripheral neuropathy at baseline. Multivariable logistic regression was used to examine the associations of PN with potential risk factors (including age, sex, nadir CD4⁺ T-cell count, history of d-drug exposure, and blood glucose levels) and neurofilament light (NfL) levels. Almost a quarter of the 585 participants reported peripheral neuropathy during the study period (median of 44 months). Peripheral neuropathy was independently associated with age (adjusted odds ratio [aOR] was 1.35, 95% CI: 1.20–1.52; additional 5 years), history of d-drugs exposure (aOR 1.88, 95% CI: 1.12–3.16), height (aOR 1.19, 95% CI: 1.05–1.35; additional 5 cm), nadir CD4⁺ T-cell count (aOR 1.10, 95% CI: 1.00–1.20; 50 cells fewer), and metabolic syndrome (aOR 2.31, 95% CI: 1.27–4.20), but not plasma NfL (Schuldt et al., 2023).

Typical DSPN symptoms include symmetric spontaneous and evoked tingling, numbness, stabbing sensations, and burning predominantly in the feet and progressing to the upper extremities (Figure 28.2) (Cornblath and McArthur, 1988; DeVivo et al., 2000; Price et al., 1999; Wulff and Simpson, 1999a). In research cohorts, DPSN may be detected in the absence of clinical symptoms if one of the following signs manifests bilaterally: diminished ability to recognize vibration and reduced sharp-dull discrimination in the feet and toes or reduced ankle reflexes. Not all people with DSPN experience neuropathic pain, however. Although 57% of the over 1,500 CHARTER cohort participants were diagnosed with DSPN, only 38% reported neuropathic symptoms (Ellis et al., 2010). Risk factors for neuropathic pain differed from risk factors for DSPN itself and included past d-drug use and higher rather than lower CD4⁺ T-cell nadir (Ellis et al., 2010).

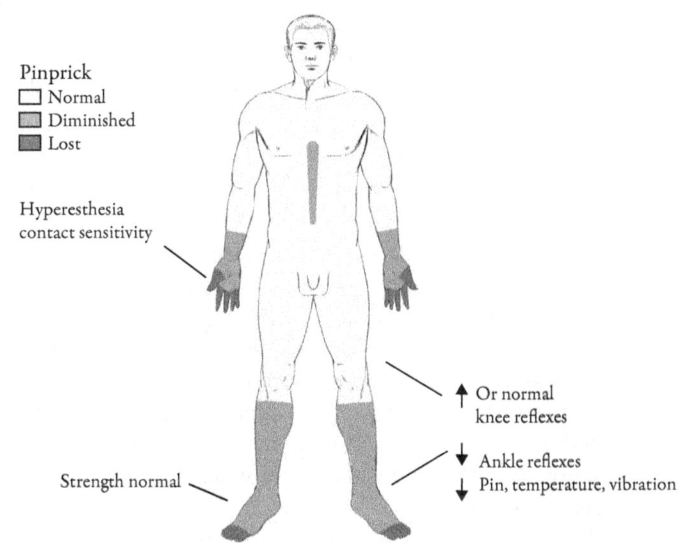

Figure 28.2 Typical signs and symptoms of distal sensory polyneuropathy.

DSPN is the result of damage to and loss of both large- and small-caliber sensory nerve fibers, with macrophage infiltration in the dorsal root ganglia and along the nerve trunks (Keswani et al., 2002). Activation of macrophages and the production of proinflammatory cytokines appear to play significant roles in the neuropathogenesis of DSPN (Pardo et al., 2001). Secreted viral proteins such as the envelope glycoprotein 120 (gp120) may also contribute to HIV-induced neurotoxicity (Keswani et al., 2003). DNA damage in the mitochondria of distal axons may add to the distal degeneration of sensory nerve fibers (Lehmann et al., 2011). Sural nerve biopsies obtained from patients with ATN have shown severe axonal destruction, prominent in unmyelinated fibers (Dalakas and Cupler, 1996). Prominent mitochondrial abnormalities have more significantly been noted in association with NRTIs, supporting the suggestion that neuronal mitochondrial damage underlies ATN (Chen et al., 1991). Further support for this concept is derived from in vitro observations of graded inhibition of mitochondrial γ-DNA polymerase by different NRTIs (Martin et al., 1994). The d-drugs are the most potent inhibitors of this enzyme in vitro (Martin et al., 1994), whereas zidovudine, lamivudine, abacavir, emtricitabine, and tenofovir have only minimal effects. Mitochondrial DNA content in lymphocytes, however, does not correlate with the presence of ATN (Simpson et al., 2006).

The differential diagnosis of DSPN/ATN includes other toxic neuropathies caused by other medications commonly used for PWH, such as metronidazole, dapsone, vincristine, isoniazid (DeVivo et al., 2000), and fluoroquinolones (Cohen, 2001), as well as diabetes mellitus, vitamin B_{12} deficiency, diffuse infiltrative lymphocytosis syndrome (DILS), alcohol-related neuropathy, hepatitis C, and uremia (DeVivo et al., 2000; Williams et al., 2002).

Both DSPN and ATN are usually diagnosed on clinical grounds. One study reported that a brief screening examination performed at a single center by trained nonphysicians correlated well with the diagnosis of DSPN made by an experienced neurologist (Marra et al., 1998). In a multicenter study, however, nonphysician neurological findings were less reliable (Simpson et al., 2006). Nerve conduction studies can be useful, typically showing axonal neuropathy with absent or reduced sensory nerve action potentials, although they might be normal either in mild cases or when the neuropathy is restricted to small fibers (DeVivo et al., 2000). Punch skin biopsies have been used to identify reduced densities of unmyelinated nerve fibers in HIV-associated sensory neuropathies. Skin biopsy analysis is now available in some settings, and is particularly helpful either when symptoms of burning pain are more prominent than actual neurologic signs or when a nonorganic cause of sensory symptoms is suspected (Polydefkis et al., 2002). A quantitative sudomotor axon reflex test may also be performed to document small-fiber neuropathy. In a study of 102 PWH, autonomic dysfunction was present in 62% of participants (Robinson-Papp et al., 2013). Sural nerve biopsy is rarely indicated except when mononeuritis multiplex is suspected, because this entity raises the specter of vasculitis.

Diagnosis of neurotoxic neuropathy can be confirmed by withdrawal of the suspected neurotoxin and monitoring for attenuation of symptoms. However, recent data indicate that exposure to d-drugs may cause a permanent neuropathy even years after drug exposure (Schuldt et al., 2023).

Treatment of HIV sensory neuropathies is primarily aimed at removing neurotoxins and managing pain and discomfort. One study showed that 40% of PWH have severe pain, with a numeric pain rating scale of 5 or greater out of 10, and 90% experience some pain (Smyth et al., 2007). Experiencing neuropathic pain appears to increase the risk of unemployment and experiencing dependence in instrumental activities of daily living (Ellis et al., 2010). In addition, neuropathic pain itself, but not the severity of neuropathic pain, is associated with current major depressive disorder and greater severity of depressive symptoms (Ellis et al., 2010).

Although there is no FDA-approved treatment for pain caused by HIV-associated DSPN, various pain-modifying agents have been used for HIV sensory neuropathies, including antidepressants, anticonvulsants, and narcotics. In mild neuropathies, over-the-counter treatments such as acetaminophen can be helpful (DeVivo et al., 2000; Wulff and Simpson, 1999a). One randomized control study demonstrated evidence of efficacy for topical capsaicin 8% (Simpson et al., 2008). Night splints may also be useful in the management of neuropathic pain with the improvement of sleep (Sandoval et al., 2010). Pain-modifying anticonvulsants and antidepressants have been useful clinically (DeVivo et al., 2000; Wulff and Simpson, 1999a) and can improve quality of life and function for many people with HIV-associated sensory neuropathies (Simpson, 2003). However, placebo-controlled trials for the treatment of neuropathic pain have shown no significant benefit from amitriptyline, low-dose topical capsaicin, pregabalin, gabapentin, subcutaneous recombinant human nerve growth factor, subcutaneous prosaptide, intranasal peptide T, or lamotrigine (Phillips et al., 2010). Lamotrigine did show some superiority to placebo in the neurotoxic ARV-exposed stratum as a secondary outcome measure of the study. Although placebo-controlled trials have been negative, tricyclic antidepressants (e.g., desipramine and amitriptyline) can occasionally be useful. Sedation is common with some, particularly amitriptyline, so these agents are more useful for control of nighttime neuropathic pain. Daytime sedation can generally be avoided by using small doses and escalating slowly. Use of opioid agonists must be approached with caution because of the prevalence of risk factors for aberrant prescription opiate use (Chou et al., 2009). Alternative treatments include acupuncture and hypnosis (Dorfman et al., 2013). Further management details are provided by Verma and colleagues (2004).

CONSIDERATIONS FOR RESOURCE-LIMITED SETTINGS

A study of DSPN in seven resource-limited settings estimated DSPN incidence in PWH who were ART-naive and had a $CD4^+$ T-cell count <300 cells/mm^3 compared to people without HIV and in PWH with viral suppression on 1 of 3 ARV regimens. A total of 860 PWH were enrolled from Brazil, India, Malawi, Peru, South Africa, Thailand, and Zimbabwe. Before initiating combination ART, 21.3% of PWH had DSPN compared with 8.5% of people without HIV. PWH with DSPN were more likely to report inability to work and depression than PWH without DSPN. Overall prevalence of DSPN among PWH virally suppressed on ART decreased from 20.3% at week 48 to 15.3% at week 144 and finally to 10.3%, at week 192. Incident DSPN was seen in 127 PWH. Longitudinally, DSPN was more likely in older individuals and PWH with fewer years of education ($P = .03$). There was no significant association between ART regimen and DSPN (Vecchio et al., 2020).

INFLAMMATORY DEMYELINATING POLYNEUROPATHY

Joseph S. Kass

LEARNING OBJECTIVE

Discuss the clinical features, differential diagnosis, and management of acute and chronic inflammatory demyelinating polyneuropathy in PWH.

WHAT'S NEW?

The differential diagnosis of acute inflammatory demyelinating polyneuropathy (AIDP) includes disorders of the spinal cord, such as transverse myelitis, acute spinal cord compression, and acute infarction of the spinal cord; disorders affecting anterior horn cells, including poliomyelitis and West Nile virus; acute peripheral neuropathies such as tick paralysis, porphyria, Lyme disease, and lead or arsenic poisoning; and neuromuscular junction disorders such as botulism, myasthenia gravis, or Lambert–Eaton myasthenic syndrome.

KEY POINTS

- Acute inflammatory demyelinating polyneuropathy (AIDP) and chronic inflammatory demyelinating polyneuropathies (CIDP) are not common HIV-associated peripheral neuropathies. Their cause is autoimmune-induced inflammation and breakdown of peripheral nerve myelin.
- AIDP has a rapid onset and progression, and often develops during acute HIV infection or before immunosuppression has evolved.
- AIDP/CIDP in PWH is not associated with the classic CSF albuminocytological dissociation expected in people without HIV. PWH often have CSF lymphocytic pleocytosis.
- AIDP is treated with either plasmapheresis or intravenous immunoglobulin, and with ganciclovir/foscarnet/cidofovir if CMV is detected as a causative agent.
- CIDP is treated with corticosteroids or intermittent courses of either plasmapheresis or intravenous immunoglobulin that may be continued long term until a therapeutic response is seen.

Peripheral neuropathy is the most common neurologic manifestation in PWH and can manifest in a number of ways: distal symmetric polyneuropathy, inflammatory polyneuropathy (AIDP/CIDP), mononeuritis multiplex, autonomic neuropathy, progressive polyradiculopathy (Wulff and Simpson, 1999b; Wulff et al., 2000). Whereas distal symmetric polyneuropathy (DSPN) is the most common presentation and can occur secondary to direct HIV infection or as a side effect of NRTIs (Parry et al., 1997; Wulff et al., 2000), inflammatory demyelinating neuropathies in PWH are much less common (Leger et al., 1989).

Inflammatory demyelinating polyradiculoneuropathies are classified as either acute or chronic based on the duration of symptom progression. AIDP, also known as Guillain–Barré syndrome (GBS), is defined as a progressive, usually ascending weakness with hyporeflexia or areflexia and with symptoms nadiring by 4 weeks. In contrast, CIDP is classified by progressive proximal and distal weakness and sensory loss with symptom progression for longer than 8 weeks.

The association between inflammatory polyneuropathies and HIV was first reported in 1985 by Lipkin et al. (1985). AIDP typically occurs during acute or early HIV infection before seroconversion has evolved (Markarian et al., 1998; Mishra et al., 1985; Wulff and Simpson, 1999b). In patients with relatively intact immune function, AIDP may be the first clinical manifestation of HIV infection (Parry et al., 1997). The Miller–Fisher variant of GBS, characterized by ataxia, ophthalmoplegia, and areflexia, has been reported in advanced HIV infection, with elevated anti-GQ1b antibody titer despite severe immunosuppression (Hiraga et al., 2007). GBS has also been reported as a manifestation of immune reconstitution syndrome in PWH treated with combination ART who experience a dramatic increase in $CD4^{+}$ T-cell counts (Piliero et al., 2003; Rauschkaa et al., 2003). CIDP generally occurs later during the advanced stage of HIV infection (Verma and Bradley, 2000, Verma, 2001).

PATHOGENESIS

Both AIDP and CIDP are thought to be due to an underlying autoimmune inflammatory response against peripheral nerve myelin-associated antigens, resulting in the breakdown of peripheral nerve myelin (Radziwill et al., 2002). Rarely, HIV infection has been reported in association with an acute axonal motor neuropathy, where the pathology is thought to be associated with an immune response against the peripheral nerve axon (Dardis, 2015; Goldstein et al., 1993; Jadhav et al., 2014; Wagner et al., 2007).

CLINICAL FEATURES

AIDP is frequently associated with a preceding illness, such as upper respiratory infection or acute enterocolitis. AIDP commonly presents with paresthesias, followed by back pain, ascending symmetric weakness, and decreased or absent reflexes. Frank numbness is not common, but neuropathic pain is very common. Patients may also experience facial weakness, ophthalmoplegia, and autonomic dysfunction (commonly labile blood pressures and tachycardia). CIDP can present with progressive or relapsing proximal and distal weakness, sensory loss, and absent reflexes. Pain is a less common presentation (Dimachkie and Barohn, 2014).

CEREBROSPINAL FLUID ANALYSIS

CSF is characteristically acellular in AIDP in PWH. Protein levels may be normal during the first week of the illness but will increase within 2–3 weeks of symptom onset. Elevated CSF protein has been associated mainly with increased permeability of the blood–CSF barrier (Winer, 2001). However, AIDP seen with HIV infection may be associated with lymphocytic pleocytosis. In a study of 10 patients with HIV-associated AIDP, CSF white blood cell count ranged from 2 to 17 cells/mm^3 (Brannagan, 2003). The presence of increased protein in the CSF is useful for diagnosis, and a lymphocytic CSF pleocytosis (10–50 cells/mm^3) distinguishes HIV-associated inflammatory demyelinating neuropathies from those without HIV infection (Wulff and Simpson, 1999b). However, the absence of CSF pleocytosis does not rule out HIV infection, and hence HIV testing is warranted for all patients with AIDP (Brannagan, 2003). In addition, either elevated CSF protein or elevated white blood cell counts may be found in PWH even in the absence of an autoimmune neuropathy (Marshall et al., 1988). Generally, CSF pleocytosis is suggestive of either inflammatory/infectious etiology or underlying malignancy. Markedly elevated cell counts or the presence of CSF polymorphonuclear granulocytes in a patient whose clinical presentation appears typical of either AIDP or CIDP should alert the provider to consider alternative diagnoses (Hughes, 1991). Enterovirus myelitis, West Nile myelitis, European tick-borne encephalitis virus, and herpes virus infection (CMV, VZV, EBV, and HSV-1 and -2) may show an initial polymorphonuclear pleocytosis. Lyme disease and HIV infection need to be considered with a lymphocytic pleocytosis (Rauschkaa et al., 2003).

In a series of 10 patients with HIV and GBS, study authors reported that the mean CD4$^+$ T-cell count was 367 cells/mm^3 (range, 55–800 cells/mm^3). An acute polyradiculoneuropathy in PWH with CD4$^+$ T-cell count of less than 50 cells/mm^3 may be secondary to CMV infection, and empiric ganciclovir may be indicated (Brannagan and Zhour, 2003).

ELECTROPHYSIOLOGY

Diagnosis is aided by nerve conduction studies showing features of demyelination—that is, slowing of nerve conduction velocities, prolonged distal latencies, temporal dispersion, conduction block, and prolonged F-wave latencies.

BIOPSY

Nerve biopsies are rarely performed to diagnose AIDP or CIDP, but biopsy may be considered if the clinical or physiologic picture is atypical. Pathology includes macrophage-mediated segmental demyelination and an inflammatory infiltrate (Cornblath et al., 1987).

DIFFERENTIAL DIAGNOSIS

The differential diagnosis of AIDP includes disorders of the spinal cord such as transverse myelitis, acute spinal cord compression, and acute infarction of the spinal cord (which in the initial phases may present with flaccid areflexia below the level of the lesion because of spinal shock); disorders affecting anterior horn cells, including poliomyelitis and West Nile virus; acute peripheral neuropathies such as tick paralysis, porphyria, Lyme disease, and lead or arsenic poisoning; and neuromuscular junction disorders such as botulism, myasthenia gravis, or Lambert–Eaton myasthenic syndrome (Wakerly and Yuki, 2015). TB, toxoplasmosis, HSV-2, syphilis, and lymphoma can also present with signs and symptoms of polyradiculitis.

In individuals with subacute/chronic neuropathy and HIV with CD4$^+$ T-cell counts of less than 50 cells/mm^3, mononeuritis multiplex, distal symmetric polyneuropathy (DSPN), and CMV-related polyradiculomyelitis or polyradiculitis need to be considered in the differential diagnosis. CMV polyradiculitis (or polyradiculomyelitis if the infection involves not only the nerve roots but also the spinal cord) typically presents as an ascending weakness beginning in the lower extremities with areflexia, sensory loss, and weakness. Patients typically experience urinary retention and decreased anal sphincter tone. MRI of the spine with contrast demonstrates enhancement of the nerve roots, typically involving the cauda equina. Nerve conduction studies will show low compound muscle action potentials and mildly slowed conduction velocity corresponding to axonal involvement. Electromyography will show acute denervation with spontaneous activity and decreased recruitment. CSF studies in CMV polyradiculitis usually reveal a polymorphonuclear-predominant pleocytosis, elevated protein, and decreased glucose levels. CSF PCR for CMV DNA can confirm the diagnosis.

CMV infection of the peripheral nervous system may also manifest as an asymmetric multifocal neuropathy, observed in PWH who have low CD4$^+$ T-cell counts. Infection affects individual peripheral nerves, with the radial, ulnar, peroneal, and lateral cutaneous nerves of the thigh being the most commonly involved nerves (Anders and Goebel, 1999). Rapid progression has been reported and can become confluent (Robinson-Papp, 2009b), mimicking acute or subacute polyneuropathy. Electrodiagnostic studies of the nerves show multifocal sensory and motor nerve dysfunction in an axonal pattern with acute denervation. CSF studies may or may not be positive for CMV DNA PCR, and nerve biopsy may also fail to reveal CMV. Empiric treatment is warranted when clinical suspicion is high, especially in the setting of concomitant CMV infection affecting other organs. Treatment involves either ganciclovir or foscarnet as the first-line option. The differential diagnosis should include mononeuritis multiplex in PWH with high CD4$^+$ T-cell counts, hepatitis C with cryoglobulinemia, mononeuritis multiplex owing to vasculitis in association with B-cell lymphoma, and distal sensory polyneuropathy associated with either HIV or ART with d-drugs.

TREATMENT

AIDP is treated with either high-dose IVIG therapy or plasmapheresis. These treatments enhance recovery and arrest clinical progression (Cornblath et al., 1987; Hadden et al., 1998; Plasma Exchange/Sandoglobulin Guillain–Barré Syndrome Trial Group, 1997). IVIG and plasma exchange have been shown to be equally effective in treating AIDP in patients without HIV (Plasma Exchange/Sandoglobulin Guillain–Barré Trial Group, 1997; van der Meche et al., 1992). In 2015, researchers reported improvement in CD4$^+$ and CD8$^+$ T-cell counts and HIV-1 RNA levels in PWH treated with IVIG for HIV-associated GBS (Rosca et al., 2015). Because of the possibility of CMV polyradiculomyelitis or polyradiculitis, patients with severe immunosuppression (CD4$^+$ T-cell counts <50 cells/mm^3) should be treated with intravenous ganciclovir, foscarnet, or cidofovir, or a combination of these, in addition to the standard treatment. CIDP is treated with oral prednisone, pulse intravenous high-dose methylprednisolone or dexamethasone, or intermittent courses of plasmapheresis or IVIG. A randomized controlled study confirmed the benefit of prednisone in HIV-related CIDP, although this treatment approach may worsen immunosuppression (Lindenbaum et al., 2001). Acute relapses in CIDP are treated with either IVIG or plasmapheresis.

PROGNOSIS

Initial clinical course and response to pharmacological treatment in AIDP is similar in patients with or without HIV (Verma, 2001). Schreiber and colleagues (2011) reported on a patient with GBS as the initial presentation of HIV infection who recovered fully using IVIG and rehabilitation without initiation of ART, suggesting that patients with GBS early in the course of HIV infection may have similar outcomes to people without HIV who have GBS. Compared to people without HIV, people with HIV-associated GBS may experience relapses and may be more likely to develop CIDP (Brannagan, 2003). With CIDP, although treatment can halt disease progression and facilitate peripheral nerve remyelination, there is evidence that unrecoverable secondary axonal damage can occur in some cases (Hughes, 1991).

NEUROLOGICAL COMPLICATIONS OF PWH WITH CMV INFECTION

Joseph S. Kass

LEARNING OBJECTIVE

Discuss the clinical syndromes, differential diagnosis, and management of neurological complications of cytomegalovirus (CMV) infection in PWH.

KEY POINTS

- Cytomegalovirus (CMV) CNS disease occurs late in the course of HIV, and it may involve different parts of the CNS.
- Diagnosis is based on clinical findings, results of imaging, and virologic markers.
- Treatment should be started empirically while awaiting CSF CMV DNA PCR results.

Cytomegalovirus (CMV), a member of the herpesvirus family, is a frequent opportunistic viral infection in PWH and occurs when the $CD4^+$ T-cell count is less than 100 cells/mm^3, attributable to reactivation of latent infection. CMV infection of the nervous system accounts for fewer than 1% of CMV infections in PWH (McCutchan, 1995) and often develops concurrently with other, more common CMV extraneural disease manifestations such as retinitis or gastrointestinal involvement. Clinical syndromes of CMV infection in the nervous system include encephalitis, polyradiculomyelitis, polyradiculitis, and multifocal neuropathy (Anders and Goebel, 1999). Although these syndromes are uncommon, recognition, treatment with antivirals, and restoring immune response are paramount to reduce the risk of death.

CMV encephalitis is the most common manifestation of CNS infection owing to CMV. CMV encephalitis has been reported to occur even while patients are on treatment with ganciclovir for extra-CNS disease (Bermann and Kim, 1994). Clinically, infection can present as diffuse encephalitis, ventriculoencephalitis, or focal encephalitis. Diffuse encephalitis develops over several weeks and thus presents subacutely with memory loss, attention and concentration difficulties, and delirium. Focal neurological deficits may also be seen. Pathologically, microglial nodules may be found in the cortex, brainstem, cerebellum, and basal ganglia, but occur most commonly in gray matter (Morgello et al., 1987). On neuroimaging, MRI may show a variety of patterns. The brain may appear normal, or it may show hyperintense T2 lesions in the areas described previously and nodular lesions with or without enhancement on T1 postcontrast images (Maschke et al., 2002).

Ventriculoencephalitis presents with lethargy, confusion, cranial nerve deficits, ataxia, and focal neurological deficits, and it sometimes occurs concomitantly with CMV polyradiculitis. Ventriculoencephalitis may be more insidious in onset and have a poorer prognosis (Maschke et al., 2002). Pathologically, necrotizing lesions are seen in the ventricular system, and imaging shows periventricular enhancement with or without ventriculomegaly.

The third and least common type of CMV encephalitis is focal encephalitis, and it presents with focal neurological deficits corresponding to a cerebral mass lesion. MRI will show ring-enhancing lesions with surrounding edema.

CSF PCR for CMV DNA confirms the diagnosis of CMV encephalitis. The CSF may also show pleocytosis with either a polymorphonuclear or a mononuclear predominance, along with elevated protein and decreased glucose levels. Viral culture is rarely positive. The detection of other viruses often confounds the diagnosis; thus, the index of suspicion must be based on the presentation and imaging findings in the context of profound immunosuppression. The differential diagnosis for CMV encephalitis must include HIV encephalitis, PML (progressive multifocal leukoencephalopathy), and neurosyphilis. When CMV encephalitis presents as a ring-enhancing lesion, the differential diagnosis expands to other etiologies known to present similarly, such as toxoplasmosis, primary CNS lymphoma, and tuberculous meningitis with tuberculomas (Offiah and Turnbull, 2006).

CMV polyradiculitis (or polyradiculomyelitis if the infection involves not only the nerve roots but also the spinal cord) typically presents as an ascending weakness beginning in the lower extremities with areflexia, sensory loss, and weakness. People typically experience urinary retention and decreased anal sphincter tone. MRI of the spine with contrast demonstrates enhancement of the nerve roots, typically involving the cauda equina. Nerve conduction studies will show low compound muscle action potentials and mildly slowed conduction velocity corresponding to axonal involvement. Electromyography will show acute denervation with spontaneous activity and decreased recruitment. CSF studies in CMV polyradiculitis usually reveal a polymorphonuclear-predominant pleocytosis, elevated protein, and decreased glucose levels. CSF PCR for CMV DNA can confirm the diagnosis.

The differential diagnosis of CMV polyradiculitis includes GBS, which may be clinically indistinguishable and only differentiated on nerve conduction studies showing a more demyelinating pattern (Corral et al., 1997). Other opportunistic infections, including TB, toxoplasmosis, and HSV-2, can present in a similar manner. Syphilis and lymphoma can also cause polyradiculitis.

Treatment for CMV encephalitis and CMV polyradiculitis/polyradiculomyelitis is similar. Induction treatment with either intravenous ganciclovir or foscarnet is the usual first-line option. In some cases of severe encephalitis, combination treatment with both ganciclovir and foscarnet has been used (Portegies et al., 2004; Silva et al., 2010). Cidofovir can be used as an alternate treatment option. Empiric treatment of CMV infection is often advised because CSF results may be delayed. Maintenance treatment with ganciclovir has been recommended, but the duration of treatment has not been well studied. Of note, patients with CMV polyradiculitis/polyradiculomyelitis have been shown to be more responsive to treatment compared to patients with CMV encephalitis (Cinque et al., 1998).

The most fully characterized CMV infection of the peripheral nervous system is an asymmetric multifocal neuropathy, observed in PWH who have low $CD4^+$ T-cell counts. Infection affects individual peripheral nerves, with the radial, ulnar, peroneal, and lateral femoral cutaneous nerve of the thigh most commonly involved (Anders, 1999). Rapid progression has been reported and can become confluent (Robinson-Papp, 2009a), mimicking a polyneuropathy. Electrodiagnostic studies of the nerves show multifocal sensory and motor nerve dysfunction in an axonal pattern with acute denervation. CSF studies may or may not be positive for CMV DNA PCR, and nerve biopsy may also fail to reveal CMV. Empiric treatment is warranted when clinical suspicion is high, especially in the setting of concomitant CMV infection affecting other organs. Treatment is also with either ganciclovir or foscarnet as the first-line option. The differential diagnosis should include mononeuropathy multiplex in PWH and high $CD4^+$ T-cell counts, hepatitis C with cryoglobulinemia, mononeuropathy multiplex owing to vasculitis in association with B-cell lymphoma, and distal sensory polyneuropathy (DSPN) associated with either HIV or ARV treatment (ATN) with dideoxynucleoside NRTIs.

INTRACRANIAL LESIONS

Joseph S. Kass

LEARNING OBJECTIVE

Discuss the clinical presentation, differential diagnosis, and treatment of intracranial lesions in PWH.

WHAT'S NEW?

Because of concern for drug-drug interactions, particularly in PWH receiving ART, most clinicians favor levetiracetam as the first-line pharmacotherapy for managing seizures. In the setting of status epilepticus, fosphenytoin, levetiracetam, and valproate appear to have equal efficacy. Enzyme-inducing antiseizure medications (ASMs) should be avoided in people on ART regimens that include protease inhibitors (PIs) and non-nucleoside reverse transcriptase inhibitors (NNRTIs).

KEY POINTS

- HIV-related focal intracranial lesions generally occur in PWH with $CD4^+$ T-cell counts less than 200 cell/mm^3.
- The most common focal mass lesion is toxoplasmosis. The use of prophylactic agents such as trimethoprim–sulfamethoxazole can decrease the incidence of toxoplasmic encephalitis.
- Primary CNS lymphoma (PCNSL) is the most common HIV-related brain neoplasm seen in PWH. On imaging studies, it is usually a solitary intracranial mass lesion in the setting of a negative toxoplasmosis serology.
- Progressive multifocal leukoencephalopathy (PML) on neuroimaging is characterized by nonenhancing lesions of the white matter involving the subcortical U-fibers without edema or mass effect.
- PWH may also develop mass lesions typical of people without HIV, so the differential diagnosis of focal intracranial lesion in PWH should include both HIV-related and non-HIV-related pathologies.

Intracranial mass lesions are common neurologic findings and account for as much as half of the neurologic disorders seen in PWH. Although intracranial mass lesions typically occur in PWH with advanced immunosuppression (CD^+ T-cell counts <200 cells/mm^3), an intracranial lesion can occasionally be the initial presenting symptom of AIDS. Intracranial lesions in PWH can be broadly categorized into three groups: opportunistic infections, neoplasms, and cerebrovascular disease (American Academy of Neurology (AAN), 1998).

The clinical presentation of intracranial lesions varies depending on the underlying etiology. Typical presenting clinical symptoms include alteration in level of awareness or consciousness as well as focal neurologic deficits. In resource-rich settings such as the United States, the most common etiologies include toxoplasmosis, PCNSL, bacterial and fungal abscesses, and PML. Additional differential diagnoses include primary brain tumor, brain metastasis from systemic cancer, tuberculoma, and lesions of fungal origin. Differentiating among this large array of conditions can be challenging. In people with large lesions with mass effect and impending herniation, open biopsy with decompression is recommended. Achieving the correct diagnosis is paramount to managing the causal pathogen in a timely and approach manner. This requires a knowledge-based diagnostic algorithm that accounts for the relative frequency of various types of intracranial lesions. Figure 28.3 provides a useful process of differential considerations based on level of immunosuppression, typical clinical and radiographic presentations, management options, and prognosis with or without empirical treatment (AAN, 1998).

Toxoplasmic encephalitis (TE) is the most common cause of space-occupying intracranial focal mass lesions in

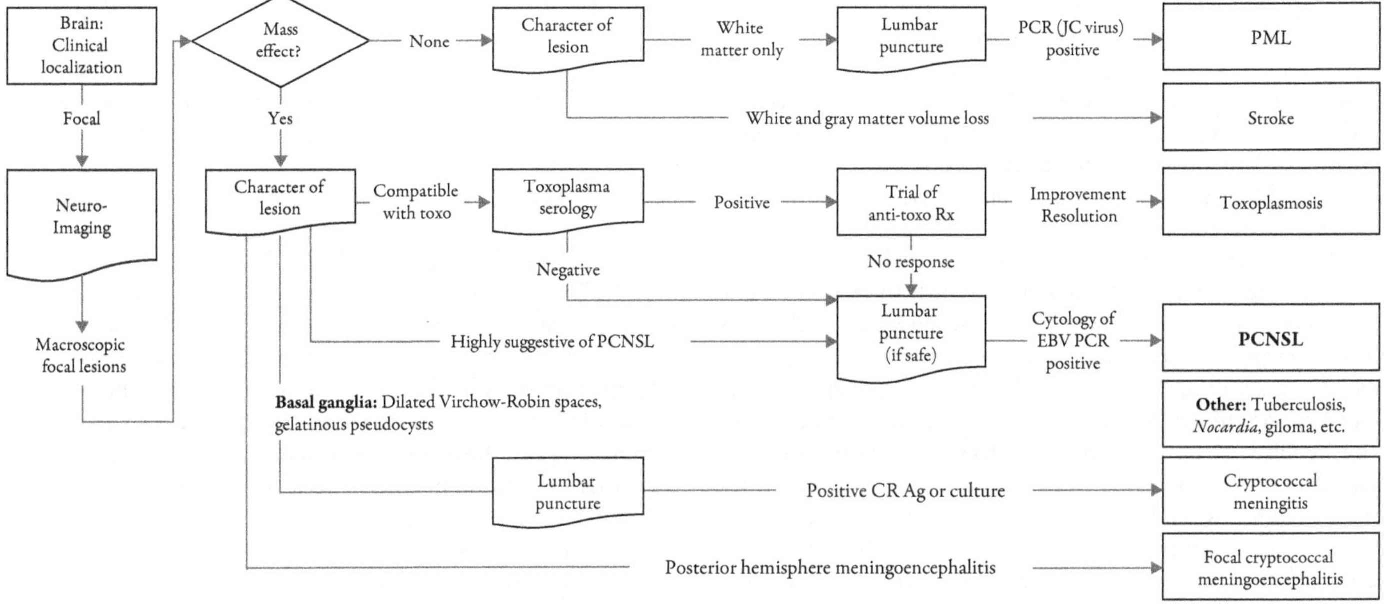

Figure 28.3 General algorithm for diagnostic evaluation of focal brain disease. SOURCE: Adapted from American Academy of Neurology (AAN). 1998;50:21–26.

PWH and typically results from reactivation of latent infection of *Toxoplasma gondii*, an obligate intracellular parasite (AAN, 2000a). In the United States, the incidence of TE has declined with widespread use of prophylaxis agents such as trimethoprim–sulfamethoxazole and ART in PWH (AAN, 1998).

TE often presents with subacute changes in level of consciousness, fever, headaches, seizures, and focal neurologic deficit. It should be suspected in any PWH and an intracranial mass lesion, especially if the patient has a CD^+ T-cell count of less than 100 cells/mm^3, is not receiving toxoplasmosis prophylaxis, and has immunoglobulin G antibodies to *T. gondii* (AAN, 2000a). Investigative studies such as CSF analysis, *Toxoplasma* serology, or imaging studies do not always provide a definitive diagnosis. Performing a lumbar puncture is often contraindicated because mass effect from the lesion increases the risk of herniation. In cases in which CSF is obtained, analysis frequently shows a nonspecific mild mononuclear pleocytosis with elevated protein. CSF PCR can detect *T. gondii* with high specificity (100%) but variable sensitivity (30%–50%) (AAN, 2002). Consequently, whereas a positive *Toxoplasma* PCR result is highly suggestive of the diagnosis, a negative result does not exclude it.

Imaging studies can also provide supportive information. MRI with and without contrast has greater sensitivity than contrast-enhanced CT, especially for detecting multiple lesions, subcortical lesions, and posterior fossa involvement. However, neither imaging modality alone is sufficient to make a diagnosis because there is no pathognomonic radiographically distinguishing feature of toxoplasmosis compared to PCNSL. Toxoplasmosis typically presents as multiple, homogeneous, ring-enhancing lesions with cerebral edema and mass effect. It has a predilection for the basal ganglia and corticomedullary junction, with involvement of both white and gray matter (AAN, 2000a). Although a solitary mass lesion with edema is often observed in PCNSL, it can also be seen in toxoplasmosis (AAN, 2000a). Thallium single-photon emission computed tomography (SPECT) and positron emission tomography (PET) can be useful in distinguishing toxoplasmosis from lymphoma. Lymphoma has increased thallium uptake on SPECT and hypermetabolism of glucose and methionine on PET. *Toxoplasma* is hypometabolic on PET and does not show uptake of thallium (AAN, 2000a). As a result of the limitations of these investigative modalities, the diagnosis of toxoplasmosis is often presumptive. Individuals with typical clinical presentations and radiographic findings are treated empirically for toxoplasmosis for 2 weeks, and a positive clinical and radiographic response supports the diagnosis. Open or stereotactic brain biopsy can yield a definitive diagnosis; however, an empiric treatment approach with assessment for response eliminates the morbidity and rare mortality risk of the procedure. However, biopsy should not be delayed in PWH who do not improve with empirical management, have large mass effect with impending herniation, and require a rapid definitive diagnosis.

First-line anti-*Toxoplasma* treatment includes sulfadiazine, pyrimethamine, and folinic acid (leucovorin) (AAN, 2000a). Folinic acid must be given to counteract myelosuppression from pyrimethamine. The duration of acute therapy is at least 6 weeks before beginning secondary prophylaxis (chronic suppressive therapy) with pyrimethamine, leucovorin, and sulfadiazine. Recrudescence occurs in up to 30% of cases, typically in patients with poor adherence to secondary prophylaxis, but occasionally in individuals with high levels of adherence (AAN, 2000a). In patients with sulfa allergy or intolerance, clindamycin (plus pyrimethamine and leucovorin) is a reasonable alternative to sulfadiazine, although clindamycin use is associated with a slightly increased incidence of recrudescence. In the case of intolerance to both sulfadiazine and clindamycin, alternatives include high-dose trimethoprim–sulfamethoxazole, and atovaquone. Atovaquone is less well tolerated because of gastrointestinal side effects. Clinical improvement should occur within the first 10–14 days of treatment, and typically occurs prior to radiographic evidence of improvement (which may be noted within 2–3 weeks of treatment initiation). Lack of improvement within the first 2 weeks should raise suspicion for an alternative diagnosis.

The use of adjunctive corticosteroids, such as dexamethasone, should be brief and implemented only in very particular circumstances, such as when there is radiographic evidence of midline shift or impending herniation, signs of critically elevated intracranial pressure, or clinical deterioration within the first 48 hours of therapy. Under these circumstances, the benefits of steroids outweigh the many risks of steroid administration. Steroids may also serve to confound the diagnosis for several reasons. Steroids can improve clinical presentation, making it difficult to distinguish between the anti-inflammatory effects of the steroids and the therapeutic effectiveness of empiric anti-toxoplasmosis treatment. In addition, steroid-associated anti-inflammatory actions affect the radiographic presentation by decreasing the intensity of contrast enhancement and surrounding edema, thus interfering with reliable comparative interpretation of subsequent radiographic images. Steroids can also complicate the pathological diagnosis of PCNSL if a biopsy is needed, rendering the biopsy falsely negative for the presence of lymphoma. Aside from more acute steroid complications such as avascular necrosis, hyperglycemia, and psychiatric symptoms, the prolonged use of steroids may also render the patient susceptible to other opportunistic infections.

An important differential diagnosis is PCNSL, which (along with systemic non-Hodgkin's lymphoma, Kaposi's sarcoma, and invasive cervical carcinoma) is one of the four AIDS-defining neoplasms. PCNSL is commonly seen in PWH with $CD4^+$ T-cell counts of less than 50 cells/mm^3 and is rarely the initial presenting symptom of AIDS. The pathogenesis of AIDS-related PCNSL is strongly related to the reactivation of latent Epstein–Barr virus (EBV) infection. The clinical presentation is very similar to TE, with symptoms such as encephalopathy, impaired cognitive function, seizures, and focal neurologic deficits such as aphasia and hemiparesis. Investigative studies such as CSF analysis and imaging are often utilized. As with TE, lumbar puncture is at times contraindicated because of a heightened risk of herniation owing to mass effect from the lesion. CSF analysis, particularly cytology, can be helpful, but it has a very low sensitivity. PCR assay of CSF for EBV DNA (which has a sensitivity greater than 80% and a specificity greater than 95%) can be diagnostic. As with TE, MRI often provides higher diagnostic yield than CT scan, but CT with contrast remains useful, particularly in people who have a contraindication to MRI. PCNSL can present with single or multiple well-defined rings or patchy enhancing lesions with edema and mass effect. It often involves supratentorial regions such as the corpus callosum and periventricular or periependymal areas (PCNSL in AIDS) (AAN, 2000b). As previously mentioned, SPECT and PET can be useful in differentiating lymphoma from other etiologies, including TE. Although PET and SPECT have limited sensitivity, they have high specificity. A diagnosis is often made using a combination of CSF cytology, toxoplasmosis serologic testing, failure of trial of empirical antibiotics usually for treatment of TE, and positive CSF PCR for EBV DNA; if necessary, a brain biopsy may be obtained (AAN, 2000b). Open or stereotactic brain biopsy is typically required prior to induction chemotherapy, which is the current mainstay treatment for PCNSL. Whole-brain radiation therapy (WBRT) consolidation in patients with responsive disease appears to prevent further neurologic progression or produce reversal of deficits. However, the treatment plan should be informed by an individual's overall health status. There can be spread of lymphoma with involvement of the eyes; therefore, a complete ophthalmologic examination, including a slit-lamp examination, should be performed (AAN, 2000b).

Other etiologies of intracranial mass lesions include other neoplasms, cerebrovascular disease, and other infections. Kaposi's sarcoma may rarely manifest as an intracranial lesion. PWH may also develop brain lesions unrelated to immunocompromised status, such as glioma or metastatic disease.

In addition to TE, PWH may develop parasitic, fungal, or bacterial infections that present as a mass lesion. Most of these infections present with meningitis and focal neurological signs and symptoms related to the presence of a mass lesion. Although neurocysticercosis (NCC) is not more common in PWH, the incidence of HIV infection is significant in countries where NCC is endemic. Coinfection has been rarely reported, but concomitant infection with HIV, NCC, and an additional pathogen have been reported. Furthermore, in the setting of immunocompromise, interpretation of imaging findings may be particularly difficult. On imaging studies, the appearance of NCC varies depending on the stage of infection. MRI is favored over CT scan, especially for evaluation of intraventricular and cisternal/subarachnoid cysts as well as cystic degeneration and pericystic inflammatory reaction (Serpa et al., 2007).

Common bacterial mass lesions include abscess from *Mycobacterium tuberculosis*, *Nocardia*, *Listeria monocytogenes*, and *Treponema pallidum*. In resource-limited settings, particularly in highly endemic areas such as Southeast Asia and Africa, tuberculous meningitis is common. Because of its proclivity for the basal meninges, tuberculous meningitis often presents clinically with multiple cranial neuropathies and hydrocephalus (AAN, 2000a). Neuroimaging may show masses, which are often tuberculomas. Intracranial tuberculomas can be seen on MRI as hypointense or isointense with gadolinium contrast enhancement owing to varying amounts of caseous necrosis. This variable appearance of intracranial tuberculoma is attributed to the changing nature of the granulomatous lesion (Park and Song, 2008). The diagnosis of tuberculous meningitis can be challenging and requires a combination of CSF analysis, including culture for TB, acid-fast bacilli stain, and TB PCR, along with a clinical evaluation for disseminated TB.

Common etiologies of fungal abscesses include *Cryptococcus neoformans*, *Candida albicans*, aspergillosis, mucormycosis, histoplasmosis, and coccidioidomycosis. Of these fungi, cryptococcosis is the most common opportunistic fungal infection in PWH and arises from an acquired infection from *C. neoformans*, an encapsulated yeast. Neuroimaging, usually a contrast-enhanced brain MRI, may show cryptococcomas—multiple enhancing lesions of various sizes, most often seen within perivascular spaces. These lesions usually resolve completely with treatment. A definitive diagnosis is made by a positive CSF culture for *C. neoformans*, a positive CSF India ink stain, or a reactive CSF cryptococcal antigen test. For additional information, see Chapter 19, "Opportunistic Infections."

PML is characterized by multifocal areas of demyelination, often in subcortical and periventricular areas, and arises because of reactivation of the human polyomavirus JC virus (JCV) infecting oligodendroglia in the setting of advanced immunosuppression. On imaging studies, the lesions do not typically enhance with contrast and do not produce edema or mass effect. The subcortical U-fibers are involved. However, in the setting of IRIS, PML can present with contrast enhancement, focal edema, and mass effect on MRI with contrast (Tan et al., 2009).

PWH with intracranial lesions are at heightened risk of developing seizures. Antiseizure medications (ASMs) should not be given for routine prophylaxis to PWH with a CNS mass lesion because not all individuals with CNS lesions will develop seizures. However, once a person experiences a seizure, chronic ASM administration is appropriate. In 2012, the AAN issued an evidence-based guideline for clinicians about ASM selection for PWH (Birbeck et al., 2012). Most of the recommendations in this guideline were rated as having weak evidence.

The AAN guideline recommends avoiding enzyme-inducing AMS (EI-ASMs) in people whose ART includes either a PI or NNRTI because pharmacokinetic interactions may result in virologic failure (Birbeck et al., 2012). Phenobarbital, phenytoin, and carbamazepine are commonly used EI-ASMs, and phenobarbital, although rarely used in resource-rich countries, is the mainstay of seizure management in resource-limited settings where HIV is highly prevalent. The guideline identifies circumstances in which specific dose adjustments to ART should be made when certain ASMs are used concomitantly. For example, PWH concurrently on phenytoin and lopinavir/ritonavir may need a 50% dosage increase in lopinavir/ritonavir to maintain adequate serum levels of the PI to ensure virologic control. Patients coadministered atazanavir/ritonavir and lamotrigine may require a 50% increase in lamotrigine dose to maintain adequate serum levels of the ASM and achieve seizure control. Patients taking both zidovudine and the P450 inhibitor valproic acid may require a zidovudine dose reduction to maintain unchanged zidovudine levels (Birbeck et al., 2012). Although not specifically recommended in the guideline, ASMs that bypass hepatic metabolism and are renally excreted, such as levetiracetam, are often favored for patients on ART given their lack of drug-drug interactions. Although previously either intravenous phenytoin or fosphenytoin was the recommended treatment for status epilepticus, one study comparing three intravenous ASMs—levetiracetam (60 mg/kg), fosphenytoin (20 mg/kg), and valproic acid (40 mg/kg)—for the treatment of benzodiazepine-refractory status epilepticus in both children and adults determined that each medication had similar efficacy (Kapur et al., 2019). Although this study was not specific for PWH, etiologies of status epilepticus varied, and the results of this study should be applicable to PWH presenting with a mass lesion causing status epilepticus.

Using the approach discussed in this chapter, common etiologies of intracranial mass lesion can be systemically evaluated in order to make a diagnosis and institute therapy. In settings with limited resources where advanced neuroimaging, CSF PCR, and biopsy are unavailable, clinical findings on history and physical examination, combined with the prevalence of infectious etiologies, should guide the diagnosis and subsequent empiric therapeutic interventions.

REFERENCES

Aberle SW, Aberle JH, Steininger C, et al. Quantitative real time PCR detection of varicella-zoster virus DNA in cerebrospinal fluid in patients with neurological disease. *Med Microbiol Immunol.* 2005;194:7–12.

American Academy of Neurology (AAN). Evaluation and management of intracranial mass lesions in AIDS: report of the Quality Standards Subcommittee of the American Academy of Neurology. *Neurology.* 1998;50:21–26.

AAN. Opportunistic and fungal infections of the central nervous system. *Neurol Continuum.* 2002;8(3):125.

AAN. Opportunistic infections: toxoplasmosis: the neurologic complications of AIDS. *Neurol Continuum.* 2000a;6(5):128–149.

AAN. Primary central nervous system lymphoma in AIDS: the neurologic complications of AIDS. *Neurol Continuum.* 2000b;6(5):177–185.

Anders HJ, Goebel FD. Neurological manifestations of cytomegalovirus infection in the acquired immunodeficiency syndrome. *Int J STD AIDS.* 1999;10:151–161.

Anderson AM, Muñoz-Moreno JA, McClernon DR, et al. Prevalence and correlates of persistent HIV-1 RNA in cerebrospinal fluid during antiretroviral therapy. *J Infect Dis.* 2017;215(1):105–113.

Antinori A, Arendt G, Becker JT, et al. Updated research nosology for HIV-associated neurocognitive disorders. *Neurology.* 2007;69(18):1789–1799.

Banerjee S, McCutchan JA, Ances BM, et al. Hypertriglyceridemia in combination antiretroviral-treated HIV-positive individuals: potential impact on HIV sensory polyneuropathy. *AIDS.* 2011;25(2):F1–F6.

Banks LT, Geraci A, Liu M, et al. A natural history of HIV myelopathy in the HAART era. *Neurology.* 2002;58:A441.

Barichello T, Rocha Catalão CH, et al. Bacterial meningitis in Africa. *Front Neurol.* 2023;14:822575.

Beardsley J, Wolbers M, Kibengo FM, et al. Adjunctive dexamethasone in HIV-associated *Cryptococcal mengitis. N Engl J Med.* 2016;374(6):542–554.

Bermann SM, Kim RC. The development of cytomegalovirus encephalitis in AIDS patients receiving ganciclovir. *Am J Med.* 1994;96:415–419.

Bhigjee AI, Madurai S, Bill PL, et al. Spectrum of myelopathies in HIV seropositive South African patients. *Neurology.* 2001;57:348–351.

Birbeck G, French J, Perucca E, et al. Evidence-based guideline: antiepileptic drug selection for people with HIV/AIDS: report of the Quality Standards Subcommittee of the American Academy of Neurology and the Ad Hoc Task Force of the Commission on Therapeutic Strategies of the International League Against Epilepsy. *Neurology.* 2012;78(2):139–145.

Boisse L, Gill MJ, Power C. HIV infection of the central nervous system: clinical features and neuropathogenesis. *Neurol Clin.* 2008;26:799–819.

Boulware DR, Meya DB, Muzoora C, et al. Timing of antiretroviral therapy after diagnosis of cryptococcal meningitis. *N Engl J Med.* 2014;370:2487–2498.

Brannagan TH 3rd, Zhou Y. HIV associated Guillain–Barré syndrome. *J Neurol Sci.* 2003;208(1–2):39–42.

Candy S, Chang G, Andronikous S. Acute myelopathy or cauda equine syndrome in HIV positive adults in a tuberculosis endemic setting: MRI, clinical, and pathologic findings. *AJNR.* 2014;35(8):1634–1641.

Carvalhal A, Gill MJ, Letendre SL, et al. Central nervous system penetration effectiveness of antiretroviral drugs and neuropsychological impairment in the Ontario HIV Treatment Network Cohort Study. *J Neuroviral.* 2016;22(3):349–357.

Charlier C, Perrodeau E, Leclercq A, et al. Clinical features and prognostic factors of listeriosis: the MONALISA national prospective cohort study. *Lancet Infect Dis.* 2017;17(5):510–519.

Chen CH, Vazquez-Padua M, Cheng YC. Effect of anti-human immunodeficiency virus nucleoside analogs on mitochondrial DNA and its implication for delayed toxicity. *Mol Pharmacol.* 1991;39(5):625–628.

Cherner M, Masliah E, Ellis RJ, et al. Neurocognitive dysfunction predicts postmortem findings of HIV encephalitis. *Neurology.* 2002;59(10):1563–1567.

Childs E, Lyles R, Selnes OA, et al. Plasma viral load and CD4+ lymphocytes predict HIV-associated dementia and senory neurology. *Neurology.* 1999;52:607–613.

Cho T, Vaitkevicius H. Infectious myelopathies. *Continuum.* 2012;18(6):1351–1373.

Chong J, Di Rocco A, Tagliati M, et al. MR findings in AIDS-associated myelopathy. *Am J Neuroradiol.* 1999;20(8):1412–1416.

Chou R, Fanciullo GJ, Fine PG, et al. Opioids for chronic noncancer pain: prediction and identification of aberrant drug-related behaviors: a review of the evidence for an American Pain Society and American Academy of Pain Medicine clinical practice guideline. *J Pain.* 2009;10(2):131–146.

Cinque P, Cleator GM, Weber T, et al. Clinical review diagnosis and clinical management of neurological disorders caused by cytomegalovirus in AIDS patients. *J Neuro Virol.* 1998;4:120–132.

Cohen JS. Peripheral neuropathy associated with fluoroquinolones. *Ann Pharmocother.* 2001;35(12):1540–1547.

Cornblath DR, McArthur JC. Predominantly sensory neuropathy in patients with AIDS and AIDS-related complex. *Neurology.* 1988;38(5):794–796.

Cornblath DR, McArthur JC, Kennedy PGE, et al. Inflammatory demyelinating peripheral neuropathies associated with human T-cell lymphotropic virus type III infection. *Ann Neurol.* 1987;21:32040.

Corral I, Quereda C, Casado JL, et al. Acute polyradiculopathies in HIV-positive patients. *J Neurol.* 1997;244:499–504.

Dalakas MC, Cupler EJ. Neuropathies in HIV infection. *Baillieres Clin Neurol.* 1996;5(1):199–218.

Dal Pan GJ, Berger JR. Spinal cord disease in human immunodeficiency virus infection. In Berger JR, Levy RM, eds., *AIDS and the Nervous System.* 2nd ed. Philadelphia: Lippincott-Raven; 1997:173–187.

Dal Pan GJ, Glass JD, McArthur JC. Clinicopathologic correlations of HIV-1-associated vacuolar myelopathy: an autopsy-based case–control study. *Neurology.* 1994;44(11):2159–2164.

DeBiasi RL, Tyler KL. Molecular methods diagnosis of viral encephalitis. *Clin Microbiol Rev.* 2004;17(4):903–925.

DeVivo DC, Percy AK, Chiriboga CA, et al. Neuromuscular disorders in HIV-1 infection. *Continuum.* 2000;6:73–76.

Dimachkie MM, Barohn RJ. Distal myopathies. *Neurol Clin.* 2014;32(3):817–842.

Di Rocco A. Diseases of the spinal cord in human immunodeficiency virus infection. *Semin Neurol.* 1999;19:151–155.

Di Rocco A, Simpson DM. AIDS-associated vacuolar myelopathy. *AIDS Patient Care STDs.* 1998;12(6):457–461.

Dorfman D, George MC, Schnur J, et al. Hypnosis for treatment of HIV neuropathic pain: a preliminary report. *Pain Med.* 2013;14:1048–1056.

Edén A, Fuchs D, Hagberg L, Nilsson S, Spudich S, Svennerholm B, Price RW, Gisslén M. HIV-1 viral escape in cerebrospinal fluid of subjects on suppressive antiretroviral treatment. *J Infect Dis.* 2010;202(12):1819–1825.

Ellis R, Deutsch R, Heaton RK, et al. Neurocognitive impairment is an independent risk factor for death in HIV infection: San Diego HIV Neurobehavioral Research Center Group. *Arch Neurol.* 1997;54(4):416–424.

Ellis RJ, Marquine MJ, Kaul M, et al. Mechanisms underlying HIV-associated cognitive impairment and emerging therapies for its management. *Nat Rev Neurol.* 2023;19(11):668–687.

Ellis RJ, Rosario D, Clifford DB, et al. Continued high prevalence and adverse clinical impact of human immunodeficiency virus-associated sensory neuropathy in the era of combination antiretroviral therapy: the CHARTER Study. *Arch Neurol.* 2010;67(5):552–558.

Erdem H, Senbayrak S, Gencer S, et al. Tuberculosis and brucellosis meningitis differential diagnosis. *Travel Med Infect Dis.* 2015;13(2):185–191.

Erlandson KM, Perez J, Abdo M, et al. Frailty, neurocognitive impairment, or both in predicting poor health outcomes among adults living with human immunodeficiency virus. *Clin Infect Dis.* 2019;68(1):131–138.

Evans SR, Ellis RJ, Chen H, et al. Peripheral neuropathy in HIV: prevalence and risk factors. *AIDS.* 2011;25(7):919–928.

Gallegos C, Tobolowsky F, Nigo M, Hasbun R. Delayed cerebral thrombosis in adults with bacterial meningitis: a novel complication of adjunctive steroids? *Crit Care Med.* 2018;46(8):e 811–e814.

Gambarin KH, Hamill RJ. Management of increased intracranial pressure in cryptococcal meningitis. *Curr Infect Dis Rep.* 2002;4(4):332–338.

Goldstein JM, Azizi SA, Booss J, et al. Human immunodeficiency virus-associated motor axonal polyradiculoneuropathy. *Arch Neurol.* 1993;50:1316–1319.

Hadden RD, Cornblath DR, Hughes RA, et al.; Plasma Exchange/Sandoglobulin Guillain–Barré Syndrome Trial Group. Electrophysiological classification of Guillain–Barré syndrome: clinical associations and outcome. *Ann Neurol.* 1998;44(5):780–788.

Hamada Y, Watanabe K, Aoki T, et al. Primary HIV infection with acute transverse myelitis. *Intern Med.* 2011;50:1615–1617.

Hammond ER, Crum RM, Treisman GJ, et al. The cerebrospinal fluid HIV risk score for assessing central nervous system activity in persons with HIV. *Am J Epidemiol.* 2014;180(3):297–307.

Handley G, Pankow S, Dien Bard J, et al. Distinguishing cytomegalovirus meningoencephalitis from other viral central nervous system infections. *J Clin Virol.* 2021;142:104936.

Hasbun R, Eraso J, Ramireddy S, et al. Screening for neurocognitive impairment in HIV individuals: the utility of the Montreal Cognitive Assessment Test. *J AIDS Clinic Res.* 2012;3:10.

Hasbun R, Rosenthal N, Balada-Llasat JM, et al. Epidemiology of meningitis and encephalitis in the United States, 2011–2014. *Clin Infect Dis.* 2017;65(3):359–363.

Hiraga A, Kuwabara S, Nakamura A, et al. Fisher/Guillain–Barré overlap syndrome in advanced AIDS. *J Neurol Sci.* 2007;258(1–2):148–150.

Hughes RA. Inflammatory neuropathy: sixth meeting of the Peripheral Neuropathy Association. St. Catherine's College, Oxford, England, August 14–18, 1990. *Neurology.* 1991;41(5):758–759.

Huis in't Veld D, Sun HY, Hung CC, Colebunders R. The immune reconstitution inflammatory syndrome related to HIV co-infections: a review. *Eur J Clin Microbiol Infect Dis.* 2012;31(6):919–927.

Jacks A, Wainwright D, Salazar L, et al. Neurocognitive deficits increase lack of retention-in-care among older adults with newly diagnosed HIV infection. *AIDS.* 2015;29(13):1711–1714.

Jadhav S, Agrawal M, Rathi S. Acute motor axonal neuropathy in HIV infection. *Indian J Pediatr.* 2014;81:193.

Jarvis JN, Lawrence DS, Meya DB, et al. Single-dose liposomal amphotericin B treatment for cryptococcal meningitis. *N Engl J Med.* 2022;386(12):1109–1120.

Johnson TP, Nath A. Biotypes of HIV-associated neurocognitive disorders based on viral and immune pathogenesis. *Curr Opin Infect Dis.* 2022;35(3):223–230.

Johnson TP, Patel K, Johnson KR, et al. Induction of IL-17 and nonclassical T-cell activation by HIV-Tat protein. *Proc Natl Acad Sci USA.* 2013;110:13588–13593.

Kallianpur AR, Hulgan T. Pharmacogenetics of nucleoside reverse-transcriptase inhibitor-associated peripheral neuropathy. *Pharmacogenomics*. 2009;10(4):623–637.

Kapur J, Elm J, Chamberlain JM, et al. Randomized trial of three anticonvulsant medications for status epilepticus. *N Engl J Med*. 2019;381:2103–2113.

Keswani SC, Pardo CA, Cherry CL, et al. HIV-associated sensory neuropathies. *AIDS*. 2002;16(16):2105–2117.

Keswani SC, Polley M, Pardo CA, et al. Schwann cell chemokine receptors mediate HIV-1 gp120 toxicity to sensory neurons. *Arch Neurol*. 2003;54(3):287–296.

Leger JM, Bouche P, Bolgert F, et al. The spectrum of polyneuropathies in patients infected with HIV. *J Neurol Neurosurg Psychiatry*. 1989;52(12):1369–1374.

Lehmann HC, Chen W, Borzan J, et al. Mitochondrial dysfunction in distal axons contributes to human immunodeficiency virus sensory neuropathy. *Arch Neurol*. 2011;69(1):100–110.

Leisman RM, Strasburg AP, Heitman, AK. et al. Evaluation of a commercial multiplex molecular panel for diagnosis of infectious meningitis and encephalitis. *J Clin Microb*. 2018;56(4):1927–1917.

Lescure FX, Moulignier A, Savatovsky J, et al. CD8 encephalitis in HIV-positive patients receiving cART: a treatable entity. *Clin Infect Dis*. 2013;57(1):101–108.

Letendre S. Central nervous system complications in HIV disease: HIV-associated neurocognitive disorder. *Top Antivir Med*. 2011;19(4):137–142.

Letendre S, Fitzsimons C, Ellis R, et al. Correlates of CSF viral loads in 1221 volunteers of the CHARTER Cohort. Abstract 172. Paper presented at the 17th Conference on Retrovirus and Opportunistic Infections. San Francisco, CA; February 16–19, 2010.

Lindenbaum Y, Kissel JT, Mendell JR. Treatment approaches for Guillain–Barré syndrome and chronic inflammatory demyelinating polyradiculopathy. *Neurol Clin*. 2001;19(1):187–204.

Lipkin WI, Parry G, Kiprov D, et al. Inflammatory neuropathy in homosexual men with lymphadenopathy. *Neurology*. 1985;35(10):1479–1483.

Lopez Castelblanco R, Lee M, Hasbun R. Epidemiology of bacterial meningitis in the US: a population-based study. *Lancet Infect Dis*. 2014;14:813–819.

Lucas SB, Wong KT, Nightingale S, Miller RF. HIV-associated CD8 encephalitis: A UK case series and review of histopathologically confirmed cases. *Front Neurol*. 2021;12:628296.

Ma B, Vigil K, Hasbun R. HIV testing in adults presenting with CNS infections. *Open Forum Infect Dis*. 2020 Jun;7(6):ofaa217.

Maggiolo F, Airoldi M, Kleinloog HD, et al. Effect of adherence to HAART on virologic outcome and on the selection of resistance-conferring mutations in NNRTI- or PI-treated patients. *HIV Clin Trials*. 2007;8(5):282–292.

Manns A, Hisada M, La Grenade L. Human T-lymphotropic virus type I infection. *Lancet*. 1999;353(9168):1951–1958.

Markarian Y, Wulff EA, Simpson DM. Peripheral neuropathy in HIV disease. *AIDS Clin Care*. 1998;10(12):89–91, 93, 98.

Marra C, Maxwell CL, Smith SL, et al. Cerebrospinal fluid abnormalities in patients with syphilis: association with clinical and laboratory features. *J Infect Dis*. 2004;189(3):369–376.

Marra CM, Boutin P, Collier AC. Screening for distal sensory peripheral neuropathy in HIV-positive persons in research and clinical settings. *Neurology*. 1998;51(6):1678–1681.

Marshall DW, Brey RL, Cahill WT, et al. Spectrum of cerebrospinal fluid findings in various stages of human immunodeficiency virus infection. *Arch Neurol*. 1988;45:954–958.

Martin F, Taylor GP. Prospects for the management of human T-cell lymphotropic virus type 1-associated myelopathy. *AIDS Rev*. 2011;13(3):161–170.

Martin JL, Brown CE, Matthews-Davis N, et al. Effects of antiviral nucleoside analogs on human DNA polymerases and mitochondrial DNA synthesis. *Antimicrob Agents Chemother*. 1994;38(12):2743–2749.

Maschke M, Kastrup O, Diener HC. CNS manifestations of cytomegalovirus infections diagnosis and treatment. *CNS Drugs*. 2002;16(5):303–315.

McArthur JC, Brew BJ, Nath A. Neurological complications of HIV infection. *Lancet Neurol*. 2005;4(9):543–555.

McCutchan JA. Cytomegalovirus infections of the nervous system in patients with AIDS. *Clin Infect Dis*. 1995;20(4):747–754.

Métral M, Darling K, Locatelli I, et al. The Neurocognitive Assessment in the Metabolic and Aging Cohort (NAMACO) study: baseline participant profile. *HIV Med*. 2020;21(1):30–42.

Mind Exchange Working Group. Assessment, diagnosis, and treatment of HIV-associated neurocognitive disorder: a consensus report of the Mind Exchange Program. *Clin Infect Dis*. 2013;56(7):1004–1017.

Mishra BB, Sommers W, Koski CL, et al. Acute inflammatory demyelinating polyneuropathy in the acquired immune deficiency syndrome. *Ann Neurol*. 1985;18:131–132.

Modi G, Ranchhod J, Hari K, et al. Non-traumatic myelopathy at the Chris Hani Baragwanath Hospital, South Africa: the influence of HIV. *QJM*. 2011:104:697–703.

Molloy S, Kanyama C, Heyderman RS, et al. Antifungal combinations for treatment of cryptococcal meningitis. *N Engl J Med*. 2018;378(11):1004–1017.

Moore RD, Wong WM, Keruly JC, et al. Incidence of neuropathy in HIV-positive patients on monotherapy versus those on combination therapy with didanosine, stavudine and hydroxyurea. *AIDS*. 2000;14(3):273–278.

Morgello S, Cho ES, Nielsen S, et al. Cytomegalovirus encephalitis in patients with acquired immunodeficiency syndrome: an autopsy study of 30 cases and a review of the literature. *Hum Pathol*. 1987;18:289–297.

Mukerji SS, Misra V, Lorenz D, et al. Impact of antiretroviral regimens on cerebrospinal fluid viral escape in a prospective multicohort study of antiretroviral therapy-experience human immunodeficiency virus-1- infected adults in the United States. *Clin Infect Dis*. 2018;67(8):1182–1190.

Nagel MA, Forghani B, Mahalingam R, et al. The value of detecting anti-VZV IgG antibody in CSF to diagnose VZV vasculopathy. *Neurology*. 2007;68(13):1069–1073.

Nesher L, Hadi CM, Salazar L, et al. Epidemiology of meningitis with a negative CSF Gram-stain: underutilization of available diagnostic tests. *Epidemiol Infect*. 2016;144(1):189–197.

Nhantumbo AA, Comé CE, Maholela PI, et al. Etiology of meningitis among adults in three quaternary hospitals in Mozambique, 2016–2017: the role of HIV. *PLoS One*. 2022;17(5):e0267949.

Offiah CE, Turnbull IW. The imaging appearances of intracranial CNS infections in adult HIV and AIDS patients. *Clin Radiol*. 2006;61:393–401.

Opintan JA, Awadzi BK, Biney IJK, et al. High rates of cerebral toxoplasmosis in HIV patients presenting with meningitis in Accra, Ghana. *Trans R Soc Trop Med Hyg*. 2017;111(10):464–471.

Osiro S, Salomon N. Varicella-zoster (VZV) multifocal vasculopathy in a patient with systemic lupus erythematosus—a diagnostic and treatment dilemma. *IDCases*. 2017;8:81–83.

Pardo CA, McArthur JC, Griffin JW. HIV neuropathy: insights in the pathology of HIV peripheral nerve disease. *J Peripheral Nerv Syst*. 2001;6(1):21–27.

Park H, Song Y. Multiple tuberculoma involving the brain and spinal cord in a patient with miliary pulmonary tuberculosis. *J Korean Neurosurg Soc*. 2008;44(1):36–39.

Parry O, Mielke J, Latif AS, et al. Peripheral neuropathy in individuals with HIV infection in Zimbabwe. *Acta Neurol Scand*. 1997;96(4):218–222.

Patel AK, Patel KK, Gohel S, et al. Incidence of symptomatic CSF viral escape in HIV infected patients receiving atazanavir/ritonavir-containing ART: a tertiary care cohort in western India. *J Neurovirol*. 2018:24(4):498–505.

Perfect JR, Dismukes WE, Dromer F, et al. Clinical practice guidelines for the treatment of cryptococcal disease: 2010 update from the Infectious Diseases Society of America. *Clin Infect Dis*. 2012;50:291–322.

Petito CK, Vecchio D, Chen YT. HIV antigen and DNA in AIDS spinal cords correlate with macrophage infiltration but not with vacuolar myelopathy. *J Neuropathol Exp Neurol*. 1994;53(1):86–94.

Phillips TJ, Cherry CL, Cox S, et al. Pharmacological treatment of painful HIV-associated sensory neuropathy: a systematic review and meta-analysis of randomised controlled trials. *PLoS One.* 2010;5(12):e14433.

Piliero PJ, Fish DG, Preston S, et al. Guillain–Barré syndrome associated with immune reconstitution. *Clin Infect Dis.* 2003;36(9):e111–e114.

Pillat MM, Bauer ME, de Oliveira AC, et al. HTLV-1-associated myelopathy/tropical spastic paraparesis (HAM/TSP): still an obscure disease. *Cent Nerv Syst Agents Med Chem.* 2011;11(4):239–245.

Plasma Exchange/Sandoglobulin Guillain–Barré Syndrome Trial Group. Randomised trial of plasma exchange, intravenous immunoglobulin, and combined treatments in Guillain–Barré syndrome. *Lancet.* 1997;349:225–230.

Polydefkis M, Yiannoutsos CT, Cohen BA, et al. Reduced intraepidermal nerve fiber density in HIV-associated sensory neuropathy. *Neurology.* 2002;58(1):115–119.

Portegies P, Solod L, Cinque P, et al. EFNS Task Force guidelines for the diagnosis and management of neurological complications of HIV infection. *Eur J Neurol.* 2004;11:297–304.

Price RW, Yiannoutsos CT, Clifford DB, et al. Neurological outcomes in late HIV infection: adverse impact of neurological impairment on survival and protective effect of antiviral therapy. AIDS Clinical Trial Group and Neurological AIDS Research Consortium Study Team. *AIDS.* 1999;13(13):1677–1685.

Radziwill AJ, Kuntzer T, Steck AJ. Immunopathology and treatments of Guillain–Barré syndrome and of chronic inflammatory demyelinating polyneuropathy. *Rev Neurol (Paris).* 2002;158(3):301–310.

Rauschkaa H, Jellingerb K, Lassmannc H, et al. Guillain–Barré syndrome with marked pleocytosis or a significant proportion of polymorphonuclear granulocytes in the cerebrospinal fluid: neuropathological investigation of five cases and review of differential diagnoses. *Eur J Neurol.* 2003;10:479–486.

Reimer-McAtee M, Ramirez D, McAtee CL, et al. Correction to: Encephalitis in HIV-infected adults in the antiretroviral therapy era. *J Neurol.* 2023;270(9):4582.

Robertson KR, Smurzynski M, Parsons TD, et al. The prevalence and incidence of neurocognitive impairment in the HAART era. *AIDS.* 2007;21:1915–1921.

Robinson-Papp J, Gonzalez-Duarte A, Simpson DM, et al. The roles of ethnicity and antiretrovirals in HIV-associated polyneuropathy: a pilot study. *J Acquir Immune Defic Syndr.* 2009a;51(5):569–573.

Robinson-Papp J, Sharma S, Simpson DM, et al. Autonomic dysfunction is common in HIV and associated with distal symmetric polyneuropathy. *J Neurovirol.* 2013;19:172–180.

Robinson-Papp J, Simpson DM. Neuromuscular diseases associated with HIV-1 infection. *Muscle Nerve.* 2009b;40(6):1043–1053.

Rolfes MA, Hullsiek KH, Rhein J, et al. The effect of therapeutic lumbar punctures on acute mortality from cryptococcal meningitis. *Clin Infect Dis.* 2014;59(11):1607–1614.

Rosca EC, Albarqouni L,Simu M. Montreal cognitive assessment (MoCA) for HIV-associated neurocognitive disorders. *Neuropsychol Rev.* 2019: 29(3):313–327.

Rosca EC, Rosca O, Simu M. Intravenous immunoglobulin treatment in a HIV-1 positive patient with Guillain–Barré syndrome. *Int Immunopharmacol.* 2015;29(2):964–965.

Rosenow JM, Hirschfeld A. Utility of brain biopsy in patient with acquired immunodeficiency syndrome before and after introduction of highly active antiretroviral therapy. *Neurosurgery.* 2007;61(1):130–141.

Sandoval R, Runft B, Roddey T. Pilot study: does lower extremity night splinting assist in the management of painful peripheral neuropathy in the HIV/AIDS population? *J Int Assoc Phys AIDS Care (Chic).* 2010;9(6):368–381.

Schifitto G, McDermott MP, McArthur JC, et al.; Dana Consortium on the Therapy of HIV Dementia and Related Cognitive Disorders. Incidence of and risk factors for HIV-associated distal sensory polyneuropathy. *Neurology.* 2002;58(12):1764–1768.

Schreiber AL, Norbury JW, DeSousa EA. Functional recovery of untreated human immunodeficiency virus-associated Guillain–Barré syndrome: a case report. *Ann Phys Rehabil Med.* 2011;54:519–524.

Schuldt AL, Bern H, Hart M; PIVOT Study Team. Peripheral neuropathy in virologically suppressed people living with HIV: evidence from the PIVOT Trial. *Viruses.* 2023;16(1):2.

Serpa JA, Moran A, Goodman JC, Giordano TP, White AC. Neurocysticercosis in the HIV era: a case report and review of the literature. *Am J Trop Med Hyg.* 2007;77(1):113–117.

Shahani L, Salazar L, Woods SP, Hasbun R. Baseline neurocognitive functioning predicts viral load suppression at 1-year follow-up among newly diagnosed HIV infected patients. *AIDS Behav.* 2018;22(10):3209–3213.

Shukla B, Aguilera EA, Salazar L, Wootton SH, Kaewpoowat Q, Hasbun R. Aseptic meningitis in adults and children: diagnostic and management challenges. *J Clin Virol.* 2017;94:110–114.

Silva CA, Penalva de Oliveira AC, Vilas-Boas L, et al. Neurologic cytomegalovirus complications in patients with AIDS: retrospective review of 13 cases and review of the literature. *Rev Inst Med Trop Sao Paulo.* 2010;52(6):305–310.

Simpson DM, Brown S, Tobias J; NGX-4010 C107 Study Group. Controlled trial of high-concentration capsaicin patch for treatment of painful HIV neuropathy. *Neurology.* 2008;70:2305–2313.

Simpson JK 3rd. Chronic neuropathic pain. *N Engl J Med.* 2003;348(26):2688–2689.

Simpson DM, Kitch D, Evans SR, et al. HIV neuropathy natural history cohort study: assessment measures and risk factors. *Neurology.* 2006;66(11):1679–1687. doi:10.1212/01.wnl.0000218303.48113.5d

Smyth K, Affandi JS, McArthur JC, et al. Prevalence of and risk factors for HIV-associated neuropathy in Melbourne, Australia 1993–2006. *HIV Med.* 2007;8:367–373.

Sulaiman T, Medi S, Erdam H, et al. The diagnostic utility of the "Thwaites' system" and "lancet consensus scoring system" in tuberculosis vs. non-tuberculosis subacute and chronic meningitis: multicenter analysis of 395 adult patients. *BMC Infect Dis.* 2020;20(1):788.

Tagliati M, Grinnell J, Godbold J, et al. Peripheral nerve function in HIV infection: clinical, electrophysiologic, and laboratory findings. *Arch Neurol.* 1999;56(1):84–89.

Tan K, Roda R, Ostrow L, McArthur J, Nath A. PML-IRIS in patients with HIV infection: clinical manifestations and treatment with steroids. *Neurology.* 2009;72(17):1458–1464.

Thao LTP, Heemskerk AD, Geskus RB, et al. Prognostic models for 9-month mortality in tuberculous meningitis. *Clin Infect Dis.* 2018;66(4):523–532.

Thwaites GE. The management of suspected encephalitis. *BMJ.* 2012;344:e3489.

Tirbaboshi J, Arkaitz I, Saye H, et al. Total and unbound bictegravir concentrations and viral suppression in cerebrospinal fluid of human immunodeficiency virus-infected patients. *J Infect Dis.* 2019;221(9):1425–1428.

Triunfo M, Vai D, Montrucchio C, et al. Diagnostic accuracy of new and old cognitive screening tools for HIV-associated neurocognitive disorders. *HIV Med.* 2018;19:455–464.

Tunkel AR, Glaser CA, Bloch KC, et al. The management of encephalitis: clinical practice guidelines by the Infectious Diseases Society of America. *Clin Infect Dis.* 2004;47(3):303–327.

Tyor WR, Glass JD, Baumrind N, et al. Cytokine expression of macrophages in HIV-1-associated vacuolar myelopathy. *Neurology.* 1993;43(5):1002–1009.

U.S. Department of Health and Human Services (USDHHS), Panel on Antiretroviral Guidelines for Adults and Adolescents. Guidelines for the use of antiretroviral agents in HIV-1-infected adults and adolescents. https://clinicalinfo.hiv.gov/en/guidelines/hiv-clinical-guidelines-adult-and-adolescent-arv/whats-new. Published September 12, 2024a. Accessed September 18, 2024.

USDHHS, Panel on Opportunistic Infections in HIV-positive Adults and Adolescents. Guidelines for the prevention and treatment of opportunistic infections in HIV-positive adults and adolescents: recommendations from the Centers for Disease Control and Prevention, the National Institutes of Health, and the HIV Medicine Association of the Infectious Diseases Society of America. https://clinicalinfo.hiv.gov/sites/default/files/guidelines/documents/adult-adolesc

ent-oi/guidelines-adult-adolescent-oi.pdf. Published August 15, 2024b. Accessed August 31, 2024.

Valcour VG. Evaluating cognitive impairment in the clinical setting: practical screening and assessment tools. *Top Antivir Med.* 2011c;19(5):175–180.

Valcour V, Paul R, Chiao S, et al. Screening for cognitive impairment in human immunodeficiency virus. *Clin Infect Dis.* 2011a;53(8):836–842.

Valcour V, Sithinamsuwan P, Letendre S, et al. Pathogenesis of HIV in the central nervous system. *Curr HIV/AIDS Rep.* 2011b;8(1):54–61.

Van der Meche FG, Schitz PI; Dutch Guillain–Barré Study Group. A randomized trial comparing intravenous immune globulin and plasma exchange in Guillain–Barré syndrome. *N Engl J Med.* 1992;326(17):1123–1129.

Vecchio AC, Marra CM, Schouten J, et al. Distal sensory peripheral neurology in human immunodeficiency virus type1-positive individuals before and after antiretroviral therapy initiative in diverse resource-limited settings. *Clin Infect Dis.* 2020;71(1):158–165.

Veltman JA, Bristow CC, Klausner JD. Meningitis in HIV-positive patients in sub-Saharan Africa: a review. *J Int AIDS Soc.* 2014;17:19184.

Verma A. Epidemiology and clinical features HIV-1 associated neuropathies. *J Peripheral Nerv Syst.* 2001;6(1):8–13.

Verma A, Bradley WG. HIV-1 associated neuropathies. *CNS Spectrums.* 2000;5(5):66–67.

Verma S, Estanislao L, Mintz L, et al. Controlling neuropathic pain in HIV. *Curr HIV/AIDS Rep.* 2004;1(3):136–141.

Vigil KJ, Salazar L, Hasbun R. Community-acquired meningitis in HIV-infected patients in the United States. *AIDS Patient Care STDs.* 2018;32(2):42–47.

Wagner JC, Bromber MB. HIV infection presenting with motor axonal variant of Guillain–Barré syndrome. *J Clin Neuromusc Disord.* 2007;9:303–305.

Wakerly BR, Yuki N. Mimics and chameleons in Guillain–Barré and Miller–Fisher syndromes. *Practical Neurol.* 2015;15:90–99.

Wang SX, Ho EL, Grill M, et al. Peripheral neuropathy in primary HIV infection associates with systemic and CNS immune activation. *J Acquir Immune Defic Syndr.* 2014;66(3):303–310.

Webb AJ, Borrelli EP, Vyas A, et al. The effect of antiretroviral therapy with high central nervous system penetration on HIV-related cognitive impairment: a systematic review and meta-analysis. *AIDS Care.* 2023;35(11):1635–1646. doi:10.1080/09540121.2022.2098231

Williams D, Geraci A, Simpson DM. AIDS and AIDS-treatment neuropathies. *Curr Headache Rep.* 2002;6(2):125–130.

Winer JB. Guillain–Barré syndrome. *J Clin Pathol.* 2001;54:381–385.

World Health Organization (WHO). Guidelines for diagnosing, preventing and managing cryptococcal disease among adults, adolescents and children living with HIV. https:// www.who.int/publications/i/item/9789240052178. Published June 27, 2022. Accessed September 12, 2024.

Wulff EA, Simpson DM. Neuromuscular complications of the human immunodeficiency virus type 1 infection. *Semin Neurol.* 1999a;19(2):157–164.

Wulff EA, Simpson DM. Neuromuscular complications of HIV-1 infection. *Curr Infect Dis Rep.* 1999b;1(2):192–197.

Wulff EA, Wang AK, Simpson DM. HIV-associated peripheral neuropathy: epidemiology, pathophysiology and treatment. *Drugs.* 2000;59(6):1251–1260.

Yousem DM, Grossman RI. *The Requisites: Neuroradiology.* 3rd ed. Philadelphia: Mosby; 2010:209.

29.

CARDIOVASCULAR DISEASE

Jarrett K. Sell and Jonathan J. Nunez

LEARNING OBJECTIVES

- Discuss the pathophysiology of cardiovascular disease (CVD) and myocardial infarction (MI) in people with HIV (PWH).
- Describe the associations between chronic HIV infection as it relates to an increased risk of CVD, MI, heart failure, stroke, peripheral arterial disease, and sudden cardiac death (SCD).
- Discuss the association of specific antiretroviral therapies (ART) and cardiovascular risk.
- Assess CVD risk in PWH by application of the American Heart Association/American College of Cardiology (AHA/ACC) atherosclerotic cardiovascular disease (ASCVD) 10-year risk calculator.
- Describe recommendations for the use of statin therapy as primary prevention of atherosclerotic cardiovascular disease in people with HIV
- List medical therapies, including statins and non-statins, to lower the risk of CVD and MI in PWH.
- Discuss lifestyle interventions, including diet, exercise, weight loss, and smoking cessation, to lower the risk of CVD and MI in PWH.

WHAT'S NEW?

- The REPRIEVE trial showed that participants with HIV infection and low-to-moderate CVD risk who received pitavastatin had a 35% lower risk of major adverse cardiovascular event than those who received placebo.
- Modeling studies continue to show that the ACC/AHA calculator appears to underestimate the risk of CVD in PWH.
- Recent systemic reviews and meta-analyses show worse clinical outcomes after hospitalization for heart failure and acute coronary syndromes in PWH.
- A 2022 systemic review and meta-analysis found that PCSK9 inhibitors may reduce non-fatal MI and stroke in adults at very high or high cardiovascular risk who are receiving maximally tolerated statin therapy or are statin-intolerant, but not in those with moderate and low cardiovascular risk.
- The current evidence suggests that the net benefit of aspirin for primary prevention is small and may be considered only in those aged 40–59 years with a 10% or greater 10-year CVD risk and a low risk of bleeding.
- Recent data continue to highlight the differential effect of specific antiretroviral (ARV) classes on weight, with integrase strand transfer inhibitors (INSTIs) having the biggest effect on weight gain, and women being most affected by weight gain.
- There is growing evidence that nicotine-containing e-cigarettes may be beneficial in aiding smoking cession.

KEY POINTS

- PWH are at increased risk for CVD, including MI, stroke, heart failure (HF), and SCD.
- The excess risk of CVD has been linked to the double burden of a high prevalence of traditional risk factors (e.g., DM, HTN, and smoking) and HIV-specific risk factors (e.g., inflammation, immune activation, immune suppression, and viremia).
- Some ART is thought to increase CVD risk through elevation of lipids levels, weight gain, and other mechanisms, although this is less commonly seen in the modern treatment era.
- PWH should be screened regularly for known CVD risk factors, including hypertension, diabetes mellitus, dyslipidemia, and cigarette smoking.
- ART modification solely to improve lipid profiles in PWH may be considered but should not compromise virologic or immunologic control.
- PWH should be assessed for 10-year CVD risk by using the ACC/AHA risk calculator. In people without known CVD and a 10-year ASCVD risk <20% who are between the ages of 40 and 75, DHHS recommends initiation of [at least] moderate-intensity statin therapy for people whose 10-year ASCVD risk estimates are 5% to <20%. When 10-year risk estimates are <5%, DHHS favors initiation of [at least] moderate-intensity statin therapy.
- In general, statin therapies are recommended for primary and secondary prevention of CVD, and additional cholesterol-lowering medications may be indicated for select high-risk patients. Additional interventions which

- have been proven to lower the risk of CVD and MI include diet, exercise, smoking cessation, and the use of antihypertensive medications.
- Given the high prevalence of smoking among PWH (>33%), treatment for tobacco use disorder should routinely be offered to all candidates.
- Gains in life expectancy for PWH owing to successful ART will be lost if management of CVD is not optimized, through a focus on modifiable CVD risk management and prevention strategies.

INTRODUCTION

There is considerable evidence that PWH are at increased risk for CVD, including MI and stroke. Epidemiological studies have consistently found higher rates of CVD, especially MI and stroke, among PWH compared to HIV-negative persons (Freiberg et al., 2013; Grinspoon et al., 2023; Kovacs et al., 2022; Rao et al., 2019). Despite access to life-preserving ART, further studies in the United States and globally continue to highlight the greater burden of coronary artery disease in PWH, even when accounting for viral suppression (Hsue and Waters, 2019; Metkus et al., 2015; Post et al., 2014; Shah et al., 2018).

Most of these studies acknowledge a higher prevalence of known traditional risk factors for CVD among PWH and typically adjust for confounding variables. Cigarette smoking, in particular, is several-fold greater in PWH compared to the general population. After accounting for such traditional risks, significant differences between PWH and people without HIV generally persist—although the more factors that are added to these models, the greater the attenuation between HIV infection and CVD (Post et al., 2014; Rao et al., 2019). Other factors, including poor diet, sedentary lifestyle, substance use, and even stress and psychiatric disorders, can increase the risk of CVD and may account for the excess CVD burden among PWH. However, data on these confounders are not typically collected (Khambaty et al., 2016; White et al., 2015).

There are also biologically plausible explanations for higher CVD risk accompanying HIV infection. Higher levels of markers of immune activation and inflammation among PWH with suppressed viremia have been observed, and a correlation between such markers and adverse events suggest infection-related pathogenic mechanisms for CVD in PWH (Deeks et al., 2013; Hunt, 2012; Scherzer et al., 2018). In addition, the increased risk of cardiovascular disease in PWH who are virally suppressed could be associated with reservoirs of infected cells. ART prevents HIV from spreading and infecting new cells, but does not eliminate cells that are already infected with the HIV virus; thus the virus persists (McLaughlin et al., 2020). Moreover, although ART has been found to consistently reduce surrogate markers for inflammation, endothelial dysfunction, and immune activation, observational studies indicate that some specific antiretroviral medications may contribute to CVD. It remains unclear if such associations are affected by confounding variables and, if truly contributing, what the mechanisms are that lead to CVD. The heightened risk for CVD in PWH, regardless of etiology, requires healthcare providers to be diligent in assessing CVD risk and intervening, when appropriate. Newer information has made it increasingly clear that the care of PWH requires not only chronic viral suppression, but also early recognition and management of CVD risk factors (Rao et al., 2019). More research is greatly needed to elucidate the mechanisms of HIV-associated CVD and therapeutic strategies to mitigate these risks.

EVIDENCE OF EXCESS RISK FOR CARDIOVASCULAR DISEASE IN HIV

One of the largest initial epidemiological studies examining differential rates of CVD among PWH and HIV-negative persons was conducted within a registry of patients receiving care in Boston that included 3,851 PWH and 1,044,589 HIV-negative patients (Triant et al., 2007). The difference in acute MI rates between PWH and people without HIV was significant, with a relative risk (RR) of 1.75 (95% confidence interval [CI]: 1.51–2.02; $p < 0.0001$), adjusting for age, gender, race, hypertension, diabetes, and dyslipidemia (Triant et al., 2007).

Similar studies of MI and stroke incidence were conducted by the Kaiser Permanente system in California (Klein et al., 2014; Klein et al., 2015). Rates of both conditions were historically higher for PWH compared to HIV-negative members. However, a convergence over time was observed in the rates of MI and stroke experienced by PWH compared to HIV-negative patients. Improved detection and management of CVD risk factors plus better treatment of HIV infection are hypothesized to account for the decline in CVD rates in this cohort. Similar declines in the rates of CVD over the past decade were reported from cohorts in Europe and British Columbia (Cheung et al., 2016; Hatleberg et al., 2016).

One analysis from the Veterans Aging Cohort Study (VACS) that included 81,000 participants (33% HIV-positive) found that PWH veterans had twice the risk of acute MI compared to those who were HIV-negative (Paisible et al., 2015). However, it also found a low prevalence of optimization of cardiac health in this high-risk population, including blood pressure control, treatment of hyperlipidemia, and smoking cessation. This alone may account for the increased risk of MI, and not HIV infection.

A 2018 systematic review by Shah included data from 80 longitudinal studies of 793,635 PWH and a total follow-up of 3.5 million person-years. Authors reported a 2.16 RR of MI and stroke in PWH compared to HIV-negative individuals (Shah et al., 2018). This is comparable to the RR of 2.48 with hypertension and 2.95 with smoking found in the multinational INTERHART study (Yusuf et al., 2004). In addition to an increased risk of MI in PWH, a 2024 systemic review and meta-analysis found that clinical outcomes after acute coronary syndromes (ACS) or revascularization were worse for PWH, with a significantly higher risk for all-cause mortality

(RR 1.64), major adverse cardiovascular events (RR 1.11), recurrent ACS (RR 1.83), and admissions for new heart failure (RR 3.39) (Haji et al., 2024). A 2021 observational cohort of veterans from the VACS also showed that HIV infection was associated with increased sudden cardiac death (SCD) risk (hazard ratio [HR] 1.14; 95% CI: 1.04–1.25), adjusting for possible confounders, and this risk was greatest for those with CD4$^+$ counts <200 cells/mm^3 or viral load >500 copies/mL (Freiberg et al., 2021). Despite some variance in data from observational cohorts, the preponderance of these studies from the United States, Europe, and sub-Saharan Africa support the fact that PWH indeed have an excess risk of CVD, including MI, stroke, HF, and SCD.

Beyond cohort studies, pathophysiological evidence of excess CVD accompanying HIV infection has been found. Relatively high levels of inflammation within the aorta, possibly mediated by monocyte activation, were demonstrated by fluorodeoxyglucose positron emission tomography (FDG-PET) scanning in a small study of ART-receiving PWH without known CVD compared to uninfected controls with similar CVD risks. These data were later correlated with vulnerable coronary plaques (Subramanian et al., 2012; Tawakol et al., 2014). Similarly, a larger cross-sectional study, the Multicenter AIDS Cohort Study (MACS), examined coronary calcium scores and coronary plaque morphology in PWH and HIV-negative MSM and found that plaque was highly prevalent in both groups (Post et al., 2014). After adjustment for major confounders, there remained a higher prevalence of plaque in PWH (prevalence ratio [PR] 1.13; 95% CI: 1.04–1.23), who were also more likely to have noncalcified plaques (the most vulnerable to rupture) (PR 1.25; 95% CI: 1.10–1.43). Older age was associated with noncalcified plaque in PWH but not in HIV-negative men. This factor seemed to drive the overall differences between groups. Adjustment for additional confounders reduced the association between HIV infection and noncalcified plaques.

In 2020, a San Francisco cohort study examined the association between cell-associated HIV RNA and DNA and development of carotid plaque over time among 152 PWH virologically suppressed on ART (McLaughlin et al., 2020). The median age of patients was 47 years old, and they were living with HIV, on average, for 13 years. The latent HIV reservoir is a group of immune cells infected with HIV but not actively producing new viruses; as they are not producing new copies of viruses, ART has no effect on them. Levels of HIV RNA and DNA were checked with blood samples, and ultrasound was performed to monitor carotid intima-media thickness (CIMT). During follow-up, there was an association between CIMT and levels of HIV RNA ($p = 0.47$) and HIV DNA ($p = 0.042$). However, when taking into account traditional risk factors, the association was not statistically significant. Yet, when looking at the formation of new carotid artery plaques, there was a statistically significant relationship between HIV RNA and DNA levels ($p = 0.008$ and $p = 0.02$). These results suggest that decreasing the HIV reservoir size, which can occur with prompt initiation of ART in persons with newly acquired infection, may decrease inflammation and reduce atherosclerosis.

The concept of HIV causing "accelerated" aging with CVD and other conditions (e.g., bone disease, frailty) possibly occurring earlier in PWH has been countered by data from the U.S. Veterans Administration Aging Cohort and a large HIV case-control study from Denmark (Althoff et al., 2015; Rasmussen et al., 2015). In both groups, excess risk of CVD with HIV infection was observed. However, this was detected at similar ages in HIV-positive and HIV-negative persons, and, over time, there was no observed increase in overall risk for PWH. In the North American NA-ACCORD cohort, the attributable risk of type 1 MI was much greater for PWH who smoked, had hypertension, or elevated lipid levels as opposed to lower CD4$^+$ T-cell counts, elevated plasma HIV RNA level, or a diagnosis of AIDS (Althoff et al., 2017). Consequently, modeling studies have found that interventions that target the management of blood pressure, glucose, and lipid levels, as well as smoking cessation, may have a much greater clinical impact than earlier initiation of HIV treatment or avoidance of ART that has been associated with risk of CVD (Smit et al., 2018).

In recent years it has also become apparent that heart failure (HF) is more common in PWH. In the Kaiser Permanente HIV-Heart Study, the rate of incident HF was compared between 39,000 PWH and over 387,000 matched controls (1:10) without HIV infection. Incident HF was higher among PWH (4% vs. 3%) with a hazard ratio indicating a 66% greater risk in the fully adjusted model that accounted for coronary syndrome events, suggesting an independent mechanism independent of atherosclerosis (Go et al., 2018). A 2020 study found that women with HIV had a higher incidence of myocardial fibrosis and subsequent reduced diastolic function (also referred to as HF with reduced ejection fraction) (Zanni et al., 2020). In addition, a retrospective cohort study evaluated HIV infection and variation in HF risk by age, sex, and ethnicity, and key findings noted the adjusted risk of HF in PWH seemed stronger in younger patients (aged 21–41 years), women, and Asian/Pacific Islander adults (Go et al., 2022). A 2024 systemic review and meta-analysis also found that PWH who were hospitalized with heart failure had a higher risk of all-cause death (HR: 1.20, 95% CI: 1.15–1.25), increased risk of HF-associated readmission (HR: 1.34, 95% CI: 1.03–1.75), and increased risk of all-cause readmission (HR: 1.27, 95% CI: 1.10–1.46) (Zhou et al., 2024), highlighting health disparities in clinical outcomes in PWH who have HF.

PROPOSED MECHANISMS

While traditional and non-HIV-related factors appear to drive much of the CVD events among PWH, factors related to HIV infection and its treatment may also play a role. Overall, the pathogenesis of atherosclerosis in the setting of HIV infection is likely more complex than the current level of understanding. Numerous mechanistic studies have examined the association between CVD (i.e., plaque, coronary calcium, arterial inflammation, and endothelial dysfunction) and markers of inflammation, immune activation, and microbial translocation across the gut (Deeks et al., 2013; Hunt, 2012). Using FDG-PET imaging, aortic wall inflammation was significantly correlated with markers of monocyte and macrophage activation, suggesting that these cell lines play a role in the observed changes. HIV-specific proteins not only drive endothelial dysfunction, but also influence adhesion molecule stimulation, leading to the efflux of cholesterol in macrophages contributing to foam cell formation, which contributes greatly to atherosclerosis development (Hudson et al., 2024). The monocyte activation marker soluble CD163 was also correlated with a noncalcified coronary plaque in men and women with HIV and well-controlled viral loads.

In the MACS coronary imaging study, as in most other cohorts, smoking rates were higher among PWH and were strongly associated with coronary plaque (Kelly et all, 2016). That smoking interacts with HIV and aging to accelerate CVD was observed by an examination of carotid intima-media thickness, suggesting that HIV infection modifies the effect of smoking and age on cardiovascular health (Fitch et al., 2013). In a related analysis, smoking and obesity were each significantly associated with levels of inflammatory markers, including interleukin-6 (IL-6), sCD14, and sTNFR-I and -II (Krishnan et al., 2014). Similar findings linking smoking and inflammation were seen in the SUN cohort of PWH (Cioe et al., 2015). In that study, heavy alcohol intake was also associated with elevations of the coagulation marker D-dimer.

Data from another study suggests that T-cell activation and inflammation may contribute to the development of vascular disease (Hsue et al., 2010). They have also suggested that HIV proteins, including transactivator of transcription (TaT) and negative factor (Nef), may induce inflammation and endothelial dysfunction (Hsue et al., 2019). Residual immune activation secondary to incomplete control of HIV infection (despite undetectable viremia), coinfections (e.g., cytomegalovirus and hepatitis C virus), and irreversible translocation of microbial products across an altered gut lumen occur in PWH. They are thought to promote a proinflammatory milieu that is proatherogenic (Deeks et al., 2013; Hsue et al., 2019). Early studies examining the potential promise of anti-inflammatory interventions have not been successful. For example, a 2021 randomized trial of colchicine (an anti-inflammatory agent) did not show improved coronary endothelial function, which is a predictor of CVD, in PWH and no history of CAD (Hays et al., 2021).

Several studies have also shown that the risk of CVD among PWH is likely correlated with immunodeficiency—specifically, nadir $CD4^+$ T-cell count or low $CD4^+$ T-cell counts (Drozd et al., 2015). Nadir $CD4^+$ T- cell count has been linked to CIMT and arterial stiffness (Hsue et al., 2019). Two cohort studies found that low $CD4^+$ T-cell counts were associated with incident MI (Hsue et al., 2019). In the NA-ACCORD cohort, lower current $CD4^+$ T cells, as well as a history of AIDS and detectable plasma HIV RNA levels, were predictors of primary MI. Collectively, it appears that markers of immune damage and viremia are predictive of or related to CVD clinical events. However, the mechanisms linking damage to the immune system from HIV to atherosclerosis remain to be elucidated (Figure 29.1).

People living with HIV can also present with a variety of cardiac manifestations, including heart failure and myocardial disease. The pathogenesis of HF in the setting of HIV infection remains unclear. One hypothesis is that HIV acts directly on the myocardium, as well as indirectly via inflammation and autoimmunity (Fung et al., 2016; Remick et al., 2014). Some ARV drugs, including nucleoside reverse transcriptase inhibitors (NRTIs), in this theoretical model may contribute to pathogenesis. Data from the REPRIEVE trial found that PWH who underwent cardiac MRI had an increased prevalence of myocardial steatosis (i.e., increased myocardial triglyceride content), which predisposes to diastolic dysfunction and HF risk (Nelian et al., 2020). It was also found that for PWH in this study, advanced age, low nadir $CD4^+$ T-cell count, and body mass index (BMI) ≥ 25 kg/m^2 were all associated with HF.

THE EFFECT OF ART ON CVD

Multiple retrospective studies and several prospective studies have evaluated the impact of ART on CVD, and, as in epidemiological studies, these are often challenged by factors that confound analyses and/or lack an appropriate control group. Historically, one prevailing thought was that ART increases CVD risk due to its negative effects on lipid levels (especially LDL-C and triglycerides), which was commonly seen with older ritonavir-boosted protease inhibitors. Recently, an increasing focus on weight gain with contemporary ART is driving new evaluations to determine the correlation between ARVs and CVD disease.

The most persuasive data on the issue of ART-related CVD risk comes from the D:A:D cohort. This is a large, ongoing, prospective, observational study of PWH in Europe, the United States, and Australia. In 2003, D:A:D investigators first reported the incidence of MI to be increased significantly with prolonged exposure to combination ART (Friis-Moller et al., 2003). The adjusted risk rate per year of ART exposure ranged from 0.32 for no ART use to 2.93 for at least 6 years of ART use. The initial association between ART and MI was mainly driven by protease inhibitor (PI) therapy—specifically lopinavir-ritonavir and indinavir (D:A:D Study Group, 2007; Sabin et al., 2014). D:A:D data reported in 2018 found that ritonavir-boosted darunavir was associated with a 51% relative increased risk of MI and 49% increased risk of stroke over a 5-year period (Ryom et al., 2018). However, a more recent study from the French Hospital Database found no significant association between MI and exposure to darunavir or atazanavir (Costagliola et al., 2020). Another study also found that the boosted PI atazanavir was not associated with an increased MI risk. This may be due to the indirect hyperbilirubinemia that occurs with atazanavir, as other studies found a cardio-protective effect of higher bilirubin levels in the blood. This is further corroborated by a retrospective analysis from the VA cohort, which found that veterans with and without HIV infection with elevated bilirubin levels had lower rates of CVD and HF after adjustment for traditional risk factors (Marconi et al., 2018).

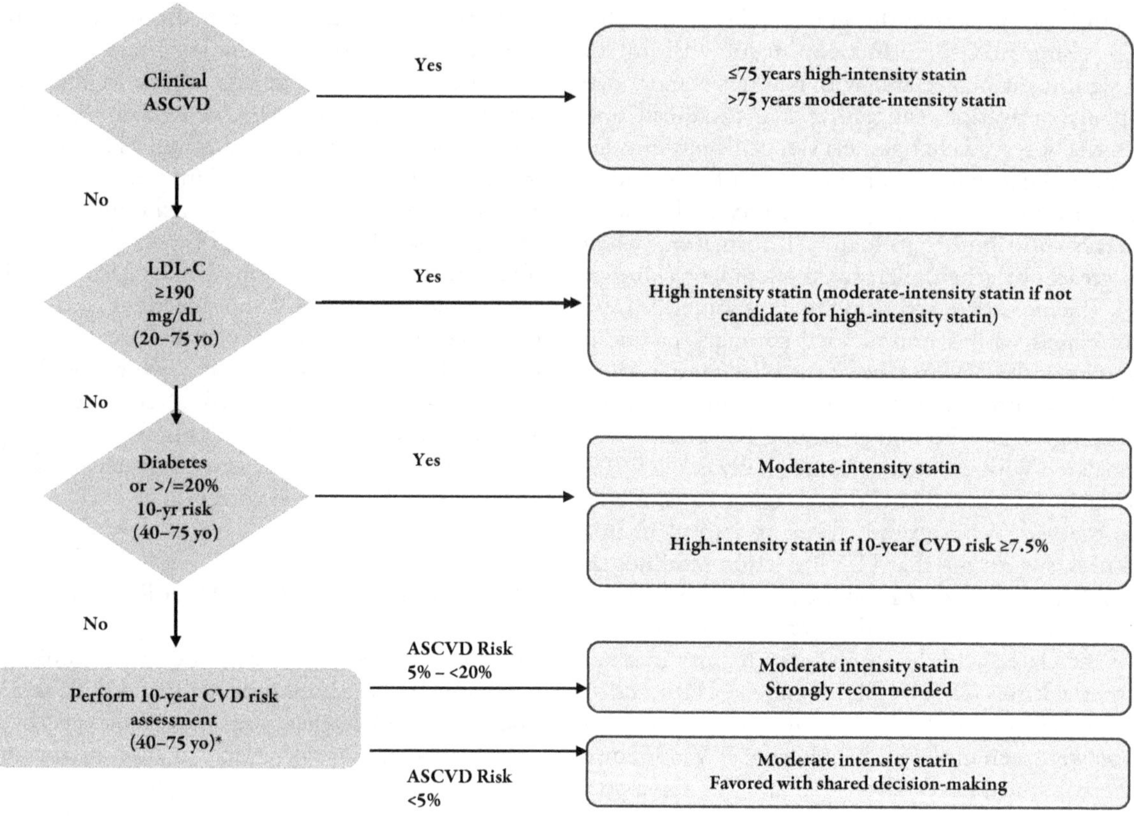

Figure 29.1 Statin Therapy in PWH SOURCE: Adapted from Stone NJ, et al. 2014 Jun 24;129(25 Suppl 2):S46-8] [published correction appears in Circulation. 2015 Dec 22;132(25):e396.); Grundy SM, et al. *Circulation.* 2019;139(25):e1046–e10812018; and Panel on Antiretroviral Guidelines for Adults and Adolescents. Statin Therapy in People with HIV. Department of Health and Human Services. https://clinicalinfo.hiv.gov/en/guidelines/hiv-clinical-guidelines-adult-and-adolescent-arv/statin-therapy-people-hiv. February 27, 2024. Updated September 12, 2024. Accessed July 29, 2024.
***Note: Data insufficient to recommend for or against statin therapy as primary prevention of ASCVD in those <40 years old with a<20% 10-year risk.**
Abbreviations: ASCVD = atherosclerotic cardiovascular disease; LDL-C = lipoprotein cholesterol; yo = years old

An earlier link between the NRTI abacavir and MI from the D:A:D cohort ushered in a series of subsequent investigations that have reached mixed conclusions. Possible biomolecular mechanisms for this association have been sought and include increased platelet reactivity and/or endothelial cell and leukocyte interactions induced by abacavir, but these mechanisms remain unproven (Baum et al., 2011; De Pablo et al., 2012). Another study of PWH switching from abacavir to tenofovir alafenamide fumarate (TAF) found changes in platelet reactivity and collagen interaction, again suggesting that abacavir causes platelet dysfunction. Investigators note that this could explain the findings of an association between abacavir and CVD (Mallon et al., 2018). A 2021 administrative health plan analysis looked at CVD risk associated with 14 different ART combinations and found that persons taking abacavir-lamivudine-darunavir had the highest incidence rate (IR 11/1000; 95% CI: 7.4–16.0) of acute MI (Dorjee et al., 2021). Per the latest U.S. Department of Health and Human Services and International Antiretroviral Association (IAS)-USA HIV treatment guidelines, abacavir should generally be avoided (DHHS, 2024; Gandhi et al., 2023). As HIV therapy evolves and exposures to new agents accumulate, D:A:D investigators and other cohorts will regularly reexamine the risks associated with CVD events.

There has been recent interest in whether INSTIs are associated with increased CVD incidence. The multicenter RESPOND cohort included over 32,000 PWH from Europe, Argentina, and Australia. Participants were followed to the first cardiovascular event, including MI, stroke, or an invasive cardiovascular procedure (e.g., stenting or angioplasty). After controlling for underlying risk factors such as hypertension, dyslipidemia, diabetes, and chronic kidney disease, findings suggested that the risk of a cardiovascular event almost doubles during the first 6 months after starting an INSTI-inclusive regimen (Neesgaard et al., 2022). This risk continued in the first 2 years of exposure but was not seen in those with more than 2 years of treatment. Contrary to these findings, no other randomized clinical trials have reported an increase in CVD incidence in persons starting an INSTI. Thus, more studies are needed to confirm if there is a risk and if that risk is applicable to other populations globally.

Further, there are other proposed mechanisms whereby ART may increase CVD risk in PWH. There is continued concern for weight gain on INSTIs and tenofovir alafenamide-containing regimens. Although more studies are needed to understand the mechanisms involved, the promotion of weight gain may lead to more insulin resistance and dyslipidemia (Lake and Trevillyan, 2021). As noted in the

Table 29.1 2017 ACC/AHA GUIDELINES FOR DIAGNOSIS AND MANAGEMENT OF HYPERTENSION

BP CATEGORY	SYSTOLIC BP		DIASTOLIC BP	TREATMENT OR FOLLOW-UP
Normal	<120 mmHg	and	<80 mmHg	Evaluate yearly; encourage healthy lifestyle changes to maintain normal BP
Elevated	120–129 mmHg	and	<80 mmHg	Recommend healthy lifestyle changes and reassess in 3–6 months
Hypertension stage 1	130–139 mmHg	or	80–89 mmHg	Assess the 10-year risk for heart disease and stroke using the atherosclerotic cardiovascular disease (AVSCD risk calculator): • If risk is <10%, start with healthy lifestyle recommendations and reassess in 3–6 months. • If risk is >10% or the patient has known clinical CVD, diabetes mellitus, chronic kidney disease, recommend lifestyle changes, and BP-lowering medication (one medication); reassess in 1 month for effectiveness of medication therapy. • If goal is met after 1 month, reassess in 3–6 months. • If goal is not met after 1 month, consider different medication or titration and continue monthly follow-up until control is achieved.
Hypertension stage 2	≥140 mmHg	or	≥90 mmHg	Recommend healthy lifestyle changes and BP-lowering medication (two medications of different classes); reassess in 1 month for effectiveness. • If goal is met in 1 month; reassess in 3–6 months. • If goal is not met after 1 month, consider different medications or titration and continue follow-up until control is achieved.

Source: Adapted from Whelton et al., 2018a.

ADVANCE trial, participants taking tenofovir alafenamide, emtricitabine, and dolutegravir were noted to have greater weight gain, risk of metabolic syndrome, and clinical obesity. Nearly 1 in 5 women developed metabolic syndrome, and just under half developed clinical obesity within 4 years of treatment (Chandiwana et al., 2024; Sokhela et al., 2024)

Providers should also be aware of potential drug-drug interactions that could contribute to QT prolongation, which is associated with SCD. At least one study found that PWH have a four-times higher risk of SCD compared to those without HIV (Tseng and Foisy, 2012) (Table 29.1).

SCREENING AND ASSESSING CARDIOVASCULAR RISK

Given the higher risk of CVD among PWH, the standard of care includes baseline screening for traditional risk factors and appropriate attention to their management. This includes blood pressure measurement, weight, and body mass index (BMI). Recommended baseline laboratory parameters include a lipid panel (total cholesterol, high-density lipoprotein [HDL]-C, low density lipoprotein [LDL]-C, triglycerides) and fasting blood glucose level or hemoglobin A1C. Baseline renal and hepatic function should also be measured. Clinicians should assess diet, level of cardiovascular activity, and family history. After ART initiation, PWH should have a lipid profile repeated approximately 3 months after stabilizing on HIV therapy. If baseline and subsequent values are normal, then yearly lipid measurements are recommended (Aberg et al., 2014; Thompson et al., 2021). Risks for CVD and dyslipidemias should generally be managed according to the most recent ACC/AHA guidelines (Grundy et al., 2018; Reiter-Brennan et al., 2020). Evidence overwhelmingly suggests that the effects of cigarette smoking on CVD are magnified in PWH. Therefore, there is a particular urgency for HIV providers to ask PWH about smoking and to incorporate evidence-based interventions to facilitate smoking cessation into their practice (see later discussion).

In the past, CVD risk was usually assessed via the Framingham Heart Study risk calculator. Older studies have used this in PWH and found that it generally performed well in assessing 10-year CVD risk. However, in retrospect, Framingham likely significantly underestimated actual CVD risk for PWH (Law et al., 2006). The newer 10-year CVD risk AHA/ACC calculator has become the standard of care in the United States (Grundy et al., 2018) (Box 29.1). Similar to the Framingham risk calculator, the ACC/AHA calculator appears to underestimate the risk of CVD in PWH (Regan et al., 2015; Soares et al., 2023; Thompson-Paul et al., 2015; Triant et al., 2018). More prospective data validating these tools in PWH are needed to develop a risk calculator that includes HIV-specific factors, traditional CVD risk factors, and the ability to stratify individuals based on sex. In 2023, the American Heart Association (AHA) also developed a new CVD risk predictor, PREVENT (Predicting Risk of cardiovascular disease

Box 29.1 KEY RECOMMENDATION FOR REDUCING THE RISK OF ATHEROSCLEROTIC CARDIOVASCULAR DISEASE (ASCVD) THROUGH CHOLESTEROL MANAGEMENT

- In all patients, regardless of age, emphasize a heart-healthy lifestyle to reduce ASCVD risk. In young adults 20–39 years of age, an assessment of lifetime risk facilitates the clinician–patient risk discussion.
- In all patients ≥40 years of age, consider an appropriate dose (moderate- or high-intensity) statin based on prior cardiovascular events and calculated 10-year cardiovascular risk to further lower CVD risk.
- In very-high-risk patients (history of multiple major ASCVD events or one event and multiple risk factors), with an LDL-C of >70 mg/dL on maximal statin therapy, consider adding ezetimibe. In patients whose LDL-C remains ≥70 mg/dL on maximally tolerated statin and ezetimibe, adding a PCSK9 inhibitor is reasonable following a clinician–patient discussion about the net benefit, safety, and cost.
- In patients with severe primary hypercholesterolemia (LDL-C level ≥190 mg/dL), begin high-intensity statin therapy without calculating 10-year ASCVD risk. If the LDL-C level remains ≥100 mg/dL, adding ezetimibe is reasonable. If the LDL-C on statin plus ezetimibe remains ≥100 mg/dL and the patient has multiple factors that increase the risk of ASCVD events, a PCSK9 inhibitor may be considered.
- Assess adherence and response to lifestyle changes and cholesterol-lowering medications with repeat lipid measurement 4–12 weeks after statin initiation, repeated every 3–12 months.

Source: Adapted from DHHS, 2024; Grundy SM, et al. *Circulation*. 2019; 139(25):e1182–e1186; Reiter-Brennan et al. *Cleve Clin J Med*. 2020;87(4):231–239.

EVENTs) (https://professional.heart.org/en/guidelines-and-statements/prevent-calculator). PREVENT has not yet been studied in PWH but attempts to include additional metabolic and renal factors to provide a more holistic prediction model. While PREVENT omits race, the prediction model includes BMI, estimated glomerular filtration rate (eGFR), and (optionally) glycosylated hemoglobin (A1C), urinary albumin-to-creatinine ratio, and zip code. Initial comparison of PREVENT with the AHA/ACC calculator suggests that PREVENT risk estimates are lower than other estimates (Anderson et al., 2024). Additional factors to consider that have not been captured in some risk calculators include: evidence of metabolic syndrome, metabolic-associated liver disease, low CD4$^+$ cell count, viremia, hepatitis C coinfection, and polysubstance use (e.g., alcohol and/or stimulant use), all which could increase the CVD risk.

Several biomarkers of coagulation and inflammation have been studied for their potential role in predicting CVD events in PWH. Some of these include the highly sensitive C-reactive protein (hsCRP), D-dimer, IL-6, and fibrinogen. Combined data from three cohorts of PWH found that IL-6 and D-dimer were independently associated with risk of serious non-AIDS events or death. Another study found that biomarkers in PWH can be clustered into a "cardiac phenotype" for risk stratification (Sherzer et al., 2018). People with high levels of CRP, IL-6, and D-dimer had a higher prevalence of pulmonary hypertension and a 3-fold increase in mortality over approximately 7 years of follow-up. In contrast, one study of PWH without CVD and CD4$^+$ counts >500 cells/mm^3 found that traditional risk factors (i.e., race, age, gender, BMI, diabetes, and smoking) and not baseline levels of IL6 or hsCRP were associated with prevalence and incidence of HTN (Ghazi et al., 2020). Other biomarkers under investigation include adiponectin and GlycA. Adiponectin increases insulin sensitivity, and in one study of PWH, lower adiponectin levels were found in cases of ART-associated lipodystrophy and were associated with subclinical CAD (McGettrick and Mallon, 2022). GlycA, although not currently measurable in most clinical labs, may be a more accurate biomarker of several other CVD-associated processes. For example, increased GlycA levels were associated with other subclinical markers of CVD such as presence of coronary artery calcium, coronary stenosis, and plaque burden (Tibuakuu et al., 2019). Clustering of these biomarkers may help identify at-risk PWH and target appropriate therapies to prevent or limit cardiovascular events.

INTERVENTIONS AND MANAGEMENT

Currently there is no robust evidence to determine if CVD risk management in PWH should differ from management in the general population. Modifiable risk factors, including diabetes, dyslipidemia, hypertension, obesity, and cigarette smoking, are important in PWH, likely more so than for the general population. Since the ACC/AHA risk calculator may underestimate the risk of heart disease in PWH, some experts believe clinicians should adjust the calculated risk upward by 1.5 to 2 times (So-Amah et al., 2020). Regardless, risk-based assessment for CVD in PWH remains a rational starting point to guide lifestyle counseling, medical therapy (mainly statins), and other potential risk-reduction interventions (Grundy et al., 2019).

Continued emphasis on effective ART with durable viral suppression should remain the primary objective, even in the presence of CVD risk factors or established CAD. Data from the SMART study, as well as the ATHENA cohort, found that ongoing viremia and incomplete immune recovery increase the risk of cardiovascular events (Lundgren et al., 2015; Van Lelyveld et al., 2012). In addition, a National Institutes of Health (NIH)–sponsored study of over 6,500 PWH found that immunologic control was the most important HIV-related factor associated with acute MI (Triant et al., 2010).

Because of their potential effects on cholesterol (and thus CVD risk), ART selection should take into consideration a PWH's individual risk factors. Some ART combinations, such as ritonavir-boosted PIs, may increase lipid subsets, including LDL-C and triglycerides. The pharmacological booster cobicistat appears to increase LDL-C (similar to ritonavir) and leads to minor changes in triglycerides. The NRTI abacavir increases LDL-C and triglycerides, whereas tenofovir disoproxil fumarate (TDF) has been observed to lower LDL-C (Tungsiripat et al., 2010). As noted earlier, abacavir has been associated with an increased risk of CVD and MI in some studies (Dorjee et al., 2018; Dorjee et al., 2021; SMART, 2008). In clinical trials, the NRTI tenofovir alafenamide (TAF) increased fasting lipid parameters (TC, HDL, direct LDL, and TGs) compared to TDF and has been associated with weight gain (Sax et al., 2014). The INSTIs raltegravir, dolutegravir, elvitegravir, and bictegravir have not been found to significantly affect lipid levels (Dorjee et al., 2018).

In PWH with moderate to severe dyslipidemia and increased CVD risk, switching ART to a regimen with less effect on cholesterol and/or triglycerides is recommended by the DHHS and IAS-USA guidelines. However, this should not be done at the expense of compromising virologic control. In the SPIRAL study, participants with stable HIV disease were switched from a ritonavir-boosted PI-based regimen to raltegravir, leading to significant improvement in lipid profiles (Martinez et al., 2010). In the SPIRIT study, changing from a ritonavir-boosted PI plus dual nucleoside regimen to rilpivirine plus TDF/emtricitabine led to significant reductions in LDL cholesterol (Palella et al., 2014). In the MARCH study, participants who were switched from a boosted PI to maraviroc had significant reductions in mean TC over 96 weeks (Pett et al., 2018). Lastly, in the NEAT 022 study, all PWH over the age of 50 years and those over 18 with a 10-year CVD risk score of >10% were switched from a ritonavir-boosted PI to dolutegravir (DTG). At 48 weeks, participants who had been switched to DTG had significant improvements in TC and other lipid fractions (Gatell et al., 2017).

Management of lipid disorders in PWH should follow guidelines established for the general population. Attention should be paid to the potential for drug-drug interactions between lipid-lowering and ART. There are several published cholesterol guidelines, but most U.S. providers follow those of AHA/ACC (Figures 29.2, 29.3, and Box 29.2). The most recent U.S. recommendations for the management of cholesterol are based on several factors, including 10-year risk of ASCVD, presence of diabetes mellitus, baseline LDL-C levels, and chronic inflammatory conditions, including HIV infection (Grundy et al., 2018). The AHA/ACC guidelines note that if ASCVD risk is uncertain, coronary artery calcium (CAC) may be used to determine indication for statin therapy (Grundy et al., 2018). These guidelines consider HIV to be a "risk-enhancing" factor which may influence starting medical therapy at a lower 10-year risk threshold than in the general population.

STATIN THERAPY

The recommended therapy for CVD risk reduction for most PWH is a 3-hydroxy-3-methylglutaryl coenzyme A reductase inhibitor or statin. These agents are very effective in lowering TC and LDL-C but vary in potency and drug interactions. Multiple clinical trials support the role of statins for primary and secondary ASVCD prevention (Grundy et al., 2018). Intensity of therapy should be determined by baseline risk and comorbidities (see Table 29.2). Preferred statins for

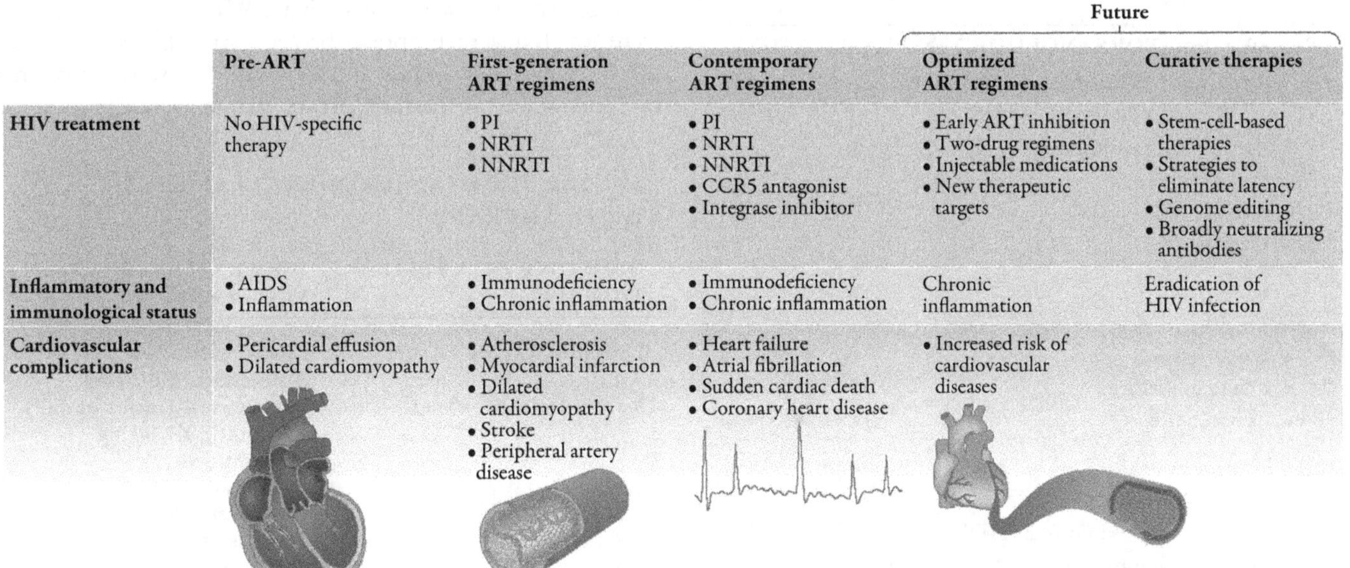

	Pre-ART	First-generation ART regimens	Contemporary ART regimens	Optimized ART regimens (Future)	Curative therapies (Future)
HIV treatment	No HIV-specific therapy	• PI • NRTI • NNRTI	• PI • NRTI • NNRTI • CCR5 antagonist • Integrase inhibitor	• Early ART inhibition • Two-drug regimens • Injectable medications • New therapeutic targets	• Stem-cell-based therapies • Strategies to eliminate latency • Genome editing • Broadly neutralizing antibodies
Inflammatory and immunological status	• AIDS • Inflammation	• Immunodeficiency • Chronic inflammation	• Immunodeficiency • Chronic inflammation	Chronic inflammation	Eradication of HIV infection
Cardiovascular complications	• Pericardial effusion • Dilated cardiomyopathy	• Atherosclerosis • Myocardial infarction • Dilated cardiomyopathy • Stroke • Peripheral artery disease	• Heart failure • Atrial fibrillation • Sudden cardiac death • Coronary heart disease	• Increased risk of cardiovascular diseases	

Figure 29.2 Overview of changes in HIV treatment and HIV-associated cardiovascular diseases. SOURCE: Hsue PY, et al. *Nat Rev Cardiol.* 2019;16(12):745–759.
Abbreviations: ART = antiretroviral therapy; CCR5 = C-chemokine receptor type 5; NRTI = nucleoside reverse transcriptase inhibitor; NNRTI = non-nucleoside reverse transcriptase inhibitor; PI = protease inhibitor.

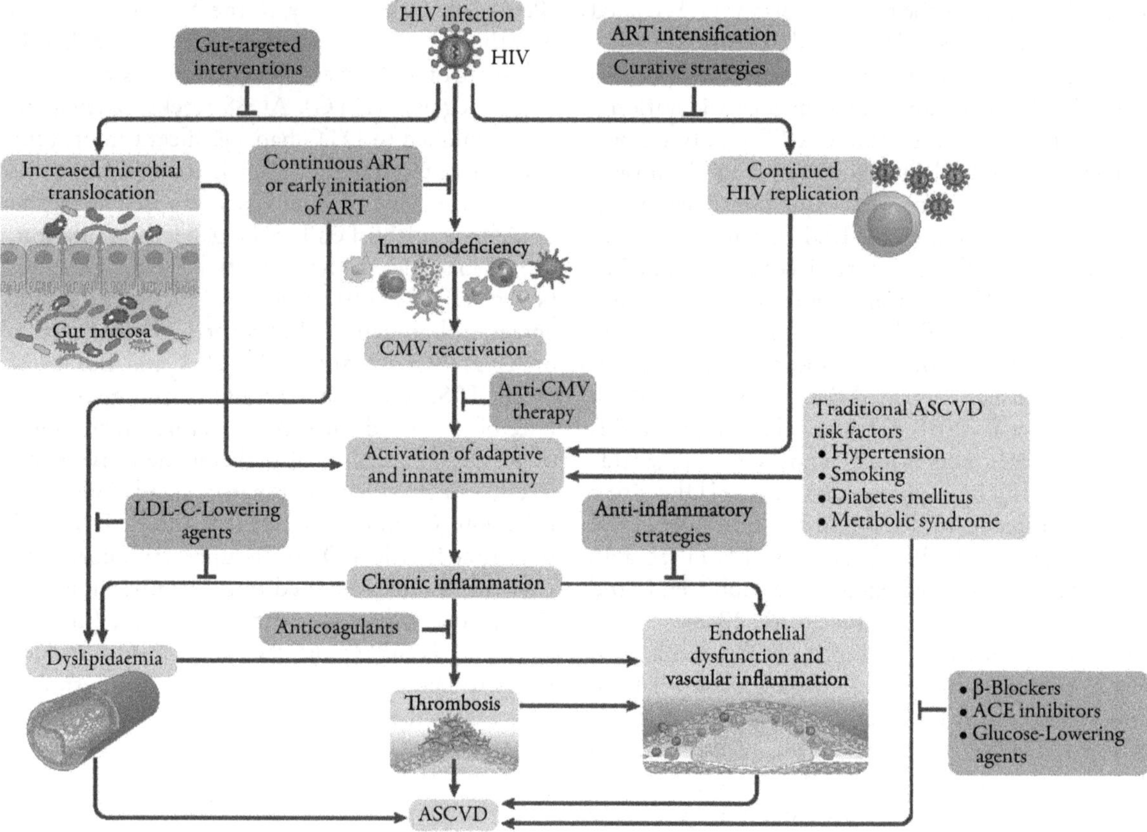

Figure 29.3 Pathophysiology and management of HIV-associated atherosclerotic cardiovascular disease. SOURCE: Hsue PY, et al. *Nat Rev Cardiol.* 2019;16(12):745–759.
Abbreviations: ACE = angiotensin converting enzyme; ART = antiretroviral therapy; ASCVD = atherosclerotic cardiovascular disease; CMV = cytomegalovirus; LDL-C = lipoprotein cholesterol.

PWH include pravastatin, fluvastatin, atorvastatin, rosuvastatin, and pitavastatin. Of note, simvastatin and lovastatin should not be used in individuals taking PIs: they are metabolized by the cytochrome P3A4 isoenzyme, and inhibition of this enzyme system results in elevated statin levels with an increased risk of rhabdomyolysis and hepatic toxicity. Conversely, the non-nucleoside reverse transcriptase inhibitor (NNRTI) efavirenz reduces simvastatin and lovastatin levels and thus decreases efficacy of these drugs.

Prior studies have shown that PWH and ASCVD risk were less likely to be prescribed a statin (Blackman et al., 2020), making it important to assess for statin hesitancy or intolerance. Secondary effects that may result in statin

Box 29.2 FACTORS INCLUDED IN THE AHA/ACA RISK CALCULATOR

10-Year ASCVD Risk: Pooled Cohort Equation

Demographics

- Age (40–79 years)
- Gender
- Race

History

- Hypertension
- Diabetes mellitus
- Tobacco use

Measurements

- Total cholesterol
- High-density lipoprotein (HDL)
- Systolic blood pressure
- Diastolic blood pressure

Adapted from https://tools.acc.org/ascvd-risk-estimator-plus/#!/calculate/estimate/.

Table 29.2 HIGH- AND MODERATE-INTENSITY STATIN THERAPY

HIGH-INTENSITY STATIN THERAPY	MODERATE-INTENSITY STATIN THERAPY
Lowers LDL-C *by* ~ ≥50%	Lowers LDL-C *by* ~30%–49%
Atorvastatin 40–80 mg	Atorvastatin 10–20 mg
Rosuvastatin 20–40 mg	Fluvastatin 40 mg twice daily
	Fluvastatin XL 80 mg
	Lovastatin 40 mg[a]
	Pitavastatin 1–4 mg
	Pravastatin 40–80 mg
	Rosuvastatin 5–10 mg
	Simvastatin 20–40 mg[a]

LDL-C = low-density lipoprotein cholesterol.

[a] Should not be used with protease inhibitors.

Source: Adapted from Grundy SM, *Circulation.* 2019;139(25):e1182–e1186.

intolerance include fatigue, myalgias, and myopathy, which can result in elevation of creatinine kinase (CK). Myalgias are reported by about 15% of persons taking statins, but most do not have elevations in CK (Guyton et al., 2014). In PWH who report myalgias, it may be prudent to rule out other causes of muscle-related symptoms such as hypothyroidism, vitamin B_{12}, or other inflammatory musculoskeletal disorders. Re-challenging a statin-intolerant person with a different agent or alternative dosing strategy (e.g., once a week dosing) can also be considered (Backes et al., 2017).

Historically, there was concern for hepatoxicity with early statins, but in 2012 the U.S. Food and Drug Administration (FDA) removed the recommendation for routine monitoring of liver function tests in individuals on statin therapy. Hepatic transaminase levels can be checked at baseline to exclude other hepatic pathology, and then repeated only as clinically indicated thereafter. For PWH with chronic HBV or HCV, it is prudent to monitor hepatic transaminases at least biannually.

In the 2023, results from the long anticipated Randomized Trial to Prevent Vascular Events in HIV (REPRIEVE), which randomly assigned 7,769 PWH and low-to-moderate risk of CVD to pitavastatin or placebo, demonstrated that pitavastatin lowered the incidence of major adverse cardiovascular events (hazard ratio, 0.65; 95% confidence interval [CI], 0.48 to 0.90; $p = 0.002$) over a median follow-up of 5.1 years (Grinspoon et al., 2023). This study found a 35% lower rate of major CV events (e.g., MI, stroke) and a slightly higher incidence of diabetes in those who received statin therapy. This benefit was shown even in persons with demographic background, comorbidities, and laboratory values reflecting low to moderate cardiovascular risk. All participants had a 10-year ASCVD risk score <15% (mean 4.5%) and the majority had LDL <160 mg/dL (median 108 mg/dL). Moreover, the participants were on stable ART and 88% had suppressed viral load with no prior history of atherosclerotic coronary vascular disease and no prior use of stains.

In response to the REPRIEVE findings, the U.S. Department of Health and Human Services clinical HIV guidelines were updated in collaboration with the AHA and ACC to recommend moderate-intensity statin therapy with pitavastatin 4 mg, atorvastatin 20 mg or rosuvastatin 10 mg for those with 10-year ASCVD risk of 5%–20%. (DHHS, 2024). For those with 10-year ASCVD risk <5%, moderate-intensity statin therapy may also be considered, while the benefits of statin therapy for those less than 40 years of age is unknown. High-intensity statin therapy (atorvastatin 40-80mg or rosuvastatin 20–40 mg) remains recommended for those with 10-year ASCD risk ≥20% or with LDL ≥190 mg/dL.

FIBRIC ACID DERIVATIVES

In PWH who have hypertriglyceridemia, defined as a fasting serum level >150mg/dL, lifestyle management, including weight loss and exercise, is initially recommended. Historically, elevated triglyceride levels were seen in PWH taking boosted protease inhibitors, but incidence has declined with diminished use of PIs. In PWH who are intolerant to statins or continue to have elevated triglycerides on a statin, fibric acid derivatives, including gemfibrozil (which has more drug interactions and risk of muscle toxicity) or fenofibrate, may be considered for primary prevention of CVD in PWH with high triglyceride levels (150–499 mg/dL) and borderline (5%–7.4%) or intermediate (7.5%–19.9%) risk. They are generally recommended in PWH with severe triglyceride levels (≥500 mg/dL) (Oh et al., 2020). These drugs have little impact on other lipid parameters, including HDL-C, LDL-C, and apolipoprotein B (apo-B). Data from D:A:D suggests a very minor association between elevated triglycerides and MI, and therefore the D:A:D: study group concluded that use of fibrates alone to lower triglycerides is unlikely to have a major impact on the incidence of MI (D:A:D, 2011).

Current ACC/AHA treatment guidelines do not recommend fibrates for dyslipidemia (Grundy et al., 2018). They cite a lack of data supporting an effect on CVD outcomes and note that their role in the primary prevention of CVD is less clear as it relates to a reduction in triglyceride levels. They note that for adults with fasting triglycerides of 500 mg/dL or greater, and especially fasting triglycerides of 1,000 mg/dL or more, it is important to identify and address causes of hypertriglyceridemia. If triglycerides are persistently elevated or increasing, a very-low-fat diet, avoidance of refined carbohydrates and alcohol, and consumption of food rich in omega-3 fatty acids are recommended. Fibrates are recommended as first-line treatment for management of PWH who are at risk for triglyceride-induced pancreatitis, which includes those with a prior history of pancreatitis or triglycerides >1,000 mg/dL (Berglund et al., 2012; Grundy et al., 2018). A Cochrane review from 2016 concluded that there is "moderate quality" evidence suggesting that fibrates lower the risk of CVD and coronary events in primary prevention, but the absolute risk reduction was less than 1% (Jakob et al., 2016). The ACCORD study specifically showed that HIV-negative patients with diabetes did not see a reduction in adverse cardiovascular events when fenofibrate was added to simvastatin (The ACCORD Study Group, 2010). ACC/AHA guidelines state that the combination of gemfibrozil with a statin should be avoided because of an increased risk for myopathy (Grundy et al., 2018).

EZETIMIBE

Ezetimibe is a drug that selectively inhibits gastrointestinal cholesterol absorption within the small intestine. Overall, this drug is safe, usually well tolerated, and effective in reducing LDL-C by an additional 12%–19% when taken with a statin therapy. Ezetimibe is neither a cytochrome P450 inhibitor nor a cytochrome P450 inducer, so metabolism with other drugs, including ART, is not a concern (Sizar et al., 2020). However, ezetimibe should not be used in PWH with moderate or severe hepatic impairment.

Studies have been performed in PWH to examine ezetimibe as both monotherapy and adjunctive therapy for lipid management, but did not specifically assess CVD outcomes (Grandi et al., 2014; Leyes et al., 2014; Nirmala et al., 2022; Saeedi et al., 2015; Wohl et al., 2008). A study from Thailand that included PWH on a PI plus a statin for at least 6 months found the addition of ezetimibe 10 mg/day produced a significant decline in mean serum TC, LDL, and TGs (Boonthos et al., 2018). Moreover, there were no adverse events or abnormal lab parameters noted. The IMPROVE-IT trial demonstrated that ezetimibe significantly reduced the risk of major cardiovascular events in a group of high-risk patients without HIV who had known CVD and already low LDL-C levels. In this trial, there was an absolute risk reduction of 2% in the cardiovascular event rate (32.7% vs. 34.7%) with the addition of ezetimibe in patients on simvastatin compared to those on simvastatin monotherapy (Cannon et al., 2015; Hammersley and Signy, 2017).

The 2018 ACC/AHA guidelines, as well as the National Institute for Care Excellence (NICE) guidelines from the United Kingdom, only recommend ezetimibe monotherapy for primary hyperlipidemia in patients for whom a statin is contraindicated or if they cannot tolerate statin therapy (Grundy et al., 2018; NICE, 2016). This is based on the lack of CVD outcome trials of ezetimibe monotherapy. A 2017 U.S. update on non-statin therapies suggests the addition of 10 mg/day of ezetimibe in patients for whom additional lowering of LDL-C is desired (Lloyd-Jones et al., 2017). The current U.S. guidelines note that it is "reasonable" to add ezetimibe in very high-risk patients with an LDL-C of greater than 70 mg/dL despite maximal statin therapy (Grundy et al., 2018). In a similar manner, the NICE guidelines from the United Kingdom and the European Society of Cardiology support ezetimibe as add-on therapy in "high or very high-risk patients" who fail to meet specific LDL targets. A randomized trial in 2022 showed that a moderate-intensity statin plus ezetimide was noninferior to a high-intensity statin for reducing the combination of cardiovascular death, major cardiovascular events, or nonfatal stroke (Kim et al., 2022).

OMEGA-3 FATTY ACIDS

Three to five grams per day of omega-3 fatty acids (DHA/EPA or "fish oil") generally produce a 30%–50% reduction in triglyceride levels. Low cost, tolerability, and lack of drug-drug interactions have made these agents historically attractive for use in the general population and PWH. In December 2019, the FDA approved the omega-3 drug icosapent ethyl as adjunctive therapy to reduce the risk of CVD in adults with triglycerides >150 mg/dL. Patients considering icosapent ethyl should have either established CVD or diabetes and two or more additional CVD risk factors. It is the first approved drug of this class to reduce CVD risk among patients with elevated triglycerides but as an add-on to maximally tolerated statin therapy (Oh et al., 2020). It is also considerably more expensive than OTC generic omega-3 fatty acid formulations.

There are data, including a recent meta-analysis of nine clinical trials ($n = 578$), evaluating the effect of omega-3 fatty acids on lipid patterns in PWH on ART (Fogacci et al., 2020). Overall findings suggest that omega-3s significantly reduced triglycerides and increased HDL cholesterol without affecting LDL or TC levels. They also noted the lack of adverse events with omega-3s. Another systematic review and meta-analysis of patients with baseline TG levels of greater than 200 mg/dL found the average combined reduction in TGs in patients taking omega-3 fatty acids was −114 mg/dL (Vieira and Silveira, 2017). Several other studies have looked at use of fish oil supplements in PWH to assess effects on inflammatory biomarkers and oxidative stress (both have potential relationships to CVD), but found either no change or no clinical benefit (Amador-Licona et al., 2016, Oliveira et al., 2015; Swanson et al., 2018).

The relationship between circulating TG levels and atherosclerosis is still unclear. Current U.S. cholesterol guidelines cite a lack of any randomized controlled trials (RCTs) evaluating omega-3s and no proof of beneficial CVD outcomes. They may prevent pancreatitis in patients with severe triglyceride elevations (>1,000 mg/dL) but have been associated with some adverse events, including gastrointestinal upset and infrequent skin conditions (rash and pruritus). Data from the British ASCEND trial found that 1 g of omega-3 fatty acid daily did not reduce nonfatal MI or stroke, TIA, or CVD death compared to an olive-oil placebo (8.9% vs. 9.2%) (Bowman et al., 2018). Two recent Cochrane reviews addressed the benefits of omega-3 fatty acids, including fish and plant-based sources (Abdelhamid et al., 2018; Abdelhamid et al., 2020). These note that increasing intake of these compounds "probably slightly reduces the risk of coronary heart disease and CVD events but has little or no effect on all-cause CVD mortality." Several studies of omega-3 fatty acids and icosapent ethyl have shown an increased risk of atrial fibrillation (Gaba et al., 2022; Kalstad et al., 2021; Nicholls et al., 2020). Therefore, omega-3 fatty acids may be considered only for select patients primarily with elevated triglycerides and high cardiovascular risk after discussion of the known risks and benefits.

PCSK9 INHIBITORS

There are currently two FDA-approved PCSK inhibitors, alirocumab and evolocumab, which are specifically indicated for the treatment of high LDL cholesterol. These medications are humanized monoclonal antibodies that inactivate proprotein convertase subtilisin-kexin type 9 (PCSK9) (Shahreyar et al., 2018). This inactivation results in decreased LDL-receptor degradation, increased recirculation of the receptor to the surface of hepatocytes, and consequent lowering of LDL cholesterol levels in the bloodstream (Everett et al., 2015). These drugs have been shown to lower LDL cholesterol by approximately 60% in patients on statin therapy and are generally safe and well tolerated. They are administered as a subcutaneous injection either every 2 weeks or once a month.

Several studies provide evidence that PCKS9 inhibitors reduce CVD events when added to statin therapy (Giugliano et al., 2017; Sabatine et al., 2017). A 2017 Cochrane study showed that PCSK9 inhibitors may slightly reduce risk of CVD events in patients with a history of CVD (Schmidt et al., 2017). Although these agents originally came on the market at $14,000 per year, they have been reduced to about $6,000 per patient/year. The use of PCSK9 inhibitors remains limited to high-risk ASCVD patients—that is, those with familial hypercholesterolemia or with known ASCVD who need further lowering of LDL despite maximal statin and ezetimibe therapy (Grundy et al., 2018; Lloyd-Jones et al., 2017). A 2022 systemic review and meta-analysis found that PCSK9 inhibitors may reduce non-fatal MI and stroke in adults at very high or high cardiovascular risk who are receiving maximally tolerated statin therapy or are statin-intolerant, but not in those with moderate and low cardiovascular risk. (Khan et al., 2022).

Of note, PSCK9 levels are elevated in PWH, and in ART-naive patients are positively associated with immunodeficiency and severity of HIV disease (Boccara et al., 2017). However, the role of PSCK9 inhibitor treatment on HIV prognosis remains unknown. In a small study of 19 PWH treated with evolocumab, an improvement in coronary blood flow was found (Leucker et al., 2020). The BEIJERINCK Study, a randomized trial comparing monthly evolocumab to placebo in 464 PWH and dyslipidemia on maximally tolerated statin therapy, found a 57% reduction in LDL levels (Boccara et al., 2020a, 2020b).

BEMPEDOIC ACID

Bempedoic acid was approved by the FDA in 2020 for use in combination therapy. This drug lowers LDL cholesterol through ATP citrate lyase inhibition. It is administered as a prodrug and then converted to its active form by enzymes found only in the liver and not in muscles, which is thought to lower risk of muscle toxicity. In clinical trials, it lowered LDL cholesterol by about 17% when combined with a moderate or high-intensity statin (Ray et al., 2019). A randomized trial of 301 patients at high risk of CVD showed that a combination of bempedoic acid and ezetimibe, when added to maximally tolerated statins, significantly lowered LDL by 38% when compared with placebo (Ballantyne et al., 2020). A 2023 study of 4,206 high-risk patients without HIV or known CVD who reported statin intolerance were randomized to receive 180 mg/day of bempedoic acid or placebo: the study found that cardiovascular events (first occurrence of cardiovascular death, nonfatal myocardial infarction [MI], nonfatal stroke, or coronary revascularization) was lower with bempedoic acid than placebo (5.3% vs. 7.6%; adjusted hazard ratio, 0.70) after a median of 39.9 months (Nissen et al., 2023). This adds to the growing list of options for statin-intolerant patients. Bempedoic acid may increase serum uric acid levels and risk of tendon rupture, and tolerability is comparable to ezetimibe. Approximately 11% of patients discontinue use because of adverse effects, which can include muscle spasms, arthralgias, and diarrhea (Ballantyne et al., 2020). Pending further data, this drug is mainly recommended as add-on therapy for patients who need further LDL-C lowering despite optimal use of a statin and ezetimibe. An advantage over the PCSK9 inhibitors is that it can be given orally and is less expensive. There are currently no data on bempedoic acid in PWH.

ASPIRIN

Aspirin (acetylsalicylic acid or ASA) has been recommended by healthcare providers for the prevention of CVD and associated clinical events, including MI and stroke. Recent CDC surveillance data found that 27% of U.S. adults were taking aspirin for primary prevention, and 74.9% for secondary CVD prevention (Wall et al., 2018). While the benefit of aspirin has been clearly demonstrated for people with established CVD, the risk–benefit equation is more complex in primary prevention of CVD and related clinical outcomes such as MI. Aspirin irreversibly inhibits cyclooxygenase-1 (COX-1) and blocks the formation and release of thromboxane A2, a strong platelet activator. The COX-1 enzyme is also responsible for producing prostaglandins that protect gastric mucosa; thus patients taking aspirin may be susceptible to gastrointestinal bleeding. Risk factors for GI bleeding with aspirin include higher dose and longer duration of use, history of gastrointestinal ulcers, bleeding disorders, renal failure, advanced liver disease, and thrombocytopenia. Other factors that increase the risk for bleeding with low-dose aspirin use include concurrent anticoagulation with warfarin, direct-acting anticoagulants (DOACs), or the use of nonsteroidal anti-inflammatory drugs (NSAIDs).

The evidence for aspirin for *primary prevention* of CVD, MI, or stroke remains limited, with very little published data on its use in PWH (O'Brien et al., 2013; Suchindran et al., 2014). With the last update in 2022, the U.S. Preventive Services Task Force (USPSTF) downgraded aspirin for primary prevention to a "C" grade recommendation (see Box 29.3) (Davidson et al., 2022). Current evidence suggests that the net benefit of aspirin for primary prevention is small and may be considered in those aged 40–59 years with a 10% or greater 10-year CVD risk (http://tools.acc.org/ASCVD-Risk-Estimator) and a low risk of bleeding. The USPSTF recommends against starting aspirin for primary prevention in those over 60 years of age, giving this a "D" grade recommendation. However, guidelines do not clearly

Box 29.3 U.S. PREVENTIVE SERVICES TASK FORCE (USPSTF) RECOMMENDATIONS FOR ASPIRIN THERAPY

ADULTS aged 40–59 years with a ≥10% 10-year CVD risk

The USPSTF suggests that the net benefit of aspirin for primary prevention is small and may be considered in those 40–59 years of age with a 10% or greater 10-year CVD risk and a low risk of bleeding (level of evidence = C).

ADULTS aged 60 years and older

The USPSTF recommends against starting aspirin for primary prevention of CVD in adults aged 60 years and older (level of evidence = D).

CVD = cardiovascular disease.
Source: Adapted from Davidson KW, et al. *JAMA*. 2022;327(16): 1577–1584.

provide recommendations on continuation or discontinuation of aspirin for primary prevention in those already taking it. The optimal dose of aspirin is not known, but 75–100 mg is the most commonly recommended dose.

Several recently completed primary prevention trials provide updated guidance regarding the use of aspirin. The Aspirin in Reducing Events in the Elderly trial included 19,000 patients aged 70 years and older from Australia and the United States who took 100 mg of aspirin daily or placebo (McNeilet al., 2018). During almost 5 years of follow-up, low-dose aspirin use resulted in a significantly higher risk of major hemorrhage and did not significantly lower risk of cardiovascular disease. In addition, all-cause mortality was higher in the aspirin group. The Aspirin to Reduce Risk of Initial Vascular Events (ARRIVE) trial from Europe randomly assigned more than 12,500 adults with presumed moderate CVD risk to aspirin 100 mg/day or placebo. During 5 years of follow-up there was no reduction in CVD events by intent-to-treat analysis (Gaziano et al., 2018). There was a 19% relative reduction in the composite endpoint of CVD events in patients who took ASA but also a doubling in the rate of GI bleeding (0.5% in absolute terms). The ASCEND trial, conducted in the United Kingdom, included 15,480 patients aged ≥40 years old with diabetes and without CVD who were randomized to aspirin 100 mg/day or placebo. After a mean follow-up of 7.4 years, the frequency of the primary endpoint (composite of nonfatal MI, nonfatal stroke, TIA, or death from any vascular cause) was 8.5% with aspirin and 9.6% with placebo. The minor benefit of aspirin came at the expense of more major bleeding events (Bowman et al., 2018). A recent systemic review also found that low-dose aspirin (<100mg/day) was associated with a small decrease in major cardiovascular events (odds ratio [OR] 0.90; 95% CI: 0.85–0.95) and a small increase in major bleeding (OR 1.44; 95% CI: 1.32–1.57) (Guirguis-Blake et al., 2022).

The AHA/ACC guidelines note that low-dose aspirin may be considered among select adults aged 40–70 years who are at higher ASCVD risk but not at increased bleeding risk. They additionally note that aspirin should not be administered for the primary prevention of ASCVD among adults of any age who are at increased risk of bleeding (Arnett et al., 2019).

For *secondary prevention*, numerous studies have evaluated the role of aspirin in acute treatment of cardiac events and secondary prevention of CVD (Jones, 2018). Robust data demonstrate that low-dose aspirin (75–100 mg/day) effectively reduces the risk of vascular event recurrence in patients with a history of a previous MI, stroke, or TIA by approximately 20%. There has been FDA-approved labeling for this indication since the 1980s (Paikin and Eikelboom, 2012). Because of this consistently reported benefit, which has been found to outweigh the risk of major bleeding, aspirin therapy for secondary prevention remains standard clinical practice.

BLOOD PRESSURE CONTROL

Hypertension has become more prevalent as PWH age. It is a major CVD risk factor and strongly associated with CAD, stroke, HF, and renal disease. Prevalence varies with different PWH cohorts but is estimated to range from 10% to 50% (Boccara, 2017). The global incidence of adult PWH with hypertension is estimated to be 35%, compared to 30% of HIV-negative adults (Fahme et al., 2018). The CDC's Medical Monitoring Project found that 42% of PWH had hypertension (n = 8,631), but only 49% had their blood pressure controlled (Olaiya et al., 2018). In a recent study of Medicaid enrollees (n = 3456), the prevalence of comorbidities increased from the fourth year to the first year of entry into care; these included cardiovascular disease (28%–40%), hypertension (24%–37%), and hyperlipidemia (12%–17%) (DerSarkissian et al., 2020).

Factors associated with elevated blood pressure in PWH appear similar to those of the general population and include older age; male sex; African American, African, and Caribbean ethnicities; higher BMI; diabetes; and chronic kidney disease. Although less commonly seen than in the past, lipodystrophy and metabolic syndrome have also been associated with hypertension in adult PWH (Fahme et al., 2018). Older studies of blood pressure changes in the D:A:D study and one U.S. cohort found no evidence that ART increased the risk of hypertension (Medina-Torne et al., 2012; Thiebault et al., 2005). Conversely, other studies have implicated both PIs and duration of ART as being associated with hypertension (Boccara, 2017). In the RESPOND consortium, integrase and protease inhibitors were associated with a higher incidence of hypertension than NNRTIs (Byonanebye et al., 2022; Byonanebye et al., 2024). Some researchers also believe that immune activation and chronic inflammation contribute to the pathophysiology of hypertension in PWH (van Zoest et al., 2017).

It is appropriate to screen and manage hypertension in adult PWH per current national guidelines (Elton et al., 2018). It should be noted, however, that current ACC/AHA hypertension guidelines (Whelton et al., 2018) have been controversial and not collectively endorsed by all professional societies. The 2017 recommendation is for a diagnosis of "hypertension" rather than "prehypertension" for adults with a systolic BP of 130 mmHg or greater. They also recommend pharmacotherapy treatment for "high-risk" people with hypertension. These include people with existing CVD or a calculated 10-year CVD risk of 10% or greater, or another high-risk condition such as chronic kidney disease or diabetes (Whelton et al., 2018a). The European AIDS Clinical Society (EACS) has also recommended a treatment threshold of systolic BP >130 mmHg and diastolic BP >80 mmHg (EACS, 2023). Some feel that by following the most recent ACC/AHA guidelines, a large number of people will be subject to medical treatment with little or no benefit in terms of CVD risk reduction and mortality (Bell, 2018; Brunstrom and Carlberg, 2018). They believe the threshold for treating hypertension should remain at 140 mmHg. Regardless, for those for whom medical therapy is deemed necessary, it is important to be aware of potential drug-drug interactions between ART and antihypertensive agents. Moreover, clinical management should consider frailty, comorbidities, and psychosocial factors and ideally should be individualized (Oliveros et al.,

2020). Nonpharmacologic therapies, including the Dietary Approaches to Stop Hypertension (DASH) diet, sodium intake restriction, and regular exercise, all play a role for most patients. Unfortunately, there have not been any large-scale studies of specific blood pressure–lowering medications in adult PWH. Small studies of renin-angiotensin antagonists show very favorable results, and many adult PWH will likely need two or more medications to reach recommended blood pressure goals (Fahme et al., 2018).

It is worth noting that a recent study from Spain found that patients who took their blood pressure medications at bedtime had a significant decrease in CVD events compared to morning dosing (Hermida et al., 2020). Better outcomes were seen for MI, coronary revascularization, and stroke over a 6-year follow-up of 1,752 patients. In addition, there were no differences in adverse events, including hypotension and sleep disturbances, between the two groups.

SMOKING CESSATION

Smoking prevalence is remarkably high in many PWH cohorts, usually much higher than in the general population (Johnston et al., 2021), with 33.6% of PWH reporting current smoking in one study (Frazier et al., 2018). Therefore, smoking cessation remains a very important part of CVD risk reduction for PWH. There is also an increased risk of lung cancer in PWH, which is directly influenced by smoking as well as immunosuppressive and inflammatory processes (Sigel et al., 2017). The D:A:D study found that smoking cessation in PWH decreased the incident RR for MI from 3.73 in the first year of smoking cessation to 2.07 after 3 years of not smoking (Petoumenos et al., 2011). Another study estimated that smoking cessation in PWH could prevent 38% of acute MIs (Althoff et al., 2017).

Tobacco cessation may significantly reduce AHA/ACA risk scores by 50% or greater. Counseling, including the "5 A strategy" (ask, advise, assess, assist, arrange follow-up), has proved successful (DeSocio et al., 2020). In addition, pharmacologic interventions, including nicotine replacement, bupropion, and varenicline, are all effective therapies to assist PWH with smoking cessation (see Box 29.4). The USPSTF recommends a combination of behavioral interventions and pharmacotherapy for all people who smoke (Patnode et al., 2021). Recent guidelines recommend varenicline over a nicotine patch or bupropion and for most people with tobacco use disorder in whom treatment is initiated (Krist et al., 2021). Dual therapy with varenicline plus a nicotine patch is also an option, although the evidence for combination treatment is limited (Leone et al., 2020). There is also growing interest in using nicotine containing e-cigarettes to aid in smoking cessation, with growing evidence of benefit from randomized trials and a 2024 Cochrane review (Auer et al., 2024; Lindson et al., 2024; Lin et al., 2024) The duration of these therapies (beyond the traditional 12 weeks) can be extended on an individual basis if clinically indicated.

A large multinational study of over 8,000 adult smokers evaluated the safety of varenicline, bupropion, and 21-mg nicotine patches. There was a very low incidence of cardiovascular events (< 0.5%) during 12 weeks of treatment and after 12 additional weeks of follow-up (Benowitz et al., 2018). These data support these therapies by themselves or in combination.

Box 29.4 RECOMMENDATIONS FOR TREATING TOBACCO USE DISORDER

- Tobacco use disorder can be safely and effectively treated with counseling and pharmacotherapy.
- Varenicline is *strongly* recommended over nicotine patches and bupropion as first-line treatment because of higher abstinence rates and fewer adverse events with varenicline.
- In patients with comorbid psychiatric conditions, varenicline is *strongly* recommended as first-line treatment as trials did not show an excess of neuropsychiatric events.
- Even in patients who are pre-contemplative about abstaining from tobacco, varenicline is still *strongly* recommended as it doubles the likelihood of abstinence.
- The combination of varenicline plus a nicotine patch is recommended over varenicline monotherapy for patients who are ready to quit, although there is low-quality evidence to support this.
- When treatment is initiated, extended-duration therapy (>12 weeks) is strongly recommended over standard (6–12 week) regimens.
- Combination nicotine replacement therapy (NRT) (particularly combining short-acting and long-acting forms) is more effective than use of a single form of NRT alone.
- Efficacy of electronic cigarettes is growing and may be an option to aid in smoking cessation for select patients.

Source: Adapted from Leone FT, et al. *Am J Respir Crit Care Med.* 2020; 202(2):5–31.
Krist AH, et al. *JAMA.* 2021;325(3):265–279.

Among PWH, a study from France found varenicline significantly more effective than placebo in helping maintain continuous abstinence at 48 weeks (Mercie et al., 2018). A Cochrane review of 12 studies assessing the effectiveness of interventions (behavioral and pharmacotherapy) to motivate and assist tobacco use cessation in PWH found moderate evidence that combined interventions were effective for long-term abstinence (Pool et al., 2016). Authors concluded that tobacco cessation should be offered to all PWH, as even non-sustained periods of abstinence are beneficial. In addition, office-based interventions that include focus groups, dedicated time to address smoking cessation as part of the clinic visit, and periodic phone follow-ups have shown efficacy in helping PWH stop smoking (Cropsey et al., 2019; Pacek et al., 2021).

NONPHARMACOLOGICAL INTERVENTIONS (DIET AND EXERCISE)

The process of atherosclerosis is thought to begin at a young age and progresses over many decades before clinical CVD (e.g., acute coronary syndromes, stable or unstable angina, and MI) becomes evident. As noted earlier, this progression appears to be accelerated in PWH due to chronic infection, inflammation, and some ART-related factors. Lifestyle modifications, including a healthy diet, regular physical activity, maintaining a normal BMI, limited alcohol use, and not smoking, have been associated with CVD risk improvement (Ozemek et al., 2020).

Regarding physical activity, the ACC/AHA guidelines for both cholesterol and hypertension both recommend that adults should be advised to engage in aerobic physical activity for 3–4 sessions per week, lasting on average 40 minutes/session and involving moderate-to-vigorous-intensity activity (Grundy et al., 2018; Whelton et al., 2018b). This can lead to improvements in TC, LDL-C, HDL-C, blood glucose, and blood pressure—and ultimately lower 10-year and lifetime risk of CVD and subsequent clinical events.

Several studies have found variable results in terms of exercise in PWH. One systematic review found that a low level of physical activity in PWH was consistently associated with older age, lower educational level, lower CD4$^+$ count, exposure to ART, and the presence of lipodystrophy. Other important barriers were the presence of pain and depression (Vancampfort et al., 2018). A more recent and encouraging study found that 12–24 weeks of cardiovascular and resistance exercise significantly reduced total and visceral fat in PWH 50–75 years old (Jankowski et al., 2020). As PWH are living longer, it is important for providers to encourage engagement in multiple aspects of a healthy lifestyle, including regular physical activity.

ACKNOWLEDGMENTS

The authors would like to acknowledge the contributions to previous editions of this chapter by David Wohl, MD, and Jeffery Kirchner, MD.

REFERENCES

Abdelhamid AS, Brown TJ, Brainard JS, et al. Omega-3 fatty acids for the primary and secondary prevention of cardiovascular disease. *Cochrane Database Syst Rev.* 2018;7(7):CD003177. Published 2018 Jul 18. doi:10.1002/14651858.CD003177.pub3

Abdelhamid AS, Brown TJ, Brainard JS, et al. Omega-3 fatty acids for the primary and secondary prevention of cardiovascular disease. *Cochrane Database Syst Rev.* 2020;3:CD003177. http//:doi: 10.1002/14651858.CD003177.pub5

Aberg JA, Gallant JE, Ghanem KG, et al. Primary care guidelines for the management of persons infected with HIV: 2013 update by the HIV Medicine Association of the Infectious Diseases Society of America. *Clin Infect Dis.* 2014;58(1):1–34.

Althoff KN, McGinnis KA, Wyatt CM, et al. Comparison of risk and age at diagnosis of myocardial infarction, end-stage renal disease, and non-AIDS defining cancer in PWH versus uninfected adults. *Clin Infect Dis.* 2015;60:627–638.

Althoff KN, Palella FJ, Gebo K, et al. Impact of smoking, hypertension and cholesterol on myocardial infarction in HIV+ adults. Abstract 130. CROI 2017. Boston, MA; 2017.

Amador-Licona N, Díaz-Murillo TA, Gabriel-Ortiz G et al. Omega 3 fatty acids supplementation and oxidative stress in HIV-seropositive patients: a clinical trial. *PLoS One.* 2016;11(3):e0151637.

Anderson TS, Wilson LM, Sussman JB. Atherosclerotic cardiovascular disease risk estimates using the predicting risk of cardiovascular disease events equations. *JAMA Intern Med.* 2024;184(8):963–970. doi:10.1001/jamainternmed.2024.1302. PMID: 38856978; PMCID: PMC11165411.

Arnett DK, Blumenthal RS, Albert MA, et al. ACC/AHA guideline on the primary prevention of cardiovascular disease: a report of the American College of Cardiology/American Heart Association Task Force on Clinical Practice Guidelines. *Circulation.* 2019;140(11):e596–e646.

Auer R, Schoeni A, Humair JP, et al. Electronic nicotine-delivery systems for smoking cessation. *N Engl J Med.* 2024;390(7):601–610.

Backes JM, Russinger JF, Gibson CA, Moriarity PM. Statin-associated muscle symptoms: managing the highly intolerant. *J Clin Lipidol.* 2017;11(1):24–33.

Ballantyne CM, Laufs U, Ray KK, et al. Bempedoic acid plus ezetimibe fixed-dose combination in patients with hypercholesterolemia and high CVD risk treated with maximally tolerated statin therapy. *Eur J Prev Cardiol.* 2020;27(6):593–603.

Baum PD, Sullam PM, Stoddart CA, et al. Abacavir increases platelet reactivity via competitive inhibition of soluble guanylyl cyclase. *AIDS.* 2011;25(18):2243–2248.

Bell KJ. Incremental benefits and harms of the 2017 American College of Cardiology American Heart Association High Blood Pressure Guideline. *JAMA Intern Med.* 2018;178(6):755–757.

Benowitz NL, Pipe A, West R et al. Cardiovascular safety of varenicline, bupropion, and nicotine patches in smokers: a randomized controlled trial. *JAMA Intern Med.* 2018;178(5):622–631.

Berglund L, Brunzell JD, Goldberg AC, et al. Evaluation and treatment of hypertriglyceridemia: an Endocrine Society clinical practice guideline. *J Clin Endocrinol Metab.* 2012;97(9):2969–2989.

Blackman AL, Pandit NS, Pincus KJ. Comparing rates of statin therapy in eligible patients living with HIV compared to uninfected patients. *HIV Med.* 2020;21(3):135–141.

Boccara F. Cardiovascular health in an aging HIV population. *AIDS.* 2017;31(Suppl 2):S157–S163.

Boccara F, Ghislain M, Meyer L, et al. Impact of protease inhibitors on circulating PCSK9 levels in PWH antiretroviral-naïve patients from an ongoing prospective cohort. ANRS-COPANA Study Group. *AIDS.* 2017;31(17):2367–2376.

Boccara F, Kumar P, Caramelli B, et al. Evolocumab treatment in patients with HIV and hypercholesterolemia/mixed dyslipidemia: BEIJERNICK study design and baseline characteristics. *Am Heart J.* 2020a; 220:203–212.

Boccara F, Kumar PN, Caramelli B, et al. Evolocumab in HIV-Infected patients with dyslipidemia: primary results of the randomized, double-blind BEIJERINCK study. *J Am Coll Cardiol.* May 26, 2020;75(20):2570–2584. doi:10.1016/j.jacc.2020.03.025

Boonthos K, Puttilerpong C, Penssuparp T. Short-term efficacy and safety of adding ezetimibe to current regimen of lipid-lowering drugs in PWH Thai patients treated with protease inhibitors. *Japan J Infect Dis.* 2018;71:220–224.

Bowman L, Marion Mafham M, Wallendszus K, et al. Effects of aspirin for primary prevention in persons with diabetes mellitus: the ASCEND Study Collaborative Group. *N Engl J Med.* 2018;379:1529–1539.

Brunstrom M, Carlberg B. Association of blood pressure lowering with mortality and cardiovascular disease across blood pressure levels: a systematic review and meta-analysis. *JAMA Intern Med.* 2018;178(1):28–36.

Byonanebye DM, Polizzotto MN, Maltez F, et al. Associations between change in BMI and the risk of hypertension and dyslipidaemia in people receiving integrase strand-transfer inhibitors, tenofovir alafenamide, or both compared with other contemporary antiretroviral regimens: a multicentre, prospective observational study from the RESPOND consortium cohorts. *Lancet HIV.* 2024;11(5):e321–e332.

Byonanebye DM, Polizzotto MN, Neesgaard B, et al. Incidence of hypertension in people with HIV who are treated with integrase inhibitors versus other antiretroviral regimens in the RESPOND cohort consortium. *HIV Med.* 2022;23(8):895–910.

Cannon C, Blazing M, Giugliano R, et al. Ezetimibe added to statin therapy after acute coronary syndromes. *N Engl J Med.* 2015;372:2387–2397.

Chandiwana NC, Siedner MJ, Marconi VC, et al. Weight gain after HIV therapy initiation: pathophysiology and implications. *J Clin Endocrinol Metab.* 2024;109(2):e478–e487.

Cheung CC, Ding E, Sereda P, et al. Reductions in all-cause and cause-specific mortality among PWH individuals receiving antiretroviral therapy in British Columbia, Canada: 2001–2012. *HIV Med.* 2016; 17(9):694–701.

Cioe PA, Baker J, Kojic EM, et al. Elevated soluble CD14 and lower D-dimer are associated with cigarette smoking and heavy episodic alcohol use in persons living with PWH. *J Acquir Immune Defic Syndr.* 2015;70(4):400–405.

Costagliola D, Potard V, Lang S, et al. Is the risk of myocardial infarction in people with HIV associated with atazanavir or darunavir? A nested case-control study within the French hospital database on HIV. *J Infect Dis.* 2020;221(4):516–522.

Cropsey KL, Bean MC, Haynes L et al. Delivery and implementation of an algorithm for smoking cessation treatment for people with HIV and AIDS. *AIDS Care Psych Soc Aspect of AIDS/HIV.* 2019;2:223–229.

Data Collection on Adverse Events of Anti-HIV Drugs (D:A:D) Study Group. Class of antiretroviral drugs and the risk of myocardial infarction. *N Engl J Med.* 2007;356:1723–1735.

D:A:D Study Group. The impact of fasting on the interpretation of triglyceride levels for predicting myocardial infarction risk in HIV-positive individuals: the D:A:D study. *J Infect Dis.* 2011;204(4):521–525.

Davidson KW, Barry MJ, Mangione CM, et al. Aspirin use to prevent cardiovascular disease: US Preventive Services Task Force recommendation statement. *JAMA.* 2022;327(16):1577–1584.

De Pablo C, Orden S, Calatayud S, et al. Differential effects of tenofovir/emtricitabine and abacavir/lamivudine on human leukocyte recruitment. *Antivir Ther.* 2012;17(8):1615–1619.

Deeks S, Lewin SR, Havlir DA. The end of AIDS: HIV infection as a chronic disease. *Lancet.* 2013; 283(9903):1525–1533.

DerSarkissian M, Bhak RH, Oglesby A, et al. Retrospective analysis of comorbidities and treatment burden among patients with HIV infection in a US Medicaid population. *Curr Med Res Opin.* 2020;36(5):781–788.

DeSocio GV, Ricci E, Maggi P, et al. Is it feasible to impact on smoking habits in PWH patients? *J Acquir Immune Defic Syndr.* 2020;83(5):496–503.

Dorjee K, Choden T, Baxi SM, et al. Risk of cardiovascular disease associated with exposure to abacavir among individuals with HIV: a systematic review and meta-analyses of results from seventeen epidemiologic studies. *Int J Antimicrob Agents.* 2018;52(5):541–553.

Dorjee K, Desai M, Choden T, et al. Acute myocardial infarction associated with abacavir and tenofovir based antiretroviral drug combinations in the United States. *AIDS Res Ther.* 2021;18(1):57.

Drozd DR, Kitahata MM, Althoff KN, et al. Incidence and risk of myocardial infarction (MI) by type in the NA-ACCORD. Abstract 748. CROI 2015. Seattle, WA; 2015.

European AIDS Clinical Society. Prevention of cardiovascular disease. https://eacs.sanfordguide.com/prevention-non-infectious-co-morbidities/cardiovascular-disease/eacs-prevention-of-cvd. October 2023. Accessed July 29, 2024.

Everett BM, Smith RJ, Hiatt WR. Reducing LDL with PCSK9 inhibitors: the clinical benefit of lipid drugs. *N Engl J Med.* 2015;373:1588–1591.

Fahme SA, Bloomfield GS, Peck R. Hypertension and PWH adults: novel pathophysiologic mechanisms. *Hypertension.* 2018;72:44–55.

Fitch KV, Looby SE, Rope A, et al. Effects of aging and smoking on carotid intima-media thickness in HIV-infection. *AIDS.* 2013;27(1):49–57.

Fogacci F, Strocchi E, Veronesi M, et al. Effect of omega-3 polyunsaturated fatty acids treatment on lipid pattern of HIV patients: a meta-analysis of randomized clinical trials. *Mar Drugs.* 2020;18(6):292.

Frazier EL, Sutton MY, Brooks JT, et al. Trends in cigarette smoking among adults with HIV compared with the general adult population, United States: 2009–2014. *Prev Med.* 2018;111:231–234.

Freiberg MS, Chang CC, Koller LH, et al. HIV infection and the risk of acute myocardial infarction. *JAMA Intern Med.* 2013;173(8):614–622.

Freiberg MS, Duncan MS, Alcorn C. HIV Infection and the risk of World Health Organization-defined sudden cardiac death. *J Am Heart Assoc.* 2021;10(18):e021268.

Friis-Moller N, Sabin C, Weber R, et al. The Data Collection on Adverse Events of Anti-HIV Drugs (D:A:D) Study Group. *N Engl J Med.* 2003;349:1993–2003.

Fung G, Luo H, Qiu Y, Yang D, et al. Myocarditis. *Circ Res.* 2016;118(3):496–514.

Gaba P, Bhatt DL, Steg PG, et al. Prevention of cardiovascular events and mortality with icosapent ethyl in patients with prior myocardial infarction. *J Am Coll Cardiol.* 2022;79(17):1660–1671.

Gandhi RT, Bedimo R, Hoy JF, et al. Antiretroviral drugs for treatment and prevention of HIV infection in adults: 2022 recommendations of the International Antiviral Society-USA Panel. *JAMA.* 2023;329(1):63–84.

Gatell JM, Assoumou L, Moyle G, et al. Switching from a ritonavir-boosted protease inhibitor to a dolutegravir-based regimen for maintenance of viral suppression in patients with high cardiovascular risk. *AIDS.* 2017;31:2503–2514.

Gaziano JM, Brotons C, Coppolecchia R. Use of aspirin to reduce the risk of initial vascular events in patients at moderate risk of cardiovascular disease. (ARRIVE): a randomized double-blind placebo-controlled trial. *Lancet.* 2018;392:1035–1046.

Ghazi L, Baker JV, Sharma S, et al. Role of inflammatory biomarkers in the prevalence and incidence of hypertension among HIV-positive participants in the START trial. *Am J Hypertens.* 2020;33(1):43–52.

Giugliano RP, Keech A, Murphy SA. Clinical efficacy and safety of evolocumab in high-risk patients receiving a statin: secondary analysis of patients with Low LDL cholesterol levels and in those already receiving a maximal-potency statin in a randomized clinical trial. *JAMA.* 2017;2(12):1385–1391.

Go AS, Horberg M, Reynolds K, et al. HIV infection independently increases the risk of developing heart failure: the HIV HEART study. Abstract THAB0103. AIDS 2018: 22nd International AIDS Conference. Amsterdam, Netherlands; July 23–27, 2018.

Go AS, Reynolds K, Avula HR, et al. Human immunodeficiency virus infection and variation in heart failure risk by age, sex, and ethnicity: the HIV HEART Study. *Mayo Clin Proc.* 2022;97(3):465–479.

Grandi AM, Nicolini E, Rizzi L, et al. Dyslipidemia in HIV-positive patients: a randomized, controlled, prospective study on ezetimibe\+ fenofibrate versus pravastatin monotherapy. *J Int AIDS Soc.* 2014;17:19004.

Grinspoon SK, Fitch KV, Zanni MV, et al.; REPRIEVE Investigators. Pitavastatin to prevent cardiovascular disease in HIV infection. *N Engl J Med.* 2023 Aug 24;389(8):687–699.

Grundy SM, Stone NJ, Bailey AL, et al. 2018 AHA/ACC guideline on the management of blood cholesterol: a report of the American College of Cardiology/American Heart Association Task Force on Clinical Practice Guidelines. *Circulation.* 2019;139(25):e1182–e1186. doi:10.1161/CIR.0000000000000698. [Published correction appears in Circulation. 2023 Aug 15;148(7):e5. doi:10.1161/CIR.0000000000001172]. *Circulation.* 2019;139(25):e1082–e1143. doi:10.1161/CIR.0000000000000625

Guirguis-Blake JM, Evans CV, Perdue LA, Bean SI, Senger CA. Aspirin use to prevent cardiovascular disease and colorectal cancer: updated evidence report and systematic review for the US Preventive Services Task Force. *JAMA.* 2022;327(16):1585–1597.

Guyton JR, Bays HE, Grundy SM, et al. An assessment of the Statin Intolerance Panel: 2014 update. *J Clin Lipidol.* 2014;8(3 Suppl):S72–S81.

Haji M, Capilupi M, Kwok M, et al. Clinical outcomes after acute coronary syndromes or revascularization among people living with HIV: a systematic review and meta-analysis. *JAMA Netw Open.* 2024 May 1;7(5):e2411159.

Hammersley D, Signy M. Ezetimibe: an update on its clinical usefulness in specific patient groups. *Ther Adv Chronic Dis*. 2017;8(1):4–11.

Hatleberg CI, Ryom L, El-Sadr W, et al. Improvements over time in short-term mortality following myocardial infarction in HIV-positive individuals. *AIDS*. 2016;30(10):1583–1596.

Hays AG, Schär M, Barditch-Crovo P, et al. A randomized, placebo-controlled, double-blinded clinical trial of colchicine to improve vascular health in people living with HIV. *AIDS*. 2021;35(7):1041–1050.

Hermida RC, Crespo JJ, Domingues-Sardina M, et al. Bedtime hypertension treatment improves cardiovascular risk reduction: the Hygia Chronotherapy Trial. *Eur Heart J*. 2020;41(48):4565–4576.

Hudson JA, Ferrand RA, Gitau SN, et al. HIV-associated cardiovascular disease pathogenesis: an emerging understanding through imaging and immunology. *Circ Res*. 2024;134(11):1546–1565.

Hsue PY, Waters DD. HIV infection and coronary heart disease: mechanisms and management. *Nat Rev Cardiol*. 2019;16(12):745–759.

Hunt PW. HIV and inflammation: mechanisms and consequences. *Curr HIV/AIDS Rep*. 2012;9(2):139–147.

Jakob T, Nordmann AJ, Schandelmaier S, et al. Fibrates for primary prevention of cardiovascular disease events. *Cochrane Database Syst Rev*. 2016;11(11):CD009753.

Jankowski CM, Mawhinney S, Wilson MP, et al. Body composition changes in response to moderate or high-intensity exercise among older adults with or without HIV infection. *JAIDS*. 2020;85(3):340–345.

Johnston PI, Wright SW, Orr M, et al. Worldwide relative smoking prevalence among people living with and without HIV. *AIDS*. 2021;35(6):957–970.

Jones R, Arps K, Davis DM. Clinician guide to the ABCs of primary and secondary prevention of atherosclerotic cardiovascular disease. https://www.acc.org/latest-in-cardiology/articles/2018/03/30/18/34/clinician-guide-to-the-abcs. Published April 2018. Accessed September 3, 2022.

Kalstad AA, Myhre PL, Laake K, et al. Effects of n-3 fatty acid supplements in elderly patients after myocardial infarction: a randomized, controlled trial. *Circulation*. 2021;143(6):528–539.

Kelly SG, Plankey M, Post WS, et al. Associations between tobacco, alcohol, and drug use with coronary artery plaque among HIV-infected and uninfected men in the Multicenter AIDS Cohort Study. *PLoS One*. 2016:e0147822.

Khambaty T, Stewart JC, Gupta SK, et al. Association between depressive disorders and incident acute myocardial infarction in human immunodeficiency virus-infected adults: Veterans Aging Cohort Study. *JAMA Cardiol*. 2016;1(8):929–937.

Khan SU, Yedlapati SH, Lone AN, et al. PCSK9 inhibitors and ezetimibe with or without statin therapy for cardiovascular risk reduction: a systematic review and network meta-analysis. *BMJ*. 2022;377:e069116.

Kim BK, Hong SJ, Lee YJ, et al. Long-term efficacy and safety of moderate-intensity statin with ezetimibe combination therapy versus high-intensity statin monotherapy in patients with atherosclerotic cardiovascular disease (RACING): a randomized, open-label, non-inferiority trial. *Lancet*. 2022;400:380.

Klein DB, Leyden WA, Chao CR. No difference in the incidence of myocardial infarction for HIV+ and HIV– individuals in recent years. *Clin Infect Dis*. 2015;60(8):1278–1285.

Klein DB, Marcus JL, Leyden WA, et al. Infection and immunodeficiency as risk factors for ischemic stroke. Abstract 741. CROI 2014. Boston, MA; 2014.

Kovacs L, Kress TC, Belin de Chantemèle EJ. HIV, combination antiretroviral therapy, and vascular diseases in men and women. *JACC Basic Transl Sci*. 2022;7(4):410–421.

Krishnan S, Bosch RJ, Rodriguez B, et al. Correlates of inflammatory biomarkers one year after suppressive ART. Abstract 757. CROI 2014. Boston, MA; 2014.

Krist AH, Davidson KW, Mangione CM, et al. Interventions for tobacco smoking cessation in adults, including pregnant persons: US Preventive Services Task Force recommendation statement. *JAMA*. 2021;325(3): 265–279.

Lake JE, Trevillyan J. Impact of Integrase inhibitors and tenofovir alafenamide on weight gain in people with HIV. *Curr Opin HIV AIDS*. 2021;16(3):148–151.

Law M, Friis-Moller N, El-Sadr WA, et al. The use of the Framingham equation to predict myocardial infarctions in PWH patients: comparison with observed events in the D:A:D study. *HIV Med*. 2006;7:218–230.

Leone FT, Zhang Y, Evers-Casey S, et al. Initiating pharmacologic treatment in tobacco-dependent adults: an official American Thoracic Society Clinical Practice guideline. *Am J Respir Crit Care Med*. 2020;202(2):5–31.

Leucker TM, Gerstenblith G, Schär M. Evolocumab, a PCSK9-monoclonal antibody, rapidly reverses coronary artery endothelial dysfunction in people living with HIV and people with dyslipidemia. *J Am Heart Assoc*. 2020;9(14):e016263.

Leyes P, Martinez E, Larrousse M, et al. Effects of ezetimibe on cholesterol metabolism in PWH patients with protease inhibitor-associated dyslipidemia: a single-arm intervention trial. *BMC Infect Dis*. 2014;11(14):497.

Lin HX, Liu Z, Hajek P, et al. Efficacy of electronic cigarettes vs varenicline and nicotine chewing gum as an aid to stop smoking: a randomized clinical trial. *JAMA Intern Med*. 2024;184(3):291–299.

Lindson N, Butler AR, McRobbie H, et al. Electronic cigarettes for smoking cessation. *Cochrane Database Syst Rev*. 2024;1(1):CD010216. Published 2024 Jan 8. doi:10.1002/14651858.CD010216.pub8

Lloyd-Jones DM, Morris PB, Ballantyne CM, et al. Focused update of the 2016 ACC expert consensus decision pathway on the role of non-statin therapies for LDL-cholesterol lowering in the management of atherosclerotic cardiovascular disease. *J Amer Coll Cardiol*. 2017;70(14):1785–1822.

Lundgren JD, Babiker AG, Gordin F, et al. Initiation of antiretroviral therapy in early asymptomatic HIV Infection. *N Engl J Med*. 2015;373(9):795–807.

Mallon P, Winston A, Post F, et al. Platelet function upon switching to TAF vs continuing ABC: a randomized sub study. Abstract 80. CROI 2018. Boston, MA; 2018.

Marconi VC, Duncan MS, So-Armah K, et al. Bilirubin is inversely associated with cardiovascular disease among HIV-positive and HIV-negative individuals in VACS (Veterans Aging Cohort Study). *J Am Heart Assoc*. 2018;7(10):e007792.

Martinez E, Larrousse M, Llibre JM, et al. Substitution of raltegravir for ritonavir-boosted protease inhibitors in PWH patients: the SPIRAL study. *AIDS*. 2010;24(11):1697–1707.

McGettrick P, Mallon PWG. Biomarkers to predict cardiovascular disease in people living with HIV. *Curr Opin Infect Dis*. 2022;35(1):15–20.

McLaughlin MM, Ma Y, Scherzer R, et al. Association of viral persistence and atherosclerosis in adults with treated HIV infection. *JAMA Netw Open*. 2020;3(10):e2018099.

McNeil JJ, Nelson MR, Woods RL, et al. Effect of aspirin on all-cause mortality in the healthy elderly. *N Engl J Med*. 2018;379(16):1519–1528.

Medina-Torne S, Ganesan A, Barahona I, et al. Hypertension is common among PWH persons, but not associated with HAART. *J Int Assoc Physicians AIDS Care (Chic)*. 2012;11(1):20–25.

Mercie P, Arsandaux J, Katalama C, et al. Efficacy and safety of varenicline for smoking cessation in people living with HIV I France (ANRS 144 Inter-ACTIV): a randomized controlled phase 3 clinical trial. *Lancet HIV*. 2018;5(3):126–135.

Metkus TS, Brown T, Budoff M, et al. HIV infection is associated with an increased prevalence of coronary noncalcified plaque among participants with a coronary artery calcium score of zero: Multicenter AIDS Cohort Study (MACS). *HIV Med*. 2015;16(10):635–639.

Neesgaard B, Greenberg L, Miró JM, et al. Associations between integrase strand-transfer inhibitors and cardiovascular disease in people living with HIV: a multicentre prospective study from the RESPOND cohort consortium. *Lancet HIV*. 2022;9(7):e474–e485.

Neilan TG, Nguyen KL, Zaha VG, et al. Myocardial steatosis among antiretroviral therapy treated people with HIV participating in the REPRIEVE Trial. *J Infect Dis*. 2020;222(Suppl 1):S63–S69.

NICE. Ezetimibe for treating primary heterozygous familial and non-familial hypercholesterolemia. Guide TA385. http://nice.org.uk/guidance. Published 2016. Accessed August 15, 2024.

Nicholls SJ, Lincoff AM, Garcia M, et al. Effect of high-dose omega-3 fatty acids vs corn oil on major adverse cardiovascular events in patients at high cardiovascular risk: the STRENGTH randomized clinical trial. *JAMA*. 2020;324(22):2268–2280.

Nirmala N, Avendano EE, Morin RA. Effectiveness of ezetimibe in human immunodeficiency virus patients treated for hyperlipidaemia: a systematic review and meta-analysis. *Infect Dis (Lond)*. 2022;54(2):99–109.

Nissen SE, Menon V, Nicholls SJ, et al. Bempedoic acid for primary prevention of cardiovascular events in statin-intolerant patients. *JAMA*. 2023;330(2):131–140.

O'Brien S, Montenont E, Hu L, et al. Aspirin attenuates platelet activation and immune activation in HIV-1-infected subjects on antiretroviral therapy: a pilot study. *J Acquir Immune Defic Syndr*. 2013;63(3):280–288.

Oh RC, Trivette ET, Westerfield, KL. Management of hypertriglyceridemia: common questions and answers. *Am Fam Phys*. 2020;102(6):347–354.

Olaiya O, Weiser J, Zhou W, et al. Hypertension among persons living with HIV in medical care in the United States: Medical Monitoring Project 2013–2014. *Open Forum Infect Dis*. 2018;5(3):ofy028.

Oliveira JM, Rondo PH, Lima LR, et al. Effects of low dose fish oil on inflammatory markers of Brazilian PWH adults on antiretroviral therapy: a randomized parallel, placebo-controlled trial. *Nutrients*. 2015;7(8):6520–6528.

Oliveros E, Patel H, Kyung S, et al. Hypertension in older adults: assessment, management and challenges. *Clin Cardiol*. 2020;43(2): 999–107.

Ozemek C, Erlandson KM, Jankowski CM. Physical activity and exercise to improve cardiovascular health for adults living with HIV. *Prog Cardiovasc Dis*. 2020;63(2):178–183.

Pacek LR, Holloway AD, Cropsey KL, et al. Cigarette smoking and cessation-related interactions with health care providers in the context of living with HIV: focus group study findings. *J Assoc Nurses AIDS Care*. 2021;32(2):e14–e19.

Paikin JS, Eikelboom JW. Cardiology patient page: aspirin. *Circulation*. 2012;125(10):e439–e442.

Paisible AL, Chang CH, So-Armah KA, et al. HIV infection, cardiovascular disease risk factor profile, and risk for acute myocardial infarction. *J AIDS*. 2015;68:209–216.

Palella FJ Jr, Fisher M, Tebas P, et al. Simplification to rilpivirine/emtricitabine/tenofovir disoproxil fumarate from ritonavir-boosted protease inhibitor antiretroviral therapy in a randomized trial of HIV-1 RNA-suppressed participants. *AIDS*. 2014;28(3):335–344.

Panel on Antiretroviral Guidelines for Adults and Adolescents. Guidelines for the use of antiretroviral agents in adults and adolescents with HIV. Department of Health and Human Services. https://clinicalinfo.hiv.gov/en/guidelines/adult-and-adolescent-arv. Updated February 27, 2024. Accessed July 29, 2024.

Panel on Antiretroviral Guidelines for Adults and Adolescents. Statin Therapy in People with HIV. Department of Health and Human Services. https://clinicalinfo.hiv.gov/en/guidelines/hiv-clinical-guidelines-adult-and-adolescent-arv/statin-therapy-people-hiv. February 27, 2024. Updated September 12, 2024. Accessed July 29, 2024.

Patnode CD, Henderson JT, Coppola EL, et al. Interventions for tobacco cessation in adults, including pregnant persons: updated evidence report and systematic review for the US Preventive Services Task Force. *JAMA*. 2021;325(3):280–298. doi:10.1001/jama.2020.23541

Petoumenos K, Worm S, Reiss P, et al.; D:A:D Study Group. Rates of cardiovascular disease following smoking cessation in patients with HIV infection: results from the D:A:D study. *HIV Med*. 2011;12(7):412–421.

Pett SL, Amin J, Horban A, et al. Week 96 results of the randomized, multicenter Maraviroc Switch (MARCH) Study. *HIV Med*. 2018;19:65–71.

Pool ER, Dogar O, Lindsay RP, et al. Interventions for tobacco use cessation in people living with HIV and IADS. *Cochrane Database Syst Rev*. 2016;13(6):CD011120.

Post WS, Budoff M, Kingsley L, et al. Associations between HIV infection and subclinical coronary atherosclerosis. *Ann Intern Med*. 2014;160:458–467.

Rao SG, Galaviz KI, Hawkins GC, et al. Factors associated with excess myocardial infarction risk in PWH adults: a systemic review and meta-analysis. *J Acquir Imune Defic Syndr*. 2019;81(2):224–230.

Rasmussen LD, May MT, Kronborg G, et al. Time trends for risk of severe age-related diseases in individuals with and without HIV infection in Denmark: a nationwide population-based cohort study. *Lancet HIV*. 2015;2(7):e288–e298.

Ray KK, Bays HE, Catapano AL, et al.; CLEAR Harmony Trial. Safety and efficacy of bempedoic acid to reduce LDL cholesterol. *N Engl J Med*. 2019;380(11):1022–1032.

Regan S, Meigs JB, Massaro J, et al. Evaluation of the ACC/AHA CVD risk prediction algorithm among PWH patients. Abstract 751. CROI 2015. Seattle, WA; 2015.

Reiter-Brennan C, Osei AD, Iftekhar Uddin SM, et al. ACC/AHA lipid guidelines: personalized care to prevent cardiovascular disease. *Cleve Clin J Med*. 2020;87(4):231–239.

Remick J, Georgiopoulou V, Marti C, et al. Heart failure in patients with human immunodeficiency virus infection: epidemiology, pathophysiology, treatment, and future research. *Circulation*. 2014;129(17):1781–1789.

Ryom L, Lundgren JD, El-Sadr W, et al. Cardiovascular disease and use of contemporary protease inhibitors: the D:A:D international prospective multicohort study. *Lancet HIV*. 2018;6:e291–e300.

Sabatine MS, Giugliano RP, Keech AC, et al. Evolocumab and clinical outcomes in patients with cardiovascular disease. *N Engl J Med*. 2017;376:1713–1722.

Sabin C, Reiss P, Ryom L, et al. Is there continued evidence for an association between abacavir and myocardial infarction risk? Abstract 747. CROI 2014. Boston, MA; 2014.

Saeedi R, Johns K, Frohlich J, et al. Lipid-lowering efficacy and safety of ezetimibe combined with rosuvastatin compared with titrating rosuvastatin monotherapy in HIV-positive patients. *Lipids Health Dis*. 2015;14:57.

Sax PC, Zolopa A, Eleon R. Tenofovir alafenamide vs. tenofovir disoproxil fumarate in single tablet regimens for initial HIV-1 therapy: a randomized phase 2 study. *J Acquir Immune Defic Syndr*. 2014;67(1):52–58.

Scherzer R, Shah SJ, Secemsky E, et al. Association of biomarker clusters with cardiac phenotypes and mortality in patients with HIV infection. *Circ Heart Fail*. 2018;11(4):e004312.

Schmidt AF, Pearce LS, Wilkins JT, et al. PCSK9 monoclonal antibodies for the primary and secondary prevention of cardiovascular disease. *Cochrane Database Syst Rev*. 2017;10(10):CD011748.

Shah ASV, Stelze D, Lee KK, et al. Global burden of atherosclerotic vascular disease in people living with HIV: systematic review and meta-analysis. *Circulation*. 2018;138:1100–1112.

Shahreyar M, Salem SA, Nayyar M. Hyperlipidemia: management with proprotein convertase subtilisin/kexin type 9 (PCSK9) inhibitors. *J Am Board Fam Med*. 2018;31(4):628–634.

Sigel K, Makinson A, Thaler J. Lung cancer in persons with HV. *Curr Opin HIV AIDS*. 2017;12(1):31–38.

Sizar O, Nassereddin A, Talati R. Ezetimibe. [Updated 2023 Aug 28]. In: StatPearls [Internet]. Treasure Island (FL): StatPearls Publishing; 2025 Jan-. Available from: https://www.ncbi.nlm.nih.gov/books/NBK532879/

Smit M, van Zoest RA, Nichols BE, et al. Cardiovascular disease prevention policy in human immunodeficiency virus: recommendations from a modeling study. *Clin Infect Dis*. 2018;66(5):743–750.

So-Armah K, Benjamin LA, Bloomfield GS, et al. HIV and cardiovascular disease. *Lancet HIV*. 2020;7:e279–e293.

Soares C, Kwok M, Boucher KA, et al. Performance of cardiovascular risk prediction models among people living with HIV: a systematic review and meta-analysis. *JAMA Cardiol*. 2023;8(2):139–149.

Sokhela S, Venter WDF, Bosch B, et al. Final 192-week efficacy and safety results of the ADVANCE trial, comparing 3 first-line antiretroviral regimens. *Open Forum Infect Dis*. 2024;11(3):ofae007.

Strategies for Management of Antiretroviral Therapy (SMART)/ INSIGHT/D:A:D Study Groups. Use of nucleoside reverse transcriptase inhibitors and risk of myocardial infarction in PWH patients. *AIDS*. 2008;22:F17–F24.
Stone NJ, Robinson JG, Lichtenstein AH, et al. 2013 ACC/AHA guideline on the treatment of blood cholesterol to reduce atherosclerotic cardiovascular risk in adults: a report of the American College of Cardiology/American Heart Association Task Force on Practice Guidelines [published correction appears in Circulation. 2014 Jun 24;129(25 Suppl 2):S46–8] [published correction appears in Circulation. 2015 Dec 22;132(25):e396. doi: 10.1161/ CIR.0000000000000346.]. *Circulation*. 2014;129(25 Suppl 2):S1–S45. doi:10.1161/01.cir.0000437738.63853.7a
Subramanian S, Tawakol A, Burdo TH, et al. Arterial inflammation in patients with HIV. *JAMA*. 2012;308:379–386.
Suchindran S, Regan S, Meigs JB, et al. Aspirin use for primary and secondary prevention in human immunodeficiency virus (HIV)-infected and HIV-uninfected patients. *Open Forum Infect Dis*. 2014;1(3):ofu076.
Swanson B, Keithley J, Baum L, et al. Effects of fish oil on HIV-related inflammation and markers of immunosenescence: a randomized clinical trial. *J Altern Complement Med*. 2018;24(7):709–716.
Tawakol A, Lo J, Zanni MV, et al. Increased arterial inflammation relates to high-risk coronary plaque morphology in PWH patients. *J Acquir Immune Defic Syndr*. 2014;66(2):164–171.
The Accord Study Group. Effects of combination lipid therapy in type 2 diabetes mellitus. *N Engl J Med*. 2010;362:1563–1574.
Thiebaut R, El-Sadr W, Friis-Moller N, et al.; D:A:D Study Group. Predictors of hypertension and changes in blood pressure in PWH patients. *Antiviral Ther*. 2005;10:811–823.
Thompson MA, Horberg MA, Agwu AL, et al. Primary care guidance for persons with human immunodeficiency virus: 2020 update by the HIV Medicine Association of the Infectious Diseases Society of America. *Clin Infect Dis*. 2021 Dec 6;73(11):e3572–e3605.
Thompson-Paul A, Buchacz K, Wei S, et al. Evaluation of the ACC/AHA CVD risk prediction algorithm among PWH patients. Abstract 747. CROI 2015. Seattle, WA; 2015.
Tibuakuu M, Fashanu OE, Zhao D, et al. Glyc A, a novel inflammatory marker, is associated with subclinical coronary disease. *AIDS*. 2019;33(3):547–557.
Triant V, Lee H, Hadigan C, et al. Increased acute myocardial infarction rates and cardiovascular risk factors among patients with human immunodeficiency virus disease. *J Clin Metab*. 2007;92(7):2506–2512.
Triant V, Perez J, Regan S, et al. Cardiovascular risk prediction functions underestimate risk in HIV infection. *Circulation*. 2018;137(21):2203–2214.
Triant V, Regan S, Lee H, et al. Association of immunologic and virologic factors with myocardial infarction rates in the U.S. health care system. *J Acquir Immune Defic Syndr*. 2010;55(5):615–619.
Tseng A, Foisy M. Important drug-drug interactions in PWH persons on antiretroviral therapy: an update on new interactions between HIV and non-HIV drugs. *Curr Infect Dis Rep*. 2012;14(1):67–82.
Tungsiripat M, Kitch D, Glesby MJ, et al. A pilot study to determine the impact on dyslipidemia of adding tenofovir to stable background antiretroviral therapy: ACTG 5206. *AIDS*. 2010;24(11):1781–1784.
Vancampfort D, Mugisha J, Richards J, et al. Physical activity correlates in people living with HIV/AIDS: systematic review of 45 studies. *Disabil Rehabil*. 2018;40(14):1618–1629.
Van Lelyveld SF, Gras L, Kesselring A, et al. ATHENA national observational cohort study: Long-term complications in patients with poor immunological recovery despite virological successful HAART in Dutch ATHENA cohort. *AIDS*. 2012;26(4):465–474.
van Zoest RA, van den Born BH, Reiss P. Hypertension in people living with HIV. *Curr Opin HIV AIDS*. 2017; 12(6):513–522.
Vieira AD, Silveira GR. Effectiveness of n-3 fatty acids in the treatment of hypertriglyceridemia in HIV/AIDS patients: a meta-analysis. *Cien Saude Colet*. 2017;22(8):2659–2669.
Wall HK, Ritchey MD, Gillespie C, et al. Vital signs: prevalence of key cardiovascular disease risk factors for million hearts 2022—United States, 2011–2016. *MMWR*. 2018;67:983–991.
Whelton PK, Carey RM, Aronow WS, et al. 2017 ACC/AHA/AAPA/ ABC/ACPM/AGS/APhA/ASH/ASPC/NMA/PCNA executive summary of the guideline for the prevention, detection, evaluation, and management of high blood pressure in adults: executive summary: a report of the American College of Cardiology/American Heart Association Task Force on Clinical Practice Guidelines. *Circulation*. 2018a;138(17):e426–e483.
Whelton, PK, Carey, RM, Aronow, WS, et al. 2017 ACC/AHA/AAPA/ ABC/ACPM/AGS/APhA/ASH/ASPC/NMA/PCNA guideline for the prevention, detection, evaluation, and management of high blood pressure in adults: a report of the American College of Cardiology/American Heart Association Task Force on Clinical Practice Guidelines. *J Am Coll Cardiol*. 2018b;71:e127–e248.
White JR, Chang CC, So-Armah KA, et al. Depression and HIV infection are risk factors for incident heart failure among veterans: VACS. *Circulation*. 2015;132(17):1630–1638.
Wohl D, Waters D, Simpson R, et al. Ezetimibe alone reduces low-density lipoprotein cholesterol in PWH patients receiving combination antiretroviral therapy. *Clin Infect Dis*. 2008;47:1105–1108.
Yusuf S, Hawken S, Ounpuu S, et al. Effect of potentially modifiable risk factors associated with myocardial infarction in 52 countries (The INTERHEART Study): case-control study. *Lancet*. 2004;364:937–952.
Zanni MV, Awadalla M, Toibio M, et al. Immune correlates of diffuse myocardial fibrosis and diastolic dysfunction among aging women with human immunodeficiency virus. *J Infect Dis*. 2020; 221:1315–1320.
Zhou Y, Zhang X, Gao Y, et al. Risk of death and readmission among individuals with heart failure and HIV: A systematic review and meta-analysis. *J Infect Public Health*. 2024 Jan;17(1):70–75.

30.

NON-OPPORTUNISTIC PULMONARY COMPLICATIONS

Priyanka Chakrabarti

LEARNING OBJECTIVE

Review and characterize the pulmonary complications related to HIV infection in order to provide early and accurate diagnosis and treatment.

KEY POINTS

NONSPECIFIC INTERSTITIAL PNEUMONITIS

- Nonspecific interstitial pneumonitis (NSIP) encompasses several lymphocytic pulmonary syndromes, including follicular bronchiolitis, lymphocytic bronchiolitis, lymphocytic interstitial pneumonitis (LIP), and diffuse infiltrative $CD8^+$ lymphocytosis syndrome (DILS).
- People with HIV (PWH) may be asymptomatic or present with subacute dyspnea, nonproductive cough, and fever in a person with $CD4^+$ T-cell counts greater than 200 cells/mm^3. X-ray findings are nonspecific, but characteristically show bilateral reticulonodular "interstitial" infiltrates.
- The diagnosis of NSIP requires histologic confirmation by biopsy. The optimal treatment remains unclear.
- Routine vaccinations, avoiding tobacco smoke and pollutants, and early antiretroviral therapy (ART) initiation can improve outcomes.

LYMPHOCYTIC INTERSTITIAL PNEUMONITIS

- Lymphocytic interstitial pneumonitis (LIP) is a common respiratory complication of HIV infection in children but a rare complication in adults with HIV.
- It presents with slowly progressive dyspnea and nonproductive cough. X-ray findings are nonspecific but characteristically show bilateral reticulonodular "interstitial" infiltrates with a basal lung predominance.
- The diagnosis requires histologic confirmation by biopsy.
- ART has been used successfully for treatment.

PULMONARY ARTERIAL HYPERTENSION

- The prevalence of pulmonary arterial hypertension (PAH) is higher in PWH compared to the general population.
- Clinical presentation is similar to the general population, with progressive dyspnea, nonproductive cough, chest pain, and occasionally syncope or presyncope. These symptoms should prompt timely evaluation to facilitate early diagnosis.
- Diagnosis is often first suggested by chest radiograph revealing prominent pulmonary arteries or by electrocardiogram. Right heart catheterization is the standard for establishing a diagnosis.
- Potential therapies for HIV-associated PAH include ART, oxygen, diuretics, and directed therapy. Prostanoids (epoprostenol, treprostinil, and iloprost), endothelin receptor antagonists (bosentan), and phosphodiesterase-5 inhibitors (sildenafil) are used in persons with HIV-associated PAH and have improved mortality.

CHRONIC OBSTRUCTIVE PULMONARY DISEASE

- The prevalence of chronic obstructive pulmonary disease (COPD) is higher in PWH compared to the general population and may be due to multiple overlapping and interacting mechanisms.
- Diagnosis and management of COPD for PWH is similar to that for the general population, with smoking cessation being the most important area for prevention and intervention.

NONSPECIFIC INTERSTITIAL PNEUMONITIS

Nonspecific interstitial pneumonitis (NSIP) is a form of idiopathic interstitial pneumonitis that has increased prevalence with the use of certain medications, autoimmune diseases, and HIV (Flaherty, 2024). The overall prevalence of NSIP is unknown. It was found in 48% of asymptomatic PWH in the 1980s (Ognibene et al., 1988) and in 38% of PWH and pulmonary symptoms or abnormal imaging studies (Suffredini et al., 1987).

The etiology of NSIP is unknown. Evidence suggests that immune dysregulation may contribute, and thus the prevalence of NSIP has declined with the use of combination ART (Collins et al., 2019). In one analysis, NSIP was found in 7% of PWH admitted for interstitial lung disease since the introduction of ART (Wolff et al., 2001).

NSIP encompasses several lymphocytic pulmonary syndromes in PWH: follicular bronchiolitis, lymphocytic bronchiolitis, lymphocytic interstitial pneumonitis (LIP), and diffuse infiltrative CD8⁺ lymphocytosis syndrome (DILS). Histologically, it is characterized by the presence of perivascular and peribronchial interstitial lymphocytes, plasma cells, and macrophages; however, these are also found along the pleura and interlobar fibrous septate (Travis et al., 1992).

Clinical symptoms are minimal or nonexistent; subacute dyspnea, nonproductive cough, and fever have been reported (Suffredini et al., 1987). Physical exam may reveal crackles. Chest radiograph and high-resolution CT may show diffuse ground glass or reticular opacities. Pulmonary function testing typically shows a restrictive defect and low diffusing capacity (Flaherty, 2024). A definitive diagnosis is made by histology of lung tissue.

There are no specific guidelines for treatment in PWH, and the condition can remain stable for many years or regress on its own. Theoretically, ART may improve its symptoms, but there is no systematic clinical evidence to support this theory. A study conducted in South Africa showed that decreased lung function remained for 2 years in adolescents with HIV despite being on ART. Routine pneumococcal, influenza vaccination along with early ART initiation can reduce the risk of developing chronic lung disease and optimize lung health by preventing lung infections. Avoiding tobacco smoke and optimizing nutrition can also improve outcomes (WHO, 2021).

HIV LYMPHOCYTIC INTERSTITIAL PNEUMONITIS

Lymphocytic interstitial pneumonitis (LIP) is a rare histopathologic disease that accounts for 40% of lung diseases in children with AIDS but only 1%–2% of lung diseases in adults with HIV (Anderson and Lee, 1988; Stover et al., 1985). A higher prevalence was noted in women based on trans-bronchial biopsy (van Zyl-Smit et al., 2015).

Histologically, LIP is characterized by diffuse infiltration with polyclonal lymphocytes and occasionally plasma cells and histiocytes into the alveolar septae and along lymphatic vessels (Halprin et al., 1972). Type II pneumocyte hyperplasia and germinal centers within lymphoid follicles are commonly found. Biopsies show CD8⁺ and CD20⁺ cells predominance. Fibrosis may develop in advanced cases.

Although the etiology of LIP is not clear, it has been suggested that Epstein–Barr virus (EBV) may play a role. EBV DNA has been found in fragments of lung tissues taken from children with LIP (Reddy et al., 1998). In contrast, other studies have not shown any difference in the frequency of EBV detection in lung biopsies when comparing adult PWH with LIP and control groups (van Zyl-Smit et al., 2015). HIV itself may play a role in the pathology of LIP, as has been demonstrated in a transgenic mouse model in which HIV induced a lymphoid interstitial pneumonitis syndrome (Hanna et al., 1998). HIV RNA copies have been amplified from lung biopsy samples of PWH and LIP, and HIV-specific IgG is frequently present in the bronchoalveolar lavage fluid (Resnick et al., 1987). A predominant CD8⁺ T-cell infiltrate was found on histology in PWH and LIP (van Zyl-Smit et al., 2015). Human T-lymphotropic virus type I (HTLV-I) has been linked to LIP in Japan (Setoguchi et al., 1991).

The clinical presentation of LIP is similar in adults and children. Cough is the predominant symptom associated with slowly progressive dyspnea, which is usually present for several months. Fever, chest pain, weight loss, and arthralgias have also been reported. Physical exam may be normal or reveal crackles. Children may have clubbing, salivary gland enlargement, lymphadenopathy, and hepatosplenomegaly.

Chest x-rays are normal or show bilateral reticular or nodular opacities. Focal areas of confluent pulmonary opacifications have been described, as well as pulmonary cysts and patchy consolidations (the latter being less common). Chest CT shows diffuse ground-glass opacities with small nodules (2–3 mm) in a peribronchovascular distribution (Pitcher et al., 2010). Like other diffuse interstitial lung diseases, spirometry typically shows decreased total lung capacity and decreased diffusing capacity.

There is no consensus regarding the optimal treatment for LIP in PWH. Corticosteroids at a dosage of 1 mg/kg/d are recommended. However, in several case reports, ART has been demonstrated to be effective by itself (Garcia Lujan et al., 2004; Innes et al., 2004; Ripamonti et al., 2003).

DIFFUSE INFILTRATIVE CD8⁺ LYMPHOCYTE SYNDROME

Diffuse infiltrative CD8⁺ lymphocytosis syndrome (DILS) is a rare multisystemic syndrome characterized by CD8⁺ T-cell lymphocytosis associated with a CD8⁺ T-cell infiltration of multiple organs. It is primarily characterized by parotid gland enlargement, xerophthalmia, xerostomia, and interstitial pneumonitis. Respiratory clinical manifestations include nonproductive cough and dyspnea. Diffuse lymphadenopathy, hepatosplenomegaly, lymphocytic gastritis, and seventh cranial nerve palsy have also been described.

Histologic examination demonstrates visceral lymphocytic infiltration that could be a direct consequence of the large amount of CD8⁺ T-cells. Lymphoid follicles with CD8⁺ germinal centers are seen in salivary and parotid glands biopsies. HIV has been detected in macrophages within the germinal center of lymphoid tissues; therefore, ART plays a major role in treatment. Immunosuppression with steroids is also recommended.

PULMONARY ARTERIAL HYPERTENSION

Pulmonary arterial hypertension (PAH) is a rare complication in PWH, found in about 1 out of every 200 cases (Mehta et al., 2000). However, PAH has a higher prevalence among PWH compared to the general population. Overall prevalence was reported to be 0.5% in earlier studies (Speich et al., 1991) and has generally remained the same in the combination ART era (Opravil and Sereni, 2008; Sitbon et al.,

2008; Zuber et al., 2004). However, with increased use of ART, PWH are now presenting with common cardiac and pulmonary illnesses leading to PAH rather than direct HIV-associated PAH (Cerrato et al., 2013). There is an average of at least 2 years between diagnosis of HIV and presentation of PAH symptoms (Mehta et al., 2000).

The occurrence of PAH in PWH does not appear to be related to $CD4^+$ T-cell count, and no clear risk factors have been identified. One small study reported that chronic hepatitis C, substance use, and female sex increased the risk of developing PAH by 3-fold (Quezada et al., 2012). In a series that compared PAH in PWH and PAH in participants without HIV, PWH were significantly younger and had milder disease (50% vs. 75% had New York Heart Association functional class III or IV, respectively) (Petipretz et al., 1994).

The clinical presentation of PWH and PAH is similar to that of people without HIV. Symptoms are related to right heart dysfunction and include progressive shortness of breath, pedal edema, nonproductive cough, fatigue, syncope, and chest pain. Physical exam may reveal increased intensity of the pulmonary second heart sound, third and fourth sound gallop, tricuspid and pulmonary regurgitation murmurs, elevated jugular venous pressure, and peripheral edema.

Chest radiographs may show cardiomegaly and an enlarged pulmonary artery but clear lung fields. A transthoracic echocardiogram shows signs of right ventricle pressure overload, including systolic flattening of the interventricular septum and hypertrophy of the ventricle wall. The tricuspid regurgitant jet velocity can be used to calculate an estimated pulmonary artery systolic pressure (ePASP) which is elevated in PAH.

Right heart catheterization is the standard for diagnosing PAH, assessing severity, and monitoring response to treatment. PAH is defined by a mean PAP of 25 mmHg or higher, a mean pulmonary capillary wedge pressure of 15 mmHg or less, and a normal or reduced cardiac output (Galie et al., 2009). A thorough evaluation should be done to exclude other causes of pulmonary hypertension.

Treatment of HIV-associated PAH is similar to that of PAH in people without HIV. Treatment is guided by the World Health Organization (WHO) functional classification for PAH, which is based on symptomology and functional limitations. PWH should be counseled against smoking. PAH-directed therapy includes endothelin receptor antagonists, phosphodiesterase inhibitors, and prostacyclin pathway agonists. Although there are no controlled clinical trials, prostanoids (epoprostenol, treprostinil, and iloprost), endothelin receptor antagonists (bosentan), and phosphodiesterase-5 inhibitors (sildenafil) have been used in HIV-associated PAH and have been shown to improve symptoms and hemodynamic parameters. Caution should be taken with the use of these medications in PWH because of possible important drug interactions, particularly with protease inhibitors and cobicistat.

Oxygen is recommended if arterial blood partial pressure of oxygen (PaO_2) is 60 mmHg or less. Diuretics reduce the right ventricular preload and are recommended in PWH with right heart failure. The role of digoxin is controversial; however, it has been shown to improve cardiac output in PWH with acute right ventricular dysfunction attributable to PAH. Anticoagulation is not routinely recommended in PWH as there is no direct data of its benefit. Calcium channel blockers are not recommended in HIV-associated PAH. Observational data show the efficacy of vasoreactivity in only a small number of PWH and PAH and very limited long-term response. Although there is no conclusive evidence of the effect of ART on the progression of HIV-associated PAH, it is recommended to start ART in all PWH with PAH regardless of the $CD4^+$ T-cell count. ART has been demonstrated to cause improvements in pressure gradient over time and to significantly reduce the risk of death in PWH and PAH.

PAH is an independent risk factor for death among PWH (Opravil and Sereni, 2008). However, with the advent of ART and the new treatment modalities, the overall survival rate at 1 year is 88% and 72% at 3 years (Degano et al., 2010).

CHRONIC OBSTRUCTIVE PULMONARY DISEASE

Given the increasing longevity attributed to effective ART and high rates of tobacco use, chronic obstructive pulmonary disease (COPD) has become a common and important condition among PWH affecting mortality, with prevalence estimates ranging from 3.4% to over 40% (Bigna et al., 2018; Fitzpatrick et al., 2018). Mechanisms contributing to the development of COPD include oxidative stress, immune activation, systemic inflammation, cellular senescence/accelerated aging, altered lung microbiome, and endothelial dysfunction, all of which may be heightened with HIV infection (Byanova et al., 2023). Factors such as these may explain the earlier and more rapid decline in lung function that has been observed among some PWH compared to the general population, even after accounting for tobacco use and other known risk factors.

Currently there are no differences in screening guidelines and diagnostic criteria for PWH compared to the general population, and most major clinical practice guidelines do not recommend routine general screening for asymptomatic individuals. The 2024 GOLD guidelines recommend spirometry to screen high-risk people for COPD at the time they are undergoing lung cancer screening or when incidental lung abnormalities are found on imaging that are consistent with COPD (e.g., air trapping, airway wall thickening, mucous plugging) (GOLD, 2024). For PWH suspected of having COPD, optimal diagnostic testing includes full pulmonary function tests with pre- and post-bronchodilator spirometry, total lung capacity, and lung volumes if spirometry is abnormal, and measurement of diffusing capacity for carbon monoxide.

Management of COPD for PWH is similar to that for the general population, and includes interventions such as inhaler pharmacotherapy, pulmonary rehabilitation, vaccinations, and smoking cessation, among others. For people receiving inhaled corticosteroids, special attention is warranted if ritonavir and cobicistat-inclusive ART combinations will be (or are concurrently being) used, given the risk of Cushing's syndrome. For PWH treated with ritonavir or cobicistat, beclomethasone is preferred. Smoking cessation remains the most impactful intervention and should be recognized as a priority for HIV care providers. Evidence suggests that multiple behavioral and pharmacologic strategies should be offered, tailored to individual needs, integrated with mental health and substance use services, and delivered across multiple sessions, with regular follow-up to support ongoing quit efforts (Hoang et al., 2024; Ledgerwood and Yskes, 2016; Mouscou-Jackson et al., 2014).

RECOMMENDED READING

Konstantinidis I, Crothers K, Kunisaki KM, et al. HIV-associated lung disease. *Nat Rev Dis Primers*. 2023;9(1):39. doi:10.1038/s41572-023-00450-5

Leung JM. HIV And Chronic Lung Disease. *Curr Opin HIV AIDS*. 2023;18(2):93–101. doi:10.1097/COH.0000000000000777

REFERENCES

Anderson V, Lee H. Lymphocytic interstitial pneumonitis in pediatric AIDS. *Pediatr Pathol*. 1988;8:417–421.

Bigna JJ, Kenne AM, Asangbeh SL, Sibetcheu AT. Prevalence of chronic obstructive pulmonary disease in the global population with HIV: a systematic review and meta-analysis. *Lancet Glob Health*. 2018;6(2):e193–e202.

Byanova KL, Abelman R, North CM, et al. COPD in people with HIV: epidemiology, pathogenesis, management, and prevention strategies. *Int J Chron Obstruct Pulmon Dis*. 2023;18:2795–2817.

Collins B, Mulhall P, Travaline J. Nonspecific interstitial pneumonia in a patient with HIV. *SN Comprehensive Clinical Medicine*. 2019;1:203–204.

Cerrato E, D'Ascenzo F, Biondi-Zoccai G, et al. Cardiac dysfunction in pauci symptomatic human immunodeficiency virus patients: a meta-analysis in the highly active antiretroviral therapy era. *Eur Heart J*. 2013;34(19):1432–1436.

Degano B, Guillaume M, Savale L, Montani D, et al. HIV-associated pulmonary arterial hypertension: survival and prognostic factors in the modern therapeutic era. *AIDS*. 2010;24:67–75.

Fitzpatrick ME, Kunisake KM, Morris A. Pulmonary disease in HIV-infected adults in the era of antiretroviral therapy. *AIDS*. 2018;32(3):277–292.

Flaherty, KR. Causes, clinical manifestations, evaluation, and diagnosis of nonspecific interstitial pneumonia. *UpToDate*. https://www.uptodate.com/contents/causes-clinical-manifestations-evaluation-and-diagnosis-of-nonspecific-interstitial-pneumonia. Published April 8, 2024. Accessed August 30, 2024.

Galie N, Hoeper M, Humbert M. Guidelines for the diagnosis and treatment of pulmonary hypertension. *Eur Heart J*. 2009;30:2493–2537.

Garcia Lujan R, Echave-Sustaeta J, Garcia Quero C, et al. Lymphoid interstitial pneumonia resolved through antiretroviral therapy in an adult infected by human immunodeficiency virus. *Arch Bronconeumol*. 2004;40:537–539.

Global Initiative for Chronic Obstructive Lung Disease. Strategy for prevention, diagnosis and management of COPD (GOLD). 2024 Report. https://goldcopd.org/2024-gold-report/. Published 2024. Accessed September 1, 2024.

Halprin G, Ramirez J, Pratt O. Lymphoid interstitial pneumonia. *Chest*. 1972;62:418–423.

Hanna Z, Kay DG, Cool M et al. Transgenic mice expressing human immunodeficiency virus type 1 in immune cells develop a severe AIDS-like disease. *J Virol*. 1998;72:121–132.

Hoang THL, Nguyen VM, Adermark L, Albarez GG, Shelley D, Ng N. Factors influencing tobacco smoking and cessation among people living with HIV: a systematic review and meta-analysis. *AIDS Behav*. 2024;28(6):1858–1881.

Innes A, Huang L, Nishimura S. Resolution of lymphocytic interstitial pneumonitis in an HIV infected adult after treatment with HAART. *Sex Transm Infect*. 2004;80:417–418.

Ledgerwood DM, Yskes R. Smoking cessation for people living with HIV/AIDS: a literature review and synthesis. *Nicotine Tob Res*. 2016;18(12):2177–2184.

Mehta NJ, Khan IA, Mehta RN, Sepkowitz DA. HIV-related pulmonary hypertension. *Chest*. 2000;118(4):1133–1141.

Moscou-Jackson G, Commodore-Mensah Y, Farley J, DiGiacomo M. Smoking-cessation interventions in people living with HIV infection: a systematic review. *J Assoc Nurses AIDS Care*. 2014;25(1):32–45.

Ognibene F, Masur H, Rogers P, et al. Nonspecific interstitial pneumonitis without evidence of *Pneumocysitis carinii* in asymptomatic patients infected with human immunodeficiency virus (HIV). *Ann Intern Med*. 1988;109:874–879.

Opravil M, Sereni D. Natural history of HIV-associated pulmonary arterial hypertension: trends in the HAART era. *AIDS*. 2008;22:35–40.

Petipretz P, Brenot F, Azarian R. Pulmonary hypertension in patients with human immunodeficiency virus infection: comparison with primary pulmonary hypertension. *Circulation*. 1994;89:2722–2727.

Pitcher R, Beningfield S, Zar H. Chest radiographic features of lymphocytic pneumonitis in HIV-infected children. *Clin Radiol*. 2010;65:150–154.

Quezada M, Martin-Carbonero L, Soriano V, et al. Prevalence and risk factors associated with pulmonary hypertension in HIV-infected patients on regular follow-up. *AIDS*. 2012;26:1387–1392.

Reddy A, Lyall E, Crawford D. Epstein–Barr virus and lymphoid interstitial pneumonitis: an association revisited. *Pediatr Infect Dis J*. 1998;17:82–83.

Resnick L, Pitchenik A, Fisher E, et al. Detection of HTLVIII/LAV specific IgG and antigen in bronchoalveolar lavage fluid from two patients with lymphocytic interstitial pneumonitis associated with AIDS related complex. *Am J Med*. 1987;82:553–556.

Ripamonti D, Rizzi M, Maggiolo F, et al. Resolution of lymphocytic interstitial pneumonia in a human immunodeficiency virus infected adult following the start of highly antiretroviral therapy. *Scand J Infect Dis*. 2003;35:348–351.

Setoguchi Y, Takahashi S, Nukiwa T, et al. Detection of human T-cell lymphotropic virus type I-related antibodies in patients with lymphocytic interstitial pneumonia. *Am Rev Respir Dis*. 1991;144:1361–1365.

Sitbon O, Lascoux-Combe C, Delfraissy JF, et al. Prevalence of HIV-related pulmonary arterial hypertension in the current antiretroviral therapy era. *Am J Respir Crit Care Med*. 2008;177:108–113.

Speich R, Jenni R, Opravil M, et al. Primary pulmonary hypertension in HIV infection. *Chest*. 1991;100:1268–1271.

Stover D, White D, Romano P, et al. Spectrum of pulmonary diseases associated with the acquired immune deficiency syndrome. *Am J Med*. 1985;78:429–437.

Suffredini A, Ognibene F, Lack E, et al. Nonspecific interstitial pneumonitis: a common cause of pulmonary disease in the acquired immunodeficiency syndrome. *Ann Intern Med*. 1987;107:7–13.

Travis W, Fox C, Devaney K. Lymphoid pneumonitis in 50 adult patients infected with the human immunodeficiency virus: lymphocytic interstitial pneumonitis versus nonspecific interstitial pneumonitis. *Hum Pathol*. 1992;23:529–541.

van Zyl-Smit RN, Naidoo J, Wainwright H, et al. HIV associated lymphocytic interstitial pneumonia: a clinical, histological and radiographic study from an HIV endemic resource-poor setting. *BMC Pulm Med*. 2015;15:38–44.

Wolff AJ, O'Donnell AE. Pulmonary manifestations of HIV infection in the era of highly active antiretroviral therapy. *Chest*. 2001;120(6):1888–1893.

World Health Organization (WHO). Consolidated guidelines on HIV prevention, testing, treatment, service delivery and monitoring: Recommendations for a public health approach. https://www.who.int/publications/i/item/9789240031593. Published July 16, 2021. Accessed August, 30, 2024.

Zuber J, Calmy A, Evison J. Pulmonary arterial hypertension related to HIV infection improved hemodynamics and survival associated with antiretroviral therapy. *Clin Infect Dis*. 2004;38:1178–1185.

31.

RENAL COMPLICATIONS

Patricia Carr Reese and Umar Farooq

LEARNING OBJECTIVES

- Describe the broad pathologic spectrum of renal disease in people living with HIV (PWH), including medication-induced renal injury.
- Explain the importance of screening and monitoring PWH for chronic kidney disease (CKD), along with the indications for nephrology referral and renal biopsy.
- Select appropriate ART regimens based on a patient's renal function and comorbidities.
- Describe treatment options for PWH with end-stage renal disease (ESRD), including dialysis and solid organ transplant.

WHAT'S NEW?

- The most common current causes of CKD in PWH are noninfectious comorbidities (NICM), specifically hypertension, vascular disease, and diabetes.
- Despite the 2015 HIV Organ Policy Equity (HOPE) Act, disparities in renal transplantation remain for Black/African-American communities and PWH.

KEY POINTS

- PWH continue to have an increased risk of developing CKD. Because of ART availability, the most common etiologies of kidney disease have changed over the course of the epidemic: from HIV-associated nephropathy (HIVAN) to renal complications from NICM such as diabetes, hypertension, hepatitis coinfection, tobacco use, and aging in general. Evidence consistently demonstrates preservation of renal function with ART in PWH.
- PWH are eligible for both renal dialysis and renal transplant.
- Tenofovir disoproxil fumarate (TDF) can impair renal function and should be changed to an alternative regimen in PWH with or at risk for renal disease. Integrase inhibitors (INSTIs) can increase serum creatinine because of inhibition of renal organic cation transporter 2 (OCT2), but do not cause direct nephrotoxicity.
- All PWH should be monitored on a regular basis for CKD. Screening at least yearly for proteinuria and eGFR is recommended for those who are clinically stable and virologically suppressed on ART.

EPIDEMIOLOGY OF RENAL DISEASE IN PEOPLE WITH HIV

Although the incidence of HIV-associated nephropathy (HIVAN) has greatly declined since the beginning of the HIV epidemic, the overall prevalence of kidney disease in PWH has increased as a result of improved survival. With improved life expectancy and increased age-related metabolic abnormalities, chronic kidney disease (CKD) is a significant comorbidity in PWH. The change in the spectrum of kidney disease is being driven by traditional risk factors, including obesity, diabetes, hypertension, smoking, the use of nephrotoxic medications, and aging of the HIV population (Heron et al., 2020a; Waheed and Atta, 2014).

Despite widespread use of ART, PWH remain at a higher risk of renal insufficiency, cardiovascular disease, and overall mortality than matched cohorts of HIV-negative people (Kalayjian, 2011; Mallipattu et al., 2014). Up to 30% of PWH are at risk of developing proteinuria—a key marker of kidney disease. Moreover, cross-sectional cohorts from Europe, Asia, and North America have demonstrated high rates of CKD in PWH, with about 6% of PWH having stages 3–5 CKD (Post and Holt, 2009). Based on another large sample of U.S. veterans, the incidence rate of end-stage renal disease (ESRD) in Black PWH is even higher than that of patients with diabetes (incidence rates per 1,000 person-years [py]: 71.1 for HIV, 59.9 for diabetes mellitus, and 27.9 for individuals with neither HIV nor diabetes) (Choi et al., 2007). Compared to the general population, PWH have a 16-fold higher risk of requiring renal replacement therapy.

PATHOGENESIS

The *ApoL1* gene, which encodes a factor to lyse the parasite *Trypanosoma brucei*, is the key susceptibility allele in HIVAN and other kidney diseases in the APOL1 nephropathy spectrum. HIV-RNA localizes to podocytes and tubular epithelial cells in the kidney, suggesting a direct role of the virus in kidney disease. Further, the role of viral proteins is supported by animal studies. The HIV regulatory protein *nef* and HIV accessory protein *vpr* are overexpressed in mice reproducing the HIVAN phenotype (Cohen et al., 2017).

Kidney disease is a major cause of mortality from non-AIDS-related conditions in PWH, along with malignancies, cardiovascular disease, and liver disease (Ryom et al., 2019a). Renal pathology in PWH was originally reported in 1984 and was called "acquired immune deficiency syndrome (AIDS) nephropathy" (Rao et al., 1984). The histopathology on kidney biopsy of these cases showed a collapsing type of focal and segmental glomerulosclerosis, and the clinical presentation was that of proteinuria, usually nephrotic, and rapid progression to ESRD. Subsequently, HIVAN became more commonly recognized as a major cause of kidney disease in PWH. In the United States, the incidence of HIVAN peaked in the mid-1990s and dropped significantly after the introduction of highly active antiretroviral therapy (HAART) by the late 1990s (Ross and Klotman, 2002). More recent data show the annual incidence of ESRD in PWH in the United States is now about 800–900 cases per year (Cohen et al., 2017).

RISK FACTORS FOR NEPHROPATHY

Risk factors for the development of kidney disease in PWH include Black race, diabetes mellitus, hypertension, hepatitis C coinfection, cardiovascular disease, and family history of CKD (Mocroft et al., 2015; Naicker and Fabian, 2010). In addition, individuals with advanced undiagnosed and/or untreated HIV infection with $CD4^+$ T-cell counts of less than 200 cells/mm^3 and active viral replication are at high risk for developing HIVAN (Bige et al., 2012; Lescure et al., 2012).

GENETIC PREDISPOSITION

The major genetic risk factor for developing HIVAN and non-HIVAN focal segmental glomerulosclerosis (FSGS) in persons of African descent is the presence of polymorphisms in the apolipoprotein 1 (*APOL1*) gene, which is located on chromosome 22 (Genovese et al., 2010; Lescure et al., 2012; Tzur et al., 2010). *APOL1* encodes a serum factor that lyses *Trypanosoma brucei*. Thus, selective mutations in Africans to counter an endemic parasite may have contributed to the current rates of HIVAN and FSGS in Black populations. Two *APOL1* risk alleles, G1 and G2, are associated with the increased susceptibility for the development of HIVAN and other types of kidney disease collectively termed *APOL1* nephropathy (Friedmam and Pollak, 2021; Genovese et al., 2010; Papeta et al., 2011). It is hypothesized that *APOL1* risk variants create pores in cell membranes within the kidney much like they do in trypanosomal organelles, but other studies suggest that overexpression of risk variants leads to mitochondrial dysfunction and injury. There is still no consensus on the molecular mechanism of *APOL1* nephropathy (Friedman and Pollak, 2021). In PWH who carry the two *APOL1* risk alleles, this alone can explain 35% of HIVAN cases and 18% of FSGS cases (Kopp et al., 2011). Two risk variants confer an odds ratio of approximately 7–10 for hypertension-associated ESRD, 17 for FSGS, 29 for HIVAN in the United States, and 89 for HIVAN in Africa. These data suggest that these diseases have some overlapping mechanism of pathogenesis (Friedman and Pollak, 2021). *APOL1* homozygosity, present in 13% of the general Black American population, was noted in more than 60% of Black Americans with HIVAN and non-HIVAN FSGS (Kopp et al., 2011).

In animal models, HIV gene expression within kidney cells is required for the development of HIVAN (Bruggeman et al., 1997). Even in people with HIVAN and undetectable plasma HIV-RNA levels, proviral DNA can be found in the renal tissue (Izzedine et al., 2011). This implies that the kidney acts as a separate compartment from blood, allowing HIV to replicate in the kidney even in PWH who achieve viral suppression in their plasma with treatment (Medapalli et al., 2011). HIV induces apoptosis of cells in addition to causing cytopathic effects. These effects, in combination with cytokine release, are thought to play a role in the development of HIVAN (see Box 31.1).

Box 31.1 RISK FACTORS AND ETIOLOGIES OF CKD IN PWH

1. **Host genetic susceptibility**
   a. *APOL1* G1 and G2 risk variants
   b. ABCC2/4 variants
   c. Sickle cell trait
2. **Sociodemographic factors**
   a. Age
   b. Race/ethnicity
   c. Illicit drug use
   d. Socioeconomic status
3. **Exposures and comorbid noninfectious conditions and their treatment**
   a. Diabetes—obesity
   b. Recurrent or severe AKI
   c. Hypertension
   d. Cardiovascular disease
   e. Malignancies
4. **Coinfections**
   a. Hepatitis B or C virus
   b. Tuberculosis
   c. Syphilis
   d. Parasitic infection
5. **Underlying etiology of CKD**
   a. FSGC
   b. HIVAN
   c. Immune complex disease
   d. Diabetic nephropathy
   e. Tubulointerstitial disease
   f. ART-related nephropathy

Source: Adapted from Swanepoel CR, et al. *Kidney Int.* 2018;22(6):84–100.

MARKERS OF KIDNEY INJURY

Markers of kidney injury include an elevated serum creatinine, proteinuria, glycosuria, and an increased fractional excretion of uric acid (Makris and Spanou, 2016). Risk factors for proteinuria include older age, Black race, insulin resistance, hypertension, and a low $CD4^+$ T-cell count (Heron et al., 2020a). The presence of albuminuria and overt proteinuria is also associated with increased cardiovascular morbidity and mortality in women initiating ART (Wyatt et al., 2011).

ASSESSMENT OF KIDNEY FUNCTION

Like the general population, kidney damage in PWH is assessed by using creatinine-based estimates of glomerular filtration rate (eGFR) with the Cockroft–Gault equation, Modification of Diet in Renal Disease, and CKD Epidemiology Collaboration (CKD-EPI) equation, but none of these estimates has been systematically validated in PWH.

In 2021, the NKF and the ASN Task Force recommended use of the CKD-EPI creatinine equation refit without the race variable in all laboratories in the United States, in acknowledgment that race as used in the eGFR equation is a social and not biologic construct (Delgado et al., 2021). They also recommended higher utilization of the CKD-EPI eGFR-cystatin C (eGFRcys) and eGFR creatinine-cystatin C (eGFRcr-cys_r) refit without race for improved accuracy of diagnosis and clinical decision-making (Inker et al., 2021). Cystatin C is an alternative marker of eGFR that does not depend on muscle mass and is more sensitive for kidney damage than creatinine-based formulas. Its role in diagnosis and as a prognostic marker in PWH remains to be defined. Dragović and colleagues (2018) found that cystatin C may be elevated in PWH with metabolic syndrome. Out of 89 PWH in their cross-sectional study, 33 individuals with metabolic syndrome had a statistically significantly higher cystatin C level compared to those without. Notably, there were no significant differences with respect to $CD4^+$ level, time on ART, smoking status, or HBV/HCV status. Another study found that cystatin C may assist in clarifying the clinical significance of plasma creatinine fluctuations after dolutegravir initiation, particularly in people at elevated risk for development of renal disease (Palich et al., 2018).

PATHOLOGIC SPECTRUM OF KIDNEY DISEASE

PWH can develop multiple forms of renal disease, including acute kidney injury (AKI), HIVAN, HIV immune complex kidney disease (HIVICK), thrombotic microangiopathy (TMA), and medication-induced nephrotoxicity. However, kidney disease in PWH has been evolving over time with increased ART usage, viral suppression, and longer life expectancy in PWH. This has increased the prevalence of traditional CKD risk factors in PWH, broadening the spectrum of renal disease etiologies (see Box 31.2) (Swanepoel et al., 2018). In one large academic center, renal biopsies from 437 PWH (80% on ART) were re-evaluated to reassess spectrum of disease. This cohort of biopsies from 2010–2018 showed the most common pathology to be immune complex

Box 31.2 HIV-RELATED KIDNEY DISEASES

I. Glomerular dominant

- a. Immune complex-mediated glomerular disease (ICGN)
  - i. IgA nephropathy
  - ii. Lupus nephritis
  - iii. Membranous nephropathy
  - iv. Membranoproliferative pattern glomerulonephritis
  - v. Bacterial infection-related glomerulonephritis
  - vi. ICGN with no etiology other than HIV
  - vii. Other immune complex diseases in the setting of HIV
- b. Podocytopathies
  - i. Classic HIVAN
  - ii. FSGS-NOS in the setting of HIV
  - iii. Minimal-change disease in the setting of HIV
  - iv. Other podocytopathy in the setting of HIV
- c. Other glomerular diseases
  - i. Diabetic nephropathy
  - ii. AA amyloidosis
  - iii. Pauci-immune GN

II. Tubulointerstitial dominant

- a. Tenofovir toxicity
- b. Tubulointerstitial injury in the setting of classic HIVAN
- c. Acute tubular injury or acute tubular necrosis (associated with ART vs. other drugs)
- d. Tubulointerstitial nephritis (associated with ART vs. other drugs)
- e. Renal parenchymal infection by bacterial, viral, or fungal pathogens
- f. Immunologic dysfunction-related tubulointerstitial inflammation
  - i. DILS
  - ii. IRIS
- g. Other tubulointerstitial inflammation in the setting of HIV

III. Vascular dominant

- a. Thrombotic microangiopathy in the setting of HIV
- b. Arteriosclerosis and/or cholesterol emboli
- c. Infarction

IV. Other conditions, in the setting of HIV infection

- a. Diabetic nephropathy
- b. Age-related nephrosclerosis

Source: Adapted from Swanepoel CR, et al. *Kidney Int.* 2018;22(6):84–100.

glomerulonephritis (17%), follow by diabetic nephropathy (16%), HIVAN (14%), tenofovir-associated nephrotoxicity (13%), focal segmental glomerulosclerosis—not otherwise specified (FSGS-NOS) (12%), and global glomerulosclerosis-NOS (9%). Regarding the trends seen during this 9-year time frame, tenofovir nephrotoxicity decreased, while FSGS-NOS and diabetic nephropathy increased. In contrast, the same institution in 1987 reported that HIVAN made up for 76% of kidney biopsies in PWH, followed by immune complex glomerulonephritis (ICGN) (9%) and interstitial nephritis (6%). Researchers also showed that serologies and clinical syndromes, except Fanconi syndrome (which is associated with tenofovir toxicity), were not predictive of biopsy findings (Kudose et al., 2020). Therefore, renal biopsy remains an important diagnostic strategy for some PWH with kidney disease to determine the underlying renal pathology, as treatment strategies often differ based on histopathologic findings.

ACUTE KIDNEY INJURY

Poor nutritional status, dehydration, polypharmacy, and less commonly, opportunistic infections, in PWH predispose to development of AKI, with incidence rates of 2.7 to 6.9 per 100 person-years (py) (Campos et al., 2016). Higher incidence of AKI is also associated with advanced age, diabetes mellitus, CKD, acute or chronic liver failure, $CD4^+$ T-cell counts of less than 200 cells/mm^3, HIV-1 RNA levels greater than 10,000 copies/mL, and hepatitis coinfection (Wyatt et al., 2006). Common causes of AKI in PWH are similar to those in people without HIV, with pre-renal states and acute tubular necrosis accounting for about one-third of cases. Less common causes of AKI in PWH include obstruction from lymphadenopathy related to malignancy, tumor lysis syndrome, and polyoma virus-induced renal dysfunction. Regardless of the etiology, short- and long-term mortality is increased in AKI in PWH, by as much as 5-fold. In one study from Portugal of 489 hospitalized PWH, mortality was 27.3% in people with AKI versus 8% for people without AKI (Campos, 2016). In another study of 433 PWH who were hospitalized, at 1, 2, and 5 years of follow-up, the cumulative probability of death in those with AKI was 21%, 25%, and 31%, respectively, compared to 10%, 13%, and 16.5% in patients without AKI (Lopes et al., 2013).

HIV-ASSOCIATED NEPHROPATHY

HIVAN is the most aggressive form of kidney disease associated with HIV infection and generally presents in patients with advanced HIV infection who exhibit rapidly declining GFR and significant proteinuria. The incidence of HIVAN significantly declined after the widespread use of ART, but it remains a cause of ESRD, most often seen in young Black PWH. HIVAN is pathologically characterized by a collapsing form of focal and segmental sclerosis, prominent tubular microcysts, and tubulointerstitial inflammation (D'Agati et al., 1989). Focal segmental glomerulosclerosis—not otherwise specified (FSGS-NOS) has become a more common finding in renal biopsies in the ART era (Kudose et al., 2020). A subset of patients with FSGS-NOS are believed to have an attenuated form of HIVAN given similar median severity of tubular atrophy, interstitial fibrosis, and inflammation to HIVAN cases. Additionally, many samples had presence of tubuloreticular inclusions, tubular microcysts, and moderate foot-process effacement seen in HIVAN. Differentiation between FSGS-NOS and attenuated HIVAN is difficult to evaluate without molecular studies addressing viral infection of renal epithelia, infiltrating leukocyte phenotype, and dysregulation of host-signaling pathways. However, patients with FSGS-NOS tend to be older, hypertensive, with cardiovascular disease, and usually on ART (Kudose et al., 2020).

IMMUNE COMPLEX GLOMERULONEPHRITIS AND HIV IMMUNE COMPLEX DISEASE OF THE KIDNEY

Various immune complex kidney diseases have been reported in patients with HIV-1 infection, such as postinfectious glomerulonephritis, membranoproliferative glomerulonephritis, membranous nephropathy, immunoglobulin A nephropathy, and lupus-like glomerulonephritis, and previously they were collectively referred to as HIV immune complex disease of the kidney (HIVICK) (Balow, 2005; Kalayjian, 2011). In 2017, Kidney Disease: Improving Global Outcomes (KDIGO) replaced the term HIVICK in favor of a more descriptive pattern of immune complex disease because of lack of certainty of HIV-associated causality in most cases. The previously eluted glomerular immune deposits with specific anti-HIV antibodies in previous HIVICK cases were found in research settings and were not replicable in routine clinical pathology laboratories. Therefore, the transition away from collectively naming all immune complex disease as HIVICK was to encourage workup of secondary and possibly treatable causes of immune complex deposition (Swanepoel et al., 2018). In a review of renal biopsies in PWH, immune complex glomerulonephritis (ICGN) was the most prevalent finding (Kudose et al., 2020). Further, in those 75 cases of ICGN, 79% had an identifiable etiology other than HIV infection. Of the remaining 21%, two-thirds were not on ART, raising suspicion for true HIVICK in those cases.

TUBULOINTERSTITIAL DISEASE

Renal tubulointerstitial disease can include HIVAN, which has a tubulointerstitial component in addition to a glomerular component. Tenofovir and protease inhibitor (PI) toxicity can also play a role and will be discussed later in this chapter. PWH are also at risk for tubular injury due to the same etiologies seen in the general population such as toxic, ischemic, septic, and hypovolemic insults. Antibiotics, proton pump inhibitors, and other medications can cause tubulointerstitial nephritis in the general and HIV population as well. However, two rare but notable causes of tubulointerstitial injury are ones that involve immune dysfunction from HIV and are characterized by prominent $CD8^+$ T-cell infiltrates (Swanepoel, 2018). Diffuse infiltrative lymphocytosis syndrome (DILS) affects the kidneys 10% of the time as a result of a hyperimmune reaction against HIV. Immune reconstitution inflammatory syndrome (IRIS) rarely involves the kidney but may occur in patients with advanced HIV infection after ART initiation, unmasking a subclinical infectious process.

NONINFECTIOUS COMORBIDITIES

Currently, the most common causes of CKD in PWH are noninfectious comorbidities (NICM), specifically hypertension, vascular disease, and diabetes (Heron et al., 2020a). Hypertension can independently cause secondary FSGS but may also compound glomerular disease caused by HIV itself. Two primary drivers of comorbid hypertension are tobacco use and obesity. Both risk factors are relevant, as the prevalence of tobacco use among PWH is 2–3 times that of the general U.S. population (Park et al., 2016). Additionally, although exact causal mechanisms are unknown, tenofovir alafenamide (TAF) and INSTIs, especially dolutegravir and bictegravir, have been found to lead to weight gain in multiple studies (Sax et al., 2020).

Progressive vascular disease may occur in PWH from a direct effect of HIV on renal vasculature but is also associated with dyslipidemia and chronic inflammation (Heron, 2020a). Thrombotic microangiopathy (TMA) is a rare complication of HIV-1 infection, with an incidence of isolated renal TMA of 0.3% (Becker et al., 2004). It manifests as thrombocytopenia and microangiopathic hemolytic anemia, with or without fever and neurological deficits. Opportunistic infections, high plasma HIV viral load, low $CD4^{+}$ counts, and various drugs used in advanced HIV disease can all contribute to development of TMA. In the post–combination ART era, atherosclerotic disease has become the dominant vascular causes of kidney disease in PWH. Management should focus on modifiable risk factors, including lifestyle management, smoking cessation, lipid-lowering agents, and ART (Swanepoel et al., 2018).

Diabetes is 4 times more prevalent and associated with worse treatment outcomes in PWH compared to the general population (Heron et al., 2020a). Multiple studies, including the 31,072-participant Veterans Aging Cohort Study, have demonstrated a synergistic effect between HIV and diabetes, leading to more rapid CKD progression in PWH and diabetes compared to persons with either condition alone (Feng et al., 2021; Medapalli et al., 2012). Taken together, NICMs are a substantial contributor to CKD among PWH, and their importance will only grow as the cohort of PWH ages. Chronic inflammation, even low levels in patients with undetectable viral loads, contribute to more rapid aging in PWH, compared to age-matched counterparts not living with HIV (McCutcheon et al., 2024). This is demonstrated by earlier aging-associated epigenetic DNA methylation patterns and accelerated shortening of telomeres in PWH. These changes lead to earlier kidney dysfunction in PWH. ART mitigates but does not eliminate these impacts. This is further complicated by the polypharmacy required to treat these comorbid conditions, and the drug-drug interactions that ensue, especially among individuals requiring regimens that include boosted protease inhibitors (PIs).

TREATMENTS

Specific recommendations regarding therapy of the conditions noted above are limited because of the lack of prospective randomized controlled trials. Most of the treatment options, including supportive care, ART, renin–angiotensin–aldosterone system inhibitors, and corticosteroids, are based on retrospective studies and nonrandomized trials.

ANTIRETROVIRAL THERAPY (ART)

Multiple observational studies have supported the benefit of ART in slowing the progression or reversing renal disease in persons with HIVAN. In an older Johns Hopkins Clinic cohort of 4,000 PWH, ART was associated with a 60% risk reduction for HIVAN, with 6.8 and 26.4 episodes per 1,000 py in PWH who did or did not receive ART, respectively (Lucas et al., 2004). In addition, no persons in the Hopkins cohort developed HIVAN when ART was initiated before the development of AIDS.

Consistent evidence demonstrates preservation of renal function with ART in HIV populations. In the Strategies for Management of Antiretroviral Therapy (SMART) study, continuous antiretroviral therapy versus episodic use of ART was evaluated in 5,472 PWH with $CD4^{+}$ T-cell counts of more than 350 cells/μL. In the continuous use group, fewer persons developed renal disease compared to the episodic use group (0.2 vs. 0.1 events/100 py) (SMART, 2006). In addition, in a prospective, multicenter cohort involving 1,776 PWH, ART intervention in persons with CKD stage 2 or greater and low $CD4^{+}$ T-cell counts led to an average increase of 9.2 mL/min/1.73 m^2 in GFR at a median follow-up of 160 weeks. These results were magnified in those with a lower baseline GFR and greater decreases in viral load (Longenecker et al., 2009).

ANGIOTENSIN-CONVERTING-ENZYME INHIBITORS AND ANGIOTENSIN II BLOCKADE

Multiple randomized controlled trials in patients with CKD from the general population have demonstrated the efficacy of angiotensin-converting-enzyme (ACE) inhibitors and angiotensin receptor blockers (ARBs) in decreasing proteinuria, slowing the progression of kidney disease, and reducing the incidence of cardiovascular disease and death. Increasing evidence in the general population highlights the benefits of ACE inhibitors and ARBs in preventing progression to dialysis, even in those with more advanced kidney disease. A 2024 meta-analysis found that patients with CKD stage 4 or 5 who started ACE inhibitors or ARBs were significantly less likely to progress to dialysis (12% vs. 17% annually; number needed to treat, 20), but mortality was similar (~3% annually) (Ku et al., 2024).

However, data regarding their use in PWH is limited. An older study of 18 PWH with biopsy-proven HIVAN, of whom 9 persons were treated with captopril, had an enhanced renal survival compared to the control group (mean renal survival, 156 ± 71 vs. 37 ± 5 days) (Kimmel et al., 1996). In another study of 44 patients with biopsy-proven HIVAN, patients treated with ACE inhibitors had significantly less progression to ESRD compared to those without therapy (14% vs. 100% at 5 years) (Wei et al., 2003). Based on these results and data from non-HIV-specific populations, ACE inhibitors or ARBs are recommended for PWH with CKD and glomerular diseases in the absence of contraindications to these medications (Swanepoel et al., 2018). The 2023 European AIDS Clinical Society (EACS) in particular recommends ACE inhibitors or ARBs for PWH who have hypertension or proteinuria (EACS, 2023).

CORTICOSTEROIDS

In patients with HIVAN, older studies found that tubulointerstitial inflammation improves after treatment with steroids (Briggs et al., 1996). However, there are no randomized trials to support steroid use in this population. In a retrospective cohort study of 21 patients, of which 13 received corticosteroids, the relative risk for progressive renal failure with corticosteroid treatment at 3 months was 0.20 ($p < 0.05$) (Eustace et al., 2000). This association remained significant despite adjustment in logistical regression analyses for baseline creatinine; 24-hour proteinuria; CD4$^+$ count; history of intravenous drug use; hepatitis B coinfection; and hepatitis C coinfection (Eustace et al., 2000). However, there were 18 infections in corticosteroid-treated patients compared to 8 in the non-corticosteroid-treated group. Larger studies are needed to further clarify the value of steroids in patients with HIV-related kidney disease but, in the post-ART era, are unlikely to be performed. Based on older data noted above, some experts would still recommend a short course of corticosteroid therapy in those with a new diagnosis of HIVAN (Atta et al., 2008; Fine et al., 2008). Risk of adverse effects, including glucose intolerance, bone disease, and further immunosuppression, must always be weighed against the benefits when steroids are used in PWH.

NOVEL MEDICAL THERAPIES

As mentioned above, diabetes is 4 times more prevalent and associated with worse treatment outcomes in PWH compared to the general population. The new conceptual framework of the four pillars of CKD treatment in diabetes, which include angiotensin receptor blockers (ARBs) or ACE inhibitors, sodium-glucose cotransporter-2 (SGLT2) inhibitors, mineralocorticoid receptor antagonists (MRAs), and glucagon-like peptide-1 (GLP-1) agonists, has not been studied specifically in PWH, but they are likely to confer similar benefits for PWH and diabetes (Agarwal and Fouque, 2023). More studies are needed to see if PWH who have CKD but do not have diabetes could benefit from the same treatments.

Direct-acting antivirals (DAA) for treatment of hepatitis C (HCV) have been available since 2011; however, their use has dramatically increased in recent years. Both hepatitis B and C are highly associated with CKD, can independently cause glomerulonephritis, and also potentiate the impacts of HIV on the kidney (Heron et al., 2020a). Regression of kidney disease in patients with HIV-HCV coinfection can be seen with successful management of both conditions. Worldwide, 25%–30% of PWH are coinfected with HCV, so increased use of highly effective DAAs could have a significant impact on CKD among PWH (Kupin, 2017).

RENAL REPLACEMENT THERAPY (DIALYSIS)

Compared to the general population, PWH have a 2- to 20-fold higher incidence of requiring renal replacement therapy (Campos et al., 2016). This number varies depending on patient populations and geographic location. Historically, overall survival of PWH on dialysis was worse compared to that of the general ESRD population, mainly because of increased risk of infections (Atta et al., 2007). Older age, lower serum albumin level, lower CD4$^+$ T-cell count, and lack of ART have all been associated with poor survival in PWH undergoing hemodialysis or peritoneal dialysis. It appears that the incidence of ESRD has plateaued, but the prevalence of PWH undergoing dialysis in the United States has increased, likely due to aging of the HIV population (Cohen et al., 2017). Survival among PWH receiving dialysis is now similar to persons without HIV disease (Campos et al., 2016; Razzak et al., 2015). Peritoneal dialysis is also an option for some PWH. In one study of 70 PWH on continuous peritoneal dialysis, there was no increase in technique failure rates or catheter patency compared to people without HIV at 1 year, although the rate of hospital admission and all-cause mortality was higher in PWH (Ndlovu and Assounga, 2017).

RENAL TRANSPLANTATION

Renal transplantation was previously contraindicated in PWH because of the concern of immunosuppressive agents in persons with an impaired immune system. However, data now show that renal transplantation is both safe and effective in PWH (Blumberg and Rogers, 2019; Locke et al., 2015; Zheng et al., 2019). Initially, renal transplantation in PWH was performed without induction therapy. However, the use of antithymocyte globulin as induction therapy is associated with a 2.6-fold lower risk of rejection, as shown in a study of 516 PWH (Locke et al., 2014). Many of the agents used in post-transplantation immunosuppression have antiretroviral properties. Mycophenolate mofetil has virostatic properties through depletion of guanosine nucleosides necessary for the viral life cycle. Calcineurin inhibitors (tacrolimus and cyclosporine) selectively inhibit infected cell growth, and sirolimus disrupts infective viral replication through suppression of antigen-presenting cell function.

Currently undergoing investigation is how donor *APOL1* status affects outcomes, due to reports suggesting increased rates of kidney failure after donation from high-risk *APOL1* genotypes. Recipient *APOL1* status does not appear to affect graft survival, which suggests that renal *APOL1*, and not circulating *APOL1* derived from the liver, is the main driver of *APOL1* kidney disease (Freedman et al., 2015). There are limited data from large prospectively designed trials, but the *APOL1* Long-Term Kidney Transplantation Outcomes Network (APOLLO) study is currently underway (Freedman et al., 2019). Additional evaluation is needed to determine causality to the *APOL1* donor kidney. This would help donor and recipient education regarding the risks and benefits of *APOL1* high-risk kidney donation (versus remaining on dialysis). A more comprehensive analysis is needed to change allocation and outcomes of kidney transplantation (Friedman and Pollak, 2021).

PWH considered eligible for renal transplant should have a $CD4^+$ T-cell count greater than 200 mm^3 and an undetectable viral load while on a stable ART regimen. There is concern for drug-drug interactions between some antiretroviral drugs and immunosuppressive agents. This is especially true for ritonavir or cobicistat-boosted protease inhibitors (PI) that are metabolized through the cytochrome P450 system. Thus, although kidney transplantation is effective in PWH, it requires close monitoring of drug levels and rejection risk.

The HOPE Act was signed into law in November 2013 and implemented in 2015. This legislation allows for the transplantation of kidneys and other organs from donors with HIV to HIV-positive recipients to increase the donor pool, shorten wait time, and make transplantation a viable option for a greater number of patients with ESRD (Cohen et al., 2017). Early outcomes from a multicenter pilot program following 75 PWH who received a kidney from deceased HIV-positive donors have been excellent, with 100% patient survival and 92% graft survival, no differences in 1-year mean eGFR, HIV breakthrough, infectious hospitalizations, or opportunistic infections (Durand et al., 2021; Klitenic et al., 2021). Despite this opportunity for expanded access, an evaluation of demographic and clinical characteristics from the U.S. Renal Data system found that HIV positive status and Black race were independently associated with a lower likelihood of being placed on a transplant waitlist (Shelton et al., 2023). Similarly, a large Canadian study demonstrated a significantly lower likelihood of transplantation among PWH despite no significant difference in allograft failure risk (Hosseini-Moghaddam et al., 2024). Additional details on solid organ transplantation in PWH can be found in Chapter 24, "Solid Organ Transplantation in People with HIV."

RECOMMENDED READING

Heron JE, Bagnis CI, Gracey DM. Contemporary issues and new challenges in chronic kidney disease amongst people living with HIV. *AIDS Res Ther*. 2020;17(1):11.

Wojciechowski D, Ghandi RT, Rosales IA. Case 11-2019: a 49-year-old man with HIV infection and chronic kidney disease. *N Engl J Med*. 2019; 380:1464–1472.

ANTIRETROVIRAL THERAPY-RELATED KIDNEY COMPLICATIONS

ART has been known for many years to cause both acute and chronic kidney injury. This was seen early in the epidemic with several of the PIs, particularly indinavir sulfate. Later it was found that tenofovir disoproxil fumarate (TDF) could cause AKI and proximal, sometimes irreversible, tubular dysfunction. Other agents, as will be discussed below, are not inherently nephrotoxic but can increase serum creatinine levels by blocking tubular secretion. Lastly, with the aging of the HIV population and associated comorbidities, polypharmacy related to ART and medications for other comorbid conditions can increase the risk of acute and chronic kidney disease in PWH.

NUCLEOS(T)IDE REVERSE TRANSCRIPTASE INHIBITORS

TDF is a nucleotide reverse transcriptase inhibitor that is used in PWH and has been associated with CKD. It is cleared by the kidneys via active proximal tubular secretion and glomerular filtration. Because of high renal toxicity rates of its acyclic nucleotide predecessors adefovir and cidofovir, both of which cause AKI and proximal tubular toxicity, there was initial concern regarding the potential renal toxicity of TDF. Early studies did not reveal significant toxicity related to TDF, but after FDA approval, case reports emerged of Fanconi syndrome, kidney injury, and diabetes insipidus (Gaspar et al., 2004; Karras et al., 2003). The active ingredient of TDF is tenofovir (TFV), and nephrotoxicity is proportional to plasma TFV concentrations. TFV undergoes glomerular filtration and active secretion by the renal proximal tubule cells (PTC) via the organic anion transporter pathway. As it accumulates in the renal PTC, TFV alters DNA expression of endothelial nitric oxide synthase, the sodium-phosphorous cotransporter, sodium/hydrogen exchanger 3, and aquaporin 2. TFV toxicity is manifested as intense renal vasoconstriction, phosphaturia, proximal tubular acidosis, polyuria, and impaired urine-concentrating ability (Novick et al., 2017). Proximal tubular dysfunction, which may manifest as a Fanconi syndrome or a limited defect, is the most common manifestation of mitochondrial disease and supports the hypothesis that tenofovir exposure causes mitochondrial dysfunction (Kalyesubula and Perazella, 2011). Fanconi syndrome is characterized by proximal tubular kidney dysfunction, with decreased tubular reabsorption and subsequent urinary wasting of phosphate, glucose, amino acids, bicarbonate, and sodium. This solute loss leads to acidosis, bone disease, and electrolyte abnormalities. When proximal renal tubulopathy is suspected, European guidelines recommend checking serum phosphate, glucose, bicarbonate, uric acid and potassium and urinary phosphate, glucose, pH, uric acid, and potassium (EACS, 2023). Most patients do not develop full Fanconi syndrome but instead manifest primarily with urinary phosphate wasting and, hence, hypophosphatemia in most cases (Waheed and Atta, 2014). This may occur in isolation or in conjunction with AKI. Urinary phosphate wasting is a more sensitive marker of TDF-induced nephrotoxicity because hypophosphatemia is not present in all cases.

Of patients on TDF, 1%–2% will need to stop treatment because of tubulopathy (Hamzah et al., 2017). Risk of development of TDF-induced nephrotoxicity is cumulative, and patients with low $CD4^+$ T-cell counts, advanced age, lower body weight, higher baseline serum creatinine, and those on a PI are most at risk (Heron et al., 2020a; Mocroft et al., 2016).

A long-term follow-up of 23,905 PWH in the Data Collection on Adverse Events of Anti-HIV Drugs (D:A:D) study cohort who initiated antiretrovirals with normal eGFR (>90 mL/min/1.73 m^2) showed a significant increase in the development of CKD with exposure to tenofovir, ritonavir-boosted atazanavir, and ritonavir-boosted lopinavir, but not to other ritonavir-boosted PIs or abacavir (Mocroft et al., 2015). These findings are consistent with previous studies in the cohort and add to the expanding literature on the long-term effects of antiretroviral agents on the kidney.

Tenofovir alafenamide (TAF) is a prodrug of TDF which has potent anti-HIV-1 activity and higher intracellular concentration in peripheral blood mononuclear cells compared to TDF, while maintaining lower plasma concentration (Markowitz et al., 2014). TAF has an increased stability and mean 91% lower plasma concentration of TFV compared to TDF. Additionally, TFV released from TDF undergoes active renal secretion via organic anion transporters (OAT1 and OAT3), leading to higher exposure of renal proximal tubules to TFV and potential for toxicity. Unlike TDF, TAF does not interact with renal transporters OAT1 and OAT3, and, therefore, it may be safer (Bam et al., 2014). An integrated analysis of 26 clinical trials confirmed these differences also impact clinical outcomes, as there were no episodes of proximal tubular nephropathy among patients taking TAF, compared to 10 cases among patients taking TDF (p <.0.001) and fewer discontinuations because of renal side effects among those on TAF compared to TDF (3/6360 vs. 14/2962, p <0.001) (Gupta et al., 2019).

In a randomized controlled trial of PWH who had achieved virologic suppression <50 copies/mL on a TDF-based regimen with a GFR of 50 mL/min/1.73 m^2 or higher, patients were randomly assigned to continue the same ART or were switched to a TAF-based regimen (in combination with elvitegravir, cobicistat, and emtricitabine). The TAF-containing regimen led to continued viral suppression with improvement in bone mineral density and renal function (Mills et al., 2016). Other "switch" studies have also found that laboratory markers of moderately/severely increased proteinuria improved after patients were changed from TDF- to TAF-based ART (Schwarze-Zande et al., 2020). Pilkington and colleagues (2020) completed a meta-analysis of 14 trials evaluating TAF and TDF safety and efficacy when boosted or not boosted. They found that TAF, when boosted by ritonavir or cobicistat and appropriately dose-reduced because of the "boosting" effect these agents have on it, provided a statistically significant improvement in efficacy over dose-unadjusted TDF as part of a boosted ART regimen (p = 0.0004). Of note, this was due almost entirely to increased levels of TFV in the blood, resulting in increased renal side effects occurring with dose-unadjusted TDF given with ritonavir or cobicistat. Virologic efficacy and adverse effects of TAF compared to TDF as part of unboosted ART regimens demonstrated no significant differences in efficacy or adverse effects. Although uncommon, two case reports show that accumulation of TFV from TAF can still be sufficient to cause mitochondrial dysfunction (Bahr and Yarlagadda, 2019; Novick et al., 2017). A more recent case report describes the development of acute proximal renal tubulopathy (PRT) in a patient previously stable on TAF with the addition of gentamycin. This highlights the potential for expected drug-drug interactions that may be observed now that TAF is used more widely (Heron et al., 2020b).

Based on current knowledge of TDF toxicities, there is no absolute consensus regarding the monitoring of kidney function in patients on tenofovir-based ART regimens. Most experts recommend the combination of an every-3-month urine dipstick for glycosuria and proteinuria (the earliest clinical signs of PRT), along with an every-3-months eGFR-based approach. Some advocate for periodic monitoring of additional markers of renal function in all patients on tenofovir regardless of GFR (Fine and Gallant, 2013; Holt et al., 2014). Although the renal toxicity of TDF is mostly reversible upon cessation of this drug, patients often do not achieve their pre-TDF CrCl levels (Waheed and Atta, 2014). The safety of TAF use after TDF-induced PRT is supported by a prospective study in which 31 individuals with TDF-induced PRT and eGFR >30 mL/min/1.73 m^2 were switched to TAF and followed for 96 weeks (Campbell et al., 2024). At the end of observation, all individuals remained on TAF, and none had recurrence of glycosuria or PRT. With the increased availability of TAF-containing single-tablet ART regimens, the use of TDF in the United States has significantly declined. Clinicians should be vigilant regarding monitoring patients for renal toxicity, and consider early ART modification when toxicity is identified.

PROTEASE INHIBITORS

Currently, PIs are used less frequently given the availability of newer and safer antiretroviral drugs, but they still have a role for some PWH, especially those with significant HIV drug resistance. Two PIs, indinavir (IDV) and atazanavir (ATV), can cause urolithiasis. This was most frequently seen with indinavir, one of the first PIs approved by the FDA in 1996, but has also been observed with other PIs (Huynh et al., 2011; Rockwood et al., 2011). With expanded use, indinavir was also associated with progression of CKD. This drug is rarely used in the United States, so its toxicity has become more of historical importance (McLaughlin et al., 2018).

Several studies found nephrotoxicity associated with atazanavir use after its approval in 2003. The largest included 22,603 D:A:D cohort participants with normal baseline kidney function (eGFR >90 mL/min/1.73 m^2) (Mocroft et al., 2010). A decline in eGFR by more than 20 to less than 70 mL/min/1.73 m^2 was associated with the use of tenofovir with ritonavir-boosted atazanavir. An earlier study of the EuroSIDA cohort (a subset of the D:A:D cohort) found similar results in a smaller study of PWH. In a study of a large Veterans Health Administration population, Scherzer and colleagues (2012) showed an association between atazanavir use and rapid GFR decline. The formation of kidney stones with atazanavir use has been well described (Chan-Tack et al., 2007). Therefore, a plausible mechanism for the potential toxicity may be related to the predilection for atazanavir to crystallize in renal interstitial tissues and urine. With many studies confirming an association of nephrotoxicity with atazanavir, close monitoring of renal function in patients taking this PI is recommended. If a decline in GFR or other evidence of nephrotoxicity is noted, it should be discontinued. If a PI is needed to maintain viral suppression, switching to darunavir is recommended (McLaughlin et al., 2018). Additional analyses from the D:A:D cohort demonstrated that DRV/r was not associated with an increased risk of CKD (Ryom et al., 2019b). This is likely to be the case for DRV/c as well, but this was not specifically analyzed.

INTEGRASE STRAND TRANSFER INHIBITORS

Integrase strand transfer inhibitors have become the most commonly used class of drugs to treat HIV infection because of their efficacy, safety, and tolerability. Raltegravir (RAL) was the first FDA-approved integrase strand transfer inhibitor (INSTI), and several studies assessed its effect on renal function. In a retrospective study of 29 PWH started on RAL there was noted a small but nonsignificant increase in serum creatinine (Lindeman et al., 2016). The authors concluded there was no evidence of direct nephrotoxicity, but the increases were likely due to inhibition of renal OCT2.

In a similar fashion, it was subsequently found that another INSTI, dolutegravir, inhibits the tubular secretion of creatinine through the OCT2 pathway at the basolateral membrane of the proximal tubular cells (Rathbun et al., 2014). This raises serum creatinine concentration without affecting the actual GFR. A phase 1 study included 34 healthy individuals who received 50 mg of dolutegravir twice daily or placebo for 14 days (Koteff et al., 2013). Participants received iohexol, which is freely filtered, and para-aminohippurate (PAH) on days 1, 7, and 14, to see if dolutegravir impacted GFR or renal blood flow. Additional tubular function biomarkers, including albumin, cystatin C, and total protein, were also measured. The authors determined that dolutegravir reversibly increased serum creatinine levels by 10%–14% but did not impact renal blood flow or glomerular filtration. This is also seen with bictegravir. As this low-level and transient rise in serum creatinine is due to the temporary effect of membrane transporter inhibition, it is generally not considered to be renal toxicity.

In the SPRING-1 and SPRING-2 clinical trials of treatment-naive PWH, a noticeable rise in serum creatinine was noted in participants who received dolutegravir without any significant clinically adverse effects (Raffi et al., 2013; Stellbrink et al., 2013). The rise in creatinine was typically seen in the first week of therapy, then stabilized thereafter. In the VIKING trial, a similar pattern was noted for PWH who had developed resistance to RAL and were switched to dolutegravir (Eron et al., 2013).

Elvitegravir, another INSTI, is primarily metabolized by the liver into two metabolites. A very small amount is excreted unchanged in the urine (McLaughlin et al., 2018). It is therefore not believed to present any risk of nephrotoxicity. However, it is coadministered with cobicistat, so small increases in serum creatinine in patients taking cobicistat-boosted elvitegravir have been reported (Imaz and Podzamczer, 2017).

Bictegravir is a second-generation INSTI that is currently widely used in the United States and developing countries in both treatment-naive and experienced patients. It has been evaluated in several large phase 3 clinical trials. Co-formulated bictegravir, emtricitabine, and tenofovir alafenamide were compared to dolutegravir-based combination ART in two noninferiority trials (Gallant et al., 2017; Sax et al., 2017). In these studies, the estimated GFR declined by −7.0 mL/min/1.73 m^2 in the bictegravir arm and −11.3 mL/min/1.73 m^2 in the dolutegravir arm at week 48, but there were no patient discontinuations because of kidney-related adverse events and no cases of tubulopathy.

Several subsequent studies evaluated the efficacy and safety of switching to a bictegravir-based regimen from either a dolutegravir-based or PI-based regimen (Daar et al., 2018; Molina et al., 2018). There were no discontinuations of therapy because of renal adverse effects. Changes in serum creatinine, serum eGFR, and urinary markers such as albumin-to-creatinine ratio were also not significant.

PHARMACOKINETIC ENHANCERS

Several antiretrovirals are co-formulated with cobicistat, a potent inhibitor of cytochrome 3A. Cobicistat increases serum levels of specific antiretroviral agents and allows once-daily dosing of these drugs (Johnson and Saravolatz, 2014). Although cobicistat has no inherent nephrotoxicity, it inhibits the cationic renal transporter MATE1 (multidrug and toxin extrusion protein-efflux) at the apical membrane of the proximal tubular cells, which blocks tubular secretion of creatinine (see Figure 31.1) (Lepist et al., 2011). This leads to an increase in plasma creatinine concentration without any effect on the actual GFR. This finding was evaluated in a study of 36 patients in which cobicistat use was associated with an increase in serum creatinine and an approximately 10 mL/min/1.73 m^2 decrease in eGFR. The decrease in eGFR was reversible upon discontinuation of the medication, thus highlighting that this drug has no adverse effect on the actual GFR (German et al., 2010). The timing of the increase in creatinine and subsequent resolution after discontinuation of cobicistat was consistent with altered proximal tubular creatinine secretion.

HIV-1 CAPSID INHIBITORS

Lenacapavir is a novel, first-in-class, long-acting agent recently approved for heavily treatment-experienced patients with multidrug resistance. Pharmacokinetic studies support the

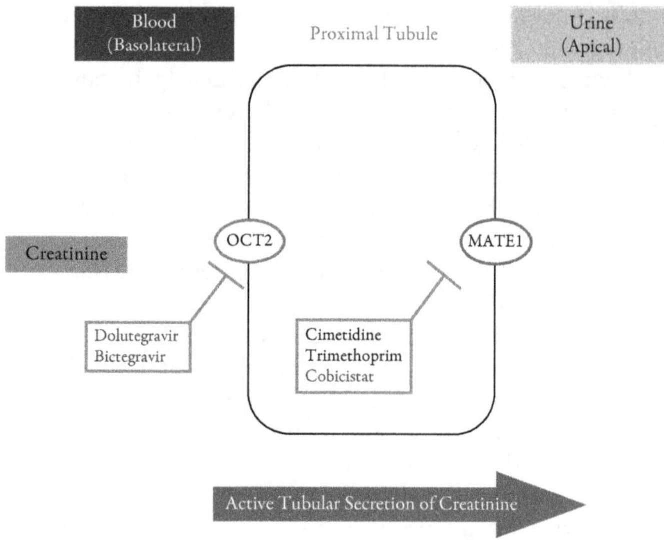

Figure 31.1 Effect of drugs on creatinine secretion. Inhibition of creatinine transporter by drugs shown will result in increase in serum creatinine without GFR effects. Model for effect of tested drugs on creatinine secretion. BCRP = breast cancer resistance protein; MATE = multidrug and toxin extrusion protein; MRP = multidrug resistance protein; OCT = organic cation transporter; OCTN = organic cation/ergothioneine transporter; Pgp = P-glycoprotein. SOURCE: From Lepist EI, et al. Abstract A1-1724. Presented at the 51st Interscience Conference on Antimicrobial Agents and Chemotherapy (ICAAC). Chicago, IL; September 17–20, 2011.

safety of lenacapavir in patients with mild, moderate, and significant kidney disease (Jogiraju et al., 2024).

DOSE ADJUSTMENT OF ART IN RENAL INSUFFICIENCY

Most non-nucleoside reverse transcriptase inhibitors (NNRTIs), integrase inhibitors, and PIs do not require dose modification in CKD or ESRD and can therefore be safely used. The class of NRTIs requires the most attention to determine appropriate renal dosing at various levels of renal insufficiency/impairment. Useful references for selecting ART in the setting of renal impairment include the DHHS Appendix B, Table 12, Antiretroviral Dosing Recommendations in Adults with Renal or Hepatic Insufficiency (DHHS, 2024) and the EACS table on ARV Dosing: Renal Impairment (EACS, 2023). TDF alone or co-formulated with other antiretroviral agents should be avoided in PWH with a CrCl level of less than 50 mL/min and stopped in those with declining eGFR. There may be instances in which other options are not available, and dose adjustments with TDF, including medication administration 3 times weekly, can be considered. In general, the availability of TAF makes this less of a clinical issue for most patients taking tenofovir as part of their ART regimen.

Data gathered from the OPERA cohort now support expanded use of full-dose, 300 mg daily, lamivudine in PWH and an eGFR between 30 and 49 mL/min/1.73 m^2 (Mounzer et al., 2021). Per manufacturer recommendations, patients with this eGFR should receive a dose adjustment to 150 mg daily. Patients receiving full-dose versus adjusted-dose lamivudine experienced more gastrointestinal symptoms and moderate lab abnormalities. However, there were no significant differences in the incidence of lactic acidosis, paresthesia, peripheral neuropathy, pancreatitis, rhabdomyolysis, anemia, neutropenia, thrombocytopenia, nausea, or severe laboratory abnormalities by lamivudine dose (full-dose 300 mg vs. adjusted-dose 150 mg daily, IRR 1.51, 95% CI: 0.59–3.92). Reduced doses of lamivudine are not available in single-tablet regimens, so continued use of full-dose lamivudine at a lower eGFR has a direct impact on pill burden and, subsequently, medication adherence. Clinicians should monitor for side effects if continuing full-dose lamivudine at lower eGFRs, but this is a viable and patient-centered option.

PWH who are taking combination single-tablet regimens often will require separation of the component drugs for individual dosing if they have a decline in renal function. However, a small study (n = 55) found that once-daily single-tablet, elvitegravir/cobicisistat/emtricitabine/tenofovir alafenamide was effective in maintaining virologic suppression in PWH on chronic hemodialysis over 96 weeks of follow-up (Eron et al., 2019). It was well tolerated and associated with improved patient satisfaction. The combination of bictegravir/emtricitabine/tenofovir alafenamide has also been evaluated in a small study of 6 patients on hemodialysis without demonstrated harm (Sidman and Ondrush, 2023). Larger studies would be helpful to determine the best combination regimens in PWH on hemodialysis.

CKD SCREENING AND MONITORING IN PERSONS WITH HIV

Chronic kidney disease may have a prolonged asymptomatic period; therefore, all PWH should be monitored regularly for CKD. Appropriate diagnosis and management of other risk factors for CKD, including diabetes and hypertension, should also be part of routine care for all PWH. In 2017, the Kidney Disease: Improving Global Outcomes (KDIGO) organization made specific recommendations regarding screening and monitoring for renal dysfunction in persons with HIV (Swanepoel, 2018). They noted that kidney disease risk stratification should be considered when choosing an ART regimen, stating that "Standard ART" as recommended by treatment guidelines may be used in those with "low risk" for CKD (eGFR >90 mL/min/1.73 m^2, uPCR <200 mg/g, <50 years of age). Avoidance of potentially nephrotoxic ART agents (e.g., TDF, indinavir, atazanavir, and lopinavir) is recommend in those with "high risk" for CKD (eGFR <70 mL/min/1.73 m^2, uPCR >500 mg/g, >60 years of age, HCV coinfection, DM, uncontrolled HTN, or CVD). Yearly screening of PWH for proteinuria and eGFR is recommended for PWH who are clinically stable and virologically suppressed on ART by the IDSA/HIVMA 2020 Primary Care Guidelines (Thompson et al., 2021), especially people who are at increased risk for developing kidney disease (e.g., Black/African-American patients, CD4$^+$ cell counts <200 cells/µL, viral load >4,000 copies/mL, diabetes mellitus, hypertension, or hepatitis C virus coinfection). Proteinuria can be further quantified by urine albumin to creatinine ratios or urine protein to creatinine ratios. Those at higher risk should have assessment of eGFR screening for proteinuria at least twice per year. All PWH should have renal function reassessed at baseline, then at 1 month after ART modification. People on TDF with a ritonavir or cobicistat-boosted PI should be assessed 2–4 times per year with eGFR, proteinuria, serum phosphorus, urinalysis, and fractional excretion of phosphate (Swanepoel et al., 2018). After review of potentially nephrotoxic medications in PWH with proteinuria and/or advancing renal failure, consider renal ultrasound evaluation to assess for evidence of renal parenchymal disease and referral to nephrology.

RECOMMENDED READING

Wearne N, Davidson B, Blockman M, Swart A, Jones ES. HIV, drugs and the kidney. *Drugs Context.* 2020; 9:2019-11-1. doi:10.7573/dic.2019-11-

REFERENCES

Agarwal R, Fouque D. The foundation and the four pillars of treatment for cardiorenal protection in people with chronic kidney disease and type 2 diabetes. *Nephrol Dial Transplant.* 2023;38(2):253–257.

Atta MG, Fine DM, Kirk GD, et al. Survival during renal replacement therapy among African Americans infected with HIV type 1 in urban Baltimore, Maryland. *Clin Infect Dis.* 2007;45(12):1625–1632.

Atta MG, Lucas GM, Fine DM. HIV-associated nephropathy: epidemiology, pathogenesis, diagnosis and management. *Expert Rev Anti Infect Ther.* 2008;6(3):365–371.

Bahr NC, Yarlagadda SG. Fanconi syndrome and tenofovir alafenamide: a case report. *Ann Intern Med.* 2019;170(11):814–815.

Balow JE. Nephropathy in the context of HIV infection. *Kidney Int.* 2005;67(4):1632–1633.

Bam RA, Birkus G, Babusis D, et al. Metabolism and antiretroviral activity of tenofovir alafenamide in CD4\+ T-cells and macrophages from demographically diverse donors. *Antivir Ther.* 2014;19(7):669–677.

Becker S, Fusco G, Fusco J, et al. HIV-associated thrombotic microangiopathy in the era of highly active antiretroviral therapy: an observational study. *Clin Infect Dis.* 2004;39(Suppl 5):S267–S275.

Bige N, Lanternier F, Viard JP, et al. Presentation of HIV-associated nephropathy and outcome in HAART-treated patients. *Nephrol Dial Transplant.* 2012. 27(3):1114–1121.

Blumberg EA, Rogers CC; American Society of Transplantation Infectious Diseases Community of Practice. Solid organ transplantation in the HIV-infected patient: guidelines from the American Society of Transplantation Infectious Diseases Community of Practice. *Clin Transplant.* 2019;33(9):e13499.

Briggs WA, Tanawattanacharoen S, Choi MJ, et al. Clinicopathologic correlates of prednisone treatment of human immunodeficiency virus-associated nephropathy. *Am J Kidney Dis.* 1996;28(4):618–621.

Bruggeman LA, Dikman S, Meng C, et al. Nephropathy in human immunodeficiency virus-1 transgenic mice is due to renal transgene expression. *J Clin Invest.* 1997;100(1):84–92.

Campbell L, Barbini B, Cromarty B, et al.; FANTA trial team. Safety of tenofovir alafenamide in people with HIV who experienced proximal renal tubulopathy on tenofovir disoproxil. *AIDS.* 2024 Jul 15;38(9):1442–1445.

Campos P, Ortiz A, Soto K. HIV and kidney diseases: 35 years of history and consequences. *Clin Kidney J.* 2016;9(6):772–781.

Chan-Tack KM, Truffa MM, Struble KA, et al. Atazanavir-associated nephrolithiasis: cases from the US Food and Drug Administration's Adverse Event Reporting System. *AIDS.* 2007;21(9):1215–1218.

Choi AI, Rodriguez RA, Bacchetti P, et al. The impact of HIV on chronic kidney disease outcomes. *Kidney Int.* 2007;72(11):1380–1387.

Cohen SD, Kopp JB, Kimmel PL. Kidney diseases associated with human immunodeficiency virus infection. *N Engl J Med.* 2017;377(24):2363–2375.

Daar ES, DeJesus E, Ruane P, et al. Efficacy and safety of switching to fixed-dose bictegravir, emtricitabine, and tenofovir alafenamide from boosted protease inhibitor-based regimens in virologically suppressed adults with HIV-1: 48-week results of a randomised, open-label, multicenter, phase 3, non-inferiority trial. *Lancet HIV.* 2018;5(7):347–356.

D'Agati V, Suh J, Carbone L, et al. Pathology of HIV-associated nephropathy: a detailed morphologic and comparative study. *Kidney Int.* 1989;35(6):1358–1370.

Delgado C, Baweja M, Crews DC, et al. A unifying approach for gfr estimation: recommendations of the NKF-ASN Task Force on reassessing the inclusion of race in diagnosing kidney disease. *J Am Soc Nephrol.* 2021;32(12):2994–3015.

Dragović G, Srdić D, Al Musalhi K, et al. Higher levels of cystatin C in HIV/AIDS patients with metabolic syndrome. *Basic Clin Pharmacol Toxicol.* 2018;122:396–401.

Durand CM, Zhang W, Brown DM, et al. A prospective multicenter pilot study of HIV-positive deceased donor to HIV-positive recipient kidney transplantation: HOPE in action. *Am J Transplant.* 2021;21(5):1754–1764.

Eron JJ, Clotet B, Katlama C, et al. Safety and efficacy of dolutegravir in treatment-experienced subjects with ratlegravir-resistant HIV type 1 infection: 24-week results of the VIKING study. *J infect Dis.* 2013;207(5):740–748.

Eron JJ, Lelievre JD, Kalayjian R. Longer-term safety and efficacy of elvitegravir/cobicistat/emtricitabine/ tenofovir alafenamide in virologically suppressed adults living with HIV and ESRD on chronic hemodialysis. *Open Forum Infect Dis.* 2019;6(S-2);864.

European AIDS Clinical Society. Guidelines on kidney disease: definition, diagnosis and management. https://eacs.sanfordguide.com/prevention-non-infectious-co-morbidities/renal-complications/kidney-disease. Published 2023. Accessed July 31, 2024.

Eustace JA, Nuermberger E, Choi M, et al. Cohort study of the treatment of severe HIV-associated nephropathy with corticosteroids. *Kidney Int.* 2000;58(3):1253–1260.

Feng J, Bao L, Wang X, et al. Low expression of HIV genes in podocytes accelerates the progression of diabetic kidney disease in mice. *Kidney Int.* 2021;99(4):914–925.

Fine DM, Gallant JE. Nephrotoxicity of antiretroviral agents: is the list getting longer? *J Infect Dis.* 2013;207(9):1349–1351.

Fine DM, Perazella MA, Lucas GM, et al. Kidney biopsy in HIV: beyond HIV-associated nephropathy. *Am J Kidney Dis.* 2008;51(3): 504–514.

Freedman BI, Julian BA, Pastan SO, et al. Apolipoprotein L1 gene variants in deceased organ donors are associated with renal allograft failure. *Am J Transplant.* 2015;15(6):1615–1622.

Freedman BI, Moxey-Mims MM, Alexander AA, et al. *APOL1* Long-Term Kidney Transplantation Outcomes Network (APOLLO): design and rationale. *Kidney Int Rep.* 2019;5(3):278–288.

Friedman DJ, Pollak MR. APOL1 nephropathy: from genetics to clinical applications. *Clini J Am Soc Nephrol.* 2021;16(2):294–303.

Gallant JE, Lazzarin A, Mills A, et al. Bictegravir, emtricitabine, and tenofovir alafenamide versus dolutegravir, abacavir, and lamivudine for initial treatment of HIV-1 infection (GS-US-380-1489): a double-blind, multicentre, phase 3, randomised controlled non-inferiority trial. *Lancet.* 2017;390(10107):2063–2072.

Gaspar G, Monereo A, Garcia-Reyne A, et al. Fanconi syndrome and acute renal failure in a patient treated with tenofovir: a call for caution. *AIDS.* 2004;18:351–352.

Genovese G, Friedman DJ, Ross MD, et al. Association of trypanolytic ApoL1 variants with kidney disease in African Americans. *Science.* 2010;329(5993):841–845.

German P, Warren D, West S, et al. Pharmacokinetics and bioavailability of an integrase and novel pharmacoenhancer-containing single-tablet fixed-dose combination regimen for the treatment of HIV. *J AIDS.* 2010;55(3):323–329.

Gupta SK, Post FA, Arribas JR, et al. Renal safety of tenofovir alafenamide vs. tenofovir disoproxil fumarate: a pooled analysis of 26 clinical trials. *AIDS*. 2019;33(9):1455–1465.

Hamzah L, Jose S, Booth JW, et al. Treatment-limiting renal tubulopathy in patients treated with tenofovir disoproxil fumarate. *J Infect*. 2017;74(5):492–500.

Heron JE, Bagnis CI, Gracey DM. Contemporary issues and new challenges in chronic kidney disease amongst people living with HIV. *AIDS Res Ther*. 2020a;17(1):11.

Heron JE, Bloch M, Vanguru V, et al. Renal proximal tubulopathy in an HIV-infected patient treated with tenofovir alafenamide and gentamicin: a case report. *BMC Nephrol*. 2020b;21(1):339.

Holt SG, Gracey DM, Levy MT, et al. A consensus statement on the renal monitoring of Australian patients receiving tenofovir based antiviral therapy for HIV/HBV infection. *AIDS Res Ther*. 2014;11:35.

Hosseini-Moghaddam SM, Kang Y, Bota SE, Weir MA. Renal transplantation in HIV-positive and HIV-negative people with advanced stages of kidney disease: equity in transplantation. *Open Forum Infect Dis*. 2024;11(5):ofae182.

Huynh J, Hever A, Tom T, et al. Indinavir-induced nephrolithiasis three and one-half years after cessation of indinavir therapy. *Int Urol Nephrol*. 2011;43(2):571–573.

Imaz A, Podzamczer D. Tenofovir alafenamide, emtricitabine, elvitegravir and cobicistat combination therapy for the treatment of HIV. *Expert Rev Anti Infect Ther*. 2017;15(3):195–209.

Inker LA, Eneanya ND, Coresh J, et al. New creatinine- and cystatin c-based equations to estimate GFR without race. *N Engl J Med*. 2021;385(19):1737–1749.

Izzedine H, Acharya V, Wirden M, et al. Role of HIV-1 DNA levels as clinical marker of HIV-1-associated nephropathies. *Nephrol Dial Transplant*. 2011;26(2):580–583.

Jogiraju V, Weber E, Hindman J, et al. Pharmacokinetics of long-acting lenacapavir in participants with hepatic or renal impairment. *Antimicrob Agents Chemother*. 2024;68(4):e0134423.

Johnson LB, Saravolatz LD. The quad pill, a once-daily combination therapy for HIV infection. *Clin Infect Dis*. 2014;58(1):93–98.

Kalayjian RC. Renal issues in HIV infection. *Curr HIV AIDS Rep*. 2011;8(3):164–171.

Kalyesubula R, Perazella MA. Nephrotoxicity of HAART. *AIDS Res Treat*. 2011;2011:562790.

Karras A, Lafaurie M, Furco A, et al. Tenfovir-related nephrotoxicity in human immunodeficiency virus-infected patients: three cases of renal failure, Fanconi syndrome, and nephrogenic diabetes insipidus. *Clin Infect Dis*. 2003;36:1070–1073.

Kimmel PL, Mishkin GJ, Umana WO. Captopril and renal survival in patients with human immunodeficiency virus nephropathy. *Am J Kidney Dis*. 1996;28(2):202–208.

Klitenic SB, Levan ML, Van Pilsum Rasmussen SE, Durand CM. Science over stigma: lessons and future direction of HIV-to-HIV transplantation. *Curr Transplant Rep*. 2021;8(4):314–323.

Kopp JB, Nelson GW, Sampath K, et al. Genetic variants in focal segmental glomerulosclerosis and HIV-associated nephropathy. *J Am Soc Nephrol*. 2011;22(11):2129–2137.

Koteff J, Borland J, Chen S, et al. A phase 1 study to evaluate the effect of dolutegravir on renal function via measured iohexol and PAH clearance in healthy subjects. *Br J Clin Pharmacol*. 2013;75:990–996.

Ku E, Inker LA, Tighiouart H, et al. Angiotensin-converting enzyme inhibitors or angiotensin-receptor blockers for advanced chronic kidney disease: a systematic review and retrospective individual participant-level meta-analysis of clinical trials. *Ann Intern Med*. 2024;177(7):953–963.

Kudose S, Santoriello, Bomback AS, et al. The spectrum of kidney biopsy findings in HIV-infected patients in the modern era. *Kidney Int*. 2020;97(5):1006–1016.

Kupin WL. Viral-associated GN: hepatitis C and HIV. *Clin J Am Soc Nephrol*. 2017;12(8):1337–1342. doi:10.2215/CJN.04320416

Lepist EI, Murray BP, Tong L, et al. Effect of cobicistat and ritonavir on proximal renal tubular cell uptake and efflux transporters. Abstract A1-1724. Presented at the 51st Interscience Conference on Antimicrobial Agents and Chemotherapy (ICAAC). Chicago, IL; September 17–20, 2011.

Lescure FX, Flateau C, Pacanowski J, et al. HIV-associated kidney glomerular diseases: changes with time and HAART. *Nephrol Dial Transplant*. 2012;27:2349–2355.

Lindeman TA, Dugan JM, Sahloff EG. Evaluation of serum creatinine changes with integrase inhibitor use in HIV-1 infected adults. *Open Forum Infect Dis*. 2016;3(2):1–3.

Locke JE, James NT, Mannon RB, et al. Immunosuppression regimen and the risk of acute rejection in HIV-infected kidney transplant recipients. *Transplantation*. 2014;97(4):446–450.

Locke JE, Mehta S, Reed RD, et al. l A national study of outcomes among HIV-infected kidney transplant recipients. *J Am Soc Nephrol*. 2015;26(9):2222–2229.

Longenecker CT, Scherzer R, Bacchetti P, et al. HIV viremia and changes in kidney function. *AIDS*. 2009;23(9):1089–1096.

Lopes JA, Melo MJ, Raimundo M, et al. Long-term risk of mortality for acute kidney injury in HIV-infected patients: a cohort analysis. *BMC Nephrol*. 2013;14:32.

Lucas GM, Eustace JA, Sozio S, et al. Highly active antiretroviral therapy and the incidence of HIV-1-associted nephropathy: a 12-year cohort study. *AIDS*. 2004;18(3):541–546.

Makris K, Spanou L. Acute kidney injury: definition, pathophysiology, and clinical phenotypes. *Clin Biochem Review*. 2016;37(2):85–98.

Mallipattu SK, Salem F, Wyatt CM. The changing epidemiology of HIV-related chronic kidney disease in the era of antiretroviral therapy. *Kidney Int*. 2014;86(2):259–265.

Markowitz M, Zolopa A, Squires K, et al. Phase I/II study of the pharmacokinetics, safety and antiretroviral activity of tenofovir alafenamide, a new prodrug of the HIV reverse transcriptase inhibitor tenofovir, in HIV-infected adults. *J Antimicrob Chemother*. 2014;69(5):1362–1369.

McCutcheon K, Nqebelele U, Murray L, et al. Cardiac and renal comorbidities in aging people living with HIV. *Circ Res*. 2024;134(11):1636–1660.

McLaughlin MM, Guerrero AJ, Merker A. Renal effects of non-tenofovir antiretroviral therapy in patients living with HIV. *Drugs Context*. 2018;7:1–15.

Medapalli RK, He JC, Klotman JP. HIV-associated nephropathy: pathogenesis. *Curr Opin Nephrol Hypertens*. 2011;20(3):306–311.

Medapalli RK, Parikh CR, Gordon K, et al. Comorbid diabetes and the risk of progressive chronic kidney disease in HIV-infected adults: data from the Veterans Aging Cohort Study. *J Acquir Immune Defic Syndr*. 2012;60(4):393–399.

Mills A, Arribas JR, Andrade-Villanueva J, et al. Switching from tenofovir disoproxil fumarate to tenofovir alafenamide in antiretroviral regimens for virologically suppressed adults with HIV-1 infection: a randomised, active-controlled, multicentre, open-label, phase 3, non-inferiority study. *Lancet Infect Dis*. 2016;16(1):43–52.

Mocroft A, Kirk O, Reiss P, et al. Estimated glomerular filtration rate, chronic kidney disease and antiretroviral drug use in HIV-positive patients. *AIDS*. 2010;24(11):1667–1678.

Mocroft A, Lundgren JD, Ross M, et al. Cumulative and current exposure to potentially nephrotoxic antiretrovirals and development of chronic kidney disease in HIV-positive individuals with a normal baseline estimated glomerular filtration rate: a prospective international cohort study. *Lancet HIV*. 2016;3(1):e23–e32.

Mocroft A, Lundgren JD, Ross M, et al.; D:A:D Study Group Royal Free Hospital Clinic Cohort, Insight Study Group, Smart Study Group and Espirit Study Group. Development and validation of a risk score for chronic kidney disease in HIV infection using protective cohort data from the D:A:D study. *PLoS Med*. 2015;12(3):e1001809.

Molina JM, Ward D, Brar I, et al. Switching to fixed-dose bictegravir, emtricitabine, and tenofovir alafenamide from dolutegravir plus abacavir and lamivudine in virologically suppressed adults with HIV-1: 48-week results of a randomised, double-blind, multicentre, active-controlled, phase 3, non-inferiority trial. *Lancet HIV*. 2018;5(7):357–365.

Mounzer K, Brunet L, Wyatt CM, et al. To dose-adjust or not to dose-adjust: lamivudine dose in kidney impairment. *AIDS*. 2021;35(8):1201–1208.
Naicker S, Fabian J. Risk factors for the development of chronic kidney disease with HIV/AIDS. *Clin Nephrol*. 2010;74(Suppl 1):S51–S56.
Ndlovu KCZ, Assounga A. Continuous ambulatory peritoneal dialysis in patients with HIV and end-stage renal failure. *Perit Dial Int*. 2017;37(3):321–330.
NovickT K, Choi MJ, Rosenberg AZ, et al. Tenofovir alafenamide nephrotoxicity in an HIV-positive patient. *Medicine*. 2017;96(36):e8046.
Palich R, Tubiana R, Abdi B, et al. Plasma cystatin C as a marker for estimated glomerular filtration rate assessment in HIV-1-infected patients treated with dolutegravir-based ART. *J Antimicrob Chemother*. 2018;73(7):1935–1939.
Panel on Antiretroviral Guidelines for Adults and Adolescents. Guidelines for the use of antiretroviral agents in adults and adolescents with HIV. Department of Health and Human Services. https://clinicalinfo.hiv.gov/en/guidelines/adult-and-adolescent-arv. Updated February 27, 2024. Accessed July 31, 2024.
Papeta N, Kiryluk K, Patel A, et al. APOL1 variants increase risk for FSGS and HIVAN but not IgA nephropathy. *J Am Soc Nephrol*. 2011;22(11):1991–1996.
Park LS, Hernández-Ramírez RU, Silverberg MJ, Crothers K, Dubrow R. Prevalence of non-HIV cancer risk factors in persons living with HIV/AIDS: a meta-analysis. *AIDS*. 2016;30(2):273–291.
Pilkington V, Hughes SL, Pepperrell T, et al. Tenofovir alafenamide vs. tenofovir disoproxil fumarate: an updated meta-analysis of 14 894 patients across 14 trials. *AIDS*. 2020;34(15):2259–2268.
Post FA, Holt SG. Recent developments in HIV and the kidney. *Curr Opin Infect Dis*. 2009;22(1):43–48.
Raffi F, Rachlis A Stellbrink HJ, et al. Once-daily dolutegravir versus raltegravir in antiretroviral-naïve adults with HIV-1 infection: 48-week results from the randomized, double-blind, non-inferiority SPRING-2 Study. *Lancet*. 2013;381(9868):735–743.
Rao TK, Filippone EJ, Nicastri AD, et al. Associated focal and segmental glomerulosclerosis in the acquired immunodeficiency syndrome. *N Engl J Med*. 1984;310(11):669–673.
Rathbun RC, Lockhart SM, Miller MM, et al. Dolutegravir, a second-generation integrase inhibitor for the treatment of HIV-1 infection. *Ann Pharmacother*. 2014;48(3):395–403.
Razzak CS, Workeneh BT, Montez-Rath ME, et al. Trends in the out-comes of end-stage renal disease secondary to HIV-associated nephropathy. *Nephrol Dial Transplant*. 2015;30:1734–1740.
Rockwood N, Mandalia S, Bower M, et al. Ritonavir-boosted atazanavir exposure is associated with an increased rate of renal stones compared with efavirenz, ritonavir-boosted lopinavir and ritonavir-boosted darunavir. *AIDS*. 2011;25(13):1671–1673.
Ross MJ, Klotman PE. Recent progress in HIV-associated nephropathy. *J Am Soc Nephrol*. 2002;13(12):2997–3004.
Ryom L, Dilling Lundgren J, Reiss P, et al. Use of contemporary protease inhibitors and risk of incident chronic kidney disease in persons with human immunodeficiency virus: the Data Collection on Adverse Events of Anti-HIV Drugs (D:A:D) study. *J Infect Dis*. 2019b;220(10):1629–1634.
Ryom L, Lundgren JD, Law M, et al. Serious clinical events in HIV-positive persons with chronic kidney disease. *AIDS*. 2019a;33(14):2173–2188.
Sax PE, Erlandson KM, Lake JE, et al. Weight gain following initiation of antiretroviral therapy: risk factors in randomized comparative clinical trials. *Clin Infect Dis*. 2020;71(6):1379–1389.
Sax PE, Pozniak A, Montes ML, et al. Co-formulated bictegravir, emtricitabine, and tenofovir alafenamide versus dolutegravir with emtricitabine and tenofovir alafenamide, for initial treatment of HIV-1 infection (GS-US-380-1490): a randomised, double-blind, multicentre, phase 3, non-inferiority trial. *Lancet*. 2017;390(10107):2073–2082.
Scherzer R, Estrella M, Li Y, et al. Association of tenofovir exposure with kidney disease risk in HIV infection. *AIDS*. 2012;26(7):867–875.
Schwarze-Zander C, Piduhn H, Boesecke C, et al. Switching tenofovir disoproxil fumarate to tenofovir alafenamide in a real-life setting: what are the implications? *HIV Med*. 2020;21(6):378–385.
Shelton BA, Becker DJ, MacLennan PA, et al. Racial disparities in access to the kidney transplant waitlist among people with human immunodeficiency virus. *AIDS Patient Care STDs*. 2023;37(8):394–402.
Sidman EF, Ondrush NM. Utilization of bictegravir/emtricitabine/tenofovir alafenamide in patients with end-stage renal disease on hemodialysis. *Am J Health Syst Pharm*. 2023;80(9):e92–e97.
Stellbrink HJ, Reynes J, Lazzarin A, et al. Dolutegravir in antiretroviral-naive adults with HIV-1: 96-week results from a randomized dose-ranging study. *AIDS*. 2013;27(11):1771–1778.
Strategies for Management of Antiretroviral Therapy (SMART) Study Group. CD4\+ count-guided interruption of antiretroviral treatment. *N Engl J Med*. 2006;355(22):2283–2296.
Swanepoel CR, Atta MG, D'Agati, et al. Kidney disease in the setting of HIV infection: conclusions from a Kidney Disease: Improving Global Outcomes (KDIGO) Patient Controversies Conference. *Kidney Int*. 2018;22(6):84–100.
Thompson MA, Horberg MA, Agwu AL, et al. Primary Care guidance for persons with human immunodeficiency virus: 2020 update by the HIV Medicine Association of the Infectious Diseases Society of America. *Clin Infect Dis*. 2021;73(11):e3572–e3605.
Tzur S, Rosset S, Shemer R, et al. Missense mutations in the APOL1 gene are highly associated with end stage kidney disease risk previously attributed to the MYH9 gene. *Hum Genet*. 2010;128(3):345–350.
Waheed S, Atta MG. Predictors of HIV-associated nephropathy. *Expert Rev Anti-Infect Ther*. 2014;12(5):555–563.
Wei A, Burns G, Williams CM, et al. Long-term renal survival in HIV-associated nephropathy with angiotensin-converting enzyme inhibition. *Kidney Int*. 2003;64(4):1462–1471.
Wyatt CM, Hoover DR, Shi Q, et al. Pre-existing albuminuria predicts AIDS and non-AIDS mortality in women initiating antiretroviral therapy. *Antiviral Ther*. 2011;16(4):591–596.
Wyatt CM, Winston J. Renal disease in patients with HIV. *Curr Infect Dis Rep*. 2006;8(1):76–81. doi:10.1007/s11908-006-0038-0
Zheng X, Gong L, Xue W, et al. Kidney transplant outcomes in HIV-positive patients: a systematic review and meta-analysis. *AIDS Res Ther*. 2019;16(1):37.

32.

ENDOCRINE DISORDERS AND METABOLIC COMPLICATIONS IN HIV

Daniel Lee

CHAPTER GOAL

Upon completion of this chapter, the reader should be able to:

- Describe the spectrum of prevalent endocrine and metabolic complications affecting people with HIV (PWH).
- Explain the mechanisms and clinical management of endocrine and metabolic diseases in PWH.
- Discuss the mechanism and clinical management of body weight changes (weight loss and weight gain) and body composition changes (lipodystrophy).

WHAT'S NEW?

- Non-alcoholic fatty liver disease, now referred to as metabolic dysfunction-associated steatotic liver disease (MASLD), remains prevalent among PWH.
- Although incidence and prevalence of HIV-associated wasting and lipodystrophy are lower in the contemporary ART era, these conditions still exist in some PWH.
- Weight gain in people with well-controlled HIV infection has become more concerning as people continue to age with HIV.

KEY POINTS

- The endocrine and metabolic complications of HIV infection are changing, with newer phenomena emerging as PWH live longer.
- HIV infection, ARVs, and other factors play a role in the development of endocrine and metabolic disorders.
- MASLD is particularly prevalent in PWH and has potential downstream consequences if not diagnosed and addressed appropriately.
- HIV-associated wasting and lipodystrophy are less common in the contemporary ART era, but providers should remain aware of these conditions and recommended treatment strategies.
- Weight gain in PWH has become a growing concern, given associated cardiometabolic risks.

INTRODUCTION

With the advent of effective antiretroviral (ARV) therapeutic regimens, HIV infection has become a chronic disease. People with HIV (PWH) have longer life expectancies and are developing endocrine and metabolic abnormalities that are prevalent among aging adults. The underlying etiology of these disorders can be attributed to multiple factors, including the effects of HIV itself, antiretroviral therapies (ART), inflammation, endothelial and immune dysfunction, and mitochondrial dysfunction. Since endocrine disorders often develop insidiously, clinical suspicion and appropriate testing are necessary for accurate diagnosis and management, which should include the participation of an endocrinologist when possible. New emerging phenotypes are being observed, with an increase in the incidence and prevalence of metabolic diseases such as central obesity, metabolic syndrome, and fatty liver disease. Weight gain has been more commonly reported, while HIV-associated lipodystrophy and HIV-associated wasting appear less commonly. There are also reports of "premature or accelerated aging," in which relatively younger PWH develop geriatric complications typically seen in people without HIV who are 20–30 years older. These include physical decline, mitochondrial dysfunction, muscle weakness, inflammation, endothelial dysfunction, insulin resistance, and cognitive decline. This chapter describes historical and current perspectives on endocrine and metabolic disorders in HIV infection, including alterations in body weight and body composition, and discusses mechanisms, emerging complications, and therapeutic strategies.

ENDOCRINE AND METABOLIC DISEASE IN HIV

Although HIV infection has been associated with endocrine and metabolic complications since the 1980s, these complications have changed dynamically as a result of improvements in pharmacotherapy and increasing life span, and other unknown contributors. Of note has been an increase in cardiometabolic complications, premature/accelerated aging, fatty liver disease, and metabolic syndrome, but the underlying mechanisms for many of these disorders are still not completely understood. PWH also continue to have more conventional endocrine disorders such as diabetes, thyroid disease, adrenal and pituitary conditions, bone disease, and gonadal disorders.

Elevations in inflammation and abnormalities in immune function in PWH could be contributing in part to some of these disorders; elevated proinflammatory cytokines and abnormalities in immune phenomena that affect endocrine function were observed in early studies (Merrill et al., 1989; Salim et al., 1988; Tracey and Cerami, 1990). For example, interleukin-1 (IL-1) has been shown to increase adrenocorticotropic hormone (ACTH) in cultured pituitary cells (Meyer et al., 1987; Szebeni et al., 1991). Other pituitary hormones may also be affected; effects include prolactin elevations (Parra et al., 2004) and deficient growth hormone secretion (Koutkia et al., 2004). HIV-positive mononuclear cells can increase interferon-α (Grunfeld et al., 1992) and impair glucocorticoid receptor activity (Norbiato et al., 1996), and abnormalities in IL-1 and tumor necrosis factor (TNF) can inhibit gonadal steroidogenesis (Calkins et al., 1988; Hales, 1992; Xiong and Hales, 1993).

Opportunistic infections may also contribute to the development of HIV-related endocrine disorders in people with advanced HIV infection. For example, cytomegalovirus (CMV) infection predisposes to an increased risk of developing adrenalitis (Glasgow et al., 1985). Infections caused by mycobacterial pathogens may also affect adrenal function, whereas CMV, cryptococcal, and toxoplasma infections can affect the central nervous system and manifest as pituitary disease (Giampalmo et al., 1990). CMV infection has been linked to hypernatremia, likely through a reset osmostat (Keuneke et al., 1999). *Pneumocystis jiroveci* has also been linked rarely to thyroiditis (Drucker et al., 1990).

PWH are also experiencing an increase in the incidence and prevalence of metabolic disorders including centripetal fat accumulation as in metabolic syndrome, fatty liver disease, and mitochondrial dysfunction. Underlying mechanisms remain poorly understood, and effective interventions are lacking. With early HIV treatment initiation and use of newer antiretroviral agents, HIV-associated lipodystrophy and wasting are now seen less frequently. Nevertheless, they may still be observed in some PWH and should be identified and managed appropriately. Studies are critically needed to guide relevant clinical trials to facilitate the identification of mechanisms and cultivate therapeutic strategies for these wide-ranging complications.

Although the development and clinical use of contemporary ART have led to significant morbidity and mortality benefits for PWH in general, these benefits are also associated with important metabolic complications, particularly dyslipidemia and body morphology changes ranging from lipodystrophy to central obesity in the context of metabolic syndrome. HIV providers should, therefore, be familiar with the role of ARV drugs, as prevention and early identification are key to appropriate clinical management should these ARV-related complications arise.

PROTEASE INHIBITORS

Early use of protease inhibitors (PIs) led to observations of abnormalities in total body fat distribution, most notably an increase in abdominal fat, sometimes described colloquially as the "protease paunch" (Mishriki, 1998) or "Crixivan belly" (Huff, 1997–1998). Since then, the PI class has been linked to the development of abdominal obesity and biochemical abnormalities such as severe hypertriglyceridemia, dyslipidemia, insulin resistance, and diabetes. Many PIs, including lopinavir/ritonavir, nelfinavir, amprenavir, and saquinavir, are metabolized by the hepatic cytochrome 450 CYP3A4 isoenzyme pathway. PIs have also been shown to directly impact insulin resistance. For example, indinavir can inhibit GLUT4 activity and thus impair insulin-stimulated glucose uptake and predispose to hyperglycemia (Caron et al., 2001; Murata et al., 2000). In addition to their permissive role in metabolic and glycemic abnormalities, PIs have been implicated in the development of prolactin abnormalities (Hutchinson et al., 2000) and osteomalacia (Cozzolino et al., 2003).

NUCLEOSIDE REVERSE TRANSCRIPTASE INHIBITORS

Nucleoside reverse transcriptase inhibitors (NRTIs) may induce changes in body morphology. For example, stavudine (no longer commonly used) has been linked to lipoatrophy (Saint-Marc et al., 1999). NRTIs have also been linked to the development of mitochondrial dysfunction (Mallon et al., 2005), which may manifest as glucose and lipid metabolism abnormalities (Sekhar et al., 2002; Shikuma et al., 2001).

NON-NUCLEOSIDE REVERSE TRANSCRIPTASE INHIBITORS

Non-nucleoside reverse transcriptase inhibitors (NNRTIs) are generally the most metabolically neutral class of ART. However, older reports linked them to dyslipidemia (Padmapriyadarsini et al., 2011) and fat depletion in 3T3-L1 cells (Minami et al., 2011).

INTEGRASE INHIBITORS

Integrase inhibitors have been associated with significant weight gain in some studies. NA-ACCORD, a large observational cohort study in the United States and Canada, compared 22,972 ART-naive adult PWH who initiated integrase strand transfer inhibitor (INSTI), PI, or NNRTI-based ART. Investigators found that, compared to PI and NNRTI drugs, INSTIs were associated with a high degree of weight gain (Bourgi et al., 2020a). Given increasing global use of dolutegravir, some analyses have specifically focused on this agent: weight gain has been observed among PWH on dolutegravir-based regimens (Bourgi et al., 2020b). Ongoing studies are being conducted to determine whether ART switches off INSTI-inclusive regimens lead to changes in weight.

ENDOCRINE DISORDERS IN HIV

Any endocrine or metabolic disorder can affect PWH, including diabetes, metabolic syndrome, disorders of adrenal, thyroid, pituitary, and gonadal function, and bone and dyslipidemia. Bone disorders and dyslipidemia are discussed in chapters 29 and 33, respectively.

DIABETES MELLITUS

The prevalence of diabetes mellitus (DM) is increasing in PWH worldwide, affecting several adult age groups, including people in their 30s (Mathabire Rücker et al., 2018; Tzur et al., 2015). Earlier findings, such as those from the Multicenter AIDS Cohort Study (MACS), found that exposure to ART resulted in a 14% incidence of DM in men with HIV (Brown et al., 2005). More recent publications have estimated this to be as high as 15.1%, with a relative risk of 2.4 compared to the general population (Duncan et al., 2018). One study from India found that PWH with lower $CD4^+$ T-cell counts had significantly higher glycemia and insulin resistance (Bajaj et al., 2020). A meta-analysis evaluating gestational diabetes in pregnant women with HIV found a high pooled prevalence (Biadgo et al., 2019). Although reasons for the meteoric rise in DM incidence are likely multifactorial, one meta-analysis implicated ART as potentially the single most consistent determinant of DM in PWH worldwide (Nduka et al., 2017).

While integrase strand transfer inhibitors (INSTIs) are felt to be more metabolically neutral as a class compared to older thymidine analogs and PIs, data are conflicting on whether INSTIs increase the risk of diabetes. One Medicaid database study found that PWH receiving INSTIs were 31% more likely to develop new onset diabetes or hyperglycemia within 6 months of ART initiation (O'Halloran et al., 2022). Case reports have described accelerated hyperglycemia and diabetes linked to bictegravir (Nolan et al., 2021). By contrast, a recent systematic review and meta-analysis examining the association between INSTIs and insulin resistance and incident diabetes mellitus in PWH did not find an association; in fact, INSTI therapy was associated with a lower risk of incident diabetes in multiple studies (Mulindwa et al., 2023).

Importantly, some data suggest that glycosylated hemoglobin (HbA1c) may not accurately estimate glycemia in PWH (Kim et al., 2009; Slama et al., 2014) and may be affected by particular antiretroviral agents. One MACS study found that HbA1c underestimated glycemia in men with HIV (Slama et al., 2014). Another investigation involving adults with type 2 diabetes found similar results (Kim et al., 2009). Collectively, evidence to date indicates an increase in the incidence and prevalence of DM among PWH and suggests that relying solely on HbA1c could lead to underdiagnosing and undertreating diabetes. As such, providers should carefully screen for hyperglycemia and diabetes in PWH and not rely solely on HbA1c for screening. Instead, HbA1c should be correlated with other measures of glycemic control (including fasting and prandial glucose levels) for a reliable and comprehensive assessment of glycemic status and control. For pregnant women with HIV, early screening for gestational diabetes is vital to reduce complications.

Overall DM management in PWH is similar to that in persons without HIV, and ideally involves a multidisciplinary team, including a diabetes educator, dietitian, prescribing clinician/physician, and diabetes nursing staff. Cornerstones of management include exercise, diet, and pharmacotherapy. Long-term end-organ complications such as retinopathy, nephropathy, neuropathy, and coronary artery disease may have profound impacts on quality of life as well as morbidity and mortality. Therefore, regular screening for these complications is critical for PWH with diabetes, especially people who may already be at elevated risk for ophthalmologic, cardiovascular, neurologic, and/or kidney disease due to other factors (e.g., advanced HIV and tobacco use).

ADRENAL DISORDERS

Early studies suggest the incidence of hypoadrenalism may be as high as 20% in PWH (González-González et al., 2001), and postmortem studies have shown that up to two-thirds of people with advanced HIV infection/AIDS may have adrenal involvement (Bricaire et al., 1988). Presentation of adrenal dysfunction may be subtle, and it is relatively common in hospitalized PWH (Membreno et al., 1987). Thus, a high index of clinical suspicion is needed to detect adrenal insufficiency (Mifsud et al., 2021). The etiology of adrenal hypofunction ranges from primary hypoadrenalism involving the adrenal gland, with elevations in adrenocorticotropic hormone (ACTH) levels (Villette et al., 1990), to secondary hypoadrenalism because of pituitary suppression attributable to inherent pituitary pathology or possibly suppression of the hypothalamic-pituitary-adrenal axis by exogenous steroid use (Danaher et al., 2009; Kaviani et al., 2011). Cases of hyperadrenalism with iatrogenic Cushing's syndrome have also been observed among PWH exposed to steroids administered via oral, inhaled, and parenteral routes (Gray et al., 2010; Johnson et al., 2006; Samaras et al., 2005; Yombi et al., 2008).

PWH may also develop abnormalities in the mineralocorticoid axis (Stricker et al., 1999). Women with HIV and wasting syndrome may have significant shunting of adrenal steroid metabolism away from androgenic pathways and toward cortisol production (Grinspoon et al., 2001).

THYROID ABNORMALITIES

Although earlier reports suggested that thyroid dysfunction in PWH is generally similar to the general population (Hoffman and Brown, 2007), subsequent studies found that prevalence may be much higher, with presentations spanning asymptomatic hypo- or hyperthyroidism to clinically overt disease (Micali et al., 2022). One study of 178 PWH found that 33% had evidence of thyroid dysfunction (Ji et al., 2016). Most abnormalities appear to involve a hypothyroid state, ranging from subclinical hypothyroidism (Madeddu et al., 2006; Silva et al., 2015) to clinically apparent disease (Beltran et al., 2003). Factors contributing to thyroid disorders in HIV infection include but are not limited to ARVs, infection, and immune factors.

Older ARVs may have been particularly problematic. For example, HIV-related nonautoimmune primary hypothyroidism and subclinical hypothyroidism have been linked to stavudine and decreased $CD4^+$ T-cell counts (Calza et al., 2002; Madeddu et al., 2006; Quirino et al., 2004; Silva et al., 2015). HIV-related immune system changes and other factors have also been linked to abnormal thyroid function tests. For example, $CD4^+$ T-cell counts have been inversely correlated with thyroid-binding globulin (Bourdoux et al., 1991), and diminished levels of triiodothyronine (T3) and reverse T3 with increased thyroid-binding globulin may be associated with HIV progression. ART initiation with subsequent immune reconstitution may also sometimes lead to autoimmune Graves's disease or Hashimoto's thyroiditis (Jubault et al., 2000). Finally, infection as an etiological factor for thyroid disease was more prevalent in the pre-ART era, caused by a wide variety of infectious microorganisms. In the current treatment era, these conditions may still be observed in people with uncontrolled HIV infection who are not on ART or not taking ART consistently.

The diagnostic workup for thyroid disease is similar to that in HIV-negative persons and should begin with evaluations of thyroxine and thyrotropin, with additional testing for thyroiditis antibodies when appropriate. Management of thyroid disease is also similar between PWH and the general population, and commonly used pharmacotherapies for thyroid disease typically do not have clinically significant drug-drug interactions with contemporary ART regimens.

PARATHYROID DISORDERS

Hyperparathyroidism is a condition marked by elevated secretion of parathyroid hormone. Hyperparathyroidism can be primarily due to abnormalities within the parathyroid gland itself, most often due to adenoma, primarily due to abnormalities within the parathyroid gland itself, most often due to adenoma, and rarely due to cancer. Secondary causes of hyperparathyroidism include conditions such as renal impairment and vitamin D deficiency. The etiology of primary hyperparathyroidism in PWH is similar to the general population and typically presents as hypercalcemia; this should be appropriately investigated, and definitive treatment usually involves surgical removal of the overactive parathyroid tissue. By contrast, vitamin D deficiency is reported to impact a third of PWH (Van den Bout et al., 2008) and is a common cause of secondary hyperparathyroidism (Dao et al., 2011; Mueller et al., 2010). Endocrinology consultation is generally indicated for these disorders. Antiretroviral drugs such as efavirenz have been implicated in the increased prevalence of vitamin D deficiency (Nylén et al., 2016), but other factors such as low $CD4^+$ T-cell counts and advanced AIDS may also play a role (Theodorou et al., 2014). Other ARV drugs, such as tenofovir disoproxil fumarate, have also been linked to secondary hyperparathyroidism in PWH (Noe et al., 2018).

GONADAL DYSFUNCTION

Gonadal dysfunction is common in PWH (Crum et al., 2005; Rietschel et al., 2000). In cisgender male adults with HIV, decreased testosterone levels may manifest as fatigue, muscle wasting, and sarcopenia, decreased bone density, low libido, weight loss, and decreased strength (Grinspoon et al., 1996; Wanke et al., 2000), and erectile dysfunction (Mylonakis et al., 2001). In one study of 300 PWH, 17% were found to be hypogonadal, and all PWH with low testosterone had secondary hypogonadism. Increasing age and higher body mass index (BMI) were positively correlated with hypogonadism, whereas smoking was negatively correlated (Crum-Cianflone et al., 2007). Although underlying causes are not fully understood, elevated prolactin levels have been implicated in the development of male hypogonadism (Collazos et al., 2009). Early research suggested that treatment of AIDS wasting syndrome using testosterone was associated with a sustained increase in lean mass (Grinspoon et al., 1999). However, given the emergence of data on long-term side effects of exogenous testosterone, initiation and continuation of this therapy (especially in older PWH) should involve careful monitoring of prostate-specific antigen levels, liver profiles, and hematocrit levels (De Vincentis and Rochira, 2023).

Women with HIV have increased rates of oligomenorrhea and amenorrhea. In one study, 8% of women with HIV had evidence of early menopause and 48% had anovulatory cycles, whereas women who ovulated had higher $CD4^+$ T-cell counts (Chirgwin et al., 1996). In a more recent study from Nigeria evaluating abnormalities in premenopausal women with HIV, mean serum levels of FSH, LH, progesterone, and estradiol did not differ between the follicular and luteal phase of the menstrual cycle, suggesting loss of hormonal regulation. Investigators linked these abnormalities to hypothyroidism, which could be corrected with treatment (Ukibe et al., 2017).

GYNECOMASTIA

Cisgender males with HIV have a 2.9% incidence of developing gynecomastia, which has been associated with factors such as hypogonadism, lipoatrophy, hepatitis C, and lipodystrophy (Biglia et al., 2004; Manfredi et al., 2001). The role of ARVs in gynecomastia development is controversial: some studies have found no correlation (Manfredi et al., 2001), whereas others have linked gynecomastia with PI-based regimens (Manfredi et al., 2004; Peyriere et al., 1999; Toma and Therrien, 1998). When associated with PI therapy, gynecomastia does not resolve after cessation of ART, and underlying mechanisms are not clear. Treatment of gynecomastia includes removal of any identifiable cause and, in severe cases, surgical excision.

PITUITARY DISEASE

The pituitary gland comprises the anterior pituitary (adenohypophysis) and posterior pituitary (neurohypophysis). Adenohypophyseal hormones are involved in controlling thyroid, adrenal, and gonadal function, growth, and milk secretion. Neurohypophysis primarily controls water balance and acts via the antidiuretic hormone. Many pituitary hormones are regulated by prohormones secreted by the hypothalamus and are delivered to the pituitary via a portal system through the pituitary stalk (e.g., corticotropin-releasing hormone, growth hormone-releasing hormone, thyrotropin-releasing hormone, gonadotropin-releasing hormone [GnRH], and vasopressin), with the sole exception being prolactin, which is under inhibitory control by dopamine. Therefore, pituitary disease can be caused by pathology at the level of the hypothalamus, pituitary stalk compression, or disease in the pituitary gland itself. HIV infection has a complex impact on pituitary function with many potential direct and indirect effects (Youssef et al., 2021).

GROWTH HORMONE DISORDERS

Disorders of growth hormone (GH) have been reported in PWH. HIV-associated lipodystrophy is described to involve GH deficiency with reduced pulse and amplitude of GH secretion, which may be related to an increased somatostatin tone, decreased ghrelin, and increased circulatory free fatty-acid concentrations (Koutkia et al., 2004). Children with HIV and adults with AIDS wasting syndrome have low levels of insulin-like growth factor-1 (IGF-1) and IGF binding protein 3 and increased concentrations of GH, suggesting resistance to GH (Frost et al., 1996; Pinto et al., 2000; Ratner Kaufman et al., 1997; Rondanelli et al., 2002).

PITUITARY ADRENAL DISORDERS

Iatrogenic Cushing's syndrome, together with secondary hypoadrenalism, is commonly observed in PWH receiving steroid therapy (Danaher et al., 2009; Gray et al., 2010; Johnson et al., 2006; Kaviani et al., 2011; Samaras et al., 2005; Yombi et al., 2008). This is likely caused by the effect of several ARV drugs (namely those involving ritonavir or cobicistat) on the hepatic cytochrome P450 system, which prolongs steroid half-life. This drug interaction results in elevated levels of exogenously administered steroids and ACTH suppression, and, thereby, of endogenous cortisol production, resulting in iatrogenic Cushing's syndrome together with endogenous adrenal insufficiency. Because sudden withdrawal of exogenous steroids could precipitate adrenal crisis, caution should be exercised while discontinuing steroids and a gradual taper is recommended.

PROLACTIN DISORDERS

Disturbances in basal and rhythmic prolactin secretions associated with $CD4^+$ T-lymphocytes have been reported among PWH (Parra et al., 2004). Serum prolactin elevation has been described (Collazos et al., 2002), and hyperprolactinemia in men with HIV has been linked to hypogonadism and gynecomastia (Collazos et al., 2009). Although the etiology of hyperprolactinemia is unclear, use of PIs has been implicated (Ram et al., 2004).

POSTERIOR PITUITARY DISORDERS

Posterior pituitary disorders are caused by excess secretion of antidiuretic hormone (ADH), resulting in hyponatremia, or a paucity of ADH, resulting in diabetes insipidus. In one report, 33% of people with AIDS were found to have hyponatremia, primarily owing to the syndrome of inappropriate ADH secretion (Agarwal et al., 1989). Case reports have also described the development of hypernatremia caused by diabetes insipidus due to intracranial pathology (Tavares-Bello et al., 2017).

METABOLIC DISORDERS IN HIV

METABOLIC SYNDROME

With increased longevity in PWH, there is also an increasing risk of developing metabolic syndrome, with central obesity, insulin resistance, hypertriglyceridemia, and hypertension, which could predispose to an increase cardiovascular risk (Hadigan et al., 2001). Whereas the prevalence of metabolic syndrome in PWH is 3%, people taking ART have a prevalence of 16%–18% (Samaras et al., 2007). Women with HIV appear to have an even higher burden of metabolic syndrome, with a 33% prevalence compared to 22% for women without HIV (Sobieszczyk et al., 2008).

Clinically, this translates into an increased incidence and prevalence of abdominal obesity, insulin resistance, dyslipidemia, and hypertension in PWH, all of which contribute to elevated cardiometabolic risk. Treatment involves a combination of patient education, dietary changes, physical activity and exercise, where possible, and appropriate pharmacotherapy targeting glycemic control, blood pressure, and lipids.

METABOLIC DYSFUNCTION-ASSOCIATED STEATOTIC LIVER DISEASE (FORMERLY NONALCOHOLIC FATTY LIVER DISEASE)

Liver disease is an important contributor to morbidity and mortality among PWH. Despite the success of hepatitis C direct-acting antivirals, there is an increase in the prevalence of nonalcoholic fatty liver disease (NAFLD), which has been defined as liver fat accumulation (causing fatty liver) in the absence of other causes of liver disease such as excess alcohol consumption, viral hepatitis, or other specific pathology. NAFLD ranges from simple hepatic steatosis to nonalcoholic steatohepatitis (NASH) and hepatic fibrosis, which progresses to cirrhosis and hepatocellular carcinoma. NASH is now the second most common indication for liver transplantation in the United States.

More recently, there has been a global effort to address the limitations of using the terminology of NAFLD. Critics pointed out that NAFLD did not capture disease pathophysiology completely, did not allow optimal characterization of subgroups, and the terms *nonalcoholic* and *fatty* were stigmatizing (Gawrieh et al., 2024). Thus, a consensus emerged to use *steatotic liver disease* (SLD) as the overarching term to describe hepatic steatosis of any etiology and to replace NAFLD with the term *metabolic dysfunction-associated steatotic liver disease* (MASLD) and *nonalcoholic steatohepatitis* (NASH) for metabolic dysfunction-associated steatohepatitis (MASH).

Recent studies have determined that MASLD prevalence is higher than previously appreciated in PWH, approaching 50% (Wegermann et al., 2023). In one study, the overall prevalence of SLD was 52% (subgroup prevalence was: MASLD 39%; metabolic dysfunction and alcohol-associated liver disease [MetALD] 10% and ALD 3%) (Gawrieh et al., 2024). Independent risk factors for MASLD included BMI >30 kg/m^2 (adjusted odds ratio = 17.3), followed by abdominal obesity (AOR = 4.3), BMI 25–29.9 (AOR = 4.1), and low HDL-cholesterol (AOR = 1.8). Clinically significant fibrosis was seen in 15%, advanced fibrosis in 4%, and cryptogenic SLD in 0.6%. A prior study examining PWH with transaminitis found up to a 55% prevalence of MASH (Morse et al., 2015).

Importantly, MASLD in PWH may have a more aggressive progression to MASH, as evidenced in one study which examined the clinical and histological differences between HIV-associated MASLD and primary MASLD and reported that HIV-associated MASLD was associated with increased severity of liver disease and higher prevalence of MASH (Vodkin et al., 2015). Furthermore, the presence of MASLD is linked to development of systemic inflammation, insulin resistance, diabetes, and cardiovascular disease. Conversely, MASLD is a well-recognized complication of type 2 diabetes, with reported prevalence as high as 80%–85%; given the rising incidence and prevalence of type 2 diabetes in PWH, MASLD and MASH could soon become the most significant overall metabolic complication of HIV infection. The combination of high prevalence of MASLD/MASH in PWH with increased severity of MASH makes it an extremely urgent public health concern, especially since mechanisms remain poorly understood and effective interventions are currently lacking.

ENDOCRINE AND METABOLIC COMPLICATIONS IN TRANSGENDER PWH

Transgender PWH usually receive gender-affirming hormonal therapy and could develop endocrine and metabolic complications; however, carefully conducted studies have been limited. One matched case-control study comparing transgender women to cisgender men with HIV found no differences between groups in terms of metabolic syndrome, but a higher frequency of subclinical hypothyroidism (median TSH 1.6-fold higher) associated with higher BMI and use of steroids as well as adrenal insufficiency (Pommier et al., 2019). A more recent study evaluating inflammation in cryopreserved peripheral blood monocytes from PWH found that estrogen elevated the toll-like receptor 4 activation induced by lipopolysaccharide in cisgender men with HIV, with increased monocyte activation and inflammatory cytokine production (i.e., IL-6, TNF-α); these findings could have implications for use of estrogens as feminizing therapy (Kettelhut et al., 2022), especially in relation to a higher risk of cardiovascular disease (Aranda et al., 2021). More studies are warranted to further investigate and understand endocrine and cardiometabolic risks and complications of gender affirming therapy.

METABOLIC CHANGES IN BODY WEIGHT AND BODY COMPOSITION

HIV infection has always been associated with changes in body weight and body composition. Prior to the advent of effective ART, the primary metabolic issue observed was HIV-associated wasting, which was associated with weight loss in the form of both muscle and fat loss. With early ART (i.e., first-generation PIs coupled with older NRTIs), PWH experienced an abnormal fat distribution, termed *lipodystrophy*. HIV lipodystrophy can manifest as fat loss (lipoatrophy), fat gain (lipohypertrophy), or a mixed pattern. As older ART agents were phased out and replaced by newer agents including the INSTI class, a new challenge of weight gain emerged. Scientific understanding and clinical approaches to prevent, evaluate, and manage this phenomenon are actively evolving.

HIV-ASSOCIATED WASTING

HIV-associated wasting is a classic opportunistic condition and potentially life-threatening complication traditionally seen in people with advanced AIDS (Kotler et al., 1989; Polsky et al., 2001). In 1987, HIV-associated wasting was defined by the CDC as an involuntary weight loss of at least 10% of baseline body weight plus either chronic diarrhea or chronic weakness and documented fever for at least 30 days not attributable to a concurrent illness or condition other than HIV infection itself (Centers for Disease Control, 1987). With the availability of effective ART, the prevalence of severe wasting declined significantly (Siddiqui et al., 2022a). However, even among people treated with ART, weight loss remains a strong predictor of morbidity and mortality (Tang et al., 2002). The old CDC definition is impractical and no longer relevant in current clinical practice, and a commonly used redefinition of wasting includes a 10% involuntary weight loss or BMI <20 kg/m^2 in the absence of other treatable, reversible causes of weight loss such as malignancy, infection, or anorexia (Polsky et al., 2001). Despite effective ART, HIV-associated wasting still can occur in virologically well-controlled PWH. Published reports suggest that PWH with wasting experience greater emergency department visits and hospitalizations (Siddiqui et al., 2022b), have declined in quality of life, and may be 3 times more likely to die than those without weight loss (Cordeiro et al., 2024). Initial evaluation involves a thorough history focusing on determining the cause of muscle mass decrease and weight loss; weight and BMI should be tracked longitudinally, and nutritional counseling with a registered dietician may be beneficial. Treatment of HIV-associated wasting should be individualized, as the cause(s) of wasting in each patient is unique. The only FDA-approved treatment for PWH with wasting or cachexia to increase lean body mass, increase body weight, and improve physical endurance is recombinant human growth hormone (Moyle et al., 2004).

HIV-ASSOCIATED LIPODYSTROPHY

With the arrival of combination ART, body composition abnormalities termed *HIV-associated lipodystrophy* (HAL) began to be described (Carr et al., 1998). *Lipodystrophy* is an umbrella term encompassing fat loss (lipoatrophy), fat gain (lipohypertrophy), and/or mixed presentation. Lipoatrophy may appear as diffuse loss of peripheral subcutaneous adipose tissue (SAT) or fat, most notably in the face, limbs, and buttocks. By contrast, lipohypertrophy may appear as central fat accumulation (namely, visceral adipose tissue or VAT) in the abdomen and/or fat accumulation in the dorsocervical region behind the neck. Often, these changes in body habitus were also accompanied by dyslipidemia (mainly hypertriglyceridemia) and insulin resistance. In addition to these metabolic consequences, the presence of HAL was potentially disfiguring, highly stigmatizing, and severely affected mental health and quality of life (Burgoyne et al., 2005).

The pathogenesis of HAL is complicated, multifactorial, and not completely elucidated (Bacchetti et al., 2005; Sattler, 2003; Tien and Grunfeld, 2004). Lipoatrophy is better understood and has been associated with the use of older NRTIs which caused mitochondrial toxicity in fat cells, leading to their death and subsequent lipoatrophy (Brinkman et al., 1999). Other risk factors of lipoatrophy include older age, disease severity, and host factors such as low nadir CD4 (Lichtenstein et al., 2001; Wohl et al., 2006). Although the etiology of lipohypertrophy is much more complicated, multifactorial and less well defined, the role of ART (especially PIs) has been extensively described. Other studies have suggested that increased age, higher baseline fat content, higher BMI, and low $CD4^{+}$ cell count at ART initiation are potential risk factors (Sax and Kumar, 2004; Wohl et al., 2006).

The therapeutic approach to lipoatrophy focuses on reversing cause(s) of fat loss and prevention of future fat loss. In PWH, lipoatrophy has most often been caused by mitochondrial toxicity related to use of thymidine NRTIs, such as zidovudine or stavudine. Thus, removal of these agents can (at minimum) stop further fat loss. Notably, no single therapy has been found to completely reverse lipoatrophy. Switching ART has shown partial improvement in some people (Carr et al., 2002; McComsey et al., 2004). Insulin sensitizers such as thiazolidinediones have been studied with mixed results (Wohl et al., 2006). Otherwise, reconstructive procedures such as the use of facial fillers (Moyle, 2005) may help with facial lipoatrophy; utilization is generally limited due to initial and ongoing costs of repeated procedures over time.

Given its multifactorial nature, the treatment for lipohypertrophy is less well defined and has generally focused on weight loss with the hope this will lead to loss of visceral adipose tissue (VAT). Lifestyle interventions such as improving diet and increasing exercise are always recommended but may have limited effect in reducing VAT (Cofrancesco et al., 2009). Although metformin has shown some promise in reducing VAT, rosiglitazone did not (van Wijk et al., 2005). The only treatment indicated for reduction of excess abdominal fat in people with HAL is tesamorelin (Dhillon, 2011; Falutz et al., 2010), or growth hormone-releasing factor. Tesamorelin is lipolytic and has been shown to reduce VAT preferentially over SAT, but likely requires lifelong administration, as fat accumulation may recur upon cessation. Lastly, surgical interventions may be needed for the removal of dorsocervical fat accumulation or lipomas but are of limited use for abdominal lipohypertrophy.

WEIGHT GAIN IN PWH

Long-standing untreated HIV infection has usually been associated with images of PWH with dramatic weight loss and wasting. However, initiation of effective ART often reverses the catabolic effects of untreated HIV infection, leading to a "return to health" weight gain, back to pre-illness baseline weight (Sax et al., 2020). ART may also ameliorate gastrointestinal dysfunction associated with initial HIV infection that impacts appetite, absorption, and weight. Recently, a rise in weight gain and/or obesity in PWH has been observed globally (Bailin et al., 2020; Crum-Cianflone et al., 2010; Koethe et al., 2016). Another possible reason for this trend is the overall increase in obesogenic environments (Wohl et al., 2024), with more exposure to energy-rich food choices and decreased engagement in physical activity due to more sedentary lifestyles, especially in resource-rich settings. The consequence of obesity is that it contributes to other adverse health conditions such as hypertension, type 2 diabetes, and cardiovascular disease. The impact of weight gain may be even more pronounced in PWH, given the already elevated risk of cardiovascular disease (particularly in women) (Kentoffio et al., 2022).

The collective understanding of weight gain after starting ART has changed in recent years. With the introduction of INSTIs, several analyses of large retrospective cohorts, as well as pooled clinical trial data, showed greater weight gain among those starting INSTIs compared to older, predominantly NNRTI-based regimens (Bourgi et al., 2020a; Norwood et al., 2017; Sax et al., 2020). Concerns also exist regarding the use of INSTIs with tenofovir alafenamide (TAF) leading to weight gain, as seen in the ADVANCE Study (Venter et al., 2022). A recently assembled expert panel reviewed key studies evaluating weight changes which included ART switch studies in PWH, as well as studies of ART used as pre-exposure prophylaxis, and concluded that INSTIs and TAF are not weight-enhancing, but actually weight-neutral (Wohl et al., 2024). In addition, tenofovir disoproxil fumarate (TDF) and efavirenz (EFV) were found to be weight-attenuating.

Management of weight gain in PWH is not different from people without HIV. Lifestyle changes are recommended, including both diet and exercise. General guidelines suggest limiting intake of sugar, carbohydrates, saturated fats, sodium, and alcoholic beverages (USDA and USDHHS, 2020). Increasing physical activity has the benefits of improving cardiovascular health, muscle strengthening, preventing frailty, and improving overall well-being and quality of life (Piercy et al., 2018). Thus far, ART switch trials have not consistently shown a benefit for reducing weight. For example, the DEFINE Study attempted to switch from an INSTI-based regimen to an INSTI-sparing, PI-based regimen but did not show any significant difference in weight at week 24 (Short et al., 2023). The Doravirine/Islatravir Switch Studies 017 and 018 attempted to assess switching to an INSTI and TAF-sparing regimen and also did not show any significant weight changes (McComsey et al., 2023). In obese PWH, pharmacologic therapies may be indicated, such as glucagon-like peptide-1 receptor agonists (GLP-1 RAs). Recent findings from a retrospective single-center cohort study found that use of GLP-1 RAs led to declines in weight, BMI, and hemoglobin A1c (Nguyen et al., 2024). Similarly, an observational study evaluating semaglutide in PWH showed that semaglutide was associated with significant weight loss and HbA1c reduction among PWH (Haidar et al, 2024). Although these results seem promising, one notable concern with the use of GLP-1 RAs in PWH is that any weight loss is often accompanied by muscle loss, which can be detrimental in older adults who may already be at risk for frailty and accelerated aging (Lee and Capeau, 2024).

CONCLUSION

PWH can be affected by a broad array of endocrine and metabolic abnormalities. Although the more common disorders are dyslipidemia, diabetes, metabolic syndrome, and insulin resistance, other disorders affecting bone, adrenal glands, pituitary, and thyroid function may also be present. For timely diagnosis and treatment of endocrine disorders in PWH, early referral to an endocrinologist is highly recommended. HIV-associated wasting and HIV-associated lipodystrophy are less prevalent, though still exist. Weight gain and MASLD have become the main metabolic conditions of concern in the current era.

REFERENCES

Agarwal A, Soni A, Ciechanowsky M, et al. Hyponatremia in patients with the acquired immunodeficiency syndrome. *Nephron*. 1989;53:317–321.

Aranda G, Halperin I, Gomez-Gil E, et al. Cardiovascular risk associated with gender affirming hormone therapy in transgender population. *Front Endocrinol (Lausanne)*. 2021;12:718200. doi: 10.3389/fendo.2021.718200

Bacchetti P, Gripshover B, Grunfeld C, et al. Fat distribution in men with HIV infection. *J Acquir Immune Defic Syndr*. 2005;40(2):121–131.

Bajaj S, Sonkar KK, Verma S, et al. Assessment of glycemic status, insulin resistance and hypogonadism in HIV Infected male patients. *J Assoc Physicians India*. 2020;68(8):43–46.Bailin SS, Gabriel CL, Wanjalla CN, Koethe JR. Obesity and weight gain in persons with HIV. *Curr HIV/AIDS Rep*. 2020;17(2):138–150.

Beltran S, Lescure FX, Desailloud R, et al. Increased prevalence of hypothyroidism among human immune deficiency virus-infected patients: a need for screening. *Clin Infect Dis*. 2003;37:579–583.

Biadgo B, Ambachew S, Abebe M, et al. Gestational diabetes mellitus in HIV-infected pregnant women: a systematic review and meta-analysis. *Diabetes Res Clin Pract*. 2019;155:107800.

Biglia A, Blanco JL, Martínez E, et al. Gynecomastia among HIV-positive patients is associated with hypogonadism: a case–control study. *Clin Infect Dis*. 2004;39(10):1514–1519.

Bourdoux PP, De Wit SA, Servais GM, et al. Biochemical thyroid profile in patients infected with human immunodeficiency virus. *Thyroid*. 1991;1:147–149.

Bourgi K, Jenkins CA, Rebeiro PF, et al. Weight gain among treatment-naïve persons with HIV starting integrase inhibitors compared to non-nucleoside reverse transcriptase inhibitors or protease inhibitors in a large observational cohort in the United States and Canada. *J Int AIDS Soc*. 2020a Apr;23(4):325484.

Bourgi K, Rebeiro PF, Turner M, et al. Greater weight gain in treatment-naïve persons starting dolutegravir-based antiretroviral therapy. *Clin Infect Dis*. 2020b Mar 17;70(7):1267–1274.

Bricaire F, Marche C, Zoubi D, et al. Adrenocortical lesions and AIDS. *Lancet*. 1988;1:881.

Brinkman K, Smeitink JA, Romijn JA, Reiss P. Mitochondrial toxicity induced by nucleoside-analogue reverse-transcriptase inhibitors is a key factor in the pathogenesis of antiretroviral-therapy-related lipodystrophy. *Lancet*. 1999;354(9184):1112–1115.

Brown TT, Cole SR, Li X, et al. Antiretroviral therapy and the prevalence and incidence of diabetes mellitus in the multicenter AIDS cohort study. *Arch Intern Med*. 2005;165:1179–1184.

Burgoyne R, Collins E, Wagner C, et al. The relationship between lipodystrophy-associated body changes and measures of quality of life and mental health for HIV-positive adults. *Qual Life Res*. 2005;14(4):981–990.

Calkins JH, Siegel MM, Nankin HR, et al. Interleukin-1 inhibits Leydig cell steroidogenesis in primary cell culture. *J Clin Endocrinol Metab*. 1988;123:1605–1610.

Calza L, Manfredi R, Chiodo F. Subclinical hypothyroidism in HIV-positive patients receiving highly active antiretroviral therapy. *J AIDS*. 2002;31:361–363.

Caron M, Auclair M, Vigouroux C, et al. The HIV protease inhibitor indinavir impairs sterol regulatory element-binding protein-1 intranuclear localization, inhibits preadipocyte differentiation, and induces insulin resistance. *Diabetes*. 2001;50:1378–1388.

Carr A, Samaras K, Burton S, et al. A syndrome of peripheral lipodystrophy, hyperlipidaemia and insulin resistance in patients receiving HIV protease inhibitors. *AIDS*. 1998;12(7):F51–F58.

Carr A, Workman C, Smith DE, et al. Abacavir substitution for nucleoside analogs in patients with HIV lipoatrophy: a randomized trial. *JAMA*. 2002;288(2):207–215.

Centers for Disease Control (CDC). Revision of the CDC surveillance case definition for acquired immunodeficiency syndrome. Council of State and Territorial Epidemiologists; AIDS Program, Center for Infectious Diseases. *MMWR Suppl*. 1987;36(1):1S–15S.

Chirgwin KD, Feldman J, Muneyyirci-Delale O, et al. Menstrual function in human immunodeficiency virus-infected women without acquired immunodeficiency syndrome. *J AIDS Hum Retrovirol*. 1996;12:489–494.

Cofrancesco J Jr, Freedland E, McComsey G. Treatment options for HIV-associated central fat accumulation. *AIDS Patient Care STDs*. 2009;23(1):5–18.

Collazos J, Esteban M. Has prolactin a role in the hypogonadal status of HIV-positive patients? *J Int Assoc Physicians AIDS Care (Chic)*. 2009;8(1):43–46.

Collazos J, Ibarra S, Martinez E, et al. Serum prolactin concentrations in patients infected with HIV. *HIV Clin Trials*. 2002;3:133–138.

Cordeiro SA, Lopes TCP, Boechat AL, Gonçalves RL. Weight loss and mortality in people living with HIV: a systematic review and meta-analysis. *BMC Infect Dis*. 2024 Jan 2;24(1):34.

Cozzolino M, Vidal M, Arcidiacono MV, et al. HIV-protease inhibitors impair vitamin D bioactivation to 1,25-dihydroxyvitamin D. *AIDS*. 2003;17:513–520.

Crum NF, Furtek KJ, Olson PE, et al. A review of hypogonadism and erectile dysfunction among HIV-infected men during the pre- and post-HAART eras: diagnosis, pathogenesis, and management. *AIDS Patient Care STDs*. 2005;19(10):655–671.

Crum-Cianflone NF, Bavaro M, Hale B, et al. Erectile dysfunction and hypogonadism among men with HIV. *AIDS Patient Care STDs.* 2007;21:9–19.

Crum-Cianflone N, Roediger MP, Eberly L, et al. Increasing rates of obesity among HIV-infected persons during the HIV epidemic. *PLoS One.* 2010 Apr 9;5(4):e10106.

Danaher PJ, Salsbury TL, Delmar JA. Metabolic derangement after injection of triamcinolone into the hip of an HIV-infected patient receiving ritonavir. *Orthopedics.* 2009;32(6):450.

Dao CN, Patel P, Overton ET, et al. Low vitamin D among HIV-infected adults: prevalence of and risk factors for low vitamin D Levels in a cohort of HIV-infected adults and comparison to prevalence among adults in the US general population. *Clin Infect Dis.* 2011;52:396.

De Vincentis S, Rochira V. Update on acquired hypogonadism in men living with HIV: pathogenesis, clinic, and treatment. *Front Endocrinol (Lausanne).* 2023;14:1201696.

Dhillon S. Tesamorelin: a review of its use in the management of HIV-associated lipodystrophy. *Drugs.* 2011;71(8):1071–1091.

Drucker DJ, Bailey D, Rotstein L. Thyroiditis as the presenting manifestation of disseminated extrapulmonary Pneumocystis carinii infection. *J Clin Endocrinol Metab.* 1990;71:1663–1665.

Duncan AD, Goff LM, Peters BS. Type 2 diabetes prevalence and its risk factors in HIV: a cross-sectional study. *PLoS One.* 2018;13(3):e0194199.

Falutz J, Mamputu JC, Potvin D, et al. Effects of tesamorelin (TH9507), a growth hormone-releasing factor analog, in human immunodeficiency virus-infected patients with excess abdominal fat: a pooled analysis of two multicenter, double-blind placebo-controlled phase 3 trials with safety extension data. *J Clin Endocrinol Metab.* 2010;95(9):4291–4304.

Frost RA, Fuhrer J, Steigbigel R. Wasting in the acquired immune deficiency syndrome is associated with multiple defects in the serum insulin-like growth factor system. *Clin Endocrinol.* 1996:44:501.

Gawrieh S, Vilar-Gomez E, Woreta TA, et al. Prevalence of steatotic liver disease, MASLD, MetALD and significant fibrosis in people with HIV in the United States. *Aliment Pharmacol Ther.* 2024;59(5):666–679.

Giampalmo A, Buffa D, Quaglia AC. AIDS pathology: various critical considerations (especially regarding the brain, the heart, the lungs, the hypophysis and the adrenal glands). *Pathologica.* 1990;82(1982):663–677.

Glasgow BJ, Steinsapir KD, Anders K, et al. Adrenal pathology in the acquired immune deficiency syndrome. *Am J Clin Pathol.* 1985;84:594–597.

González-González JG, de la Garza-Hernández NE, Garza-Morán RA, et al. Prevalence of abnormal adrenocortical function in human immunodeficiency virus infection by low-dose cosyntropin test. *Int J STD AIDS.* 2001;12(12):804–810.

Gray D, Roux P, Carrihill M, et al. Adrenal suppression and Cushing's syndrome secondary to ritonavir and budesonide. *S Afr Med J.* 2010;100(5):296–297.

Grinspoon S, Corcoran C, Anderson E, et al. Sustained anabolic effects of long-term androgen administration in men with AIDS and wasting. *Clin Infect Dis.* 1999;28:634–636.

Grinspoon S, Corcoran C, Lee K, et al. Loss of lean body and muscle mass correlates with androgen levels in hypogonadal men with acquired immunodeficiency syndrome and wasting. *J Clin Endocrinol Metab.* 1996;81:4051–4058.

Grinspoon S, Corcoran C, Stanley T, et al. Mechanisms of androgen deficiency in human immunodeficiency virus-infected women with the wasting syndrome. *J Clin Endocrinol Metab.* 2001;86:4120–4126.

Grunfeld C, Pang M, Doerrler W, et al. Lipids, lipoproteins, triglyceride clearance, and cytokines in human immunodeficiency virus infection and the acquired immunodeficiency syndrome. *J Clin Endocrinol Metab.* 1992;74:1045–1052.

Hadigan C, Meigs JB, Corcoran C, et al. Metabolic abnormalities and cardiovascular disease risk factors in adults with human immunodeficiency virus infection and lipodystrophy. *Clin Infect Dis.* 2001. 32(1):130–139.

Haidar L, Crane HM, Nance RM, et al. Weight loss associated with semaglutide treatment among people with HIV. *AIDS.* 2024;38(4):531–535.

Hales DB. Interleukin1 inhibits Leydig cell steroidogenesis primarily by decreasing 17α-hydroxylase/C17–20 lyase cytochrome P450 expression. *Endocrinology.* 1992;131:2165–2172.

Hoffman CJ, Brown TT. Thyroid function abnormalities in HIV infected patients. *Clin Infect Dis.* 2007;45:488–494.

Huff A. Protease inhibitor side effects take people by surprise. *GMHC Treat Issues.* 1997–1998;12(1):25–27.

Hutchinson J, Murphy M, Harries R, et al. Galactorrhoea and hyper-prolactinoma associated with protease inhibitors. *Lancet.* 2000;356:1003–1004.

Ji S, Jin C, Hoxtermann S, et al. Prevalence and influencing factors of thyroid dysfunction in HIV-positive patients. *Biomed Res Int.* 2016;3874257.

Johnson SR, Marion AA, Vrchoticky T, et al. Cushing syndrome with secondary adrenal insufficiency from concomitant therapy with ritonavir and fluticasone. *J Pediatr.* 2006;148(3):386–388.

Jubault V, Penformin F, Schillo F, et al. Sequential occurrence of thyroid autoantibodies and Grave's disease after immune restoration in severely immunocompromised human immuno-deficiency virus-1 infected patients. *J Clin Endocrinol Metab.* 2000;85:4254–4257.

Kaviani N, Bukberg P, Manessis A, et al. Iatrogenic osteoporosis, bilateral HIP osteonecrosis, and secondary adrenal suppression in an HIV-positive man receiving inhaled corticosteroids and ritonavir-boosted highly active antiretroviral therapy. *Endocr Pract.* 2011;17(1):74–78.

Kentoffio K, Temu TM, Shakil SS, Zanni MV, Longenecker CT. Cardiovascular disease risk in women living with HIV. *Curr Opin HIV AIDS.* 2022;17(5):270–278.

Kettelhut A, Bowman E, Gabriel J, et al. Estrogen may enhance Toll-like receptor 4-induced inflammatory pathways in people with HIV: implications for transgender women on hormone therapy. *Front Immunol.* 2022;13:879600. doi:10.3389/fimmu.2022.879600

Keuneke C, Anders HJ, Schlöndorff D. Adipsic hypernatremia in two patients with AIDS and cytomegalovirus encephalitis. *Am J Kidney Dis.* 1999;33(2):379–382.

Kim PS, Woods C, Georgoff P, et al. A1c underestimates glycemia in HIV infection. *Diabetes Care.* 2009;32(9):1591–1593.

Koethe JR, Jenkins CA, Lau B, et al. Rising obesity prevalence and weight gain among adults starting antiretroviral therapy in the United States and Canada. *AIDS Res Hum Retroviruses.* 2016;32(1):50–58.

Kotler DP, Tierney AR, Wang J, Pierson RN Jr. Magnitude of body-cell-mass depletion and the timing of death from wasting in AIDS. *Am J Clin Nutr.* 1989;50(3):444–447.

Koutkia P, Meininger G, Canavan B, et al. Metabolic regulation of growth hormone by free fatty acids, somatostatin, and ghrelin in HIV-lipodystrophy. *Am J Physiol Endocrinol Metab.* 2004;286(2):E296–E303.Lee D, Capeau J. Is the GLP-1 receptor agonist, semaglutide, a good option for weight loss in persons with HIV? *AIDS.* 2024;38(4):603–605.

Lichtenstein KA, Ward DJ, Moorman AC, et al. Clinical assessment of HIV-associated lipodystrophy in an ambulatory population. *AIDS.* 2001;15(11):1389–1398.

Madeddu G, Spanu A, Chessa F, et al. Thyroid function in human immunodeficiency virus patients treated with highly active antiretroviral therapy (HAART): a longitudinal study. *Clinical Endocrinology (Oxf).* 2006;64(4):375–383.

Mallon PW, Unemori P, Sedwell R, et al. In vivo, nucleoside reverse-transcriptase inhibitors alter expression of both mitochondrial and lipid metabolism genes in the absence of depletion of mitochondrial DNA. *J Infect Dis.* 2005;191(10):1686–1696.

Manfredi R, Calza L, Chiodo F. Another emerging event occurring during HIV infection treated with any antiretroviral therapy: frequency and role of gynecomastia. *Infez Med.* 2004;12(1):51–59.

Manfredi R, Calza L, Chiodo F. Gynecomastia associated with highly active antiretroviral therapy. *Ann Pharmacother.* 2001;35(4):438–439.

Mathabire Rücker SC, Tayea A, Bitilinyu-Bangoh J, et al. High rates of hypertension, diabetes, elevated low-density lipoprotein cholesterol,

and cardiovascular disease risk factors in HIV-positive patients in Malawi. *AIDS*. 2018;32(2):253–260.McComsey GA, Molina J-M, Mills AM, et al. Weight and body composition after switch to doravirine/islatravir (DOR/ISL) 100/0.75mg once daily: week 48 results from 2 randomized active-controlled phase 3 trials, MK8591A-017 (P017) and MK8591A-018 (P018). *J Int AIDS Soc*. 2023;26:e26134.
McComsey GA, Ward DJ, Hessenthaler SM, et al. Improvement in lipoatrophy associated with highly active antiretroviral therapy in human immunodeficiency virus-infected patients switched from stavudine to abacavir or zidovudine: the results of the TARHEEL study. *Clin Infect Dis*. 2004;38(2):263–270.
Membreno L, Irony I, Dere W, et al. Adrenocortical function in acquired immunodeficiency syndrome. *J Clin Endocrinol Metab*. 1987;65:482–487.
Merrill JE, Koyanagi Y, Chen ISY. Interleukin-1 and tumor necrosis factor α can be induced from mononuclear phagocytes by human immunodeficiency virus type 1 binding to the CD4 receptor. *J Virol*. 1989;63:4404–4408.
Meyer WJ, Smith EM, Richards GE, et al. In vivo immunoreactive adrenocorticotropin (ACTH) production by human mononuclear leukocytes from normal and ACTH-deficient individuals. *J Clin Endocrinol Metab*. 1987;64:98–105.
Micali C, Russotto Y, Celesia BM, et al. Thyroid diseases and thyroid asymptomatic dysfunction in people living with HIV. *Infect Dis Rep*. 2022;14(5):655–667.
Mifsud S, Gauci Z, Gruppetta M, Mallia Azzopardi C, Fava S. Adrenal insufficiency in HIV/AIDS: a review. *Expert Rev Endocrinol Metab*. 2021;16(6):351–362.
Minami R, Yamamoto M, Takahama S, et al. Comparison of the influence of four classes of HIV antiretrovirals on adipogenic differentiation: the minimal effect of raltegravir and atazanavir. *J Infect Chemother*. 2011;17(2):183–188.
Mishriki YY. A baffling case of bulging belly: protease paunch. *Postgrad Med*. 1998;104(3):45–46.
Morse CG, McLaughlin M, Matthews L, et al. Nonalcoholic steatohepatitis and hepatic fibrosis in HIV-1-monoinfected adults with elevated aminotransferase levels on antiretroviral therapy. *Clin Infect Dis*. 2015;60(10):1569–1578.
Moyle GJ. Plastic surgical approaches for HIV-associated lipoatrophy. *Curr HIV/AIDS Rep*. 2005;2(3):127–131.
Moyle GJ, Daar ES, Gertner JM, et al. Growth hormone improves lean body mass, physical performance, and quality of life in subjects with HIV-associated weight loss or wasting on highly active antiretroviral therapy. *J Acquir Immune Defic Syndr*. 2004;35(4):367–375.Mueller NJ, Fux CA, Ledergerber B, et al. High prevalence of severe vitamin D deficiency in combined antiretroviral therapy-naive and successfully treated Swiss HIV patients. *AIDS*. 2010;24:1127.
Mulindwa F, Kamal H, Castelnuovo B, et al. Association between integrase strand transfer inhibitor use with insulin resistance and incident diabetes mellitus in persons living with HIV: a systematic review and meta-analysis. *BMJ Open Diabetes Res Care*. 2023;11(1):e003136.
Murata H, Hruz PW, Mueckler M. The mechanism of insulin resistance caused by HIV protease inhibitor therapy. *J Biol Chem*. 2000;275:20251–20254.
Mylonakis E, Koutkia P, Grinspoon S. Diagnosis and treatment of androgen deficiency in human immunodeficiency virus-infected men and women. *Clin Infect Dis*. 2001;33:857–864.
Nduka CU, Stranges S, Kimani PK, et al. Is there sufficient evidence for a causal association between antiretroviral therapy and diabetes in HIV patients? A meta-analysis. *Diabetes Metab Res Rev*. 2017;33(6):e2902.
Nguyen Q, Wooten D, Lee D, et al. GLP-1 receptor agonists promote weight loss among people with HIV. *Clin Infect Dis*. 2024:ciae151.
Noe S, Oldenbuettel C, Heldwein S, et al. Secondary hyperparathyroidism in patients in Central Europe. *Horm Metab Res*. 2018;50(4):317–324.
Nolan NS, Adamson S, Reeds D, O'Halloran JA. Bictegravir-based antiretroviral therapy-associated accelerated hyperglycemia and diabetes mellitus. *Open Forum Infect Dis*. 2021 Apr 16;8(5):ofab077.
Norbiato G, Bevilacqua M, Vago T, et al. Glucocorticoids and interferon-alpha in the acquired immunodeficiency syndrome. *J Clin Endocrinol Metab*. 1996;81:2601–2606.
Norwood J, Turner M, Bofill C, et al. Brief report: weight gain in persons with HIV switched from efavirenz-based to integrase strand transfer inhibitor-based regimens. *J Acquir Immune Defic Syndr*. 2017;76(5):527–531.Nylén H, Habtewold A, Makonnen E, et al. Prevalence and risk factors for efavirenz-based antiretroviral treatment-associated severe vitamin D deficiency: a prospective cohort study. *Medicine*. 2016;95(34):e4631.
O'Halloran JA, Sahrmann J, Parra-Rodriguez L, et al. Integrase strand transfer inhibitors are associated with incident diabetes mellitus in people with human immunodeficiency virus. *Clin Infect Dis*. 2022;75(12):2060–2065.
Padmapriyadarsini C, Ramesh Kumar S, et al. Dyslipidemia among HIV-infected patients with tuberculosis taking once-daily nonnucleoside reverse-transcriptase inhibitor-based antiretroviral therapy in India. *Clin Infect Dis*. 2011;52(4):540–546.
Parra A, Reyes-Terán G, Ramírez-Peredo J, et al. Differences in nocturnal basal and rhythmic prolactin secretion in untreated compared to treated HIV-infected men are associated with CD4\+ T-lymphocytes. *Immunol Cell Biol*. 2004;82(1):24–31.
Peyriere H, Mauboussin JM, Rouanet I, et al. Report of gynecomastia in five male patients during antiretroviral therapy for HIV infection. *AIDS*. 1999;13:2167–2169.
Piercy KL, Troiano RP, Ballard RM, et al. The physical activity guidelines for Americans. *JAMA*. 2018;320(19):2020–2028.
Pinto G, Blanche S, Thiriet I, et al. Growth hormone treatment of children with human immunodeficiency virus-associated growth failure. *Eur J Pediatr*. 2000;159:937–938.
Polsky B, Kotler D, Steinhart C. HIV-associated wasting in the HAART era: guidelines for assessment, diagnosis, and treatment. *AIDS Patient Care STDs*. 2001;15(8):411–423.
Pommier JD, Laouenan C, Michard F, et al. Metabolic syndrome and endocrine status in HIV-infected transwomen. *AIDS*. 2019;33(5):855–865.
Quirino T, Bongiovanni M, Ricci E, et al. Hypothyroidism in HIV-infected patients who have or have not received HAART. *Clin Infect Dis*. 2004;38:596–597.
Ram S, Acharya S, Fernando JJ, et al. Serum prolactin in HIV infection. *Clin Lab*. 2004;50:617–620.
Ratner Kaufman F, Gertner JM, Sleeper LA, et al. Growth hormone secretion in HIV-positive versus HIV-negative hemophilic males with abnormal growth and pubertal development. The Hemophilia Growth and Development Study. *J AIDS Hum Retrovirol*. 1997;15:137–144.
Rietschel P, Corcoran C, Stanley T, et al. Prevalence of hypogonadism among men with weight loss related to human immunodeficiency virus infection who were receiving highly active antiretroviral therapy. *Clin Infect Dis*. 2000;31:1240–1244.
Rondanelli M, Caselli D, Arico M, et al. Insulin-like growth factor 1 (IGF-1) and IGF-binding protein 3 response to growth hormone is impaired in HIV-infected children. *AIDS Res Hum Retroviruses*. 2002;18:331–339.
Saint-Marc T, Partisani M, Poizot-Martin I, et al. A syndrome of peripheral fat wasting (lipodystrophy) in patients receiving long-term nucleoside analogue therapy. *AIDS*. 1999;13(13):1659–1667.
Salim YS, Faber V, Wiik A, et al. Anticorticosteroid antibodies in AIDS patients. *APMIS*. 1988;96:889–894.
Samaras K, Pett S, Gowers A, et al. Iatrogenic Cushing's syndrome with osteoporosis and secondary adrenal failure in human immunodeficiency virus-infected patients receiving inhaled corticosteroids and ritonavir-boosted protease inhibitors: six cases. *J Clin Endocrinol Metab*. 2005;90(7):4394–4398.
Samaras K, Wand H, Law M, et al. Prevalence of metabolic syndrome in HIV infected using International Diabetes Foundation and Adult Treatment Panel III criteria: associations with insulin resistance, disturbed body fat compartmentalization, elevated C-reactive protein, and hypoadiponectinemia. *Diabetes Care*. 2007;30:113–119.

Sattler F. Body habitus changes related to lipodystrophy. *Clin Infect Dis.* 2003;36(Suppl 2):S84–S90.

Sax PE, Erlandson KM, Lake JE, et al. Weight gain following initiation of antiretroviral therapy: risk factors in randomized comparative clinical trials. *Clin Infect Dis.* 2020;71(6):1379–1389.

Sax PE, Kumar P. Tolerability and safety of HIV protease inhibitors in adults *J Acquir Immune Defic Syndr.* 2004;37(1):1111–1124. Published correction appears in *J Acquir Immune Defic Syndr.* 2004 Nov 1;37(3):1434.Sekhar RV, Jahoor F, White AC, et al. Metabolic basis of HIV-lipodystrophy syndrome. *Am J Physiol Endocrinol Metab.* 2002;283(2):E332–E337.

Shikuma CM, Hu N, Milne C, et al. Mitochondrial DNA decrease in subcutaneous adipose tissue of HIV-infected individuals with peripheral lipoatrophy. *AIDS.* 2001;15:1801–1809.

Short WR, Ramgopal M, Hagins DP, et al. A prospective, randomized trial to assess a protease inhibitor–based regimen switch strategy to manage integrase inhibitor–related weight gain. *Open Forum Infect Dis.* 2023;10:ofad500.112.

Siddiqui J, Samuel SK, Hayward B, et al. HIV-associated wasting prevalence in the era of modern antiretroviral therapy. *AIDS.* 2022a;36(1):127–135.

Siddiqui J, Samuel SK, Hayward B, et al. The economic burden of HIV-associated wasting in the era of modern antiretroviral therapy. *J Manag Care Spec Pharm.* 2022b;28(10):1180-1189.

Silva GA, Andrade MC, Sugui Dde A, et al. Association between antiretrovirals and thyroid diseases: a cross-sectional study. *Arch Endocrinol Metab.* 2015;59(2):116–122.

Slama L, Palella FJ, Abraham AG, et al. Inaccuracy of haemoglobin A1c among HIV-infected men: effects of CD4 cell count, antiretroviral therapies and haematological parameters. *J Antimicrob Chemother.* 2014;69(12):2260–2267.

Sobieszczyk ME, Hoover DR, Anastos K, et al. Prevalence and predictors of metabolic syndrome among HIV-infected and HIV-uninfected women in the Women's Interagency HIV Study. *J AIDS.* 2008;48:272–280.

Stricker RB, Goldberg DA, Hu C, et al. A syndrome resembling primary aldosteronism (Conn syndrome) in untreated HIV disease. *AIDS.* 1999;13:1791–1792.

Szebeni J, Dieffenbach C, Wahl SM, et al. Induction of alpha interferon by human immunodeficiency virus type 1 in human monocyte–macrophage cultures. *J Virol.* 1991;65:6362–6364.

Tang AM, Forrester J, Spiegelman D, Knox TA, Tchetgen E, Gorbach SL. Weight loss and survival in HIV-positive patients in the era of highly active antiretroviral therapy. *J Acquir Immune Defic Syndr.* 2002;31(2):230–236.

Tavares-Bello C, Sousa Santos F, Sequiera Duarte J, et al. Diabetes insipidus and hypopituitarism in HIV: an unexpected cause. *Endocrinol Diabetes Metab Case Rep.* 2017;17–24. doi:10.1530/EDM-17-0024

Theodorou M, Serst̩é T, Van Gossum M, et al. Factors associated with vitamin D deficiency in a population of 2044 HIV-infected patients. *Clin Nutr.* 2014;33(2):274–279.

Tien PC, Grunfeld C. What is HIV-associated lipodystrophy? Defining fat distribution changes in HIV infection. *Curr Opin Infect Dis.* 2004;17(1):27–32.

Toma E, Therrien R. Gynecomastia during indinavir antiretroviral therapy in HIV infection. *AIDS.* 1998;12:681–682.

Tracey KJ, Cerami A. Metabolic responses to cachectin/TNF: a brief review. *Ann N Y Acad Sci.* 1990;587:325–331.

Tzur F, Chowers M, Agmon-Levin N, et al. Increased prevalence of diabetes mellitus in a non-obese adult population: HIV-infected Ethiopians. *Isr Med Assoc J.* 2015;17(10):620–623.

Ukibe NR, Ukibe SN, Emelumadu OF, et al. Impact of thyroid function abnormalities on reproductive hormones during menstrual cycle in premenopausal HIV infected females at NAUTH, Nnewi, Nigeria. *PLoS One.* 2017;12(7):e0176361.

Van den Bout-Van Den Beukel, C, Fievez L, Michels M, et al. Vitamin D deficiency among HIV type 1-infected individuals in the Netherlands: effects of antiretroviral therapy. *AIDS Res Hum Retrovir.* 2008;24:1375–1382.

van Wijk JP, de Koning EJ, Cabezas MC, et al. Comparison of rosiglitazone and metformin for treating HIV lipodystrophy: a randomized trial *Ann Intern Med.* 2005;143(5):337–-346. Published correction appears in *Ann Intern Med.* 2005 Nov 1;143(9):695. Dosage error in published abstract; MEDLINE/PubMed abstract corrected.

Venter WF, Bosch B, Sokhela S, et al. Final week 192 results from the ADVANCE trial: first-line TAF/FTC/DTG, TDF/FTC/DTG vs TDF/FTC/EFV. AIDS 2022. Montreal, Canada; July 29–August 2. Poster abstract PELBB01.

Villette JM, Bourin P, Doinel C, et al. Circadian variations in plasma levels of hypophyseal, adrenocortical and testicular hormones in men infected with human immunodeficiency virus. *J Clin Endocrinol Metab.* 1990;70:572–577.

Vodkin I, Valasek MA, Bettencourt R, et al. Clinical, biochemical and histological differences between HIV-associated NAFLD and primary NAFLD: a case-control study. *Aliment Pharmacol Ther.* 2015;41(4):368–378.

Wanke CA, Silva M, Knox TA, et al. Weight loss and wasting remain common complications in individuals infected with human immunodeficiency virus in the era of highly active antiretroviral therapy. *Clin Infect Dis.* 2000;31:803.

Wegermann K, Moylan C, Naggie S. Fatty liver disease: enter the metabolic era. *Curr HIV/AIDS Rep.* 2023;20(6):405–418.

Wohl DA, Koethe JR, Sax PE, et al. Antiretrovirals and weight change: weighing the evidence. *Clin Infect Dis.* 2024;79(4):999–1005. doi:10.1093/cid/ciae191

Wohl DA, McComsey G, Tebas P, et al. Current concepts in the diagnosis and management of metabolic complications of HIV infection and its therapy. *Clin Infect Dis.* 2006;43(5):645–653.Xiong Y, Hales DB. The role of the tumor necrosis factor-alpha in the regulation of mouse Leydig cell steroidogenesis. *Endocrinology.* 1993;132:2438–2444.

Yombi JC, Maiter D, Belkhir L, et al. Iatrogenic Cushing's syndrome and secondary adrenal insufficiency after a single intra-articular administration of triamcinolone acetonide in HIV-infected patients treated with ritonavir. *Clin Rheumatol.* 2008;27(Suppl 2):S79–S82.

Youssef J, Sadera R, Mital D, Ahmed MH. HIV and the pituitary gland: clinical and biochemical presentations. *J Lab Physicians.* 2021;13(1):84–90.

33.

HIV AND BONE HEALTH

Roger Bedimo

LEARNING OBJECTIVES

- Discuss the prevalence of low bone mineral density (BMD) and osteoporotic fractures in persons with HIV (PWH).
- Describe the risk factors associated with diminished BMD and fractures in PWH.
- Discuss the potential pathogenic mechanisms of decreased bone health and increased fracture risk in PWH.
- List the screening indications and diagnostic tests used to identify bone disease in PWH.
- Discuss current treatment strategies for PWH found to have low BMD or who have sustained bone fractures.

WHAT'S NEW?

- With the increased survival of PWH due to effective ART, the burden of comorbidity is significantly increasing, with 45% of PWH predicted to have two or more physical comorbidities by 2030. These include increased fracture risk.
- HIV infection and menopausal stage are independent predictors of lower BMD, and they have an additive effect on lumbar spine and total hip BMD changes.

KEY POINTS

- As survival of PWH on ART increases, non-AIDS complications account for an increasing impact on morbidity and mortality. Although incident fracture has been shown to be associated with an almost 50% greater risk of all-cause mortality in PWH, post-fracture mortality rates per 100 person-years (py) decreased significantly in the past couple of decades, likely reflecting advances in HIV care.
- Fracture prevalence is greater in PWH: incident fracture rates among PWH in the HIV Outpatient Study (HOPS) were increased nearly 3-fold compared to rates for the general U.S. population.
- PWH have an increased risk of all fractures, not only osteoporotic fractures. Asymptomatic vertebral fractures are highly prevalent among PWH over the age of 50.
- In addition to traditional factors such as age, smoking, and hepatitis C virus (HCV) infection, frailty, prolonged amenorrhea, and proteinuria, HIV disease-associated factors and ART-related factors are predictive indicators of fracture risk in PWH.
- Both HIV disease and ART increase bone turnover. This is likely the main mechanism for decreased BMD in PWH.
- ART initiation is associated with a BMD decrease of 2%–6%, with the largest decrease occurring in the first 6–12 months of treatment and stabilizing thereafter. Compared to tenofovir alafenamide (TAF), tenofovir disoproxil fumarate (TDF) is associated with a greater (approximately 2%) decline in BMD. Switching virologically suppressed PWH from TDF to TAF results in significant (approximately 2%) increases in BMD. The clinical relevance of these changes is not yet clear.
- HIV providers should maintain a greater index of suspicion for impaired bone health. Despite limited HIV-specific evidence-based recommendations regarding screening for bone disease, extrapolation of screening recommendations from the general population is reasonable. Several organizations recommend using dual-energy X-ray absorptiometry (DXA) and/or the Fracture Risk Assessment Tool (FRAX®) to aid in screening PWH at risk of fractures.
- Bisphosphonates can safely be administered to PWH, with evidence supporting durable gains in BMD, including among youth with HIV.

INTRODUCTION

With improved long-term survival among persons living with HIV (PWH), age-related comorbidities, including osteoporosis and fragility fractures, have become more prevalent (Althoff et al., 2024; Jespersen et al., 2021; Kim et al., 2021; Pramukti et al 2020; Trickey et al., 2023). There is increasing evidence that cardiovascular, renal, and bone disease and neurocognitive deficits are more common among aging PWH, with negative interactions between these comorbidities. Data from cohort and prospective randomized studies suggest that, for a multitude of reasons, PWH are at increased risk of metabolic bone disease and related fractures (Chang et al., 2021;

Zhang et al., 2022). More importantly, incident fracture has been associated with 48% greater risk of all-cause mortality among PWH in care in the United States. Thus, HIV providers should maintain a greater index of suspicion for decreased bone health in PWH, and routinely assess need for screening and fracture prevention interventions (Battalora et al., 2021).

BONE MINERALIZATION ABNORMALITIES

The World Health Organization (WHO) defines two categories of bone abnormalities based on comparison with the mean bone mineral density (BMD) of young healthy women (*T*-score): (1) osteoporosis—which refers to low bone mass and microarchitectural deterioration of bone tissue, correlating with a BMD value more than 2.5 standard deviations below the mean BMD of young adult women (BMD *T*-score < −2.5); and (2) osteopenia—which refers to low bone mass, with a BMD value between 1 and 2.5 standard deviations below the mean BMD of young adult women (−2.5 < BMD *T*-score < −1) (World Health Organization [WHO], 1994; Woolf and Pfleger, 2003). Osteomalacia is a third type of bone mineralization abnormality and refers to softening of bones due to impaired bone mineralization, typically resulting from severe vitamin D deficiency (McComsey et al., 2010; WHO, 2002). Osteonecrosis or avascular necrosis is another bone abnormality; it results from interrupted blood supply to a bone or part of a bone, commonly occurring as a complication of trauma or fracture and typically located at the articular end of a bone (WHO, 2002). Traditional risk factors for low BMD include low body mass index (BMI), history of fracture, older age, and race/ethnicity. Additional risk factors such as low testosterone, smoking, low $CD4^+$ T cell counts, low lean and fat mass, and lipodystrophy may be especially relevant for PWH. HIV itself impacts bone development in children, but initiation of antiretroviral therapy (ART) is associated with further decline in BMD and increased fracture risk (Guo et al., 2021; Rakuni et al., 2021). The long-term metabolic consequences of HIV and ART need further evaluation (see below for additional discussion). Additionally, data highlight significant differences between men and women regarding the effects of HIV on bone.

Bones are constantly being remodeled, in part to repair microfractures; thus, there is an ongoing delicate balance between bone formation and bone resorption. The rate of remodeling is measured from serum levels of bone turnover markers: these include bone formation markers such as osteocalcin and bone-specific alkaline phosphatase; and bone resorption markers such as C-terminal telopeptide. Bone strength is a function of bone density and bone quality. Bone quality refers to the rate of remodeling, microarchitecture, size, shape, amount of mineralization in the bone, and matrix quality (Yin, 2012). Microarchitecture is observed with computed tomography (CT) imaging. Mineralization quantity and matrix quality can be determined by biopsy, but this is rarely indicated. The importance of considering the microarchitecture or quality of bone was highlighted in a WIHS analysis which included 319 women with and 118 without HIV (Sharma et al., 2018). In this cohort, although BMD loss by DXA was similar between the two groups, bone microarchitecture or quality of bone was significantly worse in women with HIV. Ultimately, the effects of HIV on bone health are more complex than mere quantification by DXA alone.

LOW BONE MINERAL DENSITY IN PWH: PREVALENCE

Multiple cohort studies have found a higher than expected prevalence of low BMD in populations of adult PWH (Brown and Qaqish, 2006). Notably, studies have represented diverse populations, including ART-naive and ART-experienced PWH (Bedimo et al., 2012; Escota et al., 2016; McComsey et al., 2011). In one meta-analysis, the prevalence of osteopenia and osteoporosis was 2.4–3.4 times higher in PWH compared to HIV-uninfected adults, with differences by site (lumbar spine and hip) (Goh et al., 2018). Investigators from the Study to Understand the Natural History of HIV and AIDS in the Era of Effective Therapy (SUN), which was a prospective, observational cohort study funded by the Centers for Disease Control and Prevention (CDC), determined that low BMD at the hip and femoral neck was significantly more prevalent in PWH than in matched controls from NHANES (47% vs. 29%; $p < 0.001$). Among 653 participants (77% male, median age 41 years, median $CD4^+$ T-cell count 464 cells/mm^3; 89% with HIV RNA levels <400 copies/mL), 51% had osteopenia and 10% had osteoporosis at baseline (Escota et al., 2016). In a cohort study of Danish PWH which included a matched control group of seronegative individuals, PWH 40 years and older had higher cumulative incidence of osteoporosis. Additionally, this was more pronounced in the modern ART era than pre-HAART (Hansen et al., 2012). BMD has been shown to be lower in PWH before ART initiation, likely due to both an overrepresentation of traditional osteoporosis risk factors in PWH as well as catabolic effects of HIV infection due to uncontrolled viremia. Initiation of ART then leads to further declines in BMD which appear to stabilize over time. Given increased life expectancy with more widespread use of effective ART, more contemporary data on bone loss among PWH over the age of 65 years are critically needed, as this is the period in which fractures are generally most prevalent.

BONE HEALTH IN POSTMENOPAUAL WOMEN WITH HIV

Postmenopausal women with HIV demonstrate particularly high rates of BMD decline. In one longitudinal study, higher rates of bone decline at the spine and forearm were observed among women with HIV compared to HIV-negative women (Yin et al., 2012). Coupled with the increased prevalence of fractures among PWH overall, observations such as these have led to increased concern especially for postmenopausal women aging with HIV (Triant et al., 2008). In a recent analysis of the Women's Interagency HIV Study (WIHS), women with HIV had 5%–9% lower BMD at all sites (including the lumbar spine, femoral neck, and wrist) compared to uninfected women, and the prevalence of osteoporosis was significantly higher among women with HIV. In fully adjusted models, HIV infection and menopausal stage remained independent predictors of lower BMD, and also had an additive effect on lumbar spine and total hip BMD (Sharma et al., 2022). Investigators concluded that additional research was needed to better understand underlying mechanisms by which HIV impacts BMD and to mitigate osteoporosis and fracture risk in aging populations, especially women.

FRACTURES IN PWH: EPIDEMIOLOGY AND RISK FACTORS

Numerous studies have concluded that PWH are at greater risk of bone fractures. Early population-based analyses involving data from a large U.S. healthcare system found that fracture prevalence was greater in women and men with HIV compared to the general population (Triant et al., 2008). Specifically, PWH had a higher number of vertebral, hip, wrist, and combined fractures. Findings were consistent across age, race, and sex categories. However, no correlations could be made regarding specific risk factors due to limited data.

Several large observational studies have compared fracture incidence in PWH to that of control groups. Differences in populations, covariates, types, and definitions of fractures included (i.e., all fractures or fragility fractures whose definitions varied) were unique to each study. In one WIHS cohort of 1,728 PWH and 663 HIV-negative pre-menopausal women, rates of fractures were not increased in women with HIV compared to HIV-negative women (Yin et al., 2010). However, among women with HIV, having a history of an AIDS-defining illness was a more predictive indicator of fracture than being on ART. Between 2000 and 2006, incident fracture rates among 5,826 PWH in the HOPS study (median baseline age of 40 years, 79% male, and 73% on ART) were increased nearly 3-fold compared to rates in the U.S. general population (Young et al., 2011). Greater proportions of fractures were located at the hip, wrist, or spine in PWH, and fractures were associated with lower $CD4^+$ T-cell count nadir, longer duration of HIV diagnosis, and HIV-HCV coinfection. Results also suggested that younger PWH, particularly those between ages 25 and 54 years, are at an increased risk of fracture compared to the general population. Given these observations, authors recommended regular assessment of fracture risk for PWH and especially people with low nadir $CD4^+$ T-cell counts and other recognized risk factors. In the all-male Veterans Aging Cohort Study Virtual Cohort (VACS-VC) study, investigators reported that men with HIV were at greater risk for fragility fracture compared to HIV-negative counterparts (Womack et al., 2011). Among 119,318 men (33% PWH, 34% were 50 years or older at baseline, and 55% were Black or Hispanic), fracture risk factors included age, race, alcohol dependency, liver disease, tobacco use, and current use of corticosteroids or proton pump inhibitors.

European investigators have also studied the incidence of fragility fractures in PWH. In a comparative, sex- and age-matched Danish study involving 5,306 PWH and a general population cohort of 26,530 HIV-negative participants, PWH had an increased overall rate of fractures and increased risk of low-energy fractures, but not high-energy fractures (Hansen et al., 2012). There was a moderate increased risk of low-energy fracture in PWH undergoing ART after controlling for traditional osteoporosis risk factors (i.e., age and smoking).

In the AIDS Clinical Trials Group A5224s (a substudy of ACTG A5202), McComsey and colleagues concluded that fracture rates increased in 269 subjects during the first 2 years after ART initiation, compared to additional years of therapy. Although different BMD changes were observed between patients initiating different ART regimens, no significant differences in fracture rate were reported, although the cohort was young and follow-up was limited (McComsey et al., 2011). In a large retrospective cohort study involving 56,600 patients (95% male, mean age 45 years), osteoporotic fractures were associated with cumulative exposure to tenofovir disoproxil fumarate (TDF) and other ART (Bedimo et al., 2012). Finally, low femoral neck BMD was associated with greater risk of subsequent incident fracture among 1,006 participants of the HIV Outpatient Study (HOPS) and SUN Study Investigators (Battalora et al., 2016).

Additional analyses have highlighted underappreciated fracture types, namely asymptomatic vertebral fractures (Llop et al., 2018). In one cohort of 93 males and 35 females (mean age of 57 years), with more than 70% having low BMD at both hip and spine by DXA, 20% were found to have an asymptomatic vertebral fracture. Associated factors included older age, longer time since HIV diagnosis, and renal insufficiency. Authors concluded that routine spinal imaging with plain x-rays should be considered in aging PWH.

One recent meta-analysis of 84 studies focused on bone health and fracture risk in the setting of HIV (Starup-Linde 2020). Authors concluded that HIV infection is associated with a significant increase in incident fragility fracture (HR 1.51) and a marked increased risk of hip fracture (HR 4.05). This increased risk does not appear to be explained by differences in BMD alone or by early changes after ART initiation, thus suggesting a difference in the quality of bone or other factors related to HIV disease. HIV has consistently been associated with an approximately 2-fold increased risk of fracture, with a wide range of incident fracture rates reported among PWH: from 0.1/1,000 py to 11.3/1,000 py (Pramukti et al., 2020).

It's important to note that in addition to traditional risk factors such as older age and smoking, specific HIV-associated factors (e.g., nadir $CD4^+$ T-cell count) as well as ART-related factors are important predictive indicators of fracture risk in PWH. In the 2014 *Clinician's Guide to Prevention and Treatment of Osteoporosis*, the National Osteoporosis Foundation (NOF) included AIDS/HIV as disease risk factors for osteoporosis and fragility fractures (Battalora et al., 2014; NOF 2014).

More recent research has identified additional mediators of fracture risk in the setting of HIV.

Approximately 15%–30% of PWH have HCV coinfection, and people with HIV-HCV coinfection have a 3-fold higher fracture incidence compared to uninfected individuals,

Box 33.1 FRACTURE RISK FACTORS IN PWH: SUMMARY

Increased bone loss and fracture risk in PWH is multifactorial, likely involving the confluence of three groups of factors: the host (including genetic, behavioral, and environmental characteristics), the virus (and possible coinfections such as HCV), and ART.

1. The overrepresentation of traditional osteoporosis risk factors among PWH likely accounts for some of the fracture risk observed in this population. These include: smoking, alcohol consumption, exposure to glucocorticoids, decreased activity, lipodystrophy, vitamin D deficiency, low body weight/weight loss, hypogonadism, and chronic kidney disease. At least one genetic marker or HLA supertype, specifically HLA-DQ3, has been associated with bone density status in one cohort study of PWH (Haskelberg et al., 2014).
2. HIV-specific factors that likely contribute to increased fracture risk include increased bone turnover, evidenced by increased levels of serologic bone formation and bone resorption makers (Bedimo et al., 2016). HIV may directly affect bone cells by viral protein induction of osteoclastogenesis or by causing osteoblast apoptosis (Raynaud-Messina et al., 2018). The relationship between HIV proteins on bone loss may not be a direct effect, but rather an indirect or bystander effect through mitochondrial toxicity, oxidative stress, or effects on other cell processes (Agidigi and Kim, 2019; Liu et al., 2017). Moreover, T cell and B cell activation during HIV infection results in increased circulating cytokines, including tumor necrosis factor-α, interleukin-6 (IL-6), and RANKL, which appear to induce osteoclast bone resorption (Titanji, 2017). In a study by Hileman, elevated levels of IL-6 were associated with risk of progression to osteoporosis among PWH (Hileman et al., 2014).
3. Hepatitis C coinfection has been an overlooked fracture risk factor in PWH. Patients with coinfection have a 3-fold higher fracture incidence compared to uninfected individuals, and up to twice the fracture risk of HIV mono-infected people (Dong et al., 2014; Hansen et al., 2012; Lo Re et al., 2012; Maalouf et al., 2013).
4. ART initiation has been associated with a BMD decrease of 2%–6%, with the largest decrease occurring in the first 6–12 months of treatment and then stabilizing (Brown et al., 2009). Significant BMD loss was seen with older nucleoside agents such as zidovudine (van Vonderen et al., 2009) and has been well-documented with the use of TDF (McComsey et al., 2011; Yin, 2011). Fracture rates, both fragility and non-fragility, as noted previously, are higher in PWH and are associated with HCV coinfection and possibly ART (Bedimo et al., 2012; Maalouf et al., 2013).

and up to twice the fracture risk of HIV mono-infected people (Bedimo et al., 2012; Dong et al., 2014; Hansen et al., 2012; Lo Re et al., 2012; Maalouf et al., 2013). Despite being consistently associated with higher osteoporotic fracture risk in several reports, HCV coinfection has only been associated with further reductions in BMD among PWH in some, but not all, studies (Anastos et al., 2007; Bedimo et al., 2016; Hansen et al., 2012; Lawson-Ayayi et al., 2013; Lo Re et al., 2009; Maalouf et al., 2013; Yin, 2012; Yin et al., 2012; Young et al., 2011). These findings raise the possibility that the higher risk observed in people with chronic HCV infection might not be due to low BMD alone, but could involve other mechanism(s). In a large cohort of veterans, HIV-HCV coinfection remained a strong independent osteoporotic fracture predictor, even after controlling for cirrhosis (HR 1.31; 95% confidence interval [CI]: 1.12–1.52; p <0.001) (Maalouf et al., 2013). Therefore, severity of liver disease may only partly explain the HCV-associated increased risk of osteoporotic fracture (El-Maouche et al., 2011). Also, HIV-HCV coinfection is not associated with significantly lower femoral neck or lumbar spine BMD than HIV mono-infection, further suggesting that the mechanism(s) underlying increased fracture risk might differ between HIV and HCV (Bedimo et al., 2016). While HIV and ART are associated with increased bone turnover (which might drive decreased BMD and increased fracture risk), HCV did not increase bone turnover (Bedimo et al., 2020).

Frailty, a phenotype generally seen in geriatric populations, has been recognized to occur at an earlier age among PWH. WIHS Cohort investigators reported that frailty was not only more common among women with HIV than their HIV-negative counterparts, but it was also independently associated with time to first fracture as well as second fracture (Sharma et al., 2019). Sarcopenia, or the gradual loss of muscle mass, is a key component of frailty and has long been recognized as a complication of HIV infection.

Finally, observations from the MACS cohort have also linked proteinuria to fragility fractures. In this cohort of men with and without HIV, the presence of proteinuria (which was more common among men with HIV) conferred a 230% increased risk of fragility fracture (Gonciulea et al., 2019). Altogether, these data highlight how chronic comorbidities often cluster in PWH and can add complexity to the long-term care of people aging with HIV (see Box 33.1).

TRAJECTORIES OF BONE MINERAL DENSITY IN PWH: ROLE OF ART

In the general population, BMD peaks at approximately 22–35 years of age (Orwoll, 1995). In PWH initiating HIV treatment, BMD appears to decrease by 2%–6% during the first 1–2 years of ART (Brown et al., 2009). Thereafter, declines in BMD after the first year of ART appear to be much lower, although there are few data on long-term trajectories of BMD changes in PWH. One ACTG study followed 97 PWH (median age 40 years) for a median of 7.5 years after ART initiation and compared their BMD data to that from over 600 HIV-negative controls (Grant et al., 2016). While the rate of BMD loss after week 96 slowed among PWH, the decline in lumbar spine BMD (but not at the total hip) remained significantly greater compared to the control group. These data suggest ongoing metabolic bone disease despite ART-mediated virologic suppression.

Conversely, an analysis of 384 participants of the European UPBEAT cohort found that while there was no difference in the rate of lumbar spine BMD change between HIV-positive and HIV-negative participants, there was a trend toward greater decline in femoral neck BMD ($p = 0.08$) (Tinago et al., 2017). However, this study population was younger overall (median age 39 years); participants over 30 years of age had a greater BMD decline. Another analysis involving 4,640 PWH participants of ACTG trials showed higher osteoporotic fracture rates within the first 2 years after ART initiation. Continuation of ART was not associated with increased fracture rates (Yin et al., 2012). Again, this study population was relatively young (median age of 39 years).

The START study evaluated BMD changes among PWH with relatively preserved immune function ($CD4^+$ count >350 cells/mm^3) who underwent immediate versus delayed ART. Through 2.2 years mean follow-up, immediate ART resulted in greater BMD declines than deferred ART at the hip and spine, but only over the first year. After year 1, BMD changes were similar in the immediate and deferred groups (Hoy et al., 2017).

Overall, few studies have explored longer-term follow-up of BMD changes in PWH, but they suggest stabilization of BMD after the first year of ART. It remains unclear whether the slope of decline in BMD in aging PWH is greater than that of the general population. Low pre-treatment $CD4^+$ count and TDF use (see below) have been shown to be predictive of lower BMD at 5 years after ART initiation (Han et al., 2020). Importantly, one key gap in knowledge is that relatively few studies have explored BMD in virologically suppressed PWH several years after ART initiation, and whether the modest BMD decline with HIV and ART predicts a documented increased osteoporotic fracture risk in this population.

SPECIFIC ANTIRETROVIRALS AND BONE FRAGILITY

Changes in BMD are more pronounced with exposure to certain antiretroviral agents, namely tenofovir disoproxil fumarate (TDF), compared to other agents among both ART-naive and ART-experienced PWH (Cotter et al., 2013; Martin et al., 2009; McComsey et al., 2011; Stellbrink et al., 2011). Tenofovir alafenamide (TAF) appears to have more favorable effects on bone compared to TDF, such that TDF-containing-ART is associated with an approximately 2% greater decline in BMD compared to TAF (Arribas et al., 2017). Studies examining virologically suppressed PWH who switch from TDF to TAF have found significant (~2%) increases in BMD (Raffi et al., 2017). Overall, it is likely that regimens not containing any nucleoside reverse transcriptase inhibitors (NRTIs) are associated with smaller declines in BMD (Bedimo et al., 2014). Protease inhibitors (PIs) also contribute to bone loss, and this appears to be a class effect (McComsey et al., 2011; Moran et al., 2016).

In a large cohort of U.S. veterans (56,660 PWH; 98.1% male; mean age: 45.0 years; 31.2% with HCV coinfection), cumulative exposure to TDF was predictive of increased osteoporotic fracture risk (HR: 1.12; 1.03–1.21, $p = 0.011$) (Bedimo et al., 2012). Further, compared to boosted protease inhibitors or elvitegravir/cobicistat, the use of TDF with efavirenz (EFV) was associated with a significantly lower risk of osteoporotic fractures (LeFleur et al., 2018). This suggests that concomitant ARVs used with TDF may modify its impact on bone changes, possibly through differences in tenofovir exposure. Limited data are available regarding newer ARV agents and classes, including integrase strand transfer inhibitors (Bonfanti et al., 2020; Brown et al., 2015b, 2020).

ADDITIONAL BIOLOGIC MECHANISMS OF BONE FRAGILITY IN PWH

Treated HIV infection is associated with significant increase in bone turnover, reflected by elevations in serum levels of bone resorption markers like c-telopeptide, and bone formation markers like osteocalcin (Bedimo et al., 2016). Studies consistently indicate that ART initiation further increases bone turnover, and this is likely (at least in part) what drives BMD decline (McComsey et al., 2011; Stellbrink et al., 2010). A delicate balance exists between bone formation and bone resorption though the combined effects of osteoblasts and osteoclasts: osteoblasts form bone matrix but also influence bone resorption through the expression of RANKL, which induces osteoclast-mediated bone resorption (Boyce and Xing, 2007). Recent in vitro and animal data show that TDF (and to some extent other ARVs) decreases osteoblast formation and gene expression but does not increase bone resorption, as shown in clinical studies (Convadie et al., 2017; Olali et al., 2024). Reasons for these discrepancies are unclear.

CLINICAL MANAGEMENT

SCREENING FOR BONE DISEASE

There is limited evidence to guide recommendations specific to PWH regarding screening for bone disease; however, extrapolation of recommendations from the general population is reasonable. The National Osteoporosis Foundation (NOF) published recommendations for postmenopausal women and men aged 50 years or older (NOF, 2014). These guidelines were updated in 2022 by the Bone Health and Osteoporosis Foundation (BHOF) (Leboff et al., 2022), which is the new iteration of the NOF. Providers are advised to consult the complete set of guidelines for detail, however major recommendations are summarized here:

- Counsel patients on risk of osteoporosis and related fractures.
- Assess for secondary causes of osteoporosis.

- Advise patients on adequate calcium intake (1,000 mg/day for men aged 50–70 years; 1,200 mg/day for women ≥51 years and men ≥71 years) and maintain adequate vitamin D levels. In healthy individuals, a serum 25(OH) vitamin D level ≥20 ng/mL may be sufficient, but in the setting of known or suspected metabolic bone disease, ≥30 ng/mL is more appropriate.
- Recommend regular weight-bearing and muscle-strengthening exercise to reduce risk of falls and fractures.
- Advise against tobacco smoking and excessive alcohol consumption.
- Recommend BMD testing in women aged 65 years or older and men aged 70 years or older. For postmenopausal women and men aged 50–69 years, recommend BMD testing based on risk-factor profile.
- In postmenopausal women and men older than age 50 years who have had an adult-age fracture, diagnose and determine degree of osteoporosis.
- Initiate pharmacotherapy for patients with hip or vertebral (clinical or morphometric) fractures, regardless of BMD.
- Initiate therapy in patients with BMD *T*-scores of –2.5 or less at the femoral neck or spine by DXA, after appropriate evaluation.
- Initiate treatment in postmenopausal women and men aged 50 years or older with low bone mass (*T*-score between –1.0 and –2.5, indicating osteopenia) at the femoral neck or spine and a 10-year hip fracture probability 3% or greater, or a 10-year major osteoporosis-related fracture probability of 20% or greater based on the U.S.-adapted WHO absolute fracture risk model FRAX®.
- BMD testing performed in DXA centers using accepted quality assurance measures is appropriate for monitoring bone loss. Patients taking FDA-approved medications for low BMD should have laboratory and bone density re-evaluation after 2 years, or more frequently as indicated (Leboff et al., 2022; NOF, 2014).

In 2015, the Osteo Renal Exchange Program (OREP) published recommendations for the evaluation and management of bone disease in PWH (Brown et al., 2015a). Input on these recommendations was provided by 34 HIV specialists from 16 countries. Noting global variation in practice and subsequent difficulty in determining a single set of recommendations, use of the FRAX® risk calculator (see below) without BMD is recommended for patient assessment in resource-limited settings without access to DXA scanning. Although updates to these recommendations are anticipated as additional data emerge from observational cohorts and other analyses, recommendations may help guide clinicians in practice across many settings. Providers are advised to consult the complete list of recommendations and accompanying rationale; however, major points for PWH are summarized here:

- Avoid use of TDF or boosted protease inhibitors in PWH with low BMD or osteoporosis.
- Ensure adequate daily intake of dietary calcium for postmenopausal women and men ≥50 years of age (1,000 mg for men 50–70 years of age, or 1,200 mg for women ≥51 years of age and men ≥71 years of age).
- Supplementary vitamin D should be given to PWH with vitamin D insufficiency (<20 ng/mL [<50 nmol/L]) or deficiency (<10 ng/mL [<25 nmol/L]).
- Anti-osteoporosis treatment should be initiated for PWH using the same criteria as for the general population. However, since many anti-osteoporosis treatments lack sufficient safety and efficacy data specific to PWH, the bisphosphonates alendronate (70 mg once weekly) and zoledronic acid (5 mg yearly) are preferred.
- The need for continued bisphosphonate use should be reassessed after 3–5 years, given the risk of long-term suppression of bone turnover (which may manifest as osteonecrosis of the jaw or atypical femoral fractures).

SCREENING FOR VITAMIN D INSUFFICIENCY

Vitamin D testing and supplementation remain an area of debate and active inquiry. Various organizations and institutions have published guidance regarding vitamin D deficiency, although none are specific for PWH. The Institute of Medicine (IOM) published dietary reference intakes for calcium and vitamin D but did not provide screening recommendations or specific reference intakes for PWH (IOM, 2011). The Endocrine Society (EOS) and European AIDS Clinical Society (EACS) both recommended screening at-risk patients and those on ART and having risk factors for low vitamin D or fracture (Endocrine Society [EOS], 2011; European AIDS Clinical Society [EACS], 2023). The U.S. Preventive Services Task Force (USPSTF) and American Academy of Family Physicians state that current evidence is insufficient to assess the balance of benefits and harms regarding screening for vitamin D deficiency in asymptomatic adults (LeFevre and LeFevre, 2018). There are limited data on vitamin D supplementation in PWH, although several studies have demonstrated benefit for BMD and reduction in PTH and bone turnover markers (Havens et al., 2018a; Overton et al., 2015).

SCREENING FOR FALL RISK AND FRAILTY

Fall risk assessment tools are used to determine the probability of future falls, and typically aim to capture information on various fall risk factors. These include recent falls, medications, psychological and cognitive status, vision, mobility, ability to transfer, behaviors, activities of daily living, environment, nutrition, continence, and other factors. Screening for frailty in the office setting is reasonable and may help identify PWH at heightened risk for falls and fragility fractures.

SCREENING FOR FRACTURE RISK

FRAX®

FRAX® is an assessment tool developed by the WHO Metabolic Bone Disease Group to assess fractures with more optimal predictors of risk compared to *T*-scores (van den Bergh et al., 2010; WHO Metabolic Bone Disease Group, 2008), and is not HIV-specific. FRAX® provides 10-year probability of hip fracture and 10-year probability of a major osteoporotic fracture (hip, spine, shoulder, or forearm). Probability is estimated based on clinical risk factors and BMD values from the femoral neck. Models have been developed based on location (i.e., Asia, Europe, Middle East and Africa, North America, Latin America, and Oceania) and ethnicity. Risk factors included in the calculation tool are: age, sex, weight, height, previous fracture, parent fractured hip, current tobacco smoking, glucocorticoid exposure, rheumatoid arthritis, secondary osteoporosis, alcohol intake of 3 or more units per day, and BMD or, alternatively, *T*-score based on the NHANES III female reference data (Kanis et al., 2007).

The International Osteoporosis Foundation, NOF, American Society for Bone and Mineral Research, and International Society for Clinical Densitometry all endorse the use of FRAX® (van den Bergh et al., 2010). The NOF recommends using FRAX® for postmenopausal women and men aged 50 years or older who are not on treatment, who have not had spine or hip fractures, and who have *T*-scores between –1.0 and –2.5 SD (NOF, 2014; van den Bergh et al., 2010). If the FRAX® 10-year probability exceeds 20% for major osteoporotic fractures or 3% risk for hip fracture, NOF guidelines recommend initiating pharmacotherapy (NOF, 2014).

Increasing baseline FRAX® 10-year probability was consistently associated with increased rates of incident fractures in a large cohort of adult PWH (Battalora et al., 2014). Although FRAX® may underestimate fracture risk in PWH, the European AIDS Clinical Society (EACS) recommends FRAX® screening in all persons older than age 40 years (EACS, 2023).

DUAL-ENERGY X-RAY ABSORPTIOMETRY (DXA) AND OTHER ASSESSMENT TOOLS

Bone mineral density (BMD) measurements are typically obtained using DXA scan. Relevant measurement locations include the hip, spine, and forearm. DXA is a two-dimensional system in which the size of the specimen is directly proportional to the estimate of area density. Overestimation of BMD values obtained from larger patients has been cited as a concern (Amorosa and Tebas, 2006a). Of greater concern is that DXA, unfortunately, has not been validated for fractures among PWH. Furthermore, few data exist on younger adults except in those taking TDF for pre-exposure prophylaxis (PrEP). Additional concerns are the application of WHO definitions for osteoporosis and osteopenia to populations and skeletal sites other than those serving as the basis for the DXA correlations on which these bone abnormality definitions are described (Amorosa and Tebas, 2006b).

Although DXA is noninvasive and convenient, it does not assess bone condition, bone structure, or bone quality, a factor directly linked to load-bearing strength. It has been suggested that DXA may underestimate fracture risk in PWH (Ofotokun and Weitzmann, 2011). One study demonstrated that approximately 50% of postmenopausal women without HIV experiencing a fracture did not meet the clinical definition of osteoporosis based on DXA values (Nguyen et al., 2007).

Other existing BMD measurement tools may assist in the prediction of fragility fracture risk but have inherent limitations. Quantitative CT scanning (QCT) detects volumetric density and in some studies has been shown to detect a higher occurrence of osteoporosis and osteopenia (Pitukcheewanont et al., 2005). However, QCT is more expensive than DXA, requires a higher radiation dose, and is mainly used in research settings (Amorosa and Tebas, 2006a). Other tools, including quantitative ultrasound and analysis of biochemical and hormonal markers, may prove increasingly useful in the future.

Because of data indicating that modest changes in BMD have not proven to be predictive of fracture risk in PWH, researchers have investigated other means of assessing bone health. Trabecular bone score (TBS) is a novel measurement of bone microarchitecture from DXA images. A high TBS value is associated with better bone structure, whereas low TBS values indicate worse bone structure (Silva et al., 2014). TBS is a proven osteoporotic fracture predictor, even after adjusting for BMD (Leslie et al., 2015), and is now included as an independent risk factor in the FRAX® algorithm for fracture risk prediction (McCloskey et al., 2016).

Predictors of BMD and TBS were evaluated in a prospective, cross-sectional cohort study of virologically suppressed PWH, chronic HCV, HIV-HCV coinfection, and uninfected controls. In a linear regression, despite both infections being associated with decreased BMD, only HCV, but not HIV, was associated with lower TBS score. Also, people with HIV-HCV coinfection had lower TBS scores than HIV-mono-infected, HCV-mono-infected, and uninfected subjects. Neither the use of TDF nor HCV viremia, nor the severity of liver disease, was associated with lower TBS (Bedimo et al., 2018). This suggests that microstructural abnormalities underlie some of the higher fracture risk in HCV infection in PWH and the general population. TBS has also been used to compare specific ARV agents. In one recent study, despite significant differences in changes in BMD between the TDF and abacavir (ABC), there were no differences in TBS changes after initiation of TDF or ABC (Bedimo et al., 2020).

The BHOF recommends DXA screening for osteoporosis in the general population for women aged 65 years or older and men aged 70 years or older, regardless of clinical risk factors (LeBoff et al., 2022a). They also recommend that women in menopausal transition and men aged 50–69 years with clinical risk factors for fracture, such as HIV, should also be screened. Men and women aged 50 years or older who have had a fracture and for persons with other established risk factors, including rheumatoid arthritis or glucocorticoid use, should be screened (LeBoff et al., 2022). The BHOF does not provide HIV-specific guidelines for DXA screening.

After initial DXA screening, the BHOF suggests that "less frequent BMD testing may be warranted as follow-up for patients with initial T-scores in the normal or slightly below normal range (osteopenia) and for patients who have remained fracture free on treatment" (LeBoff et al., 2022). In a 2012 study of 5,000 HIV-negative women >67 years old and without osteoporosis who were followed with BMD for 15 years, the time interval during which at least 10% of women developed osteoporosis was greater than 15 years for those with normal baseline BMD and 5 years for those with baseline moderate osteopenia (Gourlay et al., 2012). Another study in 3,650 men >65 years old followed for 15 years found that only 2.5% of men without osteoporosis at baseline transitioned to a T-score less than −2.5 (Ensrud et al., 2022). These studies suggest that routine BMD testing every several years is not necessary in people with baseline normal BMD. Increasing initial screening of all patients at risk is therefore more likely to identify patients at greatest fracture risk than rescreening low-risk individuals.

The Infectious Diseases Society of America (IDSA) and HIV Medicine Association (HIVMA) recommend baseline DXA screening in HIV-positive postmenopausal women and men aged 50 years or older, based on expert opinion (Thompson et al., 2021). Following baseline DXA, IDSA/HIVMA guidelines recommend periodic monitoring of risk factors for premature bone loss. Risk factors to consider include white race, small body habitus, sedentary lifestyle, cigarette smoking, alcohol use disorder, phenytoin therapy, corticosteroid therapy, hyperparathyroidism, vitamin D deficiency, thyroid disease, and hypogonadism. The European AIDS Clinical Society (EACS) guideline recommends DXA screening for any patient with one or more of the following conditions, preferably prior to initiation of ART (EACS, 2023):

- Postmenopausal women
- Men aged 50 years or older
- History of low-impact fracture or high risk for falls
- Clinical hypogonadism
- Those with high fracture risk (i.e., >20% 10-year major osteoporotic fracture risk based on FRAX® assessment without DXA)
- Oral glucocorticoid use (minimum 5mg/day prednisone equivalent for >3 months).

Adherence to recommended measures and their effectiveness in preventing fractures in PWH have not been fully evaluated. Among a national cohort of nearly 5 million male U.S. veterans, there were only 11.5 primary prevention screenings per 1,000 py, a rate far below even the rate of fragility fractures in the same population (15.6 events/1,000 py) (LeFleur et al., 2016). In PWH, bisphosphonate therapy results in significant improvements in BMD, but the efficacy of these measures in reducing osteoporotic fracture incidence needs further evaluation (McComsey et al., 2007; Mondy et al., 2005).

THERAPEUTIC INTERVENTIONS FOR LOW BMD

Providers caring for PWH with low BMD and associated complications should consider multiple factors. These include patient profile, age, risk factor reduction interventions, potential for drug-drug interactions, underlying hepatic or renal disease, and likelihood of medication adherence. Endpoints of randomized controlled trials examining the efficacy and safety of osteoporosis treatments typically include hip fractures, any fracture, clinical and/or radiological vertebral fractures. One important caveat is that the majority of data are based on postmenopausal women, with findings usually then generalized to all persons, and then to PWH.

IDENTIFY AND TREAT SECONDARY CAUSES OF LOW BONE MINERAL DENSITY

For persons with abnormal DXA scans (*T*-scores of 1 or less) or with a history of a fragility fracture, clinicians should evaluate and address secondary causes of osteoporosis. This particularly includes cases in which vitamin D deficiency or phosphate wasting are observed, as these conditions can cause osteomalacia or bone mineralization deficiency and may be difficult to differentiate from osteoporosis based on DXA scans (Yin et al., 2012).

BEHAVIORAL AND LIFESTYLE ADVICE

Several lifestyle factors, including being sedentary and cigarette smoking, are associated with low BMD and/or fractures in the general population. Modification of diet to optimize calcium and vitamin D intake, increasing weight-bearing exercise, and smoking cessation are prudent in general but are especially important among persons at increased risk of low BMD or fractures. In addition, because excess alcohol consumption (>3 units/day) and substance use are associated with fracture risk, strategies to limit or abstain from alcohol consumption/substance use should be discussed with patients.

SPECIFIC TREATMENTS FOR BONE LOSS

Vitamin D and Calcium Supplementation

Vitamin D deficiency is common among PWH and may contribute to low BMD and fractures. Although there are no standardized guidelines for vitamin D and calcium repletion or supplementation, the IOM published a report in 2011 providing dietary recommendations for calcium and vitamin D (IOM, 2011). It suggests 1,000 mg/day of calcium for most adults aged 19–50 years and for men up to age 71 years. No more than 1,200 mg/day of calcium is suggested for women over age 50 years and for men and women aged 71 years or older (IOM, 2011).

Specific to PWH, a study in 2014 (ACTG A5280) evaluated the effect of high-dose vitamin D_3 (4,000 IU/day) plus calcium supplementation (1,000 mg/day calcium carbonate) on BMD in 142 PWH (90% male, with mean age 33 years and mean 25(OH) vitamin D level 23 ng/mL) with DXA scanning done at baseline and again 48 weeks after initiating EFV/FTC/TDF. Vitamin D/calcium supplementation mitigated BMD loss particularly at the total hip (Overton et al., 2015). The effect of vitamin D supplementation has subsequently been corroborated by others. Havens and colleagues conducted a randomized controlled trial of high-dose vitamin D among 214 young PWH (median age 22 years); 50,000 units of vitamin D monthly was associated with a significant increase in lumbar spine BMD (1.2% increase vs. no change in the placebo arm). No effect was seen on hip BMD. The group receiving vitamin D also experienced a significant decline in PTH and bone turnover markers (Havens et al., 2018b). A 2022 systemic review and meta-analysis also found that vitamin D and calcium supplementation in PWH and people on TDF-containing PrEP correlated with a significant increase in BMD in the spine and hip (standardized mean difference 0.43; 95% CI: 0.25–0.61, $p = 0.009$) (Bi et al., 2022). Individuals taking 4,000 IU/day of vitamin D obtained the highest BMD improvement.

Assuming minimal sun exposure in geographic regions of the United States and Canada, the IOM suggests 600 IU/day of vitamin D for most persons aged 1–70 years and 800 IUs for persons aged 71 years or older (IOM, 2011). These recommendations are not specific to PWH. However, it may be reasonable to monitor 25-hydroxy vitamin D levels in this population and to recommend supplementation in situations of ART initiation and continued therapy if vitamin D levels are low (Overton et al., 2015; Yin et al., 2012).

Unfortunately, more recent evidence from the large, randomized VITAL trial in 2022 did not show that vitamin D supplements prevented fractures in 26,000 relatively healthy, U.S. HIV-negative adults >50 years old who were randomized to take 2,000 IU of vitamin D_3 or placebo daily (LeBoff, 2022). During an average follow-up of 5 years, there was no difference in total fractures, nonvertebral fractures, or hip fractures, and vitamin D supplementation did not prevent fractures even in subgroups with baseline 25-OH vitamin D levels <24 ng/mL or <12 ng/mL.

Testosterone Replacement

Testosterone deficiency is relatively common in men with HIV, especially in the aging population, and is associated with a decrease in BMD. One study identified the BMD benefits of testosterone supplementation in a cohort of men living with and without HIV (Grant et al., 2019). Testosterone use was more frequently reported in HIV-positive men compared to HIV-negative men (4% vs. 2%, $p < 0.001$). In the overall study population, testosterone use was associated with significantly higher BMD at both the lumbar spine and hip when compared to men not receiving testosterone. Given potential adverse effects associated with exogenous testosterone use, clinicians should assess the risks and benefits of testosterone replacement in PWH with low BMD and low serum testosterone levels.

Bisphosphonates

Currently, there are no specific guidelines for the treatment of BMD disorders among PWH. As noted earlier, diagnosis and management of bone disease for PWH generally follow guidance for the general population. The BHOF currently recommends pharmacologic treatment for postmenopausal women and men aged 50 or older with hip or vertebral fractures or a *T*-score of −2.5 or less at the femoral neck or spine after evaluation to exclude secondary causes (LeBoff et al., 2022). In addition, patients with a *T*-score between −1.0 and −2.5 at the femoral neck or spine and 10-year probability fracture by FRAX® of 3% or greater at the hip or 10-year probability of 20% or greater for any osteoporosis-related fracture should be considered for treatment.

Bisphosphonates inhibit osteoclast resorption; studies among HIV-negative populations indicate that these medications can reduce vertebral and nonvertebral fractures by 25%–50%. They are indicated for the prevention and treatment of osteoporosis and other bone diseases, including Paget's disease (U.S. Food and Drug Administration, 2013). The American College of Physicians and the Endocrine Society recommend bisphosphonates as initial treatment for osteoporosis (Eastell et al., 2019; Qaseem et al., 2023).

The effectiveness of these antiresorptive therapies in PWH has been evaluated in numerous randomized controlled trials. Earlier studies evaluated patients with *T*-scores not within the osteoporotic range (Bolland et al., 2007; Guaraldi et al., 2004; Huang et al., 2009; McComsey et al., 2007; Mondy et al., 2005). One trial included patients with *T*-scores of less than −2.5 (Rozenberg et al., 2012). Overall, results showed significant increases in BMD at the lumbar spine in all six studies and a large increase at the hip in three (Bolland et al., 2007; Huang et al., 2009; McComsey et al., 2007).

One analysis evaluated use of the intravenous bisphosphonate, zoledronic acid, to mitigate bone loss associated with ART (Hoy et al., 2018). This study included subjects on TDF who had low BMD and randomized them to a switch from TDF or administration of a single dose of zoledronic acid or placebo. Zoledronic acid was found to be safe and well tolerated and was associated with a greater increase in BMD at the hip and lumbar spine (4.6% vs. 2.6% and 7.4% vs. 2.9%, respectively).

Longer-term data have been published confirming the beneficial effect of bisphosphonates among PWH. One group reported BMD data from 25 men with HIV 11 years after receiving 2 doses of intravenous zoledronate. Their BMD remained significantly higher at the lumbar spine (3.7%), total hip (3.7%), and femoral neck (5.0% higher) compared to those given placebo. Bone turnover markers remained lower in the treatment arm as well, suggesting that the effect of the bisphosphonate was mediated through reduced bone turnover (Bolland et al., 2019). These results were corroborated by another randomized trial of zoledronate which followed 63 PWH with bone loss for 3 years after treatment. Participants who received a single dose of zoledronate experienced an 11% increase in BMD at the lumbar spine at 3 years, compared to a 4.3% loss in the placebo arm. More modest differences were seen in the femoral neck and total hip, but these changes were not statistically significant (Ofotokun et al., 2020).

One pediatric study evaluated the use of alendronate in children and adolescents with perinatally acquired HIV and with low BMD for age. Fifty-two youths (ages 11–24 years) were randomized to weekly alendronate or placebo for 2 years. The therapy was well-tolerated with similar adverse events in both groups and no cases of osteonecrosis or non-healing fractures. The group receiving alendronate experienced 20% BMD gains in the lumbar spine at 1 year vs. 7% in the placebo arm, with similar differences in the whole-body BMD (Jacobson et al., 2020). Taken as a whole, these data suggest that bisphosphonates are safe and effective for use in PWH. In general, adverse effects of bisphosphonates include osteonecrosis of the jaw (<1 case per 100,000 py of exposure) and subtrochanteric fractures or atypical femoral shaft fractures (uncommon in patients with less than 5 years of treatment) (Yin et al., 2012). Although bisphosphonates should only be administered to patients with appropriate indications (and the FDA recommends stopping treatment after 5 years), some experts believe that HIV providers should generally maintain a low threshold to consider bisphosphonates in PWH given their increased risk of low BMD and fractures.

OTHER OSTEROPOROSIS TREATMENTS

Other osteoporosis treatments include bone anabolic agents, parathyroid and parathyroid-related peptide analogs (abaloparatide and teriparatide), RANKL inhibitors (denosumab), sclerosin inhibitors (romosozumab), and selective estrogen receptor modulators (SERMs). For most postmenopausal women with osteoporosis, bisphosphonates are the initial agents, and others will be used only when there is intolerance to bisphosphonates or if they were ineffective. Most data on treatment of PWH with osteoporosis are on bisphosphonates, with little data regarding other modalities. Teriparatide, which is a recombinant form of PTH that stimulates osteoblasts, can be used for people who do not respond to bisphosphonates. However, no data exist on its efficacy in PWH (Yin et al., 2012). Denosumab, a monoclonal RANKL antibody, blocks the RANKL/RANKL interaction but may increase the likelihood of infection. For this reason, more data are needed to determine the safety of denosumab in PWH (NOF, 2014; Yin et al., 2012). Hormone replacement therapy including estrogen and raloxifene may be appropriate in some women with HIV, but the benefits may be countered by increased risk of malignancy, thrombotic events, and cardiovascular disease.

COMPARATIVE EFFICACY AND SAFETY OF OSTEOPOROSIS TREATMENTS

Several recently published systematic reviews and meta-analyses of randomized controlled trials of postmenopausal women in the general population compared the efficacy and safety of different osteoporotic treatments and reported slightly different results. Ayers et al. concluded that bisphosphonates, denosumab, abaloparatide, teriparatide, and romosozumab, followed by alendronate, all reduce clinical fractures in postmenopausal females with osteoporosis (Ayers et al., 2023). Teriparatide was less efficacious for hip fractures. In women at very high risk for fracture, sequential use of romosozumab, then alendronate, was more effective for clinical fracture reduction than alendronate alone (RR = 0.74; 95% CI: 0.63 to 0.89). Abaloparatide and teriparatide were associated with increased withdrawals due to adverse effects; longer duration bisphosphonate use may increase atypical femoral fractures and osteonecrosis of the jaw risk, although these events were rare. Conversely, one study showed that bone anabolic treatments were more effective than bisphosphonates in the prevention of clinical and vertebral fractures (Handel et al., 2023). Finally, Kobayashi and colleagues showed that, in comparison to bisphosphonates, denosumab was significantly associated with fewer vertebral fractures (RR = 0.54; 95% CI: 0.31–0.93), less withdrawal due to adverse events (RR = 0.49; 95% CI: 0.34–0.71), more cardiovascular events, and more infections (Kobayashi et al., 2024).

ROLE OF ANTIRETROVIRAL THERAPY SELECTION AND SWITCHING

As described previously, there is good evidence that ART with TDF is associated with a greater (approximately 2%) decline in BMD compared with TAF, and switching from TDF to TAF may lead to modest BMD recovery (Arribas et al., 2017; Mills, 2016; Sax, 2014). The clinical relevance of these changes remains unclear. Because TDF is associated with greater initial loss of BMD compared to other antiretrovirals, the U.S. Department of Health and Human Services adult HIV treatment guidelines recommend avoiding TDF in patients with osteoporosis (USDHHS Guidelines, 2024a).

Limited data exist on the efficacy of ART switch strategies with regard to improved bone health outcomes. HIV providers should generally avoid TDF or ritonavir-boosted protease inhibitors in patients at risk for bone loss. Some older, short-term studies found that switching virologically suppressed patients to abacavir or raltegravir resulted in improvement in BMD compared to TDF (Haskelberg et al., 2012; Yin, 2012). For many PWH at risk for osteoporosis, TAF is the preferred nucleoside analogue to use (rather than TDF). For management of children/youth with HIV experiencing ART-associated osteopenia and osteoporosis, the DHHS pediatric guidelines recommend the following:

- Consider ART modification (e.g., switch from TDF to TAF, and/or from protease inhibitors to rilpivirine or an unboosted INSTI whenever possible).
- Supplement with vitamin D_3 to raise serum 25-OH-vitamin D concentrations to >30 ng/mL. There is no clear benefit to administering daily supplemental vitamin D_3 doses that are >4,000 IU. If patients are

receiving a daily dose of vitamin D_3 that is >4,000 IU, consider monitoring levels of 25-OH-vitamin D.

In summary, the field of metabolic bone disease in PWH remains a critical area of research, especially as PWH approach the seventh and eighth decades of life and beyond. Additional data from clinical trials and long-term observational cohorts are needed to identify the best preventive, screening, and treatment strategies for osteoporosis and fragility fractures for PWH.

REFERENCES

Agidigbi TS, Kim C. Reactive oxygen species in osteoclast differentiation and possible pharmaceutical targets of ROS-mediated osteoclast diseases. *Int J Mol Sci*. 2019;20:3576. doi:10.3390/ijms2014357

Althoff KN, Stewart C, Humes E, et al. The forecasted prevalence of comorbidities and multimorbidity in people with HIV in the United States through the year 2030: a modeling study. *PLoS Med*. 2024;21(1):e1004325.

Amorosa V, Tebas P. Bone disease and HIV infection. *Clin Infect Dis*. 2006a;42(1):108–114.

Amorosa V, Tebas P. Reply to Rojo and Ramos and to Vignolo et al. *Clin Infect Dis*. 2006b;43(1):113–114.

Anastos K, Lu D, Shi O, et al. The association of bone mineral density with HIV infection and antiretroviral treatment in women. *Antivir Ther*. 2007;12(7):1049–1058. doi:10.1177/135965350701200701

Arribas JR, Thompson M, Sax PE, et al. Brief report: randomized, double-blind comparison of Tenofovir Alafenamide (TAF) vs Tenofovir Disoproxil Fumarate (TDF), each coformulated with Elvitegravir, Cobicistat, and Emtricitabine (E/C/F) for initial HIV-1 treatment: Week 144 results. *J Acquir Immune Defic Syndr*. 2017;75(2):211–218. doi:10.1097/QAI.0000000000001350

Ayers C, Kansagara D, Lazur B, et al. Effectiveness and safety of treatments to prevent fractures in people with low bone mass or primary osteoporosis: a living systematic review and network meta-analysis for the American college of physicians. *Ann Intern Med*. 2023;176(2):182–195. doi:10.7326/M22-0684

Battalora L, Armon C, Palella F, et al. Incident bone fracture and mortality in a large HIV cohort outpatient study, 2000–2017, USA. *Arch Osteoporos*. 2021;16(1):117. doi:10.1007/s11657-021-00949-y.

Battalora L, Buchacz K, Armon C, et al. Low bone mineral density is associated with increased risk of incident fracture in HIV-infected adults. *Antivir Ther*. 2016;21(1):45–54.

Battalora LA, Young B, Overton ET. Bones, fractures, antiretroviral therapy and HIV. *Curr Infect Dis Rep*. 2014 Feb;16(2):393.

Bedimo RJ, Adams-Huet B, Nguyen V, et al. Changes in bone microarchitecture with abacavir—lamivudine versus tenofovir disoproxil fumarate—emtricitabine in adults living with HIV. *AIDS*. 2020;34(11):1687–1689. doi:10.1097/QAD.0000000000002592

Bedimo R, Cutrell J, Zhang S, et al. Mechanisms of bone disease in HIV and hepatitis C virus: impact of bone turnover, tenofovir exposure, sex steroids and severity of liver disease. *AIDS*. 2016;30(4):601–608. doi:10.1097/QAD.0000000000000952

Bedimo RJ, Drechsler H, Jain M, et al. The RADAR study: week 48 safety and efficacy of RAltegravir combined with boosted DARunavir compared to tenofovir/emtricitabine combined with boosted darunavir in antiretroviral-naive patients. Impact on bone health. *PLoS One*. 2014;9(8):e106221. doi:10.1371/journal.pone.0106221

Bedimo R, Maalouf NM, Zhang S, et al. Osteoporotic fracture risk associated with cumulative exposure to tenofovir and other antiretroviral agents. *AIDS*. 2012 Apr 24;26(7):825–831.

Bedimo RJ, Adams-Huet B, Poindexter J, et al. The differential effects of human immunodeficiency virus and hepatitis C virus on bone microarchitecture and fracture risk. *Clin Infect Dis*. 2018;66(9):1442–1447.

Bi X, Liu F, Zhang X, et al. Vitamin D and calcium supplementation reverses tenofovir-caused bone mineral density loss in people taking ART or PrEP: A systematic review and meta-analysis. *Front Nutr*. 2022bi;9:749948

Bolland MJ, Grey AB, Horne AM, et al. Annual zoledronate increases bone density in highly active antiretroviral therapy-treated human immunodeficiency virus-infected men: a randomized controlled trial. *J Clin Endocrinol Metab*. April 2007 Apr;92(4):1283–1288.

Bolland MJ, Horne AM, Briggs SE, et al. Effects of intravenous zoledronate on bone turnover and bone density persist for at least 11 years in HIV-infected men. *J Bone Miner Res*. 2019;34:1248–1253.

Bonfanti P, De Vito A, Ricci E, et al. Bone safety of dolutegravir-containing regimens in people living with HIV: results from a real-world cohort. *Infect Drug Resist*. 2020;13:2291–2300.

Boyce BF, Xing L. The RANKL/RANK/OPG pathway. *Curr Osteoporos Rep*. 2007;5(3):98–104. doi:10.1007/s11914-007-0024-y

Brown TT, Hoy J, Borderi M, et al. Recommendations for evaluation and management of bone disease in HIV. *Clin Infect Dis*. 2015a;60:1242–1251.

Brown TT, McComsey GA, King MS, et al. Loss of bone mineral density after antiretroviral therapy initiation, independent of antiretroviral regimen. *J Acquir Immune Defic Syndr*. 2009; 51:554–561.

Brown TT, Moser C, Currier JS, et al. Changes in bone mineral density after initiation of antiretroviral treatment with tenofovir disoproxil fumarate/emtricitabine plus atazanavir/ritonavir, darunavir/ritonavir, or raltegravir. *J Infect Dis*. 2015b;212(8):1241–9. Erratum in: *J Infect Dis*. 2020;221(12):2083–2084.

Brown TT, Qaqish RB. Antiretroviral therapy and the prevalence of osteopenia and osteoporosis: a meta-analytic review. *AIDS*. 2006 Nov 14;20(17):2165–2174.

Chang CJ, Chan YL, Pramukti I, et al. People with HIV infection had lower bone mineral density and increased fracture risk: a meta-analysis. *Arch Osteoporos*. 2021;16(1):47.

Conradie MM, van de Vyver M, Andrag E, et al. A direct comparison of the effects of the antiretroviral drugs Stavudine, Tenofovir and the combination Lopinavir/Ritonavir on bone metabolism in a rat model. *Calcif Tissue Int*. 2017;101(4):422–432. doi:10.1007/s00223-017-0290-3

Cotter AG, Vrouenraets SM, Brady JJ, et al. Impact of switching from zidovudine to tenofovir disoproxil fumarate on bone mineral density and markers of bone metabolism in virologically suppressed HIV-1 infected patients; a substudy of the PREPARE study. *J Clin Endo Metab*. 2013;98(4):1659–1666. doi:10.1210/jc.2012-3686

Dong HV, Cortés YI, Shiau S, Yin MT. Osteoporosis and fractures in HIV/hepatitis C virus coinfection: a systematic review and meta-analysis. *AIDS*. 2014;28(14):2119–2131. doi:10.1097/QAD.0000000000000363

Eastell R, Rosen CJ, Black DM et al. Pharmacological management of osteoporosis in postmenopausal women: an Endocrine Society clinical practice guideline. *J Clin Endocrinol Metab*. 2019;104(5):1595–1622.

El-Maouche D, Mehta SH, Sutcliffe C, et al. Controlled HIV viral replication, not liver disease severity associated with low bone mineral density in HIV/HCV co-infection. *J Hep*. 2011;55(4):770–776. doi:10.1016/j.jhep.2011.01.035

Endocrine Society (EOS). Clinical guidelines: evaluation, treatment and prevention of vitamin D deficiency: an Endocrine Society clinical practice guideline 2011. http://press.endocrine.org/doi/pdf/10.1210/jc.2011-0385. Published 2011. Accessed December 14, 2015.

Ensrud KE, Lui LY, Crandall CJ, et al. Repeat bone mineral density screening measurement and fracture prediction in older men: a prospective cohort study. *J Clin Endocrinol Metab*. 2022;107(9):e3877–e3886.

Escota GV, Mondy K, Bush T, et al. High prevalence of low bone mineral density and substantial bone loss over 4 years among HIV-infected persons in the era of modern antiretroviral therapy. *AIDS Res Human Retrov*. 2016;32(1):59–67. doi:10.1089/aid.2015.0158 Pub 15 Sep 2015.

European AIDS Clinical Society (EACS). Guidelines, version 12.0. https://eacs.sanfordguide.com/. Published October 2023. Accessed October 2023.

FRAX®. Fracture risk assessment tool. https://frax.shef.ac.uk/FRAX/. Web version 1.4.7. The University of Sheffield, UK. Accessed August 29, 2024.

Goh SSL, Lai PSM, Tan ATB, Ponnampalavanar S. Reduced bone mineral density in human immunodeficiency virus-infected individuals: a meta-analysis of its prevalence and risk factors. *Osteoporos Int.* 2018 Mar;29(3):595–613.

Gonciulea A, Wang R, Althoff KN, et al. Proteinuria is associated with increased risk of fragility fracture in men with or at risk of HIV infection. *J Acquir Immune Defic Syndr.* 2019;81(3):e85–e91.

Gourlay ML, Fine JP, Preisser JS, et al; Study of Osteoporotic Fractures Research Group. Bone-density testing interval and transition to osteoporosis in older women. *N Engl J Med.* 2012;366(3):225–233.

Grant PM, Kitch D, McComsey GA, et al. Long-term bone mineral density changes in antiretroviral-treated HIV-infected individuals. *J Infect Dis.* 2016 Aug 15;214(4):607–611. PMID: 27330053.

Grant PM, Li X, Jacobson LP, et al. Effect of testosterone use on bone mineral density in HIV-infected men. *AIDS Res Hum Retroviruses.* 2019;35(1):75–80.

Guaraldi G, Orlando G, Madeddu G, et al. Alendronate reduces bone resorption in HIV-associated osteopenia/osteoporosis. *HIV Clin Trials.* 2004 Sep–Oct;5(5):269–277.

Guo F, Song X, Li Y, et al. Longitudinal change in bone mineral density among Chinese individuals with HIV after initiation of antiretroviral therapy. *Osteoporos Int.* 2021;32(2):321–332.

Han WM, Wattanachanya L, Apornpong T, et al. Bone mineral density changes among people living with HIV who have started with TDF-containing regimen: a five-year prospective study. *PLoS One.* 2020;15(3):e0230368. doi:10.1371/journal.pone.0230368

Handel MN, Cardoso I, von Bulow C, et al. Fracture risk reduction and safety by osteoporosis treatment compared with placebo or active comparator in postmenopausal women: systematic review, network meta-analysis, and meta-regression analysis of randomised clinical trials. *BMJ.* 2023;381:e068033. doi:10.1136/bmj-2021-068033

Hansen AB, Gerstoft J, Kronborg G, et al. Incidence of low and high-energy fractures in persons with and without HIV infection: a Danish population-based cohort study. *AIDS.* 2012;26(3):285–293. PMID: 22095195.

Haskelberg H, Cordery DV, Amin J, et al. HLA alleles association with changes in bone mineral density in HIV-1-infected adults changing treatment to tenofovir–emtricitabine or abacavir–lamivudine. *PLoS One.* March 28, 2014;9(3): e93333.

Haskelberg H, Hoy JF, Amin J, et al. Changes in bone turnover and bone loss in HIV-infected patients changing treatment to tenofovir–emtricitabine or abacavir–lamivudine. *PLoS One.* 2012;7(6):e38377.

Havens PL, Stephensen CB, Van Loan MD; Adolescent Medicine Trials Network for HIV/AIDS Interventions (ATN) 109 Study Team. Vitamin D3 supplementation increases spine bone mineral density in adolescents and young adults with human immunodeficiency virus infection being treated with tenofovir disoproxil fumarate: a randomized, placebo-controlled trial. *Clin Infect Dis.* 2018a Jan 6;66(2):220–228. PMID: 29020329.

Havens PL, Long D, Schuster GU; Adolescent Medicine Trials Network for HIV/AIDS Interventions (ATN) 117 and 109 Study Teams. Tenofovir disoproxil fumarate appears to disrupt the relationship of vitamin D and parathyroid hormone. *Antivir Ther.* 2018b Sep 27. doi:10.3851/IMP3269. PMID: 30260797.

Hileman CO, Labbato DE, Storer NJ, et al. Is bone loss linked to chronic inflammation in antiretroviral-naïve HIV-infected adults? A 48-week matched cohort study. *AIDS.* 2014 Jul 31;28(12):1759–1767.

Hoy JF, Grund B, Roediger M, et al. Immediate initiation of antiretroviral therapy for HIV infection accelerates bone loss relative to deferring therapy: findings from the START bone mineral density substudy, a randomized trial. *J Bone Miner Res.* 2017;32(9):1945–1955. doi:10.1002/jbmr.318

Hoy JF, Richardson R, Ebeling PR; ZEST Study Investigators. Zoledronic acid is superior to tenofovir disoproxil fumarate-switching for low bone mineral density in adults with HIV. *AIDS.* 2018 Sep 10;32(14):1967–1975. PMID: 29927785.

Huang J, Meixner L, Fernandez S, et al. A double-blinded, randomized controlled trial of zoledronate therapy for HIV-associated osteopenia and osteoporosis. *AIDS.* 2009 Jan 2;23(1):51–57.

Institute of Medicine (IOM). *Dietary Reference Intakes for Calcium and Vitamin D.* Washington, DC: National Academies Press; 2011. http://iom.nationalacademies.org/~/media/Files/Report%20Files/2010/Dietary-Reference-Intakes-for-Calcium-and-Vitamin-D/Vitamin%20D%20and%20Calcium%202010%20Report%20Brief.pdf. Accessed December 14, 2015.

Jacobson DL, Lindsey JC, Gordon C, et al. Alendronate improves bone mineral density in children and adolescents perinatally infected with human immunodeficiency virus with low bone mineral density for age. *Clin Infect Dis.* 2020; 71:1281–1288.

Jespersen NA, Axelsen F, Dollerup J, et al. The burden of non-communicable diseases and mortality in people living with HIV (PLHIV) in the pre-, early- and late-HAART era. *HIV Med.* 2021;22(6):478–490.

Kanis JA, on behalf of the World Health Organization Scientific Group. *Assessment of Osteoporosis at the Primary Health-Care Level: Technical Report.* World Health Organization Collaborating Centre for Metabolic Bone Diseases, University of Sheffield, UK; 2007: Printed by the University of Sheffield. https://www.shef.ac.uk/FRAX®/pdfs/WHO_Technical_Report.pdf. Accessed December 14, 2015.

Kobayashi T, Morimoto T, Ito K, et al. Denosumab vs. bisphosphonates in primary osteoporosis: a meta-analysis of comparative safety in randomized controlled trials. *Osteoporos Int.* 2024;35(8):1377–1393. doi:10.1007/s00198-024-07118-0

Kim JH, Noh J, Kim W, et al. Trends of age-related non-communicable diseases in people living with HIV and comparison with uninfected controls: a nationwide population-based study in South Korea. *HIV Med.* 2021;22(9):824–833.

Lawson-Ayayi S, Cazanave C, Kpozehouen A, et al. Chronic viral hepatitis is associated with low bone mineral density in HIV-infected patients, ANRS CO 3 Aquitaine Cohort. *Journal of Acquired Immune Deficiency Syndromes.* 2013;62(4):430–435. doi:10.1097/QAI.0b013e3182845d88

LeBoff MS, Greenspan SL, Insogna KL, et al. The clinician's guide to prevention and treatment of osteoporosis [published correction appears in *Osteoporos Int.* 2022 Oct;33(10):2243. doi:10.1007/s00198-022-06479-8.]. *Osteoporos Int.* 2022;33(10):2049–2102. doi:10.1007/s00198-021-05900-y

LeFevre ML, LeFevre NM. Vitamin D screening and supplementation in community-dwelling adults: common questions and answers. *Am Fam Physician.* 2018 Feb 15;97(4):254–260.

LaFleur J, Bress AP, Myers J, et al. Tenofovir-associated bone adverse outcomes among a US national historical cohort of HIV-infected veterans: risk modification by concomitant antiretrovirals. *Infect Dis Ther.* 2018;7(2):293–308. doi:10.1007/s40121-018-0194-1

Liu Z, Xiao Y, Torresilla C, Rassart E, Barbeau B. Implication of different HIV-1 genes in the modulation of autophagy. *Viruses.* 2017; 9:389. doi:10.3390/v9120389

Llop M, Sifuentes WA, Bañón S, et al. Increased prevalence of asymptomatic vertebral fractures in HIV-infected patients over 50 years of age. *Arch Osteoporos.* 2018;13(1):56.

Lo Re V 3rd, Guaraldi G, Leonard MB, et al. Viral hepatitis is associated with reduced bone mineral density in HIV-infected women but not men. *Aids.* 2009;23(16):2191–2198. doi:10.1097/QAD.0b013e32832ec258

Lo Re V 3rd, Volk J, Newcomb CW, et al. Risk of hip fracture associated with hepatitis C virus infection and hepatitis C/human immunodeficiency virus coinfection. *Hepatology.* 2012;56(5):1688–1698. doi:10.1002/hep.25866

Maalouf NM, Zhang S, Drechsler H, et al. Hepatitis C co-infection and severity of liver disease as risk factor for osteoporotic fractures among HIV-infected patients. *J Bone Miner Res.* 2013; 28(12):2577–2583.

Martin A, Bloch M, Amin J, et al. Simplification of antiretroviral therapy with tenofovir-emtricitabine or abacavir-Lamivudine: a randomized, 96-week trial. *Clin Infect Dis.* 2009;49(10):1591–1601. doi:10.1086/644769

McCloskey EV, Oden A, Harvey NC, et al. A meta-analysis of trabecular bone score in fracture risk prediction and its relationship to FRAX. *J Bone Min Res.* 2016;31(5):940–948. doi:10.1002/jbmr.2734

McComsey GA, Kendall MA, Tebas P, et al. Alendronate with calcium and vitamin D supplementation is safe and effective for the treatment of decreased bone mineral density in HIV. *AIDS.* 2007;21(18):2473–2482.

McComsey GA, Kitch D, Daar ES, et al. Bone mineral density and fractures in antiretroviral-naive persons randomized to receive abacavir–lamivudine or tenofovir disoproxil fumarate–emtricitabine along with efavirenz or atazanavir–ritonavir: Aids Clinical Trials Group A5224s, a substudy of ACTG A5202. *J Infect Dis.* 2011; 203(12):1791–1801.

McComsey GA, Tebas P, Shane E, et al. Bone disease in HIV infection: a practical review and recommendations for HIV care providers. *Clin Infect Dis.* 2010;51(8):937–946.

Mills A, Arribas JR, Andrade-Villanueva J, et al. Switching from tenofovir disoproxil fumarate to tenofovir alafenamide in antiretroviral regimens for virologically suppressed adults with HIV-1 infection: a randomised, active-controlled, multicentre, open-label, phase 3, non-inferiority study. *Lancet Infect Dis.* 2016;16(1):43–52.

Mondy K, Powderly WG, Claxton SA, et al. Alendronate, vitamin D, and calcium for the treatment of osteopenia/osteoporosis associated with HIV infection. *J Acquir Immune Defic Syndr.* 2005;38(4):426–431.

Moran CA, Weitzmann MN, Ofotokun I. The protease inhibitors and HIV-associated bone loss. *Curr Opin HIV AIDS.* 2016;11(3):333–342.

National Osteoporosis Foundation (NOF). *Clinician's Guide to Prevention and Treatment of Osteoporosis.* Washington, DC: National Osteoporosis Foundation; 2014.

Nguyen ND, Eisman JA, Center JR, Nguyen TV. Risk factors for fracture in nonosteoporotic men and women. *J Clin Endocrinol Metab.* 2007;92(3):955–962. doi:10.1210/jc.2006-1476

Ofotokun I, Weitzmann MN. HIV and bone metabolism. *Discov Med.* 2011;11(60):385–393.

Ofotokun I, Collins LF, Titanji K, et al. Antiretroviral therapy-induced bone loss is durably suppressed by a single dose of zoledronic acid in treatment-naive persons with human immunodeficiency virus infection: a phase IIB trial. *Clin Infect Dis.* 2020;71(7):1655–1663.

Olali AZ, Wallace J, Gonzalez H, et al. The anti-HIV drug abacavir stimulates beta-catenin activity in osteoblast lineage cells. *JBMR Plus.* 2024;8(5):ziae037. doi:10.1093/jbmrpl/ziae037

Orwoll ES, Klein RF. Osteoporosis in men. *Endocr Rev.* 1995 Feb;16(1):87–116.

Overton ET, Chan ES, Brown TT, Tebas P, et al. Vitamin D and calcium attenuate bone loss with antiretroviral therapy initiation: a randomized trial. *Ann Intern Med.* 2015;162(12):815–824.

Pitukcheewanont P, Safani D, Church J, et al. Bone measures in HIV-1 infected children and adolescents: disparity between quantitative computed tomography and dual-energy X-ray absorptiometry measurements. *Osteoporosis Int.* 2005;16(11):1393–1396.

Pramukti I, Lindayani L, Chen YC et al. Bone fracture among people living with HIV: A systematic review and meta-regression of prevalence, incidence, and risk factors. *PloS One.* 2020;15:6: e0233501.

Qaseem A, Hicks LA, Etxeandia-Ikobaltzeta I, et al. Pharmacologic treatment of primary osteoporosis or low bone mass to prevent fractures in adults: a living clinical guideline from the American College of Physicians. *Ann Intern Med.* 2023;176(2):224–238. Erratum in: *Ann Intern Med.* 2023;176(6):882–884.

Raffi F, Orkin C, Clarke A, et al. Brief report: long-term (96-Week) efficacy and safety after switching from tenofovir disoproxil fumarate to tenofovir alafenamide in HIV-infected, virologically suppressed adults. *J Acquir Immune Defic Syndr.* 2017;75(2):226–231. doi:10.1097/QAI.0000000000001344

Raynaud-Messina B, Bracq L, Dupont M, et al. Bone degradation machinery of osteoclasts: An HIV-1 target that contributes to bone loss. *Proc Natl Acad Sci U S A.* 2018;115(11): E2556–E2565.

Rozenberg S, Lanoy E, Bentata M, et al. Effect of alendronate on HIV-associated osteoporosis: a randomized, double-blind, placebo-controlled, 96-week trial (ANRS 120). *AIDS Res Hum Retroviruses.* 2012;28(9):972–980.

Rukuni R, Rehman AM, Mukwasi-Kahari C, et al. Effect of HIV infection on growth and bone density in peripubertal children in the era of antiretroviral therapy: a cross-sectional study in Zimbabwe. *Lancet Child Adolesc Health.* 2021;5(8):569–581.

Sax PE, Zolopa A, Brar I, et al. Tenofovir alafenamide vs. tenofovir disoproxil fumarate in single tablet regimens for initial HIV-1 therapy: a randomized phase 2 study. *J Acquir Immune Defic Syndr.* 2014;67(1):52–58.

Sharma A, Ma Y, Tien PC, et al. HIV infection is associated with abnormal bone microarchitecture: measurement of trabecular bone score in the Women's Interagency HIV Study. *J Acquir Immune Defic Syndr.* 2018;78(4):441–449.

Sharma A, Shi Q, Hoover DR, et al. Frailty predicts fractures among women with and at-risk for HIV: results from the Women's Interagency HIV Study. *AIDS.* 2019;33:455–463.

Sharma A, Hoover DR, Shi Q, et al. Human immunodeficiency virus (HIV) and menopause are independently associated with lower bone mineral density: results from the Women's Interagency HIV Study. *Clin Infect Dis.* 2022;75(1):65–72.

Silva BC, Leslie WD, Resch H, et al. Trabecular bone score: a noninvasive analytical method based upon the DXA image. *J Bone Miner Res.* 2014;29(3):518–30. Erratum in: *J Bone Miner Res.* 2017;32(11):2319.

Starup-Linde J, Rosendahl SB, Storgaard M, Langdahl B. Management of osteoporosis in patients living with HIV: a systematic review and meta-analysis. *J Acquir Immune Defic Syndr.* 2020;83(1):1–8.

Stellbrink HJ, Orkin C, Arribas JR, et al. Comparison of changes in bone density and turnover with abacavir-lamivudine versus tenofovir-emtricitabine in HIV-infected adults: 48-week results from the ASSERT study. *Clin Infect Dis.* 2010;51(8):963–972. doi:10.1086/656417.

Thompson MA, Horberg MA, Agwu AL, et al. Primary care guidance for persons with human immunodeficiency virus: 2020 update by the HIV Medicine Association of the Infectious Diseases Society of America. *Clin Infect Dis.* 2021;73(11):e3572–e3605.

Tinago W, Cotter AG, Sabin CA, et al. Predictors of longitudinal change in bone mineral density in a cohort of HIV-positive and negative patients. *AIDS.* 2017;31(5):643–652. doi:10.1097/QAD.0000000000001372

Titanji K. Beyond antibodies: B cells and the OPG/RANK-RANKL pathway in health, non-HIV disease and HIV-induced bone loss. *Front Immunol.* 2017;8:1851.

Trickey A, Sabin CA, Burkholder G, et al. Life expectancy after 2015 of adults with HIV on long-term antiretroviral therapy in Europe and North America: a collaborative analysis of cohort studies. *Lancet HIV.* 2023 May;10(5):e295–e307.

Triant VA, Brown TT, Lee H, et al. Fracture prevalence among human immunodeficiency virus (HIV)-infected versus non-HIV-infected patients in a large US healthcare system. *J Clin Endocrinol Metab.* 2008;93(9):3499–3504.

U.S. Department of Health and Human Services (USDHHS), Panel on Antiretroviral Guidelines for Adults and Adolescents. Guidelines for the use of antiretroviral agents in HIV-1-infected adults and adolescents. Last updated February 27, 2024a. Accessed August 28, 2024.

U.S. Department of Health and Human Services (USDHHS), Panel on Antiretroviral Therapy and Medical Management of Children Living with HIV. Guidelines for the use of antiretroviral agents in pediatric HIV Infection. Table 17j. Department of Health and Human Services. https://clinicalinfo.hiv.gov/en/guidelines/pediatric-arv. Published June 27, 2024b. Accessed August 28, 2024.

U.S. Food and Drug Administration. Bisphosphonates. http://www.fda.gov/search?s=Bisphosphonates&sort_bef_combine=rel_DESC. Published August 29, 2024. Accessed August 29, 2024.

van den Bergh JP, van Geel TA, Lems WF, et al. Assessment of individual fracture risk: FRAX® and beyond. *Curr Osteoporosis Rep.* 2010 Sep;8(3):131–137.

van Vonderen MG, Lips P, van Agtmael MA, et al. First line zidovudine/lamivudine/lopinavir/ritonavir leads to greater bone loss compared to nevirapine/lopinavir/ritonavir. *AIDS.* 2009 Jul 17;23(11):1367–1376.

Womack JA, Goulet JL, Gibert C, et al. Increased risk of fragility fractures among HIV infected compared to uninfected male veterans. *PloS One*. 2011;6(2):e17217.
Woolf AD, Pfleger B. Burden of major musculoskeletal conditions. *Bull World Health Organization*. 2003;81(9):646–656.
World Health Organization (WHO). WHO manual of diagnostic imaging. http://apps.who.int/iris/bitstream/10665/42457/1/9241545550_eng.pdf. Published 2002. Accessed August 29, 2024.
World Health Organization (WHO). WHO Technical Report Series 843: assessment of fracture risk and its application to screening for postmenopausal osteoporosis. Report of a WHO Study Group. *World Health Organ Tech Rep Ser*. 1994; 843:1–129. PMID: 7941614.
Yin M. Bone loss in HIV: virus, host or ART. Paper presented at the Conference on Retroviruses and Opportunistic Infections (CROI), Seattle, WA; March 5–8, 2012.
Yin MT, Overton ET. Increasing clarity on bone loss associated with antiretroviral initiation. *J Infect Dis*. June 15, 2011;203(12):1705–1707.
Yin MT, Shi Q, Hoover DR, et al. Fracture incidence in HIV-infected women: results from the Women's Interagency HIV Study. *AIDS*. 2010 Nov 13;24(17):2679–2686.
Yin MT, Zhang CA, McMahon DJ, et al. Higher rates of bone loss in postmenopausal HIV-infected women: a longitudinal study. *J Clin Endocrinol Metab*. 2012 Feb;97(2):554–562.
Young B, Dao CN, Buchacz K, et al. Increased rates of bone fracture among HIV-infected persons in the HIV Outpatient Study (HOPS) compared with the US general population, 2000–2006. *Clin Infect Dis*. 2011 Apr 15;52(8):1061–1068.
Zhang T, Wilson IB, Zullo AR, et al. Hip fracture rates in nursing home residents with and without HIV. *J Am Med Dir Assoc*. 2022;23(3):517–518.

34.

SUBSTANCE USE AND HIV

Thanh Thuy Truong

INTRODUCTION

The relationship between substance use and HIV infection is complex and encompasses all aspects of the HIV care continuum, including prevention/transmission, screening and diagnosis, engagement in care, and treatment. Substance use can increase the likelihood of exposure to HIV via needle-sharing or impairing judgment linked to risky sexual behaviors. Among men who have sex with men (MSM), substance use is associated with an increased risk of HIV infection, particularly binge drinking, crack/cocaine, methamphetamine, and inhalant use. In a 2024 Centers for Disease Control and Prevention (CDC) report, although HIV infections have decreased by 12% overall during 2018–2022, substance use is still a major driver of new infections (CDC, 2024). Among people with HIV (PWH), substance use can impact ART adherence and engagement in care. Irregular follow-up, poor adherence to antiretroviral therapy (ART), and risk of acquiring other sexually transmitted infections (STIs) and hepatitis C all increase morbidity and mortality (Cofrancesco et al., 2008; Stern et al., 2018).

Biological, psychological, and social factors influence the relationship between substance use disorders (SUD) and HIV infection. The risk of substance use involves interactions between genes and the environment. Approximately 40%–60% of vulnerability to addiction can be attributable to genetic variance. For example, in alcohol use disorder (AUD), while some genes have been associated with susceptibility to excess alcohol consumption, polymorphisms in alcohol metabolizing enzymes like alcohol dehydrogenases ADH1B and ALDH2 are protective against AUD (Chen et al., 1999). Moreover, developmental changes across the life span are associated with behavior changes that may alter the propensity for the development of SUDs. For example, during adolescence, normal behaviors of novelty-seeking, risk-taking, and sensitivity to peer pressure may result in experimenting with legal and illegal substances. Adolescent brains have not completed development in areas involved in executive function, which is necessary for regulating impulses and emotions. Not surprisingly, notable rates of use for most substances occur between the ages of 18 to 24 years, prior to the full development of frontal lobes and functional networks (Miller et al., 2019). Adolescent neurological development is also more vulnerable to long-term effects of chronic drug and alcohol exposure and can increase the risk of developing SUDs later in life. This interaction between biological and psychological development leads to risky behaviors such as having multiple partners and inconsistent condom use (Hillfors et al., 2007). Socioeconomic disadvantage, limited education, and unstable housing also contribute to unsafe sexual practices and limited access to preventive measures, thus increasing the prevalence of HIV in these populations (Millett et al., 2007).

Psychiatric illnesses and substance use are separate and additive risk factors for HIV infection. Psychiatric illnesses are more prevalent in PWH. For example, personality disorders are highly represented among PWH, likely owing to traits such as impulsivity and maladaptive coping strategies to stress that perpetuate risky behaviors. Similarly, PWH are more likely to have chronic psychiatric disorders such as anxiety or depression, whether resulting from HIV infection of neural tissue, or a distinct comorbidity (Stern et al., 2018). One study revealed that people with a "dual diagnosis" of mental illness and substance use disorder have an HIV prevalence of 4.7% versus 2.4% for people with a substance use disorder diagnosis alone. Further, unhealthy substance use is associated with a host of medical sequelae (liver disease, infection, diabetes, cardiovascular disease, and neurocognitive changes) that add to the many potential medical complications associated with HIV. Unfortunately, inconsistent adherence to medical treatment compounds these problems (Moore, 2008; Sullivan, 2011). Therefore, a comprehensive approach to care is important for people with multiple diagnoses. Despite advancements in the diagnosis and treatment of HIV (Bhaskaran et al., 2008), stigma, shame, and motivational challenges continue to be significant barriers to care for PWH and SUD.

Early detection and intervention for both HIV and SUD can save lives and change the trajectory of chronic disease. Routine voluntary HIV testing in all persons aged 13–64 is recommended by the CDC (Branson et al., 2006). A comprehensive and harm-reduction-oriented approach involving information-sharing and collaboration with patients regarding therapeutic decisions is critical. Ongoing risky substance use should prompt evaluation for potential referral to substance use treatment services, and relapse prevention should be discussed at each patient encounter (CDC, 2003). Providers should also perform routine HIV lab monitoring and counsel PWH on opportunistic infection prevention as indicated. Limited resources in some areas may not allow for an interdisciplinary team approach, but, if possible, providers with HIV and SUD experience and expertise should be involved.

LEARNING OBJECTIVES

- Discuss issues, implications, screening/diagnosis, and treatment of substance use disorders (SUDs) in people with HIV.
- Describe the bidirectional interactions between HIV and unhealthy substance use.
- Recognize unhealthy substance use in PWH.
- Outline potential initial approaches to SUD treatment in PWH.

WHAT'S NEW?

The chapter has been updated to reflect the terminology of the fifth edition of the *Diagnostic and Statistical Manual of Mental Disorders, Text Revision* (American Psychiatric Association, 2022). Given evolving practices in SUD treatment, more thorough and specific therapeutic modalities and recommendations are included.

DIAGNOSIS AND TREATMENT OF SUBSTANCE USE DISORDERS

SCREENING AND DIAGNOSIS

Prior to conducting screening, assessment, or treatment planning, providers should evaluate their personal beliefs and attitudes toward PWH with SUD. Many patients may have complex needs, and this may elicit difficult feelings that can be emotionally and physically demanding on healthcare providers and other clinic staff. Examining countertransference reactions and biases such as homophobia and fear of infection can help decrease burnout and facilitate a stronger therapeutic alliance with patients. Providers must be comfortable discussing sensitive topics such as sex, substance use, shame, and trauma. Cultural competency is also important because people from different ethnic groups, socioeconomic classes, genders, and cultures have varying levels of comfort in discussing these topics. For example, asking personal questions about substance use and sexual behaviors may feel intrusive and disrespectful to some Asian and Pacific Islander individuals. Approaching screening with the least intrusive question initially may help facilitate more detailed information-sharing later in the assessment. HIV disproportionately affects African Americans, and many may hold deep mistrust of healthcare systems because of the historical exploitation of their community by medical institutions. Providers should be aware of social, economic, and political issues, such as institutional racism, that continue to affect the African American community. Working with lesbian, gay, bisexual, transgender, and queer (LGBTQ+) populations requires understanding and sensitivity, as this population often faces stigma, trauma, low self-esteem, and lack of family and social support. Another key population that needs special consideration is women. Women present differently and occasionally at later stages in the HIV disease process compared to men. Factors such as identity (e.g., as a caregiver), stigma (e.g., "unfit mother"), shame, and guilt over having HIV may play a major role in a woman's care decisions. Lastly, while it may be helpful to consider the common experiences of any particular group, providers should always seek to understand each individual's unique experience.

Although there are specific criteria for the diagnosis of SUD and physiologic dependence (American Psychiatric Association, 2022), assessing the impact of a substance requires a comprehensive evaluation to understand the individual's lived experience. Historically, addiction was viewed as a voluntary moral failing by the individual, which led to stigmatization that has been a significant barrier to appropriate care. In recent decades, research has advanced our understanding of the profound drug effects on neural networks involved in reward processing, motivation, and behavioral and emotional regulation that result in compulsive drug-seeking behaviors. Definitions of SUD in the literature now reflect biological, psychological, and social factors. After reviewing several definitions, one practical definition adopted by the European Monitoring Centre for Drugs and Drug Addiction (EMCDDA) is "a repeated powerful motivation to engage in a purposeful behavior that has no survival value, acquired as a result of engaging in that behavior, with significant potential for unintended harm" (West, 2013). The severity of substance use varies between individuals and encompasses low-risk, hazardous, and harmful addiction levels. Generally, an SUD is diagnosed when the use of a substance results in an impairment of functioning in multiple areas (occupational, social, and recreational), loss of control over intake, and the presence of a negative emotional state during abstinence.

The Screening, Brief Intervention, and Referral to Treatment (SBIRT) approach for tobacco and alcohol use disorders has demonstrated significant benefits in reducing use across a variety of clinical settings. Routine screening of all adults and pregnant women for alcohol and tobacco use is recommended by the U.S. Preventive Services Task Force (USPSTF) (Campos-Outcalt, 2016). A variety of screening tools for unhealthy alcohol and illicit drug use are available through the National Institute on Alcohol Abuse and Alcoholism (NIAAA), the National Institute on Drug Abuse (NIDA), and other governmental agencies. The single question, "How many times in the past year have you used an illegal drug or used a prescription medication for nonmedical reasons?" has been shown to accurately identify substance use. A response of at least one time is positive for unhealthy use. To prescreen for any alcohol use, asking, "Do you sometimes drink beer, wine, or other alcoholic beverages?" can gently prepare the person for more detailed questions about unhealthy use. For heavy drinking, the question: "How many times in the past year have you had five or more (for men) or four or more (for women) drinks in a day?" is sensitive and specific for identifying unhealthy alcohol use in primary care settings (NIAAA, 2024). A positive screen prompts further assessment of severity and impact on the individual's functioning to determine risk level. Differentiating between at-risk use and SUD is relevant to guide clinical recommendations for treatment. Brief interventions such as advice and motivational interviewing may be appropriate for at-risk use, whereas more extensive follow-up and referral to an addiction specialist would be suitable for PWH meeting criteria for an SUD. Screening is best accompanied by laboratory studies such as urine toxicology for drugs as clinically indicated. A standard urine toxicology screen is not likely to detect synthetic opioids, so separate screening with confirmation is often needed for the detection of fentanyl, hydrocodone, and oxycodone. For alcohol use, direct biomarkers such as urine ethyl glucuronide (EtG) and ethyl sulfate (EtS) can be used to assess for alcohol use up to 80 hours after drinking. The direct biomarker phosphatidylethanol (PEth) can detect moderate to heavy alcohol consumption within the past 30–60 days with 100% specificity because only PEth can form with alcohol use. Consumption of 2–4 drinks several days per week would elevate PEth to above 0.03 µmol/L (Finanger et al., 2022). Indirect alcohol markers include serum carbohydrate-deficient transferrin (CDT-20), mean corpuscular volume (MCV), and gamma-glutamyltransferase (GGT). Elevations of these markers suggest chronic heavy drinking, but they are not specific to alcohol use.

TREATMENT

GENERAL PRINCIPLES

Successful treatment of PWH with SUD commonly involves challenges and requires a multimodal approach. Chronic drug exposure leads to long-lasting neurological and behavioral changes that contribute to relapse (also sometimes referred to as "return to use"), which can feel frustrating and demoralizing for PWH and care team members. Taking the approach of chronic disease management (such as diabetes or hypertension) with an expected long-term care model represents a shift in ideology toward harm reduction, rather than complete abstinence. This involves recognizing that the illness will likely include periods of recovery and relapse, depending on adherence and treatment efficacy; this reframe may help PWH and treatment teams approach care rationally. Rather than failure, a "relapse" can be framed as a temporary setback as part of trial and error in achieving an effective care regimen. Some individuals may not be able to achieve abstinence despite appropriate treatment; thus setting attainable goals such as reducing frequency and severity of use and relapse can improve overall functioning. Clarifying and communicating these expectations to PWH and the treatment team can improve outcomes and retention in treatment (McLellan et al., 2000). The combination of psychosocial and pharmacological interventions is strongly recommended to target different facets of addiction. When possible, the use of an interdisciplinary team with psychiatry, primary care, social work, substance use counselors, and case management is ideal for supporting the individual in their recovery and preventing return to use.

General principles of effective SUD treatment include easy access to care, collaborating with the person to create a plan that addresses their individual needs, monitoring for relapse, and treating psychiatric and medical comorbidities. Screening for HIV, hepatitis B and C, tuberculosis, and other infectious diseases should be readily available. On-site availability of HIV screening/testing increases the likelihood of acceptance and receipt of results (NIDA, 1999). Even when individuals present for acute intoxication or withdrawal management, this can be viewed as an entry into treatment. Care providers should establish rapport with each person and encourage them to engage in recommended addiction services. The appropriate treatment setting depends on the PWH's insight, physical and emotional ability to engage in care, and availability of necessary treatment (e.g., opioid agonist therapy). Hospitalization is recommended for PWH who are a danger to themselves or others because of intoxication or acute psychiatric disorder, who need intensive withdrawal management, or who have life-threatening medical conditions. Residential treatment programs are ideal for PWH who have fluctuating insight and need a highly structured and supportive environment. Partial hospitalization and intensive outpatient programs can be considered for persons who transition out of residential or hospital settings to a lower level of care, but still need close monitoring to manage risk of relapse. PWH who have a history of relapse after treatment completion or have plans to return to high-risk environments would be best continued in a highly structured setting. Finally, for PWH who demonstrate insight into their SUD and have high adherence to treatment and low severity of symptoms, outpatient programs are an appropriate, cost-effective option. Outpatient programs vary from low to high intensity, many of which have a multimodal approach that involves individual and group therapy and mental health and medical treatment (Miller et al., 2019).

THERAPY

Various psychotherapies have been shown to be effective for the treatment of SUD by helping PWH modify behaviors, feelings, thoughts, and social contexts that drive compulsive substance use. Therapeutic intervention can increase motivation, improve mood, and build a strong social support network, all of which improve chances of recovery and prevent relapse. Motivational enhancement therapy is used to help PWH address ambivalence about substance use and engage in treatment. Motivational interviewing techniques enhance motivation and commitment to change or maintaining progress. Cognitive behavioral therapy (CBT) has demonstrated efficacy in relapse prevention by helping individuals identify and correct behaviors and thoughts that precede cravings and increase the risk of relapse. Studies have demonstrated retention of CBT skills at least a year after discharge from treatment (Carroll et al., 1994). Individual counseling focuses on reducing or stopping substance use, addresses various areas of impaired functioning, and connects PWH to community resources such as 12-step programs (e.g., Alcoholics Anonymous, Narcotics Anonymous) or Self-Management and Recovery Training recovery for patients who prefer science-based and secular programs. Supportive expressive psychotherapy has also been shown to improve outcomes among PWH with cocaine and opioid use disorders that are comorbid with psychiatric disorders (Woody, 1995). Another strategy that increases the duration of abstinence is voucher-based reinforcement therapy, where people are provided with a voucher that can be exchanged for retail goods and services consistent with a substance-free lifestyle each time they provide a drug-free urine sample. These voucher-based treatment approaches may be combined with individual, group, and family counseling, vocational counseling, and pharmacologic treatment.

PHARMACOLOGICAL MANAGEMENT

TOBACCO/NICOTINE

Tobacco use is higher among PWH than the general population, with the prevalence of cigarette smoking ranging from 40% to 70%. PWH are also less likely to quit smoking compared to other adults. Smoking and related illnesses account for significant mortality and morbidity in PWH, as it leads to reduced life expectancy, lung cancer, and other respiratory illnesses, lower $CD4^+$ T-cell counts, higher viral loads, and lower quality of life compared to nonsmokers (Miles et al., 2019). PWH who smoke are also more likely to engage in risky substance use and have decreased adherence to ART. E-cigarettes, also known as electronic nicotine delivery systems (ENDS), have become more popular in the general population and among PWH. While they are not without risks, ENDS are generally associated with lower respiratory symptoms than smoked tobacco, but using both smoked tobacco and ENDS is associated with a higher incidence of respiratory symptoms than either alone (Reddy et al., 2021). There are many reasons for tobacco/nicotine use, including self-medication for emotional distress (i.e., depression and anxiety), improved concentration, weight control, and peer connection. Not surprisingly, tobacco cessation in PWH decreases the risk of cardiovascular disease, cancer, and pulmonary conditions. PWH who quit smoking upon entering HIV care at age 40 extend their life by 4.6–5.7 years of life, even in the setting of incomplete ART adherence (Reddy et al., 2016). PWH who successfully quit tobacco generally report a higher quality of life with a lower burden of mental and physical symptoms (Ledgerwood and Yskes 2016; Reddy et al., 2022).

All PWH using tobacco should be offered interventions to reduce or quit smoking. Screening, Brief Intervention, and Referral to Treatment (SBIRT) or even a single session of motivational interviewing is effective in reducing the number of cigarettes per day. Clinicians may share information about smoking cessation and provide advice. Many PWH may have a fatalistic view of HIV and believe that smoking cessation is inconsequential to their overall health. Treating psychiatric conditions such as anxiety and depression would increase confidence in PWH to quit smoking. Importantly, pharmacotherapy with FDA-approved medications such as nicotine replacement therapy, bupropion, and varenicline has demonstrated efficacy in reducing tobacco use among PWH and should be offered as first-line alongside therapeutic interventions (Quinn et al., 2020; Reddy et al., 2022). Medications should be continued for several weeks (i.e., 12–24) after last use, depending on craving and cessation progress. National and state quit lines provide support and coaching in between appointments for smoking cessation. In the United States, the number 1-800-QUIT-NOW connects the individual to their state quit line. In addition, Smokefree.gov created free smartphone applications (QuitGuide and QuitStart) to help individuals track their cravings and progress. Lastly, transcranial magnetic stimulation (TMS) is a noninvasive treatment that has been FDA-cleared for smoking cessation. A small pilot trial found that the intermittent theta burst (iTBS) protocol in TMS decreased cigarette craving in PWH compared to sham iTBS (Rakesh et al., 2024). This is a promising option, especially for people who do not tolerate medications or need adjunctive intervention.

ALCOHOL

Excessive use of alcohol, especially binge drinking, is an important risk factor for HIV infection. Alcohol intoxication is linked to risky sexual behaviors (e.g., not using a condom or multiple partners) that increase the risk of infection. AUD also leads to poorer treatment outcomes due to ART nonadherence and medical morbidities like liver and cardiovascular disease.

Intoxication/Withdrawal

Alcohol intoxication is characterized by reversible psychological and behavioral changes that occur after alcohol consumption. A blood alcohol concentration of 0.08 is the limit for legal intoxication. However, significant impairment may occur at much lower levels in some PWH (i.e., younger or medically/mentally ill), while others may be functional at much higher levels because of tolerance. Intoxication is associated with physical symptoms of nausea, vomiting, and neurological impairment (i.e., slurred speech, incoordination, and ataxia). Overdose can result in respiratory depression, hypotension, hypothermia, profound central nervous system depression, coma, and death. Management of intoxication and overdose is supportive and may include IV fluids and airway protection to prevent aspiration. The presence of other forms of alcohol, such as methanol, and other substances like opioids and benzodiazepines, should prompt adjustments to the clinical management. Clinicians should be on high alert for a possible thiamine deficiency in PWH with AUD, which can precipitate Wernicke's encephalopathy and Korsakoff psychosis. Thiamine 100–200 mg (IV or IM preferred) should thus be given before glucose to avoid central pontine myelinolysis. For behavioral dysregulation not responsive to verbal de-escalation, antipsychotics such as haloperidol (e.g., 2–5 mg IV/IM/PO) and olanzapine may be considered. Benzodiazepines are commonly used to treat agitation but should be used with caution as they can further disinhibit the person and worsen agitation and respiratory depression.

Alcohol withdrawal begins within 6–24 hours of abstinence or a substantial reduction in the amount of alcohol use. Early symptoms include anxiety, irritability/restlessness, insomnia, nausea, headache, diaphoresis, and fine tremor. PWH may experience visual, auditory, and tactile hallucinations that characterize alcoholic hallucinosis. Alcoholic hallucinosis may occur independently of other withdrawal symptoms. Alcohol withdrawal seizures may occur within 12–48 hours after the last drink, sometimes earlier. For most people, withdrawal does not progress beyond mild-to-moderate symptoms that remit after 48 hours. For a minority of individuals, withdrawal can progress to delirium tremens (DTs), which is characterized by autonomic dysfunction (tachycardia, fever, hypertension) and delirium. Without proper management, DTs can be life-threatening. Pharmacologic treatment of alcohol withdrawal typically involves benzodiazepines. Selection of the benzodiazepine should consider pharmacokinetics, abuse potential, and presence of hepatic injury. For example, longer-acting agents (diazepam, chlordiazepoxide) have a smoother withdrawal course but carry higher risks of excessive sedation in some individuals (e.g., elderly). For PWH with significant hepatic dysfunction, a benzodiazepine that does not undergo first-pass metabolism (lorazepam, oxazepam) is preferred. Phenobarbital can be used in PWH who are not responding to benzodiazepines. Other agents that have shown efficacy and are well tolerated include anticonvulsants such as gabapentin, carbamazepine, and valproate (Minozzi et al., 2010). However, there are limited data on their ability to prevent DTs and withdrawal seizures. They may be added as augmenting agents, but benzodiazepines remain the first-line treatment.

PHARMACOTHERAPY FOR ALCOHOL USE DISORDER

Treatment for AUD involves medications that reduce the reinforcing effects of alcohol or deter use by causing adverse reactions when alcohol is consumed. Commonly used agents are summarized below:

- **Naltrexone** is a μ-opioid receptor antagonist that reduces the reinforcing effects of alcohol. This results in decreased craving as well as disruption of the euphoric feelings associated with alcohol intoxication. Naltrexone has been shown to reduce alcohol consumption and prevent relapse to heavy drinking (Miller et al., 2019). Naltrexone use is contraindicated in PWH with significant liver disease (acute hepatitis and liver failure); therefore, all PWH with these risks should have liver function tested prior to initiation. Monitoring for liver toxicity is recommended in PWH who may have concurrent liver disease from substance use, concurrent hepatitis infection, or liver impairment from ART. Naltrexone is often well tolerated and does not have documented interactions with ART. However, naltrexone should be avoided in individuals who require opioids for pain management or are in acute opioid withdrawal. PWH can be started on oral naltrexone at 50–100 mg/day. It is also available in IM formulation at doses of 380 mg every 4 weeks. Common early side effects (nausea and other gastrointestinal symptoms, headache, dizziness) are usually mild and transient. For the IM formulation, swelling, pain, and other injection site reactions may occur. For patients who prefer to not take naltrexone daily, naltrexone as needed ("targeted naltrexone") for craving or anticipated heavy drinking is effective to reduce the number of drinks during drinking days and mean drinks per day. Targeted naltrexone has also been shown to be effective in reducing binge drinking in individuals who do not meet the criteria for alcohol use disorder and reduces HIV-associated sexual risk behaviors in sexual- and gender-minority men (Santos et al., 2022).
- **Acamprosate** reduces alcohol use via modulation of glutamate neurotransmission and increase in γ-aminobutyric acid (GABA) activity. It has been shown to reduce alcohol consumption and increase the duration of abstinence (Stern et al., 2018). It is generally well tolerated and safe in PWH with impaired liver function. However, because it is excreted renally, dose adjustments may be needed in persons with renal failure. Acamprosate is FDA-approved at a dosage of 1,998 mg/day in divided doses (666 mg capsule 3 times daily). Its frequent dosing is a barrier to using this medication in many people. Common side effects are often mild and transient and include gastrointestinal (e.g., nausea, diarrhea) and dermatological symptoms (e.g., itching). Acamprosate carries a warning for a possible increase in suicidal behavior. However, many of these events occurred in the context of alcohol relapse, and no consistent pattern of relationship between the clinical course of recovery from AUD and the emergence of suicidality was identified (Forest Pharmaceuticals, 2004).
- **Disulfiram** discourages drinking by causing an adverse physical reaction with alcohol consumption. It acts by inhibiting acetaldehyde dehydrogenase, which prevents the metabolism of acetaldehyde, a byproduct of alcohol metabolism. Increased acetaldehyde concentration causes temporary flushing, sweating, palpitations, hypotension, nausea, and vomiting. Severe reactions have resulted in cardiovascular compromise and death. Because of these effects, it is often used for select PWH who are highly motivated or are closely supervised for compliance and abstinence. The daily dose is limited to 250–500 mg/day, owing to more adverse effects at higher doses. Disulfiram should not be administered to anyone who has not abstained from alcohol for at least 48 hours. It should also be avoided in PWH with a history of cardiovascular disease (e.g., myocardial infarction), end-stage liver disease, or in pregnant women. Caution should be used in PWH with a history of psychosis because of disulfiram's inhibition of dopamine dehydroxylase, which may increase dopamine concentrations and exacerbate psychotic symptoms. In PWH, disulfiram is often avoided because of a potential interaction with ART. However, a 2014 study indicated that there was

no significant increase in adverse symptoms compared to baseline with coadministration of disulfiram and common ARVs (i.e., ritonavir). With close monitoring, disulfiram should still be considered in some PWH to deter alcohol use (McCance-Katz et al., 2014).

- **Anticonvulsants** are commonly used off-label in treatment of AUD. Among these are gabapentin, topiramate, carbamazepine, and divalproex, all of which have demonstrated efficacy in reducing drinking and/or relapse in placebo-controlled trials. These medications have different mechanisms of action, though it is likely that they work for AUD by antagonism of glutamate receptors and potentiation of GABA receptors (Miller et al., 2019). Because of cognitive side effects, slow titration of topiramate is recommended (i.e., increase by 25 mg every week). Gabapentin has demonstrated efficacy in reducing cravings, amount consumed, and alcohol withdrawal symptoms at 900–1,800 mg/day in divided doses (Anton et al., 2020). Gabapentin may be additionally helpful for PWH with chronic pain. However, clinicians should regularly assess for potential misuse and tolerability.

OPIOIDS

Use of opioid-based drugs (e.g., heroin, morphine, oxycodone, and fentanyl), particularly injection drug use, has long been associated with HIV infection and transmission. Opioids act on μ receptors and activate the reward system in the central nervous system, resulting in euphoria and dependence. The risk of developing an opioid use disorder (OUD) has been shown to be even higher in people who also have psychiatric illness and chronic pain. Depression in people who inject drugs has been linked to increased rates of sharing needles and other equipment/paraphernalia, resulting in a greater risk for HIV infection. It is, therefore, crucial to treat both the psychiatric disorders and the behavioral risk factors in people who inject drugs (Ruiz, 2014).

The U.S. Opioid Epidemic and HIV

OUD has emerged as one of America's most pressing public health concerns, prompting greater consideration of how this growing epidemic could be impacting the transmission and treatment of HIV and other blood-borne infections, such as hepatitis C (HCV). In 2016, 2.1 million Americans were estimated to have an OUD, with nearly 12 million Americans estimated to have misused opioids during the preceding year (SAMHSA, 2017). Apart from the heightened morbidity and mortality associated with opioid overdose, this epidemic also places affected individuals at additional risk of acquiring and transmitting infectious diseases during the course of their addiction. Research shows that people who misuse opioids commonly move from oral use to inhalation to injection use as they build tolerance to the drug's effects and require more potent concentrations to achieve their desired level of intoxication (Peters, 2016). Moreover, it is estimated that 10%–20% of people who misuse prescription opioids move on to inject either opioids or heroin (Van Handle, 2016). Given the long-standing association between injection drug use and transmission of HIV and HCV via needle-sharing, public health providers must necessarily remain vigilant in hopes of identifying co-occurring trends in these epidemics. One such instance was documented in 2015, in Scott County, Indiana, where opioid use was implicated in an HIV outbreak that resulted in 181 individuals being diagnosed with HIV, most of whom were coinfected with HCV (Van Handle, 2016). This incident was integral in prompting the Centers for Disease Control and Prevention (CDC) to identify 220 jurisdictions that might be equally vulnerable to similar co-occurring outbreaks, with similar limited access to care (Van Handle, 2016). Targeted interventions such as these must be undertaken not only in hopes of preventing and rapidly identifying subsequent epidemics but also as a means of ensuring that individuals with comorbid OUD and HIV have adequate access to both medications for OUD (MOUD) and ART. In 2016, a systematic review and meta-analysis of 4,685 articles and 32 studies revealed that MOUD was associated with a 69% increase in recruitment into ART, a 54% increase in ART coverage, a 2-fold increase in ART adherence, a 23% decrease in the odds of attrition, and a 45% increase in odds of viral suppression (Low, 2016). Taken together, these striking statistics illustrate the importance of substance use recovery in both preventing HIV transmission and improving the overall quality of life and treatment for persons with HIV and OUD. It is imperative that individuals with opioid dependence are screened early for HIV/HCV, and promptly referred for OUD treatment to reduce morbidity and mortality and mitigate the public health impact of these epidemics.

MANAGEMENT OF OPIOID USE DISORDER

Intoxication/Withdrawal

Acute intoxication with opioids is characterized by euphoria, slurred speech, sedation, and analgesia. Physical signs include miosis, constipation, respiratory depression, and sedation. Overdoses result in respiratory arrest, cardiovascular compromise, coma, and death. Naloxone, a short-acting opioid antagonist, at doses of 0.5–2 mg IM/IV is used in all cases of suspected opioid overdose. Multiple doses may be required in the presence of fentanyl and other synthetic opioids. In severe cases, ICU care is required.

Opioid withdrawal is extremely uncomfortable and a reason for continued use in many individuals. Symptoms usually begin 8–12 hours after the last dose. Early symptoms include yawning, sweating, rhinorrhea, lacrimation, and irritability. More severe symptoms such as gastrointestinal disturbance (abdominal cramps, diarrhea, vomiting), insomnia, tachycardia, and hypertension may occur 24–36 hours after the last dose. People on methadone (long half-life) may have a more protracted withdrawal lasting 2–4 weeks. This initial withdrawal phase is often followed by symptoms lasting for weeks or months. This "protracted abstinence syndrome" includes depressed mood, low energy, poor sleep, and anhedonia.

Animal studies have implicated serotonin dysfunction in the development of this syndrome, which may respond to selective serotonin reuptake inhibitors (SSRIs) (Goeldner et al., 2011).

Initial treatment of OUD consists of a period of withdrawal management, which can be assisted by use of opioid agonists (e.g., methadone, buprenorphine) and/or supportive care for specific symptoms. Opioid agonists rapidly relieve withdrawal symptoms and may be continued for long-term management or tapered. Supportive care regimens may include acetaminophen/nonsteroidal anti-inflammatory drugs (NSAIDs) for muscle aches, α2-adrenergic agonists (clonidine, guanfacine, lofexidine) for autonomic symptoms, ondansetron for nausea, dicyclomine for abdominal cramps, and lorazepam for anxiety/insomnia. Rapid and ultrarapid withdrawal protocols use an opioid antagonist to precipitate withdrawal, and then manage symptoms with supportive treatments (e.g., sedation procedures, anesthesia in ultrarapid protocol, and clonidine). These protocols have a limited role as they carry significantly higher risks and are no more effective than the standard withdrawal management paradigms. Of note, while withdrawal management is an important aspect, they are not sufficient for OUD management. All patients must be appropriately linked to OUD treatment, which may include MOUD and psychosocial treatments. Opioid agonist treatment (OAT) with buprenorphine and methadone is associated with reduced overdose and opioid-related morbidity in people with and without HIV compared to other interventions (Cernasev et al., 2020; Wakeman et al., 2020).

PHARMACOTHERAPY FOR MAINTENANCE OF OPIOID USE DISORDER

Methadone

Developed in the 1960s, methadone is a μ-receptor agonist and a weak N-methyl-D-aspartate (NMDA) receptor antagonist that is very effective for treating OUD. Methadone has been shown to decrease the use of intravenous opioid drugs and communicable disease transmission by modifying behaviors such as intravenous drug use (Lollis, 2000). In the United States, methadone treatment is provided in specialized opioid treatment programs (OTPs), which require federal licensing and certification. OTP clinics also provide counseling, drug testing, and vocational training/assistance. Studies have shown that methadone doses in the range of 20–40 mg/d are effective in suppressing symptoms of withdrawal, but they may not be effective in reducing or stopping symptoms of craving (Strain, 1993a, 1993b). Maintenance doses are carefully titrated to each individual's needs (generally 60–120 mg/day).

Clinicians must be aware of the potential need to increase monitoring of PWH because of side effects and drug-drug interactions. Methadone prolongs QT/QTc intervals and increases the risk of torsade de pointes; therefore, close monitoring is required in persons who are taking other QT interval-prolonging drugs. Several antiretroviral drugs induce CYP540 enzymes and may decrease serum methadone levels; they include lopinavir/ritonavir, efavirenz, nevirapine, doravirine, and abacavir. If such medication combinations are required, methadone doses may need to be increased to adequately manage withdrawal and cravings. Methadone has been shown to inhibit the glucuronidation of zidovudine, resulting in increased plasma levels and a higher risk of zidovudine toxicity. Other medications with drug-drug interaction potential include the anticonvulsants carbamazepine and phenytoin, as well as some antibiotics, such as rifampin. The combination of central nervous system (CNS) depressants such as benzodiazepines with methadone may lead to severe CNS and respiratory depression. In general, caution should be used when combining these medications with methadone. Methadone has been shown to be safe during pregnancy (especially relative to opioid use or withdrawal) and breastfeeding. Newborns exposed to methadone may experience neonatal abstinence syndrome, which consists of blotchy skin coloring (mottling), diarrhea, high-pitched crying, excessive sucking, fever, hyperactive reflexes, increased muscle tone, irritability, poor feeding, and, in rare cases, seizures.

Buprenorphine and Buprenorphine plus Naloxone

Buprenorphine is a partial agonist to the μ-opioid receptor and antagonist at the κ-opioid receptor. As a partial agonist, buprenorphine's effects plateau at higher doses. It has a higher binding affinity to the μ-opioid receptor than most opioids, which allows it to displace or block other opioids from binding to the receptor. Therefore, PWH on buprenorphine will likely not feel greater euphoric effects from taking other opioids (i.e., heroin, oxycodone), which adds protection against overdose. In addition, buprenorphine may precipitate withdrawal in people with opioid exposure. The inclusion of naloxone in the buprenorphine/naloxone co-formulation is meant to reduce abuse potential by antagonizing buprenorphine's effects when it is injected. For U.S. providers, the Consolidated Appropriations Act removes the federal requirement for practitioners to have a special waiver to prescribe buprenorphine, such that all clinicians with an active DEA registration that includes Schedule III authority may prescribe buprenorphine for OUD as permitted by applicable state law. Low doses are typically used for initiation (regardless of the person's wish to start at a higher dose) to reduce the risk of side effects and precipitation of withdrawal. Buprenorphine induction begins at 2 or 4 mg approximately 12–24 hours after the last dose of a short-acting opioid. Individuals should be experiencing opioid withdrawal as assessed by a Clinical Opiate Withdrawal Scale (COWS) score of >8. Higher COWS scores (i.e., 14) may be needed for people with fentanyl use disorder. If well tolerated and there are still signs of withdrawal, an additional 2–4 mg can be repeated 1 or 2 hours later. For outpatient/home-based inductions, generally, no more than 8 mg should be given on day 1 (occasionally higher doses are offered to people using high potency synthetic opioids/fentanyl who are initiating buprenorphine in acute care settings). Over the first week, buprenorphine can be titrated up to 16 mg/day. Over the following weeks, titration should be based on cravings and withdrawal symptoms. Although up to 32 mg/day can be used, there is little evidence at this time to suggest that maintenance doses >24 mg/day offer greater clinical advantage. Buprenorphine/naloxone's effects plateau at 32 mg/day, and higher dose have no therapeutic benefit. Overdose can still occur, and people with respiratory depression may require airway management. Other potential side effects include CNS depression and hepatitis. People with a history of traumatic brain injury should be monitored for increased intracranial pressure because all potent opioids may elevate cerebrospinal fluid pressure. Buprenorphine is metabolized by CYP450 3A4 enzyme, and there are several clinically significant drug-drug interactions. Those taking CYP450 3A4 inhibitors such as nefazodone, fluvoxamine, fluoxetine, ketoconazole, itraconazole, erythromycin, clarithromycin, grapefruit juice, and most protease inhibitors (especially ritonavir) should take reduced doses of buprenorphine.

Naltrexone

As a μ-opioid receptor antagonist, naltrexone blocks the reinforcing effects of opioids. Oral and IM formulations of naltrexone are effective for highly motivated individuals who have completed withdrawal and can maintain abstinence from opioids. Oral naltrexone should be initiated after 5–7 days of abstinence from short-acting opioids, and 7–10 days for long-acting opioids to avoid precipitating withdrawal. It can be started at 25 mg, increased to 50 mg daily, or 350 mg weekly into 3 divided doses (100 mg, 100 mg, and 150 mg). In our experience, some patients benefit from doses of naltrexone up to 100 mg daily. While oral naltrexone is not effective for most patients with OUD, the naltrexone XR (IM formulation, administered as 380 mg every 4 weeks) can improve abstinence and retention in treatment. A randomized trial comparing naltrexone XR with OAT using buprenorphine or methadone showed noninferiority of naltrexone XR in PWH for viral suppression and past 30-day opioid use. However, treatment initiation was significantly lower in the naltrexone XR group (Korthuis et al., 2022). In addition, while the IM formulation is preferred, many patients may find it cost-prohibitive (see the section on alcohol for more details on naltrexone). Baseline and periodic monitoring of liver function tests are recommended, especially in patients on higher doses. Because patients may increase the amount of opioids used to override the blockade from naltrexone, there is still a risk of opioid overdose. Discussing this possibility with patients may open a conversation about their motivations and ambivalence toward abstinence.

COCAINE/CRACK

In addition to the increased incidence of risk behaviors in people who use cocaine, studies have shown that cocaine use may have broad-ranging effects on human immunity. Regarding HIV infection, in vitro studies have shown that cocaine enhances the infection of stimulated lymphocytes. Moreover, cohort studies in the pre-and post-HAART era have linked stimulant use with increased HIV pathogenesis (Baum, 2009). It is therefore crucial to treat PWH who have cocaine use disorder.

Cocaine enhances activity of serotonin, norepinephrine, and dopamine (DA) by blocking reuptake of these neurotransmitters. Its addiction liability is thought to be secondary to increased dopamine levels in the nucleus accumbens. Cocaine effects depend on the mode of use, with smoked (crack) and intravenous administration having the quickest effects (seconds to 30 minutes; peak 15–30 minutes) and intranasal administration having slightly more delayed effects (5–90 minutes; peak 30 minutes). Mild-to-moderate intoxication produces sympathomimetic symptoms—generally increased heart rate and blood pressure, decreased appetite, insomnia, euphoria, hyper-alertness, and irritability. With severe intoxication, dilation of the pupils, severe hypertension (HTN), hyperthermia, cardiac arrhythmias/MIs, stroke, seizures, coma, and death may occur. At any level of intoxication, psychiatric symptoms may include auditory/visual/tactile hallucinations, delusions, paranoia, and aggression/violence. Individuals with severe cocaine intoxication (i.e., malignant HTN, hyperthermia, and seizure) will need medical stabilization. Phentolamine, cooling, and other supportive measures should be given for HTN crisis and hyperthermia; benzodiazepines should be given to terminate seizures and agitation. Antipsychotics may be considered for severe agitation/aggression/psychosis but should be used with caution because they increase the risk of neuroleptic malignant syndrome and seizures during stimulant intoxication.

Research into several medications for cocaine use disorder (CUD) has failed to show consistent evidence of effectiveness, but efforts are ongoing. Commonly used agents are summarized below:

- Anticonvulsants: Among anticonvulsants studied (carbamazepine, gabapentin, topiramate, lamotrigine, phenytoin, tiagabine, and vigabatrin), only topiramate showed significant treatment outcomes—it was better than placebo at maintaining 3 weeks of cocaine abstinence (Minozzi et al., 2015). Topiramate should be increased slowly (i.e., 25 mg/week) to reduce risk of cognitive impairment. Higher doses are more likely to cause impairment, which may be more pronounced in PWH who have HIV-associated neurocognitive decline.
- Stimulants: A meta-analysis of stimulants as a class showed efficacy for promoting 3 weeks of abstinence compared to placebo, especially in people with comorbid attention-deficit hyperactivity disorder (ADHD) (Castells et al., 2016). Methylphenidate may improve HIV-associated cognitive impairment and depression in PWH (Hinkin et al., 2001). When using stimulants, extended-release formulations are preferred to reduce misuse potential.
- Bupropion: This is an antidepressant that inhibits dopamine and norepinephrine reuptake; it has demonstrated therapeutic benefit in CUD. However, the response is less robust in people with severe CUD (Chan

et al., 2019). Bupropion is especially beneficial in PWH with co-occurring tobacco use disorder.

- Doxazosin: This is an α1-adrenergic receptor antagonist that has shown some promise in decreasing cocaine use at doses of 8 mg/day in a small trial (Shorter et al., 2013).
- Disulfiram: It has been studied as a potential therapeutic agent because of its inhibition of dopamine-β-hydroxylase, which prevents the conversion of dopamine to norepinephrine, thereby increasing dopamine levels. However, efficacy data have been inconsistent (Pani et al., 2010). Disulfiram is dosed at 250–500 mg/day.
- Other agents needing further study include ondansetron 4 mg twice daily (Blevins et al., 2021; Johnson et. al., 2006), and topiramate plus mixed amphetamine salts, which showed reduced cocaine use in small trials in people with high-frequency cocaine use (Chan et al., 2019).

METHAMPHETAMINE

Methamphetamine use has grown exponentially in both rural and urban areas during the past few decades. It is an extremely potent stimulant that heightens sexual arousal with reduced inhibition and judgment, increasing the risk of STI/HIV acquisition. It can be smoked, eaten, snorted, injected, or rectally inserted. It has a rapid onset and long-lasting effects (half-life of 11–12 hours). Use induces the release of newly synthesized dopamine, norepinephrine, and serotonin. It is also an indirect catecholamine and serotonin (5-HT) agonist. Like cocaine, methamphetamine can deplete dopamine stores and lead to significant symptoms of depression and, in some cases, suicidal ideation and attempts. Other symptoms that may be experienced include psychosis (lasting weeks to months), aggression, thought disorders, and gum disease. Acute intoxication is treated like cocaine intoxication with supportive care. Phentolamine, cooling, and other supportive treatments may be used for HTN crisis and hyperthermia; benzodiazepines are used for seizures and agitation. Antipsychotics may also be required to manage severe aggression/agitation. First-line treatments for methamphetamine use disorder are psychosocial and psychotherapeutic interventions, such as contingency management, and the matrix model, which includes a variety of therapies targeting use and relapse prevention. Pharmacological interventions are limited and there are currently no FDA-approved medications. Moreover, few medications have demonstrated consistent efficacy in controlled trials. The following is a summary of medications that have demonstrated some potential:

- **Antidepressants**: Mirtazapine demonstrated efficacy in the reduction of methamphetamine use and sexual risk behaviors in a small study with cis-gender men and transgender women who have sex with men (Coffin et al., 2020).
- **Antipsychotics**: Risperidone reduced methamphetamine use in small open-label trials (Meridith et al., 2007; Meridith et al., 2009). Paliperidone improved treatment retention but did not reduce use in a randomized clinical trial (Wang et al., 2019). Both antipsychotics were effective at improving psychotic symptoms. A case series of two patients taking cariprazine showed a reduction in cravings and frequency of use as well as longer time to relapse (Truong and Li, 2022). Taken together, for patients experiencing persistent methamphetamine-induced psychosis, use of long-acting injectable formulations of risperidone and paliperidone may be helpful to increase retention and engagement in treatment.
- **Anticonvulsants**: In a multicenter randomized trial, topiramate was more effective than placebo at reducing use and relapse rates, but not at promoting abstinence. Baclofen was effective at reducing use in highly adherent participants (Chan et al., 2019). Topiramate can be dosed 25–150 mg twice daily.
- **Atomoxetine 80 mg**: This is a nonstimulant medication for ADHD that inhibits the norepinephrine transporter to increase norepinephrine and dopamine (to a lower extent) in the prefrontal cortex. A small, randomized trial in patients receiving buprenorphine/naloxone for OUD showed a reduction in methamphetamine cravings and use compared to placebo. A greater reduction in depressive symptoms was shown with atomoxetine than placebo (Schottenfeld et. al., 2018). It is important for clinicians and patients to know that atomoxetine may not have instantaneous effects as do stimulants and may take a few weeks to show full benefit.
- **Stimulants**: Stimulants as a class have not shown greater efficacy than placebo. However, it is possible that the doses used in these studies were not sufficient. Among stimulants, methylphenidate has demonstrated efficacy in reducing use, cravings, and addiction severity among people with ADHD (Chan et. al., 2019). Methylphenidate may also improve cognitive symptoms in PWH. Extended-release formulations are preferred because of a lower risk of misuse.
- **Combination pharmacotherapy**: Bupropion 450 mg plus naltrexone 380 mg extended-release injectable every 3 weeks was more effective than placebo at reducing methamphetamine use in 13.6% of individuals in one multisite trial (Trivedi et al., 2021).

ECSTASY OR MOLLY (MDMA)

Dubbed the "intimacy drug," ecstasy has been shown to produce profound feelings of closeness, which may lead to high-risk sexual behavior and HIV exposure. Some studies have shown that people using ecstasy may perceive less danger of acquiring HIV/other STIs compared to nonusers (Theall, 2006). It is, therefore, critical that PWH and people who may acquire HIV are provided with information about the dangers of ecstasy use, in addition to the other known health issues that may result from its use. Currently, there is no FDA-approved medication for the treatment of MDMA use disorder, and acute management is geared toward treating life-threatening conditions such as serotonin syndrome and hyperthermia that are commonly seen among people attending "rave parties." The primary treatment of MDMA use disorder involves cognitive behavioral interventions to help modify thought patterns and help people gain skills to cope with life stressors.

CANNABIS

The legalization and shifting attitudes toward cannabis have contributed to a rapid increase in the availability and use of cannabis products. Cannabis is used by the public for recreational and medicinal purposes, the latter for a wide range of physical and mental conditions including anxiety, insomnia, and pain. In a study of 226 PWH from Canada, 97.7% reported recreational use, and 21.8% reported medicinal use for stress, anorexia, nausea, and pain. Although negative consequences were not as strongly reported as benefits, cannabis use was associated with other behaviors such as driving under the influence, ecstasy and tobacco use, paranoia, and greater financial expenditures (Harris et. al., 2014). Cognitive impairment has been well described among PWH who use cannabis. Studies examining the impact of cannabis use on ART adherence have been inconsistent (various results indicate negative, positive, or no effect). Data on the safety and benefits of cannabis use for PWH is currently inconclusive. Many experts recommend discouraging use and taking a harm-reduction approach in PWH with continued use (i.e., reducing to low-risk levels). Alternative interventions for appetite, anxiety, and sleep should be offered when indicated.

The most common cannabinoids found in the cannabis plant are delta-9-tetrahydrocannabinol (THC) and cannabidiol (CBD). THC is a partial agonist at the cannabinoid receptors CB1 and CB2, activating the receptor up to 20%. THC use is associated with euphoria, laughter, increased appetite, altered perception of time, and relaxation. Delta-8-THC has become more widely used due to being legal in many states and may not be detected on standard urine toxicology screens. On the other hand, CBD is an antagonist at CB1 receptors, a partial agonist at CB2 receptors, and does carry similar euphoric effects to THC. These cannabinoids are smoked, vaped, or consumed as edibles. Cannabis withdrawal is associated with anxiety, irritability, insomnia, and depression. The mainstay of treatment is behavioral therapies such as CBT, motivational interviewing, and motivational enhancement therapy.

There is no well-established pharmacological intervention for cannabis use disorder. Some medications showing potential benefits include gabapentin, N-acetylcysteine (NAC), and cannabidiol. Gabapentin (1,200 mg/day or higher in divided doses) has shown benefit in reducing cannabis cravings, use, and withdrawal. Gabapentin may be beneficial for PWH who have HIV-associated polyneuropathy and pain. It is also often used off-label for anxiety and AUD. However, gabapentin has misuse potential and is now a controlled substance in several states. NAC 1,200 mg twice daily showed a use reduction in adolescents aged 15–21 years, but was not better than placebo in a group of adults aged 18–50 years (Brezing and Levin, 2018). A 2020 study showed that participants receiving CBD 400 mg and 800 mg were more likely to use less cannabis and have more days abstinent (Freeman et al., 2020). However, more studies are needed to establish the safety and efficacy of CBD. A gradual transition from THC to CBD by slowly reducing THC concentration may be a harm-reduction approach for PWH who are still ambivalent about abstinence from cannabis.

MULTIPLE SUBSTANCE USE

Most people who use illicit substances use multiple substances, with tobacco/nicotine being the most common comorbid SUD. One study found that multi-substance use was present in 93.8% of people who use heroin (John et al., 2018). In our experience, multi-substance use is the rule rather than the exception in people with moderate-to-severe SUD. Overdose death rates have skyrocketed in recent years from the "speedball" combination of methamphetamine and opioids, particularly fentanyl (NIH, 2022). Multi-substance use is associated with worse treatment outcomes and higher severity SUD. Therefore, it is important to address all SUDs even when they may seem less impairing. For example, treatment of tobacco/nicotine use disorder may improve outcomes in patients with CUD (Winhusen et al., 2014). With such high rates of multi-substance use, we recommend that all patients with illicit substance use (especially stimulant and opioid use) should be provided with naloxone nasal spray for overdose prevention. In 2023, the naloxone nasal spray became available over the counter and can be obtained from pharmacies without a prescription in most states. Community-based organizations and local health departments may have it available at little to no cost. Individuals with SUD and their support persons should check their local pharmacy and health department for availability.

OTHER CONSIDERATIONS IN PWH

Interactions between substances of use and ARV agents have been reported. The toxicity of amphetamines, MDMA, meperidine, and gamma-hydroxybutyrate (GHB) is dangerously increased by ritonavir and other HIV medications that inhibit liver metabolism. Barbiturates induce the cytochrome systems responsible for metabolism of protease inhibitors (PI), non-nucleoside reverse transcriptase inhibitors (NNRTIs), maraviroc, elvitegravir, and dolutegravir, significantly decreasing their effectiveness. Oral midazolam and triazolam are contraindicated with PIs, and NNRTIs. The toxicity of ketamine and phencyclidine (PCP) is dangerously increased by PIs and etravirine.

All the agents listed for use in withdrawal management and maintenance of sobriety have utility in PWH, but special considerations include the following:

- Buprenorphine administration is office-based and more accessible. To increase treatment of OUD, recent reforms no longer require training to apply for an X-waiver and there are no longer limitations on the number of patients who may be treated with buprenorphine. However, clinicians applying for a new or renewed DEA registration will need to attest to having completed at least 8 hours of training on opioid or other substance use disorders (SAMHSA, Training requirements [MATE Act] resources, 2024). Clinically significant interactions with ART, although generally uncommon, may occur. The CYP3A4 inhibition from atazanavir, darunavir, and ritonavir can increase buprenorphine serum levels, leading to increased sedation—especially with atazanavir. The CYP3A4 inducers etravirine and nevirapine can decrease serum concentrations of buprenorphine, which may present with increased cravings and withdrawal symptoms. Fluconazole can increase the activity of buprenorphine, whereas phenobarbital, phenytoin, rifabutin, and rifampin decrease the effective amounts, but sometimes cause withdrawal symptoms. For perioperative preparation with expected moderate to severe pain, patients receiving more than 16 mg of buprenorphine should be reduced to 16 mg the day before surgery. If the patient is on 8 mg or less, they may continue buprenorphine at the same dose. For procedures with expected mild pain, no dose adjustment is needed (Quaye and Zhang, 2019).
- Bupropion decreases the seizure threshold and increases risk of seizures in individuals with weight loss or electrolyte instability. Bupropion should be avoided in these patients until weight is restored and electrolyte abnormalities are corrected.
- Disulfiram has a high risk of hepatotoxicity and may cause the disulfiram reaction with ritonavir capsules because some formulations contain alcohol. Prior to prescribing this combination, ensure that the patient is not receiving any alcohol-containing products.
- Methadone maintenance cannot be provided outside a registered clinic and has several clinically significant interactions with some ARVs. As previously discussed, blood levels of abacavir are decreased; blood level of zidovudine is increased; abacavir increases blood levels of methadone, and dose adjustment may be required to avoid sedation; efavirenz, nevirapine, darunavir, lopinavir, and ritonavir (even in boosting doses) all decrease methadone availability and may precipitate opioid withdrawal symptoms. Drug interactions with other medications frequently used in PWH have also been reported (carbamazepine, phenobarbital, phenytoin, and rifampin sharply decrease methadone levels, and fluconazole significantly increases methadone blood levels).
- Naltrexone presents challenges to individuals requiring pain control with full opioid agonists. Oral naltrexone must be stopped 72 hours prior to procedures requiring pain control requiring narcotics, while extended release (injectable) naltrexone must be stopped 30 days prior. Other methods of analgesia and anesthesia may be considered for minor procedures.
- When selecting a medication for an SUD, consider comorbid conditions that may also benefit. For example, gabapentin may be considered for comorbid pain and cannabis use disorder. Methylphenidate may be preferred for HIV-associated cognitive impairment and stimulant use disorder.

SUBSTANCE USE AND HIV IN THE CORONAVIRUS (COVID-19) PANDEMIC

The COVID-19 pandemic has placed tremendous strain on the healthcare system, creating unique challenges for individuals with SUD. The pandemic has created social isolation, anxiety, stress, and boredom that can increase the risk for substance use. Many individuals with SUD are unstably housed, incarcerated, or actively seeking drugs, putting them at greater risk for acquiring or transmitting COVID-19. As mentioned, substance use can increase exposure to HIV, which may be more likely when access to community harm-reduction resources like syringe services programs is curtailed. In addition, people with SUD and comorbid medical conditions may be more likely to develop severe COVID-19 illness (for example, pulmonary complications may be more severe for PWH who smoke and vape tobacco and marijuana). Individuals with OUD may be vulnerable to hypoxemia with concurrent opioid use and respiratory infections. Methamphetamine can cause lung damage from constriction of blood vessels and pulmonary hypertension. People with ongoing substance use should be encouraged to practice harm-reduction behaviors such as using protective equipment (e.g., masks) when seeking drugs, practicing physical distancing when using, and using sterile needles when injecting. Providers should be aware that trauma is prevalent; depending on an individual's history, recommended interventions such as mask-wearing may elicit traumatic memories such as feelings of suffocation and helplessness. Providers attuned to these issues may be able to guide people to find solutions to practice safe behaviors.

Telehealth services have expanded in response to the COVID-19 pandemic, allowing easier access to care. Scheduled medications such as buprenorphine for OUD may be prescribed via telehealth as long as clinicians are adhering to federal and state guidelines. Collaboration between individuals and providers is key to determining if telehealth or in-person treatment is best, although many PWH with ongoing substance use may require frequent in-person visits for comprehensive evaluation, exam, and urine toxicology screens. PWH who are stable may be appropriate for a hybrid of telehealth and in-person management. Many clinics have adopted a hybrid telehealth/in-person model to provide care for different SUD populations. Whenever possible and appropriate, telehealth should be utilized if transportation and other barriers are impeding treatment. Providers are encouraged to check the CDC, SAMHSA, NIDA, and other trusted organizations for updates on recommendations and evolving clinical evidence.

SUMMARY

Substance use and SUDs are common in PWH, and require early and aggressive diagnosis and treatment, both to minimize further HIV transmission through ungoverned risk behaviors and to maximize the ability of the individual to fully participate in their care. Successful management decreases morbidity and mortality from both conditions. Adequate treatment of substance use can improve adherence (to clinic visits and ART). These principles apply even more stringently in people with "triple diagnosis"—SUD, psychiatric disorders, and HIV. As with any treatment process, success involves establishing a collaborative alliance—a therapeutic relationship between treatment staff and patients. This sets the stage for honest communication, mutual respect of boundaries, and continued participation in treatment (on both sides) despite temporary setbacks and challenges. Integrated treatment of SUD and HIV (or SUD, mental illness, and HIV in the case of triple diagnosis) offers distinct advantages for people with complex needs experiencing multiple barriers to participation. Substance use alone is not a contraindication to ART.

RECOMMENDED READING

The ASAM national practice guideline for the treatment of opioid use disorder: 2020 focused update. *J Addict Med.* 2020;14(2S Suppl 1):1–91. Erratum in: *J Addict Med.* 2020;14(3):267.

Clinical Guideline Committee (CGC) Members; ASAM Team; AAAP Team; IRETA Team. The ASAM/AAAP clinical practice guideline on the management of stimulant use disorder. *J Addict Med.* 2024;18(1S Suppl 1):1–56.

Miller SC, Fiellin DA, Rosenthal RN, Saitz R. *The ASAM Principles of Addiction Medicine.* Philadelphia: Wolters Kluwer; 2019.

SAMHSA. Prevention and treatment of HIV among people living with substance use and/or mental disorders. https://store.samhsa.gov/product/Prevention-and-Treatment-of-HIV-Among-People-Living-with-Substance-Use-and-or-Mental-Disorders/PEP20-06-03-001. n.d. Accessed November 19, 2022.

REFERENCES

American Psychiatric Association. *Diagnostic and Statistical Manual of Mental Disorders, Text Revision.* 5th ed. Washington, DC: APA Press; 2022.

Anton RF, Latham P, Voronin K, et al. Efficacy of gabapentin for the treatment of alcohol use disorder in patients with alcohol withdrawal symptoms: a randomized clinical trial. *JAMA Intern Med.* 2020;180(5):728–736.

Baum MK, Rafie C, Lai S, et al. Crack-cocaine use accelerates HIV disease progression in a cohort of HIV-positive drug users. *J AIDS.* 2009;50(1):93–99.

Bhaskaran K, Hamouda O, Sannes M, et al. Changes in the risk of death after HIV seroconversion compared with mortality in the general population. *JAMA.* 2008;300(1):51–59.

Blevins D, Seneviratne C, Wang X.-Q, Johnson BA, Ait-Daoud N. A randomized, double-blind, placebo-controlled trial of ondansetron for the treatment of cocaine use disorder with post hoc pharmacogenetic analysis. *Drug Alcohol Depend.* 2021;228:109074.

Brezing CA, Levin FR. The current state of pharmacological treatments for cannabis use disorder and withdrawal. *Neuropsychopharmacology.* 2018;43(1):173–194.

Branson BM, Handsfield HH, Lampe MA, et al. Revised recommendations for HIV testing of adults, adolescents, and pregnant women in health-care settings. *MMWR Recomm Rep.* 2006;55(RR-14):1–17.

Campos-Outcalt D. 8 USPSTF recommendations FPs need to know about. *J Fam Pract.* 2016;65:338–342.

Carroll K, Rounsaville B, Nich C, et al. One-year follow-up of psychotherapy and pharmacotherapy for cocaine dependence: delayed emergence of psychotherapy effects. *Arch Gen Psychiatry.* 1994;51:989–997.

Castells X, Cunill R, Pérez-Mañá C, Vidal X, Capellà D. Psychostimulant drugs for cocaine dependence. *Cochrane Database Syst Rev.* 2016; 2016(9):CD007380.

Centers for Disease Control and Prevention (CDC). Estimated HIV incidence and prevalence in the United States, 2018–2022. HIV Surveillance Supplemental Report 2024;29(no. 1). https://www.cdc.gov/ hiv-data/nhss/estimated-hiv-incidence-and-prevalence.html. Published May 2024. Accessed August 2024.

Centers for Disease Control and Prevention (CDC). Incorporating HIV prevention into the medical care of persons living with HIV: recommendations of CDC, the Health Resources and Services Administration, the National Institutes of Health, and the HIV Medicine Association of the Infectious Diseases Society of America. *MMWR Recomm Rep.* 2003;52(RR-12):1–24.

Cernasev, Alina, Veve MP, Cory TJ, et al. Opioid use disorders in people living with HIV/AIDS: a review of implications for patient outcomes, drug interactions, and neurocognitive disorders. *Pharmacy.* 2020;8(3):168.

Chan B, Freeman M, Kondo K, et al. Pharmacotherapy for methamphetamine/amphetamine use disorder—a systematic review and meta-analysis. *Addiction.* 2019; 114(12):2122–2136.

Chen CC, Lu R-B, Chen Y-C, et al. Interaction between the functional polymorphisms of the alcohol metabolism genes in protection against alcoholism. *Am J Hum Genet.* 1999;65:795–807.

Coffin PO, Santos G-M, Hern J, et al. Effects of mirtazapine for methamphetamine use disorder among cisgender men and transgender women who have sex with men: a placebo-controlled randomized clinical trial. *JAMA Psychiatry.* 2020;77(3):246.

Cofrancesco J Jr, Scherzer R, Tien PC, et al. Illicit drug use and HIV treatment outcomes in a US cohort. *AIDS.* 2008;22:237–245.

Finanger T, Einar AV, Spigset O, et al. Identification of unhealthy alcohol use by self-report and phosphatidylethanol (PEth) blood concentrations in an acute psychiatric department. *BMC Psychiatry.* 2022;22(1):286.

Forest Pharmaceuticals. *Campral (Acamprosate calcium) delayed release tablets [product information].* St. Louis, MO: Forest Pharmaceuticals; 2004.

Freeman TP, Hindocha C, Baio G, et al. Cannabidiol for the treatment of cannabis use disorder: a phase 2a, double-blind, placebo-controlled, randomised, adaptive Bayesian trial. *Lancet Psychiatry.* 2020; 7(10):865–874.

Goeldner C, Lutz PE, Darcq E, et al. Impaired emotional-like behavior and serotonergic function during protracted abstinence from chronic morphine. *Biol Psychiatry.* 2011;69(3):236–244.

Harris GE, Dupuis L, Mugford GJ, et al. Patterns and correlates of cannabis use among individuals with HIV/AIDS in Maritime Canada. *Can J Infect Dis Med Microbiol.* 2014;25(1):e1–e7.

Hillfors DD, Iritani BJ, Miller WC, et al. Sexual and drug behavior patterns and HIV and STD racial disparities: the need for new directions. *Am J Public Health.* 2007;97(1):125–132.

Hinkin CH, Castellon SA, Hardy DJ, Farinpour R, Newton T, Singer E. Methylphenidate improves HIV-1–associated cognitive slowing. *J Neuropsychiatry Clin Neurosci.* 2001;13(2):248–254.

John WS, Zhu H, Mannelli P, Schwartz RP, Subramaniam GA, Wu L-T. Prevalence, patterns, and correlates of multiple substance use disorders among adult primary care patients. *Drug Alcohol Depend.* 2018;187:79–87.

Johnson BA, Roache JD, Ait-Daoud N, et al. A preliminary randomized, double-blind, placebo-controlled study of the safety and efficacy of ondansetron in the treatment of cocaine dependence. *Drug Alcohol Depend.* 2006;84(3):256–263.

Korthuis PT, Cook RR, Foot CA, et al. Association of methamphetamine and opioid use with nonfatal overdose in rural communities. *JAMA Netw Open*. 2022;5(8):e2226544.

Ledgerwood DM, Yskes R. Smoking cessation for people living with HIV/AIDS: a literature review and synthesis. *Nic Tob Res*. 2016 Dec;18(12):2177–2184.

Lollis CM, Strothers HS, et al. Sex, drugs and HIV: does methadone maintenance reduce drug use and risky sexual behavior? *J Behav Med*. 2000;23(;6):545–557.

Low AJ, Mburu G, Welton NJ, et al. Impact of opioid substitution therapy on antiretroviral therapy outcomes: a systematic review and meta-analysis. *Clin Infect Dis*. 2016;63(8):1094–1104.

McCance-Katz EF, Gruber VA, Beatty G, et al. Interaction of disulfiram with antiretroviral medications: efavirenz increases while atazanavir decreases disulfiram effect on enzymes of alcohol metabolism. *Am J Addict*. 2014;23(2):137–144.

McLellan AT, Lewis DC, O'Brien CP, Kleber HD. Drug dependence, a chronic medical illness: implications for treatment, insurance, and outcomes evaluation. *JAMA*. 2000;284:1689–1695.

Meredith CW, Jaffe C, Cherrier M, et al. Open trial of injectable risperidone for methamphetamine dependence. *J Addict Med*. 2009;3(2):55–65.

Meredith CW, Jaffe C, Yanasak E, Cherrier M, Saxon AJ. An open-label pilot study of risperidone in the treatment of methamphetamine dependence. *J Psychoactive Drugs*. 2007;39(2):167–172.

Miles DRB, Bilal U, Hutton HE, et al. Tobacco smoking, substance use, and mental health symptoms in people with hiv in an urban HIV clinic. *J Health Care Poor Underserved*. 2019;30(3):1083–1102.

Mille, SC, Fiellin DA, Rosenthal RN, Saitz R. *The ASAM Principles of Addiction Medicine*. Philadelphia, PA: Wolters Kluwer; 2019.

Millett GA, Flores SA, Bakeman R. Explaining disparities in HIV infection among Black and white men who have sex with men: a meta-analysis of HIV risk behaviors. *AIDS*. 2007;21(15):2083–2091.

Minozzi S, Amato L, Vecchi S, et al. Anticonvulsants for alcohol withdrawal. *Cochrane Database Syst Rev*. 2010;3:CD005064.

Minozzi S, Cinquini M, Amato L, et al. Anticonvulsants for cocaine dependence. *Cochrane Database Syst Rev*. 2015;4:CD006754.

Moore RM, Gebo KA, Lucas GM, et al. Rate of co-morbidities not related to HIV infection or AIDS among HIV-positive patients by CD4 count and HAART use status. *Clin Infect Dis*. 2008;47(8):1102–1104.

National Institute on Alcohol Abuse and Alcoholism. Helping patients who drink too much: a clinician's guide. www.niaaa.nih.gov/health-professionals-communities/core-resource-on-alcohol. Accessed August 19, 2024.

National Institute on Drug Abuse. Principles of Drug Addiction Treatment: *A Research based Guide. 3rd ed. Rockville,* MD: NIDA (NIH Publication No. 12–4180), 1999:2–5.

National Institute on Drug Abuse. Overdose Death Rates. Available at: https://nida.nih.gov/research-topics/trends-statistics/overdose-death-rates. Accessed March 24, 2025.

New York State Department of Health AIDS Institute. *Substance Use in Patients with HIV/AIDS*. Albany: New York State Department of Health; 2009.

Pani PP, Trogu E, Vacca, R, Amato L, Vecchi S, Davoli M. Disulfiram for the treatment of cocaine dependence. *Cochrane Database Syst Rev*. 2010;1:CD007024.

Peters P, et al. HIV infection linked to injection use of oxymorphone in Indiana, 2014–2015. *N Engl J Med*. 2016;375:229–239.

Quaye ANA, Zhang Y. Perioperative management of buprenorphine: solving the conundrum. *Pain Med*. 2019;20(7):1395–1408.

Quinn MH, Bauer AM, Flitter A, et al. Correlates of varenicline adherence among smokers with HIV and its association with smoking cessation. *Addict Behav*. 2020;102:106151.

Rakesh G, Adams TG, Morey RA, et al. Intermittent theta burst stimulation and functional connectivity in people living with HIV/AIDS who smoke tobacco cigarettes: a preliminary pilot study. *Front Psychiatry*. 2024;15:1315854.

Reddy KP, Kruse GR, Lee S, et al. 2022. Tobacco use and treatment of tobacco dependence among people with human immunodeficiency virus: a practical guide for clinicians. *Clin Inf Dis*. 2022;75(3):525–533.

Reddy KP, Parker RA, Losina E, et al. Impact of cigarette smoking and smoking cessation on life expectancy among people with HIV: a US-based modeling study. *Infect Dis*. 2016;214(11):1672–1681.

Reddy KP, Schwamm E, Kalkhoran S, et al. Respiratory symptom incidence among people using electronic cigarettes, combustible tobacco, or both. *Am J Respir Crit Care Med*. 2021;204(2):231–234.

Ruiz P, Strain EC. Psychiatric complications of HIV-1 infection and drug abuse. In: *The Substance Abuse Handbook*. Philadelphia: Lippincott Williams & Wilkins; 2014: 392–402.

Santos GM, Ikeda J, Coffin P, et al. Targeted oral naltrexone for mild to moderate alcohol use disorder among sexual and gender minority men: a randomized trial. *Am J Psychiatry*. 2022;179(12):915–926.

Schottenfeld RS, Chawarski MC, Sofuoglu M, et al. Atomoxetine for amphetamine-type stimulant dependence during buprenorphine treatment: a randomized controlled trial. *Drug Alcohol Depend*. 2018;186:130–137.

Shorter D, Lindsay JA, Kosten TR. The alpha-1 adrenergic antagonist doxazosin for treatment of cocaine dependence: a pilot study. *Drug Alcohol Depend*. 2013;131(1–2):66–70.

Stern TA, Freudenreich O, Smith FA, Fricchione G, Rosenbaum JF. *Massachusetts General Hospital Handbook of General Hospital Psychiatry*. Philadelphia: Elsevier; 2018.

Strain EC, Stitzer ML, Lisbon IA, et al. Dose–response effects of methadone in the treatment of opioid dependence. *Ann Intern Med*. 1993a;119:23–27.

Strain EC, Stitzer ML, Lisbon IA, et al. Methadone dose and treatment outcome. *Drug Alcohol Depend*. 1993b;33:105–117.

Substance Abuse and Mental Health Services Administration (SAMHSA). 2016 National survey on drug use and health. https://www.samhsa.gov/data/sites/default/files/NSDUH-FFR1-2016/NSDUH-FFR1-2016.pdf. Published September 2017. Accessed August 19, 2024.

Substance Abuse and Mental Health Services Administration (SAMHSA). Training requirements (MATE Act) resources. https://www.samhsa.gov/medications-substance-use-disorders/training-requirements-mate-act-resources. Updated April 11, 2024. Accessed August 19, 2024.

Sullivan LE, Goulet JL, Justice AC, et al. Alcohol consumption and depressive symptoms over time: a longitudinal study of patients with and without HIV infection. *Drug Alcohol Depend*. 2011;117:158–163.

Theall KP, Elifson KW, Sterk CE. Sex, touch, and HIV risk among ecstasy users. *AIDS Behav*. 2006;10(2):169–178.

Trivedi MH, Walker R, Ling W, et al. Bupropion and naltrexone in methamphetamine use disorder. *N Engl J Med*. 2021;384(2):140–153.

Truong TT, Li B. Case series: cariprazine for treatment of methamphetamine use disorder. *Am J Addict*. 2022;31(1):85–88.

Van Handle M, et al. County-level vulnerability assessment for rapid dissemination of HIV or HCV infections among persons who inject drugs, United States. *J AIDS*. 2016;73(3):323–331.

Wakeman SE, Larochelle MR, Ameli O, et al. Comparative effectiveness of different treatment pathways for opioid use disorder. *JAMA Netw Open*. 2020;3(2):e1920622

Wang G, Ma L, Liu X, et al. Paliperidone extended-release tablets for the treatment of methamphetamine use disorder in Chinese patients after acute treatment: a randomized, double-blind, placebo-controlled exploratory study. *Front Psychiatry*. 2019;10:656.

West R. Models of addiction. *EMCDDA Insights*. European Monitoring Centre for Drugs and Drug Addiction (EMCDDA), Spain. 2013. ISSN 2314-9264: 22–26.

Winhusen TM, Kropp F, Theobald J, Lewis DF. Achieving smoking abstinence is associated with decreased cocaine use in cocaine-dependent patients receiving smoking-cessation treatment. *Drug Alcohol Depend*. 2014;134:391–395.

Woody GE, McLellan AT, Luborsky L, et al. Psychotherapy in community methadone programs: a validation study. *Am J Psychiatry*. 1995;152(9):1302–1308.

Wu Z, McGoogan JM. Characteristics of and important lessons from the coronavirus disease 2019 (COVID-19) outbreak in China: summary of a report of 72 314 cases from the Chinese Center for Disease Control and Prevention. *JAMA*. 2020;323(13):1239–1242.

35.

PSYCHIATRIC DISORDERS AND HIV

Richa Vijayvargiya and Elizabeth David

LEARNING OBJECTIVES

- Discuss the bidirectional relationship between HIV infection and psychiatric disorders.
- Recognize symptoms suggesting the presence of a psychiatric condition.
- Describe general principles of mental health treatment and identify when specific intervention by mental health professionals is advised.

WHAT'S NEW?

- This chapter reflects terminology from the *Diagnostic and Statistical Manual of Mental Disorders, Text Revision* (DSM-5-TR) (American Psychiatric Association, 2022) and highlights recent research confirming the ongoing close association between HIV and psychiatric symptoms/conditions.

KEY POINTS

- Mental illness is a risk factor for acquiring HIV and may also develop as a consequence of HIV infection.
- Careful diagnosis of psychiatric disorders among people with HIV (PWH) is essential given their impact on mental well-being and health outcomes, including adherence to antiretroviral therapy, disease progression, and overall mortality.
- Referral to a psychiatrist may be an important step in ensuring an accurate mental health diagnosis and appropriate treatment plan development for PWH experiencing psychiatric symptoms.
- It is important to consider sociocultural factors when conceptualizing the risk and nature of mental illness in PWH.
- The COVID-19 pandemic and the generally increasing prevalence of mental health conditions present specific challenges that influence the mental health of PWH.

INTRODUCTION

From the earliest recognized AIDS-related deaths in 1981 to the commencement of combination antiretroviral therapy (ART) in the mid-1990s to the well-tolerated, effective regimens available today, HIV has remained an epidemic in constant evolution. It is now a treatable chronic condition, and issues of HIV-associated dementia and rapid death by opportunistic infections have generally been replaced by concerns related to "premature" aging and slow neurological decline, and questions of optimizing adherence to treatment. Issues that have not changed include the tremendous psychosocial burden to individuals and their families/loved ones, economic costs, as well as factors of stigmatization and marginalization of people with HIV. Many PWH were already stigmatized before acquiring HIV. The prevalence of HIV infection is much higher in gay/bi/transgender populations, people of color, people who use drugs, people in correctional settings, people experiencing homelessness, people with histories of physical and emotional trauma, and people with mental illness (Whetten et al., 2008). For some people, HIV infection then adds to the burden through associated psychological manifestations (e.g., demoralization, depression, mania, anxiety, insomnia, and neurocognitive deficits), disturbances in appearance with advanced HIV (e.g., wasting, lipodystrophy, and Kaposi's sarcoma) and overall impacts on chronic health and daily functioning (e.g., development of kidney disease, diabetes, sexual dysfunction, and chronic pain), and through tremendous losses (e.g., loved ones/people close to them, independence, health, employment, and sense of control). From the earliest days of the epidemic, it has been recognized that psychiatric disorders and HIV are closely related (Hoffman, 1984), with some estimates of comorbidity as high as 50%–70% (Blashill et al., 2011; Gaynes et al., 2008; Lang et al., 2023). The rates of depression and anxiety in PWH increased from 2008 to 2018, reflecting trends in the general population (Lang et al., 2023). PWH also faced unique challenges during the early years of the COVID-19 pandemic: a substantive portion of PWH experienced worsened mental health due to numerous factors, including social isolation from physical distancing, worry about acquiring COVID-19, fear of increased vulnerability to COVID-19 infection due to HIV, financial implications, and triggering themes of large-scale infectious disease (Parisi et al., 2022).

Psychiatric disorders in and of themselves are potentially lethal conditions, with increased rates of suicide and increased rates of illness and death from other conditions, including cancer, diabetes, and cardiovascular and cerebrovascular disease. They are associated with tremendous costs in terms of quality of life, lost productivity, and treatment. In combination with HIV-related conditions, these issues are magnified.

Addressing complex mental health issues is central to the prevention, diagnosis, and treatment of HIV-related disorders. Psychiatric illness is both a risk factor for disease and a barrier to adequate treatment. Substance use and the presence of a "triple diagnosis" (i.e., HIV, substance abuse, and mental illness) have been particularly problematic (see Chapter 34, "Substance Use and HIV"). People who are chronically mentally ill are overrepresented in this population, and providers serving individuals with a "triple diagnosis" often must navigate challenges in reaching and treating people due to homelessness/unstable housing, medical mistrust, and the often unstructured nature of individuals' day-to-day lives. Survivors of physical and emotional trauma are a key population increasingly recognized as both vulnerable to HIV infection and challenging to treat. They often engage in "high-risk" behaviors and may be slow to establish trusting relationships with healthcare providers. Psychiatric disorders in PWH may also be complicated and challenging to treat, as highlighted in one NA-ACCORD study, which demonstrated that 24% of PWH were found to have a comorbidity of two or more mental illnesses (Lang et al., 2023). In addition to these issues of primary mental illness, secondary mental health problems (e.g., those caused by the virus and/or its treatment) are also important to identify and address.

PSYCHIATRIC DISORDERS AND HIV INFECTION

The interaction between HIV and psychiatric disorders is complex. According to a recent population-based study, PWH have been found to have a significantly increased risk of experiencing mental health disorders overall compared to people without HIV (adjusted hazard ratio 1.63). Specifically, depression, anxiety, and serious mental illness among PWH were associated with adjusted hazard ratios of 1.94, 1.38, and 2.18, respectively (Gooden et al., 2022). In the NA-ACCORD cohort, the prevalence of major depressive disorder, anxiety, and bipolar disorder were 2.3, 4.9, and 2.4 times higher, respectively (Lang et al., 2023). For many individuals, the psychiatric condition is a preexisting one, predisposing to HIV infection through behavioral factors and risk environments (e.g., condomless sex, having multiple sex partners of unknown status, and sharing drug use equipment) (Meade et al., 2012; Prince et al., 2012; Rhodes, 2002). Individuals with preexisting psychiatric illness often engage in risky behaviors with little thought or fear of consequences. This relates to increased emotional immaturity and impulsivity (as in bipolar disorder, personality disorders, anxiety conditions, and post-traumatic stress disorder [PTSD]); poor contact with reality (as in schizophrenia and other psychotic conditions); denial and disinhibition (as in substance use disorders); cognitive dysfunction (as in major neurocognitive disorders and dementia); active thoughts of self-harm (as in depression); and victimization or impaired judgment (Kent and Blumenfield, 2011; Owe-Larsson et al., 2009). Barriers to treatment, such as distrust of authority (including fear of legal consequences), poor communication skills, limited access to services or resources (including financial and transportation resources), lack of motivation, and unstructured lifestyle, all result in poor overall healthcare delivery and delayed diagnosis of all health issues. Establishing a diagnosis of mental health issues is frequently challenging, and adherence to treatment is frequently impacted by these same factors.

Even for PWH without psychiatric disorders, the diagnosis of a serious and highly stigmatized chronic medical condition may carry significant emotional, psychological, and social impacts. Freud (1910) stated that emotional health involves the ability to integrate and balance aspects of love, work, and play. PWH are subject to harmful stigmas which may exacerbate stress and contribute to mental health disorders. In a study of 201 PWH in the United States, over one-third had experienced verbal stigma because of HIV in the prior 3 months (Reif et al., 2021). In her landmark work, Kubler-Ross (1969) discussed trauma associated with serious medical illness and the individual's response to it through repetitive processes of denial, anger, bargaining, and depression before (ideally) reaching a degree of acceptance. Healthcare teams may see the negative aspect of this emotional upheaval in its behavioral correlates: unrealistic anger at clinical staff, equally unrealistic expectations of outcomes, guilt, fear, increased substance use, demoralization/hopelessness/amotivation, poor adherence to treatment, suicidal thoughts/suicide, and helplessness/neediness. In response, providers can help by building a positive and supportive treatment alliance that facilitates communication, acknowledges the significant cost to the individual, tolerates some of the stress-related behaviors, and does not take these behaviors personally but also sets limits of appropriateness. Timely referral to a psychiatrist or a psychotherapist is essential when stress becomes distress, and behavior goes beyond acceptable limits of appropriateness, or when individuals become dangerous to themselves or others.

HIV enters the central nervous system (CNS) very early in the course of systemic infection, and the brain becomes an important site of damage in PWH (Ho et al., 1985). This causes some PWH to develop neurological and psychological symptoms through mechanisms that are posited to relate to functional disturbances in inflammatory processes. Activated circulating monocytes introduce the virus across the blood–brain barrier, and CNS macrophages, microglia, and astrocytes each become infected, releasing cytokines and chemokines that lead to neuronal cell damage (Williams et al., 2014). Evidence also suggests a disturbance in glutamate functioning within the CNS, with increased extracellular glutamate leading to excitotoxicity (Vazquez-Santiago et al., 2014). Accelerated aging from HIV infection and HIV-associated treatments, damage caused by opportunistic infections or comorbid medical conditions (e.g., hepatitis C virus), and concomitant substance use also play important roles (Gannon et al. 2011). AIDS-associated mania and a continuum of neurocognitive deficits from very subtle to frank and debilitating dementia are well-defined psychiatric syndromes directly related to the presence of the virus, but depression, insomnia, and anxiety are examples of some mental health symptoms that result from the infection itself. This aspect of

HIV disease progression seems to be less amenable to ART compared to the more peripheral manifestations (Heaton et al., 2010), although antiretroviral agents with higher levels of CNS penetration may promote improvement in some functions (Cysique et al., 2004). Unfortunately, agents capable of crossing the blood–brain barrier are also the medications most likely to have psychiatric symptomatology as a side effect of use.

Regardless of etiology, the presence of psychiatric symptoms and substance use is generally associated with poorer outcomes in PWH—lower levels of treatment adherence, slower virologic suppression, diminished quality of life, increased morbidity and mortality, and increased utilization of medical services (Arashiro et al., 2023; Blashill et al., 2011; Carrico et al., 2011; Leserman, 2008; Nel and Kagee, 2011; Pence et al., 2007). Adequate treatment of psychiatric illness, however, improves outcomes across all categories (Cook et al., 2006; Horberg et al., 2008; Mellins et al., 2009; Walkup et al., 2008). In fact, among a population of men who have sex with men in Taiwan, PWH who receive treatment with antidepressant medication were shown to have a similar rate of adherence to antiretroviral medication compared to PWH without depression (Yen et al. 2022). Of note, although most of the literature cited in this chapter relates to adult PWH, the diagnostic descriptions and treatments can, for the most part, be applied to adolescents and children (Benton, 2010; Rao et al., 2007).

TREATMENT OF PSYCHIATRIC DISORDERS IN PWH

Careful diagnosis is essential given the complex interaction between psychiatric illness, HIV infection, substance use, comorbid medical conditions, and side effects of medications. Psychiatric illness cannot be diagnosed if these other medical factors play the primary role in causing symptoms (i.e., delirium), and psychiatric medications will seldom be of benefit in those scenarios. The following brief descriptions are based on the criteria from DSM-5-TR (American Psychiatric Association, 2022). The context of HIV infection results in no appreciable changes from the usual clinical manifestations of psychiatric disorders, with the possible exception of AIDS mania. Equally, pharmacological and nonpharmacological approaches to the treatment of psychiatric illness in the context of HIV infection do not drastically differ from those used for people without HIV. Some PWH do appear to have some increased sensitivity to the side effects of antipsychotic drugs, even absent of antiretroviral treatment (Hriso et al., 1991; Kelly et al., 2002; Ramachandran et al., 1997). Because many psychopharmacologic agents are metabolized by the same elements of the cytochrome P450 isoenzyme system that metabolize protease inhibitors (PIs) and non-nucleoside/nucleotide reverse transcriptase inhibitors (NNRTIs), there were some fears several years ago that they could not be used concomitantly. In fact, however, there are surprisingly few clinically significant interactions, except as specifically noted in the following sections. As in all clinical situations, a "start low and go slow" philosophy is generally warranted, and the relative risks and benefits of treatment must be carefully weighed.

STRESS AND ADJUSTMENT DISORDERS

There are multiple stressors associated with living with a serious and debilitating illness. Some kinds of emotional and behavioral reactions to this stress are normal, short-lived, and do not require treatment beyond support, reassurance, education, and therapeutic optimism. Assistance with access to resources and support networks or with informing family or significant others of the diagnosis can be "curative." Such reactions typically occur immediately after diagnosis and at periods of acute change in illness status (opportunistic infections, deteriorating $CD4^+$ T-cell count/increasing HIV RNA levels, initiation of ART, and onset of other comorbid medical complications) or in social circumstances (loss and financial problems). Typically, individuals with these acute stress reactions are able to attribute the onset and nature of their symptoms to specific life events. They can also be distracted from their emotions and symptoms and are capable of feeling pleasure and interest in other things. *Adjustment reactions* (normal responses to stressful circumstances) are typically treated with supportive counseling and psychotherapy. It is only when stress reactions—anger, worry, guilt, sadness, and insomnia—are sustained for months, reach a point that they interfere with normal life functioning, or actually threaten survival (substance abuse, high-risk activities, and self-destructive thoughts/behaviors) that they require intervention. *Adjustment disorders* may also respond to support and psychotherapy, but they may necessitate psychiatric medications and/or hospital admission. The specific medication used depends on the symptoms being manifested. A complex of sadness, guilt, and insomnia frequently responds to the use of antidepressants, particularly the more sedating ones (sertraline and mirtazapine). Symptoms on the anxiety continuum may benefit from use of almost any medication with a sedating side effect. Low-dose trazodone or antihistamine (hydroxyzine or diphenhydramine are commonly used) can be helpful, although caution must be used because these agents tend to cause drying of mucous membranes, which can be very uncomfortable and/or exacerbate oral thrush, if present. Antihistamines should be used with caution in elderly PWH and those with dementia, as these medications can increase the risk of delirium. The use of benzodiazepines is rarely indicated (see later discussion). Because of the known relationship between stress and compromised immune function, early appropriate intervention is important (Leserman, 2008).

ANXIETY DISORDERS AND POST-TRAUMATIC STRESS DISORDER (PTSD)

This group of illnesses includes generalized anxiety disorder (i.e., persistent feelings of anxiety), phobias (i.e., irrational fear of a particular thing or behavior), panic disorder (i.e., spontaneous attacks of intense anxiety), and obsessive-compulsive disorder (i.e., intrusive anxiety-provoking thoughts that compel ritualized behaviors thought to alleviate that anxiety). PTSD (i.e., anxiety-related thoughts and behaviors connected to memories of past traumatic life experiences) was formerly included in this group, but it has been separated into its own category in DSM-5. All involve activation of the sympathetic nervous system (i.e., psychological and physiological fight–flight–freeze responses) in situationally inappropriate circumstances because there is no current emergency. Careful diagnosis requires that endocrine or other general medical disorders (especially thyroid-related conditions), substance use (including caffeine, steroids, and psychostimulants), agitated depression, dementia, and delirium be eliminated as primary etiological factors. PWH have rates of anxiety disorders greater than those of the general population (Gaynes et al., 2008; Klinkenberg et al., 2004; Martinez et al., 2002), as well as an increased incidence of past traumatic experiences (Pence, 2009). Treatment ideally consists of a combination of psychotherapy (e.g., supportive, interpersonal, mindfulness, cognitive-behavioral, biofeedback, exposure and response prevention, and flooding) and psychopharmacotherapy with antidepressants and/or antianxiety agents. Because the therapeutic benefit with antidepressants is delayed in onset, it may be useful to supplement early treatment with low-dose benzodiazepine-lorazepam or other short-acting agent for panic disorder or phobias (used as needed at the onset of panic attacks or exposure to phobic object, but no more than 3 or 4 times a day) and clonazepam or other long-acting medication for generalized anxiety. Benzodiazepines are rarely the regimen of choice for more than the first 2–4 weeks, however, and should be discontinued at the earliest practical opportunity. Some alternative treatments have also been shown to be effective, including relaxation/meditation, breath training, acupuncture, and guided imagery. All of the antidepressants except bupropion have efficacy in anxiety disorders, and selection of a specific medication should be based on safety (the serotonin and serotonin/norepinephrine reuptake inhibitors [SNRIs] are overall much safer than tricyclics or monoamine oxidase inhibitors), side effect profile (e.g., relative sedation vs. excitation; potential for gastric symptoms; appetite stimulation vs. suppression; anticholinergic effects; concerns for liver function; assistance with pain control), and past response to medications in the individual or family member. The selective serotonin reuptake inhibitors (SSRIs) can increase dream and flashback symptoms in individuals with past traumatic experiences, although small doses of prazosin can mitigate this effect. As noted previously, antianxiety agents include benzodiazepines, antihistamines, buspirone, and small doses of antidepressants (e.g., trazodone) or atypical antipsychotics (e.g., quetiapine—an off-label use). All except buspirone work by sedating the individual, and they can be taken at the onset of anxiety symptoms. Buspirone, similar to antidepressants, must be taken on a regular basis to be effective. The benzodiazepines also disinhibit behaviors, cause various degrees of cognitive impairment including amnesia and motor slowing/incoordination (a serious issue in a population already at risk for neurocognitive impairment), increase the risk of falls, and can trigger relapse or increased substance use in individuals with substance use disorders/problematic substance use. They are meant for temporary use only and can usually be discontinued when the antidepressants have become effective (2–4 weeks). A consensus survey of psychiatrists treating PWH revealed clonazepam to be the most frequently used benzodiazepine, followed by lorazepam (Freudenreich et al., 2010). Alprazolam, midazolam, and triazolam should be avoided because of their high potential for addiction and adverse interactions with antiretrovirals (ARVs). As stated previously, the guiding principle for the concomitant use of any psychopharmacologic agent with an ARV is "start low and go slow."

AFFECTIVE DISORDERS

Disorders of mood, particularly depression, are the most common psychiatric manifestations of HIV disease, with rates much higher in PWH than in the general population (Berger-Greenstein et al., 2007; Gaynes et al., 2011; Treisman and Angelinno, 2007) and increasing frequency with advancing disease (Atkinson et al., 2008). Depression hinders the treatment of PWH, thus increasing the risk of disease progression and transmission (Benton, 2008; Villes et al., 2007), and it may have direct effects on immune responses (Alciati et al., 2007). PWH are at greater risk to die by suicide compared to the general population, with about 21% reporting suicidal ideation, and 5% attempting suicide in the past year. Completed suicide is estimated to occur in about 1%–2% of PWH. Psychiatric disorders and substance use disorders both increase the risk for suicide in PWH (Brown et al., 2021). Adequate treatment, however, reverses all these trends for both depression (Horberg et al., 2008; Mellins et al., 2009; Walkup et al., 2008) and bipolar disorder (Walkup et al., 2011).

Major depression consists of a constellation of symptoms related to persistent low mood (including crying spells, guilt, low self-esteem, negative ruminations, social isolation, and loss of pleasure and interest), mental slowing (including poor attention, concentration, memory, and energy; loss of libido; and motor retardation), and changes in behavior (e.g., increased or decreased sleep or appetite). Those with severe illness may also have psychotic symptoms (i.e., hallucinations and delusions), usually with depressive content. Careful diagnosis is essential because many of these symptoms might also be caused by serious medical illness, major neurocognitive impairment (e.g., dementia and delirium), side effects of medications, substance abuse, or grief and loss. Patients who have not received regular health care or lab monitoring should receive a physical exam and basic workup to evaluate for organic causes of depression, including a complete blood count, metabolic panel, calcium, vitamin D, and thyroid stimulating hormone. More rare diagnoses suggested by history or physical exam should prompt a more specialized workup. Unlike adjustment disorders, individuals with major depression generally cannot cite a precipitating event, nor can they be distracted from their negative emotions. It is the relentless nature of the symptoms that results in the sense of hopelessness and despair, with a progressive narrowing of emotional focus until it may seem that death (i.e., suicide) is the "only way out." Treatment ideally consists of combined psychotherapy and psychopharmacology with antidepressant medications, sometimes utilizing augmenting agents (i.e., a second antidepressant from another class, lithium, testosterone, thyroid medications, psychostimulants, and mood stabilizers). Low doses of antipsychotics are indicated on a temporary basis if psychotic features are present. Ketamine in very low doses is being used in some centers, but it must be used with extreme caution in PWH on ART. Replicated evidence has shown that psychotherapeutic interventions (e.g., cognitive-behavioral therapy, stress management interventions, and supportive therapy) have moderate antidepressant effects on PWH (van Luenen et al., 2018). Alternative treatments including exercise, meditation/relaxation, acupuncture, and herbal medications have also been found to be helpful. Individuals taking St. John's wort (a popular herbal antidepressant) should be cautioned because it has significant adverse clinical interactions with multiple ARVs, anticancer drugs, anti-inflammatory agents, antibiotics, psychopharmacologic agents, cardiovascular drugs, diabetes drugs, oral contraceptives, proton pump inhibitors, statins, and asthma medications (Nicolussi et al., 2019). All of the commonly used antidepressants show efficacy in PWH, and the choice of a particular medication should be based on safety (Watkins et al., 2011), side effect profile, and past response to medications in the individual or their family member. A consensus study revealed that the SSRIs are the most common first-line drugs, with citalopram the number one choice (Freudenreich et al., 2010), although this may be changing with newer U.S. Food and Drug Administration warnings about QT prolongation associated with higher doses of this medication. The SSRIs do have an anticoagulant effect, and used long term, they can result in significant decreases in bone density. They can also cause bruxism and extrapyramidal side effects as well as sexual dysfunction. Switching drugs within a pharmacologic class is of benefit if individuals find specific side effects intolerable.

If a medication in any given class of antidepressants fails to show therapeutic benefit (after an 8- to 12-week trial of adequate doses), a switch to another class of drugs is advised because agents within any given class have similar efficacy (Warden and Rush, 2007). A switch to an SNRI (e.g., venlafaxine and duloxetine) and then to bupropion is a useful algorithm when there is treatment failure (Freudenreich et al., 2010). Particular caution is suggested in using bupropion (either as an antidepressant or in smoking cessation) in combination with older PIs (especially saquinavir or indinavir) or NNRTIs (especially efavirenz) because metabolism of bupropion can be inhibited, thus increasing the risk of seizures. Lopinavir/ritonavir, on the other hand, increases metabolism of bupropion, so bupropion doses must be increased when used with this antiretroviral combination (Hogeland et al., 2007). Mirtazapine can be particularly useful for people experiencing chronic pain, weight loss, nausea, and vomiting (especially from chemotherapy regimens). Monoamine oxidase inhibitors (MAOIs) are not generally used in PWH, and they are contraindicated for concomitant use with other antidepressants and most antipsychotics. Of note, the antibiotic linezolid is also an MAOI. All antidepressant regimens take several weeks to have therapeutic benefits, and mood symptoms may not all resolve simultaneously. For this reason, particular caution and close observation are warranted in the early weeks of treatment: if energy, motivation, and a sense of agency return before suicidal thoughts and impulses disappear, a person who has had suicidal thoughts but insufficient energy to act on them may suddenly find the energy to act. The use of antidepressants in children and younger adolescents is particularly fraught with the danger of suicide, and most antidepressant medications now carry a black box warning for this population. Inpatient psychiatric treatment is necessary if there are questions of safety, and in general, it is best to err on the side of caution in this situation. Duration of treatment is a common and important question. In the general population, an individual with a single episode of depression is generally treated for 4–6 months, whereas individuals with more than two episodes receive protracted therapy with antidepressants. Because of concurrent medical illnesses, stress, and the propensity for HIV virus to cause/exacerbate affective symptoms, long-term use of antidepressants is frequently necessary.

Bipolar disorder is defined by intermittent episodes of low (i.e., depressive) and high (i.e., hypomanic or manic) moods, each lasting days, weeks, or months and in a continuum of severity from mild to disabling. These mood swings are not a reaction to life events. The lows are identical to the depressive episodes described previously. The high episodes consist of persistent elevated mood tone (e.g., euphoric or irritable), increased energy (e.g., racing thoughts that bounce from topic to topic, little need for sleep, rapid speech, and increased libido), and an inflated sense of self-worth, and they often lead to engaging in risky behaviors. In mania, there can be frank psychosis, with delusions (usually grandiose), disorganized thinking, and hallucinations leading to severe impairment in functioning and judgment. Bipolar disorder occurs at higher rates among PWH than in the general population (DeSousa Gurgel et al., 2013). HIV prevalence is approximately 1% among patients with bipolar disorder, with bipolar disorder preceding the diagnosis of HIV in 65% of patients. The rates of adherence to ARV medication as well as psychopharmacologic medication are lower among PWH with bipolar disorder (Yalin et al., 2021).

Psychopharmacologic treatment in bipolar disorder consists of mood stabilizer medications (e.g., lithium, valproic acid, carbamazepine, lamotrigine, and "second-generation" antipsychotic medications), with antidepressants and antipsychotics added if these symptoms are prominent. Some clinicians believe that long-acting benzodiazepines can be helpful in the first days of treatment for active mania, but these agents can further disinhibit and should be used only on a short-term basis. All of these medications are effective and reasonably safe in PWH. Lithium has a very narrow window of safety, and it is eliminated by the kidney. Particular caution is therefore necessary in PWH with kidney dysfunction, diarrhea, electrolyte disturbances, or cognitive impairment, but there are no specific interactions with ARVs. Lithium can cause or exacerbate thyroid dysfunction, tremor, acne, and psoriasis. Valproic acid appears to have few clinically significant drug interactions with ARVs. However, it is metabolized by the liver, and it can increase liver enzymes and cause hyperammonemia. In addition, there is a risk of severe hepatitis, weight gain, thrombocytopenia, nystagmus, and tremor. The use of carbamazepine is more complicated: it is metabolized by the cytochrome P450 system, and it induces its own metabolism. There have been reports of clinically significant carbamazepine toxicity when used in combination with ritonavir and other potent CYP3A4 inhibitors and also of virologic failure caused by enzyme induction (Liedtke et al., 2004). In addition, carbamazepine causes a significant risk for bone marrow suppression. Lamotrigine is effective, particularly for depressive symptoms, and appears to be safe when used in combination with ART. Initiation and discontinuation of this agent must be managed very carefully because of the risk of life-threatening Stevens–Johnson syndrome. Importantly, providers should be aware that use of antidepressants without a mood stabilizer in a bipolar person can trigger a manic episode.

AIDS mania is a specific manifestation of late-stage HIV infection, rarely seen in the current combination ART era. The mood is more likely to be irritable, sullen, and withdrawn than euphoric and hyper-talkative, and there is frequently no prior personal or family history of psychiatric illness. Otherwise, symptoms are typical of mania. Episodes, however, tend to be protracted, frequently with a prodrome of progressive cognitive decline. Symptoms do not typically respond to the usual psychopharmacological approaches, nor is there spontaneous remission if the condition is left untreated. The treatment of choice is initiation of aggressive ART.

PSYCHOTIC DISORDERS

Psychotic disorders are defined by loss of contact with reality (i.e., hallucinations and delusions), as well as by varying degrees of disorganized thinking and behavior. Insight and judgment are often compromised, and it is frequently difficult to communicate clearly with individuals because they can seem lost in their own, sometimes very bizarre, world. Symptoms can be present on a temporary/episodic basis (e.g., brief psychotic episodes and schizophreniform disorder) or maybe more chronic (as in schizophrenia). Although disruption of thinking and behavior are most typical, any psychotic illnesses may involve some affective symptoms, even if only because the person recognizes that they are somehow different from others. When symptoms of an emotional nature (depression or excitation) are a prominent and invariant part of the psychosis, schizoaffective disorder must be considered. The differential diagnosis includes affective disorder with psychotic features, medical illness (psychosis secondary to a medical condition such as HIV), side effects of medications, delirium/dementia, and substance use. The recommended initial medical workup for new-onset psychosis includes a urine drug screen (although many of the newer synthetic substances do not appear on standard screening assays), serology, endocrine screen, liver function tests, and computed tomography and/or magnetic resonance imaging of the brain. Visual hallucinations are rare in primary psychiatric illness, and they should also prompt a more complete medical evaluation. People with serious chronic mental illness are at increased risk of exposure to HIV owing to factors such as homelessness, poor insight/judgment, lack of knowledge, victimization, and increased rates of substance use and other high-risk behaviors (Prince et al., 2012). Without adequate psychiatric care, psychosis is a serious barrier to medical treatment because of poor adherence, difficulties communicating with providers, and unstable lifestyle (Carrico et al., 2011). Treatment consists of control of symptoms with medications along with psychosocial support. All the antipsychotic medications work in PWH. As previously noted, some PWH, even without ARV treatment, seem to be somewhat more sensitive to the dopamine-mediated extrapyramidal side effects of these drugs. These side effects are most common with high-potency first-generation antipsychotics (i.e., haloperidol and fluphenazine). Both the first-generation and newer antipsychotics have significant risks for metabolic, cardiac (prolonged QT intervals), and endocrine side effects, and all are metabolized by the liver. They do not seem to have clinically significant interactions with ARV treatments, with the possible exception of lurasidone, but QT intervals should be closely monitored because some ARVs also have this side effect. In the consensus survey, quetiapine was the most used agent for psychosis, perhaps because it is also useful in mood stabilization and sedation (Freudenreich et al., 2010). A recent meta-analysis also revealed that quetiapine is the safest of the antipsychotic drugs to use for psychosis and behavioral modification in individuals with dementia (Kales et al., 2012). Clozapine and low-potency first-generation medications (e.g., chlorpromazine and thioridazine) are seldom used (Freudenreich et al., 2010), although certainly not contraindicated. The use of depo injections tends to result in fewer side effects than seen with daily oral formulations and can be particularly useful in individuals for whom adherence with antipsychotic medication is problematic. It is safest, however, to initiate treatment with oral medication and then switch to long-acting forms later once tolerability and response have been established.

PERSONALITY DISORDERS AND PWH

Personality can be thought of as enduring patterns of behavior, and this is partly what we refer to when we say we "know" a person—the person has somewhat predictable responses to given circumstances, a familiar emotional tone, consistent belief systems, and a well-formed sense of identity and agency. When these patterns are stable and healthy, one's responses to adversity (coping techniques) help to mitigate stress, and one can modulate emotional responses to fit the circumstances, thus maintaining a stable sense of self and others and control over one's world. In personality disorders, an individual is stuck in repetitive patterns that do not work, coping techniques that escalate stressful situations, relationship paradigms that result in little perceived support and an increasing sense of frustration by and with others, spiraling loss of emotional control, and, ultimately, the fearful recognition that one is out of control of both internal and external worlds. Borderline and antisocial personality disorders are common in populations with HIV because these individuals tend to engage in high-risk behaviors. These character pathologies also complicate treatment adherence (Gilchrist et al., 2011; Hansen et al., 2009). People with personality disorders tend to be easily frustrated, expect immediate gratification, want sure-fire/magical interventions, and demand "special" treatment from everybody. They also challenge authority and cannot structure their lives adequately and consistently.

As challenging as it can be to work with these individuals, it is important to remember that their behavior is not intentional—it is their best effort to adjust to and control their chaotic world (Groves et al., 1978). Frequently, the emotions they engender in others are only reflections of the emotional turmoil within themselves. These are individuals for whom referral to psychotherapy and the presence of a strong, consistent treatment team with a clearly delineated treatment contract are essential to preserve coherent participation in medical care. Because a person's psychological symptoms may be particularly reactive to events in the environment, switching rapidly and wildly, caution should be used in initiating medications. Although consistent use of an SSRI or a mood stabilizer may be useful, chasing symptoms with medications is contraindicated. It is generally much more useful to help individuals understand that problems may be related to their own patterns of response and behavioral choices than indicating that medication is going to provide internal peace or a sense of purpose, meaning, security, and attachment.

SUBSTANCE USE DISORDERS

For a full discussion of this topic, see Chapter 34, "Substance Use and HIV." Concurrent substance use complicates the diagnosis and treatment of all other psychiatric conditions, as well as HIV-related illnesses. These complications, as well as problems with adherence to treatment and overall morbidity and mortality, are additive in nature. It is essential that HIV care providers screen for substance use and address it consistently and aggressively.

MAJOR NEUROCOGNITIVE DISORDERS (DELIRIUM AND DEMENTIA)

HIV infection is associated with a number of CNS complications that may be temporary (i.e., delirium) or permanent (i.e., the continuum of neurocognitive deficits from asymptomatic to frank dementia). Dementia is a common manifestation of advanced HIV illness, and it is discussed in Chapter 28, "Neurologic Complications of HIV Infection." Delirium is a potentially life-threatening medical condition, generally of sudden and rapid onset and pursuing a waxing and waning course. Delirium is estimated to occur in 40%–65% of hospitalized or critically ill PWH (Gallago et al., 2011) and there is a higher risk of delirium in PWH compared to people without HIV (Akgün et al., 2023). It can manifest with any psychiatric symptom (e.g., anxiety, depression, mania, and psychosis) but most frequently includes disturbances in orientation, awareness/alertness, reality testing (e.g., hallucinations, including visual—which are very unusual in primary psychiatric conditions), communication (e.g., mumbled, incoherent speech), and motor behavior (e.g., lethargy, agitation, and picking at skin/clothing/intravenous lines). Several screening tools are used to diagnose delirium, of which the Cognitive Assessment Measurement Scale (CAMS and CAMS-ICU) is probably the most thoroughly researched.

Definitive treatment involves correction of the underlying medical condition (e.g., infection, electrolyte disturbance, medication side effects, endocrine imbalance, and intoxication). *Temporary* use of low-dose antipsychotic medications can be helpful, but they should be tapered and discontinued as the delirium resolves. Providers should avoid using any anticholinergic agents (particularly diphenhydramine and other antihistamines) and antipsychotics with prevalent anticholinergic side effects (chlorpromazine and thioridazine). Olanzapine, a sedating antipsychotic, may help with agitation but has been reported to cause, exacerbate, and/or prolong delirium in some cases. Use of benzodiazepines is also generally counterproductive, with the obvious exception of delirium caused by alcohol or benzodiazepine withdrawal. Measures that improve the individual's connection with reality can be very helpful. These include constant soft lighting (shadows are often misperceived), quiet and soothing background noise, a visible clock and/or calendar in the room, a written list of names of nursing staff and others, and repeated self-introduction of caregivers and visitors.

SEXUAL DYSFUNCTION

Sexual dysfunctions are very common in PWH. Disorders of desire (e.g., hypoactive sexual desire disorder) may be almost universal in PWH, and erectile dysfunction is very common in men with AIDS (De Vincentis et al., 2021; Shindel et al., 2011). Although certainly related to stress, depression, and uncertainties about transmitting HIV to sexual partners, it may also be the case that the virus itself, the myriad associated comorbidities (including hypogonadism, diabetes, and peripheral neuropathy), and the multiple medications used to treat all these conditions play a role (Collazos, 2007; Huntingdon et al., 2019; Moreno-Perez et al., 2010; Scanavino, 2011). The treatment of sexual dysfunction, therefore, is complex. To the degree that these disorders are due to secondary issues, efforts should be made to change those conditions. Depression, stress, and comorbid conditions can be treated, and sometimes medications can be changed or doses modified to minimize sexual side effects. Sexual counseling and therapy help teach individuals that sexual behavior and love are not always about intercourse. Medications for erectile dysfunction (e.g., sildenafil, vardenafil, and tadalafil) can be used, but doses must be reduced when given with certain ARV agents because metabolism is delayed. This increases the probability of adverse side effects from erectile dysfunction drugs, including visual changes, priapism, hypotension, and acute cardiac events. As with all medications, risks and benefits must be carefully weighed in concert with the patient.

SLEEP DISTURBANCE

Insomnia is defined as difficulty initiating and/or maintaining sleep or overall nonrestful sleep. It tends to impair daytime function, and it is even more common in PWH than in the general population. This condition has been linked to poor quality of life and nonadherence to treatment (Saberi et al., 2011). Stress and depression play a role in its etiology, and some ARVs disrupt sleep continuity (e.g., efavirenz is consistently associated with sleep disturbances, including delayed sleep initiation, impaired sleep maintenance, and vivid nightmares). However, insomnia may also be a primary symptom of viral presence, with changes in sleep architecture and decreased sleep efficiency noted even prior to the onset of any HIV/AIDS-associated symptoms (Norman et al., 1992). Prior to deciding on a management plan for insomnia, a careful sleep history should be taken, with attention paid to the presence of anxiety or ruminations before bedtime, sleep-related movement disorders or restless legs, nighttime urinary frequency, snoring or apneic episodes, sleepwalking or acting out dreams, evidence of poor sleep hygiene, or excessive fear related to not being able to fall asleep. Physical examination requires evaluation for increased neck circumference or obese body habitus, which can increase the likelihood of obstructive sleep apnea. Patients with risk factors for a primary sleep disorder, such as obstructive sleep apnea, should be considered for a sleep study.

Pharmacological treatment of insomnia includes the use of benzodiazepines, nonbenzodiazepine hypnotics, antihistamines, antidepressants, and antipsychotics. Of the benzodiazepines, clonazepam, lorazepam, oxazepam, and temazepam are relatively safe, although, as previously noted, their use in people with current or past substance use disorders is problematic. Use of alprazolam, flurazepam, quazepam, and triazolam is contraindicated with some ARVs (i.e., protease inhibitors, cobicistat) and ketoconazole and also in people with kidney or liver disease. Sustained use of benzodiazepine medications is rarely, if ever, indicated. All of the nonbenzodiazepine hypnotics (eszopiclone, zaleplon, and zolpidem) are relatively safe in PWH, although dosages of zolpidem should be reduced if used with PIs, even in boosting dosages. Dosages of all nonbenzodiazepine hypnotics should also be reduced in those with liver disease. Antihistamines (especially diphenhydramine and hydroxyzine) are typically effective, and they are safe in PWH. However, it should be remembered that some individuals have paradoxical excitatory responses to these medications. Sleep induction is an off-label use for any antidepressant or antipsychotic. Nonetheless, low-dose tricyclics (especially doxepin and amitriptyline) and mirtazapine can be very useful. Tricyclics can also help relieve neuropathic pain, which may improve sleep quality. In higher doses, all are associated with weight gain, which can be beneficial in some cases. Trazodone is frequently used to induce and maintain sleep in the general population, but its use in PWH on certain ART regimens is problematic because the final metabolism of trazodone is slowed, and untoward side effects (e.g., sleep disruption, vivid dreams, increased sedation, anxiety, and hypotension) occur. Of the antipsychotics, quetiapine and olanzapine are frequently used off-label. As previously noted, some PWH are much more sensitive to the extrapyramidal side effects of these medications. They also cause endocrine disturbances (prolactinemia) and metabolic side effects that may be cumulative with those attributed to some ARVs, such as lipodystrophy, hyperlipidemia, and insulin resistance (Omonuwa et al., 2009). Brief behavioral treatment for insomnia, a psychological modality, has also been shown to improve sleep outcomes in PWH and insomnia (Buchanan et al., 2018).

PSYCHIATRIC EFFECTS OF ANTIRETROVIRAL THERAPY

Several ARV agents have prominent psychiatric side effects that have been discussed previously. The most prominent of these psychiatric symptoms are vivid dreams and nightmares (Abers et al., 2014). Unfortunately, these issues seem to be more common, problematic, and sustained in individuals who are already vulnerable or experiencing psychiatric symptoms—that is, those with chronic mental illness. Vivid dreams and nightmares can be especially troubling for individuals with PTSD or past traumatic experiences. Although psychiatric diagnoses should not be a contraindication for the use of these agents when indicated, special caution and close follow-up are warranted. As with PTSD, low-dose prazosin can sometimes ameliorate sleep disturbances.

USE OF PSYCHIATRIC CONSULTATION

Mental health concerns are very common among PWH (Bing et al., 2001; Robertson et al., 2014). In an ideal world, mental health professionals would be integrated into every HIV care setting, and individuals suspected of having significant illness or distress could be seen rapidly and frequently after referral. In reality, this is rarely the case, and even when psychiatrists and other mental health providers are on-site, visits are commonly delayed because of the high numbers of people needing care. Referrals are most warranted and useful when key foundational elements are in place. First and foremost, the individual must be aware of and agree to mental health evaluation. Exceptions to this relate to individuals who are incapable of understanding the need for assessment and treatment, imminently dangerous to self or others, or systematically destroying themselves and their treatment/treatment team by their behavior. Beyond that, the first part of a referral decision rests on the primary problem and referring to the correct person. Certain individuals will benefit most from referrals to support groups of like-minded people with similar problems and experiences, and many people prefer this form of treatment. Although there are certainly exceptions, most psychiatrists are not the primary resource for either substance use counseling or individual/marital/group psychotherapy. The first task is handled, in general, by specific substance use counselors and by self-help groups (e.g., Alcoholics Anonymous, Narcotics Anonymous). Psychotherapy is also more frequently done by behavioral specialists other than psychiatrists (e.g., psychologists, social workers, and licensed counselors). Pain management and medical management of acute intoxication/withdrawal or "detox" and maintenance therapy to prevent return to use are also frequently handled by other caregivers. In most settings, it is possible to refer directly to these providers, who can screen for cases requiring specific psychiatric intervention. Psychologists are trained explicitly in diagnostic processes (including psychological and neuropsychological testing and screening) and in psychotherapeutic interventions. Psychiatrists, although trained in behavioral interventions and therapy techniques, are medical doctors, and they are the first-line resource for the evaluation of individuals with complex psychiatric/medical issues, individuals who will probably require psychotropic medications, and people who have not responded to conventional psychotropic medications. Although psychiatrists can be helpful in diagnosing delirium and can assist in the behavioral management of symptoms, the presence of major neurocognitive disorders (including acute intoxication) generally makes it very challenging to ascertain if there is a primary underlying psychiatric illness accompanying the current medical process. One final caveat that may be helpful is: "When in doubt, consult." Most psychiatrists would rather be included when they are not needed than absent when they could help.

CULTURAL CONSIDERATIONS IN TREATING COMORBID HIV AND PSYCHIATRIC DISORDERS

The stigma associated with HIV is very well known, as is the stigma associated with psychiatric illness, but when the two are combined, the consequences can be multiplicative and mutually reinforcing. Often it is fear of marginalization and/or discrimination that causes individuals to avoid HIV and mental health screenings and to be poorly adherent to treatment once diagnoses are established. These obstacles are further magnified when the individuals impacted by comorbid HIV and psychiatric illness belong to historically marginalized demographic groups. Whether it is because of their gender, ethnicity, or sexual orientation, individuals may encounter challenges in both navigating the healthcare system and receiving care that is uniquely suited to their needs. For instance, African and Caribbean Black women have been found to experience higher rates of HIV-related stigma and are more likely to report being marginalized or discriminated against based on racist and sexist stereotypes (Loutfy et al., 2012). This finding is of particular concern and importance in the United States, as African American women continue to be disproportionately represented among new HIV cases (CDC, 2024). Despite these statistics and the best efforts of public health clinicians, many HIV/mental health interventions lack sufficient cultural sensitivity and are, therefore, less likely to be effective across different demographic groups. A 2016 cohort study of 31,000 PWH found that while 47% of respondents had an indication for antidepressant treatment, people who identified as Black non-Hispanic, Hispanic, and other non-white ethnicities were significantly less likely to initiate antidepressant treatment than their white non-Hispanic peers (Bengtson et al., 2016). These findings suggest a strong cultural component to acceptance of mental health treatment, one that may be mediated by historical mistrust of the healthcare system and/or a reliance on alternative methods of emotional support. In 2016, respondents in a qualitative study of primary care providers who treat African American PWH reported that their patients were more likely to seek emotional support from family or their spiritual community rather than seeking formal mental health treatment (Le et al., 2016). Accordingly, interventions aimed at identifying and preventing adverse HIV and mental health outcomes in highly impacted populations should be tailored to address pervasive cultural stigmas and norms. Neither HIV treatment nor mental health treatment is a "one-size-fits-all" endeavor, and clinicians should continue to enlist the input of PWH, families, and spiritual and community leaders to develop programs that suit the diversity and cultural sensitivities of the people they seek to help and heal.

CONCLUSION

From the earliest days of the AIDS epidemic, it has been apparent that many PWH have comorbid psychiatric conditions. Individuals with psychiatric illnesses (including depression, bipolar disorders, anxiety disorders, PTSD, schizophrenia, dementia, and substance use disorders) tend to engage in behaviors that place them at increased risk for exposure to HIV. Conversely, HIV infection results in numerous psychosocial stressors that trigger or exacerbate the expression of psychological symptoms in vulnerable individuals. The virus itself precipitates changes in the CNS that may cause psychiatric manifestations. Finally, use of certain ARV agents can result in psychiatric/behavioral symptoms. In turn, the presence of these psychiatric symptoms introduces additional complexities with diagnosis and treatment of HIV-related illnesses. All PWH should be screened for the presence of psychiatric illness. Many PWH respond well to traditional psychopharmacological and psychotherapeutic approaches to mental distress and illness, and, with adequate psychiatric treatment, have good adherence and favorable response to HIV treatment.

REFERENCES

Abers MS, Shandera WX, Kass JS. Neurological and psychiatric adverse effects of antiretroviral drugs. *CNS Drugs*. 2014;28(2):131–145.

Akgün KM, Krishnan S, Tate J, et al. Delirium among people aging with and without HIV: Role of alcohol and Neurocognitively active medications. *J Am Geriatr Soc*. 2023;71(6):1861–1872. doi:10.1111/jgs.18265

Alciati A, Gallo L, Monforte AD, et al. Major depression-related immunological changes and combination antiretroviral therapy in HIV-seropositive patients. *Hum Psychopharmacol*. 2007;22(1):33–40.

American Psychiatric Association. *Diagnostic and Statistical Manual of Mental Disorders*. 5th ed. Arlington, VA: American Psychiatric Publishing; 2022.

Arashiro P, Maciel CG, Freitas FPR, et al. Adherence to antiretroviral therapy in people living with HIV with moderate or severe mental disorder. *Sci Rep*. 2023 Mar 2;13(1):3569. doi:10.1038/s41598-023-30451-z

Atkinson JH, Heaeton RK, Patterson TL, et al. Two-year prospective study of major depressive disorder in HIV-positive men. *J Affect Disord*. 2008;108:225–233.
Bengtson AM, Pence BW, Crane HM, et al. Disparities in depressive symptoms and antidepressant treatment by gender and race/ethnicity among people living with HIV in the United States. *PloS One*. 2016;11(8):e0160738.
Benton TD. Depression and HIV/AIDS. *Curr Psychiatry Rep*. 2008;10(3):280–285.
Benton TD. Psychiatric considerations in children and adolescents with HIV/AIDS. *Child Adolesc Psychiatr Clin North Am*. 2010;19(2):387–400.
Berger-Greenstein JA, Cuevas CA, Brady SM, et al. Major depression in patients with HIV/AIDS and substance abuse. *AIDS Patient Care STDs*. 2007;21:942–949.
Bing EG, Burnam MA, Longshore D, et al. Psychiatric disorders and drug use among human immunodeficiency virus-infected adults in the United States. *Arch Gen Psychiatry*. 2001;58:721–728.
Blashill AJ, Perry N, Safren SA. Mental health: a focus on stress, coping, and mental illness as it relates to treatment retention, adherence, and other health outcomes. *Curr HIV/AIDS Rep*. 2011;8(4):215–222.
Brown LA, Majeed I, Mu W, et al. Suicide risk among persons living with HIV. *AIDS Care*. 2021; 33(5):616–622.
Buchanan DT, McCurry SM, Eilers K, et al. Brief behavioral treatment for insomnia in persons living with HIV, *Behav Sleep Med*. 2018;16(3):244–258. http://doi:10.1080/15402002.2016.1188392
Carrico AW, Bangsberg DR, Weisner SD, et al. Psychiatric correlates of HAART utilization and viral load among HIV-positive impoverished persons. *AIDS*. 2011; 25(8):1113–1118.
Centers for Disease Control (CDC). HV Surveillance Supplemental Report: Estimated HIV incidence and prevalence in the United States, 2018–2022. http://stacks.cdc.gov/view/cdc/156513. Published May 21, 2024. Accessed September 3, 2024.
Collazos J. Sexual dysfunction in the highly active antiretroviral therapy era. *AIDS Rev*. 2007;9:237–245.
Cook JA, Burke-Miller J, Anastos K, et al. Effects of treated and untreated depressive symptoms on highly active antiretroviral therapy use in a US multi-site cohort of HIV-positive women. *AIDS Care*. 2006;18(2):3–100.
Cysique LA, Maruff P, Brew BJ. Prevalence and pattern of neuropsychological impairment in human immunodeficiency virus-infected/ acquired immunodeficiency syndrome (HIV/AIDS) patients across pre- and post-highly active antiretroviral therapy eras: a combined study of two cohorts. *J Neurovirol*. 2004;10(6):350–357.
De Sousa Gurgel W, da Silva Carneiro AH, Barreto Reboucas D, et al. Affective disorders study group (GETA): prevalence of bipolar disorder in a HIV-infected outpatient population. *AIDS Care*. 2013;25(12):1499–1503.
De Vincentis S, Tartaro G, Rochira V, Santi D. HIV and sexual dysfunction in men. *J Clin Med*. 2021;10(5):1088. doi:10.3390/ jcm10051088
Freud S. Five lectures on psycho-analysis. *Am J Psychol*. 1910;1–21.
Freudenreich O, Goforth HW, Cozza KL, et al. Psychiatric treatment of persons with HIV/AIDS: an HIV psychiatry consensus survey of current practices. *Psychosomatics*. 2010;51:480–488.
Gannon P, Khan MZ, Kolson DL. Current understanding of HIV-associated neurocognitive disorders pathogenesis. *Curr Opin Neurol*. 2011;24(3):275–283.
Gaynes BN, Farley JF, Dusetzina SB, et al. Does the presence of accompanying symptom clusters differentiate the comparative effectiveness of second-line medication strategies for treating depression? *Depress Anxiety*. 2011;28(11):989–998.
Gaynes BN, Pence BW, Eron JJ Jr, et al. Prevalence and comorbidity of psychiatric diagnoses based on reference standard in an HIV\+ population. *Psychosom Med*. 2008;70:505–511.
Gilchrist G, Blazquez A, Torrens M. Psychiatric, behavioral and social risk factors for HIV infection among female drug users. *AIDS Behav*. 2011;15(8):1834–1843.
Gooden TE, Gardner M, Wang J, et al. The risk of mental illness in people living with HIV in the UK: a propensity score-matched cohort study. *Lancet HIV*. 2022;9(3):172–181.
Groves, JE. Taking care of the hateful patient. *N Engl J Med*. 1978;298:883–887.
Hansen N, Vaughan E, Cavanaugh C, et al. Health-related quality of life in bereaved HIV-positive adults: relationships between HIV symptoms, grief, social support, and axis II indication. *Health Psychol*. 2009;28:249–257.
Heaton RK, Clifford DB, Franklin DR, et al. HIV-associated neurocognitive disorders persist in the era of potent antiretroviral therapy: CHARTER study. *Neurology*. 2010;75(23):2087–2096.
Ho D, Tota TR, Schooley RT, et al. Isolation of HTV-III from cerebrospinal fluid and neural tissues of patients with neurologic syndromes relate to the acquired immunodeficiency syndrome. *N Engl J Med*. 1985;313(24):1493–1497.
Hoffman, RS. Neuropsychiatric complications of AIDS. *Psychosomatics*. 1984;25:393–395.
Hogeland GW, Swindells S, McNabb JC, et al. Lopinavir/ritonavir reduces bupropion plasma concentrations in healthy subjects. *Clin Pharmacol Ther*. 2007;81(1):69–75.
Horberg MA, Silverberg MJ, Hurley LB, et al. Effects of depression and selective serotonin reuptake inhibitor use on adherence to highly active antiretroviral therapy and on clinical outcomes in HIV-positive patients. *J Acquir Immune Defic Syndr*. 2008;7(3):384–390.
Hriso E, Kuhn T, Masdeu JC, Grundman M. Extrapyramidal symptoms due to dopamine-blocking agents in patients with AIDS encephalopathy. *J Psychiatry*. 1991;148(11):1558–1561.
Huntingdon B, Muscat DM, de Wit J, et al. Factors associated with general sexual functioning and sexual satisfaction among people living with HIV: a systematic review. *J Sex Res*. 2019. http:// doi:10.1080/00224499.2019.1689379
Kales HC, Kim HM, Zivin K, et al. Risk of mortality among individual antipsychotics in patients with dementia. *Am J Psychiatry*. 2012;169:71–79.
Kelly DV, Beique LC, Bowmer MI. Extrapyramidal symptoms with ritonavir/indinavir plus risperdone. *Ann Pharmacother*. 2002;36(5):827–830.
Kent LK, Blumenfield M. Psychodynamic psychiatry in the general medical setting. *J Am Acad Psychoanal Dyn Psychiatry*. 2011;9(1):41–62.
Klinkenberg WD, Dacks SL; HIV/AIDS Treatment Adherence, Health Outcomes and Cost Study Group. Mental disorders and drug abuse in persons living with HIV/AIDS. *AIDS Care*. 2004;16(Suppl 1):S22–S42.
Kubler-Ross E. *On Death and Dying*. New York: Macmillan; 1969.
Lang R, Hogan B, Zhu J, et al. The prevalence of mental health disorders in people with HIV and the effects on the HIV care continuum. *AIDS*. 2023;37(2):259–269. doi:10.1097/QAD.0000000000003420
Le H-N, Hipolito MMS, Lambert S, et al. Culturally sensitive approaches to identification and treatment of depression among HIV infected African American adults: a qualitative study of primary care providers' perspectives. *J Depress Anxiety*. 2016;5(2):223.
Leserman J. Role of depression, stress and trauma in HIV disease progression in HIV. *Psychosom Med*. 2008;70:539–545.
Liedtke MD, Lockhart SM, Rathbun RC. Anticonvulsant and antiretroviral interactions. *Ann Pharmacother*. 2004;38(3):482–489. http:// doi:10.1345/aph.1D309
Loutfy MR, Logie CH, Zhang Y, et al. Gender and ethnicity differences in HIV-related stigma experienced by people living with HIV in Ontario, Canada. *PLoS One*. 2012;7(12):e48168.
Martinez A, Israelski BS, Walker C, et al. Posttraumatic stress disorder in women attending human immunodeficiency virus outpatient clinics. *AIDS Patient Care STDs*. 2002;98:9–17.
Meade CS, Bevilacqua LA, Key MD. Bipolar disorder is associated with HIV transmission risk behavior among patients in treatment for HIV. *AIDS Behav*. 2012;16(8):2267–2271.
Mellins CA, Havens JF, McDonnell C, et al. Adherence to antiretroviral medications and medical care in HIV-positive adults

diagnosed with mental and substance abuse disorders. *AIDS Care.* 2009;21(2):168–177.

Moreno-Pérez, O, Escoín, C, Serna-Candel C. Risk factors for sexual and erectile dysfunction in HIV-infected men: the role or protease inhibitors. *AIDS.* 2010;24:255–264.

Nel A, Kagee A. Common mental health problems and antiretroviral therapy adherence. *AIDS Care.* 2011;23(11):1360–1365.

Nicolussi S, Drewe J, Butterweck V, et al. Clinical relevance of St. John's wort drug interactions revisited. *Br J Pharm.* 2019;177(6):1212–1226.

Norman SE, Cheick AD, Freeman C, et al. Sleep disturbances in men with asymptomatic human immunodeficiency (HIV) infection. *Sleep.* 1992;15:150–155.

Omonuwa TS, Goforth HW, Preud'homme X, et al. The pharmacologic management of insomnia in patients with HIV. *J Clin Sleep Med.* 2009;5(3):251–262.

Owe-Larsson B, Sall, L, Allgulander C. HIV infection and psychiatric illness. *Afr J Psychiatry.* 2009;12(2):115–128. doi:10.4314/ajpsy.v12i2.43729

Parisi CE, Varma DS, Wang Y, et al. Changes in mental health among people with HIV during the COVID-10 pandemic: qualitative and quantitative perspectives. *AIDS and Behav.* 2022;26(6):1980–1991.

Pence BW. The impact of mental health and traumatic life experiences on antiretroviral treatment outcomes for people living with HIV/AIDS. *J Antimicrob Chemother.* 2009;63(4):636–640.

Pence BW, Miller WC, Gaynes BN, et al. Psychiatric illness and virologic response in patients initiating highly active antiretroviral therapy. *J Acquir Immune Defic Syndr.* 2007;44(2):159–165.

Prince JD, Walkup J, Akincigil A, et al. Serious mental illness and risk of new HIV/AIDS diagnosis: an analysis of Medicaid beneficiaries in eight states. *Psych Serv.* 2012;63(10):1032–1038.

Ramachandran G, Glickman L, Levenson J, et al. Incidence of extrapyramidal syndromes in AIDS patients and a comparison group of medically ill inpatients. *J Neuropsych Clin Neurosci.* 1997;9:579–583.

Rao R, Sagar R, Kabra SK, et al. Psychiatric morbidity in HIV-positive children. *AIDS Care.* 2007;19(6):828–833.

Reif S, Wilson E, McAllaster C, et al. The relationship between social support and experienced and internalized HIV-related stigma among people living with HIV in the Deep South. *Stigma and Health.* 2021;6(3):363–369.

Rhodes T. The "risk environment": a framework for understanding and reducing drug-related harm. *Int J Drug Policy.* 2002;13:85–94.

Robertson K, Bayon C, Molina JM, et al. Screening for neurocognitive impairment, depression, and anxiety in HIV-infected patients in Western Europe and Canada. *AIDS Care.* 2014;26(12):1555–1561

Saberi P, Neilands TB, Johnson MO. Quality of sleep: associations with antiretroviral nonadherence. *AIDS Patient Care STDs.* 2011;26(9):517–524.

Scanavino M de T. Sexual dysfunctions of HIV-positive men: associated factors, pathophysiology issues, and clinical management. *Adv Urol.* 2011;2011:854792. doi:10.1155/2011/854792

Shindel A, Horberg M, Smith J, et al. Sexual dysfunction, HIV, and AIDS in men who have sex with men. *AIDS Patient Care STDs.* 2011;25:41–49.

Treisman G, Angelinno A. Interrelation between psychiatric disorders and the prevention and treatment of HIV infection. *Clin Infect Dis.* 2007;45(Suppl 4):S313–S317.

van Luenen S, Garnefski N, Spinhoven P, et al. The benefits of psychosocial interventions for mental health in people living with HIV: a systemic review and meta-analysis. *AIDS Behav.* 2018;22:9–42.

Vazquez-Santiago FJ, Noel RJ Jr, Prter JT, et al. Glutamate metabolism and HIV-associated neurocognitive disorders. *J Neurovirol.* 2014;20(4):315–331.

Villes V, Spire B, Lewden C, et al. The effect of depressive symptoms at ART initiation on HIV clinical progression and mortality: implications in clinical practice. *Antivir Ther.* 2007;12:1067–1071.

Walkup J, Wei W, Sambamoorthi U, et al. Antidepressant treatment and adherence to combination antiretroviral therapy among patients with AIDS and diagnosed depression. *Psychiatr Q.* 2008;79(1):43.

Walkup JT, Akincigil A, Chakravarty S, et al. Bipolar medication use and adherence to antiretroviral therapy among patients with HIV-AIDS and bipolar disorder. *Psychiatr Serv.* 2011;62(3):313–316.

Warden D, Rush AJ. The STAR*D project results: a comprehensive review of findings. *Curr Psychiatry Rep.* 2007;9(6):449–459.

Watkins CC, Pieper AA, Treisman GJ. Safety considerations in drug treatment of depression in HIV-positive patients: an updated review. *Drug Saf.* 2011;34(8):623–639.

Whetten K, Reif S, Whetten R, et al. Trauma, mental health, distrust and stigma among HIV-positive persons: implications for effective care. *Psychosom Med.* 2008;70(5):531–538.

Williams DW, Veenstra M, Gaskill PJ, et al. Monocyte mediated HIV neuropathogenesis: mechanisms that contribute to HIV associated neurocognitive disorders. *Curr HIV Res.* 2014;12(2):85096.

Yalin N, Conti I, Bagchi S, et al. Clinical characteristics and impacts of HIV infection in people with bipolar disorders. *J Affect Dis.* 2021;294:794–801.

Yen Y, Lai H, Kuo Y, et al. Association of depression and antidepressant therapy with antiretroviral therapy adherence and health-related quality of life in men who have sex with men. *PLoS One.* 2022;17(2):0264503.

36.

HIV AND HEPATITIS COINFECTION

Karen Vigil

INTRODUCTION

Hepatitis B virus (HBV) and hepatitis C virus (HCV) are the leading causes of cirrhosis and hepatocellular carcinoma worldwide. They are transmitted perinatally or through early childhood exposure, sexual contact, and injection drug use. Approximately 10% of people with HIV (PWH) also have chronic HBV infection, and up to 30% have coinfection with HCV.

HIV AND HEPATITIS B COINFECTION

LEARNING OBJECTIVE

Discuss the epidemiology, clinical presentation, diagnosis, treatment, and complications of HBV in PWH.

WHAT'S NEW?

- HepB-CpG vaccine has shown superiority compared to HepB-alum in people with HIV and prior vaccine nonresponse.
- A tenofovir alafenamide (TAF)-based antiretroviral regimen has been demonstrated to be noninferior to a tenofovir disoproxil fumarate (TDF)-based combination among PWH and chronic HBV infection.

KEY POINTS

- PWH should have a complete evaluation for HBV infection at baseline and periodically thereafter as indicated.
- All PWH without evidence of prior immunity or current HBV infection should be vaccinated against HBV.
- People with HIV-HBV coinfection should receive treatment for both viruses, regardless of $CD4^+$ T-cell count or independent need for HBV treatment.
- HBV treatment in people with HIV/HBV-coinfection should include two active agents against HBV in the context of fully suppressive antiretroviral therapy (ART) against HIV.

CLINICAL PRESENTATION

Acute hepatitis B usually manifests 1–4 months after exposure. Approximately 30% of persons will present with icteric hepatitis and symptoms of fatigue, fever, right upper quadrant pain, and nausea, while the majority will have a subclinical presentation. Fulminant hepatitis is uncommon and develops in <0.5% of people.

Around 20% of PWH will progress to chronic HBV, compared to <10% in people without HIV. Of those, 15%–40% will progress to end-stage liver disease (ESLD) or hepatocellular carcinoma (HCC), and 25% will die because of HBV-related complications.

DIAGNOSIS AND EVALUATION

Initial testing for HBV should include serologic testing for surface antigen (HBsAg), total core antibody (HBcAb total), and surface antibody (HBsAb). HBsAg can usually be detected approximately 4 weeks after exposure. Resolution of acute HBV is characterized by negative HBsAg and the presence of HBsAb and HBcAb, but reactivation may occur following severe immunosuppression. *Chronic HBV* is defined as the presence of HBsAg detected on two occasions at least 6 months apart. *Occult HBV infection*, defined as the presence of HBcAb alone with HBV DNA viremia in the absence of HBsAg, has been found in approximately 10% of PWH in the United States. Other possible causes of isolated HBcAb are the pre-seroconversion "window phase" of acute HBV infection (between loss of HBsAg and the emergence of HBsAb), resolved hepatitis B infection with HBsAb loss, or a false positive test. Individuals with occult HBV infection are also at increased risk of HBV reactivation, cirrhosis, and HCC (Shire et al., 2004).

Persons with chronic HBV should be tested for HBe-antigen (HBeAg), HBe-antibody (HBeAb), and HBV DNA. Individuals with HBeAg usually have high HBV DNA and elevated alanine aminotransferase (ALT) levels and are at high risk of future liver complications. Seroconversion from positive HBeAg to HBeAb can imply a transition from active disease to an inactive carrier state, but this occurs less commonly in people coinfected with HIV and HBV. This inactive carrier state is also characterized by HBV DNA levels less than 2,000 IU/mL and normal ALT. These persons do remain at risk for HBV reactivation and liver disease progression but at a lower rate than that of individuals with active disease. Finally, there also exists a state of HBeAg-negative active hepatitis, resulting from mutations in the precore and core promoter regions. These individuals are at significant risk of progressive liver disease, and HBV DNA levels should be monitored regularly, with treatment instituted as recommended (Hadziyannis and Papatheodoridis, 2006).

Elevations of hepatic transaminases suggest inflammation, and hepatic synthetic function is measured by serum albumin and coagulation factors. An assessment of the degree of liver fibrosis is essential, and options for this include liver biopsy or noninvasive testing such as transient elastography or an increasing array of serum biomarker tests. Persons with cirrhosis should have HCC screening by ultrasound every 6–12 months, and all persons with cirrhosis should be comanaged with a hepatologist (Lok and McMahon, 2009).

Current HIV guidelines recommend antiretroviral treatment for all PWH; persons with HIV/HBV-coinfection should be a priority group for HIV treatment. ART must include two drugs with activity against HBV, such as tenofovir alafenamide (TAF) or tenofovir disoproxil fumarate (TDF) plus emtricitabine or lamivudine, regardless of the stage of HBV or degree of liver fibrosis (Terrault et al., 2018). This is important to consider, as currently available dual antiretroviral (ARV) regimens (lamivudine/dolutegravir, rilpivirine/dolutegravir, long-acting injectable cabotegravir/rilpivirine) should not be used for people with HIV/HBV coinfection unless specific anti-HBV drugs such as entecavir are also initiated.

HIV/HBV-COINFECTION CONSIDERATIONS

Generally, the presence of HIV/HBV coinfection worsens outcomes related to HBV. PWH are less likely to resolve acute HBV exposure and have higher levels of HBV DNA compared to those without HIV (Colin, 1999). HIV/HBV coinfection is associated with more rapid progression of HBV-related cirrhosis, HCC, and fatal hepatic failure (Thio et al., 2002). Indeed, HBV infection was associated with a relative risk of 3.73 for liver-related deaths in participants with HIV/HBV coinfection in the Data Collection on Adverse Events of Anti-HIV Drugs (D:A:D) study (Weber et al., 2006).

Because the immune response plays a key role in both HBV clearance and the immune damage associated with chronic HBV infection, coinfection with HIV impacts the course of HBV infection. HIV-induced immunosuppression increases the risk of reactivation of quiescent HBV, and initiation of ART may result in exacerbation of HBV liver disease (hepatitis flares) or fulminant hepatitis (Sulkowski et al., 2001).

Stopping ARV agents with activity against HBV (lamivudine, emtricitabine, TDF, or TAF) may lead to HBV rebound, sometimes accompanied by a severe flare and hepatocellular damage (Dore et al., 2010). Thus, when persons with HIV/HBV coinfection change ARV regimens, it is crucial to maintain agents with anti-HBV activity. If anti-HBV treatment is discontinued, serum transaminase levels should be monitored regularly; if a hepatic flare occurs, then HBV therapy should be restarted immediately because this could be life-saving (U.S. Department of Health and Human Services [DHHS], Panel on Opportunistic Infections, 2024).

HBV PREVENTION

People with HIV should be counseled about transmission risks for HBV, including sexual transmission, sharing of needles and syringes, and tattooing or body piercing. People at risk for HBV should be advised to avoid these behaviors associated with transmission (DHHS, 2024).

HBV vaccination is the most effective way to prevent HBV infection. If there is no evidence of chronic infection or previous vaccination (HBsAb <10 IU/mL), then a hepatitis B vaccination series should be administered (DHHS, 2024). Individuals who are positive for HBsAb and HBcAb have a resolved infection and do not require vaccination. Individuals with "isolated HBcAb" (see previous description) who have undetectable HBV DNA should receive a complete HBV vaccine series.

Unfortunately, HBV vaccination is less effective in PWH, with efficacy rates of approximately 65%; people with $CD4^+$ T-cell count less than 350 cells/mm^3 have even lower response rates. All nonimmune PWH should receive HBV vaccination regardless of $CD4^+$ T-cell count, and vaccination should not be deferred in persons with $CD4^+$ T-cell counts less than 350 cells/mm^3. Various revaccination strategies are available for persons who do not respond to an initial series. A repeat three-dose vaccination series or a double dose of vaccine is recommended in PWH not responding to a complete vaccination (Terrault et al., 2018). A new recombinant hepatitis B vaccine (Heplisav-B®) was approved by the FDA in 2017. Heplisav-B® (HepB-CpG) is a vaccine conjugated with the Toll-like receptor 9 agonist adjuvant CpG 1018. Two large randomized clinical studies in PWH have demonstrated higher seroprotective titers when compared to HBsAg-alum-based preparations (Engerix-B®) in vaccine-naive people and prior vaccine nonresponders (Marks et al., 2023, 2024)

GOALS OF TREATMENT

The goals of treatment for HBV infection are to achieve sustained suppression of viral replication to below detectable levels and to improve or stabilize the degree of liver disease to prevent cirrhosis, hepatic failure, and HCC. Measurements of response to therapy include the decline in HBV DNA to undetectable levels, loss of HBeAg or gain of HBeAb (termed *seroconversion*), normalization of serum ALT, and improvement in liver histology. Functional cure is represented by an undetectable HBsAg, which may reduce progression to cirrhosis and liver cancer (Sherman, 2015).

HIV TREATMENT RECOMMENDATIONS IN THE SETTING OF HBV COINFECTION

Because coinfection with HIV is associated with more rapid progression of HBV-related liver disease and evidence indicates that early HIV treatment may slow development of liver disease by improving immune function and reducing HIV-related inflammation and immune activation, current HIV treatment guidelines recommend that all persons with HIV/HBV coinfection start ART with a regimen that includes two drugs with activity against HBV (DHHS, 2024).

The Panel on Opportunistic Infections makes the following recommendations for persons with HIV/HBV coinfection (DHHS, 2024):

- Regardless of $CD4^+$ T-cell count or the need for HBV treatment, ART that includes agents active against both HIV and HBV is recommended for all persons with HIV and HBV.
- ART must include two drugs active against HBV, preferably TDF or TAF, and emtricitabine or lamivudine, regardless of the level of HBV DNA.
- Pegylated interferon-α-2a and adefovir are not recommended for people with HIV/HBV coinfection. Entecavir is not recommended to be given without suppressive ART as it may result in HIV resistance.
- In circumstances where tenofovir use is not acceptable as part of the ART regimen, the alternate recommendation is to use entecavir in addition to fully suppressive ART.
- Chronic use of lamivudine or emtricitabine as a single active agent against HBV should be avoided because of the high rate of subsequent HBV resistance.

Individuals being treated for HBV should have HBV DNA measured every 12–24 weeks. If the HBV DNA is greater than 1,000 IU/mL after 1 year, then medication adherence should be assessed, and HBV resistance testing should be considered. Viral failure and resistance are more common in PWH with HBV, primarily when lamivudine is used alone for treatment. The risk of resistance has declined with use of more potent drugs such as tenofovir and entecavir (Luetkemeyer et al., 2011). Unfortunately, even with long-term suppression of HBV DNA, the loss of HBsAg (representing a functional cure of HBV) is not common in PWH (Sherman, 2015), and indefinite treatment is usually recommended.

SPECIAL CONSIDERATIONS

Immune Reconstitution Inflammatory Syndrome

Immune reconstitution during the course of HIV/HBV treatment can lead to a severe flare of chronic HBV infection, with significant increases in hepatic transaminases, perhaps because of enhanced host immune responses against HBV. HBV-associated immune reconstitution inflammatory syndrome (IRIS) is most likely to occur during the first few weeks after starting ART and can present as acute hepatitis. Careful monitoring of hepatic transaminases after ART initiation is helpful (Audsley et al., 2011). Development of hepatic synthetic dysfunction signs, such as elevated prothrombin time or low albumin, should prompt evaluation by a hepatologist. Distinguishing between HBV-related IRIS and drug-induced liver toxicity can be challenging and may require examination of liver histology and consultation with a hepatologist. Very little information is available regarding the best treatment for HBV-related IRIS, and the decision regarding whether to continue, modify, or interrupt therapy should be individualized based on the severity of hepatic injury.

Treatment Interruptions

Because of the overlap in anti-HIV and HBV activity of emtricitabine, lamivudine, and tenofovir, treatment interruption should be avoided in HIV/HBV coinfection to avoid potentially severe flares of HBV with hepatic inflammation and necrosis. In particular, when there is a need to discontinue one of the HBV-active drugs in the HIV treatment regimen, careful follow-up of liver function tests (LFTs) is required, and initiation of a second agent with anti-HBV activity such as entecavir should be considered. If there is a need to change ART because of HIV resistance, and HBV suppression is maintained despite HIV treatment failure, the antiretrovirals with activity against HBV should be continued for HBV treatment in addition to other appropriate ARV agents.

TREATMENT OPTIONS FOR HEPATITIS B INFECTION

People with HIV/HBV coinfection should start a regimen that has activity against both viruses. The preferred antiretroviral treatment consists of the backbone regimen of TAF or TDF with lamivudine or emtricitabine. Both TDF and TAF have a high genetic barrier to HBV resistance. Monotherapy with lamivudine or emtricitabine is not recommended because of the increased possibility of developing resistance. Lifelong treatment is recommended. Discontinuation of therapy has been associated with hepatitis flares. Treatment of HBV alone is not recommended.

SUMMARY

Hepatitis B infection is a common and potentially severe comorbidity for PWH. Screening for HBV infection, vaccination, and careful assessment of chronic HBV infection are essential components of HIV care. Consideration of chronic HBV status when selecting ART is essential in optimizing the management of both infections. Monitoring for HBV treatment response and screening for complications such as cirrhosis or HCC are important components of ongoing care for persons with HIV/HBV coinfection.

HIV AND HEPATITIS C COINFECTION

LEARNING OBJECTIVE

Discuss the epidemiology, clinical presentation, diagnosis, treatment, and complications of HCV in PWH.

WHAT'S NEW?

- The World Health Organization (WHO) and the U.S. Viral Hepatitis National Strategic Plan have established the goal of eliminating HCV as a public health threat by 2030. However, only approximately one-third of people received treatment within 1 year of diagnosis.

- To decrease the incidence of new cases in the general population, individuals who develop acute HCV should be treated immediately and not wait for spontaneous resolution.

KEY POINTS

- Direct-acting antivirals (DAAs) achieve a cure of greater than 90% in PWH and chronic HCV infections.
- All PWH with HCV should be offered treatment. Drug-drug interactions, disease severity, and especially, cost considerations remain.

EPIDEMIOLOGY

As ART continues to extend the life span of PWH by decades, HIV/HCV coinfection has become an increasingly important cause of both morbidity and mortality. Liver disease has emerged as one of the leading causes of non-AIDS-related deaths in PWH (Trickey et al., 2024). HIV/HCV coinfection places a growing burden on the HIV healthcare system, as evidenced by an analysis of the Advancing Clinical Therapeutics Globally (ACTG) Longitudinal Linked Randomized Trials (ALLRT) cohort. When controlling for age, race, sex, history of AIDS-defining events, and current $CD4^+$ T-cell count and HIV RNA levels, the relative risk of hospitalization, emergency department visits, and disability days for persons with HIV/HCV versus HIV mono-infected participants was 1.8 (95% confidence interval [CI]: 1.3–2.5), 1.7 (95% CI: 1.4–2.1), and 1.6 (95% CI: 1.3–1.9), respectively. A study from the New York City Department of Health and Mental Hygiene using death certificate data showed persons with HIV/HCV coinfection to be at exceptionally high risk for premature death (median age, 52 years) compared to those with HCV alone (median age, 60 years) or those with neither virus (median age, 78 years). Decedents had an odds ratio of 2.2 for death from liver cancer and 3.1 for drug-related causes, with 53.6% of deaths attributed to HIV/AIDS and 94% occurring prematurely (defined as younger than age 65 years) (Pinchoff et al., 2014).

HCV is a single-stranded RNA virus transmitted primarily through blood exposure and, less commonly, sexual or perinatal transmission. Because HIV and HCV share similar routes of transmission, approximately one-fifth of all PWH in the United States are also infected with HCV. People who inject drugs have a higher prevalence of hepatitis C infection. It is estimated that 80% of PWH and a history of injection drug use have HCV worldwide (Platt et al., 2016). Heterosexual transmission risk is low and generally quoted as less than 1% per year, but men who have sex with men (MSM) are at elevated risk. The Swiss HIV Cohort Study showed an 18-fold increase from 1998 in cases per 100 person-years seen in MSM, with HCV seen in association with a history of condomless anal sex, history of syphilis, and chronic HBV (Wandeler et al., 2012).

CLINICAL COURSE

The most striking feature of HCV, when acquired by a PWH, is its ability to cause chronic hepatitis in as much as 90% of persons within 6 months. This occurs because of the lack of $CD4^+$ T-cell responses and significantly reduced IFN-γ ELISpot responses against HCV (Elliott et al., 2006). Between 60% and 70% of chronically infected persons will have fluctuating serum ALT levels because this enzyme is most associated with HCV liver cell injury. Less than 20% have nonspecific symptoms, including fatigue and generalized weakness. There are significant similarities and differences between HIV and HCV. Both are RNA viruses with rapid replication rates (10 trillion HCV virions vs. 10 billion HIV virions produced daily). Both are prone to frequent mutations and exist as heterogeneous quasi-species to avoid the immune system. Both viruses incite abundant but ineffective antibody responses. Although both have many reservoirs in the human body, HCV exists primarily in the cytoplasm of hepatocytes and can be eradicated from the body. HIV is integrated into the nuclei of $CD4^+$ T lymphocytes and long-lived memory T-cell reservoirs and therefore cannot be eradicated with current ART. HCV RNA levels are only broadly predictive of long-term prognosis, whereas HIV RNA is very predictive of clinical events in untreated persons.

There are six main HCV genotypes (1–6) at various prevalence rates worldwide. Genotype (GT) 1 accounts for two-thirds of cases in the United States, with GTs 2–4 occurring less commonly. Genotype 3 has more rapid progression to cirrhosis and higher rates of hepatocellular carcinoma.

DIAGNOSIS

HCV may be diagnosed earlier in asymptomatic PWH with elevated ALT/AST levels because of greater frequency of lab monitoring (Mohsen and Easterbrook, 2003). Coinfection with HIV greatly impacts the natural history of HCV infection. Individuals with HIV/HCV coinfection are less likely to spontaneously clear HCV, have increased HCV RNA, and progress more rapidly to cirrhosis and ESLD (Asselah et al., 2006). Predictors of severe liver fibrosis include age older than 40 years at the time of infection, alcohol consumption of more than 50 g/d, daily marijuana use, high body mass index, male gender, postmenopausal status, and longer duration of infection (Poynard et al., 1997). Although ART may slow this rate, it continues to exceed that seen in persons with HCV mono-infection. Low $CD4^+$ T-cell counts also appear to magnify the progression. A meta-analysis of eight studies that examined the role of HIV with HCV found that persons with HIV/HCV coinfection had approximately two times the risk of cirrhosis on liver biopsy and six times the risk of decompensated liver disease with ascites, esophageal varices, or encephalopathy compared to HCV-mono-infected individuals (Poynard et al., 1997). A Veterans Health Administration study examined 4,820 persons with HIV/HCV coinfection and 6,079 persons with HCV in care from 1997 to 2010. Hepatic decompensation was significantly greater at 10 years in the HIV/HCV group (7.4% vs. 4.8%; $p < 0.001$) (Lo et al., 2014). Approximately one-third of persons with chronic HCV will progress to cirrhosis at a median time of less than 20 years (Thomas et al., 2000). Once cirrhosis has developed, 50% will decompensate within the first 5 years, with ascites being the usual first sign. Approximately 1%–4% of people with cirrhosis will develop HCC per year. Median survival time is 35 months (compared to 65 months for those without HIV) (Beretta et al., 2011).

The average time from infection to fibrosis is shortened from 35 to 25 years in persons with HIV/HCV. Therefore, treatment should not be delayed. Deferring HCV treatment in the age of DAAs may lead to increased rates of HCC and death. Data from the SHCS and published HCV data were used for a modeling analysis that predicted the decrease in progression to cirrhosis, HCC, and death in persons with HIV/HCV. If therapy was initiated during stages F0 or F1, the percentage of liver-related deaths was 2%. However, if treatment was deferred until F3 or F4 stage, mortality increased to 7% and 22%, respectively. Further, untreated individuals remain infectious; from a public health perspective, people treated between 1 month and 1 year after diagnosis remained infectious for HCV for approximately 5 years, compared to 12 years for stage 2, 15 years for stage 3, and nearly 20 years for stage 4 (Zahnd et al., 2016).

DECISION TO TREAT

All PWH should be screened for HCV with antibody testing upon entry into care and annually thereafter for those with ongoing exposure or whenever HCV infection is suspected (Thompson et al., 2020). HCV RNA levels should be tested in all people with a positive antibody test to assess for active disease because antibodies persist for a lifetime (even in persons who have cleared the virus). Historically, infants born to mothers with HIV/HCV coinfection underwent antibody testing at/after 18 months. Recent CDC guidance has shifted to recommend nucleic acid testing as early as 2–6 months for infants with perinatal HCV exposure, to identify children in whom chronic HCV may develop if not treated (Panagiotakopoulos et al., 2023) and to improve timely linkage to services. HCV transmission may be facilitated by the presence of genital erosions related to sexually transmitted diseases. Reinfection with HCV can occur, necessitating that individuals be aware that high-risk behaviors may lead to reinfection (Danta and Dusheiko, 2008). Hepatitis A and hepatitis B status should be assessed, and vaccination against these viruses should be administered if appropriate because dual or triple infections are typically more severe (Low et al., 2008).

PWH should be treated similarly to HCV-mono-infected patients. The efficacy and safety of current DAAs are similar in PWH. However, potential drug-drug interactions should be reviewed carefully. Prior to initiating HCV treatment in persons with HIV/HCV coinfection, specific baseline lab tests should be obtained. These include a complete blood count (CBC) with platelets, hepatic function panel including ALT, AST, alkaline phosphatase, albumin, and total bilirubin, prothrombin time/international normalized ratio (PT/INR), calculated glomerular filtration rate (eGFR), and HCV RNA levels. If a nonpangenotypic DAA will be prescribed, then HCV genotype is recommended. A pregnancy test is recommended for all people of childbearing potential if ribavirin (RBV) use is planned because of its known teratogenicity. Counseling on alcohol use is key given its hepatotoxicity, and it can rapidly worsen fibrosis. Hepatitis B and hepatitis A virus vaccination should be offered to all people without evidence of exposure/immunity.

Liver fibrosis should be assessed prior to starting DAA treatment. Because of risks associated with biopsy, alternatives such as FibroScan® and FibroSURE™ have rapidly risen in popularity and acceptance in clinical practice. FibroScan® utilizes a mild-amplitude, low-frequency vibration transmitted through the liver to measure tissue "stiffness." FibroSURE™ uses six blood serum tests (α_2-macroglobulin, haptoglobin, apolipoprotein A1, γ-glutamyl transferase, ALT, and total bilirubin), along with age and gender, to generate a score that correlates with degree of liver disease. Other noninvasive biomarker formulas, such as the APRI score (which incorporates platelet counts with tests of coagulation and transaminases) and fibrosis-4 (FIB-4) may also be used to evaluate degree of fibrosis. APRI and FibroSURE™ have been validated in HIV/HCV coinfection and predict no disease versus cirrhosis accurately but are not as accurate in the mid-range of the disease spectrum (Rallon et al., 2011; Schneider and Sarrazin, 2014).

Several formulas are used to assess the degree of cirrhosis. The Child–Turcotte–Pugh score uses encephalopathy, ascites, bilirubin, albumin, and PT or INR to classify severity of cirrhosis (class A: 5–6 points; class B: 7–9 points; class C: 10–15 points). The Model for End-stage Liver Disease (MELD) score uses serum creatinine, bilirubin, and INR and two or more dialysis sessions within the previous week to predict probability of survival for persons with ESLD. This is the formula currently used for liver allocation by the United Network of Organ Sharing and predicts the 3-month mortality rate. A MELD calculator is provided on the Mayo Clinic website (http://www.mayoclinic.org/medical-professionals/model-end-stage-liver-disease/meld-model) and Hepatitis C Online curriculum (https://www.hepatitisc.uw.edu/page/clinical-calculators/meld). The HALT-C formula for predicting cirrhosis uses platelet count, INR, AST, and ALT to predict the probability of a biopsy demonstrating cirrhosis (Lok and McMahon, 2009).

ACUTE HEPATITIS C

Approximately 30% of individuals do not have detectable antibodies at the onset of acute hepatitis C symptoms. Therefore, the only reliable method to diagnose acute hepatitis C is testing for HCV RNA levels by polymerase chain reaction. A positive HCV antibody test with a history of a prior negative HCV antibody test is also indicative of recent seroconversion. More than 90% of individuals will develop antibodies by 3 months post-exposure, with less than 5% of persons with HIV/HCV (usually those with advanced immunosuppression) failing to produce detectable HCV antibodies. Acute HCV is asymptomatic in 70%–80% of cases, but cure rates are significantly higher with acute disease. It is therefore important to routinely screen people at risk for HCV infection and promptly investigate elevated hepatic transaminase levels. Acute HCV infection may present with flu-like symptoms, nausea, abdominal pain, and jaundice, and people with acute infection who are symptomatic have a higher likelihood of spontaneous viral clearance. Infrequently, severe hepatic dysfunction with transaminases up to 10 times normal is seen, but fulminant hepatitis is rare (DHHS, 2024).

Due to the high efficacy and safety of DAAs, experts recommend treating people with acute hepatitis C upon diagnosis, rather than monitoring them for spontaneous resolution. Unrestricted access to HCV therapy reduces viremia prevalence and incidence, while mathematical models indicate that scaling up DAA treatment, especially for those at high risk of transmission, can further decrease HCV incidence and prevalence.

THERAPEUTIC MODALITIES

Multiple, all-oral combinations of DAAs are now available as the recommended regimens for treatment (Table 36.1). Evidence supports treating all people with HCV unless their life expectancy is less than 12 months because of a non-liver-related condition. As such, guidelines identify PWH as "high priority" for treatment given the increased risk of fibrosis and HCC. Treatment response is similar between persons with HIV/HCV coinfection and persons with HCV monoinfection. Guidelines no longer recommend the use of Peg-IFN-α-2a or -2b and RBV for HCV treatment, given low cure rates (approximately 50%) and side-effect profiles.

For the majority of HCV treatment-naive adults without cirrhosis, monitoring of HCV RNA levels during therapy is not necessary. However, treatment interruptions are common, and there are limited data on which to guide clinical management when treatment interruptions occur: guidance from the American Association for the Study of Liver Diseases/Infectious Diseases Society of America (AALSD/IDSA, 2023) includes information on when to consider obtaining an HCV RNA during therapy to guide subsequent decision-making (https://www.hcvguidelines.org/evaluate/monitoring#incomplete-adherence). HCV RNA levels should be obtained at 12 weeks post-treatment to determine cure status (SVR12).

Drug-drug interactions increase the complexity of treating HCV for some PWH on ART, as does the presence of significant renal impairment. Currently, the preferred treatment for persons with chronic kidney disease (CKD) stage 4 or 5 (eGFR <30 mL/min or end-stage renal disease) is either sofosbuvir (400 mg)/velpatasvir (100 mg) or glecaprevir (300 mg)/pibrentasvir (120 mg). ART switches may need to occur prior to HCV treatment for some PWH, and individuals may return to their previously suppressive HIV regimen after HCV treatment is completed. Although choosing a regimen to avoid drug interactions may seem daunting, interrupting ART while on HCV treatment is not recommended.

The standard of care for HCV treatment is now oral direct-acting agents (DAAs). They are engineered to work at multiple HCV-specific sites, such as the protease and polymerase enzymes. First-generation agents, boceprevir and telaprevir, were NS3/4A protease inhibitors (PIs). Although used widely until 2012, they are no longer recommended in the

Table 36.1 CURRENT DIRECT ANTIVIRAL AGENTS FOR HEPATITIS C

DIRECT ANTIVIRAL AGENT	GENOTYPES TREATED	CLASS	GFR	COMMENTS
Elbasvir/grazoprevir	1 and 4	NS5A inhibitor\+ NS3/4A protease inhibitor	No dose adjustment in patients with renal impairment, including those on hemodialysis	NS5A testing is required in patients with GT 1a
Ledipasvir/sofosbuvir	1 to 6	NS5A inhibitor\+ nucleotide polymerase inhibitor (NS5B)	No dosage recommendation for patients with glomerular filtration rate less than 30 mL/min/1.73 m²	First fixed oral combination
Sofosbuvir/velpatasvir	1 to 6	Nucleotide polymerase inhibitor (NS5B)\+ NS5A inhibitor	No dosage recommendation for patients with glomerular filtration rate less than 30 mL/min/1.73 m²	
Sofosbuvir/velpatasvir/voxilapresvir	1 to 6	Nucleotide polymerase inhibitor (NS5B)\+ NS5A inhibitor\+ NS3/4A protease inhibitor	No dosage recommendation for patients with glomerular filtration rate less than 30 mL/min/1.73 m²	For patients who have failed therapy with a NS5A inhibitor–containing regimen
Glecaprevir/pibrentasvir	1 to 6	HCV NS3/4A protease inhibitor\+ HCV NS5A inhibitor	No dose adjustment in patients with renal impairment, including those on hemodialysis	

Source: Adapted from HCVGuidelines.org. Available at https:// www.hcvguidelines.org. Accessed September 14, 2024.

United States because more efficacious and less-toxic drugs have been developed. The second wave of HCV therapies are highly effective (including for people with HIV/HCV coinfection) and involve simple rules for use, including shorter durations of therapy, increased tolerability, and fewer drug-drug interactions.

DIRECT ACTING AGENTS: MECHANISMS OF ACTION

The HCV genome encodes 10 polyproteins, 7 nonstructural proteins, and 3 structural proteins (NS3/4A, NS5A, NS5B) that play an essential role in HCV replication and are the target of current DAA. Sofosbuvir (SOF) and simeprevir (SIM) were the initial second-generation DAAs approved in the United States. SIM was discontinued in May 2018 because of decreased utilization. However, SOF has become the cornerstone of some current combination treatments for HCV.

NS5B Polymerase Inhibitor(s)

NS5B polymerase is required for viral replication, acting as a chain terminator. SOF is a nucleotide analog inhibitor of this enzyme. The NS5B site is highly conserved among all genotypes; SOF is pangenotypic. It is given as 400 mg once daily. It is not metabolized by the CYP450 enzyme complex and thus is an ideal candidate for use in people with HIV/HCV coinfection.

NS3/4A Protease Inhibitors

Glecaprevir, grazoprevir, paritaprevir, and voxileprevir are the current DAAs available in this class. They are noncovalent inhibitors of the NS3/4A serine protease of HCV.

NS5A Inhibitors

The exact mechanism of action of the NS5A inhibitors is not completely understood. However, some studies showed that they bind to the N-terminal domain of NS5A, causing structural distortion and inhibiting both viral RNA replication and virion assembly at an early stage. Daclatasvir, elbasvir, ledipasvir, ombitasvir, pibrentasvir, and velpastavir are antivirals in this class. Daclatasvir has been discontinued from the market. All others are co-formulated in fixed-dose combinations.

FIXED-DOSE COMBINATIONS

Ledipasvir/Sofosbuvir

Ledipasvir 90 mg and sofosbuvir 400 mg (LDV/SOF) was the first interferon- and ribavirin-free once-daily, single-tablet regimen for HCV approved by the FDA in 2014.

The ION-4 study was a phase 3, multicenter, open-label trial of 335 persons with HIV/HCV coinfection. Enrolled participants had GT 1 and 4 (75% GT 1a, 23% GT 1b, and 2% GT 4), 20% had compensated cirrhosis, and 55% were treatment-experienced. SVR 12 was achieved in 96%. No difference in response rates at treatment week 12 was seen with GT 1a versus GT 1b based on sex, treatment history, concomitant ART, or cirrhosis status. Ten participants relapsed after treatment. All 10 relapse case participants were Black, with 7 having the TT allele in the gene encoding IL28B (which confers an increased risk of failure with IFN-containing regimens). In multivariate analyses, Black race alone was significantly associated with relapse. The association of lower SVR with Black race, which comprised 34% of the study population, was not seen in studies of LDV/SOB in persons with HCV-mono-infection and was not related to the CYP2B6 polymorphism, which is more common in Black persons and results in increased EFV levels (Naggie et al., 2015).

LDV/SOF increases exposure to TDF by approximately 40%. Individuals on RTV-containing regimens may experience a relative increase of 30%–60% in TDF exposure, so they were excluded from the trial, along with those on cobicistat-containing combinations. Headache (25%), fatigue (21%), and diarrhea (11%) were the most common adverse events.

Sofosbuvir/Velpatasvir

The sofobuvir 400 mg and velpatasvir 100 mg (SOF/VEL) fixed-dose combination tablet is a pangenotypic regimen approved in 2016, to be given as a once-daily for 12 weeks in persons without cirrhosis or with compensated cirrhosis. In individuals with decompensated cirrhosis, it must be used with RBV. Velpatasvir is an HCV NS5A inhibitor required for viral replication.

The ASTRAL-1 study was a randomized controlled study that evaluated 12 weeks of treatment with SOF/VEL in treatment-naive and Peg-IFN treatment-experienced individuals without cirrhosis or with compensated cirrhosis. Persons with all genotypes were included. Of 328 persons with GT 1, 98% achieved SVR12. Rates were similar in persons with compensated cirrhosis. Even in previously treatment-experienced persons with IFN-based regimens and first-generation protease inhibitors, this combination achieved more than 96% efficacy (Pianko et al., 2015).

In the ASTRAL-5 study, velpatasvir/sofosbuvir was given to 106 people with HIV/HCV coinfection, virally suppressed on ART containing raltegravir, rilpivirine, or ritonavir-boosted protease inhibitors either with tenofovir or abacavir. Genotypes 1 to 4 were included; 18% of participants had compensated cirrhosis. SVR 12 was achieved in 95% of the individuals, and therapy was well tolerated. The most commonly reported side effects were fatigue, headaches, nausea, and insomnia.

Glecaprevir/Pibrentasvir

Glecaprevir 100 mg and pibrentasvir 40 mg per tablet (GLE/PIB) is a fixed-dose combination tablet (with 3 tablets taken once a day). This combination has several advantages compared to others. It is not only pangenotypic but can also be used in persons with chronic kidney disease and is approved for 8 weeks in treatment-naive individuals with no cirrhosis, based on data from ENDURANCE-1 and ENDURANCE-3 studies.

In ENDURANCE-1 and ENDURANCE-3, out of 1,208 persons with GT 1 and 3 treated for 8 weeks, 99.1% of people with GT 1 and 95% with GT 3 achieved SVR 12 (Zeuzem et al., 2018). It is also approved for use in treatment-experienced persons for a total of 8–16 weeks based on cirrhosis stage and previously used DAAs. Of note, this combination is contraindicated in individuals with advanced cirrhosis (Child–Pugh B or C). The EXPEDITION-2 study evaluated 8 weeks of GLE/PIB in persons with HIV/HCV. Overall SVR 12 rate was 98%.

Sofosbuvir/Velpatasvir/Voxilaprevir

Sofosbuvir 400 mg, velpatasvir 100 mg, and voxileprevir 100 mg (SOF/VEL/VOX) is a pangenotypic, single-tablet, fixed-dose combination indicated for 12 weeks in persons with HCV GT 1a who have failed therapy with a NS5A inhibitor–containing regimen. Voxileprevir is a reversible potent inhibitor of the NS3/4A protease required for the cleavage of the HCV-encoded polyprotein. It is administered once daily with food. Persons with advanced liver disease (Child–Pugh B and C) should not take this regimen.

POLARIS-1 and POLARIS-4 assessed the efficacy and safety of SOF/VEL/VOX for 12 weeks in persons with HCV infection who had previously received unsuccessful treatment with DAA-based regimens. All HCV genotypes were included; 46% of individuals had cirrhosis. The most common NS5A inhibitors used in previous unsuccessful treatments were ledipasvir (55% of persons), daclatasvir (23%), and ombitasvir (13%) in POLARIS-1, while in POLARIS-4 it was sofosbuvir (85%). SVR rates were achieved by 96% and 100% of participants with GT 1a and 1b, respectively. In POLARIS-1 and POLARIS-4, 83% and 49% of participants, respectively, had baseline viral substitutions associated with resistance to NS3 inhibitors or NS5A inhibitors. SVR 12 was achieved in 97% of participants in POLARIS-1 and 100% in POLARIS-4.

In a phase 2, open-label study, 49 persons with HCV GT 1 infection who previously failed to achieve sustained virologic response on a DAA-based regimen were randomized to receive SOF/VEL/VOX with or without RBV for 12 weeks. The primary efficacy endpoint was the proportion of participants achieving SVR 12. SVR 12 was achieved by 24 of 24 persons (100%) receiving sofosbuvir/velpatasvir/voxilaprevir alone and 24 of 25 (96%) receiving the same treatment with RBV. The virological response was achieved by 13 of 13 (100%) persons without baseline resistance-associated substitutions (RASs) and by 34 of 35 (97%) with baseline RASs. No large, randomized control studies in persons with HIV/HCV coinfection have been done.

Elbasvir/Grazoprevir

Elbasvir 50 mg and grazoprevir 100 mg (ELB/GRZ) is a fixed-dose combination taken once a day with or without food for the treatment of chronic HCV GT 1 or 4 infection in adults. Treatment is typically 12 weeks. RBV is added, and treatment is extended to 16 weeks if baseline NS5A polymorphisms are found in a GT 1a person. RBV may be added in GT 1a or 1b persons who are Peg/RBV/PI-experienced. People with GT 4 who are Peg/IFN/RBV-experienced also receive 16 weeks of treatment. RBV is given in two daily doses depending on baseline NS5A polymorphisms and treatment experience. No dosage adjustment for ELB/GRZ is needed for renal impairment, including those on hemodialysis, although RBV may need adjustment per guidelines. It is contraindicated in those with Child–Pugh B or C disease. ELB/GRZ is contraindicated with OATP1B1/3 inhibitors and strong CYP3A inducers such as EFV. Other contraindicated drugs include phenytoin and carbamazepine, rifampin, and St. John's wort. Coadministration with nafcillin, ketoconazole, bosentan, modafinil, entecavir (ETV), and cobicistat-containing compounds is not recommended. The risk of ALT elevations may be increased with zidovudine (ATZ), darunavir (DRV), lopinavir (LPV), and cyclosporine. Statins also interact with ELB/GRZ. Thus, atorvastatin should not exceed 20 mg; rosuvastatin should not exceed 10 mg; and the lowest possible dose of fluvastatin, lovastatin, and simvastatin should be used. Tacrolimus levels may be increased by ELB/GRZ.

ELB/GRZ was approved for the treatment of GT 1 and 4 only based on results from the C-EDGE study. A total of 299 participants were enrolled in GT 1, 4, and 6. The SVR 12 was only 92% in persons with GT 1a, but 99% in persons with GT 1b and 100% in GT 4. Further analysis demonstrated lower SVR 12 rates in persons with baseline NS5A resistance-associated variants (at positions 28, 30, 31, and 93) associated with more than 5-fold loss in elbasvir susceptibility. Therefore, a baseline resistance test is recommended in people with GT 1a. If baseline resistance mutations are found, treatment should be extended for 16 weeks, and RBV should be added. Similarly, in the C-EDGE Coinfection trial—a phase 3, open-label trial involving 218 HCV treatment-naive HCV/HIV coinfected individuals who received ELB/GRZ one tablet daily for 12 weeks—95.0% of individuals achieved a cure, with six relapses and one reinfection (Rockstroh et al., 2015).

It should be noted that the FDA has issued a black box warning that ELB/GRZ could cause LFT elevations of more than 5 times the upper limit of normal. Therefore, it is recommended that LFTs be monitored while on treatment.

TREATMENT FAILURES

For those who fail HCV treatment, assessment for disease progression should be done every 6–12 months with a hepatic function panel, CBC, and INR. If they have cirrhosis, HCC surveillance every 6 months with ultrasound is advised, and they should be referred to a hepatologist and have endoscopic evaluation for varices. Retreatment depends on genotype, initial treatment, and reason for failure and is not within the scope of this chapter.

SUMMARY

The world of HIV/HCV coinfection is in rapid flux. Similar to HIV treatment, a combination of oral agents that disrupt the HCV virus at various sites of the life cycle has the best chance of decreasing viral replication long term and curing infection. Questions regarding optimal combination, as well as drug access and costs, will need to be addressed in the next several years if the majority of persons with HIV/HCV coinfection are to be effectively treated.

ACKNOWLEDGMENTS

The authors acknowledge Aimee Wilkin, MD, MPH, who wrote the first section of this chapter in the previous edition.

REFERENCES

AASLD-IDSA. Recommendations for testing, managing, and treating hepatitis C. https://www.hcvguidelines.org. Published 2023. Accessed July 14, 2024.

Asselah T, Rubbia-Brandt L, Marcellin P, et al. Steatosis in chronic hepatitis C: why does it really matter? *Gut*. 2006;55(1):123–130.

Audsley J, Seaberg E, Sasadeusz J, et al. Factors associated with elevated ALT in an international HIV/HBV coinfected cohort on long-term HAART. *PLoS One*. 2011;6(11):e26482.

Beretta M, Garlassi E, Cacopardo B, et al. Hepatocellular carcinoma in HIV-infected patients: check early, treat hard. *Oncologist*. 2011;16(9):1258–1269.

Colin J, Cazals-Hatem D, Loriot M, et al. Influence of human immunodeficiency virus infection on chronic hepatitis B in homosexual men. *Hepatology*. 1999;29(4):1306–1310.

Danta M, Dusheiko GM. Acute HCV in HIV-positive individuals: a review. *Curr Pharm Des*. 2008;14(17):1690–1697.

Department of Health and Human Services (DHHS), Panel on Guidelines for the Prevention and Treatment of Opportunistic Infections in Adults and Adolescents with HIV. Guidelines for the prevention and treatment of opportunistic infections in HIV-infected adults and adolescents: recommendations from the Centers for Disease Control and Prevention, the National Institutes of Health, and the HIV Medicine Association of the Infectious Diseases Society of America. https://clinicalinfo.hiv.gov/en/guidelines/adult-and-adolescent-arv. Published July 9, 2024. Accessed July 14, 2024.

Dore G, Soriano V, Rockstroh J, et al. Frequent hepatitis B virus rebound among HIV-hepatitis B virus coinfected patients following antiretroviral therapy interruption. *AIDS*. 2010;24(6):857–865.

Elliott LN, Lloyd A, Ziegler JB, et al. Protective immunity against hepatitis C virus infection. *Immunol Cell Biol*. 2006;84:239–249.

Hadziyannis S, Papatheodoridis G. Hepatitis B e antigen-negative chronic hepatitis B: natural history and treatment. *Semin Liver Dis*. 2006;26:130–141.

Lo Re V III, Kallan M, Tate J, et al. Hepatic decompensation in antiretroviral-treated patients coinfected with HIV and hepatitis C virus compared with hepatitis C virus-monoinfected patients: a cohort study. *Ann Intern Med*. 2014;160(6):369–379.

Lok AS, McMahon BJ. Chronic hepatitis B: update 2009. *Hepatology*. 2009;50(3):661–662.

Low E, Vogel M, Rockstroh J, et al. Acute hepatitis C in HIV-positive individuals. *AIDS Rev*. 2008;10(4):245–253.

Luetkemeyer A, Charlebois E, Hare C, et al. Resistance patterns and response to entecavir intensification among HIV–HBV-coinfected adults with persistent HBV viremia. *J AIDS*. 2011;58(3):e96–e99.

Marks K, Kang M, Umbleja T, et al. HepB-CpG vaccine is superior to HepB-alum in people with HIV and prior vaccine nonresponse: A5379. CROI Abstract 209. In Special Issue: Abstracts from the 2024 Conference on Retroviruses and Opportunistic Infections. *Top Antivir Med*. 2024;32(1):56

Marks KM, Kang M, Umbleja T, et al. Immunogenicity and safety of hepatitis B virus (HBV) vaccine with a toll-like receptor 9 agonist adjuvant in HBV vaccine-naïve people with human immunodeficiency virus. *Clin Infect Dis*. 2023;77(3):414–418.

Mohsen AH, Easterbrook P. Hepatitis C testing in HIV infected patients. *Sex Transm Infect*. 2003;79(1):76.

Naggie S, Cooper C, Saag M, et al. Ledipasvir and sofosbuvir for HCV in patients coinfected with HIV-1. *N Engl J Med*. 2015;373(8):705–713.

Panagiotakopoulos L, Sandul AL, Connors EE, et al. CDC Recommendations for hepatitis C testing among perinatally exposed infants and children—United States, 2023. *MMWR Recomm Rep*. 2023;72(RR-4):1–19. doi:http://dx.doi.org/10.15585/mmwr.rr7204a1

Pianko S, Flamm SL, Shiffman ML, et al. Sofosbuvir plus velpatasvir combination therapy for treatment-experienced patients with genotype 1 or 3 hepatitis C virus Infection: a randomized trial. *Ann Intern Med*. 2015;163(11):809–817.

Pinchoff J, Drobnik A, Bornschlegel K, et al. Deaths among people with hepatitis C in New York City, 2000–2011. *Clin Infect Dis*. 2014;58(8):1047–1054.

Platt L, Easterbrook P, Gower E, et al. Prevalence and burden of HCV co-infection in people living with HIV: a global systematic review and metanalysis. *Lancet Infect Dis*. 2016;16(7):797.

Poynard T, Bedossa P, Opolon P. Natural history of liver fibrosis progression in patients with chronic hepatitis C: the OBSVIRC, METAVIR, CLINIVIR, and DOSVIRC groups. *Lancet*. 1997;349(9055):825–832.

Rallon NI, Soriano V, Naggie S, et al. IL28B gene polymorphism and viral kinetics in HIV. HCV coinfected patients treated with pegylated interferon and ribavirin. *AIDS*. 2011;25(8):1025–1033.

Rockstroh JK, Nelson M, Katlama C, et al. Efficacy and safety of grazoprevir (MK-5172) and elbasvir (MK-8742) in patients with hepatitis C virus and HIV coinfection (C-EDGE COINFECTION): a non-randomised, open-label trial. *Lancet HIV*. 2015;2(8):e319–e327.

Schneider MD, Sarrazin C. Commentary: antiviral therapy of hepatitis C in 2014: do we need resistance testing? *Antivir Res*. 2014;105:64–71.

Sherman K. Management of the hepatitis B virus/HIV-coinfected patient. *Top Antivir Med*. 2015;23(3):111–114.

Shire N, Rouster S, Rajicic N, et al. Occult hepatitis B in HIV-infected patients. *J AIDS*. 2004;36(3):869–875.

Sulkowski M, Thomas D, Chaisson R, et al. Reactivation of hepatitis B virus replication accompanied by acute hepatitis in patients receiving highly active antiretroviral therapy. *Clin Infect Dis*. 2001;32(1):144–148.

Terrault N, Lok A, McMahon B, et al. Update on prevention, diagnosis, and treatment of chronic hepatitis B: AASLD 2018 hepatitis B guidance. *Hepatology*. 2018;67:1560–1599.

Thio C, Seaberg E, Skolasky R Jr, et al. HIV-1, hepatitis B virus, and risk of liver-related mortality in the Multicenter Cohort Study (MACS). *Lancet*. 2002;360(9349):1921–1926.

Thomas DL, Strathdee SA, Vlahov D. Long-term prognosis of hepatitis C virus Infection. *JAMA*. 2000;284(20):2592.

Thompson MA, Horberg MA, Agwu AL, et al. Primary care guidance for persons with human immunodeficiency virus: 2020 update by the HV Medicine Association of the Infectious Diseases Society of America. *Clin Infect Dis*. 2020;73(11)e3572–e3605.

Trickey A, McGinnis K, Gill MJ, et al. Longitudinal trends in causes of death among adults with HIV on antiretroviral therapy in Europe and North America from 1996 to 2020: a collaboration of cohort studies. *Lancet HIV*. 2024;11(3):e176–e185.

Wandeler G, Gsponer T, Bregenzer A, et al. Hepatitis C virus infections in the Swiss HIV Cohort Study: a rapidly evolving epidemic. *Clin Infect Dis*. 2012;55(10):1408–1416.

Weber R, Sabin CA, Friis-Moller N, et al. Liver-related deaths in persons infected with the human immunodeficiency virus: the D:A:D study. *Arch Intern Med*. 2006;166(15):1632–1641.

Zahnd C, Salazar-Vizcaya L, Dufour JF, et al. Modelling the impact of deferring HCV treatment on liver-related complications in HIV coinfected men who have sex with men. *J Hepatol*. 2016;65(1):26–32.

Zeuzem S, Foster GR, Wwang S, et al. Glecaprevir–pibrentasvir for 8 or 12 weeks in HCV genotype 1 or 3 infection. *N Engl J Med*. 2018;378(4):354.

37.

SEXUALLY TRANSMITTED INFECTIONS

Karen Vigil

LEARNING OBJECTIVE

Discuss the diagnosis and treatment of the most prevalent sexual transmitted infections (STIs) in people with HIV (PWH).

GENITAL ULCERS

In the United States, most young, sexually active patients who have genital, anal, or perianal ulcers have either genital herpes or syphilis, with herpes being the most prevalent. Less common causes include chancroid and donovanosis.

SYPHILIS

WHAT'S NEW?

- Since 2000, the incidence of syphilis has continued to increase, including a rise in cases of congenital syphilis. PWH and men who have sex with men (MSM) are the most affected groups.
- A new STI prevention intervention involving doxycycline taken soon after sexual exposures (i.e., DoxyPEP) is recommended for MSM, bisexual, and other men who have sex with men and transgender women with a history of at least one bacterial STI in the last 12 months.

KEY POINTS

- Syphilis incidence continues to increase and is more prevalent in PWH and MSM.
- Although clinical manifestations are generally similar to the general population, severity and complications may be more common in PWH.
- Special attention to neurologic site involvement is required, as neurosyphilis may be more common among PWH.
- Although cerebrospinal fluid (CSF) abnormalities are more likely in PWH with $CD4^{+}$ cell count ≤350 cells/mm^3 and rapid plasma regain (RPR) ≥1:32, lumbar puncture is only recommended if there are any signs or symptoms of neurologic involvement.
- Penicillin is the treatment of choice for syphilis; alternatives have not been well studied in PWH.

Syphilis is a systemic disease caused by *Treponema pallidum*. In 2022, there were 203,500 reported cases of syphilis, a 78% increase since 2017 (Centers for Disease Control and Prevention (CDC, 2024). Coinfection with HIV has been reported in as much as 50%–70% of MSM, with a high HIV seroconversion rate in patients with primary and secondary syphilis (Su and Weinstock, 2011).

PRIMARY SYPHILIS

Primary syphilis refers to the chancre: a single, painless lesion with a clean base and indurated, raised borders. Chancres appear 1 week to 1 month after exposure. They are usually in the genital area but can occur anywhere on the body, including the oral cavity (Figure 37.1).

SECONDARY SYPHILIS

Secondary syphilis is characterized by a maculopapular erythematous rash that may involve the palms and soles. It typically occurs 3 weeks to 3 months after exposure. In PWH, the rash could present in several other forms, including papulosquamous, vesicular, and pustular forms. Condyloma lata (broad-based, fleshy wart-like lesions that occur in moist, warm body areas) and lues maligna (pustular ulceronodular syphilides) are complications of secondary syphilis and are more frequent in PWH (Figure 37.2).

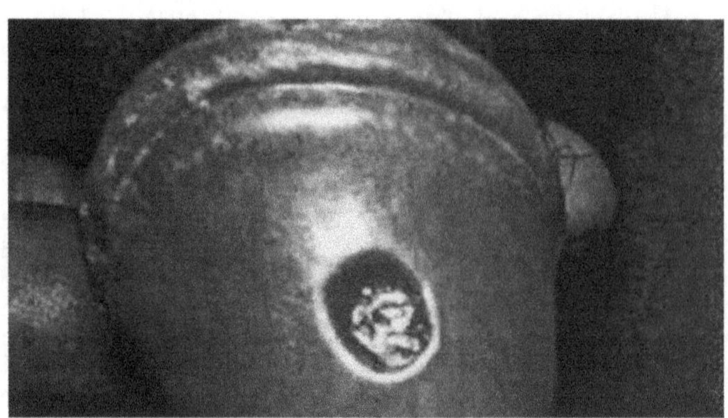

Figure 37.1 Primary stage syphilis sore (chancre) on glans of the penis. SOURCE: CDC Public Health Image Library. https://www.cdc.gov/syphilis/hcp/images/.

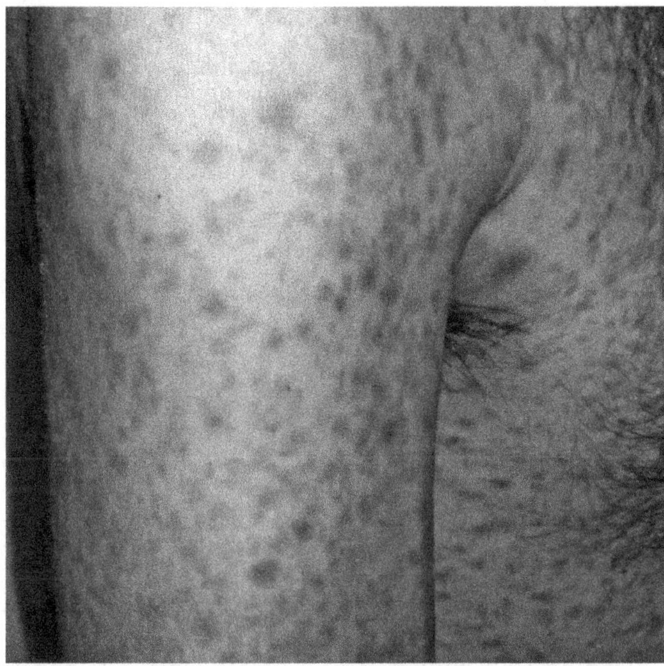

Figure 37.2 Secondary syphilis in male with HIV. SOURCE: Reproduced with permission from National HIV Curriculum (https://www.hiv.uw.edu).

LATENT SYPHILIS

Latent syphilis is defined by a positive serological test in the absence of any clinical signs or symptoms of syphilis. *Early latent syphilis* generally refers to infection acquired within the preceding year. All other forms are either late latent syphilis or latent syphilis of unknown duration. The importance of this classification relates to concerns regarding secondary transmission, which may be possible in any stage until early latent syphilis—it also determines duration of treatment.

NEUROSYPHILIS

Central nervous system (CNS) involvement may occur at any stage of syphilis. Cerebrospinal fluid (CSF) laboratory abnormalities are common in persons with early syphilis, even in the absence of neurologic signs or symptoms. No evidence exists to support variation from the recommended diagnosis and treatment for early syphilis for patients found to have such abnormalities. A CSF examination should be performed if clinical evidence of neurologic involvement is observed.

Uveitis (or other ocular syphilis manifestations) and hearing loss (or other otologic symptoms) can occur at any stage of syphilis and can be isolated or associated with neurosyphilis. Neurosyphilis can also present as CNS vasculitis. A lumbar puncture with CSF examination should be performed for anyone with cranial nerve dysfunction or neurologic symptoms, and may be considered in other scenarios (e.g., ocular symptoms and reactive syphilis serology but no ocular findings on ophthalmologic examination).

The 2021 Centers for Disease Control and Prevention (CDC) treatment guidelines (Workowski, 2021) recommend CSF examination:

- If there is evidence of neurologic symptoms
- If there are ophthalmologic or auditory signs or symptoms but examination is unrevealing
- In patients with clinical presentation of tertiary syphilis (e.g., aortitis or gumma)
- In patients with treatment failure.

CSF abnormalities are most likely in PWH with syphilis of any stage when $CD4^+$ cell count is ≤350 cells/mm^3 and a serum rapid plasma reagin titer is >1:32 (Libois et al., 2007; Marra et al., 2004). However, CSF examination has not been associated with improved clinical outcomes in the absence of neurologic signs and symptoms.

Other presentations of tertiary syphilis include cardiovascular syphilis and gummatous syphilis. Cases of rapid progression after initial infection have been reported with both entities (Maharajan and Sampath Kumaar, 2005; Weinert et al., 2008).

DIAGNOSIS

Primary chancre may be diagnosed by visualization of spirochetes under darkfield microscopic examination. This diagnostic test can only be performed from lesion exudate/tissue from anogenital and not oral lesions due to nonpathogenic spirochetes in the mouth.

Nontreponemal antigen tests (VDRL and RPR) detect antibodies to nonspecific antigens in the host after infection by *T. pallidum*. They become positive 4–6 weeks after infection or 1–3 weeks after the appearance of a primary lesion. Treponemal tests (TPHA, TPPA, and FTA-ABS) detect antibodies that react with *T. pallidum* antigens. They are confirmatory for syphilis.

The diagnosis of neurosyphilis in PWH is difficult since HIV itself causes CSF abnormalities. Classic CSF findings in neurosyphilis are lymphocytic pleocytosis, total protein elevation, and a positive VDRL test. However, it is important to note that CSF VDRL may be falsely negative in 30%–70% of cases of neurosyphilis.

TREATMENT

PWH who have early syphilis might be at increased risk for neurologic complications (Lee, 2007) and might have higher rates of serologic treatment failure with currently recommended regimens compared to people without HIV. No treatment regimens for syphilis have been demonstrated to be more effective in preventing neurosyphilis in PWH than regimens recommended for use in people without HIV (Rolfs et al., 1997). Careful and regular follow-up after therapy is essential. The recommended and alternative treatment regimens (including penicillin-allergic individuals) for syphilis in PWH are summarized in Table 37.1.

Table 37.1 RECOMMENDED AND ALTERNATIVE TREATMENT REGIMENS FOR SYPHILIS IN PWH

	RECOMMENDED REGIMEN	ALTERNATIVE REGIMEN (INCLUDING PENICILLIN-ALLERGIC PATIENTS)
Primary, secondary, and early latent syphilis	Benzathine penicillin G, 2.4 MU IM in a single dose	Doxycycline 100 mg orally twice daily for 14 days
Late latent syphilis or syphilis of unknown duration	Benzathine penicillin G, at weekly doses of 2.4 MU IM for 3 weeks	Doxycycline 100 mg orally twice daily for 28 days
Neurosyphilis	Aqueous crystalline penicillin G 18–24 MU/day, administered as 3–4 MU IV every 4 hours or continuous infusion, for 10–14 days	Procaine penicillin 2.4 MU IM once daily *plus* Probenecid 500 mg orally four times a day, both for 10–14 days

MU = million units; IM = intramuscularly; IV = intravenously.

FOLLOW-UP

PWH should be evaluated clinically and serologically for treatment failure at 3, 6, 9, 12, and 24 months after therapy. If an individual meets the criteria for treatment failure (signs or symptoms that persist or recur, or persons who have a sustained 4-fold increase in nontreponemal test titer), a lumbar puncture with CSF examination should be performed depending on sexual history or neurologic symptoms, and new treatment should be initiated. CSF examination and retreatment should be strongly considered for PWH whose nontreponemal test titers do not decrease 4-fold within 6–12 months of therapy. If the CSF examination is normal, treatment with benzathine penicillin G administered as 2.4 million units IM each at weekly intervals for 3 weeks is recommended.

PREVENTION

There is no current vaccine available to prevent syphilis. However, doxycycline taken as postexposure prophylaxis (DoxyPEP) is a recommended strategy for MSM, bisexual, and other men who have sex with men and transgender women with a history of at least one bacterial STI (syphilis, chlamydia, gonorrhea) in the last 12 months.

Findings from multiple large trials (see Table 37.2) support its use: DoxyPEP, DoxyVac, and IPERGAY found relative risk reductions in STIs, including syphilis, between 47%–66% (Luetkemeyer et al., 2023; Molina et al., 2024; and Molina et al., 2018). The only trial among cisgender women, performed in Kenya, did not find a significant decrease in bacterial STIs (Stewart et al., 2023). Appropriate drug levels as measured in hair samples were detected in only 29% of participants, suggesting that nonadherence might have played a role.

Recommended dosing is: oral doxycycline 200 mg taken as a single dose, ideally 24 hours after condomless sexual intercourse but no later than 72 hours. DoxyPEP should be prescribed along with education/counseling on additional strategies to prevent other STIs, such as immunizations (e.g., hepatitis B, human papillomavirus, mpox), condom use, and HIV pre- and postexposure prophylaxis (PrEP and PEP).

Table 37.2 RANDOMIZED CLINICAL TRIALS OF DOXYCYCLINE AS POST-EXPOSURE PROPHYLAXIS FOR SEXUALLY TRANSMITTED BACTERIAL INFECTIONS

STUDY NAME	N	POPULATION	STI RATE[1]		ABSOLUTE RISK REDUCTION
			DOXY PEP	NO DOXY PEP	
DoxyPeP USA[2]	327	MSM and transgender women taking PrEP	10.7% per quarter	31.9% per quarter	21.2% per quarter
DoxyPEP USA[2]	174	MSM and transgender women with HIV	11.8% per quarter	30.5% per quarter	18.7% per quarter
DoxyVac France[3]	502	MSM on PrEP	8.8 per 100 person-years	53.2 per 100 person-years	44 per 100 person-years
IPERGAY France[4]	232	MSM on PrEP	37.7 per 100 person years	69.7 per 100 person years	32 per 100 person years

[1] STI monitoring included syphilis, gonorrhea, and chlamydia for all studies except for DoxyVac, which included only syphilis and chlamydia.

[2] Luetkemeyer AF, et al., *N Engl J Med.* 2023;388(14):1296–1306.

[3] Molina JM, et al., *Lancet Infect Dis.* 2024;24(10):1093–1104.

[4] Molina JM, et al., *Lancet Infect Dis.* 2018;18(3):308–317.

GONORRHEA

WHAT'S NEW?

- The first isolate of multidrug-resistant *N. gonorrhoeae* (reduced susceptibility to ceftriaxone, cefixime, and azithromycin, and resistance to ciprofloxacin and penicillin) was reported in 2023 in the United States.

KEY POINTS

- Gonococcal infection remains a significant cause of urethritis, cervicitis, pharyngitis, and proctitis in sexually active PWH.
- Asymptomatic infection with gonorrhea is common at the female cervical site and male pharyngeal and rectal sites, such that routine periodic screening is required for detection.
- Nucleic acid–based testing offers high sensitivity and ease of sample collection. Patient-collected samples could be used if instructions have been provided.
- Currently recommended treatment for uncomplicated gonococcal infection is a single dose of intramuscular ceftriaxone 500 mg for people weighing <150 kg.

Gonorrhea is caused by *Neisseria gonorrhoeae*. In 2020, 677,769 cases of gonorrhea were reported to the CDC (2024)—this was a 45% increase from 2016. PWH are significantly more likely to have gonorrhea than people without HIV (Kent et al., 2005).

CLINICAL PRESENTATION

Acute urethritis is the main manifestation of gonorrhea. In men, urethral discharge—initially scant and later purulent—and dysuria are the major symptoms. The incubation period ranges from 1 to 10 days. Local complications include acute epididymitis, penile edema, penile lymphangitis, periurethral abscess, acute prostatitis, proctitis, seminal vesiculitis, infections of Tyson's and Cowper's glands, and pharyngitis. In women, gonorrhea presents as cervicitis and/or asymptomatic urethritis. Physical examination may show purulent or mucopurulent cervical, penile, or rectal exudates (Figure 37.3).

Disseminated gonococcal infection results from hematogenous dissemination of *Neisseria gonorrhoeae*. It can cause arthritis that primarily involves an asymmetric distribution in the knees, elbows, and more distal joints. A dermatitis picture with multiple discrete papules and pustules, often with a hemorrhagic component, could be present in approximately 75% of patients.

DIAGNOSIS

A gram stain of the urethral discharge reveals gram-negative diplococci in men during the first week after onset. This is less common in women. Although cultures are the gold standard for diagnosis, nucleic acid amplification tests (NAAT) in cervical swabs, urethral swabs, or urine have excellent sensitivity and specificity.

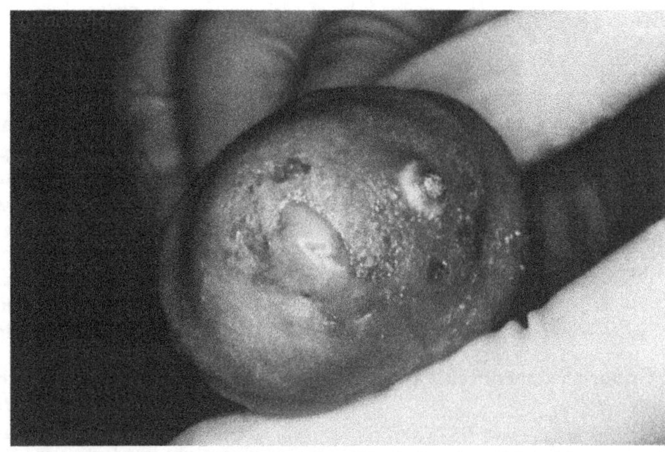

Figure 37.3 Male with a purulent penile discharge, due to gonorrhea, caused by the gram-negative bacterium, *Neisseria*. SOURCE: CDC Public Health Image Library. https://www.cdc.gov/syphilis/hcp/images/.

TREATMENT

Ceftriaxone is the standard of care for the treatment of gonorrhea. Quinolone-resistant *N. gonorrhoeae* strains are widely disseminated throughout the United States and worldwide. Treatment failure of oral cephalosporins has been reported in Asia, Europe, Africa, and Canada (Lewis et al., 2013; Unemo et al., 2012). Therefore, quinolones and oral cephalosporins are no longer recommended regimens for gonorrhea treatment in the United States. The recommended treatment regimens for gonorrhea infection in PWH are summarized in Table 37.3.

There are limited data on alternative treatment for people with cephalosporin or IgE-mediated penicillin allergy. Gentamicin 240 mg IM plus azithromycin 2 grams orally is the current recommended treatment. However, there are no data on the efficacy of this regimen to treat rectal or pharyngeal infections. Consultation with an infectious disease specialist is recommended (Kirkaldy et al., 2014).

FOLLOW-UP

If failure to ceftriaxone is suspected, culture and antimicrobial susceptibility are recommended to guide subsequent management.

CHLAMYDIA INFECTIONS

WHAT'S NEW?

- DoxyPEP is recommended for MSM, bisexual, and other men who have sex with men and transgender women with a history of at least one bacterial STI in the last 12 months.

Table 37.3 RECOMMENDED TREATMENT REGIMENS FOR GONORRHEA INFECTION IN PWH

	RECOMMENDED REGIMEN	ALTERNATIVE REGIMEN
Uncomplicated gonococcal infections of the pharynx, cervix, urethra, and rectum	**Ceftriaxone 500 mg IM as a single dose (for people who weigh <150 kg)** **Ceftriaxone 1 gram IM as a single dose (for people weighing 150 kg or more)**	**If cephalosporin allergy:** **Gentamicin 240 mg IM** ***plus*** **azithromycin 2 grams by mouth** **If ceftriaxone is not available:** **Cefixime 800 mg by mouth as single dose**
Disseminated gonococcal infection	**Ceftriaxone 1 gram IM or IV daily (duration varies and should be determined in consultation with specialist)**	—
Gonococcal meningitis and endocarditis	**Ceftriaxone 1–2 grams IV every 12 hours for 10–14 days for meningitis, and for at least 4 weeks for endocarditis**	—

IM = intramuscularly; IV = intravenously; PO = orally.

KEY POINTS

- Most *Chlamydia trachomatis* (CT) infections are asymptomatic and thus detected only by routine, periodic screening. Screening for CT is recommended for all sexually active PWH at exposed anatomic sites, at initial evaluation, and every 12 months thereafter, or more frequently as indicated by risk/exposure history.
- Nucleic acid–based testing offers high sensitivity, ease of sample collection, and use of noninvasively acquired specimens. Self-collected vaginal, meatal, and rectal swabs have comparable performance as provider-collected samples.
- Rectal CT infection is especially common among MSM; in this population, the CT subtypes that cause lymphogranuloma venereum (LGV) should be included in the differential diagnosis of those with severe symptoms of proctitis, especially when CT is found to be the cause.
- The treatment of choice for chlamydial infections is doxycycline 100 mg orally twice daily for 7 days. In patients with proctitis accompanied by bloody discharge, perianal or mucosal ulcers, and/or tenesmus, treatment may be extended for 21 days.

Chlamydia is the most commonly reported STI in the United States among men and women. In 2020, a total of 1.6 million cases of chlamydia were reported to the CDC (2024). However, underreporting might be substantial as the disease may be asymptomatic. Chlamydia infection is more frequent in younger age groups, racial/ethnic minority groups, MSM, and incarcerated populations (Burstein et al., 1998; Rietmeijer et al., 2008; Satterwhite et al., 2008). Genital and ocular chlamydial infection are caused by serotypes D to K, while serotypes L1, L2, and L3 cause lymphogranuloma venereum.

CLINICAL PRESENTATION

Chlamydia genital infection secondary to serotypes D to K could be asymptomatic or present as pharyngitis, urethritis, cervicitis, epididymitis, prostatitis, or proctitis. Pelvic inflammatory disease, perihepatitis, and infertility are long-term complications.

Serovars L1–L3 cause lymphogranuloma venereum (LGV). LGV is not endemic in the United States. Southeast Asia, the Caribbean, Latin America, and Africa are areas of more prevalence. It presents as one or more genital ulcers or papules, followed by the development of unilateral or bilateral fluctuant inguinal lymphadenopathy called buboes. Since 2003, there have been reports of outbreaks in Western Europe and in the United States of Chlamydia L2 serotype proctitis, particularly in MSM.

DIAGNOSIS

NAAT for chlamydia genital infections (by polymerase chain reaction assay or transcription-mediated amplification) is highly sensitive and specific. It can be performed on first catch urine (without the requirement of a urethral swab) as well as vaginal and rectal swabs. All sexually active women aged <25 years should be screened for chlamydia annually. Men and women who reported anal sex should also have anal swabs every year. Routine oropharyngeal screening is not recommended, but it is usually performed when screening for gonorrhea. If chlamydia is present, it should be treated similarly to other presentations.

The diagnosis of LGV is challenging. Cell culture is the only diagnostic test approved by the U.S. Food and Drug Administration, although LGV-specific molecular testing (if available) may be utilized. Serology may help with diagnosis, as titers are typically elevated during presentation. Diagnosis of LGV proctitis is even more difficult. NAAT may be used if a local laboratory has validated them. The CDC recommends that when LGV is suspected, providers should collect a specimen and send the sample to the state health department for referral to the CDC. If this is not possible, an antibiotic regimen effective against LGV should be included in empiric treatment for proctitis.

TREATMENT

The treatment of choice for chlamydia infection is doxycycline 100 mg twice a day for 7 days and 21 days for LGV. If symptoms include proctitis with bloody discharge, perianal or mucosal ulcers, or tenesmus, treatment should be extended to 21 days.

HUMAN PAPILLOMA VIRUS (HPV)

WHAT'S NEW?

Gardasil-9, a nine-valent vaccine that targets HPV types 6, 11, 16, 18, 31, 33, 45, 52, and 58, is currently the only HPV vaccine distributed in the United States. A complete three-dose series is recommended for people through age 26. PWH between the ages of 27 and 45 years might benefit from HPV vaccination and should engage in individualized discussion and collaborative decision-making with their providers.

KEY POINTS

- HPV is the most common STI in the United States. More than 200 HPV types have been identified; however, only certain strains are associated with warts and others with intraepithelial lesions and high-grade neoplasia.
- PWH have higher rates of HPV-related lesions; genital warts can be more aggressive and challenging to eradicate.

HPV is a double-stranded DNA virus that may infect the genital tract. There are over 200 types of HPV; more than 40 may infect the genital area. HPV may cause two major clinical syndromes: genital warts (condyloma acuminata) associated mainly with types 6 and 11; and epithelial cervical or anal neoplasia linked to serotypes 16 and 18 (for more information on cervical and anal neoplasia, refer to Chapter 25, "Malignancies in HIV").

HPV detection is significantly more common among PWH (Mbulawa et al., 2009), possibly due to differences in assessment and screening practices. Several studies have demonstrated that HPV increases the risk of HIV acquisition (Smith et al., 2010).

CLINICAL PRESENTATION

In most cases, HPV infection is transient, has no clinical manifestation or sequelae, and is self-limited. Genital warts typically present as single or multiple soft, fleshy, papillary or sessile, painless keratinized growths in the vulvovaginal area, penis, anus, urethra, or perineum (Figures 37.4 and 37.5). Women with HIV have a higher prevalence of genital warts, Pap smear–detected abnormalities, dysplasia, and progression to cervical cancer compared to women without HIV.

DIAGNOSIS

The diagnosis of warts is made clinically; laboratory confirmation is not typically needed. However, if the diagnosis is uncertain, a biopsy could be performed. PWH, especially MSM, have a significantly increased risk of anal cancer due to oncogenic human papillomavirus types; therefore, routine anal cytology screening in HIV care settings is recommended.

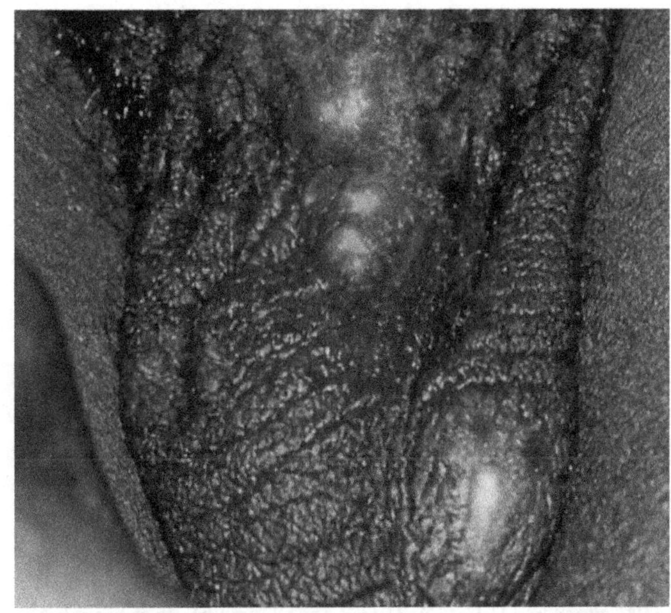

Figure 37.4 Multiple ulcerated HSV lesions on the scrotum of a man with HIV and $CD4^+$ cell count less than 50 cells/mm^3. SOURCE: Reproduced with permission from National HIV Curriculum (https://www.hiv.uw.edu).

Treatment of high-grade anal squamous intraepithelial lesions, rather than active monitoring, has been found to lower the risk of developing anal cancer (Palefsky et al., 2022).

TREATMENT

The main indications for treatment of vulvovaginal warts are bothersome symptoms and/or psychological distress. Vulvar biopsy to exclude precancerous or cancerous lesions is indicated when warts are identified in immunocompromised or postmenopausal women, when the lesions are visually atypical, or when warts fail to respond to standard therapy. The recommended treatment regimens for HPV in PWH are summarized in Table 37.4.

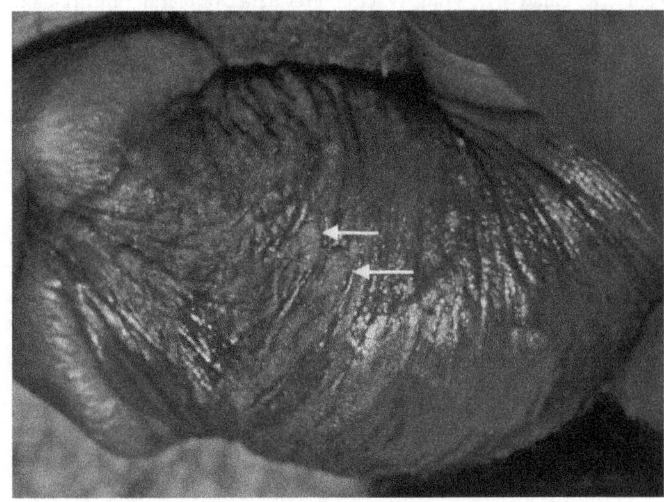

Figure 37.5 Multiple warts on shaft of penis in man with HIV. SOURCE: Reproduced with permission from National HIV Curriculum (https://www.hiv.uw.edu).

Table 37.4 **RECOMMENDED TREATMENT REGIMENS FOR HPV/WARTS IN PWH**

External genital warts, patient-applied	**Podofilox 0.5% solution or gel** *or* **Imiquimod 5% cream** *or* **Sinecatechins 15% ointment**
External genital warts, vaginal warts or anal warts, provider-administered	**Cryotherapy** *or* **Trichloroacetic acid (TCA) or bichloroacetic acid (BCA) 80%–90%** *or* **Surgical removal**

PREVENTION

Gardasil-9, a nine-valent vaccine that prevents infection with HPV types 6, 11, 16, 18, 31, 33, 45, 52, and 58, is currently the only available vaccine available in the United States.

Routine vaccination is recommended for boys and girls aged 11–12 years old, and catch-up vaccination for adults until the age of 26 years (Meites et al., 2019). Gardasil-9 is approved for use up to age 45 years. Although people over 26 may have been exposed to different HPV types, some could still be at risk of ongoing HPV infection and might benefit from immunization. Therefore, for people aged 27 through 45 years, the decision to vaccinate should be made on an individual basis.

REFERENCES

Burstein GR, Waterfield G, Joffe A, et al. Screening for gonorrhea and chlamydia by DNA amplification in adolescents attending middle school health centers: opportunity for early intervention. *Sex Transm Dis*. 1998;25:395–402. doi:10.1097/00007435-199809000-00001

Center for Disease Control and Prevention (CDC). Sexual transmitted diseases surveillance, 2022. https://www.cdc.gov/std/statistics/2022/default.htm. Published January 2024. Accessed July 14, 2024.

Kent CK, Chaw JK, Wong W, et al. Prevalence of rectal, urethral, and pharyngeal chlamydia and gonorrhea detected in 2 clinical settings among men who have sex with men: San Francisco, California, 2003. *Clin Infect Dis*. 2005;41:67–74.

Lee M, Aynalem G, Kerndt P, et al. Symptomatic early neurosyphilis among HIV-positive men who have sex with men: four cities, United States, January 2002–June 2004. *MMWR*. 2007;56:625–628.

Lewis DA, Sriruttan C, Muller EE, et al. Phenotypic and genetic characterization of the first two cases of extended-spectrum-cephalosporin-resistant Neisseria gonorrhoeae infection in South Africa and association with cefixime treatment failure. *J Antimicrob Chemother*. 2013;68:1267–1270.

Libois A, De Wit S, Poll B, et al. HIV and syphilis: when to perform a lumbar puncture. *Sex Transm Dis*. 2007;34:141–144.

Luetkemeyer AF, Donnell D, Dombrowski JC, et al. Postexposure doxycycline to prevent bacterial sexually transmitted infections. *N Engl J Med*. 2023;388(14):1296–1306.

Maharajan M, GS K. Cardiovascular syphilis in HIV infection: a case-control study at the Institute of Sexually Transmitted Diseases, Chennai, India. *Sex Transm Infect*. 2005;81:361.

Marra CM, Maxwell CL, Smith SL, et al. Cerebrospinal fluid abnormalities in patients with syphilis: association with clinical and laboratory features. *J Infect Dis*. 2004;189:369–376.

Mbulawa ZZ, Coetzee D, Marais DJ, et al. Genital human papillomavirus prevalence and human papillomavirus concordance in heterosexual couples are positively associated with human immunodeficiency virus coinfection. *J Infect Dis*. 2009;199:1514.

Meites E, Szilagyi PG, Chesson HW, et al. Human papillomavirus vaccination for adults: updated recommendations of the Advisory Committee on Immunization Practices. *MMWR*. 2019;68:698–702.

Molina JM, Bercot B, Assoumou L, et al. Doxycycline prophylaxis and meningococcal group B vaccine to prevent bacterial sexually transmitted infections I France (ANRS 174 DOXYVAC): a multicentre, open-label, randomized trial with a 2x2 factorial design. *Lancet Infect Dis*. 2024;24(10):1093–1104. doi:10.1016/S1473-3099(24)00236-6

Molina JM, Charreau I, Chidiac C, et al. Post-exposure prophylaxis with doxycycline to prevent sexually transmitted infections in men who have sex with men: an open-label randomized substudy of the aNRS IPERGAY trial. *Lancet Infect Dis*. 2018;18(3):308–317.

Palefsky JM, Lee JY, Jay N, et al. Treatment of anal high-grade squamous intraepithelial lesions to prevent anal cancer. *N Engl J Med*. 2022;386:2273–2282.

Rietmeijer CA, Hopkins E, Geisler WM, Orr DP, Kent CK. Chlamydia trachomatis positivity rates among men tested in selected venues in the United States: a review of the recent literature. *Sex Transm Dis*. 2008;35:S8.

Rolfs RT, Joesoef MR, Hendershot EF, et al. A randomized trial of enhanced therapy for early syphilis in patients with and without human immunodeficiency virus infection. The Syphilis and HIV Study Group. *N Engl J Med*. 1997;337:307–314.

Satterwhite CL, Joesoef MR, Datta SD, Weinstock H. Estimates of Chlamydia trachomatis infections among men: United States. *Sex Transm Dis*. 2008;35:S3.

Smith JS, Moses S, Hudgens MG, et al. Increased risk of HIV acquisition among Kenyan men with human papillomavirus infection. *J Infect Dis*. 2010;201:1677.

Stewart J, Oware K, Donnell D, et al.; dPEP Kenya Study Team. Doxycycline prophylaxis to prevent sexually transmitted infections in women. *N Engl J Med*. 2023;389:2331–2340.

Su JR, Weinstock H. Epidemiology of coinfection with HIV and syphilis in 34 states, United States—2009. Proceedings of the 2011 National HIV Prevention Conference. Atlanta, GA; August 13–17, 2011.

Unemo M, Golparian D, Nicholas R, et al. High-level cefixime- and ceftriaxone-resistant Neisseria gonorrhoeae in France: novel penA mosaic allele in a successful international clone causes treatment failure. *Antimicrob Agents Chemother*. 2012;56:1273–1280.

Weinert LS, Scheffel RS, Zoratto G, et al. Cerebral syphilitic gumma in HIV-infected patients: case report and review. *Int J STD AIDS*. 2008;19:62.

Workowski KA, Bachman LH, Chan PA. Sexually transmitted infections treatment guidelines, 2021. *MMWR Recomm Rep*. 2021;70:1–187.

38.

LEGAL ISSUES

Anna Kastner

ISSUES IN DISCLOSURE

LEARNING OBJECTIVE

- Discuss the healthcare provider's legal responsibilities to maintain confidentiality of patient information and make exceptions when disclosure is permitted.

WHAT'S NEW?

- Information regarding disclosure issues has remained consistent during the past several years.

KEY POINTS

- Healthcare providers have an obligation to maintain patient confidentiality.
- HIV disclosure could result in the risk of harm or criminalization for the person living with HIV.
- Healthcare providers should consult an attorney or their state laws and regulations before making any disclosures.

Information disclosed by a patient to a healthcare provider during the course of the provider–patient relationship is considered confidential. This confidentiality is essential for full and free disclosure of information so that effective counseling and therapy can be provided. Confidentiality also makes it more likely that patients will get tested for HIV and engage in care—key strategies of the federal Ending the HIV Epidemic in the U.S. initiative. In general, unless required by the law to do so, a healthcare provider is ethically barred from revealing confidential communications or information without the patient's consent.

Generally, a provider's obligation to disclose a patient's HIV status to a third party extends only to a state or local health department pursuant to state law. The health department is required to share certain information with the Centers for Disease Control and Prevention (CDC) and may also engage in partner notification or other outreach to third parties who may have been exposed to HIV. In California, Indiana, and Nebraska, providers are required to report "suspected cases" to the local health department but are not required to notify third parties who may have been exposed directly. Generally, the role of the health department is to engage in partner notification, rather than the treating provider (CDC, 2021). Partner notification has "been viewed with cautious apprehension" by advocates and people living with HIV based on concerns around confidentiality, risk of violence and criminalization, and the way that these harms are disproportionately experienced by immigrants, people of color, the LGBTQ+ community, women, people who use drugs, and sex workers (Ayala et al., 2019).

Although providers may believe that they have a "duty to warn" third parties who may have been exposed to HIV, no jurisdiction mandates this type of disclosure, and some jurisdictions explicitly prohibit this type of disclosure. For example, in Pennsylvania, Act 148 limits the sharing of HIV-related information that is obtained in the course of providing medical or social services and does not permit disclosure to a third party without written consent. This law also imposes civil liability if confidentiality is violated. Massachusetts law contains similar provisions (Massachusetts General Laws, c. 111, §70F). Even in states that do not have HIV-specific confidentiality laws, courts have held that physicians have no duty to third parties who may have been exposed to HIV by their patients (see *Santa Rosa Health Care Corporation v. Garcia*, Supreme Court of Texas, March 13, 1998).

Providers should also be aware of the ethical obligations imposed by the American Medical Association (AMA) guidelines. According to the report of the AMA, Council on Ethical and Judicial Affairs, "physicians should always consider their ethical obligations to maintain confidentiality when facing a legal requirement to disclose, and should provide the minimum information that is required by law" (AMA, 1983). This includes responding to subpoenas and providing information to state and local health departments pursuant to state law. The AMA guidelines also acknowledge that providers can advise patients on how to prevent HIV transmission but may not notify third parties about a significant threat of exposure unless specifically authorized under state law (AMA Code of Medical Ethics, 8.1, *Routine Universal Screening for HIV*). When a disclosure is made, practitioners should: "(a) restrict disclosure to the minimum necessary information; and (b) notify the patient of the disclosure, when feasible" (AMA Code of Medical Ethics, 3.2.1 *Confidentiality*, 2022).

These ethical guidelines should be considered in light of recent bio-medical advances which have ensured that virally suppressed people cannot transmit HIV through sexual contact and which empower seronegative people to have agency over their own sexual health through the use of pre- and postexposure prophylaxis (PrEP and PEP). At least one ethical decision-making model has been updated to reflect these advances and advises that HIV disclosure should never be made to consensual sexual partners (Chenneville and Gabbidon, 2020).

Healthcare providers should also consider their patient's individual situation, including issues that could put a patient at risk of harm if their HIV status is disclosed. One study has found that 24% of women living with HIV were subjected to intimate partner violence after disclosing their status to a partner (Sullivan, 2019). Additionally, disclosure could result in criminalization, as discussed in the subsequent section.

Making an unlawful disclosure could subject a provider to tort liability for unlawfully revealing confidential information. Given the legal implications of divulging a person's HIV status, healthcare providers should consult an attorney or become familiar with state laws and regulations before making any such disclosures.

PERINATAL/ADOLESCENT HIV DISCLOSURE

Complex disclosure challenges may arise during the peri/neonatal period. Local, regional, and national laws should be consulted in determining disclosure and privacy laws as they apply to the peri/neonatal period. Likewise, disclosure of HIV status to young children or adolescents is a uniquely difficult challenge. HIV status disclosure to children is quite low in sub-Saharan Africa. This may be due to several factors, including parents'/caregivers' fear of the child disclosing status to others, a lack of knowledge on how to make the disclosure, and the assessment of whether the child can cope with the psychological impact of diagnosis (Doat et al., 2019).

The World Health Organization (WHO) recommends disclosing HIV status between 6 and 12 years of age, and the American Academy of Pediatrics recommends that children are informed at "school age." The WHO guidance notes that healthcare workers are often without the support of definitive, evidence-based policies and guidelines on when, how, and under what conditions children should be informed about their own or their caregivers' HIV status (Krauss et al., 2011).

DISCLOSURE TO CHILDREN OF THEIR OWN HIV STATUS

Key conclusions of the WHO Guideline on HIV disclosure counseling for children up to 12 years of age include:

- There is evidence of health benefit (e.g., reduced risk of death) and little evidence of psychological or emotional harm from disclosure of HIV status to children with HIV. Immediate emotional reactions dissipate with time and respond to program interventions.
- Disclosure of diagnosis, as described by published researchers and by practitioners, is not an isolated event, but rather a step in the process of adjustment by the child, caregivers, and the community to an illness and the life challenges that it poses.

DISCLOSURE TO CHILDREN OF THEIR PARENTS' OR CAREGIVERS' HIV STATUS

- There is evidence of benefit to health for children (regardless of their HIV status) of caregivers with HIV if the caregiver discloses to them.
- The concerns of some caregivers that disclosure leads to increased behavioral problems in children and decreases in the quality of the relationship are not supported by children's reports about their reactions to disclosure of their caregivers' HIV status. Even by parents' reports, anticipating and preparing for the understandable initial emotional reactions can improve the child's responses, and responses improve with time. Healthcare workers are often without the support of definitive, evidence-based policies and guidelines on when, how, and under what conditions children should be informed about their own or their caregivers' HIV status.
- There appears to be no harm to caregivers when they disclose their status to their children or wards.

Considering that virally suppressed people do not transmit HIV and that interrupting the transmission cycle is critical to ending the HIV epidemic, Budhwani and colleagues examined the relationship between age of disclosure and viral load suppression by evaluating data from a pediatric HIV clinic in the southern United States. Records from cases of perinatal transmission seen between 2008 and 2018 were analyzed ($n = 61$). The preliminary findings suggest that disclosing HIV status between 10 and 12 years of age may promote viral suppression through medication adherence (Budhwani et al., 2020).

RECOMMENDED READING

American Medical Association. Code of medical ethics. https://code-medical-ethics.ama-assn.org/opinions. n.d. Accessed July 10, 2024.

American Medical Association Council on Ethical and Judicial Affairs. Report 4-I-06. https://code-medical-ethics.ama-assn.org/sites/amacoedb/files/2022-08/3.2.1%20Confidentiality%20--%20background%20reports.pdf. Published December 7, 1983. Accessed July 15, 2024.

Budhwani H, Mills L, Marefka LEB, et al. Preliminary study on HIV status disclosure to perinatal infected children: retrospective analysis of administrative records from a pediatric HIV clinic in the southern United States. *BMC Res Notes*. 2020;13:253.

Centers for Disease Control and Prevention. Sexually transmitted infections (STIs), duty to warn. https://www.cdc.gov/std/treatment/duty-to-warn.htm. Updated April 13, 2021. Accessed July 8, 2024.

Krauss B, Letteney S, de Baets A, Murugi J, Okero FA. *Guideline on HIV Disclosure Counselling for Children up to 12 Years of Age*. Geneva: World Health Organization; 2011. https://apps.who.int/iris/bitstream/handle/10665/44777/9789241502863_eng.pdf;jsessionid=27A6CA8DA056F1823129425B95692717?sequence=1. Accessed July 12, 2024.

HIV CRIMINALIZATION

LEARNING OBJECTIVE

- Describe the scope and consequences of HIV criminalization laws as well as efforts to repeal or modernize these laws.

WHAT'S NEW?

- States continue to modify their HIV criminalization statutes in keeping with advancements in treatment and prevention, although many states still have outdated laws on the books.
- Recent studies in states ranging from Ohio to Mississippi to Maryland have shown that HIV criminalization laws disproportionately impact marginalized groups living with HIV, including people of color, the LGBTQ+ community, women, and sex workers.

KEY POINTS

- HIV criminalization laws were enacted early in the HIV epidemic and often do not reflect current medical advances in HIV treatment and prevention.
- Providers should advise patients about the applicable HIV criminal laws in their state.
- Providers should be wary of requests by law enforcement for medical records and other protected health information.
- People living with HIV may consider bringing sexual partners to a medical appointment to have a provider document that they have disclosed their HIV diagnosis to their partner and to discuss prevention measures.

HIV criminalization is when people living with HIV are criminalized for conduct that would not be a crime or would be a less serious crime but for a person's HIV status. This includes criminal statutes that explicitly mention HIV, such as failing to disclose HIV status to sexual or needle-sharing partners, felony sentencing enhancement for prostitution charges, and charges for "exposure" to bodily fluids, as well as prosecutions that occur under generally applicable laws such as attempted murder, aggravated assault, or reckless endangerment. Initial funding in 1990 of the Ryan White Comprehensive AIDS Resources Emergency Act was contingent on states being able to prosecute individuals who knowingly exposed others to HIV (Mermin et al., 2021). In response, many states created new criminal statutes that specifically criminalized people with HIV.

As of 2024, 35 states still have laws that criminalize people with HIV for conduct that would not otherwise be a crime or provide sentencing enhancements for people with HIV. Five of these states require people convicted of certain HIV-related crimes to register as sex offenders. The laws for the 50 states and the District of Columbia were assessed and categorized by the CDC into four categories.

1. HIV-specific laws that criminalize or control behaviors that can potentially expose another person to HIV
2. Sexually transmitted infection (STI) and communicable, contagious, infectious disease (STI/communicable/infectious disease-specific) laws that criminalize or control behaviors that can potentially expose another person to STIs/communicable/infectious diseases. This might include HIV.
3. Sentence enhancement laws specific to HIV or STIs that do not criminalize a behavior but increase the sentence length when a person with HIV commits certain crimes
4. No specific criminalization laws.

These laws are not based on science and often apply even if HIV transmission does not occur or would be unlikely, for example in cases involving exposure to saliva. Typically, these laws also do not require proof of intent to transmit HIV. Most laws were passed before studies showed that ART reduces HIV transmission risk, and most laws do not account for HIV prevention measures that reduce transmission risk, such as condom use, ART, and PrEP.

Punishing people for behavior that is either consensual or poses no risk of HIV transmission only serves to further stigmatize already marginalized communities while missing opportunities for prevention education. The potential stigma associated with HIV criminalization laws was seen in a national study of men who have sex with men (MSM) in 2017 which found that Black MSM in states with HIV criminalization laws were more likely to report community discrimination against PWH than Black MSM in states without such laws (aPR 1.14; 95% CI: 1.02–1.29; $p = 0.02$) and intolerance toward MSM (aPR 2.02; 95% CI: 1.43–2.86; $p < 0.001$) (Baugher et al., 2021). The Williams Institute at UCLA School of Law has studied the impact of HIV criminalization laws across the country and released a report in 2024 showing that these laws are disproportionately used to criminalize women, people of color, LGBTQ+ people, and sex workers (Cisneros et al., 2024).

HIV criminalization laws also disincentivize HIV testing and engagement in care because, typically, the laws only apply if a person knows that they are living with HIV. A national survey of people living with HIV found that 69% of people surveyed believed that "laws that criminalize HIV non-disclosure, exposure and/or transmission undermine public health efforts." Respondents "who viewed public health professionals as caring more about enforcing laws that criminalize HIV transmission than about health were more than 6 times more likely to limit what they tell health care providers" (SERO Project, 2021). Additionally, these laws do not reduce HIV transmission rates. A 2017 study showed no association between HIV nor AIDS diagnosis rate and HIV criminalization laws across states, highlighting the limited efficacy of these laws in improving HIV prevention or detection (Sweeney et al., 2017). A response to the Sweeney study found that states that criminalize HIV exposure "are associated with lower proportion of HIV diagnosis and increased HIV prevalence." This suggests that these laws may exacerbate the HIV epidemic (Sah et al., 2017).

These cases highlight the tension between public health and criminal justice approaches toward disclosure and HIV transmission (Obermeyer et al, 2011). They also present an opportunity for providers to serve as expert witnesses in legal proceedings and advocate for legal reform by becoming involved with local reform coalitions and educating stakeholders, including through testimony at legislative hearings or other public bodies. "Physicians have an ethical responsibility to seek change when they believe the requirements of law or policy are contrary to the best interests of patients," as long as "the health of patients is not jeopardized and that patient care is not compromised" (AMA Code of Medical Ethics 1.2.10, *Political Action by Physicians* and 9.025, *Advocacy for Change in Law and Policy*).

National organizations and the federal government have recognized the need to update HIV criminalization laws to be consistent with current science and need for personal protection of PWH. The American Academy of HIV Medicine (AAHIVM) and its members are "opposed to laws that distinguish HIV disease from other comparable diseases or that create disproportionate penalties for disclosure, exposure, or transmission of HIV disease beyond normal public health ordinances." The AAHIVM "supports nonpunitive prevention approaches to HIV centered on current scientific understanding and evidence-based research" (AAHIVM, n.d.). The HIV Medicine Association (HIVMA) also "strongly oppose laws that criminalize transmission or non-disclosure of HIV status and other infectious diseases because of the harmful effect these laws have on individual and public health." In 2018, 20 leading HIV experts across the globe published the Expert Consensus Statement on the Science of HIV in the Context of Criminal Law, which outlines the current science regarding HIV transmission, treatment and phylogenetic analysis and "encourage[s] governments and those working in legal and judicial systems to pay close attention to the significant advances in HIV science that have occurred over the last three decades to ensure current scientific knowledge informs application of the law in cases related to HIV" (Barre-Sinoussi et al., 2018).

In the United States, the National HIV/AIDS Strategy was updated in 2021 and identifies goals for 2022–2025, which includes Goal 3.1.1:

> Strengthen enforcement of civil rights laws (including language access services and disability rights), promote reform of state HIV criminalization laws, and assist states in protecting people with HIV from violence, retaliation, and discrimination associated with HIV status, homophobia, transphobia, xenophobia, racism, substance use, and sexism.

The SERO Project is a network of PWH and their allies fighting for freedom from stigma and injustice. The SERO Project is particularly focused on ending inappropriate criminal prosecutions of people living with HIV, including for nondisclosure of their HIV status and potential or perceived HIV exposure or HIV transmission. The SERO Project is a member organization of the U.S. People Living with HIV (PLHIV) Caucus, which published *Demanding Better: An HIV Federal Policy Agenda by People Living with HIV* (US PLHIV Caucus, 2022), which lays out a road map to improve the quality of life for people living with HIV, including addressing stigma, creating a moratorium on molecular HIV surveillance, and decriminalizing HIV.

The CDC notes that since 2014, at least 12 states have modernized their HIV criminal laws: California, Colorado, Georgia, Illinois, Iowa, Michigan, Missouri, Nevada, New Jersey, North Carolina, Virginia, and Washington. Changes include removing the sex offender registry as a requirement of conviction, requiring intent to transmit, actual HIV transmission, or providing defenses for taking measures to prevent transmission such as viral suppression, condom use, and partner PrEP use.

RECOMMENDED READING

American Academy of HIV Medicine. HIV criminalization. https://aahivm.org/hiv-criminalization/. n.d. Accessed July 12, 2024.

Barre-Sinoussi F, Bekker L, Beyrer C, et al. Expert consensus statement on the science of HIV in the context of criminal law. *J Intl AIDS Soc.* 2018 Jul 25;21(7):e25161. doi:10.1002/jia2.25161

Center for HIV Law and Policy. HIV criminalization in the United States: a sourcebook on state and federal HIV criminal law and practice. http://www.hivlawandpolicy.org/sourcebook. 2024. Accessed July 8, 2024.

Mermin J, Valentine SS, McCray E. HIV criminalisation laws and ending the US HIV epidemic. *Lancet HIV.* 2021;8(1):e4–e6.

TREATING MINORS

LEARNING OBJECTIVE

- Describe legal issues related to the treatment of minors with HIV.

WHAT'S NEW?

- Information regarding the treatment of minors has remained consistent during the past several years.

KEY POINTS

- Although medical treatment of minors (persons younger than age 18 years) must generally be authorized by a parent or legal guardian, all 50 states have some exceptions that may allow minors to consent to STI testing and treatment.
- This area of law is often complex and variable. Healthcare providers unsure of their state laws and regulations should seek legal advice before treating minors for HIV.
- Providers should be aware of existing confidentiality requirements as well as the risk of inadvertent disclosure by insurance companies.

The medical care of a *minor*—defined in most states as a person younger than age 18 years—must generally be authorized by their parent or legal guardian. This usually means that a parent or guardian of a minor is required to give informed consent on behalf of the minor for most medical decisions. However, there are exceptions to this rule, and certain minors can consent to certain types of medical care without the authority of a parent or legal guardian.

CONSENT FOR STI SERVICES AND MEDICAL TREATMENT

All 50 states and the District of Columbia explicitly allow minors to consent to STI services, although 11 states require that a minor be of a certain age (generally age 12–14 years) before being allowed to consent. Thirty-two states explicitly include HIV testing and treatment in the package of STI services to which minors may consent (Guttmacher Institute, 2023). Depending on interpretation of state law, access to PrEP may also fall under STI services to which a minor can consent.

EXCEPTIONS

Almost all states have laws that authorize minors who have attained a certain status to make the majority of their own healthcare decisions. These may include minors who are married (or divorced), on active duty with the U.S. Armed Forces, emancipated by a court order, or self-sufficient such that they have attained a designated age and live away from home and manage their own financial affairs.

LAWS RELATED TO INFORMING PARENTS

Eighteen states allow healthcare providers to inform a minor's parents that he, she, or they are seeking or receiving STI services. With the exception of one state (Iowa requires that parents or guardians be notified in the case of a positive HIV test), no state requires that providers notify parents (Guttmacher Institute, 2023). In some states, healthcare providers are prohibited from telling the minor's parent(s) or legal guardian about any test-related medical care unless the minor authorizes it (e.g., see New York State Public Health Law 2785).

Providers should be aware that minors and young adults who are covered by their parents' insurance plans may lose confidentiality if their insurance company sends the parent or policy holder an Explanation of Benefits (EOB) for the treatment that the child or young adult is receiving. Fourteen states have various provisions designed to protect the confidentiality of dependents on insurance plans, and four states have specific protections for minors seeking STI treatment (Guttmacher Institute, 2023). In other jurisdictions, a patient can seek to have an EOB suppressed, but there is no guarantee that an insurance company will honor this request. Protecting the confidentiality of minors is especially important, as these disclosures could result in parents or guardians rejecting a child based on a belief about the child's gender identity, sexual orientation, or sexual activity (Nelson et al., 2023).

SEEKING LEGAL ADVICE

Healthcare providers should be aware that care of minors is an area of the law that is very complex, highly variable by state, and rife with legal risks and exposure if an incorrect decision regarding treatment is made. Therefore, it is highly advisable that healthcare providers who are unsure of the law in their state consult a lawyer before providing HIV testing or treatment to a minor. Healthcare providers must be acutely aware of the importance of consulting and obtaining the informed consent of a parent or legal guardian of the minor when required by law.

REFERENCES/RECOMMENDED READING

Centers for Disease Control and Prevention (CDC). State laws that enable a minor to provide informed consent to receive HIV and STD services. https://www.cdc.gov/hiv/policies/law/states/minors.html. Published October 25, 2022. Accessed July 9, 2024.

Kaiser Foundation. Minors' authority to consent to sexually transmitted infection (STI) services. http://kff.org/hivaids/state-indicator/minors-right-to-consent. Published September 1, 2023. Accessed July 9, 2024.

Nelson K, Skinner A, Stout C, et al. Minor consent laws for sexually transmitted infection and human immunodeficiency virus services in the United States: a comprehensive, longitudinal survey of US state laws. *Am J Public Health*. 2023;113(4):397–407.

ADVANCE PLANNING

LEARNING OBJECTIVE

- Discuss the use of durable power of attorney, advance directives, and physician orders for life-sustaining treatment for PWH.

WHAT'S NEW?

- By 2030, 70% of people living with HIV will be age 50 or older. In 2024, the regulations for the Older Americans Act defining "greatest social need" were updated to add older people living with HIV and older LGBTQ+ people to this category. This affects all levels of Older Americans Act policy, funding and planning (Administration for Community Living, 2024).

KEY POINTS

- Many people living with HIV may not have engaged in end-of-life planning, including creating a will, advance directive, or power of attorney.
- Providers can play a role in starting these discussions and sharing information with patients about their options.

By 2030, 70% of people living with HIV will be age 50 or older. People diagnosed with HIV (or any potentially life-threatening illness) face a myriad of legal concerns that affect almost every facet of their lives. At times, this may seem overwhelming to patient and provider alike. However, legal planning can greatly benefit PWH and their families. Providers can play an important role in informing patients of the benefits of planning ahead.

All providers should advise their patients to investigate and prepare three essential tools of effective legal planning:

1. A durable power of attorney for medical decision-making
2. An advance directive ("living will")
3. A will.

DURABLE POWER OF ATTORNEY

A durable power of attorney makes legal provision for someone to make decisions in a patient's stead if they are no longer able to do so. Patients should consider two such documents to best protect their legal interests: one for healthcare decisions and one for legal and financial decisions. A patient may choose a single person to fill both roles, but the responsibilities are different. A durable power of attorney for financial issues may cover any and all financial concerns or may stipulate only specific tasks, such as paying standard household expenses or filing tax returns. This should be someone the patient trusts (AIDS Law Project, 2017). A durable power of attorney for health care may cover any and all medical decisions or may stipulate that only specific decisions can be made, such as consenting to or declining any medical treatment. These documents are particularly important for couples who are not legally married, particularly same-sex couples, because without a durable power of attorney, hospitals and courts usually defer to the closest biological relative to make medical decisions.

A power of attorney may take effect immediately when a patient signs it and the healthcare or financial agent acknowledges this responsibility (AIDS Law Project, 2017). Patients must state in the document that a power of attorney is durable, or it will automatically end if the patient becomes incapacitated. In all cases, a power of attorney ends when the patient dies. Patients may choose to revoke the power of attorney at any time, either in writing or by informing medical providers (AIDS Law Project, 2017). Patients should consult an attorney in drafting a durable power of attorney to ensure that it is drawn up correctly and ensure that the person who is made power of attorney is someone they trust.

ADVANCE DIRECTIVE

An advance directive is a document in which patients provide specific instructions about the kind of health care they do or do not want in the event that they have an incapacity that makes them unable to make or communicate medical decisions. These instructions are commonly referred to as a "living will." However, there is an important distinction: living wills generally are limited to cases of terminal illness, whereas advance directives may apply to any situation in which a patient is incapacitated, even temporarily. This distinction is especially compelling regarding PWH, who may experience AIDS-related dementia or other complications that may impair rational decision-making, but they may subsequently have improved executive function as a result of ART or other interventions. However, in a large national study of PWH, fewer than half reported having advance directives. The most important factor associated with having an advance directive was whether their practitioner had discussed end-of-life issues. This study also found that providers were less likely to discuss advance directives with Black and Latino patients than with white patients, and patients who used drugs were among the least likely to obtain advance directives (Wenger et al., 2001). A more recent review of studies indicates that the presence of advance care planning is variable among people living with HIV, based on factors including socioeconomic status, health status, and practitioner resources and training (Sangarlangkarn et al., 2015). A 2019 study of 154 people living with HIV in Los Angeles and New Orleans found that only 26% of older adults had an advance directive, and 31% had a healthcare proxy (Nguyen et al., 2019). As the HIV population ages, these discussions should routinely be part of intake medical visits and should be reviewed periodically. Providers should also guard against implicit or explicit bias when discussing end-of-life decision-making.

Advance directives are valid in every U.S. state and the District of Columbia, but the specifics of the law vary from state to state. Therefore, patients who spend significant time in more than one state or who move to another state should have directives adjusted to follow each state's guidelines (Caring Connections, n.d.). In creating an advance directive, the patient should consult an expert and should attempt to answer three important questions:

- What are my goals for treatment? Among other things, patients should consider their values relative to independence, their environment, and their religious/spiritual beliefs.
- How specific should I be? No directive can cover all eventualities, but it is suggested that patients address anything that is especially important to them.
- How can I make sure that healthcare providers will follow my advance directive?

Most states give healthcare providers the right to decline to honor directives on grounds of conscience. In such cases, healthcare providers generally are obligated to refer patients to other healthcare providers who will honor the directive. It is important to ask patients about their wishes. Generally, patients need both a durable power of attorney and an advance directive. In essence, the advance directive expresses a patient's specific wishes, and the durable power of attorney grants someone the authority to execute those wishes or to make healthcare decisions that could not be anticipated by the advance directive.

PHYSICIAN ORDER FOR LIFE-SUSTAINING TREATMENT (POLST)

A POLST form, also known as a medical order for life-sustaining treatment or MOLST form, is becoming more commonly implemented as a part of advance care planning in many states. This form should be done with a healthcare provider, and it specifies medical treatments that a patient may or may not want in the event of a medical emergency or life-threatening event. In many cases it can complement the advance directive and may be more appropriate for persons with a serious illness or advanced frailty near the end of life.

WILL

A will determines what happens to a person's property after their death. Despite considerable attention to wills in the popular press, providers should not assume all patients have one—only 32% of Americans have an estate plan, a decline from 2020 (Lustbader, 2024). Without a will, the courts will distribute a person's assets according to state laws. Wills are particularly important for people with minor children because they can select a person to take care of their children if they die, once a court approves of the person (AIDS Law Project, 2017). Wills are also important in situations in which persons are not legally married to their partner because, without a will, survivors may inherit nothing and, worse, may lose personal property because they cannot prove ownership (AIDS Law Project, 2017).

Many people mistakenly believe that they do not need wills because they do not have large estates. In truth, everyone needs a will to ensure that their wishes are followed when their assets are distributed. Handwritten, unwitnessed wills (called *holographic wills*) may be valid in approximately 25 states, but formal wills are preferable. A valid, legal will must include the following elements:

- It must be typewritten, or computer generated (except holographic wills, described previously).
- The document must expressly state that it is a "Will."
- The person making the will must date and sign it.
- The will must be signed by at least two or, in some states, three witnesses who will not inherit anything under the terms of the will.

Healthcare providers should be aware that legal planning is vital for all patients but especially for PWH. By focusing on the documents discussed previously (durable power of attorney, advance directives, POLST form, and wills) and by obtaining appropriate legal advice, the planning should not be difficult or confusing.

REFERENCES/RECOMMENDED READING

Administration for Community Living. 2024 final rule to update older Americans act regulations. https://acl.gov/OAArule. Last modified June 7, 2024. Accessed July 9, 2024.

American Bar Association. Health care advance directives. https://www.americanbar.org/groups/public_education/resources/law_issues_for_consumers/directive_review/. Published March 18, 2013. Accessed July 9, 2024.

Lustbader, R. 2024 wills and estate planning study. https://www.caring.com/caregivers/estate-planning/wills-survey. Published 2024. Accessed July 9, 2024.

CIVIL RIGHTS AND DISCRIMINATION

LEARNING OBJECTIVE

- Understand how stigma and discrimination impact the lives of people living with HIV and hinder our response to the HIV epidemic.

WHAT'S NEW?

- The practice of HIV criminalization may potentially violate the Americans with Disabilities Act.

KEY POINTS

- People living with HIV are covered by the Americans with Disabilities Act, even if they are virally suppressed.
- Stigma continues to play a major role in the well-being of people living with HIV and fuels discrimination.

Stigma and discrimination continue to be major challenges to the comprehensive response necessary to address the HIV epidemic. A key focus of the HIV National Strategic Plan is to "[a]ddress stigma, discrimination, and other social and structural determinants of health that inhibit HIV prevention, testing, and care. Every person with or at risk for HIV should receive diagnostic, preventive, care, treatment, and supportive services that are non-stigmatizing, or non-discriminatory, competent, and responsive to their needs" (Department of Health and Human Services [DHHS], 2021, n.p.). Discrimination shows up in all aspects of life for people living with HIV, including relationships with friends and family, employment, housing, and even accessing basic services like nail salons. Although HIV biomedical advances continue to progress, the 2023 Gay and Lesbian Alliance Against Defamation (GLAAD) State of Stigma survey found that "Americans' discomfort interacting with those living with HIV increased" compared to the previous year. Forty-one percent of people surveyed felt "strongly/somewhat uncomfortable" interacting with a barber or hair stylist living with HIV and 32% feel "strongly or somewhat uncomfortable" interacting with a co-worker living with HIV (GLAAD, 2023, n.p.). Stigma has a profound impact on the quality of life of people living with HIV. A meta-analysis of 64 studies showed that there are "significant associations between HIV-related stigma and higher rates of depression, lower social support and lower levels of adherence to antiretroviral medications and access to and usage of health and social services" (Rueda et al., 2016). HIV stigma also intersects with other aspects of a person's identity and may be compounded by stigma associated with race, gender identity and sexual orientation, social class, immigration status, or interactions with the criminal legal system. To combat this, the National Institutes of Health are prioritizing research addressing intersectional HIV-related stigma and discrimination (Gordon and Goodenow, 2022).

The Americans with Disabilities Act (ADA) protects the rights of people living with HIV to have equal opportunity for housing, employment, government services, and public accommodations like restaurants, nail salons, and tattoo parlors. ADA protections apply to people living with HIV even if they are virally suppressed or asymptomatic. If someone believes that they have been discriminated against based on their HIV status or another disability, they can contact a local legal services organization or the Department of Justice (DOJ), Civil Rights Division. A report can be submitted to the DOJ at: https://civilrights.justice.gov. State and local antidiscrimination laws and policies may provide even stronger protections for people living with HIV than the ADA.

The practice of HIV criminalization is also potentially a violation of the Americans with Disabilities Act. In 2024, the DOJ filed a lawsuit in Tennessee arguing that the state's use of its aggravated prostitution statute, which subjects people living with HIV to harsher penalties and until 2023 required registration as a sex offender for life upon conviction, was a violation of the ADA. Although the case is still pending, the Shelby County District Attorney's Office in Memphis agreed to stop prosecuting people living with HIV for aggravated prostitution and to "cease seeking any other enhanced criminal charges or penalties on the basis of a defendant's HIV status, unless the individual's HIV posed a direct threat to the health and safety of others following an individualized assessment" (DOJ, 2024, n.p.).

The rate of people living with HIV in state and federal prisons is approximately 3 times higher than the general public in the United States (CDC, 2024). People living with HIV who are incarcerated in jails or prisons may face particular discrimination and stigma, including breaches of confidentiality as well as lack of access to medication and other healthcare services. Fear of violence can also limit an incarcerated person's willingness to disclose their HIV status or accept ART. According to a 2024 survey of LGBTQ+ people in immigration detention, "13 out of the 17 interviewees living with HIV said they were either denied medical HIV treatment or experienced some form of medical neglect" (Doubossarskaia et al., 2024). A small exploratory study in Illinois found that over 60% of the incarcerated people living with HIV who were surveyed missed doses of medication or experienced treatment interruption "because of failure to disclose their HIV status, delayed prescribing, intermittent dosing and out-of-stock medications, confiscation of medications, and medication strikes" (Culbert, 2014). Although correctional healthcare providers do not have to follow a patient's treatment plan or continue a specific medication, they are required to provide "adequate care." Providers can educate patients about their rights to adequate healthcare, if incarcerated. With a patient's consent, providers can also collaborate with defense counsel and correctional healthcare providers to ensure that treatment is not interrupted (Lambda Legal, 2010).

ACKNOWLEDGMENTS

The author would like to acknowledge the contribution of Jarrett K. Sell and Jeffrey Schouten to previous editions of this chapter.

REFERENCES

Administration for Community Living. 2024 final rule to update older Americans act regulations. https://acl.gov/OAArule. Last modified June 7, 2024. Accessed July 9, 2024.

AIDS Law Project of Pennsylvania. Your life, your decisions: wills, living wills, powers of attorney and standby guardianships. https://www.aidslawpa.org/wp-content/uploads/2020/10/Your-Life-Your-Decisions-April-2017.pdf. Published 2017. Accessed July 9, 2024.

American Academy of HIV Medicine. HIV criminalization. https://aahivm.org/hiv-criminalization/. n.d. Accessed July 12, 2024.

American Academy of HIV Medicine. Public policy platform. aahivm.org/wp-content/uploads/2019/06/policy-platform-updated-6.3.19.pdf. Updated June 3, 2019. Accessed July 12, 2024.

American Medical Association, Code on Medical Ethics, Section 3.2.1. Confidentiality. https://code-medical-ethics.ama-assn.org/sites/amacoedb/files/2022-08/3.2.1.pdf. Published August 2022. Accessed July 9, 2024.

Ayala G, Bahati M, Balan E, et al. Partner notification: a community viewpoint. *J Intl AIDS Soc*. 2019;22(S3):8.

Barre-Sinoussi F, Bekker L, Beyrer C, et al. Expert consensus statement on the science of HIV in the context of criminal law. *J Intl AIDS Soc*. 2018 Jul 25;21:e25161.

Baugher AR, Whiteman A, Jeffries WL 4th, et al. Black men who have sex with men living in states with HIV criminalization laws report high stigma, 23 U.S. cities, 2017. *AIDS*. 2021 Aug 1;35(10):1637–1645.

Budhwani H, Mills L, Marefka LEB, et al. Preliminary study on HIV status disclosure to perinatal infected children: retrospective analysis of administrative records from a pediatric HIV clinic in the southern United States. *BMC Res Notes*. 2020;13:253.

Caring Connections. Advance care planning. www.caringinfo.org/i4a/pages/index.cfm?pageid=3278. n.d. Accessed July 9, 2024.

Center for HIV Law and Policy. HIV criminalization in the United States, CHLP. https://www.hivlawandpolicy.org/resources/map-hiv-criminalization-united-states-chlp-updated-2022. Updated 2022. Accessed July 8, 2024.

Center for HIV Law and Policy. HIV criminalization in the United States: a sourcebook on state and federal HIV criminal law and practice. http://www.hivlawandpolicy.org/sourcebook. 2024. Accessed July 8, 2024.

Centers for Disease Control and Prevention (CDC). Correctional settings. https://www.cdc.gov/correctional-health/about/index.html. Updated July 3, 2024. Accessed July 12, 2024.

Centers for Disease Control and Prevention (CDC). Sexually transmitted infections (STIs), duty to warn. https://www.cdc.gov/std/treatment/duty-to-warn.htm. Updated April 13, 2021. Accessed July 8, 2024.

Chenneville T, Gabbidon K. HIV, confidentiality, and duty to protect: considerations for psychotherapists in the age of treatment as prevention, *Psychotherapy*. 2020:57(1);7.

Cisneros N, Sears B, Macklin M. Enforcement of HIV criminalization in Mississippi. Williams Institute at UCLA School of Law. https://williamsinstitute.law.ucla.edu/publications/hiv-crim-ms. February 2024. Accessed July 15, 2024.

Cisneros N, Sears B, Tentindo W. Enforcement of HIV criminalization in Ohio. Williams Institute at UCLA School of Law. https://williamsinstitute.law.ucla.edu/publications/hiv-crim-oh. February 2024. Accessed July 15, 2024.

Cisneros N, Tentindo W, Sears B, et al. Enforcement of HIV criminalization in Maryland. Williams Institute at UCLA School of Law.

https://williamsinstitute.law.ucla.edu/publications/hiv-crim-md. January 2024. Accessed July 15, 2024.

Culbert G. Violence and the perceived risks of taking antiretroviral therapy in US jails and prisons. *Intl J Prison Health*. 2014;10(2):94–110.

Department of Health and Human Services (DHHS). HIV national strategic plan: a roadmap to end the epidemic for the United States 2021–2025. https://files.hiv.gov/s3fs-public/HIV-National-Strategic-Plan-2021-2025.pdf. Published 2021. Accessed July 11, 2024.

Department of Justice (DOJ). Disability rights guide. https://www.ada.gov/resources/disability-rights-guide. Updated February 28, 2020. Accessed July 11, 2024.

Department of Justice (DOJ). Settlement agreement between the United States of America and the Shelby County District Attorney General's Office under the Americans with Disabilities Act, DJ No. 204-70-85. https://www.justice.gov/crt/media/1352376/dl. Dated May 16, 2024. Accessed July 12, 2024.

Doat AR, Negarandeh R, Hasanpour M. Disclosure of HIV status to children in sub-Saharan Africa: a systematic review. *Medicina (Kaunas)*. 2019;55(8):433.

Doubossarskaia L, Crawford B, Erfani A, et al. "No human being should be held there": the mistreatment of LGBTQ and HIV positive people in U.S. federal immigration jails. https://immigrantjustice.org/sites/default/files/content-type/research-item/documents/2024-06/2024-06-18_FINAL%20detention%20report.pdf. Published June 2024. Accessed July 11, 2024.

GLAAD. State of HIV stigma. https://glaad.org/endhivstigma/2023. Published 2023. Accessed July 11, 2024.

Gordon J, Goodenow M. Addressing HIV-related intersectional stigma and discrimination. National Institute of Mental Health. https://www.nimh.nih.gov/about/director/messages/2022/addressing-hiv-related-intersectional-stigma-and-discrimination. Published July 28, 2022. Accessed July 12, 2024.

Guttmacher Institute. Minors' access to STI services: state laws and policies. http://www.guttmacher.org/statecenter/spibs/spib_MASS.pdf. Published September 1, 2023a. Accessed July 9, 2024.

Krauss B, Letteney S, de Baets A, Murugi J, Okero FA. *Guideline on HIV Disclosure Counselling for Children up to 12 Years of Age*. Geneva: World Health Organization; 2011. https://apps.who.int/iris/bitstream/handle/10665/44777/9789241502863_eng.pdf;jsessionid=27A6CA8DA056F1823129425B95692717?sequence=1. Accessed July 12, 2024.

Lambda Legal. Your right to HIV treatment in prison and jail. https://legacy.lambdalegal.org/sites/default/files/publications/downloads/fs_your-right-to-hiv-treatment-in-prison-and-jail_1.pdf. Updated July 2010. Accessed July 12, 2024.

Lustbader, R. 2024 wills and estate planning study. https://www.caring.com/caregivers/estate-planning/wills-survey. n.d. Accessed July 9, 2024.

Massachusetts General Laws. HIV test; informed consent; disclosure of results or identity of subject of test. *MA Gen L* ch 111 § 70f (2023). https://law.justia.com/codes/massachusetts/part-i/title-xvi/chapter-111/section-70f/#. Accessed August 4, 2024.

Mermin J, Valentine SS, McCray E. HIV criminalisation laws and ending the US HIV epidemic. *Lancet HIV*. 2021;8(1):e4–e6.

Nelson K, Skinner A, Stout C, et al. Minor consent laws for sexually transmitted infection and human immunodeficiency virus services in the United States: a comprehensive, longitudinal survey of US state laws. *Am J Public Health*. 2023;113(4):397–407.

Nguyen AL, Seal D, Bruce O, et al. Caregiving preferences and advance care planning among older adults living with HIV. *AIDS Care*. 2019 Feb;31(2):243–249.

Obermeyer CM, Baijal P, Pegurri E. Facilitating HIV disclosure across diverse settings: a review. *Am J Pub Health*. 2011;101(6): 1011–1023.

Rueda S, Mitra S, Chen S, et al. Examining the associations between HIV-related stigma and health outcomes in people living with HIV/AIDS: a series of meta-analyses. *BMJ Open*. 2016;6:e011453.

Sah P, Fitzpatrick MC, Pandey A, Galvani AP. HIV criminalization exacerbates subpar diagnosis and treatment across the United States: response to the "Association of HIV diagnosis rates and laws criminalizing HIV exposure in the United States." *AIDS*. 2017; 31: 2437–2439.

Sangarlangkarn, A, Merlin, J, Tucker, R, et al. Advance care planning and HIV infection in the era of antiretroviral therapy: a review. *Top Antiviral Med*. 2015 Dec/2016 Jan;23(5):174–180.

Santa Rosa Healthcare Corp. v. Garcia, 964 S.W.2d 940 (Tex Sup Ct 1998).

Sero Project. About us. https://www.seroproject.com/about-us. n.d. Accessed July 8, 2024.

Sullivan T. The intersection of intimate partner violence and HIV: detection, disclosure, discussion, and implications for treatment adherence. *Top Antivir Med*. 2019;27(2):84.

Sweeney P, Gray SC, Purcell DW, et al. Association of HIV diagnosis rates and laws criminalizing HIV exposure in the United States. *AIDS*. 2017;31(10):1483–1488.

The White House. National HIV/AIDS strategy for the United States 2022–2025. Washington, DC. https://www.whitehouse.gov/wp-content/uploads/2021/11/National-HIV-AIDS-Strategy.pdf. Published 2021. Accessed July 12, 2024.

U.S. People Living with HIV (US PLHIV) Caucus. Demanding better: an HIV federal policy agenda by people living with HIV. https://www.pwn-usa.org/wp-content/uploads/2021/07/Networks-Policy-Agenda-FINAL.pdf. Published 2021. Accessed July 9, 2024.

Wenger NS, Kanouse DE, Collins RL, et al. End-of-life discussions and preferences among persons with HIV. *JAMA*. 2001;285:2880–2887.

39.

HIV HEALTHCARE PROGRAMS AND INSURANCE COVERAGE IN THE U.S. HEALTHCARE SYSTEM

Chauncey McGlathery

LEARNING OBJECTIVE

- Discuss the U.S. healthcare system and coverage landscape as they relate to the provision of HIV care, treatment, and prevention.

WHAT'S NEW?

Over the past couple of years, there have been several changes to HIV care environments with both positive and negative effects, including but not limited to telehealth, adoption of a "whole person" (or "status neutral") approach to services, creation of low-barrier models of care outside of traditional brick and mortar clinical settings, and a renewed emphasis on transitions of care to ensure that linkages made between settings are person-centered and robust. A number of short-term changes were made to the healthcare system in response to COVID-19 and as part of the federal government's Public Health Emergency declaration. Many of those changes have served to enhance access to care for people with HIV (PWH), such as expanded telehealth access (DHHS, 2024). However, while efforts to increase access to healthcare coverage have increased, HIV testing overall has seen a significant decline, and some PWH have fallen out of care (CDC, 2022). Although Medicaid/Children's Health Insurance Program (CHIP) enrollment rates are promising in some areas, many people in the United States still do not have adequate health insurance coverage, and eligibility determination and renewal processes are often complex processes to navigate (Corallo and Moreno, 2023).

KEY POINTS

- It has been more than 12 years since the passage of the landmark Patient Protection and Affordable Care Act (also called the Affordable Care Act [ACA]), and more than 8 years since the implementation of the Health Insurance Marketplace, which greatly expanded the availability of health coverage for PWH in the United States. However, serious challenges such as affordability and access to treatment still remain and are especially evident in states that have chosen not to expand their Medicaid coverage.
- The COVID-19 pandemic significantly undermined health insurance coverage, as broad surges in unemployment caused many to lose employer-sponsored insurance and disrupted access to care. While some of those issues have been corrected by the Biden administration and the Inflation Reduction Act, many of the variables around healthcare access—particularly for people with low incomes—will be dependent upon the particular policies and politics of the sitting administration at a given point in time. Congress has yet to pass legislation that would result in a long-term stabilization of the insurance market.

INTRODUCTION

HIV healthcare services in the United States have historically been covered by an assortment of federal, state, and local programs, such as Medicare, Medicaid, the Ryan White HIV/AIDS Program, and state and local health department–funded and/or administered programs. HIV/AIDS service organizations, local community-based organizations, federally qualified health centers, and grants from other sources also provide services for people living with HIV (PWH) who are underinsured or uninsured or who meet a certain income threshold. These programs collectively constitute the long-standing pathways to insurance coverage, care, and access to HIV-related treatment and prevention for people living with and at risk for HIV. Some programs also provide access to HIV medications, including patient assistance programs, co-pay relief, and medications for co-occurring conditions common among PWH. The system of HIV care and prevention is a patchwork largely dependent upon government funding and political will.

The 30th anniversary of the Ryan White Comprehensive AIDS Resources Emergency (CARE) Act was commemorated on August 18, 2020. The CARE Act has been reauthorized four times since it was initially signed into law and aims to accommodate new and emerging needs of PWH as well as address ongoing disparities in access to care to improve HIV-related health outcomes. Congress appropriated additional funding for the total Ryan White Program in fiscal years 2020 and 2021, though some parts have not seen notable increases in several years. Importantly, as scale-up and implementation of long-acting antiretrovirals (as treatment or prevention) continue shaping the nature of HIV care, new approaches to care engagement and retention may become necessary. Importantly, access and affordability of these newer agents have largely depended on how the patient receives healthcare coverage. Specifically, coverage across the private insurance market, Medicaid, Medicare, and state AIDS Drug Assistance Programs (ADAPs) varies and often includes prior authorization requirements or other utilization management techniques.

In 2022, the U.S. Supreme Court effectively overturned the landmark *Roe v. Wade* decision by allowing states to determine the parameters of legal abortion care. It is unknown how this ruling could impact HIV care, although it does allow for increased political reach into provider autonomy as it relates to reproductive health care. HIV healthcare providers must, therefore, remain aware of changing laws and how they may impact one's ability to provide comprehensive care and/or protect patient privacy.

NEW APPROACHES TO HIV SERVICE DELIVERY

Although the COVID-19 pandemic significantly disrupted operations for many HIV clinics and service programs, it helped to accelerate innovative models and approaches to healthcare delivery. Recent biomedical advances in HIV prevention and treatment have also emerged within the past several years (perhaps most visibly with approval of new long-acting injectable antiretroviral agents), which has prompted healthcare systems to identify, adopt, and adapt to new frameworks of care. A status-neutral approach to HIV care has continued to improve care and eliminate stigma by putting the needs of the person ahead of their HIV status (Myers et al., 2018). It also advances health equity by integrating HIV care and prevention into primary care.

Telehealth has been successfully implemented as a complementary way to deliver HIV care, although it should be noted that some populations have experienced challenges and poor outcomes with this model of care (Labisi et al., 2022). These groups include older adults, racial minorities, and people with low telehealth literacy. Barriers to telehealth include a lack of access to broadband services, compatible devices, and government regulations. Along with telehealth, mobile health clinics and other low-barrier programs have been adopted in many areas to provide care directly to individuals and communities that might not access healthcare through traditional, clinic-based services (Dombrowski et al., 2023). These have been especially useful when trying to engage with "hard-to-reach" populations or people in remote or rural areas. Low-barrier programs can effectively reach people who otherwise may not access regular care, such as people facing stigma, ostracization, discrimination, and homelessness.

Given the importance of ongoing engagement in care and reducing provider burnout, there has been a renewed emphasis on the creation of interdisciplinary care teams, as well as investment in new approaches to ensure successful transitions of care, which are frequent and may be caused by relocation, hospitalization, changes in employment/insurance coverage status, incarceration, HIV provider workforce shortages, or transitions due to aging with HIV. Interventions to improve linkage to care have been created in pediatric care, primary care, women's care, and care for persons who are incarcerated, including integrated care models. HIV-dedicated hospital teams, including clinical pharmacists, are increasingly utilized to improve ARV stewardship. More states are beginning to consider collaborative practice agreements that create a formal practice relationship between pharmacists and other healthcare practitioners; these allow pharmacists to assume responsibility for specific care functions that are aligned with their expertise and training but are otherwise beyond their typical scope of practice. Pharmacies have emerged as an important setting for new HIV testing and prevention services, as they are easily accessible in rural communities and do not require appointments. Even members of underserved populations who indicate a history of mistrust with providers often already know and trust their pharmacists. Additionally, because they are often open for longer hours than traditional clinics, pharmacies have emerged as one of the most visible areas of underdeveloped potential for pre-exposure prophylaxis (PrEP) delivery.

Importantly, systematic implementation and success of effective antiretroviral therapy (ART) requires improved access for everyone, especially priority populations like those traditionally underrepresented in the HIV workforce. Several challenges to the widespread adoption of long-acting injectable ART have been identified; these include frequent clinic visits for dose administration, injection site reactions, drug interactions, and the emergence of new HIV drug resistance if someone experiences treatment failure while receiving long-acting injectable therapy. Further research is needed to demonstrate the barriers and opportunities of long-acting agents specifically for children, adolescents, and pregnant and breastfeeding women. More information on long-acting ART is available at the Long-Acting Antiretroviral Research Resource Program (LEAP): www.longactinghiv.org. Given high levels of interest in new long-acting antiretroviral agents, it is important for healthcare systems to ensure the sustainability of their use in clinical practice.

Barring further interference by the legislatures and court systems, the new approaches described above are likely to significantly improve health outcomes for all PWH, not only for those who are currently experiencing the effects of better HIV prevention and care but also for underserved populations bearing more than their share of the burden of HIV.

AFFORDABLE CARE ACT

The ACA was signed into law by President Barack Obama and was designed to reform healthcare coverage, representing the broadest reform to the U.S. healthcare system since the 1960s. Prior to its implementation, coverage gaps and lack of access to affordable coverage impacted millions of people. When the ACA was enacted in 2010, approximately 46.5 million non-elderly Americans had no health insurance. The number dropped rapidly and reached a historic low of 27 million in 2016. The trend reversed during the Trump presidency owing to barriers erected by the administration, and approximately

1 million people became uninsured between 2017 and 2018 (KFF, 2022c). Under the Biden administration, 35 million people were able to be enrolled in coverage by the end of 2021, and the rate of uninsured people reached an all-time low (DHHS, 2022). As of early 2024, 40 states and Washington, D.C., had adopted ACA's Medicaid expansion (KFF, 2024b).

The passage of the ACA also directly affected the provision of HIV care. Reforms which had a significant impact on PWH include:

1. Prohibiting discrimination by insurers against individuals with preexisting conditions
2. Requiring that all U.S. citizens obtain health insurance coverage (this was subsequently effectively repealed, as noted above)
3. Expanding the Medicaid program to cover all individuals under 138% of the federal poverty level (FPL) (this was made optional for states by a 2012 Supreme Court ruling, see below)
4. Creating individual and small-group insurance markets ("exchanges") in each state. Along with the addition of federal tax credits for qualified individuals, these mechanisms have enabled low-income individuals to purchase more affordable insurance.

Ongoing public policy maneuvers, however, have brought about diverse changes in the availability and affordability of private insurance coverage for PWH in many cases, depending on the state of residence.

The constitutionality of various aspects of the ACA has been repeatedly challenged, even up to the U.S. Supreme Court. The most momentous of these was a 2012 decision effectively making Medicaid expansion an optional, state-by-state decision. As of 2024, 40 states and the District of Columbia have chosen to adopt Medicaid expansion in some form. The remaining 10, to date, have declined. Four of these states are located outside of the U.S. South, and the remaining 6 are southern: Florida has the second largest uninsured population (behind Texas) (Gee and Rapfogel, 2021). In its annual HIV Prevention Progress Report, the CDC, for the first time, listed "persons residing in the southern United States" as a specific population at increased risk of acquiring HIV, along with people of color, men who have sex with men, and various other groups (CDC, 2019).

Importantly, Medicaid remains the largest source of coverage for PWH in the United States, covering 42% of the population with HIV (KFF, 2023a). In states that reject Medicaid expansion, individuals who are not below the poverty line but cannot afford commercial insurance remain uninsured. Low-income adults who do not qualify for Medicaid through other qualifying categories (e.g., are not disabled, elderly, caring for children, or pregnant) are thus left without access to any affordable health coverage options whatsoever. The lack of universal Medicaid expansion at present, coupled with significant flexibility provided to state lawmakers and insurers in the state insurance markets, has left PWH in each state with insurance coverage options of widely varying value. Although the Ryan White HIV/AIDS Program (see below) is a safety net program designed to "wrap around" other forms of health coverage, it is also affected by what each state can offer to its residents living with HIV (see section on "Medicaid" below, for additional details).

In 2018, the Centers for Medicare and Medicaid Services (CMS) issued a final rule to increase the maximum use of ACA-noncompliant "short-term" insurance policies from 3 months to 364 days, thus facilitating the uptake of these policies by people who wanted or needed to buy their insurance as inexpensively as possible. Often referred to as "junk insurance," these policies usually do not cover prescription drugs, maternity care, or care for people with preexisting medical conditions. Purchasers are often not fully aware of their very limited utility at the time of purchase. On March 28, 2024, the Departments of Health and Human Services, Labor, and Treasury announced a federal rule that will limit the duration of these plans sold or issued on or after September 1, 2024. The rule will limit these plans to 3-month terms, with a maximum duration of 4 months (DHHS, 2024).

PRIVATE INSURANCE

Private health insurance in the United States is typically offered by private, for-profit, or nonprofit companies to various markets. In 2008, employment-based health insurance was the primary source of coverage for American workers (Rho and Schmitt, 2010), offered as benefits or in the form of other compensation to employees by their employers. Individual insurance plans were less common before the ACA.

Some common forms of private insurance are indemnity plans, preferred provider plans, and health maintenance organizations. With indemnity plans, individuals can generally choose any healthcare provider and have a portion of the fees paid by the insurance. With preferred provider plans, individuals must choose from a defined network of clinicians, but the clinicians are generally employed by different groups. With health maintenance plans, individuals receive care from one or a small number of clinician groups hired by the insurer.

Reimbursement to clinicians varies widely with private insurance policies, with lower rates generally paid by managed care organizations. The provider networks within insurance plans can also affect reimbursement levels, as can plan benefits, co-pays, and cost-sharing mechanisms. Coverage of particular medications and treatments varies widely under private insurance plans.

STATE INSURANCE EXCHANGES

One of the most significant accomplishments of the ACA was the creation of marketplaces for individual and small-group insurance plans in each state (Center for Consumer Information & Oversight, 2024). Each state insurance exchange is simply a market forum where private insurance companies offer various qualified health plans to residents of that state. Individuals can access the marketplace online, by phone, or in person through assistants. Potential customers also use the marketplace to determine their eligibility for Medicaid or CHIP benefits (HealthCare.gov, 2024b).

The ACA also makes tax credit subsidies available to some low- and medium-income individuals to purchase insurance through the state exchanges. Tax credits of gradated amounts are available to those with income levels between 133% and 400% FPL, and they are taken as up-front subsidies to the plan premium (HealthCare.gov, 2024c). For 2021 and 2022, the American Rescue Plan temporarily expanded eligibility for premium tax credits by eliminating the 400% FPL ceiling (IRS, 2024). To be eligible to receive the premium tax credit in 2024, individuals must have annual household income at or above 100% of the federal poverty level; not be eligible for certain types of health insurance coverage, with exceptions; file federal income tax returns; and enroll in a plan through an individual exchange (CRS, 2024).

Plans offered within the markets vary widely in cost as well as coverage and benefit design. However, all are required to provide essential health benefits as a part of the insurance package, including services within the following 10 categories: ambulatory patient services; emergency services; hospitalizations; maternity and newborn care; mental health and substance use disorder services (including behavioral health treatment); prescription drugs; rehabilitative and habilitative services and devices; laboratory services; preventive and wellness services and chronic disease management; and pediatric services (including oral and vision care) (HealthCare.gov, 2024a). In addition, all state exchange plans are required to include a minimum percentage of all the Essential Community Providers (ECPs) in a geographic area in their provider networks. ECPs are providers that serve predominately low-income, medically underserved individuals. This includes Ryan White HIV/AIDS Program providers.

MEDICAID

Medicaid has long been the essential health insurance program for people with low-income status, limited resources, and/or disability in the United States. Originally, the program covered only certain populations, such as people who were medically disabled and/or pregnant, infants, and children living in poverty. Medicaid covers inpatient, ambulatory care, and skilled nursing care. It also covers prescription medications except for persons who also have Medicare coverage ("dual eligibles"). Coverage levels, eligibility criteria, and program benefits vary widely from state to state (Medicaid.gov, Benefits, 2024a). Medicaid is financed jointly by the federal government and states and is administered by state governments in accordance with certain basic federal eligibility and benefit standards (Medicaid.gov, Financing, 2024b). At the federal level, the Medicaid program is run by the Centers for Medicare and Medicaid Services (CMS) under the U.S. Department of Health and Human Services. Medicaid is the third largest domestic program in the federal budget, after Social Security and Medicare (Rudowitz and Snyder, 2015). The federal government matches state spending for eligible beneficiaries without limit. The federal share for "traditional Medicaid"—children, parents, non-ACA expansion adults, the elderly, and people with disabilities—is based on a formula and the state's per capita income relative to other states. The design of Medicaid dictates that the government will pay a larger share of program costs in poorer states, with federal share (FMAO) varying widely by state. The ACA sought to expand the program's coverage to include all citizens below 138% FPL regardless of other categorizations (Rudowitz et al., 2021). However, this was not accepted by all states. Some states have partially expanded their Medicaid program in a variety of ways, and others have declined expansion altogether, largely for political reasons. The approximately 2.2 million eligible individuals in those states in the "coverage gap" are left with few options (KFF, 2022b).

In 2021, 41 states reported that they used capitated managed care models to deliver Medicaid services to mitigate Medicaid budgetary costs through reductions of benefits, limitations to drug formularies, and other efforts (KFF, 2022a). Some others also offer managed care–type programs to specific designated populations in an effort to reduce costs. Managed care organizations (MCOs) contract directly with the state to provide services and benefits in a variety of capacities (KFF, 2024a). Some MCOs are operated by a parent firm that also participates in the private insurance market. Traditional Medicaid programs offer provider reimbursement through fee-for-service rates that are determined by the state. MCOs make agreements for provider reimbursement based on monthly capitation rates.

MEDICARE

Medicare is the federal health insurance program for people older than 65 and for people younger than 65 with permanent disabilities in the United States. The Medicare program is also administered by CMS, and approximately one-quarter of PWH receive medical care through Medicare (KFF, 2023b). Medicare eligibility is tied to work history and contributions to Medicare through employment-based withholding. Over time, the number of PWH who use Medicare has increased because of longevity attributable to effective ART and effective treatment of multiple chronic health conditions. Medicare covers HIV testing for beneficiaries.

Since 2006, Medicare has provided prescription drug coverage under the Medicare Part D drug benefit. Most Medicare-eligible individuals can decide whether to participate through enrollment in one of several prescription drug plans that are marketed as stand-alone coverage or to rely on managed care plans ("Medicare Advantage"). When Medicare Part D was launched, Congress identified six types of prescription drugs as "protected classes" and required that they be covered by Part D plans. Antiretroviral drugs were one of the protected classes, as well as drugs used for cancer treatment, mental health treatments, and other medications that also require uninterrupted use, although that designation was under threat during the Trump administration. These protected classes were exempted from any prior authorization, step therapy, or other "utilization management" techniques that would interrupt or delay patients' access to these drugs.

Medicare Part D also includes an "exceptions and appeals" process that can be used to request coverage of drugs not covered by the plan. Individual Part D plans differ widely in terms of premiums and other cost-sharing requirements. Specifically, Medicare Part D includes a sequence of cost-sharing requirements, including an initial deductible and subsequent "out-of-pocket" costs. Most Part D plans also have a coverage gap (also referred to as the Part D "donut hole") in which, after a certain amount of the costs have been paid through the coverage plan, any additional costs become the responsibility of the individual until the costs reach the catastrophic coverage threshold (Medicare.gov, 2024a; Medicare.gov, 2024b; National Council on Aging, 2024; Medicare.gov, 2024a). At that point, nearly all costs are then covered by Medicare. The ACA closed this gap in 2020, although beneficiaries may still incur costs based on other factors.

Medicare reimbursement rates are similar to those of private insurance. Clinicians who accept Medicare reimbursement are subject to federal audits of their charts to check billed amounts against services documented.

RYAN WHITE HIV/AIDS PROGRAM

The Ryan White HIV/AIDS Program is a federal program designed specifically to ensure the provision of care, treatment, and supportive services for PWH in the United States. First enacted in 1990, it is administered by the Health Resources and Services Administration under the U.S. Department of Health and Human Services (HRSA, 2024a). Fundamentally, the Ryan White Program provides a "safety net" for healthcare services to PWH who have no other source of health coverage or are confronted with coverage limits. The program is designed to "wrap around" other forms of coverage and is—from a legal perspective—the "payer of last resort." This designation means that if an individual is eligible for any other program, they must access that coverage and benefits before accessing the Ryan White Program (HRSA, 2018).

As the third largest source of federal funding for HIV care in the United States after Medicare and Medicaid, the Ryan White Program is estimated to reach over 561,000 PWH each year (HRSA, 2021). Funding for the Ryan White Program is subject to congressional appropriation each year. In addition to federal funding, some states and localities also provide funding to their Ryan White programs through state matching funds requirements.

Part A of the Ryan White Program provides funding to Eligible Metropolitan Areas and Transitional Grant Areas hardest hit by the HIV/AIDS epidemic for a wide range of services and efforts.

Part B provides funding to states and territories (HRSA, 2023). A vitally important component is the ADAP, which is specifically funded through allocations to the states under Part B along with state funding contributions. Each state's ADAP program provides HIV-related prescription drugs to low-income individuals with limited or no prescription drug coverage (KFF, 2017). Many states also use ADAP funding to purchase health insurance and/or pay insurance premiums, co-payments, or deductibles for PWH. All ADAP programs participate in the federal 340B Program, enabling them to purchase drugs at or below the statutorily defined 340B ceiling price.

Part C of the Ryan White Program funds providers and medical clinics to deliver comprehensive medical care and treatment to PWH who have no other source for care (HRSA, 2023). Part C also funds early intervention services, ambulatory care, and primary healthcare services for PWH in underserved or rural communities and communities of color. Finally, Part C also provides planning grants and capacity grants to support organizations in the delivery of high-quality, effective HIV care.

Part D of the Ryan White Program grants support services for women, infants, children, and youth (HRSA, 2023).

Part F provides funding for a variety of initiatives, including the Special Projects of National Significance, AIDS Education & Training Centers, dental programs, and the Minority AIDS Initiative (HRSA, 2023). Part F focuses on improving overall health care, HIV care, and health outcomes for minorities, including but not limited to HIV workforce development and other innovative models of HIV care and treatment (DHHS, 2023b).

The benefits available through the ACA, together with support provided by Medicaid expansion, are now in place to provide better support to PWH which was not available when the Ryan White CARE Act was created in 1990. However, it is important to note that the number of PWH has increased over those decades and the proportion of PWHs who need services provided by these programs is climbing.

In the 30+ years since the Ryan White Program was founded, organizations have learned how to make these programs dovetail to best meet the needs of PWH in a country without universal healthcare. The early passage and development of the Ryan White CARE Act set a critical precedent for the delivery of functional, HIV-focused services. This prototype, designed in close collaboration with the people it serves, subsequently influenced the expansion of the ACA and Medicare, as these programs were similarly designed in consultation with program users. The Kaiser Family Foundation has asserted that "the Ryan White Program remains a critical component of the nation's response to HIV in the ACA era" (KFF, 2020, n.p.).

Over the past several years, the Ryan White Program has had a renewed focus on tailoring approaches to best meet the needs of highly impacted communities and addressing factors such as access to housing and transportation that directly affect clients' ability to enter and stay in care. The federal Ending the HIV Epidemic in the U.S. (EHE) initiative expands upon the vital work of the Ryan White Program to reach newly diagnosed people with HIV (as well as people with HIV who are out of care) by enhancing linkages to and engagement in care, decreasing disparities, and improving viral suppression (DHHS, 2023a). Nevertheless, the yearly appropriations process has consistently involved partisan proposals to eliminate funding for some HIV-designated initiatives in efforts to create a more austere federal funding environment.

Despite such long-standing funding-related challenges, recent Ryan White HIV/AIDS Program data highlight the following:

- Nearly 560,000 people with HIV in the United States received life-saving care, medication, and essential support services through the Ryan White HIV/AIDS Program.
- Nine out of 10 clients receiving HIV medical care were virally suppressed in 2022. This is up from 70% of clients virally suppressed in 2010 and significantly higher than 66% virally suppressed nationally.
- More than 87% of Black/African-American clients receiving HIV medical care were virally suppressed and over 91% of Hispanic/Latino clients were virally suppressed in 2022. This represents a significant increase from 63% (Black/African-American clients) and 74% (Hispanic/Latino clients) in 2010.
- Among youth and young adult clients aged 13–24 years, nearly 84% receiving HIV medical care were virally suppressed in 2022, a major increase from 47% in 2010 (DHHS, 2023a).

NETWORKS OF CARE

For HIV providers, inclusion in networks of care for health programs is of great importance. Most patients' health coverage limits them to (1) seeing only certain providers who are "in network"; (2) being charged substantially higher fees for seeing "out of network" providers; or (3) being declined services by providers not included in the network.

The ACA requires that all plans in the state exchanges include a minimum percentage of all the ECPs in a geographic area in their provider network. As indicated previously, ECPs are providers that serve predominately low-income, medically underserved individuals (KFF, 2015). This includes Ryan White HIV/AIDS Program providers.

Reimbursement rates and schedules for providers who are part of the network are set by or negotiated with health coverage issuers and entities.

PROVIDER REIMBURSEMENT

Reimbursement for medical encounters and procedures depends heavily on thorough and accurate documentation of the medical visit, diagnosis, treatment, and services as recorded and submitted through coding claims. The level of complexity and severity of the medical encounter—and thus the level of reimbursement owed—is defined by the nature of the problem(s), the number of problems at issue, the amount of time spent with the patient, and other factors. Careful documentation of these factors is required to ensure adequate and appropriate reimbursement and is also generally considered a best practice to accurately communicate a provider's clinical decision-making. Other factors that are essential to document are the specific elements of medical history, physical examination, and medical decision-making. Documenting time spent on prevention services (e.g., counseling on condom use) and promoting behavioral changes (e.g., tobacco cessation and weight loss) is also essential for accurate reimbursement of these services.

CODING

Standardized coding systems are used in the United States to process billing claims to private and public insurers. The two principal systems used for coding medical information in the United States are the International Classification of Diseases (ICD) and the Current Procedural Terminology (CPT) codes that make up the Healthcare Common Procedure Coding System (HCPCS). In general, CPT/HCPCS codes identify the services rendered, whereas ICD codes focus more on diagnoses. CPT codes are created, maintained, and trademarked by the American Medical Association (AMA, 2024).

The HCPCS was created by CMS. It is based on CPT codes but provides for two levels of coding. Level I consists of AMA's CPT codes and provides for medical services and procedures furnished by clinicians. Level I codes are numeric. Level II codes are alphanumeric and apply primarily to medical devices and non-clinician services, such as ambulatory care, immunizations, diagnostic procedures, family counseling, and services provided by other health professionals (e.g., clinical nurses, psychologists, and pharmacists) (CMS, 2024). Medicaid and Medicare services are reimbursed by CMS based on the HCPCS codes for clinician activities.

The ICD is the international standard diagnostic classification for all epidemiological, health, and clinical usage. It is a coding and classification system of diseases, symptoms, injuries, and abnormal findings. It also documents the social circumstances and external causes of injury or diseases, as classified by the World Health Organization. In the context of reimbursement, ICD codes are used in conjunction with CPT codes to classify vital records and health condition codes associated with outpatient, inpatient, medical office utilization, and hospital charges.

REFERENCES

American Medical Association (AMA). CPT coding resources. https://www.ama-assn.org/practice-management/cpt/need-coding-resources. Published May 13, 2024. Accessed July 15, 2024.

Center for Consumer Information & Oversight. State-based exchanges. https://www.cms.gov/cciio/resources/fact-sheets-and-faqs/state-marketplaces.html. Published August 28, 2024. September 11, 2024.

Centers for Medicare and Medicaid Services (CMS). Healthcare common coding procedure system. https://www.cms.gov/medicare/coding-billing/healthcare-common-procedure-system. Published August 16, 2024. Accessed September 11, 2024.

Centers for Disease Control and Prevention (CDC). HIV prevention progress report, 2019. https://www.cdc.gov/hiv/pdf/policies/progressreports/cdc-hiv-preventionprogressreport.pdf. Published 2019. Accessed July 15, 2024.

Centers for Disease Control and Prevention (CDC). HIV testing dropped sharply among key groups during first year of COVID-19 pandemic. https://www.cdc.gov/media/releases/2022/p0623-HIV-testing.html.

June 23, 2022. Accessed July 15, 2024.Corallo B, Moreno S. Analysis of recent national trends in Medicaid and CHIP enrollment. Kaiser Family Foundation. https://www.kff.org/coronavirus-covid-19/issue-brief/analysis-of-recent-national-trends-in-medicaid-and-chip-enrollment/#:~:text=Data%20show%20that%20Medicaid%2FCHIP,64.5%25%20(Figure%202). April 4, 2023. Accessed July 15, 2024.

Congressional Research Service (CRS). Health insurance premium tax credit and cost-sharing reductions. https://crsreports.congress.gov/product/pdf/R/R44425#:~:text=To%20be%20eligible%20to%20receive,plan%20through%20an%20individual%20exchange. Published February 14, 2024. Accessed July 15, 2024.

Department of Health and Human Services, U.S. (DHHS). Latest data from HRSA Ryan White HIV/AIDS program highlight nine out of ten clients with HIV are virally suppressed. December 1, 2023a. https://www.hrsa.gov/about/news/press-releases/hab-2023. Accessed July 15, 2024.

DHHS. New reports show record 35 million people enrolled in coverage related to the Affordable Care Act, with historic 21 million people enrolled in Medicaid Expansion coverage. https://www.hhs.gov/about/news/2022/04/29/new-reports-show-record-35-million-people-enrolled-in-coverage-related-to-the-affordable-care-act.html#:~:text=media%40hhs.gov-,New%20Reports%20Show%20Record%2035%20Million%20People%20Enrolled%20in%20Coverage,Enrolled%20in%20Medicaid%20Expansion%20Coverage. Published April 29, 2022. Accessed July 15, 2024.

DHHS. Public health emergency declaration. https://aspr.hhs.gov/legal/PHE/Pages/default. Published 2024. Accessed July 15, 2024.

DHHS. Short-term, limited-duration insurance and independent, noncoordinated excepted benefits coverage. https://public-inspection.federalregister.gov/2024-06551.pdf. Published July 12, 2023b. Accessed July 15, 2024.

Dombrowski JC, Ramchandani MS, Golden MR. Implementation of low-barrier human immunodeficiency virus care: lessons learned from the Max Clinic in Seattle. *Clin Infect Dis.* 2023;77(2):252–257.

Gee E, Rapfogel N. Closing the Medicaid coverage gap would save 7,000 lives each year. Center for American Progress. https://www.americanprogress.org/article/closing-medicaid-coverage-gap-save-7000-lives-year/. Published September 10, 2021. Accessed July 15, 2024.

HealthCare.gov. Essential health benefits glossary. https://www.healthcare.gov/glossary/essential-health-benefits. Published 2024a. Accessed July 15, 2024.

HealthCare.gov. Medicaid & CHIP coverage. https://www.healthcare.gov/medicaid-chip/getting-medicaid-chip/. Published 2024b. Accessed July 15, 2024.

HealthCare.gov. Premium tax credit glossary. https://www.healthcare.gov/glossary/premium-tax-credit/. Published 2024c. Accessed July 15, 2024 .

Health Resources and Service Administration (HRSA). Eligible individuals & allowable uses of funds. https://ryanwhite.hrsa.gov/sites/default/files/ryanwhite/grants/service-category-pcn-16-02-final.pdf. Published October 22, 2018. Accessed July 15, 2024.

HRSA. HIV/AIDS Bureau, Ryan White HIV/AIDS Program: about the Program. https://ryanwhite.hrsa.gov/about. Published 2024a. Accessed July 15, 2024.

HRSA. HIV/AIDS Bureau, Ryan White HIV/AIDS Program: Program parts & initiatives. https://ryanwhite.hrsa.gov/about/parts-and-initiatives. Published December 2023. Accessed July 15, 2024.

HRSA. Ryan White HIV/AIDS Program annual client-level data report. Ryan White HIV/AIDS Program services report 2020. https://ryanwhite.hrsa.gov/sites/default/files/ryanwhite/about-program/RWHAP-annual-client-level-data-report-2020.pdf. Published December 2021. Accessed July 15, 2024.

Internal Revenue Service (IRS). The Premium Tax Credit—the basics. https://www.irs.gov/affordable-care-act/individuals-and-families/the-premium-tax-credit-the-basics. Published August 22, 2024. Accessed September 11, 2024.

Kaiser Family Foundation (KFF). 10 things to know about managed care. https://www.kff.org/medicaid/issue-brief/10-things-to-know-about-medicaid-managed-care/#:~:text=As%20of%20July%202021%2C%2041%20States%20Used%20Capitated%20Managed%20Care,to%20Deliver%20Services%20in%20Medicaid. February 23, 2022a. Accessed July 15, 2024.

KFF. AIDS drug assistance programs (ADAPs). https://www.kff.org/medicaid/issue-brief/how-many-uninsured-are-in-the-coverage-gap-and-how-many-could-be-eligible-if-all-states-adopted-the-medicaid-expansion/. Published August 16, 2017. Accessed July 15, 2024.

KFF. Federal and state standards for "Essential Community Providers" under the ACA and implications for women's health. https://www.kff.org/womens-health-policy/issue-brief/federal-and-state-standards-for-essential-community-providers-under-the-aca-and-implications-for-womens-health/#:~:text=Federal%20law%20generally%20defines%20ECPs,Social%20Security%20Act%20(SSA). Published January 23, 2015. Accessed July 15, 2024.

KFF. Key facts about the uninsured population. https://www.kff.org/uninsured/issue-brief/key-facts-about-the-uninsured-population/. Published November 6, 2020. Accessed July 15, 2024.

KFF. Medicaid and people with HIV. https://www.kff.org/hivaids/issue-brief/medicaid-and-people-with-hiv/. Published March 27, 2023a. Accessed July 15, 2024.

KFF. Medicaid managed care market tracker. https://www.kff.org/statedata/collection/medicaid-managed-care-tracker/. Published 2024a. Accessed July 15, 2024.

KFF. Medicare and people with HIV. https://www.kff.org/hivaids/issue-brief/medicare-and-people-with-hiv/. March 27, 2023b. Accessed July 15, 2024.

KFF. Status of state Medicaid expansion decisions: interactive map. https://www.kff.org/medicaid/issue-brief/status-of-state-medicaid-expansion-decisions-interactive-map/. July 21, 2022b. Accessed July 15, 2024.

KFF. The Ryan White HIV/AIDS Program: the basics. https://www.kff.org/hivaids/fact-sheet/the-ryan-white-hivaids-program-the-basics/. November 3, 2022c. Accessed July 15, 2024.

KFF. The uninsured population and health coverage. https://www.kff.org/health-policy-101-the-uninsured-population-and-health-coverage/?entry=table-of-contents-trends-in-the-uninsured-rate. Published May 28, 2024b. Accessed July 15, 2024.

Labisi T, Regan N, Davis P, Fadul N. HIV care meets telehealth: a review of successes, disparities, and unresolved challenges. *Curr HIV/AIDS Rep.* 2022;19(5):446–453.

Levy M. Patient Protection and Affordable Care Act (PPACA). *Encyclopedia Britannica.* https://www.britannica.com/money/Patient-Protection-and-Affordable-Care-Act. Updated July 2, 2024. Accessed July 15, 2024.

Medicaid.gov. Benefits. https://www.medicaid.gov/chip/benefits/index.html. Published 2024a. Accessed July 15, 2024.

Medicaid.gov. Financing. https://www.medicaid.gov/chip/financing/index.html. Published 2024b. Accessed July 15, 2024.

Medicare.gov. Catastrophic coverage. https://www.medicare.gov/drug-coverage-part-d/costs-for-medicare-drug-coverage/catastrophic-coverage. Published 2024a. Accessed July 15, 2024.

Medicare.gov. Costs in the coverage gap. https://www.medicare.gov/drug-coverage-part-d/costs-for-medicare-drug-coverage/costs-in-the-coverage-gap. Published 2024b. Accessed July 15, 2024.

Myers JE, Braunstein SL, Xia Q, et al. Redefining prevention and care: a status-neutral approach to HIV. *Open Forum Infect Dis.* 2018;5(6):ofy097.

National Council on Aging. Tools & training for professionals; donut hole: who pays what in Part D." https://www.ncoa.org/article/donut-hole-part-d. Published 2024. Accessed July 15, 2024.

Rho, HJ, Schmitt J. Health-insurance coverage rates for US workers, 1979–2008. https://cepr.net/documents/publications/hc-coverage-2010-03.pdf. Published March 2010. Accessed July 15, 2024.

Rudowitz R, Snyder L. Medicaid financing: how does it work and what are the implications? Kaiser Family Foundation. http://kff.org/medicaid/issue-brief/medicaid-financing-how-does-it-work-and-what-are-the-implications/. Published May 20, 2015. Accessed July 15, 2024.

Rudowitz R, Williams E, Hinton, E, Garfield R. Medicaid financing: the basics. Kaiser Family Foundation. https://www.kff.org/report-section/medicaid-financing-the-basics-issue-brief/. Published May 7, 2021. Accessed July 15, 2024.

INDEX

For the benefit of digital users, indexed terms that span two pages (e.g., 52–53) may, on occasion, appear on only one of those pages.

Tables, figures, and boxes are indicated by an italic *t*, *f*, and *b* following the page number.

A

abacavir (ABC), 137–38
 ARV regimens, 183*t*
 baseline conditions, 184*t*
 children, 268
 cholesterol and, 411
 choosing between third drug options, 182
 combinations, 181
 drug resistance mutations (DRMs), 201*t*
 hypersensitivity reaction, 367
 principles in pregnancy, conception, and contraception, 287*t*
 reactions, 368
 toxicity and adverse effects, 273–74
 treatment in U.S., 273*t*
 treatment options for optimizing, 206, 207*t*
absorption
 drug disposition, 286
 pharmacokinetics, 141–42
acamprosate, alcohol use disorder, 469
Acanthamoeba, 376
acquired HIV drug resistance (ADR), 195
 definition, 196*t*
 epidemiology, 204
 management of, 204–5
acquired immune deficiency syndrome. *See* AIDS
ACTG 5221 (STRIDE) trial, 263
ACTG/AIDS Malignancy Consortium (AMC), 320
Activity of Daily Living (ADL), 297
acute HIV infection, 32
 recognition of, 65
 signs and symptoms of, 65*t*
acute inflammatory demyelinating polyneuropathy (AIDP). *See* inflammatory demyelinating polyneuropathy
acyclovir
 herpes simplex virus (HSV) treatment, 250, 250*t*
 varicella zoster virus, 251*t*
adjustment disorders, treatment of, 480
adjustment reactions, treatment of, 480
adolescents
 COVID-19 and emerging conditions, 94–95
 developmental issues, 92
 HIV and, 90–95
 HIV disclosure, 506
 HIV epidemiology in, 16–17
 HIV infection by race/ethnicity, 20*t*
 medical management, 92–93
 medication adherence, 94
 mental health, 94
 percentage of diagnoses of HIV by sex and transmission category, 92*f*
 percentage of diagnoses of HIV infection, 91*f*
 period of, 90
 sexual risk, 93
 substance use, 93–94
 summary of HIV care, 95
 transition to adult care, 95
adolescents with HIV (AWH), 91
adrenal disorders, people with HIV, 442
adult care, adolescents' transition to, 95
adults, HIV infection by race/ethnicity, 20*t*
advance care planning, older PWH, 301
advance directive, advance planning, 510
advance planning, 509–11
 advance directive, 510
 durable power of attorney, 510
 physician order for life-sustaining treatment (POLST), 510–11
 will, 511
 See also legal issues
ADVANCE trial, 92–93, 180–81, 408–9, 446
Advancing Clinical Therapeutics Globally (ACTG), 318, 492
adverse-effect considerations, older PWH, 298
Advisory Committee on Immunization Practices (ACIP), 75, 76
 vaccinations, 307, 334
affective disorders, treatment of, 481–83
Affordable Care Act (ACA), 83, 514, 515–16
Africa
 dissemination of HIV throughout, 6–8
 spatial dynamics showing spread of HIV-1, 6*f*
age, HIV diagnosis, 15*f*
age group HIV epidemiology, 15–17
 adolescents, 16–17
 children, 16
 older adults, 17
 young adults, 16–17
Agency for Healthcare Research and Quality (AHRQ), 122
aging and HIV
 advance care planning, 301
 adverse-effect considerations, 298
 age-related sexual changes, 302
 ART-specific clinical considerations, 298
 bone, 302
 class and drug-specific considerations for ART selection in older PWH, 299*t*
 cognition/safety concerns, 297–98
 Comprehensive Geriatric Assessment (CGA), 296–97
 comprehensive medication assessment, 299–300
 diabetes, 301
 differences in older vs. younger PWH, 295–96
 frailty, 297
 functional status, 297
 hypertension, 301–2
 malignancy, 302
 management strategy for care of older PWH, 296–301
 medication clearance considerations, 298–99
 mobility and falls, 297
 mood, 298
 multimorbidity, 296
 nutrition/weight changes, 300–1
 performing CGA, 297
 polypharmacy, 298
 problem-based management of older PWH, 301–2
 select immunizations, 302
 social/financial issues, 300
 symptom burden/pain, 301
AIDS, 260
 late-stage HIV infection, 483
 nephropathy, 428
 papular pruritic eruption (PPE) of, 366
AIDS Clinical Trials Group (ACTG), 255, 261
 tumor staging system, 318, 319*t*
AIDS Drug Assistance Programs (ADAP), 125, 126–27, 514–15
AIDS Education and Training Centers, 126–27, 130
AIDS pandemic, Kinshasa as cradle of, 6*f*, 6
AIDS-related lymphomas, World Health Organization classification, 323*b*
AIDS symptoms, persons with, 7
AIDS Treatment Network (ATN), 93–94
AIDSVAX B/E, vaccine, 231
alcohol
 intoxication/withdrawal, 468–69
 pharmacological management, 468–69
alcohol use disorder (AUD), 465
 acamprosate, 469
 anticonvulsants, 470
 disulfirma, 469–70
 naltrexone, 469
 pharmacotherapy for, 469–70
alitretinoin gel, Kaposi's sarcoma, 319
allogeneic bone marrow transplant (alloBMT), 327–28
American Academy of Family Physicians, 95, 456
American Academy of HIV Medicine (AAHIVM), 132, 191, 508
American Academy of HIV Medicine's HIV Pharmacist (AAHIVP), 130
American Academy of Neurology (AAN), 396, 399
American Academy of Pediatrics, 26, 90, 95, 278
American College of Cardiology, 301–2
American College of Obstetrics, 269
American College of Physicians, 95
American Diabetes Association (ADA), 301
American Heart Association, 301–2
American Heart Association/American College of Cardiology (AHA/ACC)
 cardiovascular disease risk, 404
 cholesterol and hypertension, 418
 factors in risk calculator, 412*b*, 412
 guidelines for diagnosis and management of hypertension, 409*t*
 screening and assessing cardiovascular risk, 409–10
 See also cardiovascular disease (CVD)
American Indian/Alaskan Native
 adults/adolescents living with HIV infection, 20*t*
 death of PWH, 20*t*
 diagnoses of HIV infection, 91*f*
 HIV infection, 15*f*
 HIV infection among MSM, 20*f*
American Pharmacists Association, 132
American Society for Bone and Mineral Research, 457
American Society of Health Systems Pharmacists, 131–32
American Society of Internal Medicine, 95
Americans with Disabilities Act (ADA), 512
American Thoracic Society, 243, 263–64
amoeba, cutaneous opportunistic infection, 376
anal cancer, screening, 283, 284*t*
Anal Cancer/HSIL Outcomes Research (ANCHOR), 283, 334
anal cytology, 66*t*
anal dysplasia
 antiretroviral therapy (ART) and, 334–35
 prevention, 334
 screening, 333–34
 treatment, 334
anal intraepithelial neoplasia (AIN)
 epidemiology of HIV-associated, 332
 screening protocol for, 333*f*
ANCHOR study, 372
angiotensin-converting-enzyme inhibitors, kidney disease, 431–32
angiotensin II blockade, kidney disease, 431–32
anogenital neoplasia
 definition, 329
 effect of ART on anal dysplasia, 334–35
 effect of ART on HIV-associated cervical dysplasia, 330
 epidemiology of HIV-associated anal intraepithelial neoplasia, 332

anogenital neoplasia (*cont.*)
epidemiology of HIV-associated cervical carcinoma, 329–30
epidemiology of HIV-associated cervical intraepithelial neoplasia, 329
epidemiology of HIV-associated squamous cell cancer of the anus, 332–33
pathogenesis of HPV in HIV infection, 329
screening, treatment, and prevention of HIV-associated anal dysplasia, 333–34
screening, treatment, and prevention of HIV-associated cervical dysplasia, 330–31
screening protocol for anal intraepithelial neoplasia (AIN), 333*f*
See also malignancies
anogenital warts, condyloma acuminatum, 371*f*, 371–72
anonymous testing, description, 54*t*
antibiotic prophylaxis, dental care, 75
antibiotics, reactions and interactions, 368–69
antibodies, neutralizing, HIV prevention, 170
antibody 3BNC117, broadly neutralizing antibody (bNAb), 224
Antibody Mediated Prevention (AMP), 232
anticonvulsants
alcohol use disorder, 470
cocaine use, 472
methamphetamine, 473
antidepressants, methamphetamine, 473
antigen seroconversion window period, 52
antineoplastic and antiretroviral therapy
cancer incidence among persons with HIV, 359
considerations for combining, 360–61
drug-disease interactions, 361
drug interactions for CYP450, 360
drug interactions for p-glycoprotein, 360
medication toxicities, 360–61
strategies for clinical management of people with cancer and HIV, 361–62
antipsychotics, methamphetamine, 473
antiretroviral (ARV) toxic neuropathy (ATN), distal symmetrical polyneuropathy (SCPN) and, 391–92
antiretroviral agents (ARVs), 137
cerebrospinal fluid activity of, 384, 385*t*
change in therapy in children, 273
in children, 272
CNS effectiveness of, 144–45
combination therapy for children, 268
dosing and coformulations, 145–47
entry inhibitors, 137, 139
FDA-approved combination ARV formulations, 146*t*
integrase strand transfer inhibitors, 137, 139
non-nucleoside reverse transcriptase inhibitors, 137, 138
novel noncurative ARV drugs, 226–27
novel PrEP ARVs and delivery methods, 168–69
nucleoside/nucleotide reverse transcriptase inhibitors, 137–38
principles in pregnancy, conception, and contraception, 287*t*
protease inhibitors, 137, 139
schematic of genetic barriers to resistance, 197*f*
specific, for treatment in United States, 273, 273*t*
suppression of HIV, 218
toxicities and adverse effects, 273–74
transplacental transfer of ARV drugs, 286
See also HIV therapy; pregnancy and ART
antiretroviral stewardship, 191
anesthesia considerations and drug interactions, 192–93
bariatric considerations for PWH, 191–92
bariatric surgery and ART, 193
hospitalization-related concerns, 190–91
perioperative care, 191–92
postoperative complications and HIV infection, 192
surgical issues, 191–92
antiretroviral therapy (ART), 1, 11–12, 23
antibiotics, 368–69
bariatric surgery and, 193
benefits in children, 274
"Berlin patient", 219
bone fragility and, 455
bone health and HIV, 460–61
bone mineral density in PWH, 454–55
combination for HIV, 478
cryptosporidiosis, 242
dose adjustment in renal insufficiency, 436
effect on cardiovascular disease (CVD), 407–9
guidelines for ART in children, 272
guidelines for initiation, 262
HIV-1 replication control, 218–19
HIV and TB coinfection, 245, 246
HIV-associated cardiovascular disease, 411*f*
HIV prevention and, 130
HIV-related primary central nervous system lymphoma (PCNSL), 322
immune reconstitution inflammatory syndrome (IRIS), 261
immunologic effects of, 39–40
initiation, 262
JC virus infection, 254
Kaposi's sarcoma, 318–19
"London patient", 219
long-acting ART (LA-ART), 105, 133
MAC and HIV, 247–48
management among transplant recipients, 308–9
microsporidiosis treatment, 243
"Mississippi baby", 219
modifying in setting of virologic suppression, 205–6
non-nuclease reverse transcriptase inhibitors (NNRTIs), 367–68, 368*f*
nucleoside reverse transcriptase inhibitor (NRTI), 368
older PWH, 298
opportunistic infections, 255
overview of, 177
persons with HIV (PWH) experiencing homelessness, 105
pharmacist enhancing efficacy and reducing errors, 132
in pregnancy, 284–91
proof of concept, 219
protease inhibitors (PIs), 368
psychiatric effects of, 485
rapid ART initiation and rapid ART reinitiation, 206–7
reactions and interactions, 367–69
renal disease and, 431
risk of non-tuberculosis-associated IRIS, 262
selection in older people with HIV (PWH), 299*t*
treatment options for optimizing, 207*t*
See also antineoplastic and antiretroviral therapy; pregnancy and ART
antiretroviral therapy (ART) treatment guidelines, 177–78, 186–87
baseline conditions, 184*t*
choosing between recommended NRTI backbones, 181–82
choosing between third drug options, 182–83
concomitant medical conditions, 185*t*
factors for consideration in ART selection, 180*t*
overview of, 177
recommended initial ART regimens, 180*b*
recommended initial regimens in certain clinical situations, 183, 183*t*
selection of initial regimen, 179–81
when to start, 178–79
when to switch or simplify ART, 184–86
antiviral agents, hepatitis C, 494*t*
Antiviral Pregnancy Registry, 163
anxiety disorders, treatment of, 480–81
APOL1 Long-Term Kidney Transplantation Outcomes Network (APOLLO) study, 433
APPROACH trial, vaccine, 232
aptamers
gene modification, 226
HIV viral life cycle, 227*f*
ASCEND trial, 265, 416
Asian
adults/adolescents living with HIV infection, 20*t*
death of PWH, 20*t*
diagnoses of HIV infection, 91*f*
HIV infection, 15*f*
HIV infection among MSM, 20*f*
Aspergillus, 369–70
aspirin, cardiovascular disease, 415*b*, 415–16
Aspirin in Reducing Events in the Elderly trial, 416
Aspirin to Reduce Risk of Initial Vascular Events (ARRIVE) trial, 416
assembly and budding, HIV viral life cycle, 227*f*
ASSERT study, 181
assessment of intervention, Ending the HIV Epidemic (EHE) initiative, 3
atazanavir (ATV), 139
absorption, 142
drug interactions, 191, 361
kidney complications, 434
pregnancy and, 285
treatment in U.S., 273*t*
treatment options for optimizing, 207*t*
atazanavir, ritonavir-boosted (ATV/r)
drug resistance mutations (DRMs), 201*t*
principles in pregnancy, conception, and contraception, 287*t*
treatment options for optimizing, 207*t*
ATHENA cohort, 410–11
atherosclerotic cardiovascular disease (ASCVD), 404
AHA/ACA risk calculator, 412*b*
cholesterol management, 410*b*, 410
pathophysiology and management of HIV-associated, 412*f*
See also cardiovascular disease (CVD)
ATLAS-2M trial, 140, 185–86, 206
ATLAS Trial, 139–40, 185–86, 206
Atomoxetine, methamphetamine, 473
atopic dermatitis and xerosis, inflammatory dermatoses in HIV, 365–66
atracurium, drug interactions, 193
Atripla (FTC/TDF/EFV), ARV formulation, 146*t*
augmentation mammoplasty, description, 100*t*
Australia, 24
azithromycin, *M. avium* complex (MAC), 248
AZT. *See* zidovudine (ZDV/AZT)

B

Bacillus Calmette-Guérin (BCG), tuberculosis, 244
Balamuthia mandrillaris, 376
bariatric surgery, antiretroviral therapy (ART) and, 193
bartonellosis
cutaneous opportunistic infection, 374
nodular bacillary angiomatosis lesion, 374*f*
Beck Depression Inventory II (BDI-II), 298
BEERS criteria, 300
behavioral health problems, disparities in health care, 86
behavioral interventions, HIV prevention, 153–54
Behavioral Risk Factor Surveillance System, 343
bempedoic acid, cholesterol therapy, 415
"Berlin patient", 219, 225
BG505 SOSIP.644, vaccine, 232
bictegravir (BIC), 139, 177
ARV-naive individuals, 286–90
children, 208–9, 268
choosing between third drug options, 182
concomitant medical conditions, 185*t*
drug resistance mutations (DRMs), 201*t*
kidney complications, 435
post-exposure prophylaxis (PEP), 166*t*, 167
pregnancy and, 285
principles in pregnancy, conception, and contraception, 287*t*
transplant recipients, 308
treatment in U.S., 273*t*
treatment options for optimizing, 207*t*
bictegravir/emtricitabine/tenofovir alafenamide, switch option, 206
Biden administration, 515–16
Biktarvy (TAF/FTC/BIC), ARV formulation, 146*t*
biological threshold, 203
biomedical interventions, HIV transmission prevention, 155–56
bipolar disorder, 482–83
bisphosphonates, bone loss and, 459–60
Black/African Americans
adults/adolescents living with HIV infection, 20*t*
death of PWH, 20*t*
diagnoses of HIV infection, 91*f*
HIV infection, 14, 15*f*
HIV infection among MSM, 20*f*
"block and lock"
HIV latency silencing, 221
viral eradication, 220
blood pressure control, cardiovascular disease, 416–17
blood supply
HIV testing, 49
safety of U.S., 154
Board of Pharmacy Specialties, 130
body contouring, description, 100*t*
body weight and composition
HIV-associated lipodystrophy, 446
HIV-associated wasting, 445–46
metabolic changes, 445–47
weight gain in PWH, 446–47
bone density scan, 66*t*
bone health and HIV, 451–52
antiretroviral therapy (ART) and bone fragility, 455

ART and bone mineral density (BMD), 454–55
behavioral and lifestyle advice, 458
biological mechanisms of bone fragility, 455
bone mineralization abnormalities, 452–55
dual-energy X-ray absorptiometry (DXA), 457–58
fracture risk factors, 453–54, 454*b*
FRAX assessment, 457
identifying/treating secondary causes of low BMD, 458
postmenopausal women with HIV, 452–53
prevalence of low mineral density, 452
role of antiretroviral therapy (ART) selection and switching, 460–61
screening for bone disease, 455–56
screening for fall risk and frailty, 456
screening for fracture risk, 457
screening for vitamin D insufficiency, 456
therapeutic interventions for low BMD, 458
treatments for bone loss, 458–60
See also bone loss treatment
Bone Health and Osteoporosis Foundation (BHOF), 455
bone loss treatment
bisphosphonates, 459–60
calcium supplementation, 458–59
osteoporosis treatment, 460
testosterone replacement, 459
vitamin D supplementation, 458–59
See also bone health and HIV
bone problems, older PWH, 302
boosting agents, selection of ART in older people with HIV (PWH), 299*t*
BPaL regimen, bedaquiline, pretomanid, linezolid, 246
Brazil, 7*f*, 24
Brazzaville, 2*f*, 6, 7*f*
breastfeeding
ARV exposure during, 208
HIV transmission to infants, 269
infant feeding counseling, 280
postpartum transmission of HIV, 270
Brief Pain Inventory-Short Form (BPI-SF), 301
British HIV Association, 186–87
broadly neutralizing antibodies (bNAbs)
HIV-1 immunotherapy, 223–24
new drugs continuing to be developed, 228*f*
brown bag review, medication reconciliation, 300
buprenorphine administration
opioid use disorder, 471–72
substance use, 475
bupropion
cocaine use, 472–73
substance use, 475
tobacco use disorder, 417
Burkitt's lymphoma (BL), 323*b*, 323–24, 327

C

Cabenuva (CAB/RPV), ARV formulations, 146*t*
cabotegravir (CAB), 139
discontinuing, 162
drug interactions, 162, 360
drug resistance mutations (DRMs), 201*t*
HIV acquisition, 209
HIV infection after, 163
pregnancy and long-acting, 285, 286–90
principles in pregnancy, conception, and contraception, 287*t*
resistance testing, 199
rilpivirine and, 139
RPV and, 179
tolerability, 162
transmitted HIV drug resistance, 203
treatment options for optimizing, 207*t*
cabotegravir, long-acting, 157, 158, 161, 179, 206, 209, 210
contraception and, 279
long-acting injectable (LAI), 137
transplant recipients, 309
treatment in U.S., 273*t*
CAB/RPV intramuscular injections, 140
calcium, supplementation, 458–59
CAMELIA study, 263
Cameroon, 5
Canadian Hypertension Education Program Guidelines, 301–2
cancer(s)
mortality, 315
risk for development, 314–15
strategies for clinical management of people with HIV and, 361–62
See also antineoplastic and antiretroviral therapy
Cancer Immunotherapy Trials Network, 346–47
Cancer Therapy Using Checkpoint Inhibitors in People Living with HIV-International (CATCH-IT) Consortium, 346–47
Candida, 260–61, 369–70
Candida albicans, 240, 370, 398–99
candidiasis
clinical presentation, 240
cutaneous opportunistic infection, 370
diagnosis, 240
epidemiology, 240
oral thrush, 370*f*
pseudomembranous, involving the tongue, 240*f*
cannabis, substance use, 474
CAPELLA trial, 140, 368
capsid inhibitor
drug resistance mutations (DRMs), 201*t*
new drugs continuing to be developed, 228*f*
carceral settings
HIV transmission in, 108
HIV treatment in resource-limited international, 107–8
release and transition to community, 108–9
testing and managing comorbid conditions with HIV in, 109
cardiac, persons with HIV (PWH), 61*t*
cardiac disease, recommended action, 185*t*
cardiovascular, health status and system review, 62*b*
cardiovascular disease, 404–5
ACC/AHA guidelines for diagnosis and management of hypertension, 409*t*
aspirin, 415*b*, 415–16
bempedoic acid, 415
blood pressure control, 416–17
diet and exercise, 417–18
effect of ART on, 407–9
evidence of excess risk for, in HIV, 405–6
ezetimibe, 413–14
factors in AHA/ACC risk calculator, 412*b*, 412
fibric acid derivatives, 413
interventions and management, 410–18
nonpharmacological interventions, 417–18
omega-3 fatty acids, 414
overview of changes in HIV treatment and HIV-associated, 411*f*
pathophysiology and management of HIV-associated ASCVD, 412*f*
proposed mechanisms, 406–7
proprotein convertase subtilisin-kexin type 9 (PCSK9) inhibitors, 414–15
recommendation for reducing the risk of atherosclerotic cardiovascular disease (ASCVD), 410*b*, 410
recommendations for treating tobacco use disorder, 417*b*, 417
screening and assessing risk, 409–10
smoking cessation, 417
statin therapy, 411–13, 412*t*
statin therapy in PWH, 407, 408*f*
cardiovascular disease (CVD), 81
care. *See* HIV care
care models, people experiencing homelessness, 103–4
CASCADE study, 179
CBC with differential, 66*t*
CCR5 antagonists, management among transplant recipients, 309
CD4+ T-cells
baseline conditions for count, 184*t*
laboratory evaluation for people with HIV, 66
latency reversal approaches, 220–21
mechanisms of decline, 36–37
memory subsets, 219
PWH and, 218–19
rendering resistant to infection, 225–26
restoring exhausted, 221–22
CD8+ T cells, restoring exhausted, 221–22
Center for Epidemiological Studies (CES-D), 298
Centers for Disease Control and Prevention (CDC), 48, 131, 263–64
AIDS-defining conditions, 314
antiretrovirals for HIV-exposed infants, 268–69
bone mineral density (BMD), 452
COVID-19 vaccination, 94
disclosure issues, 505
HIV diagnosis, 1–2
HIV screening, 49
HIV testing algorithm, 53*f*, 53
HIV testing and prevention, 109–10
HIV testing for people with HIV, 243
HIV testing laws, 51
HIV testing recommendation, 363
Medical Monitoring Project, 416
neurosyphilis, 499
opioid epidemic, 470
preventing or delaying pregnancy, 279
routine screening, 295–96
substance use, 465
transmitted HIV resistance, 203
vaccinations, 307
Centers for Medicare and Medicaid Services (CMS), 516
central nervous system (CNS)
ART medications and, 192
penetration effectiveness score of ARVs, 385*t*
cerebrospinal fluid (CBF)
activity of antiretrovirals, 384
inflammatory demyelinating polyneuropathy, 393–94
cerebrospinal fluid analysis, ART medications and, 192
cervical cancer, 314
screening, 282, 283*t*
cervical carcinoma
epidemiology of HIV-associated, 329–30
See also anogenital neoplasia
cervical dysplasia
antiretroviral therapy (ART) and HIV-associated, 330
primary prevention, 331
screening, 330–31
treatment, 331
cervical intraepithelial neoplasia (CIN)
epidemiology of HIV-associated, 329
See also anogenital neoplasia
cervical Papanicolaou (Pap) smear, 66*t*, 329
CHAMP (Control of HIV After Antiretroviral Medication Pause) study, 219
CHARTER (CNS HIV Antiretroviral Therapy Effects Research), 144–45, 391
checkpoint inhibitors, immune modulation, 221–22
chemoradiotherapy, colorectal cancer, 344
chemotherapeutic agents, drug-disease interactions, 361
chemotherapy
antiretroviral therapy (ART) interacting with, 328
systemic lymphoma, 325
chemsex, term, 154–55
chest radiography, persons with HIV (PWH), 71, 73
children
antiretrovirals (ARV) in, 272
antiretroviral therapy (ART) for, 266
benefits of therapy, 274
change in therapy, 273
disclosure of parents' or caregivers' HIV status, 506
disclosure of their own HIV status, 506
disease course, 271–72
HIV drug resistance, 208–9
HIV epidemiology in, 16
immune reconstitution inflammatory syndrome (IRIS) in, 274
natural course of HIV RNA viremia in, 271*f*
stage 3 (AIDS) classifications with perinatally acquired HIV, 16*f*
time of maternal HIV testing, 17*f*
timing of initiation of ART, 272–73
toxicities and adverse effects of ARVs, 273–74
treatment guidelines for, 272
See also infants
Children's Health Insurance Program (CHIP), 514, 516–17
Child-Turcotte-Pugh score, 493
chimeric antigen receptor T-cells, immune enhancing or modulation, 223
chlamydia, 66*t*, 501–3
clinical presentation, 502
diagnosis, 502
treatment, 502–3
See also sexually transmitted infections (STIs)
Chlamydia trachomatis, 502
chorioretinitis, cytomegalovirus (CMV), 252
chronic HBV, definition, 489
chronic inflammation
CD4+ T-cell decline, 36–37
mechanisms of, in HIV disease, 38–39
chronic inflammatory demyelinating polyneuropathy (CIDP). *See* inflammatory demyelinating polyneuropathy
chronic kidney disease (CKD), 427
noninfectious comorbidities, 431
risk factors and etiologies of, in PWH, 428*b*
screening and monitoring in PWH, 436–37
See also kidney diseases

chronic obstructive pulmonary disease (COPD), HIV infection and, 423, 425–26
cidofovir
  cytomegalovirus (CMV), 253*t*, 254
  herpes simplex virus (HSV) treatment, 250, 250*t*
cigarette smoking, lung cancer, 337
Cimduo (TDF/3TC), ARV formulation, 146*t*
circulating recombinant forms (CRFs), 28
circumcision, voluntary medical male, 167–68
cisgender women, epidemiological trends in, 13–14
cisgender women with HIV
  anal cancer screening, 283, 284*t*
  care for individuals wishing to prevent/ delay pregnancy, 279
  care for individuals with HIV wanting to become pregnant, 280
  cervical cancer screening, 282
  cervical cancer screening recommendations, 283*t*
  cervical HPV infection, 282
  contraception and pre-pregnancy care, 278–81
  gender-diverse patients, 284
  HIV serodifferent couples, 280–81
  HIV sero-positive couples, 280
  HPV vaccination, 282
  importance of family planning and pre-pregnancy care, 278–79
  infant feeding counseling, 280
  pre-pregnancy counseling for persons with childbearing potential with HIV, 279
civil rights, discrimination and, 511–12
clarithromycin, 247, 248
clinical care, people experiencing homelessness, 104–6
Clinical Care Options, 200*t*
clinical history, initial HIV visit, 63*t*
clinically significant finding, 149–50
Clinical Opiate Withdrawal Scale (COWS), 471–72
Clinical Treatment Act, 81
clinical trials
  ART and opportunistic infections, 255–56
  clinical vs. statistical significance, 149–50
  importance of diversity in, 80–81
  interpreting results, 148–50
  long-acting injectable-based regimens for multidrug-resistant HIV, 140
  long-acting injectable-based regimens for switch therapy, 139–40
  noninferiority analysis, 149
  per-protocol (PP) vs. intent-to-treat (ITT) analysis, 148–49
  phases of, 148
  potential for change, 81
  primary efficacy endpoint, 149
  women, racial and ethnic participants in, 81
  See also HIV therapy
Clinician's Guide to Prevention and Treatment of Osteoporosis, 453
clofazimine, BPaL regimen, 246
CMV. *See* cytomegalovirus (CMV)
CNS HIV Antiretroviral Therapy Effects Research (CHARTER), 144–45, 391
CNS viral escape, 383
cobicistat (COBI), 141, 142
  kidney complications, 435
  selection of ART in older people with HIV (PWH), 299*t*
  treatment in U.S., 273*t*
cobicistat-boosted darunavir (DRV/c), ARV regimens, 183*t*
cocaine/crack
  anticonvulsants, 472
  bupropion, 472–73
  disulfiram, 473
  doxazosin, 473
  stimulants, 472
  substance use, 472–73
coccidiodomycosis
  clinical presentation, 241
  diagnosis, 241
  epidemiology, 241
  treatment, 241
Cockcroft-Gault or the Modification of Diet in Renal Disease, 143
cognition concerns, older PWH, 297–98
Cognitive Assessment Measurement Scale (CAMS), 484
cognitive behavioral therapy (CBT), substance use, 467–68
coinfection/comorbidity testing, laboratory evaluation for PWH, 66*t*
colitis, cytomegalovirus (CMV), 252
collaborative drug therapy agreement (CDTA), 134
collaborative practice agreements (CPA), 130–31
colorectal cancer (CRC)
  chemoradiotherapy, 344
  clinical presentation, 343–44
  epidemiology of, in HIV, 342–43
  people with HIV, 342–45
  screening in HIV population, 343
  survival of patients with HIV and, 345
  treatment of, in HIV, 344
  treatment outcomes, 345
  See also malignancies
combination antiretroviral therapy, 34
combination pharmacotherapy, methamphetamine, 473
Combivir (AZT/3TC), ARV formulation, 146*t*
communication, disparities in healthcare, 86–87
community viral load, 13
comorbidities, antiretroviral therapy (ART) regimen, 180*t*
competence, cultural, 85
Complera (FTC/TDF/RPV), ARV formulation, 146*t*
complete metabolic panel, 66*t*
complete responses, definition, 322
Comprehensive Geriatric Assessment (CGA), 295, 296–97
comprehensive medication assessment, older people with HIV (PWH), 299–300
conception, antiretroviral (ARV) principles, 287*t*
condyloma acuminatum, cutaneous opportunistic infections, 371*f*, 371–72
Conference on Retroviruses and Opportunistic Infections (CROI), 3, 19
confidential testing, description, 54*t*
connective tissue disease, 405
CONRAD-128 study, 170
Consolidated Appropriations Act, 471–72
contact dermatitis, 405
contraception, antiretroviral (ARV) principles, 287*t*
copper IUD (Cu-IUD), preventing or delaying pregnancy, 279
coronavirus. *See* COVID-19 pandemic
corticosteroids, HIV-associated nephropathy (HIVAN), 432
counseling
  HIV status, 168*t*
  negative HIV test, 57
  partner-notification legal requirements, 57
  positive HIV test, 56–57
  post-test, 56–57
  pretest, 51–52
  See also HIV testing
COVID-19 pandemic, 12–13
  adolescents, 94–95
  ART and HIV transmission, 266
  disruptions, 12
  health disparity, 79
  HIV/STI testing, 154
  HIV testing, 51
  immunization, 75–76
  migrants with HIV, 112
  racial and ethnic disparities, 82–83
  substance use and HIV, 475
  syndemic theory, 80
  systemic racism, 83
  TB cases during, 243
  telemedicine, 68–69
  therapy access during, 177
cowpox virus, 376
CRAFFT screening tool, 93–94
creatinine
  effect of drugs on secretion, 436*f*
  pharmacokinetic enhancers, 435
criminalization, HIV, 506–8
criminal-legal-involved individuals (CLII), 106
  HIV testing and prevention, 109
  release planning, 108, 109
criminal-legal-involved populations (CLIP)
  HIV care in detention settings, 107
  HIV in, 106–10
  HIV testing and prevention, 109–10
  HIV transmission in carceral settings, 108
  HIV treatment in prisons and jails, 106–7
  HIV treatment in resource-limited international carceral settings, 107–8
  release planning: transition to community, 108–9
  testing/managing of comorbid conditions with HIV in carceral settings, 109
CRISPR/Cas9 system, genome editing, 226
Crixivan belly, 441
cryotherapy, Kaposi's sarcoma, 319
cryptococcosis
  clinical presentation, 240–41
  diagnosis, 241
  epidemiology, 240
  IRIS and ART, 261
  treatment, 241
Cryptococcus gattii, 240
  meningitis, 386
Cryptococcus neoformans, 240, 370, 398–99
  meningitis, 255–56, 386
cryptosporidiosis
  clinical presentation, 242
  diagnosis, 242
  epidemiology, 242
  treatment, 242
Cryptosporidium, 242
cultural competency
  bias in healthcare, 85–86
  patient-provider relationship, 64
Cushing's syndrome, 368, 425–26, 444
CUSTOMIZE trial, 186
cutaneous cryptococcosis
  opportunistic infection, 370
  skin lesion, 370*f*
cutaneous malignancies in HIV, 377–78
  Kaposi's sarcoma, 377
  melanoma and nonmelanoma skin cancers, 377–78
  See also malignancies
cutaneous opportunistic infections, 369–76
  amoeba, 376
  bartonellosis, 374*f*, 374
  candidiasis, 370
  condyloma acuminatum, 371*f*, 371–72
  cutaneous cryptococcosis, 370*f*, 370
  cutaneous histoplasmosis, 371
  herpes simplex, 372*f*, 372
  herpes zoster, 373*f*, 373
  methicillin-resistant *Staphylococcus aureus*, 373–74
  molluscum contagiosum, 371*f*, 371
  onchomycosis, 369–70
  oral thrush, 370*f*
  scabies, 375*f*, 375–76
  syphilis, 374*f*, 374–75, 375*f*
CYP3A4, drugs inhibiting, 360
CYP3A4 inducers, transplant recipients, 308–9
Cystoisospora belli, 242
cystoisosporiasis
  clinical presentation, 242
  diagnosis, 242
  epidemiology, 242
  treatment, 242
cytochrome P450 enzyme system (CYP450), drug interactions, 360
cytokines, immune enhancing or modulation, 222–23
cytomegalovirus (CMV), 37, 66*t*, 249, 252
  chorioretinitis, 252
  clinical presentation, 252
  CMV polyradiculopathy, 252
  colitis, 252
  dementia, 253
  diagnosis, 252
  encephalitis, 387
  esophagitis, 252
  meningitis, 387
  opportunistic infection, 441
  pneumonia, 253
  prevention/prophylaxis, 254
  retinitis, 256
  transplant infection screening, 307
  treatment, 253–54, 253*t*
  ventriculoencephalitis, 252
cytomegalovirus (CMV) infection
  characterization, 396
  encephalitis, 395
  people with HIV and, 395–96
  polyradiculitis, 395–96
  treatment, 396
  ventriculoencephalitis, 395

D

D:A:D. *See* Data Collection on Adverse Events of Anti-HIV Drugs (D:A:D) study
dapivirine, HIV acquisition, 209
dapivirine-levonorgestrel (DPV/LNG) rings, 170
darunavir (DRV), 139
  contraception and, 279
  treatment options for optimizing, 207*t*
darunavir, cobicistat-boosted (DRV/cobi), treatment options for optimizing, 207*t*
darunavir, ritonavir-boosted (DRV/r), 177
  acquired HIV drug resistance, 204–5, 205*t*
  ARV regimens, 183*t*
  baseline conditions, 184*t*
  drug resistance mutations (DRMs), 201*t*
  pregnancy, 285, 286–90
  principles in pregnancy, conception, and contraception, 287*t*
  treatment options for optimizing, 207*t*

Data Collection on Adverse Events of Anti-HIV Drugs (D:A:D) study, 407, 408, 416, 434–35, 490
deaths, HIV infection (stage 3 AIDS) by race/ethnicity, 20*t*
DEFINE Study, 446–47
delavirdine (DLV), 138
delirium, treatment, 484
Delstrigo (DOR/TDF/3TC), ARV formulation, 146*t*
dementia
  cytomegalovirus (CMV), 253
  treatment, 484
Democratic Republic of the Congo (DRC)
  mpox, 377
  origin of HIV-1, 5
  spatial dynamics showing spread of HIV-1, 6*f*
dendritic cell-based vaccines, 230, 231*t*
dental care
  antibiotic prophylaxis, 75
  bleeding risk, 74
  concurrent infections, 75
  infection risk, 74
  oral disease, 74
  oral health care, 74–75
Department of Health and Human Services (DHHS), 1–2, 13, 177
  health equity, 83
  HIV testing of newborns, 50
  infant feeding, 278
dermatologic complications of HIV
  ART drug reactions and interactions, 367–69
  cutaneous findings, 363–64
  cutaneous malignancies in HIV, 377–78
  cutaneous opportunistic infections, 369–76
  inflammatory dermatoses, 364–66
  mpox disease (formerly monkey pox), 376–77
  See also cutaneous opportunistic infections
dermatologist, indications for referral to, 364*b*
Descovy (TAF/FTC), ARV formulation, 146*t*
detention settings, HIV care in, 107
diabetes
  chronic kidney disease (CKD) and, 431
  endocrine disorder in HIV, 442
  older PWH, 301
diagnose, Ending the HIV Epidemic (EHE) initiative, 1–2
diagnostic testing, description, 54*t*
dialysis, kidney disease and, 432
didanosine (ddI), 137–38
diet and exercise, cardiovascular disease, 417–18
Dietary Approaches to Stop Hypertension (DASH) diet, 416–17
diffuse infiltrative CD8+ lymphocyte syndrome (DILS), HIV infection and, 423, 424
diffuse large B-cell lymphoma (DLBCL), 323*b*, 323
directly observed therapy (DOT), tuberculosis in PWH, 245, 246
disclosure issues
  to children of own HIV status, 506
  to children of parents' or caregivers' HIV status, 506
  legal, 505–6
  perinatal/adolescent HIV, 506
DISCOVER trial, 80, 156–57, 157*t*, 162, 182
discrimination, civil rights and, 511–12
disparities in health care
  behavioral health problems, 86
  bias in healthcare, 85–86
  creating patient-centered HIV practice, 87
  language and communication, 86–87
  religion and spirituality, 87
  sexual and gender minority patients, 86
  women and HIV, 86
distal symmetrical polyneuropathy (DSPN), 390–92
  ARV toxic neuropathy (ATN), 391–92
  considerations for resource-limited settings, 392
  HIV infection and, 390–92
  typical signs and symptoms, 391*f*
distribution, pharmacokinetics, 142
disulfiram
  alcohol use disorder, 469–70
  cocaine use, 473
  substance use, 475
diversity
  importance in clinical trials, 80–81
  patients, 84
  viral infection, 33–34
dolutegravir (DTG), 139, 177
  acquired HIV drug resistance, 204–5, 205*t*
  ART regimens, 180*b*
  ARV regimens, 183*t*
  children, 208–9
  drug resistance mutations (DRMs), 201*t*
  guidelines against use of, 179
  HIV-2 infection, 210
  HIV drug resistance, 195
  post-exposure prophylaxis (PEP), 166*t*
  pretreatment drug resistance (PDR), 210
  principles in pregnancy, conception, and contraception, 287*t*
  switching ARV therapy, 184–85
  switch option, 206
  transmitted HIV drug resistance, 203
  transplant recipients, 308
  treatment in U.S., 273*t*
  treatment options for optimizing, 207*t*
doravirine (DOR), 138
  ARV regimens, 183*t*
  chemotherapy and, 360
  choosing between third drug options, 183
  drug resistance mutations (DRMs), 201*t*
  principles in pregnancy, conception, and contraception, 287*t*
  reactions, 367–68
  transplant recipients, 308–9
  treatment in U.S., 273*t*
  treatment options for optimizing, 207*t*
Doravirine/Islatravir Switch Studies, 446–47
dorunavir (DRV), treatment in U.S., 273*t*
Dovato (3TC/DTG), ARV formulation, 146*t*
doxazosin, cocaine use, 473
DRIVE-AHEAD trials, 183
DRIVE-FOREWARD trials, 183
drug absorption, pharmacokinetics, 141–42
drug cocktails, 34
drug disposition, components of, 286*b*, 286
drug-drug interactions, pharmacists managing, 132
drug interactions, anesthesia considerations and, 192–93
drug monitoring, pharmacodynamics and, 143–45
drug resistance. *See* HIV drug resistance (HIVDR)
drug resistance mutations (DRMs), definition, 196*t*
drug targets, HIV, 29*f*
dual-affinity retargeting (DART), immune enhancing or modulation, 224
dual-energy X-ray absorptiometry (DXA), 451, 457–58
Dual Prevention Pill (DPP), 170
durable power of attorney, advance planning, 510

E
ECHO trial, 279
eclipse period, 52
eclipse phase, infection, 32, 33
ecstasy (MDMA), substance use, 473–74
efavirenz (EFV), 138, 186
  contraception and, 279
  cutaneous drug eruption, 368*f*
  drug interactions, 193
  drug resistance mutations (DRMs), 201*t*
  principles in pregnancy, conception, and contraception, 287*t*
  reactions, 367–68
  statin therapy and, 411–12
  toxicity and adverse effects, 273–74
  transplant recipients, 308–9
  treatment in U.S., 273*t*
  treatment options for optimizing, 207*t*
elbasvir/grazoprevir, HIV/HCV coinfection, 494*t*, 496
elderly. *See* older adults
electron beam radiation therapy (EBRT), prostate cancer, 341–42
electronic nicotine delivery systems (ENDS), 468
"elite" controllers
  enhanced viral control, 221
  mechanisms and consequences of virus control, 41–42
elvitegravir (EVG), 139
  drug resistance mutations (DRMs), 201*t*
  kidney complications, 435
  treatment in U.S., 273*t*
elvitegravir/cobicistat (EVG/COBI), post-exposure prophylaxis (PEP), 166*t*
emtricitabine (FTC), 137–38
  ART regimens, 180*b*
  ARV-naive individuals, 286–90
  ARV regimens, 183*t*
  choosing between third drug options, 182–83
  clinical trials with tenofovir disoproxil fumarate (TDF), 156, 157*t*
  combinations of, 181–82
  drug resistance mutations (DRMs), 201*t*
  HIV acquisition, 209
  pre-exposure prophylaxis, 159*t*
  pregnancy and, 285
  principles in pregnancy, conception, and contraception, 287*t*
  serodifferent couples, 281
  treatment in U.S., 273*t*
emtricitabine/tenofovir (FTC/TDF or TAF), 177
Ending the HIV Epidemic (EHE), 1, 48, 134, 518
  assessment of intervention, 3
  diagnose, 1–2
  four pillars, 1–3
  goals and timeline, 1
  people experiencing homelessness, 103–4
  prevent, 3
  respond, 3
  treat, 2–3
endocrine, health status and system review, 62*b*
endocrine disorders in HIV
  adrenal disorders, 442
  diabetes mellitus (DM), 442
  gonadal dysfunction, 443
  growth hormone disorders, 444
  gynecomastia, 443
  integrase inhibitors, 441
  metabolic disease in HIV, 440–41
  non-nucleoside reverse transcriptase inhibitors (NNRTIs), 441
  nucleoside reverse transcriptase inhibitors (NRTIs), 441
  parathyroid disorders, 443
  pituitary adrenal disorders, 444
  pituitary disease, 443–44
  posterior pituitary disorders, 444
  prolactin disorders, 444
  protease inhibitors, 441
  thyroid abnormalities, 442–43
  transgender PWH, 445
  See also metabolic disorders in HIV
Endocrine Society (EOS), 456
end-stage liver disease, 310
end-stage renal disease (ESRD), 427, 432
enfuvirtide (ENF), 139, 141
  CYP enzyme system, 360
  drug resistance mutations (DRMs), 201*t*
  pregnancy and, 285
  susceptibility, 199
  treatment, 273*t*
entry inhibitors (EIs)
  antiretroviral agents (ARVs), 137, 139
  CNS penetration effectiveness score, 385*t*
  drug resistance mutations (DRMs), 201*t*
  new drugs continuing to be developed, 228*f*
enzyme immunoassay (EIA), HIV testing, 52, 53*f*, 53
eosinophilic pustular folliculitis, HIV-associated, 366
epidemiology (HIV)
  adolescents, 16–17
  by age groups, 15–17
  children, 16*f*, 16, 17*f*
  by gender identity, 18*f*, 18–19
  homelessness and, 96–98
  immigrant populations, 19–21
  older adults, 17
  by region, 17–18, 18*f*
  by route of transmission, 19, 20*f*
  transgender populations, 96–98
  trends by race/ethnicity, 14, 15*f*
  trends in cisgender women, 13–14
  young adults, 16–17
Epstein-Barr virus (EBV), 424
  primary central nervous system lymphoma (PCNSL), 321
  transplant infection screening, 307
Epzicom (ABC/3TC), ARV formulation, 146*t*
esophagitis, cytomegalovirus (CMV), 252
ESPRIT study, 222
Essential Community Providers (ECPs), 517
eSTAMP trial, 56
ethnicity
  COVID-19 pandemic, 82–83
  death of persons with HIV as stage 3 (AIDS), 20*t*
  diagnoses of HIV by gender and, 18*f*, 18–19
  HIV epidemiological trends by, 14, 15*f*
  HIV infection among persons aged 13-24 years, 91*f*
  HIV pandemic, 82
  stage 3 AIDS classifications of adults and adolescents, 15*f*
etomidate, drug interactions, 193

etravirine (ETR), 138
drug interactions, 193
drug resistance mutations (DRMs), 201*t*
pregnancy and, 285
reactions, 367–68
transplant recipients, 308–9
treatment in U.S., 273*t*
European AIDS Clinical Society (EACS), 186–87, 295, 297, 333, 416–17, 456, 458
European Confederation of Medical Mycology, 264
European Monitoring Centre for Drugs and Drug Addiction (EMCDDA), 466
Evotaz (ATV/COBI), ARV formulation, 146*t*
excretion
drug disposition, 286
pharmacokinetics, 143
exhaustion, definition, 297
ezetimibe, lipid management, 413–14

F
facial feminization, description, 100*t*
fall risk, screening, 456
falls, older PWH, 297
famciclovir
herpes simplex virus (HSV) treatment, 250, 250*t*
varicella zoster virus, 251*t*
family history, initial HIV visit, 63*t*
family planning
pre-pregnancy care and, 278–79
See also cisgender women with HIV
FDA Safety and Innovation Act, 80
Federal Housing Administration, 83
Federally Qualified Health Centers (FQHCs), 81
feminizing hormone regimens
surgical procedures, 100*t*
transgender populations, 98–99
fentanyl, drug interactions, 193
fibric acid derivatives, cardiovascular disease, 413
financial issues, older people with HIV (PWH), 300
FLAIR Trial, 139, 185–86, 206
FLAMINGO study, 182
fluconazole
candidiasis treatment, 240
cryptococcosis treatment, 241
fluorodeoxyglucose-positron emission tomography (FDG-PET), 321
fluoroquinolones, *M. avium* complex (MAC), 247
fold change, 198–99
Food and Drug Administration (FDA), 80, 154
antiretroviral (ARV) drugs, 178
approved agents for HIV, 137
approved HPV vaccines, 331
ARV for infants, 268–69
blood supply, 154
diversity in clinical trials, 80–81
mechanisms for expanded access, 150
sexual risk of adolescents, 93
specimens for HPV testing, 282
SSRIs, 481–82
statin and hepatoxicity, 413
vedolizumab, 222
fosamprenavir, 139, 273*t*
foscarnet
cytomegalovirus (CMV), 253*t*, 254
herpes simplex virus (HSV) treatment, 250, 250*t*
varicella zoster virus, 251*t*
fostemsavir (FTR), 139
antiretroviral therapy, 226
drug resistance mutations (DRMs), 201*t*
HIV drug resistance, 195
pregnancy and, 285
resistance testing, 199
transplant recipients, 309
treatment in U.S., 273*t*
fracture risk, screening, 457
Fracture Risk Assessment Tool (FRAX), 451, 457
frailty, older people with HIV (PWH), 297
Frailty Index, 297
French Hospital Database, 407
French Perinatal Cohort, 291
Frontal Assessment Battery test, 382, 384
"functional cure", 219
functional status, older PWH, 297
fungal infections
candidiasis, 240
coccidiodomycosis and histoplasmosis, 241
cryptococcosis, 240–41
See also opportunistic infections (OIs)
Fusarium, 369–70
fusion, 29
fusion/entry inhibitors, HIV life cycle and drug targets, 29*f*
fusion inhibitors, CNS penetration effectiveness score, 385*t*

G
G6PD screen, 66*t*
ganciclovir
cytomegalovirus (CMV), 253*t*, 254
varicella zoster virus, 251*t*
gastroesophageal reflux disease, recommended action, 185*t*
gastrointestinal
health status and system review, 62*b*
persons with HIV (PWH), 61*t*
gay, term, 97*t*
gay, bisexual, and other men who have sex with men (GBMSM), HIV testing, 49, 50, 51
Gay and Lesbian Alliance Against Defamation (GLAAD), 511–12
GEMINI-1 and GEMINI-2 trials, 182
gender, HIV infection among persons aged 13-24 years, 91*f*
gender-affirming hormone therapy (GAHT), 98
gender dysphoria, 96
gender expression, term, 97*t*
gender identity
HIV epidemiology, 18*f*, 18–19
term, 97*t*
gene modification
excising HIV-1 provirus from host cell genome, 226
rendering host's CD4+T cells resistant to infection, 225–26
ribozymes, RNA-based interference, and aptamers, 226
strategies, 226
general testing, laboratory evaluation for PWH, 66*t*
genes, regulatory functions, 30*t*
gene therapy, 225
genetic barrier to resistance, definition, 196*t*
genetic diversity, future of HIV regional and global, 10
genitourinary
health status and system review, 62*b*
persons with HIV (PWH), 61*t*
genotypic resistance testing, 198–99
genotypic testing, HIV-1 RNA thresholds for, 199
genotyping, definition, 196*t*
Genvoya (EVG/COBI/FTC/TAF), ARV formulation, 146*t*
geographic distribution
global HIV subtype diversity, 8*f*
HIV-1 group M, 8
HIV-1 group N, 9
HIV-1 group O, 9
HIV-1 group P, 9
HIV-1 subtypes, 9*b*
HIV-2, 9–10
"Getting to Zero" campaign, people experiencing homelessness, 103–4
glecaprevir/pibrentasvir, HIV/HCV coinfection, 494*t*, 495–96
global epidemic, percentage of country populations (age 15-49) living with HIV, 11*f*
global pandemic, overview of, 10–12
glucagon-like peptide-1 receptor agonists (GLP-1 RAs), 446–47
glucose and lipid profile, 66*t*
gonadal dysfunction, people with HIV (PWH), 443
gonorrhea, 66*t*, 501
clinical presentation, 501
diagnosis, 501
follow-up, 501
male with penile discharge due to, 501*f*
recommended treatment regimens for, 502*t*
treatment, 501
See also sexually transmitted infections (STIs)
Graves's disease, 442–43
growth hormone disorders, people with HIV (PWH), 444
Guidelines for the Prevention and Treatment of Opportunistic Infections, 253
Guidelines for the Prevention and Treatment of Opportunistic Infections in Adults and Adolescents with HIV, 250
Guillain-Barré syndrome (GBS), 393
gut-associated lymphoid tissue (GALT), HIV infection, 222
gynecomastia, people with HIV (PWH), 443

H
Haemophilus influenza type b (HIB), immunization, 76
Haiti, 7*f*, 7
HAND. *See* HIV-associated neurocognitive disorder (HAND)
harm reduction, HIV prevention, 154–55
Hashimoto's thyroiditis, 442–43
head, eyes, ears, nose and throat (HEENT)
health status and system review, 62*b*
persons with HIV (PWH), 61*t*
healthcare
chest radiography and symptoms for persons with HIV (PWH), 73
dental care, 74–75
disparities in, 85–87
diversity of patients, 84
flow sheets for primary care, 71
immunizations, 75–78
importance of trust, 85
initial HIV visit, 63*t*
latent tuberculosis infection (LTBI) screening, 72
Mycobacterium tuberculosis infection screening, 72–73
preventive therapy, 73–74
providing culturally competent, 84
retention, 84
tuberculosis (TB) screening and assessment, 71–72
See also disparities in health care; immunizations
Healthcare Common Procedure Coding System (HCPCS), 519
healthcare maintenance, 63*t*, 66*t*
healthcare setting, HIV transmission in, 24–25
healthcare system
Affordable Care Act, 515–16
coding, 519
HIV in United States, 514–15
initial HIV visit, 63*t*
Medicaid, 517
Medicare, 517–18
networks of care, 519
new approaches to HIV service delivery, 515
private insurance, 516
provider reimbursement, 519
Ryan White HIV/AIDS Program, 518–19
state insurance exchanges, 516–17
health disparities, adolescents, 90–91
health disparity, definition, 82
health equity, definition, 83
Health Resources and Services Administration (HRSA), 1–2
health status, persons with HIV (PWH), 62*b*
heart and lung transplantation
candidate criteria, 307
patient and graft survival and rejection, 310
See also organ transplantation in people with HIV
hematologic, health status and system review, 62*b*
hematopoietic cell transplantation (HCT), AIDS-related non-Hodgkin's lymphoma (NHL), 327–28
hemolymphatic, persons with HIV (PWH), 61*t*
hepatitis, IRIS and ART, 262
hepatitis A virus (HAV) immunization, 76, 307
hepatitis B virus (HBV), 6–7
assessment of, 158
clinical presentation, 489
coinfection with HIV, 177, 206, 489–91
diagnosis and evaluation, 489–90
goals of treatment, 490
HBV prevention, 490
HIV and, 163
HIV/HBV-coinfection considerations, 490
HIV treatment recommendations in HBV coinfection, 490–91
immune reconstitution inflammatory syndrome (IRIS), 491
immunization, 76
IRIS and ART, 262
management and treatment, 167
recommended action for coinfection, 185*t*
susceptible individuals, 167
treatment interruptions, 491
treatment options for HBV infection, 491
vaccinations, 307
hepatitis C virus (HCV), 6–7, 306
acute hepatitis C, 493–94
clinical course, 492
coinfection with HIV, 491–97
decision to treat, 493
diagnosis, 492–93

direct antiviral agents for hepatitis C, 494t
elbasvir/grazoprevir, 494t, 496
epidemiology, 492
fixed-dose combinations, 494t, 495–96
glecaprevir/pibrentasvir, 494t, 495–96
IRIS and ART, 261, 262
ledipasvir/sofasbuvir, 494t, 495
mechanisms of action for direct acting agents, 495
NS3/4A protease inhibitors, 494t, 495
NS5A inhibitors, 494t, 495
NS5B polymerase inhibitors, 494t, 495
people with HIV/HCV coinfection, 310
post-exposure prophylaxis for, 167
sofosbuvir/velpatasvir, 494t, 495
sofosbuvir/velpatasvir/voxilaprevir, 494t, 496
therapeutic modalities, 494–95
transmission to infants, 269
treatment failures, 496
hepatitis serologies, transplant infection screening, 307
herpes simplex virus (HSV) infection
cutaneous opportunistic infection, 372
HSV-2 on female perineum, 372f
HSV-2 on male penis, 372f
transplant infection screening, 307
herpesvirus
clinical presentation, 245, 249–50
diagnosis, 245
herpes simplex virus (HSV), 249
herpes simplex virus (HSV-1 and HSV-2), 249
HSV suppressive therapy recommendations, 251t
prevention, 245
prophylaxis, 251
treatment, 245–46
treatment recommendations, 250t
herpesvirus HHV-8, pathogenesis, 324
herpes zoster, cutaneous opportunistic infection, 373f, 373
high-level resistance, 200–2
highly treatment-experienced patients, assessment and management of, 207–8
Hispanic/Latino
death of PWH, 20t
diagnoses of HIV infection, 91f
HIV infection, 14, 15f
HIV infection among MSM, 20f
Hispanic/Latinx, adults/adolescents living with HIV infection, 20t
Histoplasma capsulatum, 371
histoplasmosis
clinical presentation, 241
cutaneous opportunistic infection, 371
diagnosis, 241
epidemiology, 241
treatment, 241
HIV
dissemination throughout Africa and world, 6–8
epidemiology, 10
future of immune-based therapeutics, 42–43
future of regional and global genetic diversity, 10
global subtype diversity, 8f
immune system and, 37–38
latency reversal approaches, 220–21
latency silencing, 221
life cycle, 28, 29f
migrant and immigrant persons with, 111–13
natural history, 31
origin and entry into humans, 5–6
origin and evolution of HIV-1 and HIV-2, 5
reasons to cure, 218–19
rural populations and, 110–11
surrogate markers of, 272
testing and care continuum, 13f, 13
transmission to infants, 269
viral classification, 28
viral eradication, 220
viral life cycle, 226, 227f
viral structure, 28–29
virus production, 31
women and, 86
See also gene modification; immune-enhancing and/or modulating strategies
HIV-1
diagnosis in infants, 269
disease course in children, 271–72
distribution of subtypes, 9b
epidemic histories of groups M and O, 7
estimated global spatial dynamics of subtype B, 7f
evolution of, 5
excising provirus form host cell genome, 226
group M, 8
group N, 9
group O, 9
group P, 9
infection of children, 266
latent reservoir, 219–20
origin, 5
p24 antigen, 54
quantitative RNA assays, 54–55
spatial dynamics showing spread in Africa, 6f
HIV-1 capsid inhibitors, kidney complications, 435–36
HIV-1 reservoir, establishment and persistence of latent, 219–20
HIV-2
evolution of, 5
geographic distribution, 9–10
infection, 210
origin, 5
quantitative RNA assays, 55
HIV/AIDS, opportunistic infections (OIs) and, 239
HIV/AIDS Cancer Match Study, 282, 315, 343
HIV antibody tests, infants and children, 267
HIV-ASSIST, 200t
HIV-associated dementia (HAD), 383, 384
recommended action, 185t
HIV-associated eosinophilic pustular folliculitis, inflammatory dermatoses in HIV, 366
HIV-associated nephropathy (HIVAN), 427
HIV-associated neurocognitive disorder (HAND), 297–98, 382
cerebrospinal fluid activity of antiretrovirals, 384
clinical manifestations of, 383–84
CNS viral escape, 383
definitions of, 384
HIV protein-associated encephalopathy, 383
macrophage-mediated HIV encephalitis, 383
risk factors, 384
screening tools for cognitive impairment, 384
T-cell-mediated HIV encephalitis, 382
HIV care
complexity of PWSH care needs, 125–26
continuum of, 122–23, 123f
funding for, 126–27
hospice care, 126
interdisciplinary approach, 122
interdisciplinary team care, 123
palliative care, 126
quality improvement, 127
role of team members, 124–25, 124t
Ryan White HIV/AIDS Program (RWHAP), 126–27
stages, goals, and interventions, 124t
See also pharmacist in HIV care
HIV-CAUSAL Collaboration, 263
HIV Costs and Services Utilization Study, 86
HIV criminalization, 506–8
HIV Dementia Scale, 297–98
HIV drug resistance (HIVDR), 195–96
acquired HIVDR (ADR), 195, 204–5, 211
ART switch/simplification, 205–6
ARV resistance considerations, 205–6
calculating level of phenotypic resistance, 199f
children and youth, 208–9
genotypic and phenotypic resistance testing, 198–99
highly treatment-experienced patients, 207–8
HIV-1 RNA thresholds for genotypic testing, 199
HIV-2, 210
HIV acquisition in setting of PrEP use, 209
HIV therapeutic targets for resistance testing, 199
indications and timing, 198
interpretation of resistance testing results, 200–3
key points about, 195
mechanisms of, 196–98
mutations and impact on ARV susceptibility, 201t
next-generation sequencing, 200
pregnancy and infant feeding, 208
proviral DNA sequencing, 199–200
rapid ART initiation and rapid ART reinitiation, 206–7
resource-limited settings, 209–10
schematic indicating genetic barrier to, 197f
select resources on HIVDR clinical evaluation and management, 200t
suboptimal ART and poor ART adherence, 197f
terms and definitions, 196t
testing, 198–99
transmitted HIVDR (TDR), 195, 203–4, 211
treatment options for optimizing ART, 207t
UNAIDS "95-95-95" target, 195
HIV epidemic, priority jurisdictions for ending, 2f
HIV infection
cutaneous findings, 363–64
immune dysregulation and immunosuppression, 363
HIV latency
reversal approaches, 218, 220–21
silencing, 221
HIV Medicine Association, 131–32, 191, 458, 508
HIV National Strategic Plan, 511–12
HIV Organ Policy Equity (HOPE) Act, 306, 311, 427, 433
HIV Outpatient Study (HOPS), 453
HIV pandemic
racial and ethnic disparities, 82
syndemic theory, 80
systemic racism, 83
HIV Pharmacotherapy continuing Education Program, 130
HIV prevention, 153
behavioral interventions, 153–54
biomedical interventions for transmission, 155–56
breakthrough infection, 162–63
coinfections, 163
counseling, 168t
economic factors, 155
HIV pre-exposure prophylaxis (PrEP), 156–62
laboratory testing and management, 168t
medication interactions, 162
microbicides, 169–70
multipurpose prevention technologies (MPT), 170
new and investigational interventions for, 168–70
novel PrEP antiretrovirals and delivery methods, 168–69
physical factors, 155
post-exposure prophylaxis (PEP), 164–67
pregnancy and lactation, 163
PrEP consultation, 164
PrEP inequities, 163–64
recommended services, 168t
resistance after PrEP use, 162–63
safety of U.S. blood supply, 154
scenarios for expert PEP consultation, 169t
structural and systems-level interventions, 154–55
substance use, harm reduction, and, 154–55
tolerability and adverse effects, 162
treatment as prevention, 155
"undetectable = untransmittable", 155
vaccines and neutralizing antibodies, 170
voluntary medical male circumcision, 167–68
See also post-exposure prophylaxis (PEP); pre-exposure prophylaxis (PrEP)
HIV prevention and care, transgender populations, 101–2
HIV Prevention Trials Network (HPTN), 232
HIV protein-associated encephalopathy, 383
HIV RNA, natural course of, viremia in children, 271f
HIV RNA pretreatment, baseline conditions, 184t
HIV serology, laboratory evaluation for PWH, 66t
HIV-specific history, initial HIV visit, 63t
HIV-specific testing, laboratory evaluation for PWH, 66t
HIV Symptom Index, 301
HIV testing
algorithm, 53f, 53
blood supply screening, 49
enzyme immunoassays (EIA), 52, 53f, 53
gay, bisexual, and other men who have sex with men (GBMSM), 50
history and evolution, 48–51
home testing, 56
individual screening, 49
infants and children, 267
laboratory markers for HIV, 52f, 52
newborns, 50
perinatal screening, 50
pharmacist role in, 133–34
pretest counseling, 51–52

HIV testing (*cont.*)
rapid HIV tests, 55
resource-limited settings, 56
settings for, 55–56
strategies to improve uptake, 50–51
terminology, 54*t*
types of, 54*t*
virologic assays, 54–55
western blot, 54
See also counseling
HIV therapy
antiretroviral agents (ARVs), 137–39
ARV dosing and coformulations, 145–47
classes and mechanisms of ARVs, 137
clinical research and access programs, 148
entry inhibitors, 137, 139
FDA-approved combination ARV formulations, 146*t*
future for, 140–41
HIV viral replication, 137, 138*f*
individual person, 150
integrase strand transfer inhibitors (INSTIs), 137, 139
intermediate-size participant population, 150
interpreting clinical trial results, 148–50
key clinical trial findings, 139–40
long-acting injectable-based regimens for multidrug-resistant HIV, 140
long-acting injectable-based regimens for switch therapy, 139–40
mechanisms for expanded access, 150
non-nucleoside reverse transcriptase inhibitors (NNRTIs), 137, 138
nucleoside/nucleotide reverse transcriptase inhibitors (NRTIs), 137–38
phases of clinical trials, 148
protease inhibitors (PIs), 137, 139
widespread use, 150
See also antiretroviral agents (ARVs); clinical trials
HIVTR, (Solid Organ Transplantation in HIV: Multi-site Study) Study, 306
HIV transmission
maternal risk factors for, 271
older vs. younger people with HIV (PWH), 295–96
HIV Vaccine Trial Network, 231–32
HIV viral load (RNA), laboratory evaluation for PWH, 66*t*
HLA-B 5701, 66*t*
Hodgkin's disease, 314
holographic wills, 511
Home Access HIV-1 Test System, 56
homelessness or unstable housing
care models for people experiencing, 103–4
care of persons with HIV (PWH), 102–6
clinical care of PWH, 104–6
epidemiology of HIV and, 103
home testing
HIV self-testing (HIVST), 56
Home Access HIV-1 Test System, 56
OraQuick In-Home HIV Test, 56
Together TakeMeHome (TTMH) project, 48, 56
hormone therapy (HT)
feminizing, 98–99
gender-affirming, 96
masculinizing, 99–101
transgender populations initiating, 98
hospice care
palliative care and, 126
term, 126
hospital settings
anesthesia and drug interactions, 192–93
antiretroviral stewardship, 190–91
bariatric surgery and ART, 193
perioperative care, 191–92
postoperative complications, 192
host cell genome, excising HIV-1 provirus, 226
HPV co-testing, 66*t*
human herpesvirus (HHV-8), 254
conditions associated with, 317
discovery of, 377
pathogenesis, 317
human papillomavirus (HPV), 503–4
anal cancer screening, 283, 284*t*
cervical cancer screening, 282, 283*t*
cervical HPV infection in women with HIV, 282
clinical presentation, 503
diagnosis, 503
Gardasil-9 vaccine for, 504
HSV lesions on scrotum of man with HIV, 503*f*
immunization, 76
pathogenesis of, in HIV infection, 329
prevention, 504
recommended treatment regimens for HPV/warts in PWH, 504*t*
screening transmasculine patients, 100
treatment, 503
vaccination, 282, 307
warts on shaft of penis in man with HIV, 503*f*
See also sexually transmitted infections (STIs)
humans, entry of HIV into, 5–6
human T-cell lymphotropic virus type 1 (HTLV-1) infection, myelopathy, 389, 390
humility
bias in healthcare, 85–86
cultural, 85
patient-provider relationship, 64
HVTN 705, vaccine, 232
hyperlipidemia, recommended action, 185*t*
hypertension
ACC/AHA guidelines, 409*t*
older PWH, 301–2
hysterectomy +- oophorectomy, description, 100*t*

I
ibalizumab (IBA), 139, 141
CYP enzyme system, 360
drug resistance mutations (DRMs), 201*t*
HIV-2 infection, 210
HIV drug resistance, 195
pregnancy and, 285
resistance testing, 199
transplant recipients, 309
ibalizumab-uiyk (IBA), treatment in U.S., 273*t*
immigrant persons, HIV care of, 111–13
immigrant populations, HIV among, 19–21
Immigration and Customs Enforcement (ICE), detention facilities, 107
immigration status, federally defined, 111–12
immune check point inhibitor therapy (ICPI), malignancies in people with HIV, 345–47
immune-enhancing and/or modulating strategies, 221–25
broadly neutralizing antibodies, 223–24
checkpoint inhibitors, 221–22
chimeric antigen receptor T-cells, 223
combination strategies, 224
cytokines, 222–23
dual-affinity retargeting, 224
monoclonal antibody therapy, 223
other immunomodulatory treatments, 225
T-cell trafficking, 222
immune reconstitution inflammatory syndromes (IRIS), 190, 260
antiretroviral therapy (ART) and, 261
complication in children, 274
etiology and pathogenesis, 261
guidelines for ART initiation, 262
HIV and TB coinfection, 246
HIV/HBV coinfection treatment, 491
incidence and associated opportunistic infections, 260–61
key points, 260
MAC and HIV, 247–48
meningitis and HIV, 388
opportunistic infections, 255
pathogenesis of, 40–41
prevention, 264
progressive multifocal leukoencephalopathy (PML), 254–55
rates, 255–56
term, 260
transgender populations, 102
treatment of, 264
tuberculosis-IRIS, 263–64
immune recovery, organ transplantation in people with HIV, 311
immunization(s)
concern with, 75
coronavirus (SARS-CoV-2 or COVID-19), 75–76
Haemophilus influenza type b (HIB), 76
hepatitis A virus (HAV), 76
hepatitis B virus (HBV), 76
human papillomavirus (HPV), 76
influenza, 76
initial HIV visit, 63*t*
measles mumps rubella (MMR), 77
meningococcus, 77
Mpox (monkeypox), 77
older PWH, 302
pneumococcus, 77–78
respiratory syncytial virus (RSV), 78
tetanus, diphtheria, and pertussis (TDAP), 78
varicella virus (VAR), 77
zoster, 77
See also vaccine(s)
immunology
antiretroviral therapy (ART), 39–40
future of immune-based therapeutics, 42–43
HIV effects on system, 37–38
mechanisms and consequences of virus control in "elite" controllers, 41–42
mechanisms of CD4+ T-cell decline, 36–37
mechanisms of chronic inflammation in HIV disease, 38–39
pathogenesis of immune reconstitution inflammatory syndromes (IRIS), 40–41
role of persistent immune dysfunction during therapy, 39–40
immunomodulatory therapies, 43
immunosuppression therapy
kidney transplantation, 308
maintenance, 308
See also post-transplant management
IMPAACT P1115 trial, 271
inactivated influenza vaccine (IIV), 302
Indian Health Service (HIS), 1–2
indinavir (IDV), 139
kidney complications, 434
reactions, 368
infants
antiretrovirals for HIV-exposed, 268–69
diagnosis of HIV-1, 269
disease course, 271–72
early treatment initiation and HIV remission in HIV-exposed, 271
feeding counseling, 280
HIV drug resistance and feeding, 208
timing of HIV infection, 269–70
timing of initiation of therapy, 272–73
See also children; newborns
infection
acute, 32
establishment of HIV, 31–32
viral diversity of HIV, 33–34
infection risk, organ transplantation in people with HIV, 311
Infectious Diseases Society of America (IDSA), 131–32, 191, 263–64, 301, 302, 330–31, 458
inflammatory demyelinating polyneuropathy
acute (AIDP), 393
biopsy, 394
cerebrospinal fluid (CBF) analysis, 393–94
chronic (CIDP), 393
classification, 393
clinical features, 393
diagnosis of acute, 392–93
differential diagnosis, 394
electrophysiology, 394
HIV and, 393
pathogenesis, 393
prognosis, 395
treatment, 394
inflammatory dermatoses and HIV, 364–67
atopic dermatitis and xerosis, 365–66
HIV-associated eosinophilic pustular folliculitis, 366
papular pruritic eruption of AIDS, 366
psoriasis, 365
seborrheic dermatitis, 364
See also dermatologic complications of HIV
Inflation Reduction Act, 514
influenza, immunization, 76, 307
informed consent, CDC definition, 51
initial evaluation. *See* persons with HIV (PWH)
inmate, term, 106
insomnia, treatment of, 484–85
Institute of Medicine (IOM), 456
institutional racism, definition, 83
Instrumental Activity of Daily Living (IADL), 297
integrase inhibitors
endocrine and metabolic disease in HIV, 441
HIV life cycle and drug targets, 29*f*
integrase strand transfer inhibitors (INSTIs), 177–78
acquired HIV drug resistance, 204–5, 205*t*
antiretroviral agents (ARVs), 137, 139
children, 268
choosing between third drug options, 182–83
CNS penetration effectiveness score, 385*t*
drug interaction, 191
drug resistance mutations (DRMs), 201*t*
HIV acquisition, 209
HIV drug resistance, 197
INSTI-based regimens, 183*t*
interactions with chemotherapeutic agents, 328
kidney complications, 435
long-acting injectable (LAI), 137

management among transplant recipients, 308
new drugs continuing to be developed, 228*f*
pharmacodynamics and, 144
recommended ART regimens, 180*b*
resistance testing, 199
resource-limited settings, 210
selection, 179, 180–81
selection of ART in older people with HIV (PWH), 299*t*
switching or simplifying, 184
transmitted HIV drug resistance, 203–4
integration
HIV viral life cycle, 227*f*
reverse transcription and, 30–31
intent-to-treat (ITT) analysis, 148–49
interdisciplinary team care
HIV care, 123
importance of approach, 122
See also HIV care
interferon-γ, tuberculosis and HIV, 263
interferon gamma release assays (IGRAs), 244
Mycobacterium tuberculosis infection, 71, 73, 244, 245
INTERHART study, 405–6
intermediate resistance, 200–2
International AIDS Conference, 155, 157
International AIDS Study, 200
International Anal Neoplasia Society (IANS), 333
International Antiviral Society, 368
International Antiviral Society-USA (IAS-USA), 157–58, 178, 186–87, 200*t*
See also antiretroviral therapy (ART) treatment guidelines
International Classification of Diseases (ICD), 519
International HIV Dementia Scale, 297–98
International Osteoporosis Foundation, 457
International Prognostic Index (IPI), 324–25
International Society for Clinical Densitometry, 457
International Society for Human and Animal Mycology, 264
intracellular immunization, 225
intracranial lesions
algorithm for diagnostic evaluation of focal brain disease, 397*f*
American Academy of Neurology (AAN), 396, 399
clinical presentation, 396
common bacterial mass lesions, 398
common etiologies of fungal abscesses, 398–99
differential diagnosis, 398
imaging studies, 397
primary CNS lymphoma (PCNSL), 396, 398
progressive multifocal leukoencephalopathy (PML), 396, 399
toxoplasmic encephalitis (TE), 396–97
treatment, 397–98
See also neurological complications of HIV
intralesional chemotherapy, 319
Kaposi's sarcoma, 319
intrathecal chemotherapy, AIDS-related non-Hodgkin's lymphoma (NHL), 326
Investigational New Drug, mpox, 376–77
IPERGAY trial, 156, 157*t*
islatravir, antiretroviral therapy, 226–27
isoniazid (INH), tuberculosis in PWH, 245–46
Isospora, 242
isosporiasis. *See* cystoisosporiasis
Italian Cooperative Group AIDS and Tumors, 343–44

J
jail
HIV treatment in, 106–7
term, 106
John Cunningham virus (JCV), 249, 399
clinical presentation, 254
diagnosis, 254
IRIS and ART, 262
prevention, 254
progressive multifocal leukoencephalopathy (PML), 254
treatment, 254
Joint United Nations Programme on HIV and AIDS (UNAIDS), 10, 11–12
Juluca (RPV/DTG), ARV formulation, 146*t*

K
Kaiser Family Foundation, 85
Kaiser Permanente, 133, 405
Kaiser Permanente HIV-Heart Study, 406
Kaletra (LPV/RTV), ARV formulation, 146*t*
Kaposi, Moritz, 316
Kaposi's sarcoma (KS), 260–61, 311, 314, 316–21, 363
AIDS Clinical Trials Group (ACTG) tumor staging system, 319*t*
clinical manifestations, 317–18
cutaneous malignancy in HIV, 377
epidemiology, 316–17
impact of antiretroviral therapy (ART), 318–19
local treatment, 319
in mouth of upper gums of PWH, 378*f*
pathogenesis, 317
skin of person with HIV, 377*f*
systemic treatment, 319–20
treatment, 318–20
See also malignancies
"kick and kill", viral eradication, 220
kidney disease(s)
acute kidney injury, 430
ART-related kidney complications, 433–36
assessment of kidney function, 429
chronic kidney disease screening and monitoring in PWH, 436–37
HIV-associated nephropathy, 430
HIV immune complex disease of kidney, 430
HIV-related, 429*b*
immune complex glomerulonephritis, 430
noninfectious comorbidities, 431
pathologic spectrum, 429–31
tubulointerstitial disease, 430–31
See also renal complications
Kidney Disease: Improving Global Outcomes (KDIGO), 436–37
kidney transplantation
candidate criteria, 307
induction immunosuppression for, 308
patient and graft survival and rejection, 310
people with HIV/HCV coinfection, 310
See also organ transplantation in people with HIV
Kinshasa, cradle of AIDS pandemic, 6*f*, 6
Korsakoff psychosis, 468

L
laboratory evaluation, initial, for PWH, 65–68, 66*t*
laboratory markers, HIV testing, 52*f*, 52
laboratory testing, HIV status, 168*t*
lactation, pregnancy and, 163
Lactobacillus plantarum, 38
lamivudine (3TC), 137–38
adverse effects, 273–74
ART regimens, 180*b*
ARV regimens, 183*t*
baseline conditions, 184*t*
combinations, 181
concomitant medical conditions, 185*t*
drug resistance mutations (DRMs), 201*t*
HIV acquisition, 209
infants, 268–69
infants of PWH, 267
principles in pregnancy, conception, and contraception, 287*t*
switching ARV therapy, 184–85, 186
treatment in U.S., 273*t*
treatment options for optimizing, 206, 207*t*
lamivudine/emtricitabine, switch option, 205–6
language, patient-provider relationship, 64
language and communication, disparities in health care, 86–87
latency reversal, approaches, 220–21
latency silencing, HIV, 221
latent tuberculosis infection (LTBI)
indications for screening, 72
transplant infection screening, 307
See also tuberculosis (TB)
ledipasvir/sofosbuvir, HIV/HCV coinfection, 494*t*, 495
lefitolimod
dual bNAb treatment, 224
HIV-1 transcription, 220–21
legal issues
advance planning, 509–11
civil rights and discrimination, 511–12
confidentiality, 505
disclosure, 505–6
ethical guidelines, 505
HIV criminalization, 506–8
treating minors, 508–9
See also advance planning; minors with HIV
lenacapavir (LEN), 139, 141
antiretroviral therapy, 226
drug resistance mutations (DRMs), 201*t*
HIV-2 infection, 210
HIV drug resistance, 195
HIV prevention, 169
kidney complications, 435–36
pregnancy and, 285
resistance testing, 199
transplant recipients, 309
Leopoldville/Kinshasa, cradle of AIDS pandemic, 6*f*, 6
leronlimab, clinical trials, 223
lesbian, gay, bisexual, transgender, and queer (LGBTQ+)
discrimination, 512
disparities in health care, 86
Gay and Lesbian Alliance Against Defamation (GLAAD), 511–12
substance use, 466
lesbian/gay/bisexual/transgender/queer (LGBTQ+) communities, 62–64
levonorgestrel-containing IUD, preventing or delaying pregnancy, 279
life cycle, HIV, 28, 29*f*, 226, 227*f*
lipid rafts, 31
lipodystrophy, term, 445, 446
Listeria monocytogenes
lesions, 398
meningitis, 386
liver transplantation
candidate criteria, 307
patient and graft survival and rejection, 310
people with HIV/HCV coinfection, 310
See also organ transplantation in people with HIV
living will, advance planning, 510
"London patient", 219, 225
Long-Acting Antiretroviral Research Resource Program (LEAP), 515
long-acting cabotegravir (CAB-LA), 156, 158–61
drug interaction, 191
long-acting early viral inhibition (LEVI) syndrome, HIV prevention, 156, 158–61
long terminal repeats (LRTs), 28–29
long-term non-progressors, 41
lopinavir (LPV)
infants, 268–69
pregnancy and, 285
lopinavir, ritonavir-boosted (LPV/r)
drug resistance mutations (DRMs), 201*t*
HIV-2 infection, 210
principles in pregnancy, conception, and contraception, 287*t*
treatment in U.S., 273*t*
treatment options for optimizing, 207*t*
lower clinical threshold, 203
low-level/possible resistance, 200–2
low physical activity and energy expenditures, definition, 297
Lubumbashi, 2*f*, 6, 7*f*
lung cancer
cigarette smoking, 337
clinical presentation of, in HIV, 338
diagnosis of, in HIV, 338
epidemiology of, in HIV, 336
injection drug use (IDU), 337
non-small cell lung cancer (NSCLC), 336, 338–39
people with HIV, 336–40
risk factors associated with, in HIV, 336–38
survival of, in HIV, 339
treatment of, 338–39
See also malignancies
lymphocytic interstitial pneumonitis (LIP), HIV infection and, 423, 424
lymphoma
AIDS-related, 323*b*
See also primary central nervous system lymphoma (PCNSL); systemic lymphoma

M
macrophage-mediated HIV encephalitis, 383
magnetic resonance imaging (MRI), T-cell encephalitis, 382, 383*f*
magnetic resonance spectroscopy, 321
major neurocognitive disorders, treatment, 484
Malassezia, 366
Malassezia species, seborrheic dermatitis, 405
male circumcision, voluntary medical, 167–68
malignancies
anogenital neoplasia, 329–35
antiretroviral therapy (ART) combination, 314
cancer outcomes in PWH, 315
colorectal adenocarcinoma, 342–45
HIV-related primary central nervous system lymphoma (PCNSL), 321–22
immune check point inhibitor (ICPI) therapy, 345–47

malignancies (*cont.*)
Kaposi's sarcoma, 316–20
lung cancer, 336–39
management, 315
manifestations of AIDS epidemic, 314
older PWH, 302
organ transplantation in people with HIV, 311
people with HIV, 314–16
prostate cancer, 340–42
risk in PWH, 315
systemic lymphoma, 323–28
See also anogenital neoplasia; antineoplastic and antiretroviral therapy; colorectal cancer (CRC); cutaneous malignancies in HIV; Kaposi's sarcoma; lung cancer; primary central nervous system lymphoma (PCNSL); prostate cancer; systemic lymphoma
managed care organizations (MCOs), 517
management, HIV status, 168*t*
Many Men, Many Voices (MMMV), 93
maraviroc (MVC), 139
drug resistance mutations (DRMs), 201*t*
pregnancy and, 285
treatment in U.S., 273*t*
treatment options for optimizing, 207*t*
masculinizing hormone regimens
surgical procedures, 100*t*
transgender populations, 99–101
maternal risk factors, HIV transmission, 271
maturation inhibitors, new drugs continuing to be developed, 228*f*
MAX clinic, Seattle, 104
Mayo Clinic website, 493
Mbuji-Mayi, 2*f*, 6, 7*f*
measles mumps rubella (MMR), immunization, 77
Medicaid, 81, 83, 125, 514–17
medical care, immigrants and migrants facing barriers, 113
medical history
HIV-oriented, 60–62
initial HIV visit, 63*t*
Medicare, 514–15, 517–18
medication(s)
adolescents, 94
drug-drug interactions, 162
FDA-approved HIV pre-exposure prophylaxis (PrEP), 159*t*
initial HIV visit, 63*t*
novel noncurative antiretroviral drugs, 226–27
older PWH, 298–99
pharmacists' role in adherence, access and education, 132–33
therapy management, 132
toxicities of, 360–61
melanoma skin cancers, 377–78
meningitis
causes of, in PWH, 385*t*
immune reconstitution inflammatory syndrome (IRIS) in HIV, 388
neurologic events in early-stage HIV infection, 386
neurologic events in late-stage, advanced HIV infection, 386–88
in people with vs. without HIV, 388
in resource-limited countries, 388
meningococcal conjugate vaccine (MenACWY), 307
meningococcus, immunization, 77
mental health
adolescents, 94
people experiencing homelessness, 103, 104
psychiatric consultation, 485–86
psychiatric illness and, 479
treating comorbid HIV and psychiatric disorders, 486
men who have sex with men (MSM), 8, 10, 11
highest-risk demographic in U.S., 14
HIV route of transmission, 19
men with HIV, HPV vaccination, 329
metabolic disorders in HIV
endocrine and, 440–41
metabolic dysfunction-associated steatotic liver disease, 444–45
metabolic syndrome, 444
transgender PWH, 445
metabolic dysfunction-associated steatohepatitis (MASH), 444–45
metabolic dysfunction-associated steatotic liver disease (MASLD), 440, 444–45
metabolic syndrome, 444
metabolism
drug disposition, 286
pharmacokinetics, 142–43
methadone
opioid use disorder, 471
substance use, 475
methamphetamine
anticonvulsants, 473
antidepressants, 473
antipsychotics, 473
atomoxetine, 473
combination pharmacotherapy, 473
stimulants, 473
substance use, 473
methycillin-resistant *Staphylococcus aureus*, cutaneous opportunistic infection, 373–74
methylenedioxymethamphetamine (MDMA), substance use, 473–74
metoidioplasty, description, 100*t*
microbial translocation, 36–37
microbicides, HIV prevention, 169–70
microsporidiosis
clinical presentation, 243
diagnosis, 243
epidemiology, 242–43
treatment, 243
midazolam, drug interactions, 193
migrant and immigrant persons, HIV care of, 111–13
mild neurocognitive disorder (MND), 383, 384
Mini Mental Status Exam (MMSE), 384
minors with HIV
consent for STI services, 509
exceptions, 509
laws related to informing parents, 509
medical care of, 508–9
seeking legal advice, 509
treating, 508–9
"Mississippi baby", 219, 271
mobile care, people experiencing homelessness, 104
mobility
older PWH, 297
social determinant of health (SDH), 111–12
Model for End-Stage Liver Disease (MELD), 310, 493
molecular clocks, 6
molluscum contagiosum, cutaneous opportunistic infections, 371*f*, 371
molly (MDMA), substance use, 473–74
monoclonal antibody therapy, immune enhancing or modulation, 223
Montreal Cognitive Assessment (MoCA), 297–98, 382, 384
mood, older people with HIV (PWH), 298
mothers
postpartum transmission of HIV, 270
timing of HIV infection in children, 269–70
moxifloxacin, BPaL regimen, 246
Mpox (monkeypox)
clinical disease, 376–77
immunization, 77
IRIS and ART, 262
mRNA vaccines, 230
Multicenter AIDS Cohort Study (MACS), 321, 406, 407, 442
multicentric Castleman's Disease (MCD), 316, 317
multidrug-resistant HIV, long-acting injectable-based regimens, 140
multimorbidity
older people with HIV (PWH), 296
term, 296
multipurpose prevention technologies (MPT), HIV prevention, 170
multiracial
adults/adolescents living with HIV infection, 20*t*
death of PWH, 20*t*
diagnoses of HIV infection, 91*f*
HIV infection, 15*f*
HIV infection among MSM, 20*f*
multi-substance use, 474
mumps/measles/rubella (MMR) vaccines, 307
muscle biopsy, ART medications and, 192
musculoskeletal, health status and system review, 62*b*
mycobacterial infections, 243–48
key points, 243
learning objective, 243
Mycobacterium avium complex (MAC), 247–48
Mycobacterium kansasii, 248
Mycobacterium tuberculosis, 243–47
See also opportunistic infections (OIs)
mycobacterial tuberculosis, 387–88
Mycobacterium avium, 40, 260–61
Mycobacterium avium complex (MAC), 243
ART and, 256
clinical presentation, 247
diagnosis, 247
epidemiology, 247
IRIS and ART, 261
post-transplant infection prophylaxis, 309
prevention/prophylaxis, 248
treatment, 247–48
Mycobacterium bovis, 243–44
Mycobacterium intracellulare, 247
Mycobacterium kansasii, 243
clinical presentation, 248
diagnosis, 248
epidemiology, 248
IRIS and ART, 261
treatment, 248
Mycobacterium tuberculosis (TB), 40, 243, 260–61
anergy testing, 73
clinical presentation, 243–44
diagnosis, 244–45
epidemiology, 243
interferon gamma release assays (IGRAs), 71, 73
lesions, 398
meningitis, 255, 386
migrants and immigrants with HIV and, 112
prevention, 246–47
screening tests for, 72–73
testing frequency, 73
treatment, 245–46
tuberculin skin testing (TST), 71, 72
myelopathy, 388–90
HIV-associated vacuolar, 389
HTLV-1-associated myelopathy (HAM), 390
MRI in HIV-associated vacuolar, 389–90
people with HIV and, 388–90
tropical spastic paraparesis (TSP), 390
vacuolar myelopathy (VM), 389
See also neurological complications of HIV

N

Naegleria fowleri, 376
naltrexone
alcohol use disorder, 469
opioid use disorder, 472
substance use, 475
National Association of Chain Drug Stores Foundation, 132
National Clinician Consultation Center, 126–27, 164, 200*t*
National Coordinating Resource Center/ National AETC Support Center, 126–27
National Health Alliance, 95
National Health and Nutritional Examination (NHANES), 337–38
National HIV/AIDS Strategy (NHAS), 13, 508
National HIV Behavioral Surveillance, 50–51, 91
National HIV Behavioral Surveillance Among Transgender Women program, 18–19
National HIV Curriculum, 200*t*
National HIV Surveillance System (NHSS), 19–20, 24–25
National Institute for Care Excellence (NICE), ezetimibe monotherapy, 414
National Institute on Alcohol Abuse and Alcoholism (NIAAA), 466–67
National Institute on Drug Abuse (NIDA), 466–67
National Institutes of Health (NIH), 1–2, 80, 310, 410–11
National Kidney Foundation Kidney Disease Outcomes Quality Initiative, 143
National Lung Screening Trial, 302, 338
National Osteoporosis Foundation (NOF), 453, 455
National Perinatal HIV Hotline, 267, 280
National Rural Health Association, 111
Native Hawaiian/other Pacific Islander (NHOPI), 14
adults/adolescents living with HIV infection, 20*t*
death of PWH, 20*t*
diagnoses of HIV infection, 91*f*
HIV infection, 15*f*
HIV infection among MSM, 20*f*
natural history, HIV, 31
natural killer T (NKT) cells, 37
nausea and vomiting, drug disposition, 286
negative HIV test, 57
Neisseria gonorrhoeae, 501
Neisseria meningitides, meningitis, 386
nelfinavir (NFV), 139, 268–69
nephropathy
acquired immune deficiency syndrome (AIDS), 428
genetic predisposition, 428
risk factors for, 428
See also renal complications
nerve biopsy, ART medications and, 192

neurocognitive disorders
definitions of, 384
See also HIV-associated neurocognitive disorder (HAND)
neurologic
health status and system review, 62*b*
persons with HIV (PWH), 61*t*
neurological complications of HIV
cytomegalovirus (CMV), 395–96
distal symmetrical polyneuropathy, 390–92
inflammatory demyelinating polyneuropathy, 392–95
intracranial lesions, 396–99
meningitis, 385–88
myelopathy, 388–90
neurologic considerations, ART medications and, 192
neutralizing antibodies, HIV prevention, 170
neutralizing antibodies, broadly, HIV-1 immunotherapy, 223–24
nevirapine (NVP), 138
infants, 268–69
infants of PWH, 267
pregnancy and, 285
principles in pregnancy, conception, and contraception, 287*t*
reactions, 367–68
transplant recipients, 308–9
treatment in U.S., 273*t*
newborns
antiretroviral (ARV) prophylaxis, 267
antiretroviral therapy (ART) for, 266
high-risk, of HIV acquisition, 267
HIV testing, 50
HIV therapy, 267
low-risk, of HIV acquisition, 267
presumptive HIV therapy, 267
See also children; infants
New York State Department of Health AIDS Institute, 157–58, 164, 333–34
next-generation HIVDR testing, definition, 196*t*
next-generation sequencing, HIV drug resistance (HIVDR), 200
nicotine
management, 468
tobacco use disorder, 417
nitazoxanide, cryptosporidiosis treatment, 242
nivolumab, checkpoint inhibitors, 221–22
Nix-TB trial, HIV and TB coinfection, 246
Nocardia, lesions, 398
nonalcoholic fatty liver disease, 444–45
nonalcoholic steatohepatitis (NASH), 444–45
nonbinary, term, 97*t*
non-Hodgkin's lymphoma (NHL), 314
alternative therapies for AIDS-related, 326–27
epidemiology, 323–24
hematopoietic cell transplantation for AIDS-related, 327–28
impact of antiretroviral therapy (ART), 328
intrathecal chemotherapy for AIDS-related, 326
pathogenesis, 324
See also systemic lymphoma
noninferiority
analysis, 144–45
term, 149–50
nonmelanoma skin cancers, 377–78
non-nucleoside reverse transcriptase inhibitors (NNRTIs)
acquired HIV drug resistance, 204–5, 205*t*
antiretroviral agents (ARVs), 137, 138
children, 268
choosing between third drug options, 182–83
CNS penetration effectiveness score, 385*t*
cutaneous drug eruption by efavirenz, 368*f*
drug interactions, 193
drug resistance mutations (DRMs), 201*t*
endocrine and metabolic disease in HIV, 441
HIV drug resistance, 197
interactions with chemotherapeutic agents, 328
long-acting injectable (LAI), 137
management among transplant recipients, 308–9
NNRTI-based regimens, 183*t*
pharmacodynamics and, 144
reactions and interactions, 367–68
selection, 179
selection of ART in older people with HIV (PWH), 299*t*
switching or simplifying, 184
transmitted HIV drug resistance, 203–4
nonoccupational exposures, post-exposure prophylaxis (PEP), 165–66
non-small cell lung cancer (NSCLC), 336, 338–39
See also lung cancer
nonspecific interstitial pneumonitis (NSIP), HIV infection and, 423–24
normal cancer risk, definition, 343
North American AIDS Cohort Collaboration on Research and Design (NA-ACCORD), 315, 332–33
novel noncurative antiretroviral drugs, 226–27
nucleoside/nucleotide reverse transcriptase inhibitors (NRTIs)
acquired HIV drug resistance, 204–5, 205*t*
antiretroviral agents (ARVs), 137–38
children, 268
choosing between recommended NRTI backbones, 181–82
drug resistance mutations (DRMs), 201*t*
kidney complications, 433–34
selection, 179–80
selection of ART in older people with HIV (PWH), 299*t*
transmitted HIV drug resistance, 203
nucleoside reverse transcriptase inhibitors (NRTIs)
CNS penetration effectiveness score, 385*t*
endocrine and metabolic disease in HIV, 441
HIV drug resistance, 197
management among transplant recipients, 308
reactions and interactions, 368
nutrition changes, older people with HIV (PWH), 300–1

O
Obama, Barack, 515–16
occult HBV infection, definition, 489
occupational exposures, post-exposure prophylaxis (PEP), 164–65
Oceania, 7*f*, 8*f*, 8
Odefsey (RPV/TAF/FTC), ARV formulation, 146*t*
offender, term, 106
Ofugi's disease, 366
older adults, HIV epidemiology in, 17
Older Americans Act (2024), 509
older people with HIV (PWH). *See* aging and HIV
omega-3 fatty acids, cardiovascular disease, 414
One-Step-PrEP program, 134
onychomycosis, cutaneous opportunistic infection, 369–70
opioids
ART medications and, 192
buprenorphine and buprenorphine plus naloxone, 471–72
intoxication/withdrawal, 470–71
management of opioid use disorder, 470–71
methadone, 471
naltrexone, 472
pharmacotherapy for maintenance of opioid use disorder, 471–72
substance use, 470
U.S. opioid epidemic and HIV, 470
See also substance use
opportunistic infections (OIs), 190
candidiasis, 240
clinical trial results, 255–56
coccidiodomycosis and histoplasmosis, 241
cryptococcosis, 240–41
cryptosporidiosis and cystoisosporiasis, 242
definition, 239
fungal infections, 240–41
incidence and associated, 260–61
microsporidiosis, 242–43
mycobacterial infections, 243–48
pneumocystis pneumonia, 239–40
post-transplant infection prophylaxis, 309
protozoan/parasitic infections, 241–43
timing of antiretroviral therapy initiation, 255–56
toxoplasmosis, 241–42
viral infections, 249–55
See also cutaneous opportunistic infections; mycobacterial infections; viral infections
opt-in screening, description, 54*t*
opt-out screening, description, 54*t*
OraQuick In-Home HIV Test, 56
orchiectomy, description, 100*t*
organ transplantation in people with HIV
donors with HIV (HOPE Act), 311
heart and lung transplantation, 310
HIV Organ Policy Equity (HOPE) Act, 306, 311
kidney transplantation, 310
liver transplantation, 310
patient and graft survival and rejection, 310
persons with HIV/hepatitis C virus (HCV) coinfection, 310
post-transplant management and care, 307–9
pretransplant evaluation, 306–7
risk of infection, immune recovery and malignancy, 311
See also post-transplant management; pretransplant evaluation
orthopoxvirus, monkeypox virus, 376
Osler, Sir William, 64
osteoporosis
comparative efficacy and safety of treatments, 460
recommended action for osteopenia and, 185*t*
treatment, 460
See also bone loss treatment
Osteo Renal Exchange Program (OREP), 456

P
palliative care
hospice care and, 126
term, 126
Panel on Opportunistic Infections, 490
panobinostat, 220
Pan troglodytes, simian immunodeficiency virus (SIV), 5–6
papular pruritic eruption of AIDS, inflammatory dermatoses in HIV, 366
parathyroid disorders, people with HIV (PWH), 443
paromomycin, cryptosporidiosis treatment, 242
PARTNER-1 (Partners of People on ART: A New Evaluation of the Risks) study, 24
PARTNER-2 (Partners of People on ART: A New Evaluation of the Risks) study, 24
partner-notification legal requirements, 57
PARTNERS 1 trial, 281
past medical history, initial HIV visit, 63*t*
patient care
complexity of needs, 125–26
roles of team members, 124–25, 124*t*
See also HIV care
patient-centered medical home (PCMH) model, 87
Patient Health Questionnaire (PHQ-2), 298
Patient Protection and Affordable Care Act, 514
patient-provider relationship
cultural competency and humility, 64
language, 64
persons with HIV (PWH), 62–64
sensitive, respectful, and nonjudgmental, 62–64
patient strain, calculating level of phenotypic resistance, 199*f*
PCSK9 (proprotein convertase subtilisin-kexin type 9), cholesterol treatment, 414–15
Pediatric AIDS Clinical Trials Group, 268–69, 284–85
pediatric HIV infection, 26
Penicillium marnefii, Asian immigrants and, 113
penis, term, 96
people who inject drugs (PWID). *See* persons who inject drugs (PWID)
people with HIV (PWH). *See* persons with HIV (PWH)
Pépin, Jacques, 6–7
perinatal screening, HIV testing, 50
perinatal transmission, HIV, 26
per-protocol (PP) analysis, 148–49
persistent immune dysfunction, role of, during therapy, 39–40
personality disorders, treatment of, 483–84
personalized cognitive counseling (PCC), 93
persons who inject drugs (PWID), 3, 10
HIV transmission in, 25
persons with HIV (PWH), 13, 23
chest radiography, 71, 73
discussing initiation of therapy, 68
diversity, 79
HIV-oriented medical history, 60–62
HIV-oriented physical examination, 64–68
initial evaluation, 60
initial laboratory evaluation, 65–68, 66*t*
key clinical history elements for initial HIV visit, 63*t*
key elements in history/current health status and review, 62*b*

persons with HIV (PWH) (*cont.*)
management of, 1
patient-provider relationship, 62–64
recognition of acute and advanced HIV infection, 65
recommended physical exam, 61*t*
signs and symptoms of acute HIV infection, 65*t*
symptom screening in, 73
telehealth in HIV, 68–69
See also homelessness or unstable housing; organ transplantation in people with HIV
p-glycoprotein, drug interactions, 360
phalloplasty, description, 100*t*
pharmacist in HIV care
antiretroviral therapy (ART) efficacy, 132
enhancing prevention efforts with pre-exposure prophylaxis (PrEP), 134
enhancing treatment efficacy, 132
expanded patient care roles, 130–31
HIV testing, 133–34
implementing long-acting injectable ART (LA-ART), 133
managing drug-drug interactions and polypharmacy, 132
PrEP and postexposure prophylaxis (PEP), 130
reducing antiretroviral therapy (ART) errors, 132
settings for providing patient care, 131
skills and impact, 131–32
specialist, 130
supporting medication adherence, access, and education, 132–33
unlimited potential of, 134–35
See also HIV care
pharmacodynamics
CNS effectiveness of ARVs, 144–45
definition, 141
integrase strand transfer inhibitors, 144
non-nucleoside reverse transcriptase inhibitors (NNRTIs), 144
protease inhibitors, 143–44
therapeutic drug monitoring and, 143–45
pharmacoenhancers, ART management among transplant recipients, 309
pharmacogenomics, 145
biomarkers, 145
definition, 141, 145
pharmacokinetic boosters, interactions with chemotherapeutic agents, 328
pharmacokinetic enhancers, kidney complications, 435
pharmacokinetics
absorption, 141–42
distribution, 142
excretion, 143
factors ADME, 141
metabolism, 142–43
science of, 141
phenotypic resistance testing, 198–99, 199*f*
physical examination
HIV-oriented, 64–65
persons with HIV (PWH), 61*t*
recognition of acute and advanced HIV infection, 65
signs and symptoms of acute HIV infection, 65*t*
physician order for life-sustaining treatment (POLST), advance planning, 510–11
pituitary adrenal disorders, people with HIV (PWH), 444
pituitary disease, people with HIV (PWH), 443–44
PIVOT (Protease Inhibitor Monotherapy Versus Ongoing Triple Therapy) trial, 391
plasmid DNA expressing HIV-1 genes, T-cell vaccines, 230
pneumococcus
immunization, 77–78
pneumococcal vaccine-naive, 77
Pneumocystis jirovecii
post-transplant infection prophylaxis, 309
risk of infection, 311
thyroiditis, 441
Pneumocystis jirovecii pneumonia (PJP)
antibiotics, 368–69
IRIS and ART, 261
prophylaxis, 325
pneumocystis pneumonia (PCP), 255, 260–61
chest radiograph of PWH and, 239*f*
clinical presentation, 239
diagnosis, 240
epidemiology, 239
treatment, 240
pneumonia, cytomegalovirus (CMV), 253
point-of-care, description, 54*t*
polymerase chain reaction (PCR), Epstein-Barr virus (EBV), 321
polymorphism, definition, 196*t*
polypharmacy
older people with HIV (PWH), 298
pharmacists managing, 132
term, 298
polyradiculopathy, cytomegalovirus (CMV), 252
POP-UP low-barrier care model, San Francisco, 104
positive HIV test, 56–57
posterior pituitary disorders, people with HIV (PWH), 444
postexposure prophylaxis (PEP), 25
baseline testing and monitoring, 167
exposures scenarios for PEP initiation, 165*t*
general principles, 164*b*, 164
HIV prevention, 164–67
nonoccupational exposures, 165–66
occupational exposures, 164–65
PEP regimens for adult and adolescent exposed persons, 166*t*
recommended PEP regimens, 166–67
special considerations, 167
See also HIV prevention
postoperative complications, HIV infection and, 192
post-test counseling
negative HIV test, 57
partner-notification legal requirements, 57
positive HIV test, 56–57
post-transplant management
antiretroviral therapy (ART) among transplant recipients, 308–9
CCR5 antagonists, 309
immunosuppression therapy, 308
induction immunosuppression for kidney transplantation, 308
infection prophylaxis, 309
integrase strand transfer inhibitors (INSTIs), 308
maintenance immunosuppression, 308
newer ART agents and formulations, 309
non-nucleoside reverse transcriptase inhibitors (NNRTIs), 308–9
nucleoside reverse transcriptase inhibitors (NRTIs), 308
protease inhibitors (PIs) and pharmacoenhancers, 309
See also organ transplantation in people with HIV
post-traumatic stress disorder (PTSD), treatment of, 480–81
potential low-level resistance, 200–2
PREDICT study, 145
pre-exposure prophylaxis (PrEP), 1, 153, 156–62
assessment of HIV status prior to PrEP initiation, 160*f*, 161*f*
clinical trials and real-world effectiveness, 156–57
coinfections, 163
delivery strategies, 161–62
discontinuing, 162
FDA-approved PrEP medication options, 159*t*
HIV acquisition in setting of, 209
HIV resistance after PrEP use, 162–63
indication, 157–58
initiation of, 158
long-acting early viral inhibition (LEVI) syndrome, 158–61
medication interactions, 162
medication options, 158
monitoring, 158
pregnancy and lactation, 163
PrEP inequities, 163–64
prescribing PrEP, 158–62
select phase 3 randomized controlled trials, 157*t*
tolerability and adverse effects, 162
See also HIV prevention
pregnancy and ART, 279–80
antiretroviral (ARV) principles, 287*t*
Antiretroviral Pregnancy Registry (APR), 291
ARV exposure during, 208
ARV-naive individuals, 286–90
ARV principles in pregnancy, conception, and contraception, 287*t*
basic principles on use of ARVs, 286
components of drug disposition, 286*b*, 286
HIV drug resistance, 208
intrapartum zidovudine during labor, 291
lactation and, 163
physiologic changes during pregnancy, 285–86
pregnancy while on ART, 290
pregnancy without viral suppression, 291
transplacental transfer of ARV drugs, 286
pregnancy counseling, infant feeding, 280
pregnancy test, 66*t*
pre-pregnancy care
importance of family planning and, 278–79
individuals wishing to prevent/delay pregnancy, 279
individuals with HIV wanting to become pregnant, 280
persons of childbearing potential with HIV, 279
See also cisgender women with HIV
pretest counseling, HIV testing, 51–52
pretransplant evaluation
criteria for transplantation, 306–7
infection screening, 307
vaccinations, 307
See also organ transplantation in people with HIV
pretreatment drug resistance (PDR), 210
definition, 196*t*
PREVENIR trial, 156
Prevent, Ending the HIV Epidemic (EHE) initiative, 3
PREVENT (Predicting Risk of cardiovascular disease EVENTs), 409–10
prevention. *See* HIV prevention
Prevention Access Campaign, 155
preventive vaccines, 230–32
Prezcobix (DRV/COBI), ARV formulation, 146*t*
primary care
HIV healthcare flow sheets, 71
transgender populations, 101
primary central nervous system lymphoma (PCNSL), 314, 321–23
clinical presentation, 321–22
epidemiology, 321
role of antiretroviral therapy (ART), 322
survival, 322
treatment, 322
See also malignancies
primary efficacy endpoint, 149
prison(s)
HIV treatment in, 106–7
term, 106
private health insurance, 516
productive infection, 37
progressive multifocal leukoencephalopathy (PML)
immune reconstitution inflammatory syndrome (IRIS), 254–55
JC virus reactivation, 254
prolactin disorders, people with HIV (PWH), 444
PROMISE (Peers Reaching Out and Modeling Intervention Strategies), 25, 26
PROMISE (Promoting Maternal and Infant Survival Everywhere) trial, 208, 270
Pro-Publica analysis, 80–81
prostate cancer
clinical presentation, 341
epidemiology of, in HIV, 340
men with HIV, 340–42
risk factors for, 340–41
screening, 341
treatment and treatment outcomes, 341–42
See also malignancies
protease inhibitors (PIs)
adverse effects, 274
antiretroviral agents (ARVs), 137, 139
children, 268
choosing between third drug options, 182–83
CNS penetration effectiveness score, 385*t*
contraceptive effectiveness, 279
drug interactions, 193
drug resistance mutations (DRMs), 201*t*
endocrine and metabolic disease in HIV, 441
HIV drug resistance, 197
HIV life cycle and drug targets, 29*f*
kidney complications, 434–35
management among transplant recipients, 309
pharmacodynamics and, 143–44
PI-based regimens, 183*t*
pregnancy and long-acting ritonavir-boosted, 285
reactions and interactions, 368
ritonavir-boosted, and cholesterol, 411
selection, 179
selection of ART in older people with HIV (PWH), 299*t*
protease paunch, 441
protozoan/parasitic infections
cryptosporidiosis and cystoisosporiasis, 242
microsporidiosis, 242–43
toxoplasmosis, 241–42
See also opportunistic infections (OIs)
proviral DNA sequencing
definition, 196*t*
persons with HIV (PWH), 199–200

psoriasis, inflammatory dermatoses in HIV, 365
psychiatric
health status and system review, 62*b*
initial HIV visit, 63*t*
persons with HIV (PWH), 61*t*
psychiatric disorders, 478–79
affective disorders, 481–83
antiretroviral therapy (ART) and, 485
anxiety disorders and post-traumatic stress disorder (PTSD), 480–81
cultural considerations in treating comorbid HIV and, 486
delirium and dementia, 484
HIV infection and, 479–80
major neurocognitive disorders, 484
personality disorders and PWH, 483–84
psychotic disorders, 483
sexual dysfunction, 484
sleep disturbance, 484–85
stress and adjustment disorders, 480
substance use and, 465
substance use disorders, 484
treatment of, in PWH, 480–85
use of psychiatric consultation, 485–86
psychiatric history, initial HIV visit, 63*t*
psychiatric illnesses
recommended action, 185*t*
substance use and, 465
psychotic disorders, treatment of, 483
pulmonary, persons with HIV (PWH), 61*t*
pulmonary arterial hypertension (PAH), HIV infection and, 423, 424–25
pulmonary complications
chronic obstructive pulmonary disease (COPD), 423, 425–26
diffuse infiltrative CD8+ lymphocyte syndrome, 424
HIV lymphocytic interstitial pneumonitis (LIP), 423, 424
nonspecific interstitial pneumonitis (NSIP), 423–24
pulmonary arterial hypertension (PAH), 423, 424–25
pulmonary considerations, ART medications and, 192
PURPOSE 1 clinical trial, 80, 157, 157*t*, 169
pyrimethamine/sulfadiazine/leucovorin, toxoplasmosis treatment, 242
pyroptosis, 36

Q
qualitative HIV RNA assays, 55
quality improvement, HIV care, 127
quantitative CT scanning (QCT), 457
quasispecies, 196–97

R
race
COVID-19 pandemic, 82–83
death of persons with HIV as stage 3 (AIDS), 20*t*
diagnoses of HIV by gender and, 18*f*, 18–19
HIV epidemiological trends by, 14, 15*f*
HIV infection among persons aged 13-24 years, 91*f*
HIV pandemic, 82
stage 3 AIDS classifications of adults and adolescents, 15*f*
radiotherapy, Kaposi's sarcoma, 319
raltegravir (RAL), 139
children, 208–9
drug resistance mutations (DRMs), 201*t*
HIV-2 infection, 210
kidney complications, 435
post-exposure prophylaxis (PEP), 166*t*
principles in pregnancy, conception, and contraception, 287*t*
transplant recipients, 308
treatment in U.S., 273*t*
treatment options for optimizing, 207*t*
raltegravir HD (RAL HD), post-exposure prophylaxis (PEP), 166*t*
Randomized Trial to Prevent Vascular Events in HIV (REPRIEVE) trial, 42, 404, 413
Rapid ART, 178
rapid HIV tests, 55
Rapid Nutrition Screening for HIV disease (RNS-H), 300–1
Rapid Plasma Reagin or Venereal Disease Research Laboratory, 374–75
rapid testing, description, 54*t*
REACH trial, 169
Ready, Set, PrEP program, 3
recombinant zoster vaccine (RZV), 77, 307
older PWH, 302
reduction mammoplasty/mastectomy, description, 100*t*
region, HIV epidemiology by, 17–18, 18*f*
region of residence, HIV infection among persons aged 13-24 years, 91*f*
release planning, people from jail and prison, 108–9
religion, disparities in health care, 87
remifentanil, drug interactions, 193
renal complications
angiotensin-converting enzyme inhibitors and angiotensin II blockade, 431–32
antiretroviral therapy (ART), 431
ART-related kidney complications, 433–36
assessment of kidney function, 429
corticosteroids, 432
dialysis, 432
epidemiology of disease in PWH, 427
HIV-related kidney diseases, 429*b*
markers of kidney injury, 429
novel medical therapies, 432
pathogenesis of kidney disease, 427–28
people with HIV, 427
renal replacement therapy, 432
renal transplantation, 432–33
risk factors and etiologies of CKD in PWH, 428*b*
risk factors for nephropathy, 428
treatments for HIV and, 431–33
See also kidney diseases
renal insufficiency, antiretroviral therapy (ART) dose adjustment, 436
renal placement therapy, kidney disease and, 432
renal transplantation, kidney disease and, 432–33
REPRIEVE. *See* Randomized Trial to Prevent Vascular Events in HIV (REPRIEVE) trial
resistance, 200–2
resistance testing, laboratory evaluation for PWH, 66*t*
resistant HIV, antiretroviral therapy (ART), 197*f*
resource-limited international carceral settings, HIV treatment in, 107–8
resource-limited settings, HIV drug resistance, 209–10
respiratory, health status and system review, 62*b*
respiratory syncytial virus (RSV), immunization, 78
respond, Ending the HIV Epidemic (EHE) initiative, 3
RESPOND cohort, 408
reverse transcriptase inhibitors
HIV life cycle and drug targets, 29*f*
new drugs continuing to be developed, 228*f*
reverse transcription, HIV viral life cycle, 227*f*
reverse transcription and integration, HIV, 30–31
ribozymes, gene modification, 226
rifampin, tuberculosis in PWH, 245–46
rifamycins, *Mycobacterium kansasii* infection, 248
rilpivirine (RPV), 138, 141, 142
ARV regimens, 183*t*
baseline conditions, 184*t*
cabotegravir and, 139
chemotherapy and, 360
drug interactions, 191, 360
long-acting cabotegravir plus, 206
long-acting injectable (LAI), 137
pregnancy, 285
principles in pregnancy, conception, and contraception, 287*t*
reactions, 367–68
switching ARV therapy, 184–85
transplant recipients, 308–9
treatment in U.S., 273*t*
treatment options for optimizing, 207*t*
RING study, 157*t*
ritonavir (RTV), 193
contraception and, 279
CYP34A inhibitor, 367
infants, 268–69
lopinavir, RTV-boosted (LPV/r), 139
protease inhibitor, 142
selection of ART in older people with HIV (PWH), 299*t*
treatment in U.S., 273*t*
See also atazanavir, ritonavir-boosted (ATV/r); darunavir, ritonavir-boosted (DRV/r); lopinavir, ritonavir-boosted (LPV/r)
rituximab, systemic lymphoma, 326
RIVER study, 224
RNA interference, gene modification, 226
romidepsin, 220
Rural Health Information Hub, 111
rural populations, HIV and, 110–11
RV144 trial, vaccine, 231
Ryan White Comprehensive AIDS Resources Emergency (CARE) Act, 507, 514–15, 518
Ryan White HIV/AIDS Program (RWHAP), 2–3, 83–84, 110, 126–27, 134, 518–19
AIDS Drug Assistance Program (ADAP), 190, 518

S
safety concerns, older PWH, 297–98
SALSA study, 184–85
SALT study, 184–85
San Francisco RAPID program, 92
Sanger sequencing, definition, 196*t*
SAPiT trial, 263
saquinavir (SQV), 139
Sarcoptes scabiei, scabies, 375
SARS-CoV-2 pandemic, 3
immunization, 75–76
mRNA vaccines and, 230
vaccinations, 307
scabies
crusted (Norwegian), 375*f*, 375
cutaneous opportunistic infection, 375–76
screening
description, 54*t*
laboratory evaluation for PWH, 66*t*
Screening, Brief Intervention, and Referral to Treatment (SBIRT), 466–67, 468
Screening Tool for Older Persons' Prescriptions (STOPP), 300
Screening Tool to Alert to Right Treatment (START), 300
Scytalidium, 369–70
SEARCH Dynamic Choice HIV Prevention, 166–67
seborrheic dermatitis, inflammatory dermatoses in HIV, 364
Self-Management and Recovery Training, 467–68
serodifferent partners
HIV, 280–81
natural conception between, 281
sero-positive couples, HIV, 280
SERO Project, 508
sex assigned at birth, diagnoses of HIV infection, 92*f*
sexual and gender minority patients, disparities in health care, 86
sexual changes, age-related, older PWH, 302
sexual dysfunction, treatment of, 484
sexual history, initial HIV visit, 63*t*
sexually transmitted disease (STD), 51
sexually transmitted infections (STIs), 66*t*, 163
chlamydia infections, 501–3
genital ulcers, 498
gonorrhea, 501
human papilloma virus (HPV), 503–4
laboratory evaluation for PWH, 66*t*
syphilis, 498–500
See also gonorrhea
Sexual Maturity Rating (SMR) staging, adolescents, 90
sexual risk, adolescents, 93
sexual transmission, HIV, 23–24
"shock and kill" cure strategy, combination strategies, 224
SILCAAT study, 222
silicone, transgender populations, 102
simian-human immunodeficiency virus (SHIV) infection, 220–21
simian immunodeficiency virus (SIV), 5, 36–37, 220–21
SINGLE study, 182
skin
health status and system review, 62*b*
persons with HIV (PWH), 61*t*
sleep disturbance, treatment of, 484–85
slowness, definition, 297
smallpox, 376
SMART study, 410–11
smoking cessation, cardiovascular disease, 417
social determinants of health, 79, 81, 111–12
social history, initial HIV visit, 63*t*
social issues, older people with HIV (PWH), 300
SOCv8, gender-affirming surgery, 100–1
sofosbuvir/velpatasvir, HIV/HCV coinfection, 494*t*, 495
sofosbuvir/velpatasvir/voxilaprevir, HIV/HCV coinfection, 494*t*, 496
Solid Organ Transplantation in HIV: Multi-site Study (HIVTR), 306
See also organ transplantation in people with HIV
"soothe and snooze", HIV latency silencing, 221
SPIRIT study, 411
spirituality, disparities in health care, 87
SPRING-2 study, 182
squamous cell cancer of the anus (SCCA), 329
epidemiology of HIV-associated, 332–33

STALWART study, 222
Stanford HIV Database, 200*t*
Stanford HIVDB system, 200–2
START trials, 92, 137, 178, 190, 455
state insurance exchanges, 516–17
statin therapy
cardiovascular disease, 411–13
high- and moderate-intensity, 412*t*
people with HIV, 408*f*
statistically significance finding, 149–50
statistical significance, 149–50
status epilepticus, 384
stavudine (d4T), 137–38
steatotic liver disease (SLD), 444–45
stem cells, gene modification, 226
STEP trial, vaccine, 231
"sterilizing cure", 219
Stevens-Johnson syndrome, 273–74, 367–69
stimulants
cocaine use, 472
methamphetamine, 473
Strategies for Management of Antiretroviral Therapy (SMART) study, 431
Streptococcus pneumonia, vaccinations, 307
Streptococcus pneumoniae, meningitis, 386
stress and adjustment disorders, treatment of, 480
Stribild (EVG/COBI/FTC/TDF), ARV formulation, 146*t*
STRIDE trial, 263
Study to Understand the Natural History of HIV and AIDS in the Era of Effective Therapy (SUN), 452
Substance Abuse and Mental Health Services Administration (SAMHSA), 1–2
substance use
adolescents, 93–94
alcohol, 468–69
antiretroviral agents and, 474–75
cannabis, 474
cocaine/crack, 472–73
disorders, 484
ecstasy or molly (MDMA), 473–74
general treatment principles, 467
HIV and, in coronavirus pandemic, 475
HIV infection and, 465–66
HIV prevention, 154–55
management of opioid use disorder, 470–71
methamphetamine, 473
multiple, 474
opioids, 470
people experiencing homelessness, 104
pharmacological management, 468–74
pharmacotherapy for alcohol use disorder, 469–70
pharmacotherapy for maintenance of opioid use disorder, 471–72
screening and diagnosis of disorders, 466–67
tobacco/nicotine, 468
treatment therapies, 467–68
superiority, term, 149–50
surgical procedures, transgender populations, 100*t*
surrogate markers, HIV, 272
susceptible, 200–2
Swiss Cancer Registries, 336
Swiss HIV Cohort Study, 316–17
SWITCHMRK 1 and 2 studies, 184
switch therapy, long-acting injectable-based regimens, 139–40
SWORD-1 study, 184–85
SWORD-2 study, 184–85
Symfi (TDF/3TC/EFV), ARV formulation, 146*t*
Symfi Lo (TDF/3TC/EFV), ARV formulation, 146*t*
Symtuza (TAF/FTC/DRV/COBI), ARV formulation, 146*t*
syndemic theory, concept of, 80
syphilis, 66*t*, 498–500
cutaneous opportunistic infection, 374–75
diagnosis, 499
follow-up, 500
latent, 499
neurosyphilis, 499
prevention, 500
primary, 374*f*, 374–75, 498*f*, 498
randomized clinical trials of doxycycline, 500*t*
secondary, 374–75, 375*f*, 498, 499*f*
transplant infection screening, 307
treatment, 499, 500*t*
See also sexually transmitted infections (STIs)
syringe service programs (SSPs), 3
systemic lymphomas, 323–29
AIDS-related lymphomas, 323*b*
AIDS-related non-Hodgkin's lymphoma (NHL), 323–29
alternative therapies for AIDS-related NHL, 326–27
chemotherapy, 328
chemotherapy in pre-ART and current ART eras, 325
clinical characteristics, 324
epidemiology, 323–24
hematopoietic cell transplantation for AIDS-related NHL, 327–28
impact of ART, 328
intrathecal chemotherapy for AIDS-related NHL, 326
pathogenesis, 324
prognostic features, 324–25
regimens including rituximab, 326
treatment, 325–28
See also malignancies
systemic racism, 79
COVID-19, HIV and, 83
definition, 83
impact of, 81
systemic treatment, Kaposi's sarcoma, 319–20
Systolic Blood Pressure Intervention Trial (SPRINT), 301–2

T
TANGO study, 184–85
targeted testing, description, 54*t*
TB-PRACTECAL study, 246
T-cell activation
chimeric antigen receptor T-cells, 223
immunomodulatory treatments, 225
rendering host's CD4+T cells resistant to infection, 225–26
restoring function of exhausted, 221–22
T-cell activity, dual affinity retargeting (DART), 224
T-cell-mediated HIV encephalitis, 382
magnetic resonance imaging (MRI), 383*f*
T-cell trafficking, immune modulation, 222
T-cell vaccines, 229–30
dendritic cell-based vaccines, 230
mRNA vaccines, 230
plasmid DNA expressing HIV-1 genes, 230
viral-vector-based vaccines, 229–30
telehealth
definition, 68–69
HIV care, 515
initial evaluation of PWH, 68–69
TEMPRANO trials, 92, 137, 178, 190
tenofovir (TFV)
drug resistance mutations (DRMs), 201*t*
kidney complications, 433–34
tenofovir alafenamide (TAF), 137–38
ART regimens, 180*b*
ARV-naive individuals, 286–90
ARV regimens, 183*t*
children, 268
choosing between third drug options, 182
combinations of, 181–82
concomitant medical conditions, 185*t*
drug resistance mutations (DRMs), 201*t*
elvitegravir and, 169–70
kidney complications, 434
medication toxicity, 360–61
pre-exposure prophylaxis, 159*t*
pregnancy and, 285
pregnant individuals, 286–90
principles in pregnancy, conception, and contraception, 287*t*
rifamycins and, 243
switching ARV therapy, 186
transplant recipients, 308
treatment in U.S., 273*t*
treatment options for optimizing, 207*t*
tenofovir alafenamide/emtricitabine (TAF/FTC)
discontinuing, 162
DISCOVER trial, 156–57, 157*t*, 162
drug interactions, 162
HIV prevention, 169
post-exposure prophylaxis (PEP), 166*t*
pregnancy and lactation, 163
tolerability, 162
tenofovir disoproxil fumarate (TDF), 137–38
ART regimens, 180*b*
ARV regimens, 183*t*
cholesterol and, 411
choosing between third drug options, 182–83
clinical trials with emtricitabine (FTC), 156, 157*t*
combinations of, 181–82
concomitant medical conditions, 185*t*
drug resistance mutations (DRMs), 201*t*
kidney complications, 433–34
pre-exposure prophylaxis, 159*t*
renal function, 427
serodifferent couples, 281
switching ARV therapy, 186
tolerability of TDF/FTC, 162
toxicity and adverse effects, 274
transplant recipients, 308
treatment in U.S., 273*t*
treatment options for optimizing, 207*t*
tenofovir disoproxil fumarate/emtricitabine (TDF/FTC)
HIV prevention, 169
post-exposure prophylaxis (PEP), 166*t*
tenofovir disoproxil fumarate/lamivudine (TDF/3TC), post-exposure prophylaxis (PEP), 166*t*
tenofovir gel, microbicides, 169–70
tenofovir-levonorgestrel (TFV/LNG), 170
testing. *See* HIV testing
testosterone replacement, bone loss and, 459
tetanus, diphtheria, and pertussis (TDAP), immunization, 78
Thailand, 24
therapeutic immunization
ACTG 5197 study, 229
ANRS 093 study, 229
early vaccine trials, 228–32, 231*t*
Vacc-4x trial, 229
therapeutic vaccine trials
overview of (1990-2015), 228–32
select, 231*t*
therapy, initiation of, 68
thrombotic microangiopathy (TMA), HIV-1 infection and, 431
thymidine analogue mutations (TAMs), 196*t*, 203
thyroid abnormalities, people with HIV, 442–43
Timed Get-Up-and-God (TUG) test, 297
tipranavir (TPV), 139, 273*t*
tobacco, management, 468
tobacco cessation, cardiovascular disease, 417
tobacco use disorder, recommendations for treating, 417*b*, 417
Together TakeMeHome (TTMH) project, 48, 56
toxoplasma, 66*t*
Toxoplasma, myelopathy, 389
Toxoplasma gondii, 309, 396–97
encephalitis, 256
toxoplasmosis
brain magnetic resonance imaging (MRI) of PWH and *Toxoplasma* encephalitis, 242*f*
clinical presentation, 241
diagnosis, 241–42
epidemiology, 241
IRIS and ART, 261
meningitis, 388
post-transplant infection prophylaxis, 309
treatment, 242
trans, term, 97*t*
transcription, HIV viral life cycle, 227*f*
transgender, term, 96, 97*t*
transgender man/transmasculine person, term, 97*t*
transgender men, HIV risk and prevalence, 97–98
transgender populations
common surgical procedures, 100*t*
diagnoses of HIV, 18*f*, 18–19
endocrine and metabolic complications, 445
epidemiology, demographics, and terminology, 96–98
feminizing hormone regimens, 98–99
HIV and, 95–102
HIV care and prevention, 101–2
initiating hormone therapy, 98
masculinizing hormone regimens, 99–101
primary care, 101
silicone, 102
summary of HIV and, 102
terminology and identities, 97*t*
transgender woman/transfeminine person, term, 97*t*
transgender women
prevalence, 97
virologic suppression, 97
translation, HIV viral life cycle, 227*f*
transmission of HIV
diagnosis, 92*f*
healthcare setting, 24–25
perinatal, 26
sexual, 23–24
use of injection drugs, 25
transmitted HIV drug resistance (TDR), 195
definition, 196*t*, 203
epidemiology, 203
management of, 203–4
transsexual, term, 97*t*
travesti, term, 97*t*

treat, Ending the HIV Epidemic (EHE) initiative, 2–3
treatment, HIV prevention, 155
Treponema pallidum
lesions, 398
syphilis, 374, 499
Trichophyton megninii, onychomycosis, 369–70
Trichophyton mentagrophytes, onychomycosis, 369–70
Trichophyton rubrum, onychomycosis, 369–70
trimethoprim-sulfamethoxazole (TMP-SMX)
cryptosporidiosis treatment, 242
pneumocystic pneumonia (PMP), 240
toxoplasmosis treatment, 242
Trinidad and Tobago, 7*f*
Triumeq (ABC/3TC/DTG), ARV formulation, 146*t*
Trizivir (AZT/3TC/ABC), ARV formulation, 146*t*
tropical spastic paraparesis (TSP), 390
HTLV-1-associated myelopathy (HAM), 390
tropism testing, 66*t*
Trump, Donald, 515–16
trust, importance of, 85
Truvada (FTC/TDF), ARV formulation, 146*t*
Trypanosoma brucei
HIV-associated nephropathy (HIVAN), 428
kidney diseases, 427
tuberculin skin testing (TST), 71
screening for *Mycobacterium tuberculosis* infection, 72–73
tuberculosis, 244
tuberculosis (TB), 66*t*
indications for latent TB infection (LTBI) screening, 72
IRIS, 263–64
preventive therapy, 73–74
recommended action, 185*t*
screening and assessment, 71–72
timing of ART with TB IRIS, 263–64
transmission to infants, 269
transplant infection screening of latent TB, 307
See also Mycobacterium tuberculosis infection
Tuskegee syphilis study, 85

U
UB-421 monoclonal antibody, 223
ubiquitin proteasome system (UPS), 31
uncoating, 30
"Undetectable = Untransmittable (U = U)", 155, 164–65, 270
United Nations Programme on HIV/AIDS (UNAIDS), 1, 10, 195
United States (U.S.)
adults and adolescents living with HIV infection by race/ethnicity, 20*t*
counseling on breastfeeding for PWH, 270
deaths of persons with HIV (stage 3 AIDS) by race/ethnicity, 20*t*
HIV care continuum, 13*f*, 13
HIV diagnosis by region, 17–18, 18*f*
HIV infection by region of residence, 15*f*
HIV prevalence, incidence and deaths, 12–13
overview of HIV epidemic, 12
safety of U.S. blood supply, 154
United States Preventive Services Task Force (USPSTF), 105–6
University of Buffalo, 130
unstable housing. *See* homelessness or unstable housing
upper clinical threshold, 203
urinalysis, 66*t*
U.S. Cancer Statistics Surveillance, Epidemiology, and End Results (SEER) program, 315
U.S. Health Resources and Services Administration, telehealth definition, 68–69
U.S. National Institutes on Health (NIH), 290
U.S. Preventive Services Task Force (USPSTF), 49, 91–92, 157–58, 297–98, 302, 336, 338, 343, 456, 466–67
U.S. Public Health Service, 48–49, 85, 330–31
U.S. Scientific Registry of Transplant Recipients (SRTR), 310
U.S. Veterans Administration Aging Cohort, 406

V
vaccination(s)
Gardasil-9 for HPV, 504
hepatitis B vaccine, 490
human papillomavirus (HPV), 329
pretransplant, 307
See also immunization(s)
vaccine(s)
ChAdV63.HIVconsv prime with MVA. HIVconsv boost, 224
HIV prevention, 170
mpox, 376–77
overview of early therapeutic trials (1990-2015), 228–32
preventive, 230–32
select therapeutic trials, 231*t*
T-cell, 229–30
therapeutic and preventive, 228
vaccinia virus, 376
vacuolar myelopathy (VM), 389
HIV-associated VM, 389
MRI in HIV-associated VM, 389–90
vagina, term, 96
vaginoplasty
description, 100*t*
penile-inversion technique, 101
valacyclovir
herpes simplex virus (HSV) treatment, 250, 250*t*
varicella zoster virus, 251*t*
Valley fever, 241
vanganciclovir, cytomegalovirus (CMV), 253*t*, 254
varenicline, tobacco use disorder, 417
varicella, 66*t*
varicella vaccine, 307
varicella virus (VAR), immunization, 77
Varicella zoster, 260–61
varicella zoster virus (VZV), 249
clinical presentation, 251
cutaneous opportunistic infection, 373*f*, 373
diagnosis, 251
human herpesvirus (HHV-3), 373
IRIS and ART, 261
prevention, 252
transplant infection screening, 307
treatment recommendations, 251, 251*t*
variola virus, 376
vedolizumab, HIV study, 222
ventriculoencephalitis, cytomegalovirus (CMV), 252
vesatolimod, 220–21
Veterans Aging Cohort Study (VACS), 296, 297, 405
Veterans Aging Cohort Study Virtual Cohort (VACS-VC), 453
Veterans Health Administration, 82, 492–93
VIKING trial, 435
viral budding, 31
viral hepatitis serologies, 66*t*
viral infections
cytomegalovirus (CMV), 249, 252–54
herpes simplex virus (HSV), 249–51
human herpesvirus-8 (HHV-8), 254
John Cunningham virus (JCV), 249, 254
PML-immune reconstitution inflammatory syndrome (PML-IRIS), 254–55
varicella zoster virus, 249, 251–52
See also opportunistic infections (OIs)
viral suppression, pregnancy without, 291
viral-vector-based vaccines, T-cell vaccines, 229–30, 231*t*
virologic assays
HIV-1 p24 antigen, 54
HIV testing, 54–55
qualitative HIV RNA assays, 55
quantitative HIV-1 RNA assays, 54–55
quantitative HIV-2 RNA assays, 55
virologic synapse, infection, 32
virology
classification of HIV, 28
reverse transcription and integration, 30–31
viral accessory and regulatory protein functions, 30*t*
viral diversity, 33–34
viral entry, 29, 30*f*
viral kinetics and latency, 32–33, 33*f*
viral structure of HIV, 28–29
virus production, 31
VISCONTI study, 219
vital signs, persons with HIV (PWH), 61*t*
vitamin D
level, 66*t*
screening for insufficiency, 456
supplementation, 458–59
voluntary medical male circumcision, 167–68
vorinostat, 220
VRC01, broadly neutralizing antibody (bNAb), 224
VRX496 (Lexgenleucel-T), 226

W
weakness, definition, 297
weight changes, older people with HIV (PWH), 300–1
weight loss, definition, 297
Wernicke's encephalopathy, 468
western blot, HIV testing, 54
White
adults/adolescents living with HIV infection, 20*t*
death of PWH, 20*t*
diagnoses of HIV infection, 91*f*
HIV infection, 15*f*
HIV infection among MSM, 20*f*
wild-type HIV, antiretroviral therapy (ART), 197*f*
Wild-type lab strain, calculating level of phenotypic resistance, 199*f*
wild-type virus, definition, 196*t*
will, advance planning, 511
Williams Institute, UCLA School of Law, 507
women
bone health of postmenopausal, with HIV, 452–53
disparities in health care, 86
HIV and, 86
See also cisgender women with HIV
Women's Interagency HIV Study (WIHS), 278, 330, 452–53
women with HIV (WWH), HPV vaccination, 329
world, dissemination of HIV throughout, 6–8
World Health Organization (WHO), 10, 24, 82, 157–58, 186–87, 519
AIDS-related lymphomas (ARLs), 323*b*, 323
bone abnormalities, 452
cervical cancer screening, 330
disclosing HIV status, 506
Fungal Priority Pathogens List (FPPL), 240
global HIV pandemic, 10–11
HIV/HCV coinfection, 491
meningitis, 385
Metabolic Bone Disease Group, 457
mpox as public health emergency, 376
preventing or delaying pregnancy, 279
pulmonary arterial hypertension (PAH), 425
World Professional Association for Transgender Health, 96

X
xerosis, atopic dermatitis and, 365–66

Y
young adults, HIV epidemiology in, 16–17
youth, HIV drug resistance, 208–9

Z
zalcitabine (ddC), 137–38
zidovudine (ZDV/AZT), 137–38, 141
drug resistance mutations (DRMs), 201*t*
infants, 268–69
infants of PWH, 267
intrapartum ZDV during labor, 291
medication toxicity, 360–61
post-exposure prophylaxis (PEP), 164
pregnancy, 284–85
toxicity and adverse effects, 273–74
transplant recipients, 308
treatment in U.S., 273*t*
U.S. guidelines, 267
zoster, immunization, 77
recombinant zoster vaccine (RZV), 77
zoster vaccine live (ZVL), 77